Health & Physical

Assessment in Nursing

Fourth Edition

Cynthia Fenske, DNP, RN
Campus Dean for Nursing
Associate Professor
Concordia University Ann Arbor
Ann Arbor, Michigan

Katherine Watkins, DNP, RN, CPNP-PC, CNE
Clinical Professor
Doctor of Nursing Practice Program Coordinator
Northern Arizona University
Flagstaff, Arizona

Tina Saunders, MSN, RN, CNE, GCNS-BC
Senior Lecturer
Kent State University College of Nursing
Kent, Ohio

Donita D'Amico, MEd, RN
Associate Professor
William Paterson University
Wayne, New Jersey

Colleen Barbarito, EdD, RN
Associate Professor
William Paterson University
Wayne, New Jersey

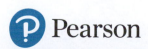

Executive Portfolio Manager: Pamela Fuller
Development Editor: Pamela Lappies
Portfolio Management Assistant: Taylor Scuglik
Vice President, Content Production and Digital Studio: Paul DeLuca
Managing Producer Health Science: Melissa Bashe
Content Producer: Michael Giacobbe
Vice President, Sales & Marketing: David Gesell
Vice President, Director of Marketing: Brad Parkins
Executive Field Marketing Manager: Christopher Barry
Field Marketing Manager: Brittany Hammond

Director, Digital Studio: Amy Peltier
Digital Producer: Jeff Henn
Full-Service Vendor: Pearson CSC
Full-Service Project Management: Pearson CSC, Dan Knott
Manufacturing Buyer: Maura Zaldivar-Garcia, LSC Communications, Inc.
Interior Designer: Studio Montage
Cover Designer: Studio Montage
Text Printer/Bindery: LSC Communications, Inc.
Cover Printer: Phoenix Color

Credits and acknowledgments borrowed from other sources and reproduced, with permission, in this textbook appear on appropriate page within text except for the following: Chapter 1 opener: Westend61/Getty Images; Chapter 2 opener: Jan Novak/123rf; Chapter 3 opener: kali9/Getty Images; Chapter 4 opener: Monkey Business Images/Shutterstock; Chapter 5 opener: KidStock/Blend Images/Corbis; Chapter 6 opener: Cultura Creative (RF)/Alamy Stock Photo; Chapter 7 opener: wavebreakmedia/Shutterstock; Chapter 8 opener: Iakov Filimonov/Shutterstock; Chapter 9 opener: wavebreakmedia/Shutterstock; Chapter 10 opener: belushi/Shutterstock; Chapter 11 opener: Terry Schmidbauer/123RF; Chapter 12 opener: Monkey Business Images/Shutterstock; Chapter 13 opener: FotoFlirt/Alamy Stock Photo; Chapter 14 opener: Andy Gin/Shutterstock; Chapter 15 opener: ferrantraite/Getty image; Chapter 16 opener: Alistair Berg/DigitalVision/Getty; Chapter 17 opener: bbernard/Shutterstock; Chapter 18 opener: bbernard/Shutterstock; Chapter 19 opener: Ariel Skelley/DigitalVision/Getty images; Chapter 20 opener: Monkey Business Images/Shutterstock; Chapter 21 opener: Rawpixel.com/Shutterstock; Chapter 22 opener: veryulissa/Shutterstock; Chapter 23 opener: Halfpoint/Shutterstock; Chapter 24 opener: Cathy Yeulet/123RF; Chapter 25 opener: Blend Images/Superstock; Chapter 26 opener: Ariel Skelley/Getty Images; Chapter 27 opener: Syda Productions/Shutterstock; Chapter 28 opener: LittlePerfectStock/Shutterstock; Cover: LittlePerfectStock/Shutterstock.

Notice: Care has been taken to confirm the accuracy of information presented in this book. The authors, editors, and the publisher, however, cannot accept any responsibility for errors or omissions or for consequences from application of the information in this book and make no warranty, express or implied, with respect to its contents.

The authors and publisher have exerted every effort to ensure that drug selections and dosages set forth in this text are in accord with current recommendations and practice at time of publication. However, in view of ongoing research, changes in government regulations, and the constant flow of information relating to drug therapy and drug reactions, the reader is urged to check the package inserts of all drugs for any change in indications of dosage and for added warnings and precautions. This is particularly important when the recommended agent is a new and/or infrequently employed drug.

Library of Congress Cataloging-in-Publication Data
Names: D'Amico, Donita, author. | Fenske, Cynthia, author. | Watkins, Katherine, author. |
  Saunders, Tina, author. | Barbarito, Colleen, author.
Title: Health & physical assessment in nursing / Cynthia Fenske, Katherine Watkins, Tina Saunders,
  Donita D'Amico, Colleen Barbarito.
Other titles: Health and physical assessment in nursing
Description: 4th edition. | Upper Saddle River, New Jersey : Pearson Education, Inc., [2020] |
  Donita's name appears first in the previous editions. | Includes bibliographical references and index.
Identifiers: LCCN 2019000240 | ISBN 9780134868172 (student edition) | ISBN 013486817X (student edition)
Subjects: | MESH: Nursing Assessment--methods | Physical Examination--nursing | Holistic Nursing--methods |
  Case Reports
Classification: LCC RT48 | NLM WY 100.4 | DDC 616.07/5--dc23
LC record available at https://lccn.loc.gov/2019000240
1 19

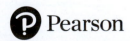

ISBN-10: 0-13-486817-X
ISBN-13: 978-0-13-486817-2

Cynthia Fenske, DNP, RN

Cynthia Fenske graduated with a BSN from Valparaiso University and an MS in Medical-Surgical Nursing from the University of Michigan. She earned her Doctor of Nursing Practice degree from Oakland University in Rochester Hills, Michigan. She was a faculty member at the University of Michigan for 32 years prior to leaving to start a nursing program at Concordia University Ann Arbor. In the classroom her teaching responsibilities include physical assessment, medical–surgical nursing, and fundamentals; in the laboratory setting she teaches physical assessment, nursing skills, and simulation.

Dr. Fenske has published articles on the use of simulation and innovative teaching strategies to assess and enhance learning. She is a faculty advocate, consultant, and trainer for Pearson Education's virtual community, The Neighborhood 2.0. Her research includes strategies to improve the development of clinical judgment and interprofessional teamwork skills through the use of simulation.

Dr. Fenske is a member of Sigma Theta Tau International Honor Society of Nursing and the State of Michigan State Board of Nursing.

Katherine Watkins, DNP, RN, CPNP-PC, CNE

Dr. Watkins earned her MSN as a Pediatric Nurse Practitioner at Yale, her post-master's certificate in Nursing Education at University of Alaska Anchorage (UAA), and her doctor of nursing practice from Northern Arizona University. She is a Clinical Professor of Nursing at Northern Arizona University in Flagstaff, Arizona. Dr. Watkins earned dual bachelor's degrees in architecture and geography and spent many years as a successful graphic designer and illustrator before coming to professional nursing and nursing education. After earning her MSN, she moved to Alaska and practiced as a pediatric primary care NP and began teaching nursing full-time at the UAA. Dr. Watkins has taught nursing education courses at all levels and in a variety of delivery formats with a particular focus on teaching nursing assessment at the pre-licensure and advanced levels.

Dr. Watkins is the coordinator for the Doctor of Nursing Practice program, is a Certified Nurse Educator, and practices part time as a primary-care pediatric NP in rural northern Arizona. She volunteers as a manuscript reviewer for *Journal of Pediatric Health Care* and on TeamPEDS of the National Association of Pediatric Nurse Practitioners.

Tina Saunders MSN, RN, CNE, GCNS-BC

Tina Saunders earned a baccalaureate degree in nursing from Youngstown State University, and a master's degree in nursing as an Adult Clinical Nurse Specialist with a specialization in gerontology from Kent State University. She has been a faculty member of the College of Nursing at Kent State University since 2006. She is the coordinator for the MSN Nurse Educator concentration and teaches in the RN-to-BSN program as well as in the Adult-Gerontology Clinical Nurse Specialist and Nurse Educator MSN program concentrations. Her clinical practice experience includes long-term care and critical care step-down nursing.

Mrs. Saunders has published an article on teach back methodology in *Orthopaedic Nursing* and has authored online RN-BSN health assessment and capstone courses for Pearson. She serves on several committees, on task forces, and in leadership positions within Kent State University at the College of Nursing. She is a member of the Delta Xi chapter of Sigma Theta Tau International, National League for Nursing, Northeast Ohio Clinical Nurse Specialists, Midwest Nursing Research Society, and Gerontological Advanced Practice Nurses Association. In addition, she serves on the editorial review board for the *Online Journal of Issues in Nursing* (OJIN).

Donita D'Amico, MEd, RN

Donita D'Amico, a diploma nursing school graduate, earned her baccalaureate degree in Nursing from William Paterson College. She earned a master's degree in Nursing Education at Teachers College, Columbia University, with a specialization in Adult Health. Ms. D'Amico has been a faculty member at William Paterson University for more than 30 years. Her teaching responsibilities include physical assessment; medical–surgical nursing; nursing theory; and fundamentals in the classroom, skills laboratory, and clinical settings. Within the university, she is a charter member of the Iota Alpha Chapter of Sigma Theta Tau International. She also serves as a consultant and contributor to local organizations.

Colleen Barbarito, EdD, RN

Colleen Barbarito received a nursing diploma from Orange Memorial Hospital School of Nursing, graduated with a baccalaureate degree from William Paterson College, and earned a master's degree from Seton Hall University. She received her Doctor of Education from Teachers College, Columbia University. Prior to a position in education, Dr. Barbarito's clinical experiences included medical–surgical, critical care, and emergency nursing. Dr. Barbarito has been a faculty member at William Paterson University since 1984, where she has taught Physical Assessment and a variety of clinical laboratory courses for undergraduate nursing students and curriculum development at the graduate level. Dr. Barbarito is a member of Sigma Theta Tau International Honor Society of Nursing and the National League for Nursing.

Thank You

CONTRIBUTORS

We extend a sincere thanks to our contributors, who gave their time, effort, and expertise so tirelessly to the development and writing of chapters and resources that helped foster our goal of preparing student nurses for evidence-based practice.

Fourth Edition Contributors

Laura Karnitschnig, DNP, RN, CPNP
Assistant Professor
Northern Arizona University, School of Nursing
Flagstaff, Arizona
Chapter 11, Psychosocial Health, Substance Use, and Violence Assessment

Previous Edition Contributors

Michelle Aebersold, PhD, RN
Clinical Assistant Professor/Clinical Associate Professor
Director of Simulation and Educational Innovation
University of Michigan
Ann Arbor, Michigan
Case Studies

L. S. Blevins, MS, MFA, ELS, RN
WilliamsTown Communications
Zionsville, Indiana

Vicki Lynn Coyle, RN, MS
Assistant Professor
William Paterson University
Wayne, New Jersey
Chapter 25, The Pregnant Woman

Dorothy J. Dunn, PhD, RN, FNP-BC, AHN-BC
Assistant Professor, School of Nursing
President, Lambda Omicron Chapter of Sigma Theta Tau
Northern Arizona University
Flagstaff, Arizona
Chapter 4, Health Disparities

Dawn Lee Garzon, PhD, APRN, BC, CPNP
Clinical Associate Professor
University of Missouri–St. Louis
Ladue, Missouri
Pediatrics content in assessment chapters

Karen Kassel, PhD, ELS
WilliamsTown Communications
Zionsville, Indiana

Sheila Tucker, MA, RD, CSSD, LDN
Executive Dietitian, Auxiliary Services
Nutritionist, Office of Health Promotion
Performance Nutritionist, Athletics
Part-time Faculty, Connell School of Nursing
Part-time Faculty, Woods College of Advancing Studies
Boston College
Boston, Massachusetts
Chapter 10, Nutritional Assessment

Linda D. Ward, PhD, ARNP
Assistant Professor
Washington State University College of Nursing
Spokane, Washington
Genetics and Genomics in Chapter 5, Interviewing and Health History

REVIEWERS

We would like to extend our deepest gratitude and appreciation to our colleagues who have given their time to help create this updated edition of our health and physical assessment textbook. These individuals helped us plan and shape our book by providing valuable feedback through the review of chapter content, art, design, and more. *Health & Physical Assessment in Nursing, Fourth Edition*, has reaped the benefit of your collective expertise, and we have improved the materials due to your efforts, suggestions, objections, endorsements, and inspiration. Those who generously gave their time include the following:

Carol S. Amis, MSN, RN, CCRN-K
Faculty, Nursing Program
Minneapolis Community & Technical College
Minneapolis, Minnesota

Jocelyn M. Dunnigan, PhD, RN, BC
Associate Professor
University of Mary, Division of Nursing
Bismarck, North Dakota

Matthew Good, MS, RD, LD
Master's of Science in Nutrition and Dietetics
President & Founder, Good Health Industries, LLC
Youngstown, Ohio

Marie P. Loisy, RN, MSN, FNP-C
Associate Professor, Nursing
Chattanooga State Community College
Chattanooga, Tennessee

Shirley MacNeill, MSN, RN, CNE
Chair, Allied Health Department
Upward Mobility LVN to ADN Nursing Program Coordinator
Lamar State College
Port Arthur, Texas

Rosemary Macy, PhD, RN, CNE, CHSE
Associate Professor
Faculty Development & Education Coordinator
School of Nursing
Boise State University
Boise, Idaho

Tonia Mailow, DNP, RN
Assistant Professor, School of Nursing
Murray State University
Murray, Kentucky

Carole A. McKenzie, PhD, CNM, RN
Associate Professor
Texas A&M University
Commerce, Texas

Jill Morsbach, RNC-MNN, MSN
Assistant Professor of Nursing
Missouri Western State University
St. Joseph, Missouri

Brenda Reed, RN, DNP, FNP-BC
Assistant Professor, Professional Practice Nursing
Texas Christian University
Harris College of Nursing & Health Sciences
Fort Worth, Texas

Christy Seckman, DNP, RN
Associate Professor
Goldfarb School of Nursing at Barnes-Jewish College
St. Louis, Missouri

Adam Strosberg, DNP, ARNP-BC
Christine E. Lynn College of Nursing
Florida Atlantic University
Boca Raton, Florida

Jennifer Wheeler, RN, MSN/Ed
Assistant Professor of Nursing
Jackson College
Jackson, Missouri

This updated edition of *Health & Physical Assessment in Nursing*, along with its comprehensive collection of digital resources, will help instructors guide pre-licensure nursing students and facilitate their learning of the art, science, and skills of health and physical assessment. The focus of this book is assessment of the whole person and recognizing the wide diversity of patients and settings where nurses practice. The professional nurse will assess the entirety of the patient experience, including the physical, emotional, cultural, and spiritual aspects of their lives. Because learning the practice of nursing is complex, this text provides a systematic and detailed look at health and physical assessment as the fundamental first step in the nursing process. We approach assessment holistically while emphasizing the scientific, evidence-based knowledge and skills needed for professional practice. We introduce concepts related to health, wellness, communication, culture, and human development to underscore the importance of health assessment as an integral part of the expanded role of the nurse.

ORGANIZATION OF THIS TEXTBOOK

Health & Physical Assessment in Nursing is composed of four units. Unit I, Foundations of Health Assessment, introduces foundations of nurses' role in comprehensive health assessment. The chapters within this unit examine the definitions and concepts important to assessment, as well as the social and cultural influences. Nursing assessment includes all of the factors that impact the patient and health. Chapter 1 describes the knowledge, skills, and processes that comprise the role of professional nurses in holistic health assessment and health promotion. Among these processes is evidence-based practice (EBP). This is introduced in Unit I, and references to evidence-based guidelines, recommendations, and practices are addressed throughout this text. The professional nurse functions within the healthcare delivery system and has a responsibility to partner with other professionals and patients to maximize health. We introduce all the steps of the nursing process, then provide a detailed explanation of assessment. Chapter 2 discusses many concepts related to health and wellness, including health promotion. This chapter also provides definitions of health and examples of several health promotion models. Chapter 3 discusses how the patient's culture, heritage, and spirituality have significant influences on the individual's health-related activities. This chapter provides an overview of cultural concepts and describes methods to incorporate and address the patient's culture, values, and beliefs in the assessment process. Chapter 4 discusses the expanded understanding of health disparities across populations. An examination of the assessment of vulnerable patient groups includes factors that place certain populations at risk for health disparities.

Unit II, Techniques for Health Assessment, introduces the fundamental skills for performing the health and physical assessment. This unit emphasizes current evidence-based nursing practice and guidelines. Chapter 5 presents the skills, knowledge, and attitudes needed to gather the subjective data through interviewing and collecting the health history. The nurse's ability to communicate effectively is essential to the interview process, and this chapter presents details of the communication process and examples of effective communication techniques. Chapter 6 covers the key principles of nursing documentation across a variety of settings. We describe techniques and equipment required for physical assessment in Chapter 7. Chapter 8 provides an in-depth explanation of the initial steps of the objective physical assessment—the general survey and measurement of vital signs. Chapters 9, 10, and 11 discuss factors that are of crucial importance to health assessment: pain; nutrition; and assessment of mental health, substance use, and violence. Each chapter describes concepts related to these areas and includes measurements, methods, and tools to guide data gathering and interpretation of findings for patients across the lifespan.

Unit III, Physical Assessment, introduces the methods and techniques that nurses use to obtain objective data. Current evidence-based practice knowledge and guidelines are highlighted throughout this unit. The chapters in Unit III are organized by body system, and each chapter begins with a review of anatomy and physiology. This is followed by a Special Considerations section with discussion of the issues the nurse must consider when collecting subjective and objective data, including health promotion; age; developmental level; and cultural, psychosocial, and emotional wellness. These highly structured chapters use a consistent format to guide students through the steps of assessment and build their skills step by step.

Unit IV, Specialized Assessment, contains three chapters that provide information about physical assessment of specialized patient groups. These chapters focus on assessment concepts and issues relevant to pregnant females; newborns, infants, children, and adolescents; and older adults. Chapter 28 presents a comprehensive overview of the complete health assessment along with a focus on hospitalized patients.

NEW CHAPTERS

Several chapters have been combined, reorganized, and amended in this edition. Completely new chapters include the following:

- Chapter 6, Documenting Your Findings, provides the rationale for accurate documentation, as well as the core principles for solid documentation. Differentiating the methods of documentation for subjective and objective data is emphasized. We also provide charting for narrative notes, problem-oriented charting, flow sheets, and more.

- Chapter 26, Newborns, Infants, Children, and Adolescents, describes the assessment of pediatric populations. This content has been brought together in this chapter, showing the changes in practices as children age.

- Chapter 27, Older Adults, presents assessment techniques and consideration for the older adult patient. Abnormal conditions related specifically to the aging process are identified.

- In Appendix C we present advanced skills that offer step-by-step instructions for some skills that, while less common, may still be performed by nurses in certain situations.

FEATURES TO HELP YOU USE THIS TEXT

Features are designed to enhance the learning process and help you use this text successfully. New features for this edition—Medical Language, Evidence-Based Practice, and the Documenting Your Findings section—are shown and described along with those from previous editions.

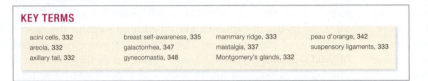

KEY TERMS

acini cells, 332	breast self-awareness, 335	mammary ridge, 333	peau d'orange, 342
areola, 332	galactorrhea, 347	mastalgia, 337	suspensory ligaments, 333
axillary tail, 332	gynecomastia, 348	Montgomery's glands, 332	

Key Terms at the beginning of chapters identify the terminology that the student encounters in conducting assessment and the pages where the student can find the definitions. Key terms are boldfaced throughout and defined in the text and in the glossary.

Knowing components of medical language can improve and enhance the learning experience. Prefixes, suffixes, and root words found in the chapter are provided in the **NEW Medical Language** features after the Key Terms to reinforce learning of these fundamental parts of medical terminology.

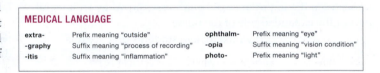

MEDICAL LANGUAGE

extra-	Prefix meaning "outside"	ophthalm-	Prefix meaning "eye"
-graphy	Suffix meaning "process of recording"	-opia	Suffix meaning "vision condition"
-itis	Suffix meaning "inflammation"	photo-	Prefix meaning "light"

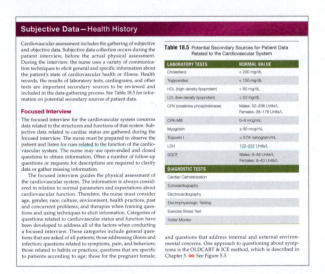

In the **Subjective Data—Health History** sections, students learn how to gather subjective data while conducting a patient interview. We provide Focused Interview Questions that ask the patient about general health, illness, symptoms, behaviors, and pain. We also provide follow-up questions to help the student gather more data from the interview, as well as rationales and supporting evidence so the student understands why the nurse must ask these questions. We provide reminders about specific communication techniques to increase student confidence and competence while performing the health assessment. A Potential Secondary Sources for Patient Data table is included in each of the assessment chapters in Unit III. The table includes laboratory tests with the normal values and other possible diagnostic tests relevant to the particular system.

In **Objective Data—Physical Assessment**, we show the student how to collect objective data and conduct a physical assessment—from the preparation of the room and gathering of equipment, to greeting the patient and the examination, to sharing findings with the patient. **Equipment** features help students prepare for the assessment by identifying the equipment needed to conduct the assessment. **Helpful Hints** boxes provide suggestions and reminders about conducting the physical assessment. We offer clinical guidance to prepare the student for the assessment and promote patient comfort.

Throughout the Objective Data–Physical Assessment section are two columns. The left-side column demonstrates step-by-step instruction for patient preparation, position, details for each technique in assessment, and the expected findings. The right-side column includes corresponding abnormal findings and special considerations, such as an alternate method, technique, or finding in relation to age, development, culture, or specific patient condition such as obesity. This format helps the student differentiate normal from abnormal findings while interpreting and analyzing data to plan nursing care. Hundreds of photos and illustrations help the student envision how to perform the techniques precisely and thoroughly. Documentation samples for each chapter are presented to help students practice this skill.

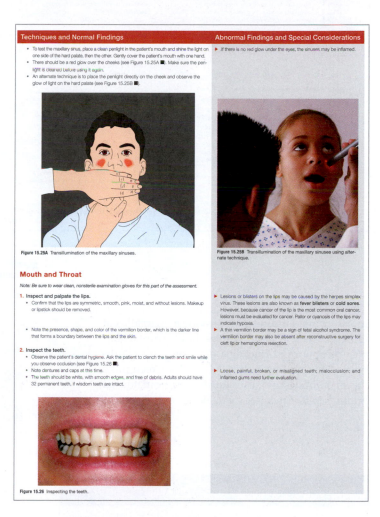

Alert! boxes remind students of specific nursing care tips or signs to be aware of when performing a physical assessment and identify critical findings that the nurse should report immediately.

ALERT! *Do not percuss or palpate the patient who reports pain or discomfort in the pelvic region. Do not percuss or palpate the kidney if a tumor of the kidney is suspected, such as a neuroblastoma or Wilms' tumor. Palpation increases intra-abdominal pressure, which may contribute to intraperitoneal spreading of this neuroblastoma. Deep palpation should be performed only by experienced practitioners.*

Familiarity with evidence-based practice information is critical for student success and nursing excellence. **NEW Evidence-Based Practice** boxes summarizing the findings of recent studies related to chapter content appear throughout the text.

Evidence-Based Practice

Concussion

- Sports injuries, specifically concussions, are a significant clinical and public health concern because of the potential long-term effects including cognitive impairment and mental health problems in some individuals (Manley et al., 2017). In addition to implementing evidence-based guidelines for recognition of concussion, researchers are looking for new ways to measure the severity of the injury and the time needed for recovery or return to play. There is a promising role for advanced brain imaging, a variety of biomarkers, and genetic testing in the assessment of concussion (McCrea et al., 2017).
- A novel method to objectively determine when an athlete can safely return to play after a concussion injury has been uncovered. Athletes who show an elevated plasma tau concentration within 6 hours of a concussive injury tend to have a prolonged return to play time (Gill, Merchant-Borna, Jeromin, Livingston, & Bazarian, 2017).
- In mild traumatic brain injury, researchers found several salivary markers that were up to 85% accurate in determining risk of prolonged post-concussion symptom risk in children (Johnson et al., 2018).

The **NEW Documenting Your Findings** sections explain the importance of documentation of assessment findings. There is a focus on the clear distinction between subjective and objective findings. Examples of findings for each body system are presented.

Documenting Your Findings

Documentation of assessment data—subjective and objective—must be accurate, professional, complete, and confidential.

Focused History (Subjective Data)

This is information from Review of Systems (ROS) and other pertinent history information that is or could be related to the patient's neurologic function.

Patient reports a change in coordination and balance. States difficulty in climbing stairs and doing usual stretching exercise routine. Denies history of head injury, seizures, migraines, or other neurologic illnesses. States no change in vision, hearing, taste, smell, sensation, or memory.

Physical Assessment (Objective Data)

Grooming and hygiene appropriate, posture erect, body language and facial expressions appropriate. Able to follow directions, complete calculations accurately, speech and language clear, abstract thinking and judgment intact. Oriented × 3. CN I–XII intact. Positive Babinski. Unable to complete tandem walk or standing on one foot without losing balance. Upper extremity coordination and RAM intact. Sensation intact to light touch, sharp/dull, temperature, vibration, stereognosis.

Patient-Centered Interaction

Source: Olena Kachmar/123RF.

Ms. Angela Carbone, age 55, comes to the Medi-Center at 10:30 a.m. with the chief complaint of left back pain. She has some nausea but denies vomiting. She complains of dysuria and gross hematuria and indicates she had a kidney stone on the right side several years ago. The following is an excerpt from the focused interview with Ms. Carbone.

Interview

Nurse: Good morning. Ms. Carbone. Are you having pain now?

Ms. Carbone: Yes, I am.

Nurse: On a scale of zero to ten with ten being the highest, how do you rate your pain?

Ms. Carbone: Now it is about four, but I'm afraid it will become ten or twelve like the last time.

Nurse: I need to ask you some questions to get information from you. Will you be able to talk to me for a few minutes?

Ms. Carbone: I think so! I'll try. I'll let you know if I can't sit any more.

Nurse: Tell me about the pain.

Ms. Carbone: I have back pain on my left side, right here (pointing to the left costovertebral area). It feels like it moves down my back but not all the time. It really hurts and is getting worse each day.

Nurse: When did the pain start?

Ms. Carbone: It started about five days ago. That's when I noticed my urine was darker than usual.

Nurse: Did you do anything to help reduce the pain?

Ms. Carbone: Not really. At first I thought I slept funny. Then my urine got darker. I tried to drink three glasses of water a day, but I became nauseated and had to stop drinking.

Nurse: Earlier you commented that you are afraid the pain will become ten or twelve like the last time. Tell me more.

Ms. Carbone: I had a kidney stone about three years ago on my right side. Now the pain is similar on the left side.

Analysis

The nurse immediately asked Ms. Carbone about her current pain status to determine her ability to participate in the interview. Throughout the interview, the nurse used open-ended questions and leading statements. These statements encouraged verbalization by the patient to explore and describe actions and feelings in detail. The open-ended questions and leading statements permitted the patient to provide detail, thereby eliminating the need for multiple closed questions.

The **Patient-Centered Interaction** feature teaches effective communication skills. It presents a brief clinical scenario and interaction between the patient and the nurse. Each Patient-Centered Interaction includes assessment cues to help the student develop strong communication skills by addressing body language, cultural sensitivity and values, language barriers, and noncompliance. These are common issues that present challenges to nurses, and the Analysis at the end of each interaction offers the student goals that the nurse must obtain with this specific patient.

In **Abnormal Findings**, we provide a vivid atlas of illustrations and photographs that feature examples of abnormal findings, diseases, and conditions. This section helps the student recognize these conditions and distinguish them from normal findings before they see them in the clinical setting.

Abnormal Findings

Abnormalities of the eye arise for a variety of reasons and can be associated with vision, eye movement, and the internal and external structures of the eye. The following sections address abnormal findings associated with the eyelids (see Table 14.2), the eye (see Table 14.3), and the **fundus** (see Table 14.4). In addition, an overview of conditions that may be associated with an impaired pupillary response is provided (see Table 14.5).

Table 14.2 Abnormalities of the Eyelids

Blepharitis
Blepharitis is inflammation of the eyelids. Staphylococcal infection leads to red, scaly, and crusted lids. The eye burns, itches, and tears.

Basal Cell Carcinoma
Usually seen on the lower lid and medial canthus. It has a papular appearance.

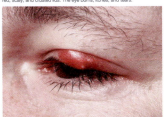

Blepharitis.
Source: Gromovataya/Shutterstock.

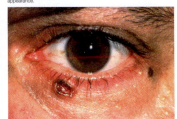

Basal cell carcinoma on lower eyelid.
Source: DR ZARA/BSIP SA/Alamy Stock Photo.

Application Through Critical Thinking

CASE STUDY

Source: logoboom/ Shutterstock.

John Jerome is a 45-year-old male who made an appointment for an annual employment physical assessment. Mr. Jerome completed a written questionnaire in preparation for his meeting with a healthcare professional. He checked "none" for all categories of family history of disease except diabetes. He indicated that he knew of no changes in his health since his last assessment.

The focused history reveals the following:

A male wearing eyeglasses entered the room; he appears his stated age of 45 yrs. He turned his head to the left and right and looked about the room before sitting across from the examiner. The patient had some redness in the sclera of both eyes. During the interview, the patient reveals that his last eye examination occurred 6 months ago, and he received a prescription for new glasses. He states that he is still having a problem with the new glasses and needs to have them checked. When asked to describe the problem, Mr. Jerome replies, "I just don't feel right with these glasses, and these are the second pair in a little over a year." He further states, "I just think I am overworking my eyes lately. I need to rest from more than ever, and I have had some headaches. I thought the glasses would help, but it hasn't gotten better." The patient denies any other problems. In response to inquiries about family history, he reports that his mother had diabetes but had no problems with her eyes. He doesn't know of any other eye problems in his family, except his mother had told him that an aunt of hers had been blind for some time. He reiterates that his only problem of late has been "this thing with my glasses, otherwise I feel fine."

The physical assessment reveals the following:

- Vital signs: BP 128/84—P 88—RR 22
- Height 6'3", weight 188 lb
- Eyeballs firm to palpation
- Moderately dilated pupils

SAMPLE DOCUMENTATION

The following information is summarized from the case study.

SUBJECTIVE DATA: Visit for annual employment physical assessment. Negative family history except diabetes. No changes in health since last assessment. Last eye assessment 6 months ago—result prescription for new glasses. Stated he was having a problem with the new glasses. "I don't feel right with them." Stated, "I think I'm overworking my eyes lately. I thought the new glasses would help, but it hasn't gotten better." History of aunt with blindness.

OBJECTIVE DATA: Turns head to left and right and looked around room before sitting across from examiner. Scleral redness bilaterally. Eyeballs firm to palpation. Pupils moderate dilation. Cupping of optic discs. Height 6'3", weight 188 lb. VS: BP 128/84—P 88—RR 22.

CRITICAL THINKING QUESTIONS

1. What conclusions would the nurse reach based on the data?
2. How was this conclusion formulated?
3. What information is missing?
4. What is the priority for this patient, and what options would apply?
5. As Mr. Jerome ages, for what age-related vision changes will he be at risk?

In the **Application Through Critical Thinking** sections, we challenge students to apply critical thinking and clinical reasoning by working through a Case Study. After a detailed patient scenario, students will answer critical thinking questions and prepare documentation.

MYLAB NURSING

MyLab Nursing is an online learning and practice environment that, in tandem with the text, helps students master key concepts, prepare for the NCLEX-RN exam, and develop clinical reasoning skills. Through a new mobile app experience, students can study Pathophysiology: Concepts of Human Disease anytime, anywhere. New adaptive technology with remediation personalizes learning, moving students beyond memorization to true understanding and application of the content. MyLab Nursing contains the following features.

Dynamic Study Modules

New adaptive learning modules with remediation personalize the learning experience by allowing students to increase both their confidence and their performance while being assessed in real time.

NCLEX-Style Questions

Practice tests with more than a thousand NCLEX-style questions of various types build student confidence and prepare them for success on the NCLEX-RN exam. Questions are organized by chapter.

Decision-Making Cases

Clinical case studies provide opportunities for students to practice analyzing information and making important decisions at key moments in patient care scenarios. These 15 unfolding case studies are designed to help prepare students for clinical practice.

Pearson eText

Student learning is enhanced both in and outside the classroom. Students can take notes, highlight, and bookmark important content, or they can engage with interactive and rich media to achieve greater conceptual understanding of the text content. Physical examination sections are enhanced by videos illustrating the steps of the processes.

RESOURCES FOR FACULTY SUCCESS

Pearson is pleased to offer a complete suite of resources to support teaching and learning, including the following:

- **TestGen Test Bank**
- **Lecture Note PowerPoints**
- **Instructor's Resource Manual**
- **Teaching Resources, including laboratory guides, laboratory activities, games, and demonstration videos**

ACKNOWLEDGMENTS

The fourth edition of this book would not have been possible without the contributions of many individuals. We especially want to thank Pamela Lappies, our development editor, who has provided invaluable support and guidance. Thanks also goes to Executive Portfolio Manager Pamela Fuller for her commitment to excellence in nursing education and dedication to shaping this updated book into the greatest possible resource for students. Special thanks goes to Portfolio Management Assistant Erin Sullivan for scheduling, supporting, and coordinating many pieces of this project.

Contents

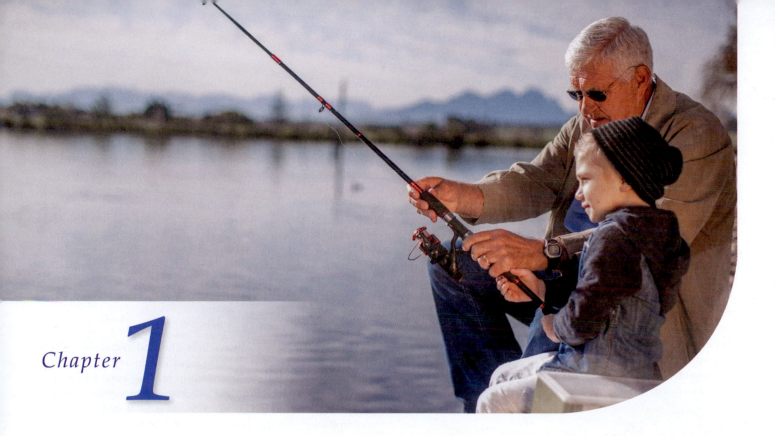

Chapter 1

Health Assessment

LEARNING OUTCOMES

Upon completion of the chapter, you will be able to:

1. Explain the roles of the professional nurse in healthcare.

2. Explain evidence-based practice and its significance in nursing.

3. Explain the steps of the nursing process.

4. Define health assessment and identify key components.

5. Apply the critical thinking process to health assessment in nursing.

6. Describe the concepts of health, wellness, and health disparities.

7. Examine how national health policy is structured to enhance individual and population health.

KEY TERMS

assessment, 4	health assessment, 5	nursing diagnosis, 5	subjective data, 4
critical thinking, 4	health disparity, 7	nursing process, 4	wellness, 7
documentation, 6	health history, 6	objective data, 4	
focused interview, 6	interpretation of findings, 5	patient record, 6	
health, 7	interview, 6	physical assessment, 6	

Introduction

The complex nature of health, wellness, and provision of care in today's healthcare system in the United States has necessitated an expansion of the role of the nurse. In the past, healthcare focused on treatment of patients' illnesses and symptoms. The focus today is on a healthcare model that emphasizes wellness, health promotion, and disease prevention. This change in focus is behind the push for nurses to develop an expanded knowledge base, greater flexibility, and the ability to work in a variety of settings and to practice to the full extent of their education and training (Institute of Medicine, 2011). Today's patients are taking a more active role in all aspects of their healthcare, from planning, screening, and decision making to choosing treatment modalities and prevention techniques. This chapter introduces the nursing process and focuses on the important first step: the foundational concepts of health and physical assessment that are the basis for the remaining chapters.

Health assessment is an integral part of the expanded role of the nurse and is performed in a variety of settings with patients across the lifespan. A broad definition of the assessment process is introduced in this chapter, whereas subsequent chapters in this unit provide detailed information in critical areas of health assessment (Health and Wellness; Cultural and Spiritual Considerations; and Health Disparities). Unit II provides detailed information regarding Techniques for Health Assessment, including Interviewing and Health History, Documentation, Techniques and Equipment, the Physical Exam, Pain Assessment, Nutrition Assessment, and Mental Health, Substance Use, and Violence Assessment. Unit III provides step-by-step guides for learning how to perform physical assessment of each body system. ∞

Role of the Professional Nurse

Nursing care is based on a foundation of education in the biologic and physical sciences, as well as the humanities and social sciences. From this foundation, the professional nurse may perform a variety of roles, including direct patient care, teaching, advocacy, and manager or coordinator of care. Using research data, standards of care, and the nursing process, the professional nurse provides competent care to individuals, families, communities, and populations. Additionally, the nurse may participate on interprofessional teams to plan and provide care for those with complex healthcare needs. The actions of the professional nurse will be directed to promote and support health and wellness, prevent injury and champion safety, and to treat and care for the ill and dying. To perform these actions, the nurse works in a variety of settings, including patients' homes, hospitals, clinics, nursing homes, schools, and workplaces. Advanced practice roles in nursing include researcher, nurse practitioner (NP), certified registered nurse anesthetist (CRNA), certified nurse midwife (CNM), and clinical nurse specialist (CNS), as well as roles in administration and education. Each of these advanced roles requires education beyond that for entry into practice; this usually means earning a master's or doctoral degree in nursing or a related field.

Regardless of the setting, the role of the professional nurse is multifaceted. Each situation requires the professional nurse to use critical thinking and the nursing process. To provide the highest quality of care, the nurse will base all actions on the foundation of scientific evidence and best clinical judgment. Brief descriptions of the roles of the nurse are provided, but remember, in any situation, a nurse may perform multiple roles.

Teacher

As a teacher, the nurse helps the patient to acquire knowledge required for health maintenance or improvement, to prevent illness or injury, to manage therapies, and to make decisions about health and treatment. Teaching occurs in all settings and for a variety of reasons and may be informal or formal. Teaching is an important intervention to promote wellness and prevent illness or injury. Teaching is used when collection and analysis of patient data reveal a knowledge deficit or a need for education about an identified risk or when the patient displays a readiness to learn to enhance health. Teaching is a critically important role for nurses in all settings. The need for learning in individuals, families, and groups arises in response to lack of knowledge about common changes or risks that occur with aging, role change and development, illness, health promotion, and disease prevention. Teaching to help people and populations avoid illness and injury is called health promotion, which is addressed in detail in Chapter 2. ∞

Caregiver

The caregiver role has always been the traditional role of the nurse. Historically, physical care was the primary focus. Today, the nurse uses a holistic approach to nursing care. Using critical thinking and the nursing process, the professional nurse provides direct and indirect care to the patient. Indirect care is accomplished with the delegation of activities to other members of the team. As patient advocate, the nurse acts as a protector. Patients are kept informed of their rights, given information to make informed decisions, and encouraged to speak for themselves. As a case manager or care coordinator, the professional nurse helps to coordinate care, participates in the interprofessional team, and plans patient outcomes within a specific time frame. Providing care, containing costs, and identifying the effectiveness of the plan are all responsibilities of the professional nurse.

Advanced Practice Roles

Health policy and legislation provide for roles in nursing that require advanced formal education and may require certification. Professional nurses function in advanced roles, including but not limited to nurse researcher; nurse practitioner (NP); certified registered nurse anesthetist; certified nurse midwife (CNM); clinical nurse specialist (CNS); hospital, healthcare agency, or academic administrator; and various types of nurse educator. A brief description of these roles is included below. Please see the Appendix C for advanced practice assessment techniques usually used by NPs, CNSs, CNMs, and other advanced practice patient care roles. ∞

Nurse Researcher   The nurse researcher identifies problems regarding patient care, designs plans of study, and develops tools. A nurse researcher may work in a clinic, hospital, or laboratory and be focused on patient care outcomes, administering treatments for a clinical trial, or collecting data to help understand population-based outcomes. The nurse performing the research adds to the body of knowledge of the profession, gives direction for future research, and improves patient care. Nurse researchers may also be engaged in continuous quality improvement projects in institutions and agencies. These advanced practice nurses may be doctorally prepared to conduct primary research or to lead in the dissemination of new evidence.

Nurse Practitioner The nurse practitioner has advanced degrees and is certified by the American Nurses Credentialing Center, American Association of Nurse Practitioners (AANP), Pediatric Nurse Certification Board, and other organizations. The NP practices independently in a variety of primary care or acute care settings. NPs typically specialize in a population, including family (FNP), geriatric (GNP), psychiatric–mental health (PMHNP), women's health (WHNP), pediatrics (PNP), or adults (ANP), as well as acuity-level acute care (AC) or primary care (PC). Nurse practitioners are clinicians who combine expertise in diagnosis and treatment of illness with a nurse's understanding of health promotion and prevention (AANP, 2017).

Nurse Anesthetist In addition to undergraduate nursing education, the CRNA has completed an accredited nurse anesthesia education program and passed a national certification examination. In collaboration with other healthcare providers, including anesthesiologists and surgeons, CRNAs provide a full range of anesthesia services. CRNAs are the sole providers of anesthesia care in most rural hospitals (American Association of Nurse Anesthetists, n.d.). CRNAs must maintain registered nurse licensure, as well as credentialing by the National Board of Certification and Recertification for Nurse Anesthetists.

Certified Nurse Midwife The American Midwifery Certification Board (AMCB) is the national certifying body for registered nurses who have earned their graduate-level education in an accredited program. A certified nurse midwife (CNM) is an advanced practice nurse who can practice independently and attends to the health and well-being of women in all ages and stages of life. Midwives provide general healthcare services; gynecologic services; family planning needs; care for pregnancy, labor, and birth; and menopause care.

Clinical Nurse Specialist Clinical nurse specialists have advanced education and degrees in a specific population of patients and/or aspect of practice. They provide direct patient care, direct and teach other team members providing care, and conduct nursing research within their area of specialization.

Nurse Administrator Today, the role of the nurse administrator, nurse leader, or nurse manager varies and may include professional titles of chief nursing officer, vice president of nursing services, supervisor, or clinical manager. The responsibilities vary and could include management of complex patient care areas, staffing, budgets, organizational and staff performance, consulting, and ensuring that the goals of the agency are being accomplished. Advanced degrees are usually required for these positions. It is common to find nurse administrators with advanced degrees in several disciplines, such as nursing and business administration (Martin & Warshawsky, 2017).

Nurse Educator The nurse educator is a nurse with advanced degrees and is employed to teach nursing in a variety of settings such as a university, community college, healthcare agency, or hospital. Teaching may include topics for pre-licensure students, nursing staff development, or continuing education for all levels of nurses. The educator is responsible for didactic and clinical teaching, curriculum development, clinical placement, and evaluation of learning.

Evidence-Based Practice

Evidence-based practice (EBP) in nursing is the use of a focused problem-solving approach to clinical decision making that involves the conscientious use of the best available scientific evidence, clinical expertise, and patient preferences and values (Melnyk & Fineout-Overholt, 2015). Evidence-based practice evolved from Florence Nightingale's work in the 1800s, through medical practice changes in the 1970s, and to the nursing profession beginning in the 1990s (Nightingale, 1969). Its origins came from Nightingale's revolutionary idea that through improvements in sanitation and nutrition, patients' health would improve. She kept records of patient conditions and outcomes before and after implementation of hygiene practices. This evidence, determined through experimentation, helped create the "best practice" guidelines for nurses in that era (Nightingale, 1969).

The modern beginnings of EBP can be traced to the 1970s and the work of Cochrane (Mackey & Bassendowski, 2017). Before his work, much of medical practice was carried out based on the individual physician's choices and assumptions. In the early 1970s systematic research studies, such as randomized controlled trials (RCT), were developed. It was discovered that many assumptions upon which medical care was implemented were unfounded. "Cochrane believed that limited resources would always be an issue within the healthcare system, and clinicians should strive to utilize only those procedures that had been proven to be the most effective" (Mackey & Bassendowski, 2017, p. 52). To be proven effective, an intervention, procedure, medication, or treatment regimen that was tested using the RCT methodology would be considered to be the highest quality evidence. In 1992, the term *evidence-based medicine* was coined and defined as "the conscientious, explicit and judicious use of current best evidence in making decisions about the care of individual patients" (Sackett, Rosenberg, Gray, Haynes, & Richardson, 1996, p. 71)

In order to provide safe, effective, and competent care, nurses must incorporate evidence from the sciences, practical research, and best practice. As a nurse, you are expected to implement changes to practices based on scientific studies showing improvement in patient outcomes, increased patient satisfaction, and other metrics. The amount of time from bench research proving a positive outcome to implementation in practice-based policy has been as long as 15 years. That time gap has shortened in recent years because of a focus on quality improvement projects led by nurses, to the implementation of practice innovations, to the recognition of excellence by organizations, and from government agencies holding hospitals and other healthcare facilities to higher standards. The faster that best evidence is disseminated, the better the quality of patient care can be. It is the job of the nurse to stay abreast of changes to practice and to the innovations in medicine and healthcare (Melnyk & Fineout-Overholt, 2015).

The EBP movement is intended to influence outcomes in healthcare through the development of best practice policies and guidelines. The Agency for Healthcare Research and Quality (AHRQ), through Evidence-based Practice Centers (EPCs) in the United States and Canada, reviews scientific literature on clinical, behavioral, organizational, and financial topics to produce evidence reports and technology assessments. The resulting evidence reports and technology assessments are used by federal and state agencies, private sector professional societies, health delivery systems, providers, payers, and others committed to evidence-based healthcare (AHRQ, n.d.). The work of the AHRQ is intended to improve healthcare through the support of research on the quality of services and patient outcomes. Further, the AHRQ translates research into practice through the provision of information needed to make critical decisions about healthcare (AHRQ, n.d.).

To promote the use of EBP and to facilitate achievement of the best possible patient outcomes, numerous clinical practice guidelines and recommendations have been developed. There are many sources for specific practice guidelines and recommendations, including the public resource: AHRQ's National Guideline Clearinghouse (https://www.guideline.gov). Nurses must make use of the best available evidence as they provide care and assist patients, families, and communities to achieve optimum health outcomes.

Nursing Process

The **nursing process** is a systematic, rational, dynamic, and cyclic process used by the nurse for assessing, planning, implementing, and evaluating care for the patient. To guide the practice of the professional nurse, the American Nurses Association (ANA) suggests the use of the *Standards of Practice* (ANA, 2015), which are based on the nursing process. The nursing process has five steps (see Figure 1.1 ■) including assessment, diagnosis,

planning, implementation, and evaluation. Nurses use the nursing process along with critical thinking skills as the basis for the implementation of safe, competent patient care. **Critical thinking** may be defined as using cognitive skills to acquire new knowledge and making judgments in the processes of delivering safe quality healthcare (Nelson, 2017). The nursing process, along with critical thinking, can be used in any setting, with patients of all ages, and in all levels of health and illness.

To ensure that nursing care is comprehensive, evidence based, and appropriate, the nursing process begins with a comprehensive and systematic assessment of the patient. **Assessment** is the gathering of complete, accurate, and relevant data about the patient. The data gathered will include information that the patient tells the nurse—**subjective data**—and information the nurse measures or observes on the patient—**objective data**. During the process of gathering the subjective data from the patient, the nurse must be attuned to what the patient says, along with the signs, symptoms, behaviors, and cues offered by the patient. This situational awareness and focused data collection will enable the nurse to create a comprehensive database about the patient. Beginning with assessment, each step of the nursing process is defined in the following sections. Although the steps of the nursing process are identified as separate steps, in practice they are interrelated and overlap to varying degrees. It should be understood that the nursing process is cyclical, and when something changes for the patient, further information should be collected, which may change the diagnoses, interventions, and outcomes. The application and effective use of the

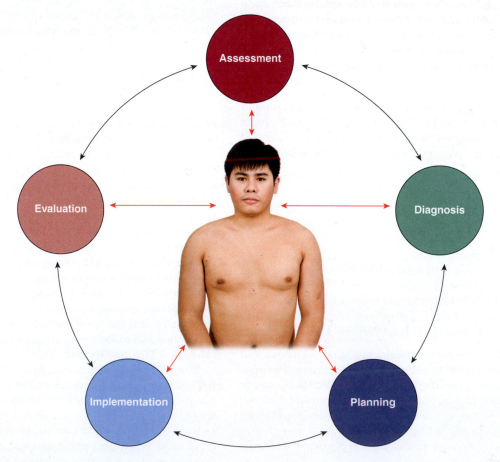

Figure 1.1 The nursing process.

nursing process is influenced by the ability of the nurse to adapt to changing conditions and to obtain comprehensive, accurate data. The comprehensive health assessment includes subjective and objective data obtained from primary or secondary sources. This information is collected to create a patient database from which a plan of care can be created that is patient centered and patient specific. This first step in the nursing process is then analyzed using the nurse's knowledge base and critical thinking skills to formulate patient-specific health goals to be addressed in the plan of care.

Assessment

Assessment, the first step of the nursing process, is the collection, organization, and validation of subjective and objective information or "data." It is imperative that the nurse understand the difference between subjective data, which consist of information that the patient experiences and reports to the nurse, and objective data, which are observed or measured by the nurse and include information that is heard, felt, seen, or sensed by the nurse. Subjective data are what the "subject" tells the nurse. Subjective data include the patient's perception of their health status, level of pain, history of health and illness, list of allergies, recall of food eaten, and medications being taken. Objective data may be found in charts and be relevant to growth and development or in laboratory values (e.g., hemoglobin, hematocrit, total cholesterol, blood glucose). Objective data also will be found upon examination of the patient and include vital signs, rate and quality of pulses, blood pressure, heart and lung sounds, skin texture, body temperature, and language development, among others. These two concepts are further examined throughout this text. This information forms a comprehensive *patient database*, which is used by the nurse to create the plan of care. The patient database describes the social, emotional, physical, and spiritual health status of the patient. Data are collected and documented in what is referred to as the patient's chart; the chart may be on paper or in the electronic health record (EHR), also known as an electronic medical record (EMR). In an assessment, the nurse gathers data about a patient by asking questions, taking measurements, and performing examinations, all in a systematic manner, which is covered in detail in this text.

Assessment begins when the nurse first encounters the patient or the patient chart. The nurse will use a variety of methods of data collection during the assessment process. The nurse will talk with the patient as well as look, listen, touch, and smell. Each sense will allow the nurse to learn different things about the patient. Each piece of information collected about a patient is important and adds to the picture of the total health status of the patient. As the assessment progresses, the answers and **interpretation of findings** will guide the nurse about what questions to ask next, and what additional information is needed.

Diagnosis

The second step of the nursing process is the formulation of a **nursing diagnosis**. The nurse uses critical thinking and applies knowledge from the sciences and other disciplines to organize, analyze, and synthesize the data. Subjective and objective data are compared with normative—expected—values and standards. All of the data, subjective and objective, are taken into consideration to determine areas where nursing intervention will support or improve health and wellness. Along with the assessment data, the nurse's knowledge base, experience, and personal characteristics influence the critical thinking process. Nursing diagnoses are relevant to patient problems and will be the focus of nursing care to reach a goal or outcome that is determined during the planning phase of the nursing process. To begin to develop nursing diagnoses, data are clustered or grouped together thematically. After analyzing and synthesizing the collected data, the nurse identifies an applicable nursing diagnosis, which is the basis for planning and implementing nursing care.

Planning

Planning is step three of the nursing process and involves identifying measurable patient goals or outcomes, setting priorities, and selecting evidence-based nursing interventions that promote achievement of the measurable patient goals or outcomes. When possible, the nurse must practice patient-centered care by including input from the patient, the family, and other involved healthcare providers. When formulating goals for nursing care, a useful mnemonic to remember is SMART. A nursing goal should always be specific, measurable, attainable, and relevant and should include a time element. These qualities are critical to the next steps of implementation and evaluation.

Implementation

Implementation is step four of the nursing process. During implementation, the nurse carries out specific, relevant nursing interventions meant to achieve the goals set in the planning phase. Implementation of evidence-based nursing interventions promotes the patient's achievement of the goals. If the nursing interventions are well thought out and specific to the patient and setting, they are more likely to be achieved. It is important to note that an intervention that works for one patient may need to be altered to work for a different patient. A thorough and comprehensive assessment will aid in the creation of patient-centered interventions.

Evaluation

The final step of the nursing process is evaluation. During this phase, the nurse evaluates the degree to which the patient has accomplished the identified goals or outcomes. If a SMART goal was developed in the planning phase, it should be easily measurable—for example, ambulation of 50 feet. Based on the evaluation, the nurse may need to revise or add to the elements of the nursing care plan—for example, revisions may include adding, changing, or discontinuing nursing diagnoses or nursing interventions.

It is important to point out that a single nursing diagnosis may generate more than one patient goal. Likewise, achievement of a single patient goal may require multiple nursing interventions.

Health Assessment

Health assessment is a process undertaken by the nurse to systematically collect subjective and objective information about a patient to create a comprehensive database for use in planning care. The focus may be to determine the patient's current or ongoing health status, to predict risks to health and well-being, or to identify health-promoting activities. The setting and context in which the assessment takes place will guide the actions of the nurse during this process. Data related to the patient's health status will be collected and will include physical, social, cultural, environmental, and emotional factors. Further information may include wellness behaviors, illness signs and symptoms, patient strengths and weaknesses, and risk factors. During the health assessment process, the nurse will use a variety of sources to gather both subjective and objective data. The nursing knowledge base along with effective communication techniques and use of critical thinking skills are essential in helping the nurse to gather the detailed, complete, and relevant data needed to formulate a plan of care to meet the needs of the patient. The three parts of the complete health assessment are the interview, the physical assessment, and documentation of the findings. Each of these components is described in detail in Chapter 5, Interviewing and Health History: Subjective Data, Chapter 6, Documentation, and Chapter 8, General Survey and Physical Exam: Objective Data. ∞ Below you will find an overview of basic considerations related to health assessment of the ambulatory patient. A focus on the hospitalized and critically ill patient may require considerably more in-depth assessment processes and will be discussed in detail in Chapter 28, Complete Health Assessment. ∞

Subjective Data: The Interview

The nurse gathers subjective data throughout the interview, which is composed of the health history and either a comprehensive or focused **interview**. The data collected will come from primary and secondary sources.

Subjective data are sometimes referred to as covert (hidden) data or as a symptom because they are perceived by the primary source—the patient—and cannot be observed by others. In some situations, secondary sources—the family members or caregivers—report subjective data based on perceptions the patient has shared with them. This information is relevant when the patient is very ill and unable to communicate, and it is required when the patient is an infant or a child.

In the interview, the nurse will systematically gather information about the patient's health history and about the current state of health.

The Health History The purpose of the **health history** is to obtain information about the patient's health in his or her own words and based on the patient's own perceptions. During the health history portion of the interview, the nurse collects biographic data, perceptions about health, past and present history of illness and injury, family history, a review of body systems, and health patterns and practices. The health history provides cues regarding the patient's health and guides further data collection. The health history is the most important aspect of the assessment process. Detailed information on how to obtain a complete health history is presented in Chapter 5, Interviewing and Health History: Subjective Data. ∞ Following up on the information presented in the history, the nurse may determine areas where further details would be useful.

This determination will lead the nurse to perform a focused interview.

The Focused Interview The **focused interview** is the portion of the interview in which the nurse asks the patient to clarify points, provide missing information, and elucidate information identified in the health history. The focused interview might zero in on one body system, for example, or on the family history of a disease. The nurse does not use a prepared set of questions but, rather, applies knowledge and critical thinking when asking specific and detailed questions or requesting descriptions of symptoms, feelings, or events. Therefore, the focused interview provides the means and opportunity to expand the subjective database regarding specific strengths, weaknesses, symptoms, or risk factors expressed by the patient or required by the nurse to begin to make reliable judgments about information and observations as part of planning care. In-depth information about the focused interview in health assessment is included in each chapter in Unit III of this text. ∞

Objective Data: Physical Assessment

The second phase of the health assessment is the **physical assessment**, the hands-on examination of the patient. Components of the physical assessment are the general survey and an examination of body systems. Objective data, observed or measured by the professional nurse during the physical assessment, will be combined with all other reliable sources of information to complete the comprehensive database on which care planning may be based. Objective data can be seen, felt, heard, or measured by the nurse—for example, skin color can be seen, a pulse can be felt, a cough can be heard, and a blood pressure can be measured. These objective data will be used in conjunction with the subjective data to complete the patient database. The accuracy of the objective data depends on the nurse's ability to systematically and consistently use evidence-based methods of data collection. Chapter 7, Physical Assessment Techniques and Equipment, and Chapter 8, General Survey and Physical Exam, provide more detailed information. ∞ Unit III includes descriptions of the physical assessment process for each body system. ∞

Documentation and Privacy

The last step in the preparation of a comprehensive patient database is **documentation**, the accurate and complete recording of all subjective and objective data collected during the interview and physical examination. The information is written or "charted" in a new patient record or added to an existing health record. This **patient record** is a legal document used to plan care, to communicate information between and among healthcare providers, and to monitor quality of care. Further, the patient record provides information used for reimbursement of services and is often a source of data for research. The patient record is reviewed by accrediting agencies to determine adherence to standards. Nursing documentation should be concise, precise, succinct, and professional; the data recorded are to be free of judgment, bias, or value statements. The types and amounts of documentation are determined by the purpose of the healthcare service and often by the setting. Chapter 6, Documentation, provides more detailed information. ∞

The documentation in the patient record must be kept confidential according to federal regulations regarding patient privacy including the Health Insurance Portability and Accountability Act (HIPAA). Regulations under this law became effective in April 2003 to create a national standard for privacy and to provide individuals with greater control over personal health information. The HIPAA regulations protect medical records and other individually identifiable health information, whether communicated in writing, orally, or electronically. Identifiable health information includes demographic data and any information that could be used to identify an individual. For further information about HIPAA regulations, contact the U.S. Department of Health and Human Services (USDHHS, 2012).

Critical Thinking

Critical thinking in nursing is a cognitive process of purposeful and rational analysis of information to enable clinical reasoning, judgment, and decision making. Key elements of critical thinking include collection of information, analysis of situation, generation of alternatives, selection of alternatives, and evaluation, as shown in Figure 1.2 ∎. Chan's (2013) systematic review of qualitative studies reported that critical thinkers demonstrate four characteristics: seek and gather information; question the quality of the data and investigate sources; examine, analyze, and evaluate data to draw conclusions; and finally, apply the theory or solution to the problem. Competence in critical thinking is central to all nursing activities and is at the core of the application of the nursing process (Perez et al., 2015). Critical thinking is more than problem solving; it is a way to apply logic and cognitive skills to the complexities of patient care. It requires nurses to avoid bias and prejudice in their approach while using all of the knowledge and resources at their disposal to assist patients in achieving health goals or maintaining well-being (Alfaro-LeFevre, 2013). The process of critical thinking parallels the nursing process in that information is gathered (assessment); problems are identified (diagnosis); goals, outcomes, or solutions are chosen (planning); interventions or possible solutions for

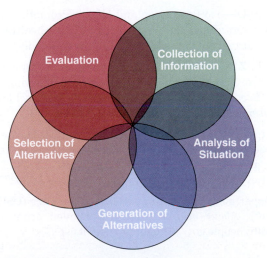

Figure 1.2 Elements of critical thinking.

meeting the goals are selected and implemented (implementation); and finally the nurse evaluates whether or not the problem is solved and determines if the interventions worked, reexamines the original problem, and determines if a new problem exists to examine (evaluation).

Health and Health Disparities

Traditionally, **health** has been thought of as the absence of disease. The terms *health* and *wellness* are often used interchangeably to describe the state when one is not sick. However, the concept of health extends beyond freedom from physical illness. When considered from a holistic approach, health include psychosocial and spiritual components as well. **Wellness** describes a state of being that is balanced, personally satisfying, and characterized by the ability to adapt and to participate in activities that enhance quality of life. Health and wellness, which incorporate personal responsibility and choices regarding lifestyle and environmental factors, are discussed in depth in Chapter 2, Health and Wellness. ∞

The nurse must understand that health, when examined from a national perspective, is more than an individual concern. Health and wellness are also considered relative to populations or groups of individuals. In the United States, the USDHHS joined the healthcare reform movement with its 1979 report entitled *Healthy People: The Surgeon General's Report on Health Promotion and Disease Prevention*. The efforts of this agency to address national concerns for health and safety continue with reports by an advisory committee to the Secretary of the USDHHS. The committee, made up of industry and academic leaders in health policy, medicine, nursing, oral health, child health, wellness, safety, and disease prevention, develops a 10-year plan, the first of which was called *Healthy People 1990*. It has revised and republished the report for the subsequent decades: 2000, 2010, and 2020. *Healthy People 2030*, which has not been released as of this writing, will contain national health promotion and disease prevention objectives based on public input, scientific knowledge, and outcome evaluation from previous years (Office of Disease Prevention and Health Promotion [ODPHP], 2017b).

The initiatives of *Healthy People*, as well as the focus on prevention and wellness, take into account the needs of a wide range of individuals and communities. An important concept when considering the health of individuals, communities, and populations is that health outcomes and conditions affect different groups in uneven ways. This is the concept of **health disparity**: "[I]f a health outcome is seen to a greater or lesser extent between populations, there is disparity. Race or ethnicity, gender, sexual identity, age, disability, socioeconomic status, and geographic location all contribute to an individual's ability to achieve good health" (ODPHP, 2017b, para. 1). What this means for nurses is recognizing that these social determinants will have an impact on the health outcomes on specific populations. The nurse, in the assessment process, is careful to understand the variety of factors that will impact the patient's health status. Disparities in healthcare are discussed in depth in Chapter 4, Health Disparities. ∞

Application Through Critical Thinking

CASE STUDY

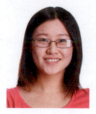

Source: Pressmaster/Shutterstock.

Mary Wong is a 19-year-old college freshman living in the dormitory. She has come to the University Health Center with the following complaints: nausea, vomiting, abdominal pain increasing in severity, diarrhea, a fever, and dry mouth. She tells you, the nurse, "I have had abdominal pain for about twelve hours with nausea, vomiting, and diarrhea." These symptoms, she tells you, "all started after supper in the student cafeteria on campus."

You conduct an interview and follow it with a physical assessment, which reveals the following: symmetric abdomen, bowel sounds in all quadrants, tender to palpation in the lower quadrants, guarding. Mary's skin is warm and moist, her lips and mucous membranes are dry.

CRITICAL THINKING QUESTIONS

1. Identify the findings as objective or subjective data.

2. What factors must be considered in conducting the comprehensive health assessment of Mary Wong? Provide a rationale.

3. How would you cluster the data you obtained from your history and physical examination of Mary?

4. Before developing a nursing diagnosis, what must you do?

REFERENCES

Agency for Healthcare Research and Quality (AHRQ). (n.d.). *Evidence-based practice centers (EPC) program overview.* Retrieved from http://www.ahrq.gov/research/findings/evidence-based-reports/overview/index.html

Alfaro-LeFevre, R. (2013). *Critical thinking, clinical reasoning, and clinical judgment: A practical approach* (5th ed.). St. Louis, MO: Elsevier.

American Association of Nurse Anesthetists (AANA). (n.d.). *Become a CRNA.* Retrieved from http://www.aana.com/ceandeducation/becomeacrna/pages/default.aspx

American Association of Nurse Practitioners (2017). *What's an NP?* Retrieved from https://www.aanp.org/all-about-nps/what-is-an-np

American Nurses Association (ANA). (2015). *Nursing: Scope and standards of practice* (3rd ed.). Silver Spring, MD: ANA.

Chan, Z. C. Y. (2013). A systematic review of critical thinking in nursing education. *Nurse Education Today, 33,* 236–240. http://dx.doi.org/10.1016/j.nedt.2013.01.007

Institute of Medicine. (2011). *The future of nursing: Leading change, advancing health.* Washington, DC: National Academies Press. http://www.nap.edu/catalog.php?record_id=12956

Mackey, A., & Bassendowski, S. (2017). The history of evidence-based practice in nursing education and practice. *Journal of Professional Nursing, 33*(1), 51–55. http://dx.doi.org/10.1016/j.profnurs.2016.05.009

Martin, E., & Warshawsky, N. (2017). Guiding principles for creating value and meaning for the next generation of nurse leaders. *Journal of Nursing Administration, 47*(9), 418–420. doi:10.1097/NNA.0000000000000507

Melnyk, B. M., & Fineout-Overholt, E. (2015). *Evidence-based practice in nursing & healthcare* (3rd ed.). Philadelphia, PA: Wolters Kluwer Health.

Nelson, A. E. (2017). Methods faculty use to facilitate nursing students' critical thinking. *Teaching and Learning in Nursing, 12,* 62–66. http://dx.doi.org/10.1016/j.teln.2016.09.007

Nightingale, F. (1969). *Notes on nursing: What it is and what it is not.* New York: Dover Books. (Original work published 1860)

Office of Disease Prevention and Health Promotion. (2017a). *HealthyPeople.gov.* Retrieved from https://www.healthypeople.gov

Office of Disease Prevention and Health Promotion. (2017b). *Disparities.* Retrieved from https://www.healthypeople.gov/2020/about/foundation-health-measures/disparities

Perez, E. Z., Canut, M. T. L., Pegueroles, A. F., Llobet, M. P., Arroyo, C. M., & Merino, J. R. (2015). Critical thinking in nursing: Scoping review of the literature. *International Journal of Nursing Practice, 21,* 820–830. doi:10.1111/ijn.12347

Sackett, D. L., Rosenberg, W. M. C., Gray, J. A. M., Haynes, R. B., & Richardson, W. S. (1996). Evidence based medicine: What it is and what it isn't. *British Medical Journal, 312,* 7023, 71–72. Retrieved from http://www.jstor.org/stable/29730277

U.S. Department of Health and Human Services (USDHHS). (2012). *About healthy people.* Retrieved from http://healthypeople.gov/2020/about/default.aspx

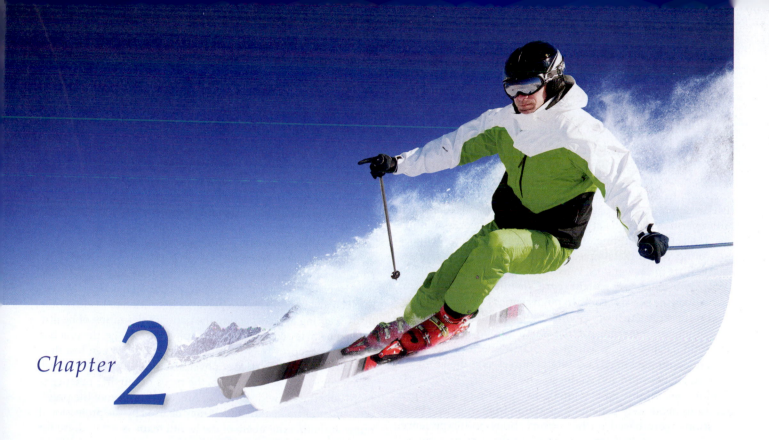

Chapter 2

Health and Wellness

LEARNING OUTCOMES

Upon completion of this chapter, you will be able to:

1. Describe the importance of nursing theory to the practice of nursing and health assessment.

2. Describe the concepts of health, wellness, and health promotion.

3. Relate perspectives of health promotion to the individual, family, and community.

4. Demonstrate how to use the nursing process to encourage health promotion.

KEY TERMS

health promotion, 12	secondary prevention, 12	wellness, 11
primary prevention, 11	tertiary prevention, 12	wellness theories, 11

Introduction

To expand on the definitions of health and wellness introduced in Chapter 1, this chapter presents an overview of the importance of nursing theory to the science and art of nursing. In addition, this chapter presents the concept of health promotion in nursing as it applies to patients, families, and communities. It is within this context that you will conduct the practice of nursing and develop a broad foundation for the use of the nursing process. This chapter introduces the notion that *how* the nursing assessment is conducted gives the nurse vital information about the patient's perceptions of health, wellness, and health promotion. In order to gather the data that will be relevant to the care of a specific patient in a specific setting, you must be able to choose an appropriate approach to the process. Having an understanding of the various ways of thinking about nursing care will enable you to choose the relevant questions to ask, to prioritize the patient's needs, and to be efficient and effective in carrying out your nursing care. The remainder of Unit I consists of an overview of cultural and spiritual considerations as they relate to health and physical assessment, and populations at risk for poor health outcomes—health disparities—are covered in depth.

Nursing Theory and Foundations

Nursing is more than a set of skills or a functional process. As a discipline and profession, it has a unique identity and is underpinned by a "commitment to values, knowledge, and processes to guide the thought and work of the discipline" (Parker & Smith, 2015, p. 4). This body of knowledge has been built over time and has at its foundation the theories of nursing. The act of explaining, describing, or predicting what goes on around you is the simplest definition of a theory. Nurses, as scientists, may wonder "Why do my patients get well?" or "Why does the young patient regress while hospitalized?" or "Why does the body become hypoglycemic?" These questions, stemming from curiosity about the phenomena nurses see happening around them, are the starting point for theorizing (McKenna, Pajnkihar, & Murphy, 2014). Modern nursing care is founded on the innate curiosity of nurses, and the testing of theories about health and wellness.

Florence Nightingale (1865), for example, developed questions about why patients were dying from infection; these questions were based on her observations and experience. She theorized that if the environment were more sanitary, soldiers would be in the best position to let nature cure them (Nightingale, 1865). This deceptively simple way of thinking is the way that theories of nursing have developed. There are many books that go into great detail about nursing theory. This chapter will introduce just a few of the common nursing theories that have been tested over time and have been shown to help nurses organize their thinking about nursing as well as the practice of nursing care.

Models of Health

The following are commonly accepted models that explain the concept of health:

- In the *clinical model*, health is defined as the absence of disease or injury. The aim of the care by the health professional is to relieve signs and symptoms of disease, relieve pain, and eliminate malfunction of physiologic symptoms.

- The *adaptive model* highlights the individual's abilities and flexibility in a challenging environment (Ebrahimi, Wilhlemson, Moore, & Jakobsson, 2012).

- The *ecologic model* developed by Leavell and Clark (1965) examines the interaction of agent, host, and environment. Health is present when these three variables are in harmony. When this harmony is disrupted, health is not maintained at its highest level and illness and disease occur.

- In the *role performance model*, health is defined in terms of an individual's ability to perform social roles (Anderson & Tomlinson, 1992). This model also includes the concept of the "sick role."

- The *eudaemonistic model* views individuals as civilized and cultured who have the capacity for continued growth. In this model, the definition of health is the fulfillment of a person's potential (Ebrahimi et al., 2012).

- The *health promotion model* defines health as the actualization of inherent and acquired human potential through goal-directed behavior, competent self-care, and satisfying relationships with others while adjustments are made to maintain structural integrity and harmony with relevant environments (Pender, Murdaugh, & Parsons, 2015).

Health is highly individualized, and the definition one develops for one's self will be influenced by many factors. These factors will include but are not to limited to age, gender, race, family, culture, religion, socioeconomic conditions, environment, previous experiences, and self-expectations.

Nurses must recognize that each patient will have personal definitions for health, illness, and wellness. Likewise, health-related behaviors will be unique for each patient. Nurses must be aware of their own personal definition of health while also accepting and respecting the patient's definition of health. When health is defined in terms of physical change, the practice focus is on improvement of physical function. When health is considered to be reflective of physical, cultural, environmental, psychologic, and social factors, the focus of nursing practice is more holistic and wide ranging. Any combination of the previously mentioned health models may be used by the professional nurse and other members of the health team as a paradigm for the design and delivery of health care.

Health, Wellness, and Health Promotion

The state of healthcare today underscores the importance of health, wellness, health promotion, disease prevention, and health maintenance. Consumers of healthcare are sophisticated and have access to a wealth of ever-expanding medical knowledge. They are more active in making healthcare decisions and want to have input on how their healthcare is delivered. As the patient now has more control regarding the planning, implementation, and evaluation of strategies and outcomes of health, so the roles of the healthcare providers, including the nurse, have expanded.

Individuals are more conscious of health and wellness than in the past and have become more proactive regarding health and healthcare practices. This requires a stronger emphasis on wellness, health promotion, and disease prevention. A national focus on prevention is supported by several governmental agencies. One is the creation in 1984 of the U.S. Preventive Services Task Force (USPSTF), an independent group of national experts in prevention and evidence-based medicine. The USPSTF makes recommendations based on the best current evidence about screenings, counseling services, and preventive medications (Agency for Healthcare Research and Quality, 2017). Another is *Healthy People 2020*, whose agenda describes 10-year national objectives for improving the health of all Americans (Office of Disease Prevention and Health Promotion [ODPCP], 2017). Each topic area is linked to objectives related to health improvement. The objectives serve as a foundation for the development of plans to improve health for both individuals and communities. Many of the plans to improve health incorporate the promotion of screening for health problems as well as implementation of preventive measures, including immunization, increased physical activity, and education regarding all aspects of health (ODPHP, 2017).

Healthy People 2020 is a comprehensive framework that includes 42 topic areas, each with objectives, interventions, and resources for achievement of the health goal. The vision of *Healthy People 2020* is to achieve "a society in which all people live long, healthy lives" (ODPHP, 2017). Goals to meet this vision include factors that influence individual and community health and wellness. You are encouraged to explore the HealthyPeople.gov website to learn more about all of the initiatives, goals, and stories related to community engagement. ∞

Definitions of Health

In 1947, the World Health Organization (WHO) presented a definition of health that remains active today: Health is "a state of complete physical, mental, and social well-being, not merely the absence of disease or infirmity" (WHO, 2018, para. 1). Although this definition is accepted and understood by most people in developed countries, there are efforts to adapt this definition to include concepts more relevant to indigenous populations across the world (Charlier et al., 2017). In addition to the accepted model of health as incorporating body, mind, and social health, the authors propose to include the concept of "equilibrium of human mankind within its environment" (p. 34). This refers to the interface between humans and the environment that may be conceptualized as "planetary health" and adds a new dimension to the historic definitions of health (Charlier et al., 2017). The traditional definition may also be of limited usefulness when referring to the health status of individuals living with chronic conditions and disabilities (Witt et al., 2017). In the definition, there is a focus on complete well-being, which may not be attainable for some individuals (Witt et al., 2017). These ideas are encouraging nurses to reexamine how they provide nursing care to the patients, families, and communities they serve and to expand the focus of nursing care beyond the traditional definitions. Some of the traditional models and definitions related to health, wellness, and health promotion described in this chapter provide evidence that nurses view health as far more than the absence of illness, disease, and symptoms.

The following traditional definitions of health reflect the work of selected nursing theorists:

- A state of being and the process of becoming whole and integrated in a way that reflects person and environment mutuality (Roy & Andrews, 1999)

- The state of a person as characterized by soundness or wholeness of developed human structures, and mental and bodily functioning that requires therapeutic self-care (Orem, 1971)

- A culturally defined, valued, and practiced state of well-being reflective of the ability to perform role activities (Leininger, 2007)

- A state of well-being and use of every power the person possesses to the fullest extent (Nightingale, 1865)

Definitions and Theories of Wellness

Wellness describes a state of life that is balanced, personally satisfying, and characterized by the ability to adapt and to participate in activities that enhance quality of life. Concepts basic to wellness include self-responsibility and decision making regarding nutrition, physical fitness, stress management, emotional growth and well-being, personal safety, and healthcare. **Wellness theories** describe ways the nurse may approach patient care. An understanding of the patient's perceptions of wellness influence the nurse's approach to patient care. When using a wellness perspective, the nurse focuses on the patient's personal strengths and abilities to enhance health. The goals of nursing care are to assist the patient to participate in health-promoting activities, prevent illness, and seek help for needs and problems. In addition, the nurse focuses on the wellness concerns of the patient and supports the patient's spiritual and end-of-life needs. Theories regarding wellness can assist nurses to clarify their perceptions of wellness. The following theories focus on wellness but also, in some cases, include prevention of illness or injury.

Dunn (1973) defined wellness for the individual as an integrated method of functioning that is oriented toward maximizing the potential of which the individual is capable. It requires the individual to maintain a continuum of balance and purposeful direction within the environment where he or she is functioning. This theory is seen as a grid with two intersecting axes. Health intersects with environment, creating four quadrants (see Figure 2.1 ■). The health axis extends from peak wellness to death, creating various degrees of health and illness. The environmental axis moves from a very favorable environment to a very unfavorable environment. This model takes into consideration the uniqueness of the individual and the influence of family and community regarding healthcare practices (Dunn, 1973).

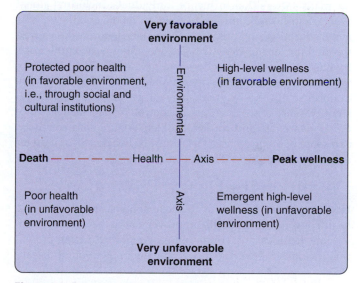

Figure 2.1 Dunn's model of wellness.

Leavell and Clark (1965) described primary, secondary, and tertiary levels of prevention in the healthcare system. In their model, actions are taken to maintain health, prevent illness, provide early detection of a disease, and restore the individual to the highest level of optimum functioning (see Figure 2.2 ■). The key word to emphasize as the focus of primary prevention is *prepathogenic*—that is, before the development of disease or pathology. Actions are taken to prevent disease, illness, or injury. **Primary prevention** implies health and a high level of wellness for the individual. Immunizations, a healthy diet, health teaching, genetic counseling, and the correct use of safety equipment at work are examples of primary prevention strategies (Leavell & Clark, 1965).

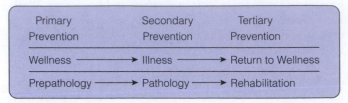

Figure 2.2 Levels of prevention.

Early diagnosis of health problems—and prompt treatment with the restoration of health—is the focus of **secondary prevention**. Emphasis is on resolving health problems and preventing serious consequences. Screenings, blood tests, x-rays, surgery, and dental care are strategies used at this level of prevention. **Tertiary prevention** is activity aimed at restoring the individual to the highest possible level of health and functioning. Rehabilitation is the focus for tertiary prevention. Strategies include use of rehabilitation centers for orthopedic and neurologic problems. Teaching the patient and family members interventions to improve coping with a chronic illness and recognition of complications are examples of tertiary prevention strategies. Table 2.1 provides examples of nursing considerations in relation to the levels of prevention.

Hattie, Myers, and Sweeney (2004) endorse a holistic model of wellness and prevention that incorporates an awareness of the many factors that influence individuals, including global events, family and community, religion, media and the government, education, and business. These outside forces are viewed through the lens of five life tasks, including work and leisure, friendship, love, self-direction, and spirituality. The life task of self-direction is influenced by personal choices about nutrition, exercise, self-care, stress management, gender identity, cultural identity, sense of worth, sense of control, realistic beliefs, emotional awareness and coping, problem solving and creativity, and sense of humor. These tasks must be in balance for individuals to attain wellness (Hattie et al., 2004).

Definitions of Health Promotion

Health promotion refers to those actions used to increase health or well-being and the improvement of the health of individuals, families, and communities. At its core, health promotion includes the work required for the prevention of disease and injury, but it also includes teaching and guidance to help patients reach the goals of optimum health. These efforts which lead to absence of illness are the activities of health promotion.

Pender et al. (2015) define *health promotion* as "behavior motivated by the desire to increase well-being and actualize human health potential" (p. 5). Examples of health promotion activities include but are not limited to health screenings and vaccinations, weight-control measures, exercise, management of stress, smoking cessation, anticipatory guidance for families, and coping with life experiences.

Perspectives on Health Promotion

The role of the nurse as teacher is often employed in the promotion of health for individuals, families, and communities. Understanding nursing theories, knowing the definitions of health and wellness, and having a comprehensive nursing knowledge base are necessary in order to help patients reach or maintain their optimum level of health. Health promotion is often part of the process of the interview—as you learn what the patient needs to know, you determine the best way to convey that information. Nurses must take into account the individual's health status or level of wellness, relevant risk factors, physical fitness, nutrition, health behaviors, and lifestyle. This information is revealed during the nursing assessment and while obtaining the health history. Health promotion is based on a patient's current health status along with an assessment of teaching needs.

Health promotion may be viewed from the perspective of the patient, the family unit, or a community or population. Individuals may have risk factors that make them vulnerable to certain conditions, illnesses, diseases, or injury. Some of these are modifiable, some are not. Those risk factors that are inherent to the individual and cannot be controlled include age, genetic factors, biologic characteristics, and family history. Individual health promotion includes the identification of lifestyle and environmental risks that influence the level of wellness, as well as promoting efforts to reduce or eliminate those risks. Families and communities can be understood to experience risk factors as well. Families in rural communities may have limited access to specialty healthcare; particular geographic areas have populations at higher risk for disease such as the Zika virus outbreak in the southern

Table 2.1 Levels of Prevention

LEVEL OF PREVENTION	FOCUS	EXAMPLES
Primary	Improving overall health	Education about diet, exercise, environmental hazards, accident protection
	Health promotion	Immunization
	Prevention of illness, injury	Assessment of risks for injury, illness
Secondary	Early identification of illness	Health screening and diagnostic procedures
		Promotion of regular healthcare examinations across the life span
	Treatment for existing health problems	Regimens for treatment of illness
Tertiary	Return to optimum level of wellness after an illness or injury has occurred	Education to reduce or prevent complications of disease
	Prevention of recurrence of problems	Referral to rehabilitation services

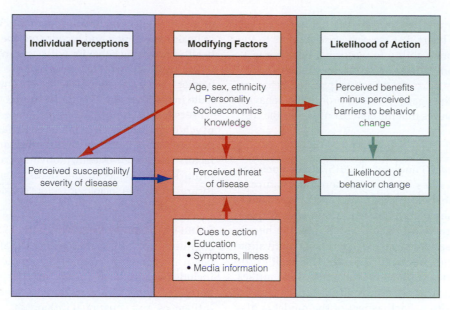

Figure 2.3 Health belief model.

United States. The following models illustrate approaches to health promotion at the individual patient level. These models may help you understand individual health behaviors and guide you in planning nursing interventions.

Health Belief Model

The *health belief model* (Rosenstock, 1974) was developed to predict who would participate in health screenings or obtain vaccinations (see Figure 2.3 ■). According to the health belief model, the following individual perceptions and beliefs influence the decision to act to prevent illness:

- One is vulnerable to an illness.
- The effects of the illness are serious.
- The behavior prevents the illness.
- The benefit of reducing a risk is greater than the cost of the preventive behavior.

Mediating variables influence individual perceptions. The first of the variables is *perceived susceptibility*—that is, the belief about the likelihood of developing an illness. *Perceived severity* is the second variable and refers to the individual's determination of how serious an illness would be. The severity includes the physical, psychologic, and social effects of illness. Another variable is the *perceived cost* of the health-promoting behavior. This refers to factors that interfere with the performance of a behavior. The individual must weigh the physical and psychologic costs versus the benefit.

The health belief model includes two constructs: (1) cues to action and (2) self-efficacy. Cues to action are internal and

external stimuli that affect the individual's motivation to participate in health-promoting activities. For example, heart disease in a family member or knowledge about the Great American Smokeout, a mass media campaign by the American Cancer Society, may motivate one to stop smoking. Self-efficacy refers to the level of self-confidence an individual has about the ability to perform or be successful in the activity.

Last, mediating factors affect the health-promoting behaviors by influencing the perceptions of vulnerability, severity, effectiveness, and cost. Mediating factors include age, gender, ethnicity, education, and economic status.

Theory of Reasoned Action/Planned Behavior

The theory of reasoned action/planned behavior is a prediction theory representing a sociopsychologic method for predicting health behavior (see Figure 2.4 ■). The theory of reasoned action/planned behavior is based on the assumptions that behavior is under volitional control and that people are rational beings. The theory holds that the intention to perform a behavior is a determinant in performance of the behavior (Ajzen, 1991).

Three variables affect the intention to perform a behavior: subjective norms, attitudes, and self-efficacy. *Subjective norms* refer to the individual's perception of what significant others believe or expect in relation to the individual's performance of a behavior. For example, whether one intends to begin a daily exercise program would be influenced by what one believes a spouse's opinion of the activity would be. *Attitudes* refer to value assigned to a particular behavior. An attitude someone

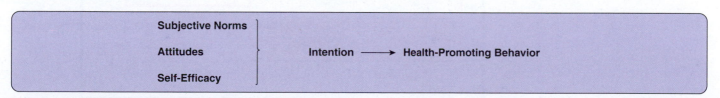

Figure 2.4 Theory of reasoned action/planned behavior.

holds may be that eliminating saturated fat from the diet is a good way to prevent heart disease. *Self-efficacy* refers to the level of confidence in one's ability to perform a behavior (e.g., feeling confident that one can avoid saturated fats in the diet). According to the theory of reasoned action/planned behavior, an individual is likely to engage in health-promoting behavior when the individual believes that the benefit outweighs the cost.

Health Promotion Model

The *health promotion model* (Pender et al., 2015) is a competence model. This model describes "the multidimensional nature of persons interacting with their interpersonal and physical environments as they pursue health" (p. 44). Along with emphasizing individual characteristics and behaviors, the health promotion model focuses on variables that impact motivation and behavioral outcomes (see Figure 2.5 ■). The health promotion model provides a framework through which nurses can develop strategies to assist individuals to engage in health-promoting activities. Each aspect of the model is discussed in the following sections of this chapter.

Individual Characteristics and Behaviors According to the health promotion model, prior related behaviors and personal factors have an effect on future behaviors. Prior related behaviors include knowledge, skill, and experience with health-promoting activities. Prior behavior can have a positive or negative effect on health promotion. When one has engaged in health promotion and recognized the benefit, it is likely that health-promoting behavior will occur in the future. Conversely, when health-promoting activities have been difficult or when barriers to participation have arisen, one is less likely to participate in health promotion in the future.

Personal factors that can influence behavior are biologic, psychologic, and sociologic. Biologic factors include age, gender, body mass index, strength, agility, and balance. Psychologic factors refer to self-esteem, motivation, and perceptions of one's health status. Socioeconomic status, education, race, and ethnicity are among the sociologic factors considered within the health promotion model.

Behavior-Specific Cognition and Affect Behavior-specific cognition and affect are variables that impact motivation to begin and continue activities to promote health. These variables include perceived benefit of action, perceived barriers to action, perceived self-efficacy, activity-related affect, interpersonal influences, and situational influences.

PERCEIVED BENEFITS OF ACTION Engagement in a particular behavior is determined by the belief that the behavior is beneficial or results in a positive outcome. Benefits may be intrinsic, such as stress reduction, or extrinsic, such as financial reward. Perceived benefits of action motivate the individual to participate in health-promoting activities.

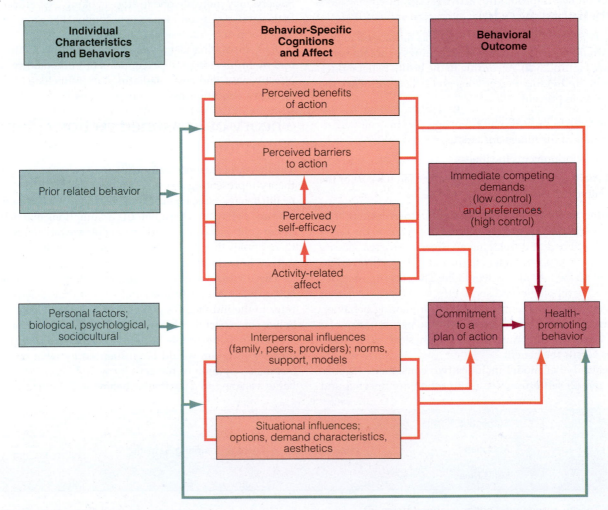

Figure 2.5 Health promotion model.

PERCEIVED BARRIERS TO ACTION Barriers to participation in health-promoting activities may be real or imagined. The barriers include perceptions about the availability, expense, convenience, difficulty, and time required for an activity. Barriers are seen as hurdles and personal costs of participating in a behavior.

PERCEIVED SELF-EFFICACY Perceived self-efficacy is a judgment of one's ability to successfully participate in a health-promoting activity to achieve a desired outcome. Individuals with high self-efficacy are more likely to overcome barriers and commit to health-promoting activity. Those with low self-efficacy have diminished efforts or cease participation in activities.

ACTIVITY-RELATED AFFECT Activity-related affect refers to subjective feelings before, during, and after an activity. The positive or negative feelings influence whether a behavior will be repeated or avoided.

INTERPERSONAL INFLUENCES Interpersonal influences are the individual's perceptions of the behaviors, beliefs, or attitudes of others. The family, peers, and health professionals are interpersonal influences on health-promoting behaviors. These influences also include expectations of others, social support, and modeling the behaviors of others.

SITUATIONAL INFLUENCES Situational influences include perceptions and ideas about situations or contexts. Situational influences on health-promoting activities include perceptions of available options, demand characteristics, and aesthetics of an environment. Access to a cafeteria offering healthy foods at work or having a gym nearby are examples of available options that promote health. Demand characteristics include policies and procedures in employment and public environments. No-smoking policies in public buildings and work environments are demand characteristics that promote health. Aesthetics refers to the physical and interpersonal characteristics of environments. Environments that are safe and interesting and promote comfort and acceptance versus alienation are factors that facilitate health promotion.

Situational influences may be direct or indirect. For example, the requirement to wear protective eyewear and gloves in a microbiology laboratory creates a direct demand characteristic—that is, employees must comply with the regulation.

COMMITMENT TO A PLAN OF ACTION Commitment to a plan of action includes two components: The first component is commitment to carry out a specific activity. The second component is identification of strategies for carrying out and reinforcing the activity. Commitment without strategies often leads to "good intentions" but results in failure to actually carry out the activity.

IMMEDIATE COMPETING DEMANDS AND PREFERENCES Competing demands are alternative activities over which the individual has little control. These demands include family or work responsibilities. Neglect of competing demands may have a more negative impact on health than nonparticipation in a planned health-promoting activity. Competing preferences are alternative behaviors over which the individual has high control. The control is dependent on the ability to self-regulate. Choosing to have lunch with a friend at the health club rather than participating in the aerobics class is an example of choosing the competing preference over the health-promoting activity. Unless an individual can recognize, address, or overcome competing demands and preferences, a plan for health promotion may unravel.

BEHAVIORAL OUTCOMES Health-promoting behavior is the expected outcome in the health promotion model. Health-promoting behaviors can lead to improved health, better functional ability, and improved quality of life across the age span. An example of application of each of the models is presented in Figures 2.6 ■, 2.7 ■, and 2.8 ■. The information is derived from the following case study.

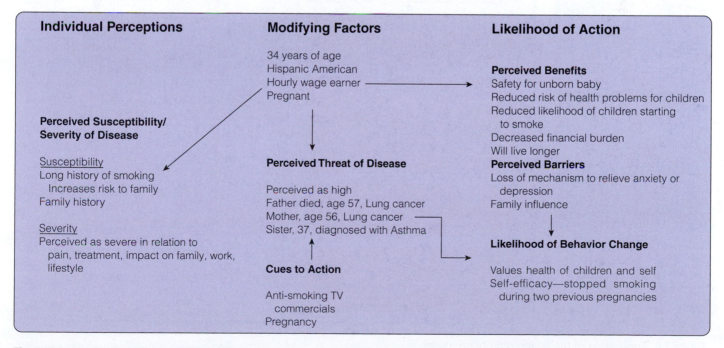

Figure 2.6 Application of the health belief model.

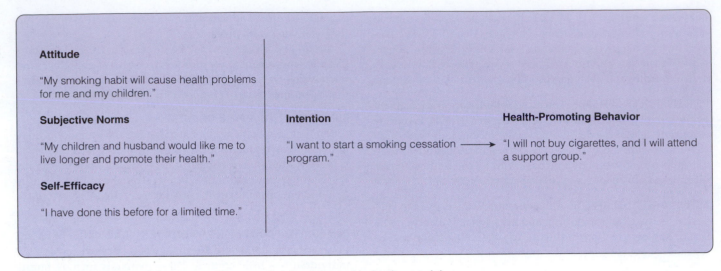

Figure 2.7 Application of the theory of reasoned action/planned behavior model.

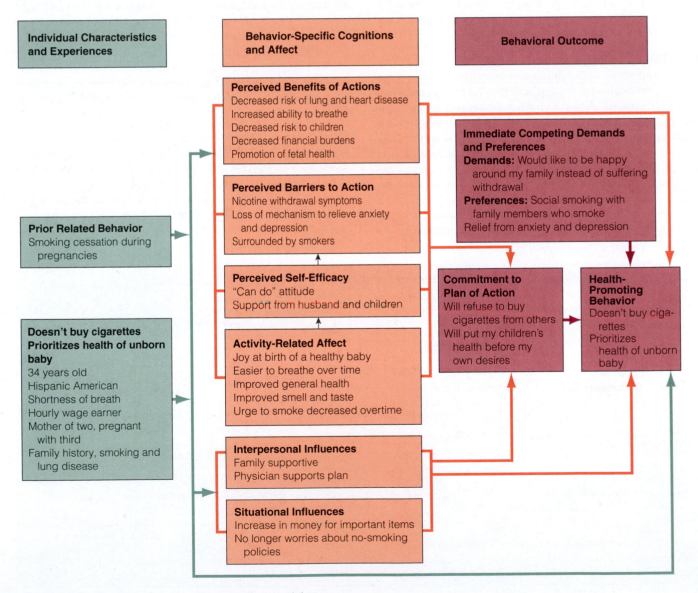

Figure 2.8 Application of the health promotion model.

CASE STUDY

Mrs. Lucia Alvarado is a 34-year-old Hispanic American. She has been a heavy smoker for the past 21 years. Both of her parents and two of her siblings also have a history of smoking. Her father died at age 57 from lung cancer, her mother was recently diagnosed with early stage lung cancer, her older sister suffers from asthma, and her younger brother often struggles with shortness of breath. Mrs. Alvarado is married and the mother of a 13-year-old boy and a 5-year-old girl. She is currently pregnant with her third child. She was able to quit smoking while she was pregnant with her first two children and plans to do the same during her current pregnancy. However, after her second pregnancy, she started smoking again. Mrs. Alvarado works as an hourly employee at a local hotel, and she often has a hard time catching her breath during repeated bending, lifting, and walking. Mrs. Alvarado realizes that her smoking habit can create physical, emotional, family, and economic problems. She frequently sees anti-smoking commercials on TV, and she knows the dangers of smoking during pregnancy, the effects of secondhand smoke on her children's health, and the reality that her children are likely to smoke if they see her smoking. She wants to use her pregnancy as a stimulus to quit smoking for good. Mrs. Alvarado will start a smoking cessation program with the support of her physician and family.

As stated, the models for health promotion guide intervention. Nurses promote positive health-promoting behaviors by emphasizing the benefits of the behaviors, assisting the patient to overcome barriers, and providing positive feedback for success. Personal factors influence health behaviors. Some of the factors such as age, gender, and family history cannot be changed. Nursing interventions will generally focus on factors that can be modified. However, it is also important to develop interventions to address factors that cannot be changed. For example, a patient with a family history of colon cancer may avoid screening programs because of fear or a belief that the development of colon cancer is inevitable. Nurses can provide support for these patients and emphasize the importance of early detection in improved outcomes in colon cancer.

Health assessment and screening provide a rich database from which the nurse can assist the patient, family, or community to identify the current health status, risks for illness or injury, strengths and weaknesses, and resources required to begin or continue appropriate health promotion activities. A variety of strategies including education, support, and modeling are used in health promotion. The nurse assists the individual to develop a plan of action and serves as a resource to guide the activity, monitor progress, and evaluate outcomes.

Health Promotion and the Nursing Process

Once a comprehensive patient database is developed from the health and physical assessment, the nurse works with the patient as the nursing process is applied in problem identification. The process continues through the development and implementation of the plans for care and is completed when the nurse and patient evaluate the outcomes. The following outlines the nursing process as related to health promotion.

Assessment

Comprehensive assessment of the patient is essential to health promotion and patient teaching. Through the health history and physical assessment, the nurse gathers information about the patient's current health status, risk factors, and predisposing factors associated with specific diseases. These risk factors are revealed through data about age, gender, race, and family history. The physical findings yield information including height, weight, and vital signs, as well as data about behaviors and lifestyle practices. Additional assessments are conducted in relation to health promotion. These include physical fitness, nutritional status, a health risk appraisal, lifestyle inventories, assessment of current stressors, and stress management strategies. Social structure assessments include family and support systems, level of education, income, roles, and other activities. Areas included in most health risk appraisals are presented in Box 2.1. Available to the nurse are a variety of tools and resources that will help in understanding assessment of patients related to health promotion. The Centers for Disease Control and Prevention (CDC) has many links for information about chronic disease tracking and prevention (CDC, 2017). Also, instructions for patient self-assessment are available in written form, in English and Spanish, and online through organizations such as the American Diabetes Association and the American Heart Association.

Diagnosis and Planning: The Plan of Care

Once data are gathered, the professional nurse works with the patient to identify current, ongoing, or potential problems, as well as strengths and supports. This information is combined with the nurse's knowledge base and critical thinking to establish patient-centered and appropriate goals. For example, problems may include obesity and smoking, and the patient goals

Box 2.1 Areas of Assessment in Health Risk Appraisal

- Demographic information (age, gender, height, weight)
- Type and amount of exercise
- Occupation
- Smoking
- 24-hour dietary history
- Family history of heart disease, diabetes, cancer
- History of screening tests according to gender and age (mammography, prostate-specific antigen [PSA] test)
- Oral hygiene and dental care history
- Immunization history
- Personal history of illness
- Safety measures (seat belt, sunscreen, condom)
- Sexual activity and reproductive history
- Use of alcohol, illicit drugs, prescription drugs
- Emotional state or mood

could be to lose a specific amount of weight and stop smoking by a specified date. Taking into account the patient strengths, supports, and challenges, the goals and priorities are established to develop a plan to meet the needs of the patient.

Implementation and Evaluation: Roles of the Professional Nurse

In implementing the plan, the nurse takes on the roles of educator, counselor, facilitator, researcher, nurturer, and role model. As educator, the nurse interprets and informs the patient of the significance of findings from all of the completed assessments. This can include subjective and objective data such as laboratory values. Education then may consist of one-on-one sessions related to specific aspects of care or preventive measures as dictated by need. The nurse provides education about specific problems, risks, treatments, or behaviors and may have to provide education about resources available to meet the needs of the patient and family.

As a counselor, the nurse creates and plans opportunities to discuss the implementation of specific activities and to review progress in behavior change or in goal attainment. The counseling role can occur in one-on-one sessions or with groups of patients involved in the same treatment, prevention, or promotion activity. In the facilitator role, the nurse may meet with the patient's family members to provide information, to encourage their participation with the patient in health-related activities, or to promote family support for the patient. As a facilitator, the nurse helps the patient and family gain access to services and facilities required to meet the identified health needs. Each of these roles may require the nurse to search for evidence-based guidelines to help the patient meet their health goals.

The nurturing role of the nurse includes providing the types and amounts of support and encouragement that will assist patients to meet their health-related goals. The nurturing role is particularly important when a patient is attempting to change or modify a behavior. The nurse models wellness and health-promoting behaviors and is willing to share experiences and difficulties in developing plans or meeting goals for healthy behaviors and lifestyles. Additionally, the nurse will identify individuals within the same culture or community who have experienced similar problems or have similar goals in relation to health promotion and wellness and with whom the patient can interact and relate to as a model.

The nurse and patient are involved in continual evaluation of progress in meeting goals. The evaluation process provides opportunities to address concerns. During evaluation, the patient has the opportunity to modify, continue, or discontinue the plan. As a result of evaluation, priorities may be reordered or the methods and tactics may be changed.

Application Through Critical Thinking

CASE STUDY

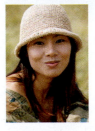

Source: Photofrenetic/Alamy Stock Photo.

You are participating in a health fair performing wellness screenings. *Gina Clark*, a 22-year-old female, approaches your table. She states that she is interested in seeing how healthy her habits are and wants to learn what suggestions you have to help her feel better about her health. Your screening findings show a blood pressure of 132/83, pulse 88, respirations 18, temperature 98.2°F, height 5 ft 4 in, and weight 190.

Gina reports that she drinks a lot of soda and eats fast food several times each week. She does not like vegetables and tends to "snack" a lot rather than sitting down for prepared meals. She states that she would like to eat better and exercise, but she never seems to find the time. She had joined a gym with a friend about a month ago but stopped going after 2 weeks when she became frustrated with sore muscles and lack of results. She would like to lose about 60 pounds and is interested in information on how to accomplish this goal. She tells you that she does not socialize much or go out with friends because she is self-conscious about her weight. Her weight, she says, makes her feel uncomfortable. She slowly leans forward and quietly tells you that she is "repulsed" by her body and does not ever want to look in a mirror or have a picture taken. She indicates that whenever she is stressed about something, she tends to eat even more. "It is like a vicious cycle. I don't know what to do."

CRITICAL THINKING QUESTIONS

1. Describe the importance of wellness in comprehensive health assessment.

2. Where does the patient see herself on the health–illness continuum?

3. What information is appropriate to share with Gina regarding healthy weight loss?

4. What guidelines around physical activity should you share with Gina?

5. How does the theory of reasoned action/planned behavior relate to Gina's situation and her intent to exercise?

REFERENCES

Agency for Healthcare Research and Quality. (2017). *U.S. Preventive Services Task Force: An introduction*. Rockville, MD: Authors. Retrieved from http://www.ahrq.gov/professionals/clinicians-providers/guidelines-recommendations/uspstf/index.html

Ajzen, I. (1991). The theory of planned behavior. *Organizational Behavior and Human Decision Processes, 50*, 179–211. Retrieved from https://doi.org/10.1016/0749-5978(91)90020-T

Anderson, K. H., & Tomlinson, P. S. (1992). The family health system as an emerging paradigmatic view for nursing. *Journal of Nursing Scholarship, 24*(1), 57–63. doi: 10.1111/j.1547-5069.1992.tb00700.x

Centers for Disease Control and Prevention (CDC). (2017). Chronic disease prevention and health promotion. Retrieved from https://www.cdc.gov/chronicdisease/index.htm

Charlier, P., Coppens, Y., Malaurie, J., Brun, L., Kepanga, M., Hoang-Opermann, V., . . . Herve, C. (2017). A new definition of health? An open letter of autochthonous peoples and medical anthropologists to the WHO. *European Journal of Internal Medicine, 37*, 33–37. Retrieved from https://doi.org/10.1016/j.ejim.2016.06.027

Dunn, H. (1973). *High-level wellness*. Arlington, VA: R. W. Beatty.

Ebrahimi, Z., Wilhelmson, K., Moore, C. D., & Jakobsson, A. (2012). Frail elders' experiences with and perceptions of health. *Qualitative Health Research, 22* (11), 1513–1523. doi:10.1177/1049732312457246

Hattie, J. A., Myers, J. E., & Sweeney, T. J. (2004). A factor structure of wellness: Theory, assessment, analysis, and practice. *Journal of Counseling & Development, 82* (3), 354–364. http://doi.org/10.1002/j.1556-6678.2004.tb00321.x

Leavell, H. C., & Clark, E. G. (1965). *Preventive medicine for the doctor in his community* (3rd ed.). New York, NY: McGraw-Hill.

Leininger, M. M. (Ed.). (2007). *Culture care diversity and universality: A theory of nursing* (2nd ed.). New York: National League for Nursing Press.

McKenna, H., Pajnkihar, M., & Murphy, F. (2014). *Fundamentals of nursing models, theories, and practice with Wiley E-Text*. West Sussex, UK: John Wiley & Sons, Ltd.

Nightingale, F. (1865). *Notes on nursing*. New York, NY: D. Appleton and Company. Retrieved from https://babel.hathitrust.org/cgi/pt?id=osu.32436010792867;view=1up;seq=11

Office of Disease Prevention and Health Promotion. (2017). *HealthyPeople.gov*. Retrieved from https://www.healthypeople.gov

Orem, D. E. (1971). *Nursing: Concepts of practice*. Hightstown, NJ: McGraw-Hill.

Parker, M. E., & Smith, M. C. (2015). *Nursing theories & nursing practice*. Philadelphia, PA: F. A. Davis Company.

Pender, N. J., Murdaugh, C. L., & Parsons, M. A. (2015). *Health promotion in nursing practice* (7th ed.). Upper Saddle River, NJ: Pearson Education, Inc.

Rosenstock, I. M. (1974). Historical origins of the health belief model. In M. H. Becker (Ed.), *The health belief model and personal health behavior*. Thorofare, NJ: Charles B. Slack.

Roy, C., & Andrews, H. (1999). *The Roy adaptation model* (2nd ed.). Stamford, CT: Appleton & Lange.

Witt, C. M., Chiaramonte, D., Berman, S., Chesney, M. A., Kaplan, G. A., Stange, K. C., . . . Berman, B. M. (2017). Defining health in a comprehensive context: A new definition of integrative health. *American Journal of Preventive Medicine, 53*(1), 134–137. http://dx.doi.org/10.1016/j.amepre.2016.11.029

World Health Organization (WHO). (2018). *Constitution of WHO: Principles*. Retrieved from http://www.who.int/about/mission/en/.

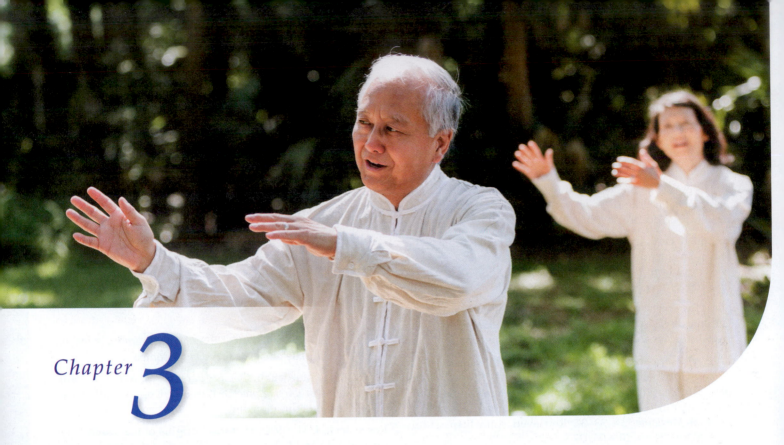

Chapter **3**

Cultural and Spiritual Considerations

LEARNING OUTCOMES

Upon completion of this chapter, you will be able to:

1. Examine the components included in the definitions of culture and spirituality.

2. Practice using terms related to culture and spirituality.

3. Describe the impact of culture and spirituality on health and wellness.

4. Demonstrate cultural and spiritual sensitivity when interacting with patients.

KEY TERMS

assimilation, 23	ethnocentrism, 22	race, 22	spiritual state, 28
cultural competence, 23	heritage, 22	religion, 28	subcultures, 21
culture, 21	heritage consistency, 22	spiritual care, 28	
diversity, 22	heritage inconsistency, 22	spirituality, 28	
ethnicity, 22	moral code, 27	spiritual distress, 28	

Introduction

The United States is made up of people of many races, ethnicities, religions, and heritages. It is expected that the diversity in the United States will continue to expand throughout this century. In 2015, 46,630,000 people living in the United States were born in other countries. Close to 26% of these immigrants came from Mexico, followed by China, India, the Philippines, and Puerto Rico, each having close to 4% (Pew Research Center, 2016). In 2014, the U.S. Census Bureau predicted that by 2060 the Asian population will have increased from 6% to 12% of the U.S. population (U.S. Census Bureau, 2014).

An individual's culture, race, religion, and ethnicity impact beliefs about health and illness and the practices related to both. The nurse must develop the ability to discover knowledge of different cultures and religions, as it is not possible to completely understand all of them. The nurse must continue to learn about other cultures and religions and bring acknowledgment of personal cultural and spiritual beliefs and values to each nurse–patient encounter.

According to the Joint Commission (2014) and the American Association of Colleges of Nursing (2008), cultural and spiritual competence are aspects of patient-centered care that will help to ensure the same high-quality care to all patients and strengthen the delivery of healthcare. Nurses need to understand how various cultural and religious groups perceive life processes, define health and illness, maintain health, determine the causes of illness, and provide care and cure. It is also important to understand how the nurse's cultural and spiritual background influence care. When nurses understand diversity, apply cultural and spiritual knowledge, and act in culturally and spiritually competent ways, they can be more effective in assessing patients, developing culturally and spiritually sensitive interventions, and influencing healthcare policy and practice.

Culture

The National Institutes of Health (NIH) describes **culture** as a combination of knowledge, beliefs, and behaviors that often are specific to racial, ethnic, geographic, social, or religious groups (National Institutes of Health (NIH), 2018). In other words, it is the total of the various practices, beliefs, traditions, customs, language, thoughts, actions, values, and rituals learned from our families by way of socialization (Spector, 2017).

Culture frames an individual's perception of health and illness. Culture influences how healthcare information is received, how symptoms are perceived, and how rights and protections are exercised. It affects what is considered to be a health problem and the type of treatment to be provided. Culture is learned generally within the family group (see Figure 3.1 ■), is shared by the majority within the culture, and changes in response to interactions with events in the external environment. Culture has also been identified as the way a population or group finds a shared meaning for information.

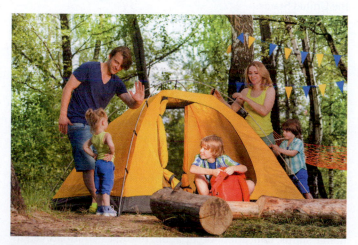

Figure 3.1 Nuclear family interaction.
Source: Sergey Novikov/Shutterstock.

Subdivisions of Culture

Culture may be divided into material and nonmaterial culture. Objects such as dress, art, utensils, and tools and the ways they are used are components of the *material culture*. *Nonmaterial culture* is composed of verbal and nonverbal language, beliefs, customs, and social structures. Cultures may be further defined as *macrocultures*, that is, national, racial, or ethnic groups within which *microcultures* exist based on age, gender, or religious affiliation. **Subcultures** exist within larger cultural groups. Subcultures are composed of individuals who have a distinct identity based on occupation, membership in a social group, or heritage. For example, professional nurses are a subculture within the larger culture of healthcare professionals and are also part of the larger American culture (see Figure 3.2 ■). Many individuals refer to themselves according to an ethnic origin, such as Italian American, Greek American, or Arab American. These individuals often form associations with others of the same ethnic origin, thereby creating a subculture within the larger American culture.

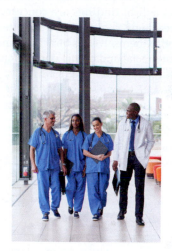

Figure 3.2 Diversity within the subculture of nursing.
Source: michaeljung/Shutterstock.

Generational subcultures also exist. At present, the impact of this phenomenon is highlighted in the workplace setting as, for the first time in United States history, individuals from five generations are working side by side. Although diversity in knowledge and experience can be beneficial, generational differences also may create significant sources of miscommunication and conflict. The five generations are categorized as follows:

- *Veterans:* Born before 1946
- *Baby boomers:* Born 1946–1964
- *Generation X:* Born 1965–1981
- *Generation Y (also called Millennials):* Born 1982–2000 (Reynolds, Bush, & Geist, 2008)
- *Generation Z:* Born 1995–2012 (Levit, 2015)

Each generation differs with regard to numerous aspects of workplace behaviors and attitudes, including views about authority, preferences regarding communication style, and knowledge of various technologies (Levit, 2015; Reynolds et al., 2008). For the nurse, the dynamic of generational subcultures is relevant both to interactions with other healthcare team members and to nurse–patient relationships.

Terms Related to Culture

The terms *culture, race,* and *ethnicity* are often used synonymously. However, these terms refer to different aspects and characteristics of populations and groups of people. These terms and others related to culture are defined in the following sections.

Race   **Race** refers to the identification of an individual or group by shared genetic heritage and biologic or physical characteristics. Members of a given race have similarities in skin color, skeletal structure, texture of the hair, and facial features. Knowledge of the differences in racial characteristics is significant in health assessment because findings are interpreted according to norms for age, gender, and race. However, gene pools are becoming increasingly diverse. Skin color is not always a clear indication of racial identity. For example, dark-skinned individuals from Pakistan, Bangladesh, and parts of India are Caucasian by racial norms as far as medical findings are concerned. Also, racial blending is increasingly common in the United States. Many individuals identify themselves as biracial or multiracial. Definitions of minority racial and ethnic populations in the United States are provided by the Office of Minority Health (OMH, 2013). In 2010, the U.S. Census Bureau identified the following categories of race:

- Hispanic, Latino, or Spanish origin
- Black or African American
- American Indian and Alaska Native
- Asian
- Native Hawaiian and Other Pacific Islander
- White (Colby & Ortman, 2015, p. 9)

Heritage   According to the UMass Amherst Center for Heritage and Society (n.d.), **heritage** is defined as "the full range of our inherited traditions, monuments, objects, and culture. Most important, it is the range of contemporary activities, meanings, and behaviors that we draw from them." **Heritage consistency** describes the extent to which one's lifestyle reflects one's traditional heritage, as well as the degree to which the individual identifies with his traditional heritage. **Heritage inconsistency** describes the adoption and implementation of beliefs and practices obtained by way of acculturation into a dominant or host culture (Berman & Snyder, 2016; Spector, 2017). See Box 3.1 for an example of a heritage assessment tool.

Ethnicity   The term *ethnic* refers to a group of people who share a common culture and who belong to a specific group. Ethnic groups are those with common social and cultural values over generations. **Ethnicity** is the awareness of belonging to a group in which certain characteristics or aspects such as culture and biology differentiate the members of one group from another. Ethnicity is defined by shared interest, ethnic heritage, religion, food, politics, or geography and nationality.

Ethnicity incorporates internal and external identification with a group. Internal identification means that one considers oneself a member of an ethnic group. For example, one may identify oneself as Arab, African, French, Irish, Italian, or

---

Box 3.1 Mini Heritage Assessment

1. Where were your parents and grandparents born?
2. In what country did they grow up?
3. If they were born and/or grew up outside the United States, when did they come to the United States?
4. If you have extended family nearby, how often do you see them?
5. If your native language is not English, how often do you read and speak in your native tongue?
6. What is your religious preference?
7. Do you belong to a religious institution? If so, how often do you attend services and activities there?
8. As an adult do you live in a neighborhood where the neighbors are the same religion and ethnic background as you?
9. Do you participate in ethnic activities and/or prepare ethnic foods?

Source: Spector, R. E. (2017). *Cultural diversity in health and illness* (9th ed.). Hoboken, NJ: Pearson.

Jamaican American. External identification means that those outside of the group perceive the person as a group member.

However, nurses must be aware that national origin is often more important to patients than broader ethnic categories—for example, "Asian American" is a recognized ethnic group, but Asian Americans are likely to identify themselves as Japanese, Filipino, Asian Indian, Korean, Vietnamese, Chinese, Hawaiian, or Samoan.

In the United States, ethnicity is often demonstrated by participation in groups that promote the heritage or traditions of the group. For example, Emerald Societies exist to promote Irish heritage; Italian American social groups promote bonds for those of Italian ancestry.

Ethnicity refers to the degree of attachment with ancestral groups, heritage, or place of birth. Some ethnic identities such as Polish or Syrian are traced to locations in which ancestors were born outside of the United States. Ethnic groups such as Cajuns or Pennsylvania Dutch evolved from geographic regions within the United States.

Ethnocentrism   **Ethnocentrism** is the tendency to believe that one's own beliefs, way of life, values, and customs are superior to those of others. Ethnocentrism creates the belief that one's own customs and values are the standard for judging the values, customs, and practices of others. Ethnocentrism can interfere with collection and interpretation of data as well as the development of plans of care to meet patient needs. Awareness of one's own cultural beliefs, values, and biases can reduce ethnocentrism and foster culturally competent care.

Diversity   **Diversity** is defined as the state of being different. Diversity occurs between and within cultural groups. Characteristics of diversity include nationality, race, color, gender, age, and religion. In addition, diversity is established by socioeconomic status, education, occupation, residence in urban versus suburban or rural areas, marital status, parental status, sexual orientation, and the time spent away from one's country of origin.

For example, Arab Americans are considered a cultural group in the United States. They share tradition as descendants of tribes of the Arabian Peninsula and share Arabic as a common language. However, diversity within this group is characterized by differences in religion, occupation, geography, and period of immigration to the United States. Many of the early Arab immigrants were from Libya and Syria and identified themselves as Christians. However, because Muslims were forbidden to emigrate, fear of deportation may have influenced their recorded statement of religious faith. These immigrants came to the United States seeking economic opportunity (Abdelhady, 2014). Later immigrants settled in urban areas of the northeastern United States and, for the most part, were self-employed or in managerial and professional occupations. In contrast, Arab immigrants after World War II were and continue to be predominantly refugees from nations undergoing political strife. They were primarily followers of the Islamic religion who settled in the midwestern and western United States and maintained strong ethnic ties to the nations from which they emigrated, including Palestine, Iraq, Lebanon, and Egypt. Many Arab immigrants sought educational degrees or were professionals who remained in the United States.

Acculturation Acculturation refers to the process of adaptation and change that occurs when members of different cultures are exposed to one another (Spector, 2017). When the host group has the most power, the host group usually applies its power to influence change among incoming cultural groups (Spector, 2017). In contrast to this unidirectional change, acculturation also may produce bidirectional change, in which the dominant and nondominant cultural groups effect changes on one another (Smokowski & Bacallao, 2011).

Assimilation **Assimilation** refers to the adoption and incorporation of characteristics, customs, and values of the dominant culture by those new to that culture. Assimilation is unidirectional in nature (Smokowski & Bacallao, 2011). For example, immigrants to the United States may assimilate over time and adopt the values of one culture over another. The assimilation process occurs more easily for those who have willingly emigrated from their native land.

Assimilation is affected by several factors including beliefs, language, age, and geography. Those who hold similar values and speak the language of the adopted country more easily assimilate. Assimilation occurs more easily in second-generation immigrants. For example, children born to Chinese parents in Western countries may adopt Western culture more easily, whereas parents tend to maintain the traditional culture. Chinese Americans living in "Chinatown" districts in large cities of the United States are more likely to maintain much of their traditional Chinese cultural practices and beliefs (Smokowski & Bacallao, 2011).

Slow assimilation has occurred in the Cuban American population. Cuban Americans have established enclaves in Miami, Florida, and Union City, New Jersey. In these enclaves, Spanish remains the predominant language in the home and in many of the workplaces. The slow assimilation to English, as well as the isolation within Cuban communities, results in strong ethnic identity and some degree of insulation from the prevailing American culture (Smokowski & Bacallao, 2011).

Cultural Competence The capacity of nurses or health service delivery systems to effectively understand and plan for the needs of a culturally diverse patient or group constitutes **cultural competence**. Spector (2017) views cultural competence as a complex combination of knowledge, attitudes, and skills used by the healthcare provider to deliver services that attend to the total context of the patient's situation across cultural boundaries. The development of cultural competence is essential to nursing. Because cultural competence develops over time through knowledge acquisition and experience, the key to developing cultural competence is to be sensitive to each patient's culture even if you are initially unfamiliar with their specific cultural beliefs. Incorporating the patient's cultural values, beliefs, customs, and practices improves the nurse's ability to gather and interpret data and to plan care appropriate to meet the needs of diverse patients.

Cultural Phenomena That Impact Healthcare

Culture and heritage influence an individual's perceptions about internal and external factors that contribute to health or cause illness, as well as the practices the individual follows to prevent and treat health problems.

In many Westernized countries, beliefs about health and illness are derived from a scientific approach. The scientific approach includes "germ theory" as applied in infectious diseases; knowledge of changes in body structures and functions associated with aging, including arthritis, menopause, and vision changes; and the understanding that diet and lifestyle choices influence health and illness. Health practices include seeking healthcare from healthcare providers who use scientific methods to diagnose and treat illness. Healthcare practices also include following recommendations for disease prevention, such as screening for risks, screening for early detection of problems, and immunization.

In many cultures, beliefs about health and illness are built around nonscientific theories, such as diseases being caused by disturbance in the hot and cold balance of the body, requiring the consumption of foods that oppose these imbalances. Other cultures believe that health is related to achieving harmony with nature. Illness is explained as disruption in harmony, which is caused by some acts on the part of the ill person or by a curse having been placed on the person.

Two factors have influenced perceptions of health and healthcare practices in the United States. The first factor is that people of all nations continue to immigrate to the United States. As a result, the beliefs and practices of these individuals, families, and groups influence the ways in which individual healthcare is managed. Many of the immigrant populations have adapted to and use the healthcare system in the United States but retain cultural practices. For example, patients of some heritages may believe that eating a healthy diet, getting proper sleep, and not going to bed with wet hair promote health. Some patients may be more likely to use home remedies for colds and headaches, including the use of honey for a sore throat and applying a wet rag to the head for headaches (Spector, 2017). Some groups are accustomed to Westernized approaches to all aspects of healthcare yet may consult an elder or use herbal treatments before seeking care and continue the use of herbs while receiving prescribed treatments (Spector, 2017). The adoption of scientific beliefs and practices is influenced by the length of time from immigration and often by the age of the patient. Conversely, the exposure to and knowledge of a variety of cultural beliefs and healthcare practices has promoted the adoption of many treatments, remedies, and therapies from those cultures by healthcare practitioners in the United States. For example, acupuncture, which is part of traditional Chinese medicine, has become a widely accepted therapy and is now used for pain relief in many modern healthcare settings, including some hospitals, although it has many other traditional uses as well (Spector, 2017).

Culture influences the patient's perceptions of healthcare providers as well. Some, for example, recognize the doctor as the head of the healthcare team and hold physicians in high regard. Others may respect healthcare professionals but fear seeking care because of concerns about confidentiality (Spector, 2017).

How nurses are viewed is often dependent on the individual's cultural view of women's roles in society as well as a lack of respect for those viewed as subservient to the physician. In many cultures, the assistance of a family member or cultural healer is sought before that of a healthcare professional. Furthermore, health-seeking behaviors are influenced by the type of illness, language barriers, and concerns that family and cultural rituals surrounding care of the sick and dying will not be respected or permitted.

From a broad perspective, categories of cultural phenomena that impact the provision of healthcare include temporal relationships, family patterns, dietary patterns, health beliefs and practices, and communication. Understanding these phenomena is essential to comprehensive health assessment and to the delivery of safe and effective nursing care. Selected examples of each of the phenomena are described in the following sections, and communication is included in Chapter 5, Interviewing and Health History: Subjective Data. ∞

Differences in language, beliefs, values, and customs exist within cultural groups. As such, cultural beliefs and behaviors are patient specific and may or may not include attributes that are generalized to a given culture. To avoid stereotyping, assessment of an individual's beliefs is essential. In every case, the patient—and the patient's beliefs—should be treated with respect.

Temporal Relationships

Temporal relationships refer to an individual's or group's orientation in terms of past, present, or future as well as clock-time orientation. Cultural variations exist in temporal orientation. For example, the temporal orientation of a patient who is a member of the Cherokee nation may be to the past. Their actions are based on tradition and respect for ancestral practices. The predominant cultures of Western countries are future-oriented as demonstrated by the propensity to invest in the future and "save for tomorrow." Individuals from Latino or Chinese cultures are more likely to be "present"—that is, concerned about the here and now. Another trait of Western cultures is concern with time in terms of abiding by the clock, schedules, and punctuality. In other cultures and groups, such as Cuban Americans, Mexican Americans, and Native Americans, clock time may not be regarded as important.

Family Patterns

Family patterns refer to the roles and relationships that exist within families. These roles and relationships include patterns for responsibilities, values, inclusion, and decision making. The roles and responsibilities of family members are often culturally specific in terms of age and gender. For example, patriarchal households, in which the male is responsible for all decisions, including those related to healthcare, are common in Appalachian, Italian, and Filipino groups. African American groups are more likely to follow matriarchal patterns.

Dietary Patterns

Nutritional intake has an impact on health from infancy through old age. The types and amounts of foods that individuals include in the diet are often culturally determined. In addition, certain foods and beverages, as well as mealtimes, are part of cultural rituals or accepted practices. For example, Americans are known for morning coffee or coffee break rituals, and those from Hispanic cultures are known to eat dinner later in the evening. Eating practices are also associated with culturally determined events or holidays. Muslims may fast (no food or drink) from dawn to sunset during the month of Ramadan. Lent is a period during which Roman Catholics may fast by eating just one full meal and two small meals on Ash Wednesday and Good Friday, and they may abstain from meat on Ash Wednesday and all Fridays until Easter. In the United States, turkey is a traditional Thanksgiving meal. Certain foods are prohibited in some religious or cultural groups. For example, Muslims and Jews are prohibited from eating pork, although some followers of those religions do not abide by that restriction. Most cultures have theories about nutrition and health; different types of foods are selected, and food preparation practices vary according to needs in relation to health and illness. In traditional Mexican, Iranian, Chinese, and Vietnamese cultures, a patient may seek a balance between hot and cold foods to prevent illness and as one of the aids for cure in certain illnesses. When a culture adheres to guidelines from the Western healthcare perspective, foods high in fat and salt may be avoided as a way to prevent heart disease and some cancers.

Box 3.2 provides questions about diet to ask patients along with the reasons for doing so.

Health Beliefs and Health Practices

There are three general categories of health beliefs: magico-religious, biomedical, and holistic health. In a magico-religious belief system, health and illness are believed to be controlled by various supernatural or spiritual forces. This type of belief system is found in Latino and West Indian cultures in which illness may be attributed to evil eye (maldyok) or voodoo (spirits that control destiny and may be contacted to cure illness). Those who hold biomedical health beliefs consider illness to be caused by germs, viruses, or a breakdown in body processes and functions, and they believe that physiologic human processes can be affected by human intervention. Individuals who follow traditional Western medical practice hold this belief.

In a holistic health belief system, one holds that human life must be in harmony with nature and that illness results from disharmony between the two. The holistic belief system is consistent with the concepts of yin and yang in the Chinese culture, the hot and cold theory of illness in some Latino cultures, and

Box 3.2 Cultural Diet Influences

MODEL QUESTIONS	RATIONALES
• Do you speak or read any other languages?	• Understanding primary and secondary languages is important for both communication and education.
• Is there anyone else you would like us to include in this nutrition conversation?	• In some cultures, a patient may defer to an elder or authority figure when answering questions about health.
• Is there any time of the year that you change your diet for cultural reasons, including religion?	• Cultural and religious beliefs and traditions can affect food choices, beliefs, and practices in many ways, from the number of meals eaten in a day to choices of foods, preparation methods, and overall food beliefs.
• Are there any foods you avoid for cultural reasons?	• Diversity exists within cultural and religious groups. It is important to avoid applying general knowledge about cultural and religious food practices to all people within a group; instead, explore individual interpretation and influences.
• What types of foods do you believe promote health or keep you well?	• Assess common dietary staples, as well as foods believed to be associated with health or symbolic benefits. Some food is thought to promote health or cure conditions. Other beliefs may be related to life-span issues, such as the proper diet during pregnancy for easy delivery or to make the "hot" condition "colder."
• Are there any foods that you would try to consume if you were sick or for certain conditions?	• Many religious groups have dietary laws that are observed differently by subgroups within the population. Consumption of kosher meats, fasting, and avoidance of certain foods such as pork, crustaceans, birds of prey, beef, or other animal products are examples.
• Do you use any health remedies or practices that are related to your culture?	• Ask about food practices and special meals for special occasions and holidays. Some religious groups fast during parts of some religious holy days.
• *For the patient with a health diagnosis or condition*: Please tell me what you think caused this condition.	• Discuss food preparation methods. A variety of cultures make similar types of dishes but prepare them differently—for example, using different fats such as bacon drippings, lard, oils, or ghee (clarified butter).
• Is there anything else that you would like me to know about your dietary practices?	• Ask about medicinal herb use because this varies among cultures and is often an important aspect of health beliefs.
• *For the patient who has immigrated*: Has your diet changed in any way since you moved here? What is different? What is the same?	• Explore to what extent any acculturation has taken place and what traditional practices have changed resulting from living in a new dominant culture. Ask whether new foods have been added along with traditional foods, whether newer or different versions of foods have been substituted, and whether any traditional foods have been omitted. In some cases, traditional diets are healthier than the diet in the new culture, and encouragement to maintain healthy traditions may be helpful.

the dimensions of the medicine wheel as accepted by some Native Americans.

Seeking healthcare for illness and disease is one health practice that is influenced by culture—by one's health beliefs, as well as economics, geography, and knowledge. In some geographic regions and areas where there is limited access to Westernized healthcare, people often rely on folk healing or folk medicine. Folk healing is generally derived from cultural traditions and includes the use of teas, herbs, and other natural remedies to treat or cure illness. In many cultures, care is sought only when all other remedies have been exhausted or when the symptoms have become severe. This custom often results in complications and prolonged illness or hospitalization. This practice in some Appalachians and older European Americans may be a result of stoicism, or it may be a result of lack of knowledge and understanding of the healthcare system or language barriers that can

occur in other cultural groups who have immigrated to the United States.

Access to healthcare impacts one's health practices as well. Those in lower socioeconomic groups or without insurance are more likely to self-medicate, use folk or family remedies, and seek episodic acute care than are those who have higher income levels and health insurance.

Ideally, the nurse should be familiar with the cultural beliefs of the groups who are most often served by a given institution or organization and should use reliable resources to obtain information about unfamiliar cultural groups. It is important to note that expertise with regard to every culture is neither expected nor needed in order to develop cultural competence. Instead, nurses must focus on patients' answers to questions in order to understand what ideas and beliefs patients hold about health and then consider how those beliefs might be implicated in treating patients.

Culture in Comprehensive Health Assessment

Comprehensive health assessment refers to obtaining subjective and objective data that are used to identify patient needs. The data are then used to develop and implement plans to meet those needs. Cultural data are essential to this process because they inform the nurse about a variety of factors and practices that impact the current and future health status of the patient. Cultural data in comprehensive assessment would include all of the cultural phenomena described in the previous section.

When conducting the assessment of culture, the nurse must be careful to avoid stereotyping—that is, the nurse must not assume because a patient looks a certain way or has a certain name that he or she belongs to or identifies with a certain cultural or religious group. For example, Mexico is considered a Catholic country, but not all Mexican people are Catholics. In addition, even if the nurse is of the same cultural or ethnic background as the patient, it cannot be assumed that the nurse's beliefs and practices are the same. The nurse and the patient may identify themselves as Hispanic. However, if the nurse relates to a Colombian culture, whereas the patient is from Cuba, the nurse must recognize that aspects of the Latin or Hispanic cultures from those areas can be quite different. A nurse who was born and raised in the United States must avoid assuming that a patient who states "I'm all American" shares the same beliefs and values. The nurse should ask patients to describe what identification with a specific culture means to them. The use of open-ended questions helps to obtain information about the meaning of the patient's statements about ethnic or cultural identity. Often the follow-up question about the family's cultural or ethnic identity can reveal areas to explore in relation to beliefs about illness or disease, diet, and relationships. For example, a patient who states "I'm all American" may reveal links with ethnic groups after further questioning by saying, "My parents are from Germany, and we eat lots of German foods, but I'm like all of my American friends."

Ethnic Identity and Culture

Information about ethnicity and culture is gathered because it enables the nurse to determine physical and social characteristics that influence healthcare decisions. Ethnicity and culture may influence a number of health-related factors for the patient. These factors include health beliefs; health practices; verbal and nonverbal methods of communication; roles and relationships in the family and society; perceptions of healthcare professionals; diet; dress and rituals; and rites associated with birth, marriage, child rearing, and death.

Information about the patient's ethnicity and culture is obtained by asking questions such as these:

- Do you identify with a specific ethnic group?
- How strong would you say that identity is?
- What language do you speak at home?
- Do you or members of your family speak a second language?
- Are you comfortable receiving information about your health in English?
- Would you like an interpreter during this interview?
- Would you like to have an interpreter during the physical examination?
- Are there rules in your culture about the ways an examination must be carried out?
- Are there rules about the gender of the person who is examining you?
- Do you need to have someone in your family participate in the interview or examination?

Information about health beliefs and practices, family, roles and relationships, cultural influences on diet, activity, emotional health, and other topics are included in other components of the health history, including the review of body systems. For example, when asking about the patient's health patterns, the nurse will gather information about cultural healing or rituals associated with health and health maintenance. Further, when asking about nutrition, the nurse will gather information about cultural influences on food selection, preparation, and consumption.

Information about ethnicity and culture can be obtained by conducting a complete cultural assessment at this point in the health history. Box 3.3 includes a "mini" cultural assessment with generalized questions and information on how to ask these questions. Box 3.4 includes the information to be obtained in a complete cultural assessment.

Box 3.3 Mini Cultural Assessment

The mini cultural assessment provides a starting point for asking patients about any cultural beliefs that would affect how you provide healthcare. Before beginning the cultural assessment, inform the patient that you will be asking questions about cultural beliefs. When asking the questions, provide examples to explain the type of information you are looking for. If the patient gives a positive answer to any of these questions, a more thorough cultural assessment should be conducted. Recording the patient's answers to these questions will be vital to providing ongoing, culturally sensitive care, especially for patients who are in the hospital for multiple shifts.

1. What is your preferred language? Would you feel more comfortable with an interpreter present?

2. Do you identify with a specific ethnic or other group? For example, do you identify as Mexican, Black, Chinese, LGBTQ . . . ?

3. Do you follow any cultural rules about how an examination should be carried out? For example, would you prefer a provider of the same sex? Are there rules about exposure of certain body parts?

4. Do you follow any cultural or spiritual practices that would affect your healthcare? For example, do you have any dietary restrictions? Do you have rituals that must be performed at certain times of the day? Do you have a spiritual leader you would like us to contact?

5. Do you prefer to have a family member present during exams or discussions about your health and treatment?

Box 3.4 Cultural Assessment

1. What racial group do you identify with?
2. What is your ethnic group?
3. How closely do you identify with that ethnic group?
4. What cultural group does your family identify with?
5. What language do you speak?
6. What language is spoken in your home?
7. Do you need an interpreter to participate in this interview?
8. Would you like an interpreter to be with you when health issues are discussed?
9. Are there customs in your culture about talking and listening, such as making eye contact or the amount of distance one should maintain between individuals?
10. How much touching is allowed during communication between members of your culture and between you and members of other cultures?
11. How do members of your culture demonstrate respect for another?
12. What are the most important beliefs in your culture?
13. What does your culture believe about health?
14. What does your culture believe about illness or the causes of illness?
15. What are the attitudes about healthcare in your culture?
16. How do members of your culture relate to healthcare professionals?
17. What are the rules about the sex of the person who conducts a health examination in your culture?
18. What are the rules about exposure of body parts in your culture?
19. What are the restrictions about discussing sexual relationships or family relationships in your culture?
20. Do you have a preference for your healthcare provider to be a member of your culture?
21. What do members of your culture believe about mental illness?
22. Does your culture prefer certain ways to discuss topics such as birth, illness, dying, and death?
23. Are there topics that members of your culture would not discuss with a nurse or doctor?
24. Are there rituals or practices that are performed by members of your culture when someone is ill or dying or when they die?
25. Who is the head of the family in your culture?
26. Who makes decisions about healthcare?
27. Do you or members of your culture use cultural healers or remedies?
28. What are the common remedies used in your culture?
29. What religion do you belong to?
30. Do most members of your culture belong to that religion?
31. Does that religion provide rules or guides related to healthcare?
32. Does your culture or religion influence your diet?
33. Does your culture or religion influence the ways children are brought up?
34. Are there common spiritual beliefs in your culture?
35. How do those spiritual beliefs influence your health?
36. Are there cultural groups in your community that provide support for you and your family?
37. What supports do those groups provide?

Spirituality

Spiritual and belief patterns reflect an individual's relationship with a higher power or with something, such as an ideal, a group, or humanity itself, that the person sees as larger than self and that gives meaning to life. The outward demonstration of spirituality may be reflected in religious practice, lifestyle, or relationships with others. A moral code is often included in one's belief patterns. A **moral code** comprises the internalized values, virtues, and rules one learns from significant others. It is developed by the individual to distinguish right from wrong. An individual's spiritual beliefs and moral code are affected by culture and ethnic background.

Spirituality impacts a person's life. Numerous studies have found that when spiritual practices are a part of a person's life, improvements are seen in their overall health, as well as an increased ability to handle stressful and life-changing events and decreased risk of mortality (Koenig, Larson, & Larson, 2001; Lucchetti, Lucchetti, & Koenig, 2011). Reliance on spiritual behaviors increases personal growth, reduces the effects of stress, and improves health during difficult life issues (Hellman, Williams, & Hurley, 2015; Park et al., 2013). Spiritual beliefs and religious practices have also been shown to have a positive impact on resilience (Murray-Swank & Pargament, 2005). Resilience occurs when people are able to adapt well in the face of adversity, including serious illness or loss of a loved one. Conversely, negative feelings about spirituality may be associated with poorer health outcomes, including depression, anxiety, anorexia, and drowsiness (Delgado-Guay et al., 2011). Negative feelings toward God, feeling punished by God, or believing that an evil force is at work in one's life has been associated with a higher incidence in mortality in older adults (Pargament, Koenig, Tarakeshwar, & Hahn, 2001).

Spiritual health has been closely linked to both emotional and physical health. When health challenges or other life difficulties occur, many people turn to their religious beliefs and practices as a means to maintain hope, gain a sense of meaning to their life, and reduce stress. Involvement in religious activities appears to enable those who are ill to cope more effectively and grow from their experiences, rather than being defeated by them (Koenig et al., 2001). Health challenges or other life difficulties often create the need for spiritual connection. Spiritual health is inextricably linked to both physical and emotional health, thus making it an important and impactful component of care. Holistic nursing care encompasses physical, psychologic, and spiritual dimensions as a means to treat the entire person rather than just the physical or emotional symptoms (Cooper, Chang, Sheehan, & Johnson, 2013).

Studies have shown that many patients desire to discuss their spiritual health with their healthcare providers during times of physical and emotional stress, such as receiving news of a serious or life-threatening diagnosis (Taylor & Mamier, 2013). The nurse and physician are not generally viewed as the primary spiritual caregivers, but their availability as a support is important. Nurses are typically the members of the healthcare team who are most physically present to patients, which may aid in the development of trust within the nurse–patient relationship, allowing the patient to feel comfortable sharing their spiritual concerns. Therefore, it is important for nurses to have the skills needed to respond to patients' spiritual concerns in an efficient, effective, and ethical manner (Baldacchino, 2015; Taylor & Mamier, 2013).

Terms Related to Spirituality

Spirituality and religion are related terms, yet they are distinctly different. Spirituality is defined as "sensitivity or attachment to religious values and things of the spirit rather than material or worldly interests" (Spirituality, n.d.). This can be contrasted with the definition of **religion**, "the body of institutionalized expressions of sacred beliefs, observances, and social practices found within a given cultural context" (Religion, n.d.). In a broader sense, spiritualty's focus is one of attunement to ideals not of this earthly realm, whereas religion has a focus on the content of one's beliefs and how those beliefs are outwardly manifested. Spirituality may be evidenced by the act of doing spiritual things such as praying or meditating, but it tends to be more abstract than religion, which promotes a creed or certain set of beliefs, rituals, and ethics (Got Truth Ministries, 2018).

Spirituality refers to the individual's sense of self in relation to others and a higher being, what one believes gives meaning to life, and what fosters hope for one's will to live. The spirit is the part of each person that controls the mind, and the mind then controls what the body does. Spirituality may be a part of a particular religion, which is an organized faith system that includes rituals, beliefs, practices, and symbols to draw people close to God, a higher power, or ultimate truth. Spirituality can be separate from a religion as it provides meaning and purpose in life, even for those who do not believe in any god or higher power. A **spiritual state** describes the person's feelings about their spirituality that can fluctuate along a continuum of well-being to spiritual distress (Baldacchino, 2015).

Spiritual care is a part of the art of nursing care. Spiritual care is defined as meeting patients' spiritual needs by way of recognizing and respecting these needs, facilitating participation in religious rituals, engaging in active listening, promoting hope, demonstrating empathy, and making referrals to other professionals, including chaplains, pastors, rabbis, priest, and imams, for example, as additional support. Caring for patients through supportive and empathetic actions can help promote a sense of well-being. The goal in spiritual care is to help patients find meaning and purpose in their life, even in the midst of illness, so the delivery of care is not the most important aspect. The heart and spirit by which the care is provided is of the utmost importance. The nurse should take an active and involved approach to meet a patient's spiritual needs, including calling in an expert in the patient's theological beliefs to clarify beliefs and conflicts.

Spiritual Distress   **Spiritual distress** can be described as an interruption in one's value system or beliefs. This disruption affects the person's entire being by threatening their sources of hope, peace, and meaning for their life. The greater the degree to which unmet spiritual needs remain unmet, the greater is the spiritual distress experienced by the patient. Spiritual distress may have a harmful effect on a patient's well-being, prognosis, and quality of life and may cause depression. Spiritual distress can and does occur frequently, especially in the case of serious illness or injury. It is important to note that not everyone will experience spiritual distress in the same way or to the same degree (Monod et al., 2010; Taylor & Mamier, 2013).

Spiritual distress can be expressed in many ways. Defining characteristics of spiritual distress include these (Caldeira, Timmins, deCarvalho, & Vieira, 2017; King et al., 2017; Selby, Seccaraccia, Huth, Kurrpa, & Fitch, 2016):

- Expressing concern about or questioning the meaning of life and death and/or the patient's belief system
- Questioning feelings of anger at or of abandonment by God or a higher power
- Feeling a sense of emptiness
- Having difficulty sleeping, having nightmares, or being afraid to sleep
- Seeking spiritual guidance
- Experiencing a change in mood or behavior such as anger, withdrawal, anxiety, crying, apathy, hostility

How should nurses respond to spiritual distress to help resolve the issues? Wright (2008) offers helpful recommendations to nurses for "softening the suffering" during periods of spiritual distress:

1. *Enter into the relationship completely committed to being present:* Be truly present and focus all your attention on the patient and the distress the patient is experiencing. Allow the patient to talk about these experiences and focus on the story rather than trying to change the subject or cheer them up.

2. *Ask the patient to share stories of suffering:* Encourage the patient to talk about the experience of the illness on all aspects of life. Ask the patient about the impact on family, marriage, work, and other things that are important to the patient. Be willing to listen and reminisce.

3. *Use active listening skills:* Listen with your heart and mind, not just with your ears. Reflect back to the patient what you heard. This provides clarity as well as an opportunity for the patient to know that his or her suffering was heard and acknowledged. Be willing to be there for the patient without feeling the need to "do something."

4. *Provide the patient with compassionate care:* Enter fully into the relationship with the patient in distress to facilitate healing through a connection built on caring. Provide a calm and relaxing setting. Treat the patient respectfully and with dignity.

5. *Acknowledge the suffering:* This can provide the patient with a chance to thrive. Do not say you understand how the patient feels because you cannot. Instead ask the patient to help you understand more clearly what this situation has meant.

6. *Help the patient explore the meanings associated with the distress:* Explore the meaning and purpose the patient believes is behind the suffering. Work with the patient to

find ways to keep desired rituals and ways of life. Help the patient and family look for ways to create memories.

7. *Offer hope:* Hope can provide confidence that may help the patient heal. Support any desire the patient may have to maintain a relationship with friends and family. Contact the patient's spiritual advisor for additional support.

Spiritual Assessment

An important area of spiritual care is a systematic approach for collecting information for a spiritual history. As previously stated, a majority of patients want their caregivers to address their spiritual concerns, so it is important that the spiritual history contain more than just a simple listing of the patient's religion.

In order for a spiritual assessment to produce usable results, certain components must be present. Box 3.5 describes sample components of a general spiritual assessment.

Spiritual History Many spiritual history tools have been developed as a means to gain a broader understanding of the patient's beliefs, values, ability to find meaning and hope during suffering, and recognition of the role of religion in their life (Taylor, Testerman, & Hart, 2014). Numerous researchers have designed formal spiritual assessment tools, including the following well-known frameworks:

- Stoll (1979) introduced direct questioning as a method to assess spirituality and incorporated four basic areas for questioning: the patient's concept of God, sources of hope and strength, religious practices, and the relationship between spiritual beliefs and health.

- McSherry and Ross (2002) described methods for assessment of spirituality and spiritual needs as including direct questioning, indicator tools, and values clarification tools.

- Anadarajah and Hight (2001) developed the use of HOPE questions as a formal spiritual assessment in the patient interview. The mnemonic *HOPE* is explained as follows: *H* refers to questions about the patient's spiritual resources, including sources of hope, meaning, love, and comfort. *O* refers to participation in or association with organized religion. *P* includes personal spiritual practices. *E* refers to the effects of healthcare and end-of-life issues.

- Hodge (2001) described a narrative framework for spiritual assessment. This qualitative instrument incorporates a spiritual history and a framework to identify spiritual strengths as summarized in Box 3.6.

The FICA Spiritual History Tool, created in 1996 by Dr. Christina Puchalski, provides an efficient way to gather the key elements about a patient's spiritual beliefs. The FICA tool consists of four domains of spiritual assessment: *Faith* and belief; the *Importance* of spirituality in a person's life; the person's spiritual *Community*; and interventions to *Address* spiritual needs during care. The questions within the FICA tool are straightforward, are easily understandable, and identify the aspects of the patient's life that provide significant spiritual support. The information obtained opens the door for nurses and other healthcare providers to discuss issues of meaning to patients, including those involving healthcare decisions (Borneman, Ferrell, & Puchalski, 2010). See Box 3.7.

Spiritual Care Competence

Spiritual care competence by the nurse or healthcare provider is a continuous and holistic process that involves several aspects. Most important, it begins with an awareness and understanding of one's own spiritual values and beliefs. It is difficult to assess and support a patient experiencing spiritual distress without being comfortable knowing how your own spirituality influences your thinking, actions, and provision of care to others. Ask yourself the following questions:

- How comfortable are you asking patients about their spiritual beliefs, practices, and needs?

- How comfortable are you praying with a patient or asking a patient if prayer is desired?

- Do you have the skills needed to develop and implement a spiritual plan of care?

- How comfortable are you assessing a patient for signs of spiritual distress?

Your answers will indicate the areas that require growth in knowledge, comfort, and action (Hellman et al., 2015; Milner, Foito, & Watson, 2016).

Spiritual competence requires the nurse to know how to complete a spiritual assessment and be comfortable doing it. This

---

Box 3.5 Sample Components of a Spiritual Assessment

- Desire to discuss spirituality or religious beliefs
- Choice of individual with whom discussion of spirituality or region is preferred (e.g., nurse, hospital chaplain, physician, or another individual)
- Life philosophy or beliefs about life
- Affiliation with religion or particular spiritual beliefs
- Importance of spirituality or religion in daily life
- Significant spiritual rituals or practices, including prayer or meditation
- Conflicts between religious or spiritual beliefs and health-related treatments

Sources: Data from Williams, Meltzer, Arora, Chung, & Curlin. (2012). Attention to inpatients' religious and spiritual concerns: Predictors and association with patient satisfaction. *Journal of General Internal Medicine, 26*(11), 1265–1271; Hodge & Horvath. (2010). Spiritual needs in health care settings: A qualitative meta-synthesis of patients' perspectives. *Social Work, 56*(4), 306–316.

Box 3.6 Narrative Spiritual Assessment

Part I. Narrative Framework—Spiritual History

Sample Interview

1. Describe your personal and family religious traditions. (Include importance of religion and religious practices.)
2. What practices were important to you in youth? How have those experiences influenced your life?
3. How would you describe your religiosity or spirituality today? Do you believe your spirituality provides strength? How?

Part II. Interpretive Framework—Evokes Spiritual Strengths

1. *Affect:* How does spirituality affect joy, sorrow, coping? What part does spirituality play in providing hope?
2. *Behavior:* What rites or rituals do you use or follow? Do you have a relationship with a religious community or leader?
3. *Cognition:* Describe your current beliefs. Do your beliefs affect the ways you deal with difficulties or impact healthcare decisions?
4. *Communion:* What is your relationship with God? How do you communicate? Does your relationship help you in difficult times?
5. *Conscience:* Describe your values. How do you determine right and wrong?
6. *Intuition:* Have you experienced spiritual hunches, premonitions, or insights?

Source: Adapted from Hodge (2001). Spiritual assessment: A review of major qualitative methods and a new framework for assessing spirituality. *Social Work, 46*(3), 203–214.

Box 3.7 FICA Spiritual History Tool©

F—Faith and Belief

"Do you consider yourself spiritual or religious?" or "Is spirituality something important to you?" or "Do you have spiritual beliefs that help you cope with stress/difficult times?" (Contextualize to reason for visit if it is not the routine history.)

If the patient responds "No," the healthcare provider might ask, "What gives your life meaning?" Sometimes patients respond with answers such as family, career, or nature.

(The question of meaning should also be asked even if people answer yes to spirituality.)

I—Importance

"What importance does your spirituality have in your life? Has your spirituality influenced how you take care of yourself, your health? Does your spirituality influence you in your healthcare decision making (e.g., advance directives, treatment, etc.)?"

C—Community

"Are you a part of a spiritual community?" Communities such as churches, temples, and mosques, or a group of like-minded friends, family, or yoga, can serve as strong support systems for some patients. Can explore further: "Is this of support to you and how? Is there a group of people you really love or who are important to you?"

A—Address in Care

"How would you like me, your healthcare provider, to address these issues in your healthcare?" (With the newer models, including diagnosis of spiritual distress, A also refers to the "Assessment and Plan" of patient spiritual distress or issues within a treatment or care plan.)

© C. Puchalski, 1996

Source: Christina M. Puchalski, MD, FICA Spiritual History Tool, adapted from The FICA Spiritual History Tool #274, *Journal of Palliative Medicine, 17*(1), 2014.

includes collecting comprehensive information that is focused on the patient's spiritual history, beliefs, needs, and concerns. The assessment data must be collected on each patient and then incorporated into the patient's plan of care so it can be disseminated to all providers working with the patient. Recognition of the signs of spiritual distress and the plan of care that includes an empathetic response to the distress should be included. Evaluation of the plan of care should be completed frequently. Nurses must be able to care for the patient's physical needs while simultaneously incorporating the patient's spirituality, values, and beliefs into the plan of care (Taylor & Mamier, 2013; Williams et al., 2012).

The nurse has an obligation to prioritize meeting the holistic needs of all patients. Therefore, knowledge of cultural, spiritual, and language differences is essential in current practice. The nurse must examine his or her own cultural and spiritual values and beliefs and reflect on their significance to encounters and interactions with patients of diverse cultures and religions. The nurse must continue to learn about a variety of cultures, religions, and languages. When language differences exist, the nurse must use all resources possible to ensure that decisions are based on accurate information. These resources include the use of translators and written materials provided in the language of the patient. Last, the nurse must seek information about community resources to meet the needs of the diverse cultural and spiritual groups for whom care is provided.

Application Through Critical Thinking

CASE STUDY

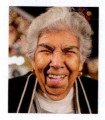

Source: Eric Raptosh Photography/Getty Images.

Rachel Wood is a nursing student doing her rotation at a clinic that provides care to patients who do not have health insurance. Today she and the other students are seeing an older Latino woman from Mexico, Mrs. Reyes, who was in the United States visiting her granddaughter and became ill. Her granddaughter, Antonia, brought her to the clinic because she does not have any health insurance. Mrs. Reyes, whose native language is Spanish, does not speak English. Antonia speaks both English and Spanish, was born in the United States, and is a citizen. Her parents came here when they were in their twenties and are very happy here in the United States. Antonia lives with her parents and brother. Her grandmother wants to see a *curandero* (a traditional Latin American healer that she normally sees in Mexico), but her granddaughter is explaining to her that there are none in this area, and they need to see the nurse practitioner in the free clinic. Antonia says to her, "That is so old-fashioned, Grandma. No one does that here." The nurse practitioner requests a translator and then proceeds to interview the patient.

CRITICAL THINKING QUESTIONS

1. What is important for the nurse to understand about the culture as it relates to Mrs. Reyes?

2. Mrs. Reyes will need discharge educational materials. What standards support ensuring that these are available in Spanish?

3. Antonia's comment to her grandmother that "No one does that (sees a curandero) here" could be an example of assimilation. Why would that be true?

4. How should the nurse approach Mrs. Reyes's request for a curandero?

5. How should the nurse interact with the translator during the patient interview?

REFERENCES

Abdelhady, D. (2014). The sociopolitical history of Arabs in the United States: Assimilation, ethnicity, and global citizenship. In S. C. Nassar-McMillan, K. J. Ajrouch, & J. Hakim-Larson (Eds.), *Biopsychosocial perspectives on Arab Americans: Culture, development, and health* (pp. 17–43). New York, NY: Springer.

American Association of Colleges of Nursing. (2008). Cultural competency in baccalaureate nursing education. Retrieved from http://www.aacnnursing.org/Portals/42/AcademicNursing/CurriculumGuidelines/Cultural-Competency-Bacc-Edu.pdf?ver=2017-05-18-143551-883

Anadarajah, G., & Hight, E. (2001). Spirituality and medical practice: Using the HOPE questions as a practical tool for spiritual assessment. *American Family Physician, 63*(1), 81–89. Retrieved from http://www.aafp.org/afp/2001/0101/p81.html

Baldacchino, D. (2015). Spiritual care education of health care professionals. *Religions, 6,* 594–613.

Berman, A., & Snyder, S. J. (2016). *Kozier and Erb's fundamentals of nursing: Concepts, process and practice* (10th ed.). Hoboken, NJ: Pearson.

Borneman, T., Ferrell, B., Puchalski, C. (2010). Evaluation of the FICA tool for spiritual assessment. *Journal of Pain and Symptom Management, 40*(2) 163–173.

Caldeira, S., Timmins, F., de Carvalho, E. C., and Vieira, M. (2017). Clinical validation of the nursing diagnosis *spiritual distress* in cancer patients undergoing chemotherapy. *International Journal of Nursing Knowledge, 28*(1), 44–52. doi:10.1111/2047-3095.12105

Campbell, Y., Machan, M., & Fisher, M. (2016). The Jehovah's Witness population: Considerations for preoperative optimization of hemoglobin. *AANA Journal (84)*3, 178–183.

Caplan, S., Escobar, J., Paris, M., Alvidrez, J., Dixon, J. K., Desai, M. M., Whittemore, R. (2013). Cultural influences on causal beliefs about depression among Latino immigrants. *Journal of Transcultural Nursing, 24*(1), 68–77.

Colby, S., & Ortman, J. (2015). Projections of the size and composition of the U.S. population: 2014–2060 Population estimates and projections. *U.S. Department of Commerce Economics and Statistics Administration U.S. Census Bureau.* Retrieved from http://www.census.gov/content/dam/Census/library/publications/2015/demo/p25-1143.pdf

Cooper, K. L., Chang, E., Sheehan, A., & Johnson, A. (2013). The impact of spiritual care education upon preparing undergraduate nursing students to provide spiritual care. *Nurse Education Today, 33,* 1057–1061.

Delgado-Guay, M., Hui, D., Parsons, H., Govan, K., De la Cruz, M., Thorney, S., & Bruera, E. (2011). Spirituality, religiosity, and spiritual pain in advanced cancer patients. *Journal of Pain and Symptom Management, 41*(6), 986–994.

Got Truth Ministries. (2018). Is there a difference between religion and spirituality? Retrieved from https://www.compellingtruth.org/difference-religion-spirituality.html

Hellman, A., Williams, W., & Hurley, S. (2015). Meeting spiritual needs: A study using the spiritual care competency scale. *Journal of Christian Nursing, 32*(4), 236–241.

Hodge, D. R. (2001). Spiritual assessment: A review of major qualitative methods and a new framework for assessing spirituality. *Social Work, 46*(3), 203–214.

Hodge, D. R., & Horvath, V. E. (2010). Spiritual needs in health care settings: A qualitative meta-synthesis of patients' perspectives. *Social Work, 56*(4), 306–316.

Joint Commission. (2014). Advancing effective communication, cultural competence, and patient-and family-centered care: A roadmap for hospitals. Retrieved from https://www.jointcommission.org/roadmap_for_hospitals

King, S., Fitchett, G., Murphy, P. E., Pargament, K. I., Harrison, D. A., & Loggers, E. T. (2017). Determining best methods to screen for religious/spiritual distress. *Supportive Care in Cancer, 25*(2), 471–479. doi:10.1007/s00520-016-3425-6

Koenig, H., Larson, D., & Larson, S. (2001). Religion and coping with serious medical illness. *Annals of Pharmacotherapy, 35,* 352–359.

Levit, A. (2015, March 28). Make way for Generation Z. *New York Times.* Retrieved from https://www.nytimes.com/2015/03/29/jobs/make-way-for-generation-z.html?_r=0

Lucchetti, G., Lucchetti, A., & Koenig, H. (2011). Impact of spirituality/religiosity on mortality: Comparison with other health interventions. *Explore, 7*(4), 234–238. doi:10.1016/j.explore.2011.04.005

McSherry, W., & Ross, I. (2002). Dilemmas of spiritual assessment: Considerations for nursing practice. *Journal of Advanced Nursing, 38*(5), 479–488.

Milner, K. A., Foito, K., & Watson, S. (2016). Strategies for providing spiritual care and support to nursing students. *Journal of Christian Nursing, 33*(4), 238–243.

Monod, S., Rachat, E., Bula, C., Jobin, G., Martin, E., & Spencer, B. (2010). The spiritual distress assessment tool: An instrument to assess spiritual distress in hospitalized elderly persons. *Geriatrics, 10,* 88. doi:10.1186/1471-2318-10-88

Murray-Swank, N. A., & Pargament, K. I. (2005). God, where are you? Evaluating a spiritually-integrated intervention for sexual abuse. *Mental Health, Religion, & Culture, 8*(3), 191–203.

National Institutes of Health (NIH). (2018). Cultural Respect. Retrieved from https://www.nih.gov/institutes-nih/nih-office-director/office-communications-public-liaison/clear-communication/cultural-respect

Office of Minority Health (OMH). (2013). *The national CLAS standards.* Retrieved from https://www.minorityhealth.hhs.gov/omh/browse.aspx?lvl=2&lvlid=53

Pargament, K., Koenig, H., Tarakeshwar, N., & Hahn, J. (2001). Religious struggle as a predictor of mortality among medically ill elderly patients: A 2-year longitudinal study. *Archives of Internal Medicine, 161*(15), 1881–1885.

Park, N., Lee, B., Sun, F., Klemmack, D., Roff, L., & Koenig, H. (2013). Typologies of religiousness/spirituality: Implications for health and well-being. *Journal of Religion and Health, 52*(3), 828–839.

Pew Research Center (2016). Origins and destinations of the world's migrants, from 1990–2015. Retrieved from http://www.pewglobal.org/2016/05/17/global-migrant-stocks/?country=US&date=2015

Religion. (n.d.). By permission. From Merriam-Webster.com © 2018 by Merriam-Webster, Inc https://www.merriam-webster.com/dictionary/religion

Reynolds, L., Bush, E. C., & Geist, R. (2008). The Gen Y imperative. *Communication World, 25*(2), 19–22.

Selby, D., Seccaraccia, D., Huth, J., Kurrpa, K., & Fitch, M. (2016). A qualitative analysis of a healthcare professional's understanding and approach to management of spiritual distress in an acute care setting. *Journal of Palliative Medicine, 19*(11), 1197–1204. doi:10.1089/jpm.2016.0135.

Smokowski, P. R., & Bacallao, M. (2011). *Becoming bicultural: Risk, resilience, and Latino youth.* New York: New York University Press.

Spector, R. E. (2017). *Cultural diversity in health and illness* (9th ed.). Hoboken, NJ: Pearson.

Spirituality. (n.d.) By permission. From Merriam-Webster.com © 2018 by Merriam-Webster, Inc https://www.merriam-webster.com/dictionary/spirituality

Stoll, R. (1979). Guidelines for spiritual assessment. *American Journal of Nursing, 79*(9), 1574–1577.

Taylor, E., & Mamier, I. (2013). Nurse responses to patient expressions of spiritual distress. *Holistic Nursing Practice, 27*(4), 213–224. doi:10.1097/HNP.0b013e318294e50a

Taylor, E., Testerman, N., & Hart, D. (2014). Teaching spiritual care to nursing students: An integrated model. *Journal of Christian Nursing, 31*(2), 94–99.

U.S. Census Bureau. (2014). *U.S. Census Bureau projections show a slower growing, older, more diverse nation a half century from now* [Press release]. Retrieved from https://census.gov/data/tables/2014/demo/popproj/2014-summary-tables.html

UMass Amherst Center for Heritage and Society. (n.d.) *What is heritage?* Retrieved from http://www.umass.edu/chs/about/whatisheritage.html

Williams, J. A., Meltzer, D., Arora, V., Chung, G., & Curlin, F. A. (2012). Attention to inpatients' religious and spiritual concerns: Predictors and association with patient satisfaction. *Journal of General Internal Medicine, 26*(11), 1265–1271.

Wright, L. (2008). Softening suffering through spiritual care practices: One possibility for healing families. *Journal of Family Nursing 14*(4), 394–411.

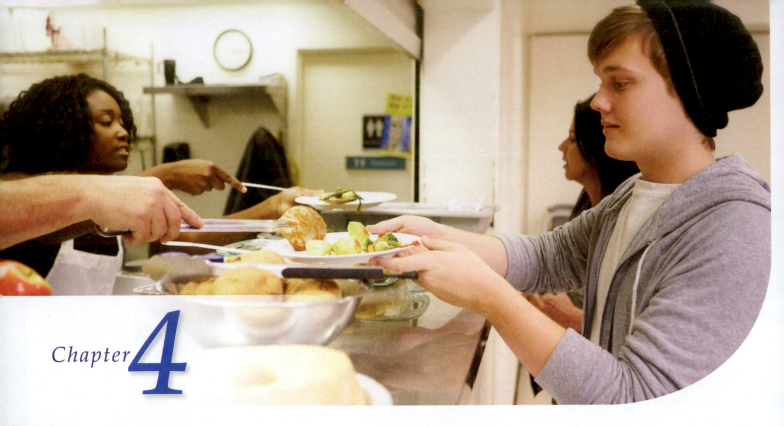

Chapter 4

Health Disparities

LEARNING OUTCOMES

Upon completion of the chapter, you will be able to:

1. Explain health disparities in relation to vulnerable patient groups and their impact on the nurse's role in health assessment.

2. Identify the factors that influence health disparities in vulnerable populations.

3. Identify strategies to reduce and eliminate health disparities.

KEY TERMS

disabilities, 37
geography, 36
health disparities, 34

health equity, 35
mixed-status family, 38

social determinants of health, 37
vulnerable populations, 35

Introduction

Health disparities have been a major concern in healthcare for many years. They negatively affect groups of people who face socioeconomic and other burdens because of a variety of factors that are discussed in detail in this chapter. This often results in decreased quality of life, lack of access to healthcare, and poorer healthcare outcomes. It is essential for the nurse to have an understanding of the causes of health disparities, the impact disparities have on caring for patients, and strategies to address and remove these barriers so that all individuals can have equal access to healthcare.

Health Disparities

Some people in the United States, as well as globally, receive less or lower quality healthcare than others because of health disparities. **Health disparities** are "preventable differences in the burden of disease, injury, violence, or opportunities to achieve optimal health that are experienced by socially disadvantaged populations" (Centers for Disease Control and Prevention [CDC], 2015, para. 1). These gaps are grouped broadly into categories such as social, economic, demographic, and geographic disadvantages (CDC, 2013; National Partnership for Action to

End Health Disparities [NPA], n.d.; World Health Organization [WHO], 2018).

Disparity within a population is identified when there are higher rates of diseases, deaths, and suffering when compared with those in the general population (National Institute on Minority Health and Health Disparities, n.d.). **Vulnerable populations** are groups of individuals who are not well integrated into the healthcare system because of age, gender, income, race, ethnicity, nativity, language, sexual orientation, gender identity, disability, geographic location, and other social risk factors. This isolation places members of these groups at risk for exclusion from necessary preventive or medical care, and thus it constitutes a potential threat to their health.

Many causes of disparities in vulnerable populations are controllable, but people within these populations often do not have the resources to be able to avoid these barriers and reach optimal health (NPA, n.d.). For example, a healthy living environment supports good health. However, many disadvantaged individuals live in housing that is older and may contain harmful mold, materials, or other substances (e.g., lead, asbestos). These individuals may also live in neighborhoods with high crime and violence that put them at risk for exposure to increased violence, causing a potential for physical injury, emotional stress, and a reduction in the ability to enjoy outdoor physical activity.

The WHO (2018) views health as a fundamental human right for all individuals. Therefore, attainment of equity is an essential goal. **Health equity** "is the absence of avoidable or remediable differences among groups of people, whether those groups are defined socially, economically, demographically, or geographically" (WHO, 2018, para. 1). Health equity means that all people have an equal opportunity to experience optimal health and healthcare (Office of Disease Prevention and Health Promotion [ODPHP], Healthy People 2020, 2017a; WHO, 2018). Although there have been some improvements toward the goal of equity, significant health disparities continue for vulnerable populations in the United States (National Quality Forum [NQF], 2017). Efforts to attain equity require a strong focus and commitment by all healthcare stakeholders to eliminate avoidable inequalities and address past and current injustices (NQF, 2017; ODPHP, Healthy People 2020, 2017a). Strategies for reducing disparities in vulnerable populations are discussed in more detail later in this chapter.

Health Disparities: Considerations for Nursing and Health Assessment

Nurses play a crucial role when performing health assessments for patients from vulnerable populations. The data from health assessments help to determine the patient's current and ongoing health status, predict risk, and identify health promotion activities. The data may assist the nurse in identifying barriers to healthcare caused by health disparities. Nurses can positively affect health disparities via interdisciplinary collaboration and by designing a plan of care with optimal health outcomes for the patient.

A focus on improving the availability and quality of care among persons who are experiencing health disparities—through patient history taking and physical examination—allows clinical interventions to become opportunities for each individual to attain his or her full health potential. For example, the Omaha System was developed for use in diverse practice settings such as public health, home health, and nurse-managed centers. It is a research-based system that documents patient assessment and nurse interventions directed toward wellness, support systems, and coping skills. Using this system identifies and categorizes teaching needs, guidance and counseling, treatments and procedures, case management, and surveillance to address health disparities of vulnerable populations (Thompson, Monsen, Wanamaker, Augustyniak, & Thompson, 2012).

Nurses also must be aware of the social factors linked to a patient's cultural identity during an assessment. Cultural competence in nursing is more than an understanding of race and ethnicity. It is an awareness and an acceptance of patients' health practices, beliefs, values, and attitudes in order to improve their health outcomes. Nurses must develop an awareness of their own cultural beliefs and cultural competence to effectively care for vulnerable individuals (NQF, 2017) (see Chapter 3, Cultural and Spiritual Considerations ∞).

Factors Influencing Health Disparities in Vulnerable Populations

The CDC (2013), in partnership with other organizations, continues to identify and address the different factors that may lead to health disparities. It assesses vulnerable populations as defined by the following:

- Race and ethnicity
- Age
- Gender
- Sexual orientation or gender identity
- Geography
- Disability status
- Socioeconomic status

Race and Ethnicity

People of color—often considered individuals of Asian, Hispanic/Latino, Black/African American, and American Indian/Alaska Native backgrounds (U.S. Department of Health and Human Services, Office of Minority Health, 2016)—make up more than 37% of the United States population (U.S. Census Bureau, 2016). Members of these communities of color tend to experience more issues with preventable diseases, death, and disabilities than do Caucasians (CDC, 2017a). These issues can be attributed to factors such as lack of access and utilization of care, as well as poor patient–provider interactions. In addition, minorities are more likely to be uninsured or underinsured and have an income below the poverty level (Artiga, Foutz, Cornachione, & Garfield, 2016). Box 4.1 gives examples of issues related to health disparities in communities of color.

Age

When performing a health assessment on a patient from the perspective of a vulnerable population, it is imperative that the nurse consider health issues that occur across the lifespan as they relate to a patient's cognitive and emotional development.

Box 4.1 Examples of Health Disparities among People of Color

- Some Asian Americans may contend with infrequent medical visits because of fear of deportation, language and cultural barriers, and lack of health insurance (U.S. Department of Health and Human Services, Office of Minority Health, 2017a).
- African Americans have the highest death rates from heart disease and stroke; the highest prevalence of hypertension, diabetes, and peritonitis; the largest HIV infection rate; and the highest death rate from homicide (National Institutes of Health, 2016).
- When compared with White individuals, African Americans are more likely to report barriers to seeing a healthcare provider because of cost (CDC, 2017b).
- Native Hawaiians/Pacific Islanders have higher rates of smoking, alcohol consumption, and obesity and have limited access to cancer prevention and screening programs (U.S. Department of Health and Human Services, Office of Minority Health, 2017c).
- Although the Indian Health Service (IHS) typically serves the health needs of the American Indian population, more than half of the people in this group do not permanently reside on reservations and have limited or no access to IHS services (U.S. Department of Health and Human Services, Office of Minority Health, 2017c).
- Factors that may contribute to poorer health outcomes among American Indians and Alaska Natives are cultural barriers, geographic isolation, inadequate sewage disposal, and economic factors (U.S. Department of Health and Human Services, Office of Minority Health, 2017c).
- There are higher rates of STDs among some communities of color compared with White individuals (CDC, 2017c).
- Hispanics/Latinos experience significantly higher rates of contracting gonorrhea, chlamydia, and syphilis when compared with White individuals, not because of ethnicity or heritage but because of social conditions (e.g., poverty, lower educational levels, lack of employment) that are more likely to affect people of color (CDC, 2017a).

Health disparities can affect individuals of certain age groups in different ways. In general, the very young and very old are often most vulnerable (Mid-America Regional Council [MARC], 2018). Examples of disparities related to certain age groups include the following:

- Infants and children who live in poverty and belong to certain communities of color, as described previously in this chapter, are at a higher risk for illness and death than infants and children in the broader population. Miller and Chen (2013) reported that childhood poverty rates in the United States have climbed steadily since the 2008 recession. Children of lower socioeconomic status may experience household crowding, inadequate nutrition, and more exposure to secondhand smoke.
- In adolescents, risky behaviors (e.g., alcohol and drug use, tobacco use, unhealthy dietary behaviors, sexual risk behaviors) are more prevalent in vulnerable populations (Thompson, Connelly, Thomas-Jones, & Eggert, 2013).
- Older adults often face unique healthcare challenges that predispose them to the need for medical care. However, accessing care can be an issue because of lack of transportation and cost (Psychology Benefits Society, 2016).

Gender

Healthcare disparities can also be addressed in the context of gender issues. Some studies have found that disparities between men and women exist in the diagnosis of certain health conditions and recommendations of treatment (Kent, Patel, & Varela, 2012). Nurses should be aware of resources to assist in reducing disparities because of gender.

For example, programs such as Well-Integrated Screening and Evaluation for Women Across the Nation (WISEWOMAN) provide low-income, under- or uninsured women with the knowledge, skills, and opportunities to improve their diet, physical activity, and other lifestyle behaviors to prevent, delay, and control cardiovascular and other chronic diseases (CDC, 2017d).

Sexual Orientation and Gender Identity

Researchers in the field of gender identity development have raised awareness that gender is not exclusively determined by an assigned sex at birth but, rather, is determined by a person's sense, belief, and ultimate expression of self (U.S. Department of Health and Human Services, Substance Abuse and Mental Health Services Administration, Center for Substance Abuse Prevention, 2012). Lesbian, gay, bisexual, and transgender (LGBT) individuals experience health disparities associated with societal stigma, discrimination, and denial of their civil and human rights (ODPHP, Healthy People 2020, 2018). High rates of psychiatric disorders, substance abuse, and suicide are linked to discrimination against individuals in this group.

It is important to routinely ask all patients questions regarding gender identity and sexuality in a way that is free of bias and demonstrates cultural competence. When addressing patients, the nurse should always ask how they identify and/or how they wish to be addressed (BWHC LGBT & Allies Employee Resource Group, 2016). One must be careful not to assume how a patient identifies him or herself. Rather, the nurse must be skillful in understanding how to build a rapport and trusting relationship with the patient and how to ask questions as part of the health history to accurately document gender and sexuality. As with many vulnerable populations, in order to ensure sensitivity to LGBT individuals, nurses must possess an awareness and understanding of the terms and definitions that are specific to the LGBT population. Table 4.1 lists terms and definitions related to gender identity.

Geography

Geographic location can have a significant impact on the health of vulnerable populations. **Geography** refers to the country, region, section, community, or neighborhood in which one was born and raised or in which one currently resides or works. Residing in a metropolitan (urban) area or residing in a rural

Table 4.1 Terms and Definitions Specific to Sexual Orientation and Gender Identity

TERM	DEFINITION
Bigender	A person whose gender identity encompasses both male and female genders. Some may feel that one identity is stronger, but both are present.
Female to Male (FTM)	A person who transitions from female to male, meaning a person who was assigned the female sex at birth but identifies and lives as a male. Also known as a transgender man.
Gender Identity	A person's internal sense of being male, female, or something else. Since gender identity is internal, one's gender identity is not necessarily visible to others.
Gender Nonconforming	A person whose gender expression is different from societal expectations related to their perceived gender.
Genderqueer	A term used by persons who may not entirely identify as either male or female.
Male to Female (MTF)	A person who transitions from male to female, meaning a person who was assigned the male sex at birth but identifies and lives as a female. Also known as a transgender woman.
Transgender	A person whose gender identity and/or expression are different from that typically associated with their assigned sex at birth. *Note: The term* transgender *has been used to describe a number of gender minorities including, but not limited to, transsexuals, cross-dressers, androgynous people, genderqueers, and gender nonconforming people.* Trans *is shorthand for* "transgender."
Transgender Man	A transgender person who currently identifies as a male (see also FTM).
Transgender Woman	A transgender person who currently identifies as a female (see also MTF).
Transsexual	A person whose gender identity differs from their assigned sex at birth.
Two-Spirit (2-S)	A contemporary term that references historical multiple-gender traditions in many First Nations cultures. Many Native/First Nations people who are lesbian, gay, bisexual, transgender, or gender nonconforming identify as Two-Spirit. In many First Nations, Two-Spirit status carries great respect and leads to additional commitments and responsibilities to one's community.

area presents geographic challenges for some individuals seeking healthcare. Individuals living in rural areas can be disproportionately affected by the physical locations of healthcare services. For example, hospitals may be farther away, the number of providers may be limited, and specialists may be unavailable. Patients with limited financial resources may be unable or reluctant to travel long distances for routine preventive care. Alternatively, for those living in urban areas, the cost of in-city transportation may pose a barrier to access to healthcare services. In either scenario, health conditions may consequently go undiagnosed or untreated and become more serious.

Disabilities

Individuals with **disabilities** are people who may be in need of healthcare services because of a variety of health concerns. They include people with mental health problems, learning disabilities, and physical disabilities or illnesses that result in a degree of dependence on others. Disabled persons are considered a vulnerable population and are at higher risk for experiencing barriers in healthcare than other members of the population. Several chronic disorders—such as asthma, congestive heart failure, chronic obstructive pulmonary disease, diabetes, and inflammatory bowel disease—can also be reasons for a person to experience disability, especially as the disease progresses.

Some disabilities can be hidden or difficult to recognize. The International Classification of Functioning, Disability and Health (ICF) provides a standard language for classifying changes in body function and structure, activity, participation levels, and environmental factors that influence health. The ICF can help assess the health and functioning activities and factors that can help or create barriers to fully participation in society (WHO, 2017a).

The World Health Organization Disability Assessment Schedule 2.0 (WHODAS 2.0) demonstrates advantages over other assessment instruments for health and disability; this assessment is short, simple to administer, and applicable across cultures and clinical and general population settings (WHO, 2017b). The instrument covers cognition, mobility, self-care, getting along with others, life activities, and participation.

The Disability and Health Data System (DHDS) is an innovative disability and health data tool that is used to identify disparities in health between adults with and without disabilities. The DHDS allows for comparing answers to questions on a state-by-state basis for the percentage of disabilities by age, sex, race/ethnicity, and veteran status; percentage of those who smoke; obesity; vaccine coverage; and preventive services (CDC, 2016). Access this comprehensive data tool for the 50 United States by using this link: www.cdc.gov/ncbddd/disabilityandhealth/dhds.html.

Socioeconomic Status

Social determinants of health are the situations in which a person is born, lives, works, and ages, as well as the systems in place to deal with illness (ODPHP, Healthy People 2020, 2017b). The CDC (2014) further defines social determinants of health as "the complex, integrated, and overlapping social structures and economic systems that are responsible for most health inequities" (para. 14). The WHO (2017a) addresses socioeconomic disparities as a major concern in the United States and globally.

Socioeconomic status (SES) is often a main contributor or compounding issue affecting health disparities in vulnerable populations. Income and education are two of the most common factors in determining SES. SES disparities within vulnerable populations have been noted in this chapter, but there are other groups of individuals who are considered vulnerable and for whom SES is often a contributing factor.

Uninsured and Underinsured   Individuals may experience issues with access to healthcare because of lack of health insurance. The amount and type of insurance coverage are also major factors in access to care and are of particular concern in younger and older adult populations (CDC, National Center for Health Statistics, 2017). In recent years, there has been an attempt to address this problem through regulations that are now a part of the Affordable Care Act (ACA). (The ACA is discussed in more detail later in this chapter.)

Maternal and Infant Health   Although women and children are discussed in the preceding sections, special consideration must be taken regarding maternal and infant health as a result of differences in SES. Maternal and infant health issues occur most commonly within racial and ethnic communities of color (particularly African Americans and Latinos) and in those living in poverty (Association of State and Territorial Health Officials, 2013; Klawetter, 2014). These issues include higher rates of infant mortality and preterm births, low birth weight, and higher rates of maternal morbidity and mortality. Access to quality care and education before conception, during pregnancy, and between pregnancies is an important step in reducing maternal and infant mortality as well as pregnancy-related complications (ODPHP, Healthy People 2020, 2017c).

Immigrants and Refugees   The foreign-born population in the United States has increased significantly over the past five decades. As of 2014, an estimated 42.4 million immigrants (legal and illegal) were living in the United States. Immigrants come to the United States from many different countries. In 2017, 40% of immigrants obtaining lawful permanent residence (LPR) in the United States included individuals from Mexico, the People's Republic of China, India, Cuba, the Dominican Republic, and the Philippines (U.S. Department of Homeland Security, 2017). This profile differs from past profiles of immigrant families that often included individuals from Europe and Canada (Pew Research Center, 2015). In addition to those obtaining LPR, the number of refugees entering the United States has steadily increased. In the past 5 years, an average of 70,000 refugees have entered the country (U.S. Department of Homeland Security, 2016). An awareness of the unique challenges and disparities in health occurring among immigrants and refugees is important for nurses and all healthcare providers. Some of the most common barriers for this population are access to healthcare; healthcare system and insurance navigation; obstacles related to culture, language and literacy; lack of transportation; and experiencing a generalized fear and mistrust of the healthcare system/providers (Hall & Cuellar, 2016).

Within the immigrant family, having "undocumented status" may cause additional stress and uncertainty, may negatively affect health outcomes and educational attainment, and may result in increased social isolation for immigrant children (Chavez, Lopez, Englebrecht, & Anguiano, 2012; U.S. Census Bureau, 2010). The U.S. Department of Homeland Security (2018) reports that 12.1 million undocumented immigrants lived in the United States in 2014. In a review of U.S. Census Bureau statistics, Capps, Fix, and Zong (2016) found that during the period of 2009–2013, five million children under the age of 18 were living with at least one unauthorized immigrant parent. With increasing numbers of children growing up in families in the United States where one or both parents are undocumented

immigrants, it becomes more important that healthcare providers understand the impact of this trend as recognized in the relatively new term "mixed-status families" (Capps et al., 2016).

The term **mixed-status family** has been defined as a family in which one or more family members are undocumented immigrants and other family members are citizens, lawful permanent residents, or immigrants with another form of temporary legal immigration status. Belonging to a mixed-status family where at least one parent is a non–U.S. citizen has its disadvantages concerning healthcare and health insurance. Illegal immigrants often are wary of applying for public health benefits for their children because they fear doing so will alert authorities about their illegal status. In addition, these families may not seek healthcare because of fear of deportation. Immigration status can also exacerbate the level of violence in an abusive relationship when the batterer uses the threat of deportation and release of information about the victim's legal status.

Another issue contributing to health disparity is the number of unaccompanied children attempting to enter the United States. Since October 2013, about 52,000 unaccompanied children from Latin America have been apprehended at the U.S.–Mexico border. Factors such as gang violence, enduring poverty, and drug trafficking have been identified as reasons why these child immigrants made the greater-than-1,500-mile journey from Guatemala, El Salvador, and Honduras to the United States. The Office of the United Nations High Commissioner for Refugees (UNHCR) agency found that of 404 children who left Latin America, at least 59 cited international protection needs from homicide, rape, poverty, police corruption, and gang violence as reasons for crossing the border. Upon entering the United States, the unaccompanied children remain vulnerable because of language barriers and no parental presence or guidance (Yu-Hsi Lee, 2014).

Incarcerated Men and Women   Once incarcerated, men and women are at higher risk for developing acute and chronic disease, mental health problem, substance abuse problem, or infectious disease over the course of their confinement (Justice and Health Connect, 2013). Although the latest report on individuals in the U.S. adult corrections system indicates a slight decrease in numbers, 6,741,400 people were estimated to be in the system at the end of 2015 (Bureau of Justice Statistics, 2015). In general, imprisoned individuals have poorer health than those who are not imprisoned, with White women standing out as having the poorest health (Nowotny, Rogers, & Boardman, 2017). In addition, when prisoners are included in statistics for national health outcomes, poorer health is noted, particularly in African American males.

Veterans   The Veterans Administration (VA) cares for a disproportionate number of disadvantaged, low-income, and vulnerable individuals. Because of vulnerable veterans' propensity for premature morbidities and mortality, they experience challenges when accessing the healthcare system, especially within the VA system itself. Older veterans, especially those with cognitive impairment, increased fragility, and limited social support, make up the fastest growing segment of the VA's patients.

Most veterans today are White males, although women, African American, Latino, and other non-White veterans represent a growing population within the VA system (U.S. Department of Veterans Affairs, n.d.). Veterans of color will make up nearly 34% of the population by 2040. It is anticipated that women will make up about 20% of this population by that time and will have specific needs and challenges related to accessing care in a previously male-oriented and -dominated system. In an attempt to be proactive and address anticipated needs of service-women, the VA conducts ongoing research and implemented a healthcare equality (HCE) workgroup along with several other programs. In its first National Veterans Health Equity report in 2016, the HCE workgroup found that when compared with White veterans, all other racial and ethnic communities of color had higher rates of mental health/substance use disorders and that mental health and substance use conditions are more prevalent in women than men (U.S. Department of Veterans Affairs, n.d.).

The VA has been effective in collecting data on specific behavioral risk factors, such as physical activity levels, smoking, and alcohol use. The information assists state and federal health officials in developing strategies for preventing and controlling health problems for the estimated 25.6 million veterans and 1.8 million active duty, reserve, and National Guard personnel in the United States. Each war has had a specific impact on the health of servicemen and servicewomen and their families. For example, health research on the Vietnam War has described the illnesses and diseases related to Agent Orange, including depression, anxiety, and posttraumatic stress disorder (PTSD). The utilization of advances in body protection during the recent warfare in Iraq and Afghanistan has yielded more injured soldiers coming home alive, but they return with traumatic brain injury (TBI) and physical disabilities, including loss of a limb or limbs. According to O'Neil et al. (2014), a history of mild traumatic brain injury (mTBI) is common among military members who served in Operations Enduring Freedom, Iraqi Freedom, and New Dawn (OEF/OIF/OND). Veterans and military members with a history of mTBI frequently reported cognitive, physical, and mental health symptoms. The findings of the study suggest that appropriate reintegration services are needed for treatment of PTSD, substance use disorders, headaches, and other difficulties veterans experienced after deployment regardless of mTBI history. Veterans who provided service to our country during wartime are an especially vulnerable population, and the nurse must recognize them as such.

Homelessness   Despite signs of improvement in the United States and throughout the world, homelessness remains a serious problem. The U.S. Department of Housing and Urban Development (HUD) (n.d.) recognizes four primary categories of homelessness for individuals and families:

- Literally homeless
- At imminent risk for homelessness
- Homeless as defined by other federal statutes
- Fleeing or attempting to flee domestic violence.

According to the National Alliance to End Homelessness (2016), more than 550,000 people were homeless in 2015. Although this is a decrease from 2014 of about 60,000 people, homelessness continues to be a significant problem that creates barriers to attaining good health and access to quality healthcare. (See Figure 4.1 ■.) The high incidence of homelessness can be attributed to numerous factors, including increased unemployment rates, lack of affordable housing, poor physical or mental health, drug and alcohol abuse, gambling, family and relationship breakdown, domestic violence, and physical and/or sexual abuse (Salvation Army, 2017). Significant health inequalities are associated with homelessness in America (Stafford & Wood, 2017). For example, homeless individuals are more likely to experience a reduction in life expectancy, increased morbidity, and increased usage of acute hospital services.

Assessment of the homeless individual or family begins with establishing trust. A nonjudgmental attitude is essential to developing rapport with all patients, including members of the homeless population. For these individuals, actual and perceived powerlessness can affect every aspect of life, including physical and mental health. For women and children, the risk for physical and emotional trauma is compounded. Homeless women are at increased risk for sexual or domestic abuse.

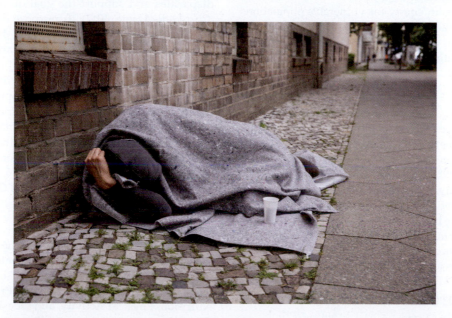

Figure 4.1 Homeless individuals often have little access to good healthcare.
Source: Andrey_Popov/Shutterstock.

Witnessing this abuse can commonly cause emotional and behavioral problems among homeless children (National Institutes of Health [NIH], 2017).

Along with physical assessment, psychosocial assessment is essential to effectively caring for members of this population. In addition to ensuring that the individual's or family's physical health needs are met, the nurse should conduct a thorough psychosocial assessment (see Chapter 5 ∞). Collaboration with other members of the healthcare team should include facilitating referrals to social services, mental health professionals, community assistance programs, and other organizations that may be able to offer assistance.

Strategies to Reduce and Eliminate Health Disparities

When caring for patients who are at higher risk for experiencing disparities, it is essential to understand the steps that are being taken to reduce disparities. Organizations such as the CDC and Agency for Healthcare Research and Quality (AHRQ) have developed reports on key disparities in the United States with priorities and recommendations for improving health disparities (AHRQ, 2015; CDC, 2013). The CDC (2013) reports that although there has been some improvement and an overall reduction in disparities, many significant gaps in health outcomes, access to care, adoption of healthy behaviors, and exposure to healthy living environments remain. AHRQ (2015) discussed significant improvements in access to care, and continued improvement in quality of care but with wide variations in relation to National Quality Strategies (i.e., effective treatment, care coordination, patient safety, person-centered care, healthy living, and care affordability). AHRQ (2013) also reported some progress in disparities related to race and socioeconomic status for access and quality, but there is a strong need for more improvement.

Several initiatives at local, state, national, and international levels have been implemented in an effort to reduce health disparities and achieve health equity for vulnerable populations. Some initiatives were addressed previously in this chapter. The following programs and organizations provide additional examples of these initiatives.

Healthy People 2020

The Office of Disease Prevention and Health Promotion (ODPHP), Healthy People 2020 (2017a) describes health disparities based on race, ethnicity, gender, sexual identity, age, disability, socioeconomic status, and geographic location. The goal of *Healthy People 2020* is to eliminate health disparities by improving access, quality, and care among identified vulnerable populations in the United States. *Healthy People* objectives aim to address ways to remove barriers causing disparities in order to assist these vulnerable individuals. It provides evidence-based interventions and resources for various vulnerable populations to assist healthcare providers in delivering optimal care.

Affordable Care Act

The Affordable Care Act (ACA) was created with the hopes of decreasing gaps in health disparities for all individuals in the United States (Adepoju, Preston, & Gonzales, 2015; Artiga, Urbi, & Foutz, 2017). ACA strategies to address disparities include better and broader data collection and reporting, equalization of care among all individuals, expansion of research focused on disparities, increased diversity in the U.S. workforce, and improved cultural competency of healthcare providers through the development of specialized programs. The ACA also set out to address disparities in preventive services and health insurance coverage.

The ACA puts patients in charge of their own healthcare. Under the ACA law, a new Patient's Bill of Rights gives Americans the stability and flexibility needed to make informed choices about their healthcare. The hallmarks of the ACA include ending of preexisting condition exclusions; increasing the age that a child is covered under a parent's insurance plan to age 26; ending lifetime limits on coverage; ensuring that premium dollars are spent on healthcare, not administrative costs; and providing preventive care coverage at no cost to the individual. Preventive healthcare services such as screenings, vaccinations, and healthy pregnancy counseling are thought to improve the health and well-being of pregnant women, promote the healthy birth of babies, and enhance overall population health (Minnesota Association for Children's Mental Health, 2018).

It was the hope of the creators of the ACA that enrollment in insurance plans under the ACA by individuals who had not had coverage in the past by 2014 would help to reduce disparities. Many low-income individuals and people of color who were not insured before ACA are now covered (Artiga et al., 2017). However, with the new presidential administration, healthcare is a key area of potential change. The impact on disparities must be monitored closely in the years to come.

National Partnership for Action to End Health Disparities

The National Partnership for Action to End Health Disparities (NPA) is the first national, community- and partnership-driven organization whose efforts address the problems of health disparities and support the goal of attaining health equity (Correa-de-Araujo, 2017). Its purpose is to "mobilize a nationwide, comprehensive, community-driven, and sustained approach to combating health disparities and to move the nation toward achieving health equity" (NPA, 2016, para. 3). The goals of the NPA in relation to health disparities are to increase awareness, strengthen leadership, improve health and healthcare outcomes for racial and ethnic minorities and other underserved individuals, improve cultural and linguistic competency, and improve availability and dissemination of data for use in healthcare practice as well as evaluation of data.

Racial and Ethnic Approaches to Community Health

Racial and Ethnic Approaches to Community Health (REACH) is a national initiative of the CDC that uses an evidence-based approach "to create healthier communities for populations experiencing chronic disease health disparities" (Centers for Disease Control and Prevention, Division of Nutrition, Physical Activity, and Obesity, CDC, 2017, para. 1). REACH supports community-based programs and culturally tailored interventions to prevent risky health behaviors such as "tobacco use, physical inactivity, and poor nutrition, and it helps to manage chronic diseases such as diabetes and heart disease among African Americans, American Indians, Hispanic/Latinos, Asian Americans, Alaska Natives, and Pacific Islanders" (Centers for Disease Prevention and Control, National Center for Chronic Disease Prevention and Health Promotion, 2017, para. 1). For example, Boston REACH: Partners in Health and Housing is an effort to improve the health of the people of Boston, especially Black and Latino residents (Boston Public Health Commission, 2016). The program's goals include improving access to and consumption of nutritious foods and beverages, increasing connections for residents to community health and social service resources, and promoting the quality of and access to smoke-free housing. To date, REACH initiatives across the United States have resulted in decreases in smoking and obesity, as well as increases in fruit and vegetable consumption and healthy behaviors (CDC, National Center for Chronic Disease Prevention and Health Promotion, 2017).

Application Through Critical Thinking

CASE STUDY

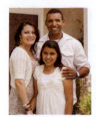

Source: Andy Dean Photography/ Shutterstock.

The Molina family immigrated to the United States 8 years ago when Roberto and Rita started a family. Roberto and Rita met and married in El Salvador and are undocumented citizens. They have one female child, Vanessa, who was born in the United States 8 years ago. Rita is pregnant with her second child. They are seeking healthcare for their growing family. Roberto works in the fields picking lettuce and has a handyman business to support his family.

CRITICAL THINKING QUESTIONS

1. Discuss how the Molina family is at risk and vulnerable.
2. What factors must be considered when performing a health history and assessment for Rita?
3. Identify health promotion activities.
4. What would be the predictors of health for the Molina family?

REFERENCES

Adepoju, O. E., Preston, M. A., & Gonzales, G. (2015). Healthcare disparities in the Post-Affordable Care Act era. *American Journal of Public Health, 105*(S5), S665–S667.

Agency for Healthcare Quality and Research (AHRQ). (2015). *2015 National Healthcare Quality and Disparities Report and 5th Anniversary Update on the National Quality Strategy.* Retrieved from https://www.ahrq.gov/sites/default/files/wysiwyg/research/findings/nhqrdr/nhqdr15/2015nhqdr.pdf

Artiga, S., Foutz, J., Cornachione, E., & Garfield, R. (2016). *Key facts on health and health care by race and ethnicity.* Retrieved from https://www.kff.org/disparities-policy/report/key-facts-on-health-and-health-care-by-race-and-ethnicity

Artiga, S., Urbi, P., & Foutz, J. (2017). *What is at stake for health and health care disparities under ACA repeal?* Retrieved from https://www.kff.org/disparities-policy/issue-brief/what-is-at-stake-for-health-and-health-care-disparities-under-aca-repeal

Association of State and Territorial Health Officials. (2013). *Disparities and inequalities in maternal and infant health outcomes.* Retrieved from http://www.astho.org/t/article.aspx?artid=8150

Boston Public Health Commission. (2016). *Boston REACH: Partners in health and housing.* Retrieved from http://www.bphc.org/whatwedo/healthy-homes-environment/healthy-homes/partners-in-health-housing/Pages/default.aspx

Bureau of Justice Statistics. (2015). *Correctional populations in the United States, 2015.* Retrieved from https://www.bjs.gov/index.cfm?ty=pbdetail&iid=5870

BWHC LGBT & Allies Employee Resource Group. (2016, May 20). *LGBT welcoming toolkit for primary care practices.* Retrieved from http://www.brighamandwomensfaulkner.org/about-us/patient-visitor-information/diversity/documents/lgbt-welcoming-toolkit.pdf

Capps, R., Fix, M., & Zong, J. (2016). *A profile of U.S. children with unauthorized immigrant parents.* Retrieved from https://www.migrationpolicy.org/research/profile-us-children-unauthorized-immigrant-parents

Centers for Disease Control and Prevention (CDC). (2013). *Health Disparities and Inequalities Report—United States, 2013.* Retrieved from https://www.cdc.gov/mmwr/pdf/other/su6203.pdf

Centers for Disease Control and Prevention (CDC). (2014). *NCHHSTP social determinants of health.* Retrieved from https://www.cdc.gov/nchhstp/socialdeterminants/definitions.html

Centers for Disease Control and Prevention (CDC). (2015). *Health disparities.* Retrieved from https://www.cdc.gov/healthyyouth/disparities

Centers for Disease Control and Prevention (CDC). (2016). *Disability and health data system.* Retrieved from http://www.cdc.gov/ncbddd/disabilityandhealth/dhds.html

Centers for Disease Control and Prevention (CDC). (2017a). *Minority health.* Retrieved from https://www.cdc.gov/minorityhealth

Centers for Disease Control and Prevention (CDC). (2017b). *African American health.* Retrieved from https://www.cdc.gov/vitalsigns/aahealth/index.html

Centers for Disease Control and Prevention (CDC). (2017c). *STD health equity.* Retrieved from https://www.cdc.gov/std/health-disparities/default.htm

Centers for Disease Control and Prevention (CDC). (2017d). *WISEWOMAN.* Retrieved from https://www.cdc.gov/wisewoman/index.htm

Centers for Disease Control and Prevention (CDC), Division of Nutrition, Physical Activity, and Obesity. (2017). *REACH.* Retrieved from https://www.cdc.gov/nccdphp/dnpao/state-local-programs/reach/current_programs/index.html

Centers for Disease Control and Prevention (CDC), National Center for Chronic Disease Prevention and Health Promotion. (2017). *REACH 2017 fact sheet.* Retrieved from https://www.cdc.gov/nccdphp/dnpao/state-local-programs/reach/pdf/REACH-overview-2017-508.pdf

Centers for Disease Control and Prevention (CDC), National Center for Health Statistics. (2017). *Health insurance and access to care.* Retrieved from https://www.cdc.gov/nchs/data/factsheets/factsheet_hiac.pdf

Chavez, J. M., Lopez, A., Englebrecht, C. M., & Anguiano, R. P. V. (2012). Exploring the impact of unauthorized immigration status on children's well-being. *Family Court Review, 50*(4), 638–649.

Correa-de-Araujo, R. (2017). Improving access and utilization of data to support research and programs intended to eliminate disparities and promote health equity. *Journal of Health Disparities Research and Practice, 9*(OMH Special Issue), 1–12. Retrieved from https://digitalscholarship.unlv.edu/cgi/viewcontent.cgi?article=1637&context=jhdrp

Hall, E., & Cuellar, N. G. (2016). Immigrant health in the United States: A trajectory toward change. *Journal of Transcultural Nursing, 27*(6), 611–626. doi:10.1177/1043659616672534

Justice and Health Connect. (2013). *Health disparities in the criminal justice system: Quick facts.* Retrieved from http://www.jhconnect.org/wp-content/uploads/2013/09/health-disparities-final.pdf

Kent, J. A., Patel, V., & Varela, N. A. (2012). Gender disparities in healthcare. *Mount Sinai Journal of Medicine, 79*(5), 555–559. doi:10.1002/MSJ

Klawetter, S. (2014). Conceptualizing social determinants of maternal and infant health disparities. *Journal of Women and Social Work, 29*(2), 131–141. doi:10.1177/0886109913516451

Mid-America Regional Council (MARC). (2018). *Vulnerable populations: Age.* Retrieved from http://www.marc2.org/healthdata/vpopulations_age.htm

Miller, G. E., & Chen, E. (2013). The biological residue of childhood poverty. *Child Development Perspectives, 7*(2), 67–73.

Minnesota Association for Children's Mental Health. (2018). *Key features of the Affordable Healthcare Act law.* Retrieved from http://www.macmh.org/2012/08/key-features-of-the-affordable-healthcare-act-law

National Alliance to End Homelessness. (2016). *The state of homelessness in America 2016.* Retrieved from http://end-homelessness.org/wp-content/uploads/2016/10/2016-soh.pdf

National Institutes of Health (NIH). (2016). *What are health disparities?* Retrieved from http://www.niaid.nih.gov/topics/minorityhealth/pages/disparities.aspx

National Institutes of Health (NIH). (2017). *Homeless health concerns.* Retrieved from http://www.nlm.nih.gov/medlineplus/homelesshealthconcerns.html

National Institute on Minority Health and Health Disparities. (n.d.). *Overview.* Retrieved from https://www.nimhd.nih.gov/about/overview

National Partnership for Action to End Health Disparities (NPA). (n.d.). *National Partnership for Action to End Health Disparities: Toolkit for community action.* Retrieved from https://minorityhealth.hhs.gov/npa/files/Plans/Toolkit/NPA_Toolkit_092617.pdf

National Partnership for Action to End Health Disparities (NPA). (2016). *Learn about the NPA.* Retrieved from https://minorityhealth.hhs.gov/npa/templates/browse.aspx?lvl=1&lvlid=11

National Quality Forum (NQF). (2017). *A roadmap for promoting health equity and eliminating disparities: The four I's for health equity.* Retrieved from https://www.qualityforum.org/Publications/2017/09/A_Roadmap_for_Promoting_Health_Equity_and_Eliminating_Disparities__The_Four_I_s_for_Health_Equity.aspx

Nowotny, K. M., Rogers, R. G., & Boardman, J. D. (2017). Racial disparities in health conditions among prisoners compared with the general population. *SSM-Population Health, 3,* 487–496. doi.org/10.1016/j.ssmph.2017.05.011

Office of Disease Prevention and Health Promotion (ODPHP), Healthy People 2020. (2017a). *Disparities.* Retrieved from https://www.healthypeople.gov/2020/about/foundation-health-measures/Disparities

Office of Disease Prevention and Health Promotion, Healthy People 2020. (2017b). *Social determinants of health.* Retrieved from https://www.healthypeople.gov/2020/topics-objectives/topic/social-determinants-of-health9

Office of Disease Prevention and Health Promotion, Healthy People 2020. (2017c). *Maternal, infant, and child health.* Retrieved from https://www.healthypeople.gov/2020/topics-objectives/topic/maternal-infant-and-child-health

Office of Disease Prevention and Health Promotion (ODPHP), Healthy People 2020. (2018). *Lesbian, gay, bisexual, and transgender health.* Retrieved from https://www.healthypeople.gov/2020/topics-objectives/topic/lesbian-gay-bisexual-and-transgender-health

O'Neil, M. E., Carlson, K. F., Storzbach, D., Brenner, L. A., Freeman, M., Quinones, A. R. . . & Kansagara, D. (2014). Factors associated with mild traumatic brain injury in veterans and military personnel: A systematic review. *Journal of the International Neuropsychological Society 20,* 249–261.

Pew Research Center. (2015). *U.S. foreign-born population trends.* Retrieved from http://www.pewhispanic.org/2015/09/28/chapter-5-u-s-foreign-born-population-trends

Psychology Benefits Society. (2016). *Starting a conversation: How can we reduce health disparities among older adults?* Retrieved from https://psychologybenefits.org/2016/07/07/how-we-can-reduce-health-disparities-among-older-adults

Salvation Army. (2017). *Why are people homeless?* Retrieved from http://www.salvationarmy.org.au/en/Who-We-Are/our-work/Homelessness/Why-are-people-homeless

Stafford, A., & Wood, L. (2017). Tackling disparities for people who are homeless? Start with social determinants. *International Journal of Environmental Research and Public Health, 14*(12), 1–12. doi:10.3390/ijerph14121535

Thompson, E. A., Connelly, C. D., Thomas-Jones, D., & Eggert, L. L. (2013). School difficulties and co-occurring health risk factors: Substance use, aggression, depression, and suicidal behaviors. *Journal of Child and Adolescent Psychiatric Nursing, 26,* 74–84.

Thompson, C. W., Monsen, K. A., Wanamaker, K., Augustyniak, K., & Thompson, S. L. (2012). Using the Omaha System as a framework to demonstrate the value of nurse managed wellness center services for vulnerable populations. *Journal of Community Health Nursing, 29,* 1–11.

U.S. Census Bureau. (2010). *The foreign-born population in the United States: 2010.* Retrieved from http://www.census.gov/prod/2012pubs/acs-19.pdf

U.S. Census Bureau. (2016). *Population estimates.* Retrieved from https://www.census.gov/quickfacts/fact/table/US/PST045216

U.S. Department of Health and Human Services, Office of Minority Health. (2016). *Minority population profiles.* Retrieved from https://minorityhealth.hhs.gov/omh/browse.aspx?lvl=2&lvlid=26

U.S. Department of Health and Human Services, Office of Minority Health. (2017a). *Profile: Asian Americans.* Retrieved from https://minorityhealth.hhs.gov/omh/browse.aspx?lvl=3&lvlid=63

U.S. Department of Health and Human Services, Office of Minority Health. (2017b). *Profile: Native Hawaiians/Pacific Islanders.* Retrieved from https://minorityhealth.hhs.gov/omh/browse.aspx?lvl=3&lvlid=65

U.S. Department of Health and Human Services, Office of Minority Health. (2017c). *Profile: American Indian/Alaskan Native.* Retrieved from https://minorityhealth.hhs.gov/omh/browse.aspx?lvl=3&lvlid=62

U.S. Department of Health and Human Services, Substance Abuse and Mental Health Services Administration, Center for Substance Abuse Prevention. (2012). *Top health issues for LGBT populations information & resource kit.* Retrieved from https://store.samhsa.gov/shin/content/SMA12-4684/SMA12-4684.pdf

U.S. Department of Homeland Security. (2016). *2016 yearbook of immigration statistics.* Retrieved from https://www.dhs.gov/sites/default/files/publications/2016%20Yearbook%20of%20Immigration%20Statistics.pdf

U.S. Department of Homeland Security. (2017). *Legal immigration and adjustment of status report fiscal year 2017, quarter 3.* Retrieved from https://www.dhs.gov/immigration-statistics/special-reports/legal-immigration

U.S. Department of Homeland Security. (2018). *Estimates of the Unauthorized Immigrant Population Residing in the United States.* Retrieved from https://www.dhs.gov/immigration-statistics/population-estimates/unauthorized-resident

U.S. Department of Housing and Urban Development (HUD). (n.d.). *Homeless assistance.* Retrieved from http://portal.hud.gov/hudportal/HUD?src=/program_offices/comm_planning/homeless

U.S. Department of Veterans Affairs. (n.d.). *Overview of VA research on health equity.* Retrieved from https://www.research.va.gov/topics/health_equity.cfm

World Health Organization (WHO). (2017a). *Social determinants of health: Key concepts.* Retrieved from http://www.who.int/social_determinants/thecommission/finalreport/key_concepts/en

World Health Organization (WHO). (2017b). *World Health Organization disability assessment Schedule 2.0.* Retrieved from http://www.who.int/classifications/icf/whodasii/en

World Health Organization (WHO). (2018). *Equity.* Retrieved from http://www.who.int/healthsystems/topics/equity/en

Yu-Hsi Lee, E. (2014). *Why kids are crossing the desert alone to get to America.* Retrieved from https://thinkprogress.org/why-kids-are-crossing-the-desert-alone-to-get-to-america-f5be4974386d

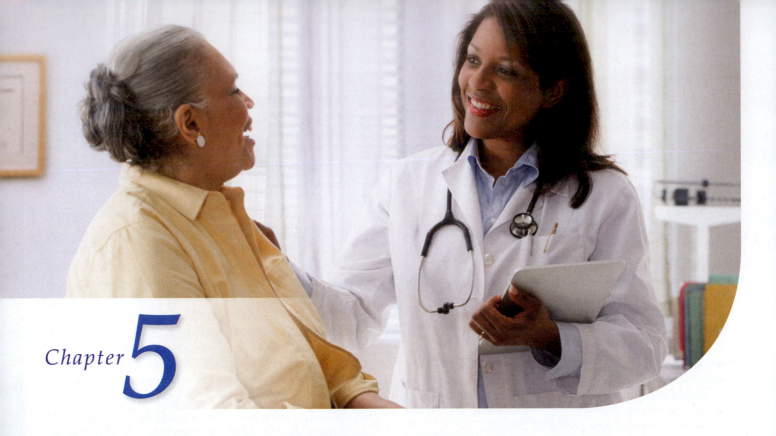

Chapter 5

Interviewing and Health History: Subjective Data

LEARNING OUTCOMES

Upon completion of this chapter, you will be able to:

1. Examine the purpose of a nursing health history in the health assessment.

2. Identify strategies that promote effective communication when conducting a health history interview.

3. Outline the professional characteristics used in establishing a nurse–patient relationship.

4. Analyze personal bias and other barriers to effective nurse–patient interaction.

5. Identify the purpose of each phase of the nursing health history interview.

6. Explain the importance of each component of the nursing health history for patients across the lifespan.

KEY TERMS

active listening, 47
attending, 47
communication, 46
concreteness, 49
decoding, 46
empathy, 49
encoding, 46

false reassurance, 49
focused interview, 52
genogram, 60
genuineness, 49
health history, 45
health pattern, 58
interactional skills, 46

interview, 51
listening, 47
paraphrasing, 48
pedigree, 60
positive regard, 49
preinteraction, 51
primary source, 45

reflecting, 48
secondary source, 45
sexual orientation, 55
summarizing, 48
transgender, 55

Introduction

In this unit, you are introduced to the knowledge, skills, and attitudes you will need to be able to perform a comprehensive health and physical assessment. This chapter details the foundational knowledge and skills needed to perform the subjective portion of the health assessment: the health history. As discussed in Chapter I, the comprehensive patient database includes subjective and objective data, which are used by the nurse to create a patient-centered plan of care. Included in this chapter are methods and skills of interviewing, nurse–patient communication techniques, and an outline of professional nursing behaviors related to interviewing, as well as barriers to effective communication. The chapter concludes with an in-depth description of the types and components of a thorough health history.

The Purpose of the Health History: Subjective Information

Health assessment typically begins with collection of information from the patient through an interview which provides an opportunity to gather detailed information about events and experiences that have contributed to a patient's current state of health. The **health history** is a detailed record of the patient's past and current health, as well as a record of perceptions about his state of wellness. The health history is gathered during the initial health assessment interview, which usually occurs during the patient's first visit to a healthcare facility and is updated with each subsequent visit. The purpose of the health history is to document the responses of the patient regarding actual and potential health concerns. Thus, the nursing health history includes several distinct sections covering past and present illnesses, family and genetic information, as well as a wellness assessment covering patient strategies and lifestyle choices. This information is used to inform the health promotion activities for complete patient-centered care.

A health history performed by the professional nurse has a different focus from the medical history performed by the physician or nonphysician provider. Although both contain subjective data, the focus of the medical history is to gather data about the cause and course of disease. Thus, the medical history focuses on the disease rather than on the patient and the patient's lifestyle practices. For example, the physician might ask a patient to relate the details of the range of motion in the left hip to determine the cause of abnormal movement and to prescribe a specific treatment. The nurse obtains the same information but uses it to determine the extent to which the patient will need support and teaching regarding ambulation and performance of activities of daily living (ADLs), such as getting dressed independently at home. The nurse and the medical provider gather the same information for different purposes. The nursing health history may produce information about a medical diagnosis, but the focus is on patient-centered care or on the patient's response to the health concern as a whole person, not just on a specific illness or condition.

Sources of Information

The health history will include an interview with the patient as well as review of pertinent data from other sources. The primary source of information for an adult health history is the interview with the patient. Other additional sources of information—secondary sources—may be included in a comprehensive health assessment.

Primary Source   The patient is usually the best and, therefore, **primary source** of information for the health history interview. The patient is the only one who can describe personal symptoms, experiences, and factors leading to the current health or wellness concern. In some situations, the patient may be unable or unwilling to provide information. For example, a patient who has had a cerebrovascular accident (brain attack or stroke) may not be able to understand what is being said or verbalize a response. The nurse carefully evaluates the patient who is unable to give accurate and reliable information and uses another source of information if indicated. Other specific types of patients may or may not be able to provide accurate and reliable information, including infants or young children; patients who are seriously ill, comatose, sedated, or in substantial pain; or individuals with developmental, cognitive, or physical disability. In some situations, the patient may be hesitant to talk to the nurse. In such situations, an adult patient is able but unwilling to provide certain types of information because of fear, anxiety, embarrassment, or distrust. Some reasons why patients may be hesitant to share information include these:

- *Fear of a terminal diagnosis:* A patient may not be ready to cope with the stress of a terminal illness and may deny its possibility.
- *Fear of undergoing further physical examination:* A patient with claustrophobia may deny problems because of fear of a magnetic resonance imaging (MRI) scan.
- *Embarrassment:* A male patient may refuse to discuss urinary problems because he fears catheterization or rectal examination.
- *Fear of legal implications:* A patient who is an alcoholic involved in a motor vehicle crash may fear revealing the addiction to alcohol.
- *Fear of losing a job:* An airline pilot may be reluctant to admit visual problems or hearing loss.
- *Lack of trust:* A patient with AIDS who wishes the diagnosis to remain private may fear a breach in confidentiality.

Exploration of reasons why a patient is hesitant, and an understanding and compassionate nurse may be able to reassure the patient that her health needs are the primary concern.

Secondary Sources   A **secondary source** is a person or record that provides additional information about the patient. The nurse uses secondary sources when the patient is unable or unwilling to communicate. Secondary sources may also be used to supplement previously obtained data. The most commonly used secondary sources are medical records and information from significant others to whom the patient has expressed thoughts and feelings about lifestyle or health status.

Although patients often share their personal experiences, feelings, and emotions with significant others, the Health Insurance Portability and Accountability Act (HIPAA) states that the nurse must obtain the patient's permission before requesting information from another person. In emergency situations, the HIPAA regulations permit the use of professional judgment and experience in solicitation of information from secondary sources when the patient is incapacitated and only in an attempt to protect the patient.

It is imperative the nurse be cautious when collecting patient data from another person as such information may be prejudiced by that person's own bias, life experience, and values and may not be a true reflection of the patient's own thinking. Every attempt must be made to validate secondary information by verifying it with the patient, by observation, or by confirming the information with at least one other source. The nurse does not seek secondary information if the patient is competent but unwilling to provide personal information and has not granted the nurse permission to explore information with secondary sources. The nurse should respect the wishes and confidentiality of the patient and attempt to obtain the information at a later time.

Documenting the Health History

Documentation of the health history, as part of the data gathered from the assessment, is the last step in the preparation of a comprehensive patient database. The accurate and complete documentation of all subjective and objective data collected during the interview and physical examination is critical in the planning, implementation, and evaluation of nursing care. The specific type of documentation will be determined by setting, purpose, and timing of the healthcare encounter. A variety of formats for documentation are available, including checklists, fill-in forms, and narrative records, among others. Like all parts of the comprehensive patient database, the health history written by the nurse becomes part of the patient record, forming a legal document. The knowledge and skills for accurate, appropriate, and professional documentation are presented in detail in Chapter 6, Documentation. ∞

Interactional Communication Skills and the Health History

During the interview to obtain the health history, the nurse uses the principles of effective communication. A basic definition of **communication** is the exchange of information between individuals. During the communication process an individual develops an idea and transmits it in the form of a message to another person. The person receiving the message perceives the message and interprets it. Once the receiver interprets the meaning, the receiver formulates a response and transmits it back to the sender as feedback. **Encoding** is the process of formulating a message for transmission to another person. To encode an idea, the sender has to choose the words, body language, signs, or symbols that will be used to convey the message. **Decoding** is the process of searching through one's memory, experience, and knowledge base to determine the meaning of the intended message. (See Figure 5.1 ∎.)

To communicate successfully, the patient must be able to accurately decode the messages the nurse sends. For example, communication may break down if the nurse uses words that the patient does not understand or behaves in a manner that is frightening to the patient. Communication may also break down if the nurse fails to decode the patient's messages accurately by not listening actively and attentively.

Interactional skills are actions that are used during the encoding and decoding processes to obtain and disseminate information, develop relationships, and promote understanding of self and others. Nurses use a variety of interactional skills during the communication process to gather assessment data from the patient, family, significant others, and other healthcare personnel. The interactional skills that are helpful during an interview include listening, attending, paraphrasing, leading, questioning, reflecting, and summarizing (see Table 5.1). The nurse uses these interactional techniques to help the patient communicate information thoroughly and also to confirm that the nurse has understood the patient's communication correctly.

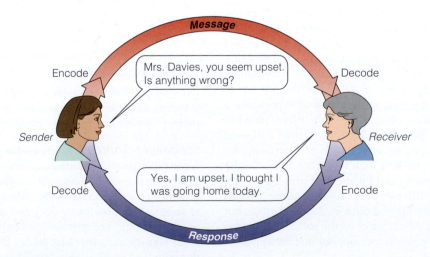

Figure 5.1 The communication process.

Table 5.1 Interactional Skills

SKILL/DEFINITION	TECHNIQUE	EXAMPLES
Attending Giving the patient undivided attention	• Use direct eye contact if appropriate for culture. Look at the patient during the conversation. • Lean toward the patient slightly. • Select quiet area with no distractions for interview. • Convey unhurried manner; avoid fidgeting and looking at watch.	• Nurse arranges with peers for no interruptions during interview. • Nurse sits facing patient, remains alert, and focuses on what patient is saying.
Paraphrasing/Clarification Restating the patient's basic message to test whether it was understood	• Listen for the patient's basic message. • Restate the patient's message in your own words. • Ask the patient if your words are an accurate restatement of the message.	*Patient:* "I toss and turn all night. Sometimes I can't get to sleep at all. I don't know why this is happening. I've always been a deep sleeper." *Nurse:* "It sounds like you're not getting enough sleep. Is that right?"
Direct Leading Directing the patient in order to obtain specific information or to begin an interaction	• Decide what area you want to explore. • Tell the patient what you want to discuss. • Encourage the patient to follow your lead.	• "Let's discuss the pain in your back." • "When did your symptoms begin?"
Focusing Helping the patient zero in on a subject or get in touch with feelings	• Use focusing when the patient strays from the topic or uses tangential speech. • Listen for themes, issues, or feelings in the patient's rambling conversation. • Ask the patient to give more information about a specific theme, issue, or feeling. • Encourage the patient to emphasize feelings when giving this information.	• "Describe how you feel when you can't sleep." • "Did you say you were angry and frustrated before you went to bed? Go over that again."
Questioning Gathering specific information on a topic through the process of inquiry	• Use open-ended questions whenever possible. Avoid using questions that can be answered with "yes," "no," "maybe," or "sometimes." • Ask the patient to express feelings about what is being discussed. • Ask questions that help the patient gain insight.	• "What did you mean when you said your back was breaking?" • "How did you feel after you talked to your boss?"
Reflecting Letting the patient know that the nurse empathizes with the thoughts, feelings, or experiences expressed	• Take in the patient's feelings from verbal and nonverbal body language. • Determine which combination of "cues" you should reflect back to the patient. • Reflect the "cues" back to the patient. • Observe the patient's response to the reflected feelings, experience, or content.	*Feelings:* "It sounds like you're feeling lonely." "It must really be frustrating not to be able to get enough sleep." *Experience:* "You're yawning. You must be tired." "You act as if you're in pain." *Content:* "You think you're going to die." "You believe the medication is helping."
Summarizing Tying together the various messages that the patient has communicated throughout the interview.	• Listen to verbal and nonverbal content during the interview. • Summarize feelings, issues, and themes in broad statements. • Repeat them to the patient, or ask the patient to repeat them to you.	"Let's review the health problems you've identified today."

Listening

Listening is paying undivided attention to what the patient says and noticing what the patient is doing. Listening is the most important interactional skill and involves interpretation of what has been said. Successful listening involves taking in the patient's whole message by hearing the words as well as interpreting body language. Successful listening is an active process requiring effort and attention on the part of the nurse and may include encouraging the patient to speak by making comments such as "I see" and "Go on." While listening to a patient, it is important to push from one's mind thoughts about the day's schedule or the next patient and to give full attention to the patient, so as not to miss some of the message. The nurse should note not only the words the patient speaks but also the tone of voice and even what the patient does not say.

For example, the woman who states "My mother died last week" and immediately moves to another topic of discussion has told the nurse a lot about how she is dealing with a death in her family. While listening, periods of silence may be a form of therapeutic communication. By remaining with the patient and allowing several seconds—or even minutes—to pass without speaking, the nurse demonstrates caring while allowing the patient time to process and potentially verbalize emotions (Berman, Snyder, & Frandsen, 2016).

Attending

Giving full attention to verbal and nonverbal messages is called **attending**. Very similar to **active listening**, which includes paying attention, showing that you are listening, and offering feedback if appropriate, attending to the patient's message is an important interactional skill. Humans use body language, or nonverbal communication, often without being aware of it. We send, receive, and interpret messages from other's body language that may include posture, gestures, or direction of gaze (Mandal, 2014). Body language and nonverbal messages also provide significant clues, including information which the patient may have omitted intentionally or unintentionally that the nurse might otherwise overlook. Because body language can send messages such as hostility, defensiveness, or confusion, the nurse attends to both verbal and nonverbal messages. Some examples of nonverbal cues include eye contact, the way a patient is dressed, accessories, and what items the patient has in the room, such as books, a rosary, or photographs. Such cues tell a significant story and add more depth to the intended message.

For the nurse, attending includes maintaining consistent, appropriate eye contact with the patient as well as using proper body positioning to demonstrate attentiveness (see Figure 5.2 ■). For example, after establishing rapport with the patient, the nurse should use body posture to reflect involvement by leaning slightly forward toward the patient (Berman et al., 2016).

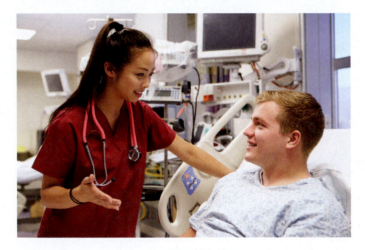

Figure 5.2 The nurse conveys attentive listening through a posture of involvement.
Source: Cathy Yeulet/123RF.

Paraphrasing

Another important interactional skill is the ability to check to make sure that the nurse has understood the patient accurately by **paraphrasing**—that is, restating the patient's basic message. For example, the patient may say "I don't really know if I should have this test." The nurse would paraphrase by saying "It sounds like you're saying you feel you don't have enough information to make the decision."

Leading

Nurses use leading skills to encourage open communication. These skills are most effective when starting an interaction or when trying to get the patient to discuss specific health concerns. Leading skills are especially helpful in getting patients to explore their feelings and to elaborate on areas already

introduced in the discussion. The leading techniques nurses commonly use when interviewing a patient include direct leading, focusing, and questioning.

Questioning

Questioning is a very direct way of speaking with patients to obtain subjective data. Questioning techniques include open-ended and closed questions. *Open-ended questions* are purposefully general and encourage the patient to provide additional information. Examples of open-ended questions include "Tell me what brought you here today" or "You said that your ankle hurts. Tell me more about that." *Closed questions* limit the patient's response to "yes," "no," or one-word answers—for example, "Were you feeling angry when your mother said that?"

Reflecting

Reflecting is repeating the patient's verbal or nonverbal message for the patient's benefit. It is a way of showing the patient that the nurse empathizes or is in tune with the patient's thoughts, feelings, and experiences. For example, Mr. Bates, a 60-year-old with diabetes, is admitted to an outpatient clinic to be evaluated for a possible amputation of his right lower leg because of gangrene. During the clinic visit, Mr. Bates sits in a chair in the examination room with his head in his hands. When the nurse begins to question him, he looks up and says "Leave me alone. Nothing you can do will help. I might as well be dead." The nurse's response might be "Mr. Bates, may I sit here for a while? I can see that you are upset" (reflecting feeling). "You must feel angry that this is happening to you" (reflecting content). This example demonstrates that thoughts, feelings, and experiences are reflected at the same time.

Summarizing

Summarizing is the process of gathering the ideas, feelings, and themes that patients have discussed throughout the interview and restating them in several general statements. Summarizing is a useful tool because it shows patients that the nurse has listened and understood their concerns. It also allows patients to know that progress is being made in resolving their health concerns and signals closure of the interview. One strategy is to read back to the patient what has been documented and then ask "Is that correct?" This allows the patient to fill in details if needed and shows he is part of the care planning process.

Professional Characteristics to Enhance the Nurse–Patient Interaction

Patients are more willing to discuss their health issues if they perceive that they are in a trusting, helping relationship and have developed a sense of rapport or mutual trust and understanding with the interviewing nurse. Carl Rogers, founder of the humanistic approach to psychology, developed the idea of patient-centered therapy (Rogers, 1957). Rogers (1957) defined the helping relationship as one "in which at least one of the parties has the intent of promoting the growth, development, maturity, improved functioning, and improved coping with life of the other"(pp. 27–32). Nurses who establish helping relationships with their patients believe that the positive aspects of the helping relationship are shared by the nurse as well as the patient. The nurse–patient relationship is the foundation of nursing care, and nurses must be vigilant to keep in mind the expectations patients have about this relationship. Professional nurses are competent, caring, and supportive and must learn to manage technical skill along with compassion and kindness (Wiechula et al., 2015).

Positive Regard

Positive regard is the ability to appreciate and respect another person's worth and dignity with a nonjudgmental attitude. Nurses who respect their patients also value their individuality and accept them regardless of race, religion, culture, ethnic background, or country of origin. Patients sense positive regard in nurses by their demeanor, attitudes, and verbal and nonverbal communication.

Empathy

Empathy is at the core of patient-centered care providing a therapeutic and supportive environment for the patient (Pehrson et al., 2015). Nurses demonstrate empathy by showing their understanding and support of the patient's experience or feelings through actions and words. Communicating an understanding of what a patient is experiencing can have healing power. Nurses must practice to learn now to accurately convey their empathy to the patients (Kelley & Kelley, 2013). Empathy allows the nurse to see the issues through the patient's eyes, fostering understanding of the patient's health concerns.

Genuineness

Genuineness is the ability to present oneself honestly and spontaneously. People who are genuine present themselves as down-to-earth and real. To be genuine, nurses must convey interest in, and focus on, the situation at hand, giving the patient their full attention. They use direct eye contact, facial expressions appropriate to the situation, and open body language. Facing the patient, leaning forward during conversation, and sitting with arms and legs uncrossed are examples of open body language. A genuine person communicates in a congruent manner, making sure that verbal and nonverbal messages are consistent. The nurse who tells a patient to "take your time" during the interview, but constantly looks at the clock, gives a mixed or incongruent message. Genuineness and congruent communication promote rapport and trust with the patient.

Concreteness

For the nurse, **concreteness** means speaking to the patient in specific terms rather than in vague generalities. For instance, saying "I need this information to help you to plan a diet to lower your cholesterol level" is more specific than "I need this information to plan your nursing care." The more specific statement promotes understanding and a sense of security in the patient. Speaking to the patient in concrete terms implies that the nurse respects the patient's ability to understand and recognizes the patient's right to know the details of the plan of care.

Barriers to Effective Patient Interaction

In some situations, the nurse may unknowingly hinder the flow of information by interacting in a way that is harmful rather than helpful. These nontherapeutic interactions interfere with the communication process by causing the patient to feel uncomfortable, anxious, or insecure. Some specific types of communication techniques that can be harmful if used during the health assessment interview are false reassurance, interrupting or changing the subject, passing judgment, cross-examination, avoidance language, euphemisms, unwanted advice, use of technical terms, and insensitivity. These techniques may not be *consciously* employed by the novice nurse. To be sure to avoid these behaviors, the nurse must develop self-awareness of tone, style, and content. This takes practice to achieve and hard work to incorporate in therapeutic interactions. Role playing and simulated clinical scenarios are ways to practice and receive feedback on communication styles.

False Reassurance

False reassurance occurs when the nurse assures the patient of a positive outcome with no basis for knowledge of this outcome. False reassurance deprives patients of the right to communicate their feelings. Examples include the nurse responding with "Everything will be all right" or "Don't worry about not being able to sleep at night. You'll be fine." False reassurance can be implied by the tone of voice used by the nurse in the communication process.

Interrupting or Changing the Subject

Interrupting the patient or changing the subject shows insensitivity to the patient's thoughts and feelings. In most cases this happens when the nurse is uncomfortable with the patient's comments and does not know how to deal with them. Patients who show extreme emotions such as anger or weeping during the interview, who ask intimate questions about the nurse's personal life, or who are sexually aggressive in the presence of the nurse may make the nurse uncomfortable during the interview. In these instances, the nurse must recognize what it is about the patient's behavior that is making her uncomfortable and deal with the situation at hand in a professional manner rather than changing the subject—for example, "Your questions about my personal life are making me feel uncomfortable. We need to talk about what is concerning you today instead."

Passing Judgment

Everyone has personal biases regarding health, wellness, and lifestyle. Nurses must carefully reflect on their own beliefs and avoid using these to judge their patients' behaviors or actions. In the interview, the nurse should work to "normalize" behaviors to obtain honest answers in the assessment—for example, ask "How many cigarettes do you smoke daily?" rather than "You don't smoke, do you?" Judgmental statements may be subtle but convey a strong message that the patient must live up to the nurse's value system to be accepted. These statements imply nonacceptance and discourage further interaction.

Cross-Examination

Asking question after question during an assessment interview may cause the patient to feel threatened, and the patient may seek refuge by revealing less information. Because all interviews include many questions, the nurse should be careful not to overwhelm the patient with an endless barrage of questions. It is helpful to pause occasionally between questions and ask how the patient is tolerating the interview so far. Encouraging patients to express their feelings about the pace and nature of the interview may help them feel more at ease.

Euphemisms

Using terms that are customarily thought to be less harsh, known as euphemisms, may also create barriers by misleading or confusing the patient and family. For example, using the term "passed away" when speaking of a patient's death may not be understood by everyone (Naik, 2013). Instead, nurses should be as direct as possible to avoid misunderstandings.

Unwanted Advice

Although one major role of the nurse is that of teacher, a novice nurse may try to offer advice about a patient's personal life. Even when it is well intentioned, unsolicited or unwanted advice is an imposition to the patient and is not professional. This is especially true when offering casual advice unrelated to the healthcare purpose of the encounter. Rather than offering such casual advice, the nurse's role is to offer expert guidance based on therapeutic principles and evidence-based practice that are intended to promote health and wellness. For example, when teaching a patient regarding smoking cessation, the nurse should focus on the facts about smoking and its physiologic effects on the patient's body rather than on telling the patient about how the nurse quit smoking "cold turkey."

Technical Terms

Whenever possible, the nurse should use lay language rather than technical terms and avoid jargon, slang, or clichés. Terms such as *anterior* and *posterior* are useful for nursing and medical personnel but are more confusing to the patient than the terms *front* and *back*. Most patients will understand the term *urinate* but not the term *void* when asked about urinary elimination. It is also best to avoid the use of initials and acronyms unless they are commonly accepted as everyday language.

Sensitive Issues and Uncomfortable Situations

Nurses often need to ask patients questions that are sensitive and personal. Timing and pacing in the interview should include starting with the less sensitive issues and building up trust and confidence between the nurse and patient. Additionally, the nurse can let the patient know that the patient may find several questions uncomfortable or embarrassing. The nurse must let the patient know that the information is needed to help with the development of the plan of care. The patient may feel uncomfortable providing information about such concerns as abuse, homelessness, emotional and psychological problems, use of drugs and alcohol, self-image, sexuality, or religion. Discomfort with these issues may cause the patient to lapse into silence. It is important to be sensitive to the patient's need for silence. The patient may need to reflect on what was said or to come to grips with emotions the question has evoked before proceeding.

The nurse also watches for nonverbal signs, such as tear-filled eyes or wringing of hands, which indicate the patient's need to pause for a moment. After a period of silence, if the patient does not resume the conversation, the nurse may need to prompt the patient by saying something like "After that, what happened?" or "You were saying. . . ." During an interview, a patient may begin to cry, and if that happens the nurse should offer tissues, let the patient cry, and wait until the patient is ready to proceed before asking additional questions. Some patients may feel that they need permission to cry. A nurse who sees that the patient is holding back tears can give the patient permission to cry by saying "I know that you are upset. It is all right to cry." If the patient reacts to questions about sensitive issues with anger, the nurse should acknowledge what the patient is feeling: "I can see that you are angry. Please tell me why." If the patient becomes angry, the nurse should acknowledge the anger and wait to resume the interview until the patient's anger dissipates.

Sometimes the nurse asking the patient sensitive questions may cause him or her to feel uncomfortable. A nurse who anticipates being uncomfortable with certain questions should take time to reflect on and come to terms with these feelings before beginning the interview. Role playing the situation with another nurse as the patient or mentally visualizing how to react in the anticipated situation will help avoid uncomfortable feelings during the interview. When asking sensitive questions, it is best to be direct and honest with the patient: "I feel uncomfortable asking you such personal questions, but I need the information to complete your plan of care." Communication strategies like these will help the nurse conduct a thorough and effective interview in these sensitive situations.

Cultural Influence and Bias

Differences in culture and the ways in which they are demonstrated have a significant impact on the interactions that occur in the nurse–patient relationship. The professional nurse must be prepared to recognize and adapt the interactional processes to adjust for cultural differences. Further, nurses must not allow their own cultural values and practices to bias the impressions of the patient or to impair the interaction.

Language may be the most noticeable indication of a difference in cultures. When the nurse's language is not the same as the patient's language, the nurse must always employ a professional medical interpreter. Other communication challenges may occur due to natural differences in communication patterns among individuals. For example, although silence or a lag in conversation may be viewed as awkward or uncomfortable for some, this practice varies widely based on several factors, including those related to cultural background. Nonverbal communication may be prioritized over talking, and healthcare providers may be expected to identify a health-related problem through instinctive reasoning as opposed to asking the patient a series of questions. Other behaviors and actions of the health history, such as note taking, might not be valued among some cultures in which history has been passed down by way of oral storytelling. In this case it may be preferable for the nurse who is gathering the patient's history to refrain from taking notes during the interview and to instead rely on memory while with the patient.

In order to provide the best care, the nurse must ask the patient for his or her guidance during the interview process and must remember that the patient is the expert on his or her culture and beliefs. Of importance to the professional nurse is maintaining an awareness of the influence of cultural background on the patient's beliefs and behaviors and seeking to recognize those potential influences for each patient. Chapter 3, Cultural and Spiritual Considerations, provides an in-depth discussion. ∞

Phases of the Health History Interview

The health history **interview** is the exchange of information between the nurse and the patient. This information, along with the data from the physical assessment, is used to develop nursing diagnoses and design the nursing care plan. Unlike other types of interviews that nurses conduct, the health history interview is a formal, planned interaction to inquire about the patient's health patterns, ADLs, past health history, current health issues, self-care activities, wellness concerns, and other aspects of the patient's health status. In most situations, nurses use a special health history tool to collect assessment data. The health history is a critical component of the comprehensive health interview.

The health assessment interview is divided into three phases: preinteraction, the initial or formal interview, and the focused interview. The first two phases provide information the nurse uses along with information from the physical assessment to develop the comprehensive patient database, formulate nursing diagnoses, and initiate the nursing care plan. The third phase, the focused interview, occurs throughout all stages of the nursing process. Its purpose is to gather, clarify, and update additional patient data as they become available.

Phase I: Preinteraction

The **preinteraction** phase is the period before first meeting with the patient. During this time, the nurse collects data from the medical record; previous health risk appraisals; health screenings; therapists, dietitians, and other healthcare professionals who have cared for, taught, or counseled the patient; and family members or friends as necessary. The nurse reviews the patient's name, age, sex, nationality, medical and social history, and current health concerns. If necessary, the nurse also reviews the latest evidence-based practice guidelines, recent research, new treatments, medications, prevention strategies, and self-care interventions that might have a bearing on the patient's care.

The nurse uses information obtained during the preinteraction phase to plan and guide the direction of the initial interview. Nurses are more likely to conduct a successful interview if they know, in advance, any patient-specific information such as communication needs including foreign language interpretation, necessary physical accommodations, or personal history of chronic or ongoing issues.

Information about the patient is not the nurse's only consideration during the preinteraction stage. During this phase, the nurse reflects on his or her own strengths and limitations and on his or her personal biases. For example, a nurse opposed to abortion may have difficulty interviewing a patient who is considering an abortion. In this situation, the nurse's anxiety could interfere with the collection of data and the provision of nursing care. Nurses should be aware of their feelings, biases, and prejudices and plan how to interact with the patient. For instance, a nurse who has had an experience similar to the patient's would need to decide whether to reveal that to the patient.

Environment The nurse chooses the setting and time before the initial interview takes place. A quiet, private place where few distractions or interruptions will occur is most conducive to a successful interview. The patient will feel more relaxed and comfortable if the area has subdued lighting, moderate temperature, and comfortable seating. Additionally, if an interview is scheduled, be sure the patient remains dressed until it is time for a physical examination. More chairs should be provided if family members or an interpreter will be present. A glass of water and tissues should be available for the patient's use. The most ideal setting is one that is private because the presence of another person might hinder the patient's ability to speak freely. If the patient is hospitalized, the nurse should hold the interview in a private conference room if one is available. The nurse can also hold the interview in the patient's room, preferably with no roommates present. If this is not possible, the nurse should select a quiet time of day for the interview, draw bedside curtains or place a screen for privacy, and use a subdued level of speech. In the home setting, a quiet room or even the backyard may be used as long as the patient is comfortable and no distractions are present.

The nurse should sit facing the patient at a comfortable distance without using a table, a computer, a desk, or any other barrier that might make communication difficult. When possible, the nurse and the patient should be on the same level. If the nurse sits in a chair that is higher than the patient's or stands at the bedside, it places the patient in an inferior position that might make the patient uncomfortable. A distance of approximately 1.5 to 4 ft between the nurse and the patient is most likely to make the patient feel at ease. Moving closer than 1.5 ft may invade the patient's intimate space, and some patients may consider this impingement on private space aggressive or seductive. Although 1.5 to 4 ft is the average distance, each person's personal space differs slightly. If the patient moves backwards in the chair, suddenly crosses arms and legs, or seems anxious, the nurse may be invading the patient's intimate space. If so, the nurse should move back until the patient seems more relaxed. An interpreter or family member who is present to assist with the interview should sit on one side of the patient so that conversation flows easily.

The interview should be scheduled at a time that is convenient for the nurse and the patient. The interview should not interfere with cooking dinner, picking up the children after school, or work. If the patient is hospitalized, the nurse takes care not to schedule the interview at the same time diagnostic tests or treatments are scheduled, during mealtimes, or during visiting hours. The interview should be postponed if the patient is in pain, has been sedated recently, is upset, or is confused.

Phase II: The Initial Interview

The initial interview is a planned meeting during which the nurse interviewer gathers information from the patient. In most cases, the nurse uses a health history form to collect the data to avoid overlooking any area of information. The nurse gathers information about every facet of the patient's health status and state of wellness at this time. The next section details these questions. These data will be used to develop tentative nursing diagnoses. In addition to providing data, the initial interview also helps establish a nurse–patient relationship based on mutual trust and gives the nurse insight into the patient's lifestyle, values, and feelings about wellness, health, and illness.

The health assessment interview is an anxiety-producing situation for most patients. In few other situations is a person required to tell a stranger such intimate details about his or her personal history, health habits, or physical and emotional problems. The nurse has a great responsibility to allay patients' fears and anxieties so that patients can communicate as effectively as possible. One way to make patients feel at ease is to address them by their title (Dr., Mrs., Mr., Ms.) and family name (last name) rather than given name (first name). It is important to ask permission to use the patient's given name because some patients may feel that the nurse is being overly familiar or inappropriate. In this case, the patient will be reluctant to divulge personal information.

The initial interview begins with the nurse describing the interviewing process, explaining its importance, and telling the patient what to expect. The nurse might say something like this: "Good morning, Mrs. Jentzen. I'm Eric Hernandez, the nurse who will be taking care of you today. To plan your care, I need some additional information. For about the next forty-five minutes I would like to find out as much as possible about you and why you are here. Because we will be talking about a variety of things, I'll be jotting down some notes as we speak. Please stop me at any time if you don't understand a question or need more information about something. Some questions have to do with personal and private areas such as your beliefs, family, income, emotions, and sexual activity. Everything we discuss will be held in strict confidence. However, you may choose not to disclose some information."

Notice several things about these introductory remarks. First, the nurse introduced himself and described the purpose of the interview in a friendly, caring tone intended to make the patient feel at ease. Second, the nurse gave the patient a time frame and said notes would be taken during the interview. This advance notice is important, because some patients become threatened or anxious when the nurse writes down information. Third, the nurse encouraged the patient to interrupt or ask questions at any point during the interview. Finally, the nurse reinforced the privacy and confidentiality of the interview.

After making the introductory comments, the nurse will begin to seek information about the patient's health status. The opening questions are purposely broad and vague to let the patient adjust to the questioning nature of the interview—for instance, "What led up to your seeking assistance with your health?" If the nurse begins the interview with a series of very specific personal questions, the patient may begin to withdraw, giving less and less information until no exchange takes place. The nurse continuously assesses the patient's anxiety level as the interview continues. Restlessness, distraction, and anger are signs that the patient perceives the interview as threatening. The nurse will elicit the best information from patients by asking carefully thought-out and clearly stated, open-ended questions throughout the interview.

After gathering sufficient information, the nurse proceeds with closure of the interview. The nurse indicates that the interview is almost at an end and gives the patient an opportunity to express any final questions or concerns—for example, "Is there anything else you would like to discuss or ask about since our time is just about at an end?" It is important to take a few minutes to summarize the information gathered in the interview and to identify key health strengths as well as concerns. The nurse should review what the patient can expect next with regard to nursing care. A final step is to thank the patient—for example, "I've appreciated your time and cooperation during the interview."

Phase III: The Focused Interview

The nurse uses a **focused interview** technique throughout the physical assessment, during treatment, and while caring for the patient. The purpose of a focused interview is to clarify previously obtained assessment data, gather missing information about a specific health concern or issue, update and identify new diagnostic cues as they occur, guide the direction of a physical assessment as it is being conducted, and identify or validate probable nursing diagnoses.

Consider the following situation:

Mr. Geoffrey Tripton is a 28-year-old stockbroker who is a new patient at the outpatient clinic. He told the nurse during the initial interview that he experiences severe abdominal pain, nausea, and bloating after eating spicy foods and that this is why he has decided to seek help. After establishing rapport with Mr. Tripton, the nurse used a focused interview to elicit the following additional information: The patient drinks at least 8 cups of coffee and smokes 1 pack of cigarettes a day, tends to forget to eat when feeling stressed, uses over-the-counter medication to treat his heartburn, and recently lost a large amount of money in the stock market. When questioned further, Mr. Tripton confirmed that his pain sometimes occurs at times when he has not eaten spicy food. He further stated that his smoking recently had doubled to 2 packs of cigarettes daily.

By using a focused interview, the nurse clarified information that had been previously obtained (the patient's abdominal pain is not associated with spicy food), included additional needed information, and identified several new cues not observed before (caffeine and nicotine intake, stress, and anxiety). It is not unusual for patients like Mr. Tripton to avoid giving complete information during the initial interview because of feelings of anxiety, distrust, discomfort, or confusion.

Nurses use the focused interview continuously to update diagnostic cues because signs, symptoms, and patient health concerns often change from moment to moment or day to day. Nurses perform most focused interviews during routine nursing care. For example, while bathing a patient who recently had surgery, the nurse focuses on the patient's discomfort by asking pertinent questions about his pain. Examples of focusing questions or statements a nurse might use in this situation to update information include "Is the pain as severe as it was yesterday?" or "Describe the pain you are experiencing now."

In some cases, the information that the nurse learns during the focused interview plays an important part in how physical assessment is performed. If the patient states that he is experiencing severe pain in the upper right quadrant of the abdomen, for example, the nurse would examine this area last. Beginning the assessment with the nontender areas permits the nurse to establish the borders of the affected area. Examination of a painful area can exacerbate symptoms, increase the pain, and force termination of the assessment process.

In Mr. Tripton's situation, the nurse's initial hypothetical nursing diagnosis was pain due to eating spicy foods, with symptoms of abdominal discomfort, nausea, and abdominal distention present. However, with the additional information obtained during the focused interview, the nurse updated the nursing diagnosis to pain as a result of nicotine and caffeine intake, stress, and missed meals, with the supporting symptoms of abdominal discomfort, nausea, and abdominal distention. Further, the nurse added a new diagnosis of anxiety because of the patient's financial losses, with supporting symptoms of chain smoking, forgetting meals, increased intake of coffee, and agitation.

The process of obtaining subjective data about patient symptoms is called symptom analysis; many nurses find it helpful to use an acronym to guide a symptom-focused interview. One acronym is OLDCART & ICE. When using the acronym, the nurse will elicit information about the onset, location, duration, characteristics, aggravating factors, relieving factors, and treatment of symptoms, as well as the impact of symptoms on ADLs, the coping strategies used to deal with symptoms, and the emotional responses to the symptoms. An explanation of the acronym appears in Figure 5.3 ■. Use of the symptom analysis in development of nursing diagnoses is covered in detail in Chapter 6, Documentation. ∞

The focused interview is used to validate probable or hypothetical nursing or collaborative diagnoses. After the initial interview, the nurse develops several hypothetical nursing diagnoses. Before making a final diagnosis, the nurse conducts a focused interview along with a physical assessment to gather additional data. These additional data are then compared with defining characteristics of the probable diagnoses to determine the most appropriate nursing diagnosis for the patient. The chapters in Unit III contain focused interview questions for each body region or system.

OLDCART & ICE Acronym
O = Onset
L = Location
D = Duration
C = Characteristics
A = Aggravating Factors
R = Relieving Factors
T = Treatment
&
I = Impact on ADLs
C = Coping Strategies
E = Emotional Response

Figure 5.3 OLDCART & ICE acronym.

Components of the Health History

The data collected during the interview are recorded in the patient's health history. The type of recording is determined by the agency or facility in which the interview is carried out. The process of writing down, entering information in a computer system, or recording is known as documentation. The patient's health history becomes part of the patient record and is a legal document, and most healthcare settings have implemented electronic systems for collecting the data, organizing them, and ensuring that the interviewer does not omit any information. A variety of terms may be used to describe the electronic system of documentation, including *electronic health record* (EHR) and *electronic medical record* (EMR). Although these two terms are sometimes used interchangeably, they are not synonymous. The EMR is focused on treatment and diagnosis and is not necessarily portable. By comparison, the EHR is designed to be portable and is broader in scope; it incorporates multidisciplinary aspects of the patient's assessment, care, and treatment. This text primarily describes use of the EHR. Documentation of the health history and physical examination is covered in detail in Chapter 6, Documentation. ∞

The format, sequencing, and organization of the nursing health history data collection vary across institutions, agencies, and facilities but generally include the components identified in Box 5.1: biographic data, history of present illness, past medical history, family medical history, psychosocial history, and review of body systems. The information gathered for each of the components of the health history serves a purpose in health assessment and in application of the nursing process for each patient. Responses to the questions asked in the health history provide specific information about the individual. The nurse will use professional judgment in determining the significance of the responses, the need for follow-up questioning, and the relevance of information to meeting the health needs of the patient.

Biographic Data

The biographic data include the patient's name and address, age and date of birth, birthplace, marital or relationship status, sex, gender identity, sexual orientation, race, religion, occupation, health insurance information, and the reliability of the source of information. When possible, the patient completes a paper form or an online document that elicits these data. Otherwise, the interviewing nurse documents it.

Ideally, to allow for a holistic approach to assessing and caring for the patient, biographic data should include information related to sexual health, including a patient's sexual orientation. However, discussion of sensitive information, including that related to sexual health and practices, requires the nurse to first establish trust and rapport with the patient. As such, this information is best discussed in person, as opposed to collecting the data by way of paper, telephone, or online questionnaire.

Biographic data provide a data set that will inform the nurse's initial clinical judgments. The biographic data will be used to relate and compare individual characteristics to established expectations and norms for physical and emotional health. Furthermore, the biographic data provide information about

BOX 5.1 Health History Format: Subjective Data

I. **Biographic Data**	Medications; Prescription and Over the Counter	Roles and Relationships
Name	III. **Past Medical History (PMH)**	Family
Address	Medical	Social Structure/Emotional Concerns
Age	Surgical	Self-Concept
Date of Birth	Hospitalization	VI. **Review of Body Systems (ROS)**
Birthplace	Outpatient Care	Skin, Hair, and Nails
Marital Status	Childhood Illnesses	Head, Neck, and Lymphatics
Sex	Immunizations	Eyes
Gender Identity	Mental and Emotional Health	Ears, Nose, Mouth, and Throat
Sexual Orientation	Allergies	Respiratory
Race	Substance Use	Breasts and Axillae
Religion	IV. **Family Medical History (FMH)**	Cardiovascular
Occupation	Immediate Family	Peripheral Vascular
Health Insurance	Extended Family	Abdomen
Source of Information/Reliability	Genogram or Pedigree	Urinary
II. **History of Present Illness (HPI)**	V. **Psychosocial History**	Male Reproductive
Reason for Seeking Care	Occupational History	Female Reproductive
Health Beliefs and Practices	Education	Musculoskeletal
Health Patterns: Lifestyle, Nutrition, Activity	Financial Background	Neurologic

social and environmental characteristics that impact physical and emotional health.

A thorough discussion of each of the pieces of information in the biographic data section of the health history is presented in the following sections.

Name and Address   The patient's name and address are generally the first pieces of biographic data to be collected. Listening to the patient state his or her name and address provides the first opportunity to assess the patient's ability to hear and speak. The patient's address reveals information about the patient's environment. The nurse will associate the environment with known health benefits and risks. For example, individuals living in crowded urban environments are at risk for problems associated with heavy vehicular traffic, including respiratory problems from exhaust. Conversely, access to a variety of healthcare facilities and services is usually greater in urban areas than in rural areas.

Age and Date of Birth   The patient's age and date of birth are requested in the biographic data. Establishing the age of the patient permits the nurse to begin evaluation of individual characteristics in relation to norms and expectations of physical and social characteristics across the age span. For example, the skin of a 20-year-old is expected to be smooth and elastic, whereas the skin of a 70-year-old would be expected to have wrinkles and decreased elasticity. The patient's age also influences behavior, communication, and dress. For example, one would expect

that the vocabulary of an 18-year-old would be greater than that of a 6-year-old. It is expected that adolescent clothing and appearance will be influenced by trends more frequently than will that of older adults.

Birthplace   The biographic data include identification of the patient's birthplace. Identification of the birthplace allows the nurse to determine the environmental and cultural factors that impacted or contributed to the patient's current state of health and well-being. For example, in the United States, individuals who are born and live in areas where coal mining accounts for much of the industry are at greater risk for respiratory diseases such as black lung and emphysema than are individuals who are born in coastal areas or mountain areas of the United States. Further, individuals born in tropical areas outside of the United States are more likely to have been exposed to parasitic diseases than are those born within the United States.

It is important to determine the length of time the patient spent in and near the place of birth and the places in which the patient lived before locating to the current residence. Cultural, environmental, and geographic characteristics of regions and nations influence the health and well-being of the inhabitants. Geographic moves force individuals to adapt and adjust to new cultural norms. Problems in development may result when frequent moves prohibit individuals from forming and maintaining attachments to family and friends. It is important to understand the characteristics of the areas in which patients were born and where they resided throughout their lives. Acquiring knowledge of the characteristics of cities, communities, and regions beyond one's own experience is difficult. For example, a nurse who was born and lived in or near New York City can describe an urban and suburban environment that encompasses a highly developed area in terms of industry, business, and entertainment, with a transportation and highway system that permits rapid travel and access to business and leisure activities, schools, and a variety of healthcare facilities. That nurse will understand that there are communities within New York City which reflect ethnic, cultural, economic, and social differences. Yet, that same nurse may not be able to describe the characteristics of locations beyond New York City. Immigrants in the United States may have knowledge about their location of origin and the region in which they now reside. However, they may not be able to describe the physical environment of regions beyond their experience. All nurses encounter patients who were born or lived in cities, regions, or countries about which the nurses have little specific knowledge. Therefore, nurses must ask patients to describe the locations where they were born or where they resided over time, using questions or statements such as the following:

- Is the place you were born in a city?
- Is the region in which you lived close to a large city?
- Tell me about the place where you were born.

To find out about the physical and environmental characteristics of each location, the nurse will include questions such as these:

- Was the area you grew up in an industrial area?
- Was the place where you were born a farming area?
- How far did you have to travel to shop or go to school or get to a healthcare facility?
- How many people reside in that city?

Marital Status Marital status is another element of the biographic data. Marital status indicates whether the patient is single, married, widowed, or divorced. To include all sexual orientations and potential relationship statuses, the nurse should ask the patient if he or she is in a partnership (or partnered) with another person. It is helpful to determine the length of the marriage, relationship, partnership, widowhood, and divorce status.

The patient's marital or relationship status provides initial information about the presence of significant others who may provide physical or emotional support for the patient. In addition, when a patient relates the loss of a significant other through death or divorce, the nurse begins to evaluate emotional responses and coping ability expected in relation to the event and length of time since the event. The nurse also considers the information in relation to expectations for an individual's stage in life.

Sex and Gender The patient's sex is an element of the biographic data and refers to the biological sex of the individual to distinguish between male and female. There are differences between males and females in terms of physical development, secondary sex characteristics, and reproduction. For example, most males have greater muscle mass than females do. Fat

distribution in the thighs, hips, and buttocks is typically seen in females in greater amounts than in males. Males develop coarse facial hair as a beard, whereas females do not. Moreover, certain health risks are associated with sexual differences. For example, although breast cancer can occur in males, it occurs more frequently in females. Osteoporosis occurs in both sexes; however, postmenopausal females are at greater risk. Adolescent males are at greater risk for injury from motor vehicle crashes than are females; however, adolescent females have a higher incidence of eating disorders than do adolescent males.

The nurse should be aware that the term *gender* refers to role, not biological sex, and is influenced by the culture to which one belongs (American Psychological Association [APA], 2011). *Gender* implies the psychological, behavioral, social, and cultural aspects of male or masculinity and female or femininity (APA, 2015).

SEXUAL ORIENTATION AND GENDER IDENTITY Sexual orientation refers to an "inherent or immutable enduring emotional, romantic, or sexual attraction to other people," whereas gender identity is defined as "one's innermost concept of self as male, female, a blend of both or neither" (Human Rights Campaign [HRC], 2017, para. 1–2). The internal sense of oneself as male or female or other is another way of understanding gender identity (Sherer, Baum, Ehrensaft, & Rosenthal, 2015). The term **transgender** describes individuals whose gender identity is different from the cultural expectations based on the sex assigned at birth. Being transgender does not imply any specific sexual orientation, and individuals may identify as straight, gay, lesbian, bisexual, or asexual, for example (HRC, 2017). It is estimated that up to 5% of the U.S. population identifies as transgender (Hyderi, Angel, Madison, Perry, & Hagshenas, 2016), and the nurse must ensure that patients feel comfortable and safe in discussing all aspects of their healthcare. There may be patients who are hesitant to discuss with healthcare providers issues related to sexual orientation or gender identity.

To provide holistic care, the nurse should seek to build trust and to create an environment that promotes discussion of all health-related issues, including those related to sexual health. Sexual practices and an individual's self-identified sexual orientation and gender identity may provide insight about a number of potential health risks.

Race *Race* refers to classification of people according to shared biologic and genetic characteristics. The nurse can begin to identify characteristics of the patient in relation to expectations, norms, and risk factors associated with race. It is important to note that there has been and continues to be a blending of racial distinctions in the United States. Many individuals identify themselves as biracial or as having mixed racial origins. Families can consist of members of any given racial background (see Figure 5.4 ■) Therefore, expectations, norms, and risks are not as clearly delineated as they have been in the past. Assessment requires the nurse to ask specifically about this aspect of a patient's biographic data.

Risk for specific conditions may be increased or decreased related to a patient's race. For example, a recent study examined the differences in cardiovascular disease risk factors for Asian Americans, who are one of the fastest-growing racial groups in

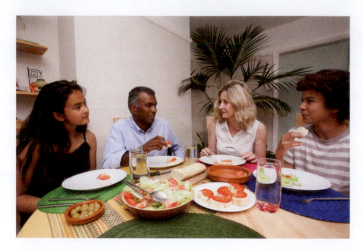

Figure 5.4 Families can consist of individuals with a variety of cultural backgrounds.

Source: Justin Hoffmann/Pearson Education Ltd.

the United States (Echeverria et al., 2017). The authors examined a large data set to determine that Asian Americans are at an increased risk of diabetes; this information will help determine appropriate teaching and screening tools.

Religion　Religion generally refers to an organizing framework for beliefs and practices and is associated with rites, rituals, and ceremonies that mark specific life passages such as birth, adulthood, marriage, and death. Religious beliefs often influence perceptions about health and illness. For example, some religions impose dietary or sleep pattern restrictions that can impact the state of health. The nurse will ask the patient the following questions or use the following statements to elicit information:

- What is your religion or religious preference?
- Tell me how your religion influences your health.
- Are there beliefs that govern your life?
- Tell me how your beliefs affect your relationships with others.

Additional information about the role of religion in the patient's life is obtained when asking about health practices and family history and when obtaining psychosocial information (see Chapter 3, Cultural and Spiritual Considerations, for a detailed discussion of cultural assessment; see Chapter 11, Mental Health, Substance Use, and Violence Assessment, for information about psychosocial assessment). ∞

Occupation　The patient's occupation is part of the biographic data; if the patient is not employed, this information is also important to learn. Information about what type of daily activities the patient engages in and where the patient spends time will help in determining whether physical, psychological, or environmental factors associated with these activities may influence the patient's health. For example, individuals who spend time in a loud warehouse may have diminished hearing acuity. Those employed in law enforcement and public safety often have an increased risk for physical injury (Lyons, Radburn, Orr, & Pope, 2017). An occupational history or profile provides information about previous, current, or potential health-related

risks and problems associated with work and workplace environments. The following are some questions to elicit information about work-related health concerns:

- What type of work is performed?
- Where does the work take place?
- How many hours are spent at work?
- How much time is involved in commuting to work?
- Does the workplace have safety guidelines in place?
- Are health services available in the workplace?
- Are health promotion programs available in the workplace?
- Does health screening occur in the workplace?
- What types of safety equipment are used in the workplace?
- Does the work environment contribute to stress?
- Does the type of work or the work schedule contribute to conflicts in family or other relationships?
- Are there risks for crime victimization or violence in the workplace?
- Is child care available at the workplace?
- Does the workplace have disaster and emergency plans?
- Does the work situation provide social support?

Health Insurance　Health prevention, health seeking, and health maintenance behaviors are influenced by the ability to pay for services. Although health insurance information usually is collected by administrative staff, it may be appropriate for the nurse to ask the patient questions regarding access to health insurance.

Health insurance alone does not indicate the patient's inclination to participate in healthcare. For example, uninsured individuals seek and receive healthcare in clinics and through other low- or no-cost means, and others are private payers for health services. Changes in national health insurance policy have significantly impacted the ability to obtain health insurance in the United States. The federal government of the United States has supported some type of national health insurance system since 1912 when President Teddy Roosevelt first suggested a program. Over the subsequent 60 years, there was an intermittent administrative push for the creation of a national health insurance fund open to all Americans. It was 1965 before the first national healthcare program was created for older Americans. Medicare was signed into law by President Lyndon B. Johnson (Anderson, 2016). Further national programs have been developed including expansions of the coverage of Medicare to include prescription drugs. Coverage for those under age 65 who are from low-income families, pregnant women, and individuals with disabilities was added under Medicaid programs. In 1997, a federally supported, state-run program, the Children's Health Insurance Program (CHIP) was created to provide health insurance and preventative care to uninsured American children. Most of these children were from working families who earned too much to be eligible for Medicaid. These programs, in addition to the Affordable Care Act of 2010, have created new ways for Americans to obtain and pay for healthcare insurance (Centers for Medicare & Medicaid Services [CMS], 2017).

Source of Information The biographic data must identify the source of the information for the health history. The usual source of information is the patient, who is the primary source (see Figure 5.5 ■). Secondary sources of information include family members, friends, healthcare professionals, and others who can provide information about the patient's health status. If the nurse and the patient do not speak the same language, or the comprehension or health literacy is compromised by a language barrier, the nurse must use a professional interpreter. The use of the interpreter must be indicated when recording the source of information. It is always preferable to use a professional interpreter rather than a patient's family member or friend to serve as an interpreter. Poor patient outcomes may result from misunderstanding (Juckett & Unger, 2014). Detailed information regarding interpreting in healthcare may be found on the website of the National Council on Interpreting in Health Care (www.ncihc.org).

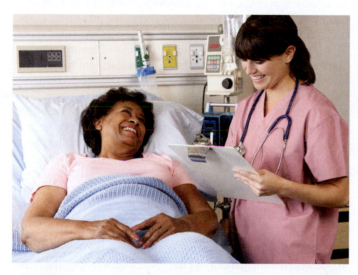

Figure 5.5 Patient serving as the primary source of assessment data.
Source: Monkey Business Images/Shutterstock.

Reliability of the Source Reliability of the source means that the person providing information for the health history is able to provide a clear and accurate account of present health, past health, family history, psychosocial information, and information related to each of the body systems. Usually the patient is considered to be the most reliable source. The nurse determines the reliability of the patient by assessing the ability to hear and speak as well as the ability to accurately recall past health-related events. For pediatric patients, the parents or guardians serve as the source of information. Secondary sources are used when the patient cannot participate in the interview because of physical or emotional problems.

History of Present Illness

The history of present illness or health includes information about all of the patient's current health-related issues, concerns, and problems. The history includes determination of the reason for seeking care as well as identification of health beliefs and practices, health patterns, health goals, and information about medication and therapies.

Reason for Seeking Care The patient usually gives the reason for seeking care when the nurse asks "Why are you seeking help today?" or "What is bothering you?" The reason for seeking care is sometimes referred to as the "chief complaint" or the "presenting problem." The nurse explores the reason for seeking care because it provides the first clues to choosing possible nursing diagnoses and sets the direction of the rest of the health history interview. It is not appropriate, however, to attempt to develop nursing diagnoses at this point. The patient has given minimal information, and no physical assessment or diagnostic testing has been performed. Instead, the nurse develops a list of statements that reflect the patient's major reasons for seeking care. Each statement is a brief, concise, and time-oriented description of the patient's concern. Here are some examples of statements describing the reason for seeking care:

- Substernal chest pain since 9:00 a.m.
- Swelling in lower legs and feet for the past 2 weeks
- Physical examination needed for football team by next Tuesday
- Weight gain of 10 lb since discontinuing daily walking regimen

The patient's own words should be used to document the reason for seeking care whenever possible—for example, "I've lost fifteen pounds in the last three weeks" or "I've lost the feeling in my right arm and hand." The nurse explores the onset and progression of each behavior, symptom, or concern the patient relates. Also, the nurse asks patients how their concern has affected their activities of daily living and what expectations they have for recovery and subsequent self-care. The answers to these questions provide valuable information about the patients' ability to tolerate and cope with the stress brought on by their health concerns and healthcare.

Health Beliefs and Practices A person's beliefs about health and illness are influenced by numerous factors, including exposure to information and personal experiences. Culture and heritage, which have a profound influence on the patient's beliefs about health and illness, are discussed in Chapter 3, Cultural and Spiritual Considerations. ∞

Healthcare information is widely available in all forms of media, through educational programs, and in literature provided by healthcare and community organizations. Many individuals use the internet as a primary source of healthcare information. The easy access to a broad scope of reliable and unreliable information about preventive and treatment services has promoted a different approach to healthcare. Patients who use a variety of information sources are more likely to be informed about recommendations for screening and preventive measures for themselves or family members according to age. Additionally, these patients are more likely to seek advertised or popular therapies they have read or heard about, to question recommended therapies, or to seek many opinions about treatment. The risks associated with the use of the internet for healthcare information are based on a patient's ability to judge the validity, currency, and scientific basis of the sources. The nurse's role includes evaluating the patient's health-related knowledge base and the accuracy of the information. In addition, the nurse should encourage the patient to use authoritative, evidence-based online resources when seeking educational health information. During any discussion about the patient's use of online health resources, the nurse should reinforce the importance of speaking with a primary care provider before making health decisions.

Health Patterns   A **health pattern** is a set of related traits, habits, or actions that affects a patient's health. The description of the patient's health patterns plays a key role in the total health history because it is how the nurse learns about a patient's lifestyle choices. Important aspects of health patterns include a patient's choices related to diet and nutrition, activity or exercise, sleep amount and quality, and the patient's pattern of accessing healthcare. These patterns may be assessed in more detail at the same time as the body system related to it is covered. For example, diet and nutrition assessment include information related to the usual diet the patient follows and any concerns they have about this area. Chapter 10, Nutritional Assessment, provides detailed information. ∞ Activity and exercise assessment should include specifics about time, intensity, and frequency of a patient's activities or exercise. A critically important area to assess is the patient's sleep pattern because sleep is critical for physical and psychological well-being (Aitken et al., 2017). For example, the number of hours a patient sleeps, the time a patient awakens and falls asleep, and the number of times a patient awakens during the night define a patient's sleep patterns. Nurses can use a variety of tools to assist patients to identify sleep problems. These include asking the patient to record a sleep diary and using a list of questions to identify sleep difficulties. These questions include the following:

- Do you snore loudly?
- Have you observed that you stop breathing or gasp for breath during sleep?
- Do you feel drowsy or fall asleep while reading, when watching TV, while driving, or in other daily activities?
- Do you have unpleasant feelings in your legs when trying to sleep?
- Are there interruptions to your sleep (pain, dreams, light, or temperature)?
- Do you have some trouble with sleep on three or more nights a week?

Health patterns also refer to the types and frequency of healthcare in which a patient participates. The nurse will ask questions related to the frequency of healthcare visits and preventive and screening measures used by the patient. For example, the nurse will ask the patient to give the dates of the last physical, dental, hearing, and eye examinations. In addition, the nurse will inquire about preventive measures such as immunizations and screenings such as mammography for breast cancer, stool examination for bleeding as a sign of rectal cancer, and laboratory screening of cholesterol and glucose levels because of their links with heart disease and diabetes.

Medications   Information about the use of medications is obtained during this part of the health history. The assessment should include a list of the prescription and over-the-counter (OTC) medications the patient is using. The nurse should determine the name, dose, purpose, duration, frequency, and desired or undesired effects of each of the medications. When the patient provides information about medications, the nurse is able to determine the patient's level of knowledge about the medication regimen, whether the patient has an understanding of the problem for which the medication has been prescribed, and whether the patient has noted or received information about the therapeutic effects of the medication. The source of the medication must be identified as well—for example: Has the medication been obtained from another country? (In an acute illness, such as a respiratory infection, medication is prescribed according to dose and duration [length of time the drug will be taken] to reduce symptoms and, ultimately, to cure the illness.) Is the patient using medication that was prescribed for someone else? (The illness may be ineffectively treated and may become worse. In addition, the medication shared with another may interact or interfere with drugs that the other individual is currently using.)

The nurse must ask about a patient's use of prescription medications; over-the-counter products; home or folk remedies; and alternative or complimentary therapies including herbs, teas, vitamins, dietary supplements, and other substances. Although the usefulness and effectiveness of herbal preparations and dietary supplements are controversial topics, and such products are not regulated by the U.S. Food and Drug Administration (FDA), individuals want control over their health and often have strong beliefs that herbal preparations and dietary supplements are natural and cause fewer side effects (Wu, Wang, Tsai, Huang, & Kennedy, 2014). The use of herbal remedies, teas, vitamins, and folk remedies can interfere with the action of some prescribed medications and can, in some instances, be harmful. For example, higher than recommended doses of vitamin E may interfere with medications including aspirin, warfarin, tamoxifen, and cyclosporine (Podszun & Frank, 2014).

When gathering information about medications, it is helpful to ask whether the patient has the container. Reading the name and dosage is called medication reconciliation, and it provides the specific information the nurse needs to make judgments about patient data. The nurse uses the medication reconciliation and history to identify any potential drug interactions and to determine if the patient requires education about medications, dosing, side effects, and interactions. It is also helpful to ask patients about categories of OTC medications. Categories may include laxatives; vitamins; herbs; pain relievers including aspirin and nonsteroidal anti-inflammatory drugs (NSAIDs); cold remedies; drops for the eyes, nose, or ears; enemas; allergy preparations; appetite stimulants or suppressants; sleep aids; and medicated lotions, creams, or ointments. Asking about each category is an efficient method to obtain a comprehensive assessment of medication use. The last category of medication information to assess is the patient's use of recreational or illegal drug use. This information may be obtained by asking "What other medications, drugs, or substances do you use?"

Past Medical History

The past medical history includes information about childhood diseases; immunizations; allergies; blood transfusions; major illnesses; injuries; hospitalizations; pregnancy; labor and childbirth; surgical procedures; mental, emotional, or psychiatric health problems; and the use of alcohol, tobacco, and other substances. The patient should describe each incident, including the date, treatment, healthcare provider, and any other pertinent information. If the patient has had a surgical procedure, the nurse elicits specific information concerning the type of surgery and postoperative course. Complicated labor and childbirths are recorded here as well as in the reproductive section of the review of the systems. Many health history forms include a checklist of the most commonly occurring illnesses or surgical procedures to help the patient recall information.

Depending on the age of the patient, the nurse might ask the patient to recall childhood illnesses or the immunization history. Having had German measles, polio, chickenpox, streptococcal throat infections, or rheumatic fever is especially significant because these diseases have sequelae that may affect the patient's health status and health concerns in adulthood. If the patient is a child, the nurse should inquire if immunizations are up to date and should verify this through immunization records. The nurse asks adult patients about their status of tetanus, pertussis, and influenza immunizations among others, as well as any vaccines required for foreign travel. The complete immunization history includes the name of the immunization, the number of doses, and the date of each dose or completion date of the series.

Information about the patient's emotional, mental, or psychiatric health should include the description of the problem. The nurse asks the patient to identify whether care was received through a healthcare provider, through a support group, from clergy or a pastor, or within the family or community. The information should include a description of the therapy or remedy, as well as the outcome of treatment. The nurse's questioning must reflect sensitivity to personal, family, and cultural reluctance to describe problems of an emotional or psychiatric nature.

The following questions or statements are used to obtain information about emotional and mental health:

- Have you ever had an emotionally upsetting experience?
- Tell me about any emotional upsets you have experienced.
- Have you ever sought assistance for an emotional problem?
- Where did you go to get assistance?
- Did the assistance help you with the problem?
- Have you ever been told that you have a mental illness or psychiatric disorder?
- What were the circumstances that led to the mental or psychiatric problem?
- What care did you receive for the mental or psychiatric problem?
- Has the care helped the problem?
- Do you take any medication for a mental or psychiatric problem?
- Are you experiencing problems now?
- What kind of help would you like to receive for the emotional, mental, or psychiatric problem?

Information about allergies and the use of illicit drugs, caffeine, alcohol, and tobacco is included in the health history.

Information about allergies should include determination of the allergy as food, drug, or environmentally occurring, including the symptoms, treatment, and personal adaptation. It is important to determine the extent of the patient's knowledge about allergens, especially when exposure to allergens can result in anaphylactic reactions. The nurse should ask the patient to describe the ways allergies are managed. The information should indicate whether a patient's allergies have been identified through testing, through confirmation of a cause by a healthcare professional, or by informal means. Eliciting information about adaptation includes identification of patient practices such as avoidance of allergens, the use of environmental controls (e.g., filters, air conditioners, or other devices) in the home or work environment, and the use of ingested remedies or medications. The information enables the nurse to begin to identify educational needs about allergies. The learning needs may include general or specific details about avoidance of allergens, methods to manage allergy symptoms, and measures to employ in severe allergic reactions. For example, the nurse may suggest that a patient obtain and wear a medical alert bracelet when severe allergies are identified.

When gathering information about the use of alcohol, tobacco, caffeine, and illicit drugs, the nurse will want to know the type, amount, duration, and frequency of use of each substance. The information is elicited whether the patient is currently using any substances or reports that she has stopped using the products. Tobacco use includes cigarettes, electronic cigarettes, vaping, cigars, and products that are chewed or inhaled as snuff. Use of any of these products has an impact on the physical health of the patient and family. Smoking has been definitively linked with lung cancer and emphysema both for the smoker and for those exposed to secondhand smoke. Alcohol abuse promotes liver disease, increases risk of injury or death in accidents, and is associated with disruptions in families.

Family Medical History

Information about the patient's family medical history, or family health history, has always been part of a comprehensive health assessment. The family medical history is a review of the patient's family to determine if any genetic or familial patterns of health or illness might shed light on the patient's current health status. Historically, this assessment focused on inherited conditions caused by a defect in a single gene or a variation in the number or structure of a particular chromosome. The importance of family medical history was to inform reproductive decision making in families affected by inherited conditions such as muscular dystrophy, cystic fibrosis, hemophilia, and other rare inherited disorders. These genetic—or inherited—conditions are caused by changes in the DNA that makes up the genes passed from parent to child. A further understanding of the whole of an organism's genes is called genomics. Since the successful completion of the Human Genome Project revealed the total human DNA sequence, called the human *genome*, medical researchers have begun to apply their understanding of this information to a wide variety of healthcare issues (National Human Genome Research Institute [NHGRI], 2016). In contrast to understanding the genetics of an individual, the definition of genomic medicine can help the nurse understand why the study of genomics is important to healthcare. "Genomic medicine is an emerging medical discipline that involves using genomic information about an individual as part of their clinical care (e.g., for diagnostic or therapeutic decision-making) and the health outcomes and policy implications of that clinical use" (NHGRI, 2016, para. 1).

The modern understanding of the influence of specific genes on common diseases such as cancer and cardiovascular disease is undisputed. Evidence of genetic or familial predisposition to breast and colon cancers has led to new treatments and earlier screenings (Evans, 2016). This knowledge makes assessment of family medical or health history very important. No longer is family medical history limited to rare inherited diseases, in fact the greatest benefit may come from establishing a basis to predict risk (or susceptibility) for common diseases such as diabetes, cancer, and heart disease. Knowing an individual's disease risk can be used to personalize healthcare, targeting interventions to those who will benefit most (Evans, 2016). If a person is found to have a family medical history of diabetes, knowledge of their genetic susceptibility may help providers create a personalized strategy for diabetes prevention and screening (Karaderi, Drong, & Lindgren, 2015). Including common diseases in family medical history assessment means that many more people at increased risk will be identified in time to tailor disease prevention and screening. Evidence-based recommendations based on family medical history of various cancers are rapidly being implemented, and this information is considered to be a critical tool for improving patient outcomes (Frank, Sundquist, Yu, Hemminki, & Hemminki, 2017).

Family medical history may be thought of as the original genetic test, and all professional nurses—regardless of academic preparation, practice setting, role, or specialty—must know how to gather the data and how to document in the patient's medical record. The documentation of the information is usually in the form of a diagram called a **genogram** or **pedigree**. The information learned from the family medical history will be critical in forming the nursing diagnoses and in planning care for the patient. Detailed information about how to document the family medical history and create a genogram is presented in Chapter 6, Documentation. ∞

Family medical history is part of the subjective nursing assessment; as such, its accuracy and completeness rely on patients' knowledge about the health of their relatives and their willingness and ability to share that information with health professionals. Sharing family medical history may raise issues of privacy and fear of discrimination. The nurse should remember that a family medical history is different from a personal health history in that it reflects information about multiple individuals, which greatly increases the risk for harm if confidentiality is broken. For example, the data collected may reveal previously undisclosed details about the patient and family, such as infertility or pregnancy termination, misattributed paternity, and mental health conditions (Hercher & Jamal, 2016). Therapeutic communication skills are particularly important when eliciting this potentially sensitive information. As in the other sections of the patient's health history interview, therapeutic communication skills must be employed to elicit accurate, detailed, and complete information.

EVIDENCE-BASED PRACTICE
Gathering the Family Health History

- Most people have a family health history (FH) of at least one common disease or health condition. This makes collection of the FH one of the best ways to use the rapidly advancing science of genetics and genomic testing for disease diagnosis, prognosis, risk prediction, prevention, and treatment (Lushniak, 2015).
- An accurate FH is critical to providing the highest quality of personalized healthcare. Even with all the advancements in genomic science and improved diagnostic precision, the FH still provides the most efficient and low-cost method of providing an individualized plan of care. FH collection tools embedded in the electronic health record are shown to improve rates of completed FHs (Hickey, Katapodi, Coleman, Reuter-Rice, & Starkweather, 2017).
- A novel tablet-based application created to capture FH data shows promise for improving risk assessment in genetic counseling. Compared with paper-based genograms or pedigrees, the software, called Proband, will require nurses and providers to practice its use to become proficient (Tipsword, White, Spaeth, Ittenbach, & Myers, 2017).

Psychosocial History

The psychosocial history includes information about the patient's living situation, educational level, financial background, roles and relationships, ethnicity and culture, family, spirituality, and self-concept. Together, these comprise a patient's social determinants of health—the conditions in which people are born, grow up, live, and work (Davis & Chapa, 2015). This information can reveal risk factors for a variety of problems related to known health disparities, such as low socioeconomic level, rural or underserved geographic locations, and low educational attainment. Determining the patient's level of education establishes expectations related to the ability to comprehend verbal and written language. These abilities are significant during the assessment process, in discussion of health problems or needs, and in education of the patient. The types of words that will be used and the choice of educational approaches and materials are influenced by the patient's abilities to read, write, and in some cases perform calculations. The patient's financial situation—that is, the ability to obtain health insurance or pay for health services—has an impact on health, health practices, and health-seeking behaviors. Low income is associated with a lowered health status and predisposition to illness. A patient may report that she now enjoys a secure financial situation. However, she may have been born and raised in poverty.

Poverty in youth is associated with poor nutrition and lack of regular medical and dental care. These deficiencies can have long-term consequences for the patient (Davis & Chapa, 2015).

The nurse will also gather information about the patient's roles and relationships, family, ethnicity and culture, spirituality, and self-concept. The nurse will ask the patient to identify a significant other and support systems. Support systems include family members, friends, neighbors, club members, clergy and church members, and members of the healthcare team. The information provides an initial impression of the family dynamics and informs the nurse of religious and spiritual needs of the patient. Determination of roles and relationships is important when planning healthcare and assisting the patient to make healthcare decisions. The nurse must respect the practices of the patient and prepare to include recognized decision makers in the planning process.

The following are questions and statements to elicit information about roles and relationships, family, and self-concept:

- Tell me about your family.
- How many people are in your family?
- Who is the head of the family?
- What is your role in the family?
- Who makes decisions about healthcare in your family?
- Who is involved in discussing health or emotional problems in your family?
- Are there certain roles for children in the family?
- Who is your significant other?
- Tell me about your support system.
- Tell me how you feel about yourself.
- How would you describe yourself to someone else?
- Tell me about your body image.

Chapter 3, Cultural and Spiritual Considerations, provides a thorough discussion of cultural considerations related to assessment. Principles of psychosocial assessment are described in Chapter 11, Mental Health, Substance Use, and Violence Assessment. ∞

Review of Body Systems

Sometimes called Review of Systems (ROS), the focus of this portion of the health history is to uncover current and past information about each body system and its organs. The nurse asks the patient about system function and any abnormal signs or symptoms, paying special attention to gathering information about the functional patterns of each system. For example, when assessing the gastrointestinal system, the nurse should ask the patient to describe digestive and elimination patterns ("How many bowel movements do you have each day?") as well as function ("Are your bowel movements usually hard or

soft?"). Open-ended questions or statements are best for eliciting information about abnormal signs or symptoms: "Describe the abdominal pain you've been experiencing. What other symptoms are associated with the pain?" The nurse carefully explores the characteristics and quality of each subjective symptom the patient identifies to obtain a total picture of each system.

Some health history formats use a cephalocaudal or head-to-toe approach for collecting data. In this approach, one considers regions of the body rather than systems. Other formats use an approach related to a nursing theory. Regardless of the method, each area of the body must be reviewed until all systems are covered in each region.

Unit III of this text provides information related to the systems of the body. ∞ Each chapter provides suggestions for questions to gather subjective data about a particular system. Focused interview questions are included and follow-up information is provided to elicit details when symptoms are reported. Examples of the types of information required for a comprehensive system review are included in the sample documentation of the health history. Box 5.2 lists the systems included in this part of the health history.

Box 5.2 Review of Body Systems

- Skin, Hair, and Nails
- Head, Neck, and Related Lymphatics
- Eyes
- Ears, Nose, Mouth, and Throat
- Respiratory System
- Breasts and Axillae
- Cardiovascular System
- Peripheral Vascular System
- Abdomen
- Urinary System
- Reproductive System
- Musculoskeletal System
- Neurologic System

Lifespan Considerations

The basic components of a health history are the same whether the nurse works with children or adults. However, for pregnant women, pediatric patients, and older adult patients, a number of variations must be incorporated into the health history. Unit IV covers in-depth the specialized assessment needs of Pregnant Female (Chapter 25), Infants, Children, and Adolescents (Chapter 26), and Older Adults (Chapter 27). ∞ These chapters present the unique lifespan considerations related to each of these patient populations.

Application Through Critical Thinking

CASE STUDY

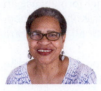

Source: Jennifer Hogan/123RF.

The nurse conducts a health history interview with Mrs. Martha Washburn, a 67-year-old African American. The following are excerpts from the health history:

"Mrs. Washburn, I am going to ask you a lot of questions before the physical assessment. I need to have correct responses, and I have to tell you, there will be a lot of them if we are to get to the root of your problem. I will use the information to develop a plan of care.

"What are you here for? Did someone come with you? I see on your chart that you have some problems with urination; are you incontinent? How long have you had the problem? You really should use the adult diapers when you go out."

The nurse includes the following questions: "What is your economic status? Do you go to church? What do you do when you are ill?

"We need information about your family, so let's start out with your parents. Are they alive? Do you have siblings?"

During the interview, Mrs. Washburn seems very anxious. She becomes quite upset when the nurse asks her about her incontinence. She tries to deny it at first and then admits it when the nurse makes reference to her medical record documentation of the problem.

The nurse completes a review of symptoms and prepares the patient for the physical examination by showing her a room and asking her to get undressed.

CRITICAL THINKING QUESTIONS

1. Critique the nurse's actions in the initial interview phase of the case study.

2. Identify the types of information sought in the questions in the case study.

3. Create alternative approaches to the interview and questioning techniques in the case study.

4. Describe your own preparation for an interview of Mrs. Washburn.

5. If Mrs. Washburn did not speak English, how would you modify the health history exam?

REFERENCES

Aitken, L. M., Elliott, R., Mitchell, M., Davis, C., Macfarlane, B., Ullman, A., . . . McKinley, S. (2017). Sleep assessment by patients and nurses in the intensive care: An exploratory descriptive study. *Australian Critical Care, 30*(2), 59–66. Retrieved from https://doi.org/10.1016/j.aucc.2016.04.001

American Psychological Association (APA). (2011). *Publication manual of the American Psychological Association* (6th ed.). Washington, DC: Authors.

American Psychological Association (APA). (2015). *APA Dictionary of psychology* (2nd ed). Washington, DC: Authors

Anderson, S. (2016). A brief history of Medicare in America. Retrieved from https://www.medicareresources.org/basic-medicare-information/brief-history-of-medicare

Berman, A., Snyder, S., & Frandsen, G. (2016). *Kozier and Erb's fundamentals of nursing: Concepts, process, and practice* (10th ed.). Hoboken, NJ: Pearson.

Centers for Medicare & Medicaid Services. (2017). *History: CMS' program history.* Retrieved from https://www.cms.gov/About-CMS/Agency-information/History

Davis, S. L., & Chapa, D. W. (2015). Social determinants of health: Knowledge to effective action for change. *The Journal for Nurse Practitioners, 11*(4), 424–429. https://doi.org/10.1016/j.nurpra.2015.01.029

Echeverria, S. E., Mustafa, M., Pentakota, S. R., Kim, S., Hastings, K. G., Amadi, C., & Palaniappan, L. (2017). Social and clinically-relevant cardiovascular risk factors in Asian American Adults: NHANES 2011-2014. *Preventive Medicine, 99*, 222–227. https://doi.org/10.1016/j.ypmed.2017.02.016

Evans, D. G. (2016). Genetic predisposition to cancer. *Medicine, 44*(1), 65–68. Retrieved from https://doi.org/10.1016/j.mpmed.2015.10.003

Frank, C., Sundquist, J., Yu, H., Hemminki, A., & Hemminki, K. (2017). Concordant and discordant familial cancer: Familial risks, proportions and population impact. *International Journal of Cancer, 140*(7), 1510–1516. doi:10.1002/ijc.30583

Hercher, L. & Jamal, L. (2016, March). An old problem in a new age: Revisiting the clinical dilemma of misattributed paternity. *Applied & Translational Genomics, 8*, 36–39. Retrieved from https://doi.org/10.1016/j.atg.2016.01.004

Hickey, K. T., Katapodi, M. C., Coleman, B., Reuter-Rice, K., & Starkweather, A. R. (2017). Improving utilization of the family history in the electronic health record. *Journal of Nursing Scholarship, 49*(1), 80–86. doi:10.1111/jnu.12259

Human Rights Campaign. (2017). Sexual orientation and gender identity definitions. Retrieved from https://www.hrc.org/resources/sexual-orientation-and-gender-identity-terminology-and-definitions

Hyderi, A., Angel, J., Madison, M., Perry, L. A., & Hagshenas, L. (2016). Transgender patients: Providing sensitive care: What to say? What to prescribe? When to refer? *Journal of Family Practice, 65*(7), 450–461. Retrieved from JFPONLINE.com.

Juckett, G., & Unger, K. (2014). Appropriate use of medical interpreters. *American Family Physician, 90*(7), 476–480. Retrieved from https://www.aafp.org/afp

Karaderi, T., Drong, A. W., & Lindgren, C. M. (2015). Insights into the genetic susceptibility to type 2 diabetes from genome-wide association studies of obesity-related traits. *Current Diabetes Reports, 15*(83), 1–12. doi:10.1007/s11892-015-0648-8

Kelley, K. J., & Kelley, M. F. (2013). Teaching empathy and other compassion-based communication skills. *Journal for Nurses in Professional Development, 29*(6), 321–324. doi:10.1097/01.NND.0000436794.24434.90

Lushniak, B. D. (2015). Surgeon general's perspectives. *Public Health Reports, 130*(1), 305. doi:10.1177/003335491513000102

Lyons, K., Radburn, C., Orr, R., & Pope, R. (2017). A profile of injuries sustained by law enforcement officers: A critical review. *International Journal of Environmental Research and Public Health, 14*(142), 1–21. doi:10.3390/ijerph14020142

Mandal, F. B. (2014). Nonverbal communication in humans. *Journal of Human Behavior in the Social Environment, 24*(4), 417–421. doi:10.1080/10911359.2013.831288

Naik, S. B. (2013). Death in the hospital: Breaking the bad news to the bereaved family. *Indian Journal of Critical Care Medicine, 17*(3), 178–181. doi:10.4103/0972-5229.117067

National Human Genome Research Institute [NHGRI]. (2016). All about the human genome project (HGP). Retrieved from https://www.genome.gov/10001772/all-about-the-human-genome-project-hgp/

Pehrson, C., Banerjee, S. C., Mann, R., Shen, M. J., Hammonds, S., Coyle, N., . . . Bylund, C. L. (2016). Responding empathically to patients: Development, implementation, and evaluation of a communication skills training module for oncology nurses. *Patient Education and Counseling, 99*, 610–616. Retrieved from https://doi.org/10.1016/j.pec.2015.11.021

Podszun, M., & Frank, J. (2014). Vitamin E-drug interactions: Molecular basis and clinical relevance. *Nutrition Research Reviews, 27*(2), 215–231. doi:10.1017/S0954422414000146

Rogers, Carl R. (1957). The necessary and sufficient conditions of therapeutic personality change. *Journal of Consulting Psychology, 21*, 95–103.

Sherer, I., Baum, J., Ehrensaft, D., & Rosenthal, S. M. (2015). Affirming gender: Caring for gender-atypical children and adolescents. *Contemporary Pediatrics, 32*(1), 16–19. Retrieved from http://www.advanstar.com/healthcare

Tipsword, M. L., White, P. S., Spaeth, C. G., Ittenbach, R. F., & Myers, M. F. (2017, December 22). Investigation of the use of a family health history application in genetic counseling. *Journal of Genetic Counseling*, 1–14. doi:10.1007/s10897-017-0196-2

Wiechula, R., Conroy, T., Kitson, A. L., Marshall, R. J., Whitaker, N., & Rasmussen, P. (2015). Umbrella review of the evidence: What factors influence the caring relationship between a nurse and patient? *Journal of Advanced Nursing, 72*(4), 723–734. doi:10.1111/jan.12862

Wu, C., Wang, C., Tsai, M., Huang, W., & Kennedy, J. (2014). Trend and pattern of herb and supplement use in the United States: Results from the 2002, 2007, and 2012 National Health Interview surveys. *Evidence-Based Complementary and Alternative Medicine, 2014*(872320), 1–7. http://dx.doi.org/10.1155/2014/872320

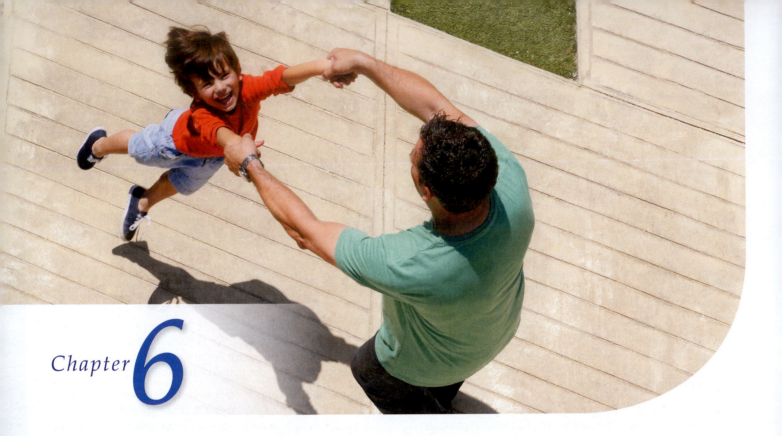

Chapter 6

Documentation

LEARNING OUTCOMES

Upon completion of this chapter, you will be able to:

1. Describe the purpose of nursing documentation.

2. List the key principles of nursing documentation.

3. Correctly document the subjective and objective findings from a comprehensive health history and physical assessment.

4. Use the correct nursing documentation format for a given setting.

KEY TERMS

anatomic planes, 68
charting, 75
confidentiality, 69
documentation, 64
electronic medical record (EMR), 64
electronic health record (EHR), 64
patient portals, 64
proband, 74
SBAR, 66
uniform language, 68

Introduction

To make use of the patient-related data collected during the assessment, the nurse must ensure that it is accurate, professional, complete, and confidential. The process of writing, recording, or storing this data is called **documentation**, and documentation also is the written evidence of the nursing care provided, the interactions between nurses and other healthcare professionals, and the results or outcomes of interventions (Selvi, 2017). Many nurses refer to the act of documenting as "charting" because they are writing in the chart. Historically, documentation consisted of handwritten notes collected in charts; often

these notes were kept in binders and stored on carts or shelves. These charts were susceptible to loss through water or fire damage, misplacement, and theft. The privacy of the patient information and patient confidentiality could only be assured by a physical lock and key. Today, although the patient chart may still be available to carry in hand, most of contemporary charting or documentation is done in a digital format using complex proprietary software resulting in the creation of the **electronic health record (EHR)**, also known as the **electronic medical record (EMR)**. Other forms of digital access to patient information include **patient portals** or web access (Kuhn, Basch, Barr, & Yackel, 2015). A patient portal is a web-based entryway for patients to access their EHR, make appointments, or communicate with their medical providers. Many primary care and specialty medical provider practices are providing this type of access to patients. The types of documentation are varied in length, format, and use; the principles that guide the creation of all nursing documentation are consistent.

Even though the forms of documentation have changed over time, the key purpose and principles of professional documentation have not. This chapter presents a comprehensive definition of documentation, its purpose in nursing and healthcare, the principles of professional documentation, and an overview with examples of some of the documentation the nurse may perform or encounter in a variety of nursing settings. The type, content, style, and formatting of documentation are often determined by the policies of the agency or facility; these varied formats may include digital or paper checklists, fill-in forms, and narrative records. The comprehensive patient database that is created from the health history and physical examination becomes part of the patient record and is a legal document.

Purpose of Nursing Documentation: Communication

The primary purpose of documentation is to communicate information between and among the health professionals involved in the immediate and ongoing care of the patient. The documentation serves as an archive of patient information related to the direct care of the patient, as well as by members of the interprofessional healthcare team, and for other intra- or interagency, legal, financial, research, or quality improvement uses. Professional nursing documentation is the accessible record of the nursing process. Without documentation, there is no record of nursing care completed, and that means it will be impossible to find out if an intervention worked (Andrews & St. Aubyn, 2015). Therefore, nurses learn early on the adage *If it is not documented, it was not done.*

Because effective communication is crucial to patient care, the nurse must adhere to the following guidelines for documentation: All nursing documentation must be accurate, professional, complete, and confidential. Nursing documentation is an activity essential to patient care and must be seen as an extension of care rather than a secondary job. The nurse must prioritize the time, energy, and care needed to perform this task (Ahn, Choi, & Kim, 2016). Accuracy in documentation is ensured through use of standard and uniform professional language, which is used to create an objective, clear, and detailed record of assessment findings.

Medical and nursing terminology used by the nurse includes standard and accepted abbreviations, symbols, and terminology and must reflect professional and organizational standards. Some common examples are listed in Box 6.1. The complete and appropriate documentation is ensured through concise, precise, succinct, and professional language and through the avoidance of judgmental or biased language. One way to avoid inaccurate perceptions is to remember to use "person-first language" so that a patient is referred to as "the patient with diabetes" rather than "the diabetic" (Selekman, 2014, p. 44).

Box 6.1	**Standard Abbreviations**
ABD	Abdomen
ADL	Activities of daily living
BP	Blood pressure
CBC	Complete blood count
CNS	Central nervous system
CVA	Costovertebral angle, cerebrovascular accident
Dx	Diagnosis
Ht	Height
Hx	History
LMP	Last menstrual period
P	Pulse
RR	Respiratory rate
T	Temperature
VS	Vital signs
WBC	White blood cell
Wt	Weight

Finally, the documentation must be accurately and completely identified; the nurse, date and time of entry, as well as the context, if appropriate, must be included in each entry. Confidentiality must be maintained by using secure documentation systems—digital or paper—and adhering to laws and policy governing transmission of patient information. These guidelines are explored in detail in the following sections.

Communication Within the Healthcare Team

Communication among those caring for a patient ensures that the patient receives timely, effective, and safe care. Using documentation that is accurate, professional, complete, and confidential enhances interprofessional communication. The interprofessional care team may include nurses, physicians, physical therapists, dieticians, discharge planners, and others. Timely and accurate documentation must be entered into the patient chart as soon as possible so that other care-team members are able to review it before performing their interventions, evaluating interventions, or writing the next set of orders. Beyond the immediate hands-on patient care, other agency-based members of the healthcare team, such as pharmacists and billing professionals, also access and use the patient care documentation. Consistent and timely entry of documentation about patient care will ensure optimum patient outcomes in all healthcare settings.

As you read the following case, consider the possible outcomes that could occur if nursing interventions are not consistently documented.

Communication Among Team Members: SBAR Communication among healthcare team members happens through written documentation. In addition, team members often share

CASE STUDY

Nurse A administers a narcotic pain medication at 10:00 a.m. in anticipation of a patient going to physical therapy at 11:00 a.m. The medication is to be administered every 6 hours. At 10:45 a.m. the physical therapist arrives, and the patient states he is in too much pain to participate. The therapist looks in the chart to see if pain medication was administered and sees no documentation for pain medication since the night before. The therapist asks Nurse B, the charge nurse, to give the patient a dose of his narcotic pain medication; she gives this dose and documents it in the chart. Later, Nurse A comes into the patient room to see how physical therapy is going and notices that the patient is very sleepy. After the session has ended, Nurse A and the charge nurse talk to each other, and they determine that Nurse A did not document the pain medication given at 10:00 a.m. The patient is monitored, the physician alerted, new orders given for a reversal medication, and Nurse A completes an incident report.

patient-related information through verbal reporting. The **S**ituation, **B**ackground, **A**ssessment, and **R**ecommendation (**SBAR**) format is commonly used in all types of healthcare agencies, institutions, and professions to guide communication.

The SBAR tool was developed in 2002 by U.S. Navy personnel as a method for communicating critical information quickly (Stewart & Hand, 2017). Since then, this tool has been taught to nurses, physicians, pharmacists, and many other providers and is shown to increase patient safety (Barnett, Nagy, & Hakim, 2017). This technique provides a simple framework for the nurse to organize information when giving a verbal report, and may be useful when planning written documentation of patient care (Institute for Healthcare Improvement, n.d.). Tools such as the SBAR and other templates and checklists may be useful to guide documentation because they prompt the nurse about which areas to include and they present a logical order or sequence to follow (Manias, Bucknall, Hutchinson, Botti, & Allen, 2017). A sample SBAR form is shown in Figure 6.1 ■; in this example the SBAR is for guiding communication between a nurse and a physician.

Future Communication with Other Professionals

An important purpose of documentation is to communicate information over time. That means keeping a record for retrieval in the future by others who may or may not be involved in direct patient care. For example, researchers may access a database of patient information in order to perform quality improvement projects on a unit or across a particular population. If the agency is involved in legal action, the documentation may be the only record of what happened to a particular patient. In addition, healthcare agencies, insurers, and other governmental entities may require access to patient care documentation in order to be paid. The general principles of documentation are the same for all types: The documentation must be accurate, professional, complete, and confidential; in addition, it must remain retrievable.

Principles of Nursing Documentation

The purpose of documentation is communication across providers in the healthcare setting. To ensure communication is accurate and effective—the right information at the right time—the nurse must adhere to the four basic principles of documentation. These principles—accuracy, professionalism, completeness, and confidentiality—are detailed in the following sections. Accurate and professional documentation that is complete supports positive patient outcomes (Chand & Sarin, 2014).

Accuracy

The most important aspect of documentation is accuracy, which means that documentation is limited to facts or factual accounts of observations rather than opinions or interpretations of observations. Accuracy of the recording of subjective data is dependent on what the patient says, whereas accuracy of objective data is based on what the nurse observes or measures. When recording subjective data, it is important to use quotation marks to record a patient's exact words rather than interpreting the statement by putting it in nursing or medical terms. For example, rather than documenting that a patient is experiencing *pain and ecchymosis of the left lateral and anterior gluteal region* the nurse should write: *patient states "my left hip is bruised and really hurts."* The nurse must remember that the patient's own words should be used to document accurately the subjective data from the health history interview. Additionally, it is best to avoid words such as *seem, apparently,* or *appears*.

In documenting the objective physical examination, accuracy dictates that the nurse use precise measurements and descriptions of the location of symptoms and physical findings. Vague, slang, or lay-person terminology should be avoided. For example, instead of writing that the patient had *a red and bumpy rash and swelling on the left foot*, the nurse should document that a patient had *scattered erythematous, maculo-papular lesions and edema on the dorsal surface of the left foot over the first through third phalanges*. Additionally, use exact measurements such as *intake of 400 mL of water* instead of *adequate water intake*. System-specific terminology and medical language are highlighted in each system chapter in Unit III of this book.

Concise, Precise, Succinct, Professional   These four terms define the requirements for ensuring accurate and complete documentation. Nursing documentation must be:

- *concise*: the information given is brief but comprehensive
- *precise*: exact and accurate in details
- *succinct*: brief and clearly expressed
- *professional*: expressed using accepted professional medical terminology, symbols, abbreviations, and acronyms.

Abbreviations and acronyms must be known and understood by those in the medical profession. It is unacceptable to create your own acronyms as this can be confusing or dangerous if the meanings are not clear. For example, a nurse may use the acronym *MS* to mean "multiple sclerosis," but it is also known to mean "morphine sulfate" or "magnesium sulfate." If the nurse is not sure of the appropriate acronym, it is best to spell out the words. The Joint Commission (TJC) (2017), an independent, nonprofit organization that accredits healthcare

SBAR report to physician about a critical situation

S	**Situation** **I am calling about** (insert patient name here) . **The patient'scode status is** (note what the patient's code status is) **The problem I am calling about is** ________________________. I am afraid the patient is going to arrest. **I have just assessed the patient personally:** **Vital signs are** : Blood pressure ____/____, Pulse ______, Respiration_____ and temperature ______ **I am concerned about the:** Blood pressure because it is over 200 or less than 100 or 30 mmHg below usual Pulse because it is over 140 or less than 50 Respiration because it is less than 5 or over 40. Temperature because it is less than 96 or over 104.
B	**Background** **The patient's mental status is:** Alert and oriented to person place and time. Confused and cooperative or non-cooperative Agitated or combative Lethargic but converant and able to swallow Stuporous and not talking clearly and possibly not able to swallow Comatose. Eyes closed. Not responding to stimulation. **The skin is:** Warm and dry Pale Mottled Diaphoretic Extremities are cold Extremities are warm **The patient is not or is on oxygen.** The patient has been on ________ (l/min) or (%) oxygen for ______ minutes (hours) The oximeter is reading ______% The oximeter does not detect a good pulse and is giving erratic readings.
A	**Assessment** **This is what I think the problem is:** (describe what you think is the problem is) **The problem seems to be cardiac infection neurologic respiratory** ____ **I am not sure what the problem is but the patient is deteriorating.** **The patient seems to be unstable and may get worse, we need to do something.**
R	**Recommendation** **I suggest or request that you** (describe what you want done). transfer the patient to critical care come to see the patient at this time. Talk to the patient or family about code status. Ask the on-call family practice resident to see the patient now. Ask for a consultant to see the patient now. **Are any tests needed:** Do you need any tests like CXR, ABG, EKG, CBC, or BMP? Others? **If a change in treatment is ordered then ask:** How often do you want vital signs? How long to you expect this problem will last? If the patient does not get better when would you want us to call again?

Figure 6.1 SBAR report.

Source: Institute for Healthcare Improvement. (n.d.). *SBAR Tool: Situation-background-assessment-recommendation.* Cambridge, MA: authors. Retrieved from http://www.ihi.org/resources/Pages/Tools/SBARToolkit.aspx

organizations across the United States, works to improve healthcare and ensure excellence in patient safety and effectiveness through the development of performance standards and certification. One area that it has targeted for improvement is communication among healthcare professionals across disciplines. To help ensure safety, TJC publishes a "Do Not Use" list of abbreviations that are not acceptable for use in healthcare documentation. Common abbreviations such as "U" for unit, "IU" for international unit, and "QD" for daily should not be used as they can be mistaken for "0," "IV," or "00" when written by hand. Another important feature addresses the use of leading or trailing zeros when writing quantities or dosages. For example, "2.0 mg" can be mistaken for "20 mg" if the decimal point is unclear or difficult to read. Other symbols are also susceptible to misinterpretation. The best practice is to write out symbols such as "greater than" or "less than" and to avoid using abbreviations for drug names and unfamiliar or infrequently used symbols. This information is periodically updated. To find the most current "Do Not Use" list go to https://www.jointcommission.org/facts_about_do_not_use_list/#.

Legal Principles The goal of nursing is to provide quality care based on nursing standards, and nursing documentation is the way to communicate to others about the care you provided. The written record or documentation will be a permanent record of your knowledge and understanding of the nursing standards of care (Neil, 2015). Because nursing documentation constitutes a legal record of nursing care, the accuracy of the charting will support nurses' testimony if called as a witness in legal proceedings. If a nurse is called on to testify about care they have given, documentation that is comprehensive, objective, and accurate will help validate the oral explanations. In addition to conveying the specifics of patient care, accurate and thorough charting may protect nurses from claims of negligence (Horowitz, 2015).

Remaining up to date on your specialty, joining and participating in professional nursing organizations, earning or maintaining certifications, and clearly understanding your job description and scope of practice are some ways to ensure that you follow current standards of care, including the following charting and documentation do's and don'ts:

Do's

- Do chart facts accurately, completely, and concisely.
- Do request training and practice to obtain new skills and update old skills.
- Do verify orders that are unclear.

- Do chart patient noncompliance (e.g., do explain why a medication was refused and what further actions you took).

Don'ts

- Don't falsify or destroy any portion of a medical record.
- Don't accept an assignment if you are unsure of your competency.
- Don't document for anyone else.
- Don't make statements or document criticisms (e.g., "Sorry, we are short staffed tonight" or "The night shift apparently never checked patient's pulse") (Horowitz, 2015).

Professionalism

Nursing documentation as a communication tool among healthcare professionals requires the nurse to use language that is commonly accepted and understood. In healthcare, professionalism is expressed by the consistent use of a **uniform language**. By using current and accepted terminology, all individuals involved in documenting any aspect of the patient's care will provide the foundation for consistent interpretation of data.

Uniform language is used for all patient data documented during the nursing process. In addition to the use of standard acronyms and abbreviations, nurses' writing must be coherent and free of errors in spelling, grammar, and structure. Professional nursing documentation requires use of specific terms to describe assessment and physical examination findings. These terms describe where on the body the condition exists, to what extent or distribution, and other descriptors such as color, texture, shape, and size.

In describing the locations on the body, terminology describes how the body is separated by **anatomic planes**—the imaginary lines separating the body into parts—referred to as the frontal plane, median plane, horizontal plane, and sagittal plane. These and additional terms for documentation of findings relative to body location are included in Table 6.1. Terminology related to color, texture, shape, size, and form are detailed in the specific body system chapters in Unit III. Consistent use of all accepted terminology will enhance nursing documentation.

Completeness

To ensure that all nursing documentation is complete, it should be done as promptly as possible; be easily readable and coherent, whether handwritten or entered electronically; and be accessible to those who require access. Documenting immediately after completion of a task, or as soon as possible, is important because recollection of details becomes difficult as time passes. One method for ensuring accuracy is to take notes about assessment details during the data collection process. This may be particularly important when recording direct patient quotes and precise information about the location of a lesion, a wound, or an abnormal finding. To maintain the patient's trust, the nurse should inform the patient that notes will be taken during the

Table 6.1 Medical Terminology: Body Locations

TERM	DEFINITION
anterior (ventral)	toward the front
caudad	toward the feet
cephalad	toward the head
deep	below the surface
distal	farthest from the center or a medial line
external	outside of
frontal plane	separating the anterior and posterior sections of the body
horizontal plane	dividing the superior and inferior parts of the body
inferior	lower
internal	inside of
lateral	farther from the midline, toward or on the side
medial	closer to the midline
median plane	separating the body into right and left halves
prone	face down
posterior (dorsal)	toward the back
proximal	closest to the center or a medial line
sagittal plane	referring to any plane parallel to the median
superior	upper
supine	face up
superficial	on or above the surface

interview or examination. These notes can then be used to remind the nurse of details revealed during the interview or physical exam process.

To ensure completeness, the nurse's name or initials should be included, along with the time and date of the entry as well as all other pertinent information. All EHR entries are digitally "stamped" with this information, and most facilities use some type of computerized documentation system to maintain that type of record. It is noteworthy that documentation in a digital format, although legible, is still vulnerable to errors or omissions. Entries in any record must be well thought out and checked for typographical errors, correct spelling, and accurate grammar before submission. Poorly written documentation can reflect carelessness on the nurse's part, and this impression may be detrimental if documentation is presented in legal proceedings. When documenting either in a paper chart or in the EHR, nurses must not leave any blank lines. To start on a subsequent line, the nurse must draw a line or type a strikethrough to ensure no other information can be inserted in the blank space.

In reviewing the documentation, if a mistake is found, the nurse must be able to audit, or revise, the entry. In handwritten notes, the error is noted by drawing a single line through it and marking it with the writer's signature, time, and date. In the digital environment, errors are marked with a time stamp that includes the nurse's identifier along with time and date. Additionally, a "reason code" may be attached to any changes made in the patient record, such as "wrong patient" or "charted in error." Further, if the nurse must document at the end of the shift something that happened earlier, the entry should note that it is a "late entry." It is illegal to document something before it is actually done.

Confidentiality and Patient Protection

Protecting the patient's rights is crucial in all healthcare settings and is assured through legislation and training. **Confidentiality** signifies that information sharing is limited to only those individuals with direct involvement in a patient's care. Security of patient information also extends to confidentiality and security of the clinical professionals' information and the agency- or organization-level information. Each nurse is responsible for institutional-level security and confidentiality policies and procedures. The basic principles of confidentiality state that data be considered appropriate for inclusion in a health record only if the specifics have direct bearing on the patient's care.

Health Insurance Portability and Accountability Act (HIPAA)

Protection of an individual's health information is regulated federally through the Health Insurance Portability and Accountability Act (HIPAA). The overarching rule is that only individuals who are directly involved with a patient's care are allowed access to that patient's health record. Regulations under HIPAA became effective in April 2003, and the penalties for failure to comply are severe. The aim of the law was to create a national standard for privacy and to provide individuals with greater control over personal health information. Healthcare providers, hospitals, and health insurance providers are required to follow policies to protect the privacy of health information, known as protected health information (PHI). The HIPAA regulations protect medical records and other individually identifiable health information, whether communicated in writing, orally, or electronically. Personally identifiable PHI includes demographic information such as age, gender, address, and name, as well as any other information that could identify an individual. Examples of the latter include photographs, x-rays, medical record numbers, and diagnoses. The nurse must take care when documenting data or discussing a patient not to inadvertently share this PHI inappropriately.

Training

In addition to general training on HIPAA, training and education for nurses regarding the technical aspects of documentation policies and procedures must be provided by the employing organization or agency (American Nurses Association [ANA], 2010). This type of training often happens during a new employee's orientation, yearly as a refresher, and when new information is disseminated. One important aspect of becoming a professional nurse is learning how policies and procedures work to allow nurses sufficient time to complete their daily documentation (ANA, 2010). Other aspects of training involve learning how to use the electronic health record system. This training also includes security training, usually from the information technology department, and covers passwords and other security.

Documenting the Comprehensive Patient Assessment

The assessment of the patient's health includes the health history interview and the physical assessment. In order to make use of the comprehensive patient database, the first step in the nursing process is complete when the information is recorded in the patient's chart or medical record. From this database, the nurse can proceed to identify nursing diagnoses, create patient-centered goals, and select nursing interventions to achieve the goals. The patient database is comprised of subjective information and objective assessment findings, and it is often called the "history and physical" (H&P). The nurse may review any notes taken during the assessment process as that will help to make the documentation accurate, professional, complete, and confidential.

Documenting the Health History: Subjective

Chapter 5, Interviewing and Health History: Subjective Data, presents the interview and history-taking process. The information documented from the interview process will provide to anyone reviewing the chart an overall picture of the patient's symptoms, concerns, and condition.

The subjective data are recorded using the words of the patient, often citing direct quotes. As the nurse uses communication skills to elicit as much detail as possible about each area and topic within the health history, notes are taken to aid in the documentation of this data. The nurse should ask the patient to explain his or her meaning of words such as *good, average, okay, normal,* and *adequate*. The nurse must be sure to record what the patient intended by use of such terms. Sample documentation of a health history is included in Box 6.2 and Box 6.3. The format of data collection tools and forms vary, depending on the facility or agency. Box 6.2 is a case study presented in narrative form. Box 6.3 represents a fill-in form for documentation of the health history. As shown in the example, quotation marks are not used because all entries are understood to be stated by the patient.

Box 6.2 Narrative Recording of the Health History

Biographic Data *Mrs. Corrina Soto, age 33, comes to the health center for a health assessment. She is employed as a graphic designer for a community-based financial institution. Mrs. Soto has insurance through Corporate Insurance Company, through her employer. It covers medical, dental, and vision care. She lives in a single-family residence at 22 Highland Avenue, Midland Park, New Jersey. Mrs. Soto lives with her husband, who she names as her emergency contact. Mrs. Soto was born on July 20, 1981, in Santa Clara, Cuba. She immigrated to the United States 9 years ago. She speaks English with an accent. Mrs. Soto can read and write in English and Spanish. Aside from her husband and in-laws, Mrs. Soto has no immediate family in the United States. She completed 16 years of schooling in Cuba, including earning a university degree in graphic design. She has no formal religious affiliations, because religious practice was not permitted in Cuba when she was there. Some of her family were "hidden" Catholics. She states, "I am happy with my life. I have made adjustments to being in the United States. I have many Cuban friends and have a close relationship with my husband's family. I like my job, except when it gets really stressful."*

Present Health Status: Reason for Seeking Healthcare *Mrs. Soto has no complaints except "weight gain and occasional headaches relieved with aspirin." The weight gain has occurred "over three years since I started dating my husband and more since we got married last year." The headaches occur "when I'm tired, stressed, or spending too much time on my computer."*

Health Beliefs and Practices *Mrs. Soto has no current health problems, except as stated above. She believes "health is important and you need to take care of yourself, but sometimes it's out of your control." When she was a child her mother used to tell her things like "no bathing when you have your period, no water at all" and she "prepared certain foods for certain illnesses and sometimes got medicines from a botanica for ailments." Since she has been covered by health insurance and encouraged by her husband, she has had regular physical, gynecologic, dental, and eye examinations, all of which have been completed annually for 3 years.*

Mrs. Soto states she "sleeps well most nights about 8 hours, unless I stay up and read." She "feels rested most mornings." She tries to exercise but finds it hard "after work and when it's cold out."

Mrs. Soto would like to lose weight to "feel healthier—my clothes would fit, and I'd feel good about myself." People in Cuba would not have a problem with this weight, but she added "I don't like it." Eating patterns include "fast foods at lunch, bread at every meal, and dessert or snacks at night."

Medications *Mrs. Soto uses oral contraceptives "for four years," without problems, and takes a multivitamin and a fish oil capsule every day. She is not undergoing any therapy and states, "I really have never needed any specific care."*

Past History, Surgeries, and Illnesses *Mrs. Soto had measles as a child. She received smallpox, polio, mumps, tetanus, and other "vaccines" as a child. She has had no major illnesses. She has never been hospitalized, received a blood transfusion, been pregnant, or had allergies. Mrs. Soto cut her lower left leg on glass as a child, had sutures, and a scar remains. She had four wisdom teeth extracted 2 years ago with no complications and "no other surgery."*

Emotional History *Mrs. Soto states, "I miss my family and get sad when I can't see them. I get frustrated when I don't understand some American ways. I'm pretty emotional. I cry over books and movies, but I haven't had a mental problem." She doesn't smoke, but her whole family smoked when she was in Cuba. "I drink some one or two glasses of wine on weekends or at dinner with my in-laws. I have never used drugs or anything like that."*

Family History *Mrs. Soto's father died at age 56 from "some type of cancer. He didn't live with us, so I don't know for sure and my mother doesn't talk about him." Her mother is 49 and has no known illnesses. She has a brother, 30, and a sister, 27. Both are "well." Her grandparents were not really known to her but were "old when they died."*

Psychosocial History–Occupation *Mrs. Soto held jobs in restaurants as a teenager in Cuba. "Since coming to America, I have worked as a graphic designer for two different employers." She states, "I have not been poor but just okay almost all my life until the last four or five years. My current employer pays very well, and I have a good retirement plan now. At home in Cuba, things are really bad, no proper food or medicine. They were better when I was there, but not like here."*

Roles and Relationships *She states, "I love my family, but I can't see them. I have friends here that are like my family. My friends were a big part of my wedding. One walked me down the aisle. I call home to Cuba, but it's hard to be far away. My husband was born and raised in the United States, but his family is originally from Mexico. We dated for two years before we got engaged. He helped me a lot, and we love each other very much. His family is like my new family. We see them a lot, they help us, and they treat me like a daughter, so it's very good."*

Ethnicity and Culture *Mrs. Soto says she will always consider herself Cuban, but "I am an American citizen now and am so much more of a gringo than my friends. I have come to like American food, especially pasta, but still make my beans and rice and other Cuban foods. My husband likes it too, but not every day. I laugh sometimes when I call my mother in Cuba and speak English sometimes."*

Spirituality *Mrs. Soto states, "I have no real religion; family and honesty are important to me. I believe in God and sometimes pray, but I really believe your family helps you when you are in need."*

Self-Concept *Mrs. Soto says of herself, "I am a good person. I worry about others. I want to have a family, with children who embrace their Cuban and Mexican heritage but who know America is their home. I take care of myself, and other than some extra pounds think I look pretty good."*

Review of Systems

Skin, Hair, and Nails

Denies problems. "I use sunscreen, shower daily, use conditioner on my hair and lotion to prevent dry skin. I would like to have a professional manicure more often, but I keep my nails looking nice."

Head and Neck

Denies problems except "occasional headache relieved by aspirin."

Eyes

Annual eye exam for 3 years. Reading glasses for "computer work."

(continued)

Box 6.2   Narrative Recording of the Health History (continued)

Ears, Nose, Mouth, and Throat

Denies problems with hearing, has "never had an official exam." Regular dental exams. Wisdom teeth extracted with no problems. No trouble eating or swallowing.

Respiratory

Denies problems. "A cold once a year." No exposure to pollutants. No history of tobacco use. Exposure to secondhand smoke from birth to 24 years of age at home. Denies cough, difficulty breathing.

Breasts and Axillae

"I have large breasts and have since I was twelve. I don't like to examine my breasts; I get scared I might find something. I do get them checked every year by the doctor." No changes, discharge, discomfort.

Cardiac

Denies problems. No history of heart disease. Never has palpitations.

Peripheral Vascular

Denies problems. "The doctor says my blood pressure is fine. I have two veiny spots on my legs, but they don't hurt. They are flat and stringy."

Gastrointestinal

Denies problems. "My bowels move every day with no problem. I get diarrhea when I'm nervous sometimes."

Urinary

Denies problems. "I pass urine five or six times a day and more if I drink more water or coffee."

Reproductive

Onset of menses age 11. "Regular every twenty-eight days for three or four days. I take birth control pills." Denies pregnancy, abortion.

Sexuality

"I'm heterosexual." "Relations are good with my husband."

Musculoskeletal

Denies problems. But "I don't get enough exercise."

Neurologic

No history of head injury, seizure, tremor, loss of consciousness. "Other than headache, I'm okay."

Box 6.3   Documentation of a Health History

Health History

Date: June 30, 2018

Name:	Corrina Soto
Address:	22 Highland Avenue, Midland Park, NJ 07432
Telephone:	201–555–0000
Age:	34
Date of birth:	July 20, 1984
Birthplace:	Santa Clara, Cuba (Sixth-largest city in Cuba, hospital, university, manufacturing. Three hours from Havana. Historic significance: Last battle site of Revolution, memorial to Che Guevara.) Came to the United States 9 years ago.
Gender:	Female
Marital status:	Married (Chris, age 34, emergency contact)
Race:	Hispanic
Religion:	None really, religious practice was forbidden in Cuba. Some family are hidden Catholics.
Occupation:	Graphic designer. Financial institution.
Health insurance:	Corporate insurance. Medical, dental, vision.
Source:	Patient
Reliability:	Reliable, alert, oriented, recall of information intact (nursing assessment).

(continued)

Box 6.3   Documentation of a Health History (continued)

Present Health/Illness

Reason for Seeking Care

Scheduled health assessment. No complaints except weight gain and occasional headaches, relieved with aspirin. Weight gain of 20 pounds over 3 years "since I started dating my husband, most since we got married last year. I get headaches when I'm stressed, tired, or read too much."

Height/Weight

5′6″/157 lbs. (71.36 kg)

Vital Signs

B/P: 128/64, HR: 72, RR: 20, T: 97.9°F

Health Beliefs and Practices

"Health is important and you need to take care of yourself, but sometimes it's out of your control. When I was younger my mother would tell me no bathing when you have your period, no water at all. My mother prepared certain foods for certain illnesses and sometimes got medicine from a botanica for ailments. All medical care was done well because it was all free."

Health Patterns

"At first in America I didn't see doctors. Because I have health insurance and my husband reminds me to make appointments, I have physician, dentist, gynecologist, and eye doctor exams. I have had them all every year for the last three years. I don't examine my breasts, but the doctor does it each year. I haven't had any vaccines since I came here, and I think my blood tests are okay. I sleep well most nights for about eight hours, unless I stay up and read. I try to exercise, but it is so hard after work and when it's cold out. Diet is crazy sometimes. I have coffee and toast in the morning. Lunch depends on my schedule, sometimes a sandwich, sometimes a salad. Dinner is probably pizza or fast food three or four times a week. I have a sweet at night. I like all kinds of foods, and I still like Cuban foods like beans, pork, and rice. I eat all kinds of American foods. I especially like pasta and bread, and I have them at almost all meals."

Medications

"I take birth control pills. I have been on them for four years. I have not had a problem. I take a vitamin "one-a-day" every day and fish oil—my doctor told me to. I take aspirin for headaches, but that's all. I don't use stuff like my mother did in Cuba and that some of my friends do."

Health Goals

"To lose weight so my clothes fit and I feel better about myself. In Cuba people would not have a problem with this weight, but I don't like it."

Past History

Childhood Illnesses

"Measles when I was little. I don't remember other illnesses."

Immunizations

"Smallpox, polio, and other vaccines like tetanus as a child. I don't remember others specifically."

Medical Illnesses

"A cold every year—but really no serious illnesses."

Hospitalization

"I've never been in the hospital."

Surgery

"Never had any except wisdom teeth. All four out two years ago because the dentist said they were packed in. I did okay."

Injury

"Cut on my leg on glass, had stitches, and have a scar by my knee."

Blood Transfusion

"Never had one."

Emotional/Psychiatric Problems

"I miss my family and get sad when I can't see them. I get frustrated when I don't understand some American ways, and I'm pretty emotional. I cry over books and movies, but I haven't had a mental problem."

Allergies

Food: "None I know of." Medication: "I don't know of any." Environment: "No, I don't have a problem."

Use of Tobacco

"I don't smoke, never have, but my family smoked when I was in Cuba."

Use of Alcohol

"I have one or two glasses of wine on weekends or at dinner with my in-laws. I don't like beer or liquor."

Use of Illicit Drugs

"I have never used drugs or anything like that."

Family History

Father

"He died at age 56 from 'some cancer.' He didn't live with us, so I don't know for sure, and my mother doesn't say."

Mother

Her mother is 49 and well.

Siblings

She has a brother, 33, and a sister, 27. Both are "well."

Grandparents

Her grandparents were not really known to her but were "old" when they died.

Box 6.3   Documentation of a Health History (continued)

Psychosocial History

Occupational History

Jobs in restaurants as a teenager in Cuba. In America—graphic designer for two employers over the past 9 years, most recently for a financial institution.

Educational Level

Completed 16 years in Cuba, including a college degree in graphic design. Speaks: English, Spanish. Reads: English, Spanish.

Financial Background

"I have not been poor but just okay for all my life until the last four or five years. My current employer pays well, and I have a good retirement plan now. Things are really bad in Cuba. No food or medicine. They were better when I was there but not like here."

Roles and Relationships

"I love my family, but I can't see them. I have friends here that are like my family. My friends were a big part of my wedding. One walked me down the aisle. I call home to Cuba, but it's hard to be far away.

Ethnicity and Culture

"I will always consider myself Cuban, but I am an American citizen now and am comfortable with American culture. I like all American things, especially food. I still make beans and rice and other Cuban foods. My husband likes Cuban and Mexican food, but not every day.

Family

"My family is in Cuba. I miss them a lot. I would like them to come here someday. My husband was born and raised here, but his parents are from Mexico. We dated for two years before we got married. He helped me a lot, and we love each other very much. His family is my new family. We see them a lot, they help us out, they treat me like a daughter, so it's very good."

Spirituality

"I have no real religion. Family and honesty are important to me. I believe in God and sometimes pray, but I really believe your family helps you when you are in need."

Self-concept

"I am a good person. I worry about others. I want to have a family with children who understand being Cuban but who believe America is a good place. I take care of myself, and except for a few pounds, I think I look pretty good."

Review of Systems

Skin, Hair, Nails

No changes, rashes, lesions, color changes, sweating. No birthmarks. Scar left knee. Shower daily, hair shampoo every other day. No use of hair dyes for 2 years. Would like professional manicure more often but keeps nails trimmed and polished.

Head, Neck, Related Lymphatics

Occasional headaches relieved by aspirin. No history of injury, seizure, tremor, dizziness. No neck swelling.

Eyes

Annual exam—no change in 2 years. Glasses for distance. Next exam—3 months. Pupils equal and reactive to light.

Ears, Nose, Mouth, and Throat

Denies hearing problems, never had specific exam. Nose patent, no injury, sense of smell intact, clear drainage with cold. No trouble eating or swallowing. Dental exam annually, last exam 1 month ago. Brushes and flosses twice daily.

Respiratory

Denies respiratory problems. A cold once a year. No exposure to pollutants. No history of tobacco use. Exposure to secondhand smoke birth to 24 years. Denies cough, difficulty breathing. No history of respiratory problems. Unsure of TB screening. Respirations regular and non-labored. Lungs clear to auscultation in all fields bilaterally.

Breasts and Axillae

Annual exam by physician. No SBE. Large breasts with no masses, lumps, or discharge.

Cardiovascular

No history of heart disease. Never has palpitations. No edema or cyanosis. Apical pulse regular to auscultation with normal S1 S2 noted. Capillary refill < 2 seconds.

Peripheral Vascular

"The doctor says my blood pressure is fine. I have two veiny spots on my legs, but they don't hurt." No peripheral edema noted. Pedal pulses palpable.

Abdomen

Denies problems. "My bowels move every day with no problem. I get diarrhea when I'm nervous sometimes." Active bowel sounds present in all quadrants. Abdomen soft and non-tender to palpation.

Urinary

Denies problems. No history of UTI. "I pass urine five or six times a day and more if I drink more."

Reproductive

On oral contraceptives. Onset menses age 11. Regular every 28 days for 3 to 4 days. Para 0. Gravida 0.

Sexual

Self-described as heterosexual. "Relations are good with my husband."

Musculoskeletal

Denies problems. "I don't get enough exercise." Range of motion—normal. Denies problems with strength.

Neurologic

"Other than headache, I'm okay." Denies falls, balance problems, memory problems. Right-handed. Alert and oriented. Can sense touch and temperature.

Documenting the Family Medical History: The Genogram

The comprehensive patient database includes the information about a patient's family medical history in order to include genetic factors in the health assessment. This information is obtained during the interview, and documentation is usually done in the form of a genogram, which is a diagram of the family relationships of the patient along with the health status of those family members (Patch, 2013). A genogram makes it easy to see patterns of health and illness across generations. In a genogram, each family member is represented by a symbol, using a circle for females and a square for males. Figure 6.2 ■ shows standardized symbols used in genograms. The family relationships of individuals are shown by lines that connect individuals. These represent genetic relationships (see Figure 6.3 ■). Each family member's health information is coded and printed below their symbol. The result is a visual representation of a family's health information in the context of genetic relationships, allowing easy identification of disease incidence and patterns of inheritance.

When documenting a family history, the information from at least three generations is included. If the **proband** (the person around whom the genogram is created) has children, often four generations are depicted. It is useful to begin with the proband and then "build" the genogram by adding the most closely related family members: first, second, and third-degree relatives (i.e., parents, siblings, and children; aunts, uncles, grandparents, grandchildren, nephews, nieces, and half-siblings; and first cousins, great-grandparents, and great-grandchildren). Depict members of each generation along the same horizontal plane. Record coded health information under each individual's symbol, including name or initials, medical condition or cause of death, infertility, pregnancy complications, and adoption status. It is important to include the age of the family member or the age at death and the age at diagnosis of chronic conditions (e.g., diabetes, heart disease, cancer, hypertension) or events such as a miscarriage or stillbirth. At the top of the genogram, indicate the ancestry (country of origin) of individuals in the originating generation. Be sure to date the genogram to facilitate future updates.

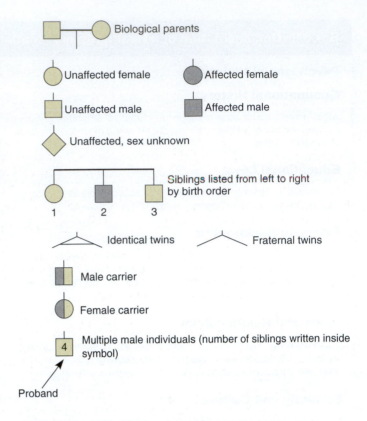

Figure 6.2 Selected standard symbols for use in drawing a genogram.

Nurses use the information in the family history to inform care planning (Patch, 2013). Formal risk assessments may be conducted by genetic specialists or nurses with specialized training to quantify the risk of having a child with a particular condition or to calculate cancer susceptibility. More commonly, genograms are examined for genetic "red flags," conditions that indicate an individual may benefit from specific genetic information or services. Nurses should be able to evaluate a genogram for genetic

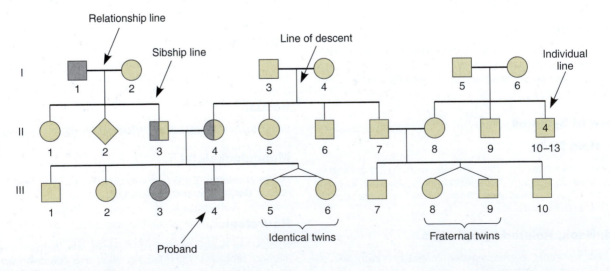

Figure 6.3 Sample three-generation genogram.

or hereditary red flags, including known genetic disorders: multiple family members with the same or related conditions; conditions in the less-often affected sex (e.g., breast cancer in a male); early age of disease onset; sudden, early, or unexpected deaths; multiple pregnancy losses; and birth defects, neurodevelopmental delays, or regressions. Upon identifying a genetic red flag, the nurse should discuss the finding with the patient and explore options for follow-up or referral (Patch, 2013).

Documenting the Physical Examination: Objective

Documentation of the physical examination findings will require the nurse to use accurate and professional terminology for body systems, directions, surfaces, and findings. The documentation of objective findings must be free of judgment and opinion. The nurse must document only what is seen, heard, palpated, counted, measured, weighed, and smelled during the physical exam. Additional objective information from laboratory or imaging reports also may be included. The nurse should choose descriptive terminology that is concise, precise, succinct, and professional. Using words that are vague or could be interpreted should be avoided. For example, a rash should be described as objectively as possible: The nurse should write *2–3 mm hyperpigmented macules scattered throughout a 10-cm × 10-cm area centered on, and surrounding, the umbilicus*, rather than *tan spots on the stomach near the belly button*. Throughout the chapters in Unit III covering each body system, vocabulary is presented to help you learn the medical terminology. Each chapter includes a section titled *Documenting Your Findings*, which presents a sample of accurate, professional, complete, and confidential documentation of the subjective and objective findings for that system.

Charting and Documentation

Because the purpose of documentation is to communicate information, the data must be accessible where and when needed by healthcare workers caring for patients. The variety of documentation formats exists to address a wide range of nursing situations. Nurses practice in hospitals, clinics, schools, and surgery centers, among others. The specific format of documentation will vary depending on the location or type of nursing. Patient information is contained in the patient chart—as mentioned earlier, this may be a paper chart or an EHR. Because patients are cared for in a variety of ways, a variety of documentation methods and formats may be in use. **Charting**, or documenting of periodic assessments of hospitalized patients, can take the form of narrative notes in the form of a paragraph, problem-oriented notes, and written or digital flow sheets.

The case study on this page presents a patient encounter with a nurse in an outpatient clinic setting. The case illustrates several formats of documentation; examples of documentation formats follow the case.

Narrative Notes

A nurse's note or progress note consists of data recorded during a visit to healthcare providers or clinics for continued management of an existing condition. These notes are generally

---

CASE STUDY

Janet Lewis, a 20-year-old female, came to the university health center. Ms. Lewis told the nurse, "I feel bloated and achy in my left side, and it has increased over the past three or four days." In response to questions about appetite, Ms. Lewis responded, "I really don't feel like eating, and I'm worried because I'm supposed to eat carefully. I recently had anemia and have been taking pills for it for a month." When asked about bowel elimination, she said, "My last BM was four days ago; it was hard pellets and dark colored." She responded to questions about gastrointestinal symptoms with the following: "I'm not nauseous, and I haven't vomited." She further reported, "I had my last period ten days ago." She told the nurse that her voiding was normal in amount and number of voids. Ms. Lewis brought her medication with her. The label read "Ferrous gluconate 300 mg by mouth three times daily." Her physician instructed her to take the medication and have a follow-up visit in 1 month.

The physical assessment revealed the presence of bowel sounds in all quadrants, dullness to percussion in the left upper and lower quadrants, firm distention, and tenderness in the left lower quadrant. There was no tenderness at the costovertebral angle (CVA). Hard, dry stool high in the rectum was identified on the rectal examination, and a sample was applied to a slide for occult blood testing. Blood was drawn for a complete blood count (CBC).

A rectal suppository was administered with a result, within 15 minutes, of a moderate amount of hard, dark stool. Ms. Lewis stated, "I feel a little better, but still achy." She was discharged to her dormitory with 30 mL of milk of magnesia (MOM) to take at bedtime. Ms. Lewis was advised to increase her fluid intake and continue to take the ferrous gluconate as ordered. She was instructed to call the health center in the morning as a follow-up measure and to call her physician to schedule a visit and to discuss her laboratory results.

The nurse provided education as follows:

- *Constipation and change in stool color are side effects of ferrous gluconate.*
- *Ferrous gluconate should be taken 2 hours after meals, with a full glass of water or juice.*
- *Increasing roughage by adding fresh fruits to the diet will help to reduce the constipation.*

---

limited to findings indicating change, progress, or problems associated with the existing condition. Although the documentation of the full health history and physical exam will be comprehensive, charting of inpatient and outpatient care may be done as a narrative note. When using narrative notes, the documentation is written in a paragraph style or format as if it is being "narrated" or told to a listener. The information may be recorded in chronologic order from initial contact through conclusion of the assessment, or in categories according to the type of data collected. The narrative record often includes professional nursing judgments made about the data, plans to address concerns, and actions taken to meet the health needs of the patient. The example narrative note refers to Ms. Lewis's visit to the university health center (see Figure 6.4 ■)

Progress Notes

Patient Data:

place patient sticker here

Date	Time	Nursing Note
10/28/2017	0730	20 year-old female seen because she "feels bloated" and has an "achiness" in her left side that has "increased over the past 3 or 4 days". She states she "really doesn't feel like eating" and that she is "worried" because she was "supposed to eat carefully" because she recently "had a problem with anemia" and has been taking pills for it for a month. She brought the medication with her. The label reads: Ferrous Gluconate 300 mg three times a day. She stated the doctor told her to take the pills until she has a return visit next month. She denies nausea and vomiting, last BM of dark hard pellets was 4 days ago. LMP 10 days ago. Voiding "normal" amount and number of voids. On exam: VS: T: 36.9, P: 88, R: 22, B/B 110/66. skin: pale, warn, dry. Abdomen: distended, BS normoactive x4, dullness to percussion LUQ and LLQ;firm, tenderness to palpation on LLQ, No CVA tenderness. Rectal exam: hard stool high in rectum, dark color. CBC drawn, stool for occult blood. Ducolax suppository administered. Result – moderate hard, dark stool after 15 minutes: "feels a little better, but still achy". Discharged to dorm with medication. Advised pt to increase fluid intake, continue Ferrous Gluconate as ordered. Education: 1. Side effects of iron: dark stool, constipation. 2. Schedule 2 hours after meals, take with full glass of water or juice. 3. Increase roughage – fruits in diet. 4. Call in AM for follow-up. 5. Call PCP for lab results. ———————————— R. Smith, RN

Figure 6.4 Narrative progress note.

Problem-Oriented Charting

Problem-oriented documentation includes the SOAP and APIE methods. The letters SOAP refer to recording **S**ubjective data, **O**bjective data, **A**ssessment, and **P**lanning. Subjective data are those reported by the patient or a reliable informant. Objective data are derived from the physical assessment, patient records, and reports. Assessment refers to conclusions drawn from the data. Planning indicates the actions to be taken to resolve problems or address patient needs (see Figure 6.5 ■ and Figure 6.6 ■). The letters APIE refer to **A**ssessment, **P**roblem, **I**ntervention, and **E**valuation. When using this method, documentation of assessment includes combining the subjective and objective data. The nurse will draw conclusions from the data, identify and record the problem or problems, and plan to address these problems. Interventions are documented as they are carried out. Evaluation refers to documentation of the response to the plan. See Figure 6.5 and Figure 6.6 for sample SOAP and APIE notes related to the health center visit of Ms. Lewis.

Flow Sheets

Documentation of health assessment data can be accomplished through the use of printed or digitally available forms, check sheets, or flow sheets. Whether in paper or electronic form, these methods of documentation are usually formatted for a specific purpose or need such as vital signs, medication administration record, intake and output, preoperative or postoperative care, and wound assessment. They may use columns or categories for

SOAP Note

Patient Data:

> place patient sticker here

Date	Time	Nursing Note
10/28/2017	0730	**S:** "I feel bloated and achy in my left side and it has increased over the past 3 or 4 days." "I really don't feel like eating." "I'm worried because I am supposed to eat carefully" because "I recently had a problem with anemia and have been taking pills for it for a months." "My last BM was 4 days ago; it was dark-colored hard pellets." "I'm not nauseous and I haven't vomited." "My last period was 10 days ago." **O:** VS: T: 36.9, P: 88, R:22, BP 110/66. Skin pale, warm, dry, Abdomen distended, BS normoactive x4, dullness to percussion LUQ and LLQ; firm, tender LLQ. No CVA tenderness. Rectal exam hard stool high in rectum, dark color. **A:** Taking ferrous gluconate 300mg TID for anemia. No history of abdominal pain, discomfort, disease. Impression: constipation. **P:** Rectal suppository and laxative, CBC, stool for occult blood. Education: medication, diet, fluid intake _____R. Smith, RN

Figure 6.5 SOAP notes.

recording data and may include lists of expected findings with associated qualifiers for ranges of normal or abnormal findings. Charts and check sheets often provide space for narrative descriptions or comments for each area assessed. Figure 6.7 ■ provides an example of a vital signs flow sheet with sample entries.

Symptom Assessment Documentation

Focused documentation of symptom assessment is intended to address a specific purpose or focus—that is, a symptom or need. A comprehensive health assessment may reveal one or more symptoms to assess further and document. The format for symptom assessment documentation is often done using the OLDCART & ICE acronym. The following example relates to Mrs. Jennifer Dellarsini, a 54-year-old computer engineer who is visiting an urgent care center for cough and discomfort lasting over a week. The nurse completed a symptom analysis using the OLDCART & ICE acronym to guide information gathering about Mrs. Dellarsini's symptom of a cough. Figure 6.8 ■ shows

the OLDCART & ICE acronym and how the nurse's use of it yields important information about Mrs. Dellarsini, her cough, and her responses to this symptom. The data from the interview regarding the characteristics of the cough guide the physical assessment to include the upper and lower respiratory systems. In addition, the information about exhaustion and disrupted activity indicates the need for assessment of oxygenation, tissue perfusion, and nutrition. Follow-up in response to patient cues throughout the physical assessment will enable the nurse to develop appropriate nursing diagnoses to guide the care for this patient.

Charting by Exception

Charting by exception is a system in which documentation in a standardized flow sheet either includes a set of defaults or the documentation is limited to exceptions from preestablished norms or significant findings. Flow sheets—either digital or paper—are available with the "normal" parameters identified. The nurse may select or chart "normal" if the patient meets all of the listed parameters. If there are exceptions, the nurse may note these only. For example, if the category is respiratory

APIE Note

Patient Data:

place patient sticker here	

Date	Time		Nursing Note
10/28/2017	0730	**A:**	*"I feel bloated and achy in my left side and it has increased over the past 3 or 4 days."*
			"I really don't feel like eating." "I'm worried because I am supposed to eat carefully" because
			"I recently had a problem with anemia and have been taking pills for it for a month."
			"My last BM was 4 days ago; it was dark-colored hard pellets." "I'm not nauseous and
			I haven't vomited." "My last period was 10 days ago." VS: T:36.9, P: 88, R:22, BP 110/66.
			Skin pale, warm, dry. Abdomen distended, tender LLQ, No CVA tenderness. Rectal exam hard
			stool high in rectum, dark. Taking ferrous gluconate 300mg TID for anemia. No history of
			abdominal pain. Impression: constipation.
		P:	*Rectal suppository and laxative at bedtime.*
			CBC, stool for occult blood. Education: medication, diet, fluid intake.
			Follow up here and with PCP.
		I:	*Ducolax suppository administered.*
		E:	*Moderate hard, dry, dark stool. "I feel a little better, but still achy."_____ R. Smith, RN*

Figure 6.6 APIE notes.

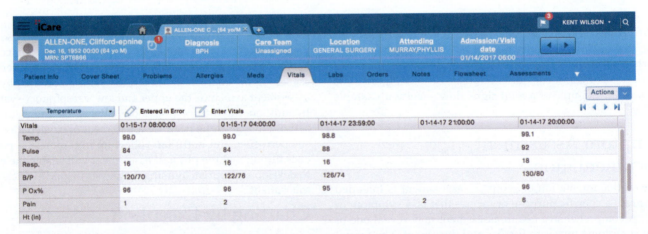

Figure 6.7 Vital signs flow sheet.
Source: RealEHRprep with ICare. Copyright © 2017 by ICare.

assessment, the normal parameters may include *Respirations 12–20; Regular rhythm; Lung sounds clear; Breathing unlabored.* If the patient had unlabored, regular, rhythmic breathing at a rate of 10 bpm with clear lung sounds, the nurse can document *within normal limits except rate 10 bpm.* It is imperative for the nurse to carefully review and understand the default data to ensure that only patient-specific data for that assessment are recorded (Arrowood et al., 2013). This type of documentation eliminates much of the repetition involved in narrative and other forms of documentation. When using this method, it is incumbent on nurses to fully understand the normal parameters to which they are comparing their patients.

OLDCART & ICE Acronym	
Symptom: Cough	
Onset	8 days ago.
Location	Mostly in my throat.
Duration	Every day, and coughing jags last 4 or 5 minutes at various times during the day and night.
Characteristics	Wet and painful, mucous comes up, it is clear, it comes on when my throat feels like it has mucous from my nose running down.
Aggravating Factors	It is worse in the morning and at night, if I exert myself too much, like rushing around to get dressed or cook.
Relieving Factors	It quiets if I sit still and drink a cup of tea.
Treatment	I have just been using cough drops and tea or warm water with lemon juice. I have taken ibuprofen for the pain.
Impact on ADLs	I am exhausted, that's why I came. I'm worried this may be more than a virus. I have not been able to do all of the things I need to do. I go to work and that's about it. I really need to do some grocery shopping and laundry, but I don't feel up to it.
Coping Strategies	I'm trying to deal with it by resting when I can. My friends encouraged me to come here.
Emotional Response	Well, I am a little worried that this could be really serious. I have to admit that the worry has not helped me relax and rest.

Figure 6.8 Documentation of the Symptom: Cough, with OLDCART & ICE.

Developing Documentation Proficiency

Development of confidence and competence in documentation is an important part of nursing education. Documentation in a patient chart or record is the way nurses communicate with the healthcare team, healthcare agencies, and one another. Whether handwritten or recorded in an EHR, the compilation and storage of information about patient assessment and care create an important resource. The data will be used in direct patient care and potentially for research purposes, in legal proceedings, or for quality improvement processes. No matter how it is used, nursing documentation must be accurate, professional, complete, and confidential. Understanding the guidelines and practicing to improve the quality of nursing documentation will enhance patient outcomes. In each chapter on body system assessment, you are provided with samples of questions to ask during the patient interview and examples of terminology to use in documenting that system. Practicing the documentation of subjective and objective data collection for body systems will guide and assist in the development of such skills. Table 6.2 shows examples of professionally written documentation with rationales.

Table 6.2 Examples of Professional Documentation

DO NOT USE	PROFESSIONAL DOCUMENTATION AND RATIONALE
Older male, demanding and grumpy	68-year-old male, avoids eye contact; loudly requesting RN change his medications. States he is angry that he has a new medication. Using terms like demanding, grumpy, and irritating to describe a patient reveals more about the nurse's attitude than the patient. In cases where the patient has a bad outcome, terms like these on a chart will call into question the kind of care the nurse provided.
Arms have normal skin color and temperature.	Upper extremities with skin color light pink Caucasian; warmer distally, cool proximally Avoid vague terms, such as fair and normal. Be clear, concise, and specific in your documentation.
Inside of nose was red and swollen.	Nares patent, turbinates erythematous and edematous Specific area of nose is described clearly; professional terminology used.
Large area of pus and red skin	5-cm × 6-cm patch of erythema with 1-cm × 1-cm area of purulent exudate at the center Precise measurement and use of medical language improve professionalism.
An orange-size lump in the right armpit	Right axillae with 15-cm spherical, firm, mobile, nontender nodule Use precise measurements in metric units to facilitate comparison with future or past data.

Application Through Critical Thinking

CASE STUDY

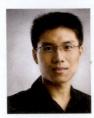

Thomas Lee is a 32-year-old marketing executive who is being seen in the clinic for headaches. He tells you that he has been having headaches for several years, that they are getting worse and more frequent, and that the medications he takes are just not helping anymore. Thomas does not have a regular primary care provider, so you tell him you are going to do a complete health history, including a genogram. You are now reviewing that information with Thomas as part of his visit. You note the following items that are of particular importance:

Source: otnaydur/
Shutterstock.

- His parents are both of Japanese descent but he was born here in the United States. His mother (age 55) has a history of migraines and depression, and his father (age 56) has heart disease and has had one MI.

- His paternal grandparents were born in Japan and moved to the United States. His grandfather died at age 85 from heart disease, and his grandmother committed suicide at age 65. It is thought she had depression, but no one in the family will discuss it because they are ashamed.

- His maternal grandparents are both alive. His grandmother is 78 and has had a stroke. His grandfather is 82 and has lung cancer and is only expected to live about 6 months.

- His sister is 34 and suffers from migraines and depression.

- His mother's sister also has migraines and depression.

CRITICAL THINKING QUESTIONS

1. Why did the nurse do an extensive health history when Thomas came in with a specific complaint?

2. What information will the nurse include on the genogram? For the patient? For the relatives?

3. What effect does the patient's ancestry have related to the conditions mentioned?

4. How does the genogram help the nurse?

5. What area would the nurse want to focus on based on the information found in the genogram?

REFERENCES

Ahn, M., Choi, M., & Kim, Y. (2016). Factors associated with the timeliness of electronic nursing documentation. *Healthcare Informatics Research*, 22(4), 270–276. https://doi.org/10.4258/hir.2016.22.4.270

American Nurses Association (ANA). (2010). *ANA's principles for nursing documentation: Guidance for registered nurses.* Silver Spring, MD: Author.

Andrews, A., & St. Aubyn, B. (2015). If it's not written down; it didn't happen . . . *Journal of Community Nursing*, 29(5), 20–22. Retrieved from http://www.jcn.co.uk

Arrowood, D., Choate, E., Curtin, E., DeCathelineau, S., Drury, B., Fenton, S., . . . Harper, M. (2013). Integrity of the healthcare record: Best practices for EHR documentation. *Journal of American Health Information Management Association*, 84(8), 58–62. Retrieved from http://www.ahima.org

Barnett, S., Nagy, M. W., & Hakim, R. C. (2017). Integration and assessment of the Situation-Background-Assessment-Recommendation framework into a pharmacotherapy skills laboratory for interprofessional communication and documentation. *Currents in Pharmacy Teaching and Learning*, 9, 794–801. doi:10.1016/j.cptl.2017.05.023

Chand, S., & Sarin, J. (2014). Electronic nursing documentation. *International Journal of Information Dissemination and Technology*, 4(4), 328–331.

Horowitz, A. C. (2015, January/February). Charting with a jury in mind. *Long-Term Living: For the Continuing Care Professional*, 10–11. Retrieved from www.ltlmagazine.com

Institute for Healthcare Improvement. (n.d.). *SBAR Tool: Situation-background-assessment-recommendation.* Cambridge, MA: Authors. Retrieved from http://www.ihi.org/resources/Pages/Tools/SBARToolkit.aspx

Kuhn, T., Basch, P., Barr, M., & Yackel, T. (2015). Clinical documentation in the 21st century: Executive summary of a policy position paper from the American College of Physicians. *Annals of Internal Medicine*, 162, 301–303. doi:10.7326/M14-2128

Manias, E., Bucknall, T., Hutchinson, A., Botti, M., & Allen, J. (2017). *Improving documentation at transitions of care for complex patients.* Sydney, Australia: Australian Commission on Safety and Quality in Health Care. Retrieved from https://www.safetyandquality.gov.au/wp-content/uploads/2017/06/Rapid-review-Improving-documentation-at-transitions-of-care-for-complex-patients.pdf

Neil, H. P. (2015, January/February). Legally: What is quality care? Understanding nursing standards. *MEDSURG Nursing*, 14–15. Retrieved from http://www.ajj.com/services/pblshng/msnj/default.htm

Patch, J. C. (2013). Identifying individuals who might benefit from genetic services and information. *Nursing Standard*, 28(9), 37–42. doi:10.7748/ns2013.10.28.9.37.e7514

Selekman, J. (2014). It's not called that anymore: Changes in medical terminology. *NASN School Nurse*, 29(1), 43–44. doi:10.1177/1942602X13508787

Selvi, S. T. (2017). Documentation in nursing practice. *International Journal of Nursing Education*, 9(4), 121–123. doi:10.5958/0974-9357.2017.00108.8

Stewart, K. R., & Hand, K. A. (2017). SBAR, communication, and patient safety: An integrated review. *MedSurgNursing*, 26(5), 297-305. Retrieved from http://www.ajj.com/services/pblshng/msnj/default.htm

The Joint Commission (2017) *Facts about the official "do not use" list of abbreviations*. Retrieved from https://www.jointcommission.org/facts_about_do_not_use_list/#

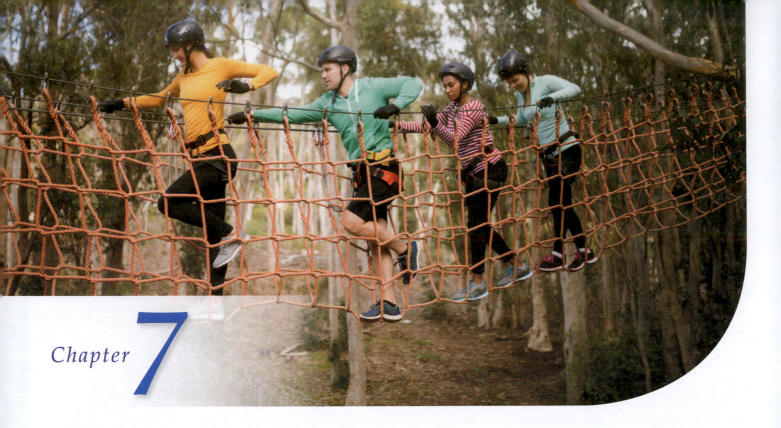

7

Physical Assessment Techniques and Equipment

LEARNING OUTCOMES

Upon completion of this chapter, you will be able to:

1. Differentiate between the four basic techniques used by the professional nurse when performing physical assessment.

2. Compare and contrast the purpose of equipment required to perform a complete physical assessment.

3. Discuss professional responsibilities related to critical thinking, patient safety and comfort, and principles of standard precautions in nursing practice.

KEY TERMS

auscultation, 86	fremitus, 84	hyperresonance, 86	pleximeter, 86
cues, 91	guarding, 84	inspection, 83	plexor, 85
dullness, 86	healthcare-associated	palpation, 83	resonance, 86
flatness, 86	infections (HAIs), 94	percussion, 85	tympany, 86

MEDICAL LANGUAGE

hyper-	Prefix meaning "high," "elevated," "above normal"
-meter	Suffix meaning "measure"
ophthalmo-	Prefix meaning "eye"
oto-	Prefix meaning "ear"

-pathic	Suffix meaning "disease," "disorder"
-scope	Suffix meaning "instrument for visual examination"
sub-	Prefix meaning "under," "below"

Introduction

Physical assessment requires hands-on examination of the patient and is an integral part of health assessment process in order to provide safe, effective, high-quality care (Douglas et al., 2016; Douglas, Windsor, & Lewis, 2015). Just as the interview and health history provide the nurse with important subjective data, the physical exam offers pertinent objective data. Together, the subjective and objective data provide essential information for the nurse to use when making decisions and caring for the patient.

This chapter introduces the physical assessment techniques and equipment necessary to obtain a thorough physical examination. In addition, professional responsibilities of the nurse in relation to health assessment are addressed.

Basic Techniques of Physical Assessment

When performing a physical assessment, the nurse will use the four basic or cardinal techniques to obtain objective and measurable data that will be included in the patient database. Recall that the patient database is a collection of subjective and objective information gathered about a patient's medical history and physical assessment findings. It is important to note that these techniques are performed in a particular order—inspection, palpation, percussion, and auscultation—with the exception of the abdominal assessment. Because percussion and palpation could alter the natural sounds of the abdomen, it is important to auscultate before performing palpation and percussion. This sequence is further discussed in Chapter 20 of this text. ∞

Inspection

Inspection is the skill of observing the patient in a deliberate, systematic manner. It begins the moment the nurse meets the patient and continues until the end of the patient–nurse interaction (see Figure 7.1 ■). Inspection always precedes the other assessment skills and is never rushed. Most novice nurses feel uncomfortable staring at the patient; nevertheless, careful scrutiny provides critical assessment data. The nurse should talk to the patient, help the patient relax before proceeding with inspection, and avoid the temptation to touch the patient. It is important to complete inspection of the patient before using any of the other techniques. However, if the patient is a child, the nurse may need to vary the approach to secure the child's attention and cooperation.

Inspection begins with a survey of the patient's appearance and a comparison of the right and left sides of the patient's body, which should be nearly symmetric. As the nurse assesses each body system or region, he or she inspects for color, size, shape, contour, symmetry, movement, or drainage. When inspecting a large body region, the nurse should proceed from general overview to specific detail. For example, when inspecting the leg, the nurse surveys the entire leg first and then focuses on each part, including the thigh, knee, calf, ankle, foot, and toes in succession. One should remember to look at the patient, listen for natural sounds, and use the sense of smell to detect odors. Use of each of the senses enhances the findings.

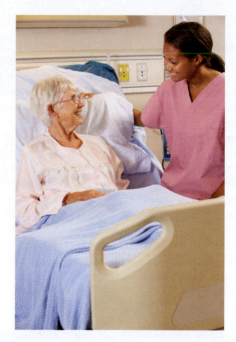

Figure 7.1 Inspection of patient.
Source: Monkey Business Images/Shutterstock.

Throughout inspection, the nurse applies the skills of critical thinking to analyze the observations and determine the significance of the findings to the general health of the patient. The nurse must know the anticipated findings regarding inspection of a body part. The nurse asks "Are the findings considered to be within normal parameters, or are they unexpected? Are the findings consistent with other diagnostic cues? What other information is needed to support this finding?"

Although the nurse will perform most of the inspection without the help of instruments, some special tools for visualizing certain body organs or regions are important. For example, the ophthalmoscope is used to inspect the inner aspect of the eye. This and other instruments used to enhance inspection are discussed later in this chapter.

Palpation

Palpation is the skill of assessing the patient through the sense of touch to determine specific characteristics of the body. These characteristics include size, shape, location, mobility of a part, position, vibrations, temperature, texture, moisture, tenderness, and edema. The approach used by the nurse to obtain these data is important. The nurse must be gentle and obtain the confidence of the patient. The hand of the nurse must be moved slowly and intentionally. The nurse must learn how much pressure to use with the examining hand during palpation. Too much pressure may produce pain for the patient. Too little pressure may not permit the nurse to perceive the data accurately. This is a skill that requires practice and is developed over time.

The hand has several sensitive areas; therefore, it is important to use the part of the hand most responsive to body structures and functions. The nurse will use the fingertips, finger pads, base of the fingers, palmar surface of the fingers, and the dorsal and ulnar surfaces of the hand (see Figure 7.2 ■).

The finger pads are used for discrimination of underlying structures and functions such as pulses, superficial lymph nodes, or crepitus. Vibratory tremors felt through the chest wall are known as **fremitus**. Fremitus can be vocal, when the patient speaks, or tussive, during coughing. Vibrations are best perceived by the examiner when using the base of the fingers (metacarpophalangeal joints). The ulnar surface of the hand, including the finger, is most sensitive to vibrations such as fremitus. The palmar aspect of the fingers is used to determine position, consistency, texture, size of structures, pain, and tenderness. The dorsal surface of the fingers is most sensitive to temperature. Remember, the dominant hand is always more sensitive than the nondominant hand. The fingertips are used in percussion and are discussed later in this chapter. During palpation, the nurse should use light, moderate, or deep pressure, depending on the depth of the structure being assessed and the thickness of the layers of tissue overlying the structure.

Light Palpation

One must always begin with light palpation. This is the safest, least uncomfortable method and allows the patient to become accustomed to the nurse's touch. Light palpation is used to assess surface characteristics, such as skin texture, pulse, or a tender, inflamed area near the surface of the skin. For light palpation, the finger pads of the dominant hand are placed on the surface of the area to be examined. The hand is moved slowly, and the finger pads, at a depth of 1 cm (0.39 in.), form circles on the skin during assessment, as demonstrated in Figure 7.3 ■.

Deep Palpation

Deep palpation is used to palpate the abdomen and organs that lie deep within a body cavity, such as the kidney, liver, or spleen, or when overlying musculature is thick, tense, or rigid, such as in obesity or with abdominal **guarding**, which is a tensing of the muscles of a particular area to protect from pain or agitation of sites impacted by injury or disease. Deep palpation is performed at a depth of 2 cm to 4 cm (approximately 0.75 in. to 1.5 in). When performing deep palpation, the nurse should use more than moderate pressure by placing the palmar surface of the fingers of the dominant hand on the skin surface (see Figure 7.4 ■). Two-handed deep palpation may also be performed. In this technique, the fingers of the nondominant hand are placed over the fingers of the dominant hand, pressing and guiding the fingers downward. Performing palpation with the two-handed approach provides extra support and pressure and allows the nurse to palpate at a deeper level.

All palpation must be used with caution; however, greatest caution must be used with deep palpation. When associated with pain, involuntary guarding or rigidity, especially in the abdomen, may be a sign of pathology. Deep palpation is contraindicated if one suspects that the rigidity is caused by inflammation or alterations in underlying organs and structures due to conditions such as dissecting aneurysms, peritonitis, or ectopic pregnancy.

Additional Considerations

Before beginning the technique of palpation, the nurse should explain to the patient what will occur. It is difficult to feel underlying structures if there is rigidity in the area to be palpated. Voluntary guarding or rigidity may occur if the patient is tense or frightened. Therefore, it is important to help the patient relax and become comfortable before proceeding. To help prevent discomfort, the nurse should

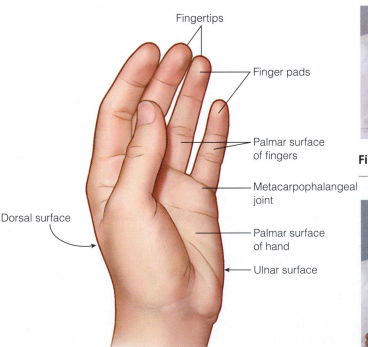

Fingertips

Finger pads

Palmar surface of fingers

Metacarpophalangeal joint

Dorsal surface

Palmar surface of hand

Ulnar surface

Figure 7.2 Sensitive areas of the hand.

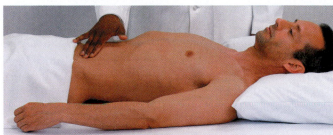

Figure 7.3 Light palpation.

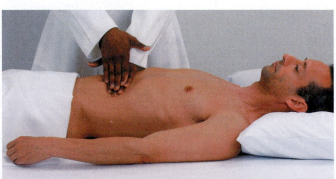

Figure 7.4 Deep palpation.

warm the hands; keep fingernails short, smooth, and trimmed; and not wear jewelry. Nonsterile gloves should be used if open skin areas or drainage were noted during inspection. Gloves may be latex or nonlatex materials, depending on the latex allergy of the nurse or the patient (National Institute for Occupational Safety and Health [NIOSH], 1998).

The nurse should proceed slowly, using smooth, deliberate movements and avoiding abrupt changes. Most patients will be more relaxed if the nurse talks to them during the examination, explaining each movement in advance. For example, during an abdominal assessment, the nurse might say "I'm going to place my hand on your abdomen next. Tell me if you feel any discomfort and I will stop right away. How does it feel when I press down in this area?" It is a good idea to touch each area before palpating it. This touch informs the patient that the examination of the area is about to begin and may prevent a startled reaction. Known painful areas of the body are usually the last areas to be palpated.

Through palpation, the nurse perceives data from the assessment and applies critical thinking. The nurse must be able to anticipate the findings regarding palpation of a body structure. Examples of critical thinking questions include these: Should light, moderate, or deep pressure be used? If so, why? Are the findings consistent with normative parameters or are they unexpected findings? Does the patient report any discomfort or pain during the process of palpation? Is there voluntary or involuntary guarding? Are the findings consistent with other diagnostic cues? What other information is needed to support this finding?

Percussion

Percussion is the third technique used by the nurse to obtain data when performing physical assessment. **Percussion** comes from the Latin word *percutire*, meaning "to strike through." Therefore, the nurse strikes through a body part with an object, fingers, or reflex hammer, ultimately producing a measurable sound. The striking or tapping of the body produces sound waves. As these waves travel toward underlying structures, they are heard as characteristic tones. The procedure is similar to a musician striking a drum, creating a vibration heard as a musical tone. Percussion is used to determine the size and shape of organs and masses and whether underlying tissue is solid or filled with fluid or air.

Three methods of percussion can be used: direct percussion, blunt percussion, and indirect percussion. The part of the body to be percussed indicates the method to be used.

Direct Percussion *Direct percussion* is the technique of tapping the body with the fingertips of the dominant hand. It is used to examine the thorax of an infant and to assess the sinuses of an adult, as illustrated in Figure 7.5 ■.

Blunt Percussion *Blunt percussion* involves placing the palm of the nondominant hand flat against the body surface and striking the nondominant hand with the dominant hand. A closed fist of the dominant hand is used to deliver the blow. This method is used for assessing pain and tenderness in the gallbladder, liver, and kidneys, as shown in Figure 7.6 ■.

Indirect Percussion *Indirect percussion* is the technique most commonly used because it produces sounds that are clearer and more easily interpreted. A hammer or tapping finger used to strike an object is called a **plexor**, derived from the Greek word

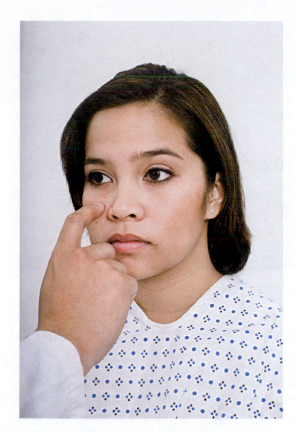

Figure 7.5 Direct percussion.

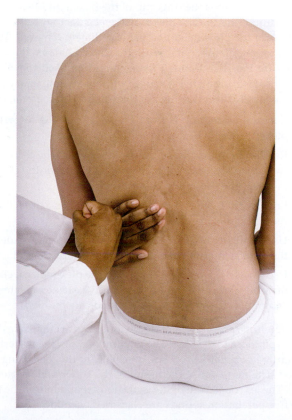

Figure 7.6 Blunt percussion.

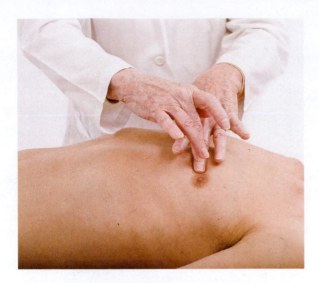

Figure 7.7 Indirect percussion.

plexis, meaning "a blow" or "to strike." **Pleximeter**, from the Greek word *metron*, meaning "measure," refers to the device that accepts the tap or blow from a hammer (see Figure 7.7 ■).

To perform indirect percussion, the hyperextended middle finger of the nondominant hand is placed firmly over the area being examined. This finger is the pleximeter. It is important to keep the other fingers and the palm of this hand raised in order to avoid contact with the body surface. Pressure from the other fingers and palm on the adjacent surface muffles tones being produced. Using only wrist action of the dominant hand to generate motion, the nurse delivers two sharp blows with the plexor. The plexor is the fingertip of the flexed middle finger of the dominant hand. The plexor makes contact with the distal phalanx of the pleximeter and is immediately removed. When the plexor maintains contact with the distal phalanx, the sound waves are muffled. Enough force should be used to generate vibrations and, ultimately, a sound, without causing injury to the patient or self. The following are some helpful percussion hints:

- Ensure that motion is from the wrist, not the forearm or plexor finger.
- Release the plexor finger immediately after the delivery of two sharp strikes, as this action will allow for the clearest, most accurate sound to be produced.
- Ensure that only the pleximeter makes contact with the body.
- Use the tip of the plexor finger, (*not* the finger pad) to deliver the blow as this will help produce the clearest sound.
- Use two strikes and then reposition the pleximeter. Delivery of more than two rapid consecutive strikes creates the "woodpecker syndrome" and sounds are muffled.

Sounds   Interpreting a percussion tone is an art that takes time and experience to develop. The amount of air in the underlying structure being percussed is responsible for the tone being produced. The more dense the tissue is, the softer and shorter the tone. The less dense the tissue is, the louder and longer the tone. The five percussion sounds are classified as follows:

- **Tympany** is a loud, high-pitched, drumlike tone of medium duration characteristic of an organ that is filled with air. It

is heard commonly over the gastric bubble in the stomach or over air-filled intestines.

- **Resonance** is a loud, low-pitched, hollow tone of long duration. It is the normal finding over the lungs.
- **Hyperresonance** is an abnormally loud, low-pitched tone of longer duration than resonance. It is heard when air becomes trapped and overinflates the lungs.
- **Dullness** is a high-pitched tone that is soft and of short duration. It is usually heard over solid body organs such as the liver or a stool-filled colon.
- **Flatness** is a high-pitched tone, very soft, and of very short duration. It occurs over solid tissue such as muscle or bone.

Percussion sounds have characteristic features the nurse learns to interpret. These features include intensity, pitch, duration, and quality.

Intensity or *amplitude* of a sound refers to the softness or loudness of the sound. The louder the sound is, the greater the intensity or amplitude of the sound. This is influenced by the amount of air in the structure and the ability of the structure to vibrate.

Pitch or *frequency* of the sound refers to the number of vibrations of sound per second. Slow vibrations produce a low-pitched sound, whereas a high-pitched sound comes from more rapid vibrations.

Duration refers to the length of time of the produced sound. This time frame ranges from very short to very long, with variation in between.

Quality refers to the recognizable overtones produced by the vibration. This will be described as clear, hollow, muffled, or dull.

Like other assessment skills, the nurse perceives data from the assessment of the patient and applies critical thinking. The nurse must be able to anticipate and identify the produced sound. Is this sound the expected sound? Is this sound considered to be within the normative range for this body part? Does the patient report any discomfort or pain during percussion? Are the findings consistent with other diagnostic cues? What other information is needed to support this finding?

Auscultation

Auscultation is the skill of listening to the sounds produced by the body. When auscultating, one uses both the unassisted sense of hearing and special instruments such as a stethoscope. Body sounds that can be heard with the ears alone include speech, coughing, respirations, and percussion tones. Many body sounds are extremely soft, and a stethoscope is needed to hear them. Stethoscopes work not by amplifying sounds but by blocking out other noises in the environment. Use of the stethoscope is described later in this chapter.

Auscultating body sounds requires a quiet environment in which the nurse can listen not just for the presence or absence of sounds but also for the characteristics of each sound. External distractions such as radios, televisions, and loud equipment should be eliminated whenever possible. The nurse should avoid auscultating over clothing, gowns, and sheets; rubbing against patients' clothes or drapes; or touching the stethoscope tubing, because these actions produce sounds that will obscure the sounds of the body. Movement of the stethoscope over thick or coarse hair on the chest or back may alter or obscure sounds. It is important to keep the patient warm, because shivering is uncomfortable and also obscures body sounds.

Many times the nurse will hear more than one sound at a time. For example, the nurse might note that a patient's respirations are loud, high-pitched, long, and raspy. It is important to focus on each sound and identify the characteristics of each sound. Closing the eyes and concentrating on each sound might help the nurse focus on the sound.

The nurse uses critical thinking with the technique of auscultation. The nurse must know the expected sound in the body region being auscultated. Is this sound considered to be within the normative range for this body region? Are unusual sounds heard? Are these findings consistent with other diagnostic cues? What other information is needed to support this finding?

Equipment

Throughout physical assessment, the nurse will use various instruments and pieces of equipment. Special equipment and the senses of the nurse are used to measure, observe, touch, and listen to sounds of the body. These will help in visualizing, hearing, and measuring data. It is the responsibility of the nurse to know how to operate and when to use all equipment in order to comply with patient safety regulations. Before beginning the physical assessment, the nurse should gather all the equipment, organize it, and place it within easy reach. Table 7.1 gives a complete list of the equipment needed for a typical screening

Table 7.1 Equipment Used During the Physical Assessment

EQUIPMENT	USED BY THE NURSE TO . . .
Computer, laptop, or tablet	Record data from the exam
Cotton balls or wisps	Test the sense of touch
Cotton-tipped applicators	Obtain specimens
Culture media	Obtain cultures of body fluids and drainage
Dental mirror	Visualize mouth and throat structures
Doppler	Obtain readings of pulse, fetal heart rate, and in special circumstances, blood pressure
Flashlight	Provide a direct source of light to view parts of the body
Gauze squares	Obtain specimens; collect drainage
Gloves	Protect the nurse and patient from contamination
Goggles	Protect the nurse's eyes from contamination by body fluids
Lubricant	Provide lubrication for vaginal or rectal examinations
Nasal speculum	Dilate nares for inspection of the nose
Ophthalmoscope	Inspect the interior structures of the eye
Otoscope	Inspect the tympanic membrane and external ear canal
Penlight	Provide a direct light source and test pupillary reaction
Reflex hammer	Test deep tendon reflexes
Ruler, marked in centimeters	Measure organs, masses, growths, and lesions
Scale	Measure the weight of the patient
Skin-marking pen	Outline masses or enlarged organs
Slides	Make smears of body fluids or drainage
Specimen containers	Collect specimens of body fluids, drainage, or tissue
Sphygmomanometer	Measure systolic and diastolic blood pressure
Stadiometer	Measure the height of the patient
Stethoscope	Auscultate body sounds
Tape measure, flexible, marked in centimeters	Measure the circumference of the head, abdomen, and extremities
Test tubes	Collect specimens
Thermometer	Measure body temperature
Tongue blade	Depress the tongue during assessment of the mouth and throat
Tuning fork	Test auditory function and vibratory sensation
Vaginal speculum	Dilate the vaginal canal for inspection of the cervix
Vision charts	Test near and far vision
Watch with second hand	Time heart rate, respirations, or bowel sounds

(continued)

SPECIAL EQUIPMENT	USE/DESCRIPTION

Goniometer

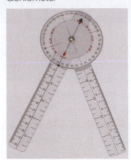

Measures the degree of joint flexion and extension. Consists of two straight arms of clear plastic usually marked in both inches and centimeters. The arms intersect and can be angled and rotated around a protractor marked with degrees. The nurse places the center of the protractor over a joint and aligns the straight arms with the extremity. The degree of flexion or extension is indicated on the protractor.

Skinfold calipers

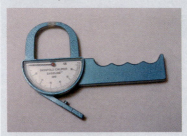

Measures the thickness of subcutaneous tissue. The nurse grasps a fold of skin, usually on the upper arm at the triceps area, waist, or thigh, keeping the sides of the skin parallel. The edges of the caliper are placed at the base of the fold and the calipers tightened until they grasp the fold without compressing it.

Transilluminator

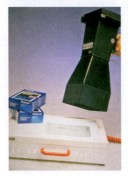

Detects blood, fluid, or masses in body cavities. Instruments manufactured for transillumination are available, or a flashlight with a rubber adapter may be used. In either case, the light beam produced is strong but narrow. When directed through a body cavity, the beam produces a red glow that reveals the presence of air or fluid. Solid material such as blood or masses will obstruct the beam of light, thus producing no glow or passage of the light beam.

Source: National Library of Medicine.

Wood's lamp

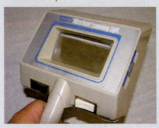

Detects fungal infections of the skin. The Wood's lamp produces a black light, which the nurse shines on the skin in a darkened room. If a fungal infection is present, a characteristic yellow-green fluorescence appears on the skin surface.

Monofilament

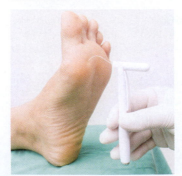

A single strand of synthetic nylon bristle used for assessing loss of peripheral nerve sensation in the feet of patients with diabetes and other neuropathic or circulatory disorders. With the patient's eyes closed, the tip of the bristle is placed over various locations of the plantar surface of the foot. The patient should be able to identify when the foot is being touched in each area.

Source: Satit Umong/123RF.

exam. Special equipment is required for assessment of several of the body systems. For example, the reflex hammer is used in the neurologic assessment and the vaginal speculum in assessment of the female reproductive system. Each chapter in Unit III of this text provides a discussion of specialized equipment and how it is used in physical assessment of a particular system. ∞

Stethoscope

The stethoscope is used to auscultate body sounds such as blood pressure, heart sounds, respirations, and bowel sounds. The stethoscope has three parts: the binaurals (earpieces), the flexible tubing, and the end piece. The end piece contains the diaphragm and the bell (see Figure 7.8 ■). To be effective in blocking out environmental noise, the binaurals should fit snugly but comfortably, sloping forward, toward the nose, to match the natural slope of the ear canals. (Most manufacturers supply different binaurals from which to choose.)

The tubing that joins the binaurals to the diaphragm and bell is thick, flexible, and as short as possible (approximately 30 cm to 36 cm, or 12 in. to 14 in.). Longer tubing may distort the sound.

The flat end piece, called the diaphragm, screens out low-pitched sounds and, therefore, is best for transmitting high-pitched sounds such as lung sounds and normal heart sounds (see Figure 7.9 ■). The nurse should place the diaphragm evenly and firmly over the patient's exposed skin. The deep, hollow end piece, called the bell, detects low-frequency sounds such as heart murmurs. It is placed lightly against the patient's skin so that it forms a seal but does not flatten to a diaphragm. Either end piece may be held against the patient's skin between the

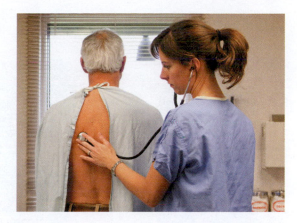

Figure 7.9 Nurse using a stethoscope to auscultate the patient's lungs. The nurse should place the diaphragm of the stethoscope evenly and firmly over the patient's exposed skin. *Source:* Heath Korvola/Getty Images.

index and middle fingers of the examiner (see Figure 7.10 ■). Friction on the diaphragm or bell from coarse body hair may cause a crackling sound easily confused with abnormal breath sounds. This problem can be avoided by wetting the hair before auscultating the area. Stethoscopes usually include an assortment of interchangeable diaphragms and bells in different sizes for different purposes—for example, smaller diaphragm pieces are used for examining children.

Doppler

A Doppler uses ultrasonic waves to detect sounds that are difficult to hear with a regular stethoscope, such as fetal heart sounds and peripheral pulses that cannot be easily palpated. Handheld Dopplers may be in the form of a stethoscope or other type of device with a speaker to listen to the blood flow (Figure 7.11 ■). It operates on a principle discovered in the 19th century by Johannes Doppler, the Austrian physicist who found that the pitch of a sound varies in relation to the distance between the source and the listener. To the listener, the pitch sounds higher when the distance from the source is small and lower when the distance from the source is great.

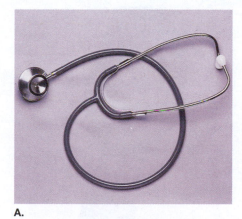

A.

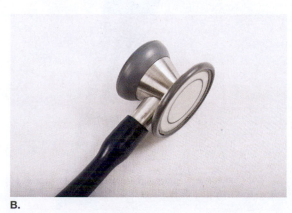

B.

Figure 7.8 A. Stethoscope with a bell and diaphragm.
B. Close-up of diaphragm (flat disc on bottom) and a bell (top).

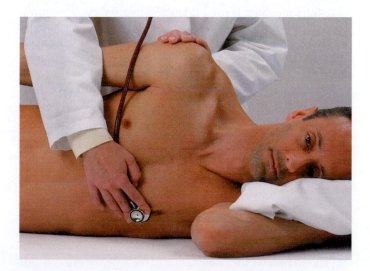

Figure 7.10 Nurse using a stethoscope.

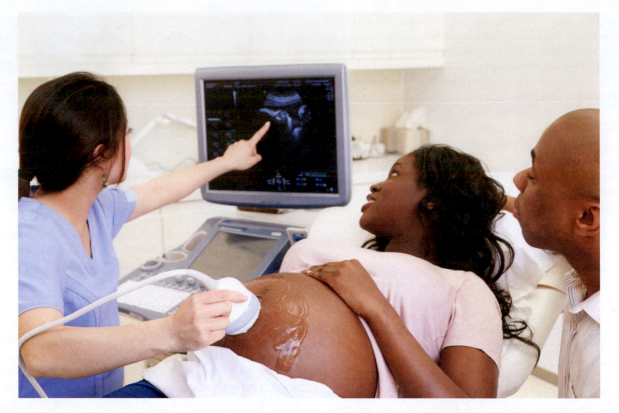

Figure 7.11 Using a Doppler ultrasound.
Source: Monkey Business Images/Shutterstock.

When using the Doppler to assess the pulse, the nurse turns it on, applies a small amount of gel to the end of the probe, or transducer (this helps to eliminate interference and friction with the skin and pick up the sound), and places the probe gently against the patient's skin over the artery to be auscultated. It is important to avoid heavy pressure because it may impede blood flow. The probe sends a low-energy, high-pitched sound wave toward the underlying blood vessel. As the blood ebbs and flows, the probe picks up and amplifies the subtle changes in pitch, and the nurse will hear a pulsing beat.

Ophthalmoscope

An ophthalmoscope is used to inspect internal eye structures. Its main components are the handle, which holds the battery, and the head, which houses the aperture selector, viewing aperture, lens selector disk, lens indicator, lenses of varying powers of magnification, and mirrors (see Figure 7.12 ■).

The light source shines light through the viewing aperture, which is adjusted to select one of five apertures (see Figure 7.13 ■):

1. The *large aperture* is used most often. It emits a large, full spot for viewing dilated pupils.

2. The *small aperture* is used for undilated pupils.

3. The *red-free filter* shines a green beam used to examine the optic disc for pallor or hemorrhaging, which appears black with this filter.

4. The *grid* allows the examiner to assess the size, location, and pattern of any lesions.

5. The *slit* allows for examination of the anterior eye and aids in assessing the elevation or depression of lesions.

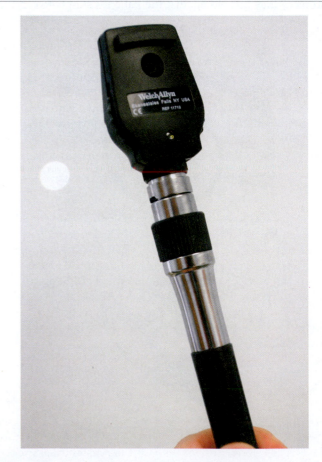

Figure 7.12 Ophthalmoscope demonstrating aperture.

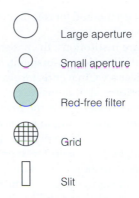

○ Large aperture

○ Small aperture

● Red-free filter

⊞ Grid

▯ Slit

Figure 7.13 Apertures of ophthalmoscope.

The lens selector dial must be rotated to bring the inner eye structures into focus. While looking through the viewing aperture, one rotates the lens selection dial to adjust the convergence or divergence of the light. At the zero setting, the lens neither converges nor diverges the light. The lens dial is moved clockwise to access the numbers in black, which range from −1 to −40. These lenses improve visualization in a patient who is farsighted. The lens dial is moved counterclockwise to access the red numbers, which range from −1 to −20. These lenses improve visualization if the patient is nearsighted. See Chapter 14 and Appendix C for a more detailed discussion of assessment of the eye. ∞

Otoscope

The otoscope is used to inspect external ear structures. The main components of the otoscope are the handle, which is similar to that of the ophthalmoscope, the light, the lens, and specula of various sizes (see Figure 7.14 ■). The specula are used to narrow the beam of light. The nurse should select the largest one that will fit into the patient's ear canal. If a nasal speculum is not available, the otoscope can be used to inspect the nose. In this case, the nurse should use the shortest, broadest speculum and insert it gently into the patient's naris. See Chapter 15 for a more detailed discussion of assessment of the ears and nose. ∞

Professional Responsibilities

Throughout all aspects of the assessment process, the nurse must apply critical thinking while providing a safe and comfortable environment for the patient. The nurse must identify cues presented by the patient and apply critical thinking to determine the relevance of these data. The safe external environment created by the nurse includes comfort, warmth, privacy, and the use of standard precautions, which will be discussed later in this chapter.

Cues

In addition to developing the skills of inspection, palpation, percussion, and auscultation, the nurse must be able to recognize the relative significance of the many visual, palpable, or auditory cues that may be present during an assessment. **Cues** are bits of information that hint at the possibility of a health problem. In other words, the nurse needs to know what to look for. To become skilled at cue recognition, nurses should cultivate

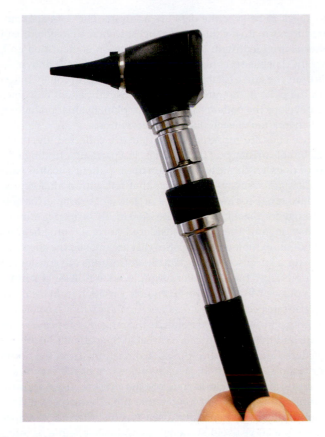

Figure 7.14 Otoscope.

their senses until they readily perceive even slight cues. For example, some things that are noticed during an initial survey or inspection of the patient may hint at an underlying health problem. Swelling (edema) of the legs provides a cue to assess for heart problems. Bruising (ecchymosis) of the skin is a cue to ask the patient about recent falls, trauma, injury, anticoagulant medication, or a bleeding problem. Grimacing, guarding (protective posture), or wincing when a patient moves or when a body part is moved during assessment are cues to examine the underlying joint and muscles for problems or masses. Cues that suggest hearing loss include not following directions, looking at the examiner's lips during conversation, or speaking in a loud voice. Asymmetry of facial expression is a cue to assess function of the cranial nerves. Odors are cues to suggest a problem with hygiene or drainage from an orifice or wound. Cue recognition develops with practice, but beginners can acquire the skill by observing an experienced nurse, by practicing on partners, and by studying the visual aids in this text.

Critical Thinking

Throughout the assessment process, the nurse gathers subjective and objective data. Recall that subjective data are reported by the patient during the interviews, and the objective data come from the physical assessment and the application of the four techniques of inspection, palpation, percussion, and auscultation. These data form the database reflecting the health status of the patient. During this process, the presented cues must be interpreted.

The interpretation of cues and other collected data uses the process of critical thinking. The nurse should be organized when collecting data; this allows the nurse to look for inconsistencies and check to be sure the data are accurate. The data are compared to normative values and ranges. Data are clustered, and patterns are identified. Missing information is identified and, after the database is completed, valid conclusions are drawn. At this time, the nurse establishes priorities of care. In collaboration with the patient, the nurse identifies desired patient outcomes and develops the patient's nursing care plan. Evaluation follows implementation of each nursing intervention.

Once cues are recognized and data are collected, the nurse must be able to interpret the findings. Is a particular finding normal, or does it indicate an alteration in the patient's health? Normal data are assessment findings that fall within an accepted standard range for a specific type of data. For example, the normal range for the adult pulse rate is 60 to 100 beats per minute. A pulse of 76 is, therefore, considered normal. Some healthy individuals exhibit characteristics that are outside the standard range for a specific type of data. Such findings are considered variations from the norm. For example, a long-distance runner with a pulse of 48 exhibits an acceptable variation from the norm for pulse rate because it is a result of regular cardiovascular conditioning. Findings that are outside the range for a specific type of data and that may indicate a threat to the patient's health are considered unexpected findings or deviations from the norm. For example, an irregular, thready pulse rate of 120 is an unexpected finding that could indicate the presence of a harmful condition. It is important to note that not all unexpected findings indicate the presence of a disease or disorder. For example, fatigue in a 20-year-old student may indicate anemia or infection, or it may be caused simply by a lack of sleep.

Providing a Safe and Comfortable Environment

Patients are more likely to discuss health problems and consent to a physical assessment if they feel they are in a safe and comfortable environment. The nurse plays a vital role in developing this environment by providing an examination space that is appropriate for the setting, ensuring maintenance of dignity and privacy for the patient, and noting special considerations for each patient. These special considerations may include personal preferences, cultural differences, or health status. The nurse must obtain patient permission to proceed, make the patient feel comfortable, and communicate with the patient throughout the physical assessment.

Setting The physical assessment may be performed in a variety of settings, including a clinic, a hospital room, a school nurse's office, a corporate health services office, or a patient's home. No matter where the location, the nurse is responsible for preparing a setting that is conducive to the patient's comfort and privacy. The examination room should be warm, private, and free from distractions and interruptions. Overhead lighting must ensure good visibility and be free of distortion. A portable lamp to highlight body surfaces and contours may be needed.

Preparation Before beginning the assessment, the nurse should thoroughly explain to the patient what is to follow and encourage the patient to ask questions. If the patient does not speak the nurse's language, it is important to secure the assistance of a translator. If the patient's hearing is impaired, the nurse

must determine the best method for communication, which may include the use of sign language.

In many healthcare institutions, the patient is asked to sign a consent form for the physical assessment, especially if invasive procedures such as a vaginal or rectal examination or blood studies are to be performed. It is the nurse's responsibility to ensure that the patient understands the procedures to be performed and that all necessary consent forms are signed.

In most cases, patients should empty their bladder before the examination. Voiding helps patients feel more comfortable and relaxed and facilitates palpation of the abdomen and pubic area. If urinalysis is to be done, the patient should be instructed in obtaining a clean-catch specimen and be given a container for the urine sample.

Privacy After ensuring that the examination room is warm, the nurse shows the patient how to put on the examination gown and leaves the patient to undress in privacy. It may be helpful to assure the patient that it is all right to leave underpants on until just before the genital assessment. Before reentering the examination room, the nurse should knock to alert the patient.

Drapes are used to preserve the patient's privacy and to provide warmth. When invasive procedures such as vaginal or rectal assessments are performed, drapes provide an aseptic field. When used properly, a drape exposes only the part of the body being examined and covers the surrounding area. Drapes are available in a variety of shapes and materials ranging from simple rectangular sheets made of linen to disposable drapes made of paper lined with waterproof plastic.

Examination Considerations To begin the assessment, the patient should be positioned on a sturdy examination table with a firm surface that is covered with a clean sheet or paper cover. Though not as efficient, a firm bed will suffice if an examination table is not available. The table must be placed to allow the nurse easy access to both sides of the patient's body. The table's height should allow the nurse to perform the examination without stooping. The nurse should also have a stool to sit on during certain parts of the examination and a small table or stand to hold the examination equipment.

During the assessment, the nurse should explain each step in advance so that the patient can anticipate the nurse's movements. Patients are more relaxed and cooperative during the procedure when they understand what is about to happen. This is also an opportunity to provide patient teaching. For example, while inspecting the patient's skin, the nurse may want to discuss the long-term effects of sun exposure. Sharing information with patients during the assessment may alleviate their anxiety, enhance their understanding, and give them a sense of partnership in their healthcare.

At times, the nurse may note an unexpected finding and want to call in another examiner to check the finding. In such instances, it is best simply to inform the patient that another examiner is being asked to check the assessment. Because the finding may be normal, it is best to avoid alarming the patient.

Special Considerations Many patients experience anxiety before and during a physical examination. These feelings may stem from fear of pain, embarrassment at being looked at and touched by a stranger, or worry about the outcome of the examination. The nurse can alleviate the patient's anxiety by approaching the examination gradually, first by communicating with the patient, then by performing simple measurements such as height, weight, temperature, and pulse, which most patients find familiar and nonthreatening. As these measurements are taken, the patient will have the opportunity to ask additional questions and to become accustomed to the nurse's presence.

The examination should be individualized according to the patient's personal values and beliefs. Some patients, for example, may request that a family member be present during the examination. Some may ask for a nurse of the same sex. Some female patients may object to breast and vaginal examinations, regardless of the gender of the examiner, and some male patients may refuse penile, scrotal, and rectal examinations. A thorough assessment of the patient's culture, religious beliefs, and environment, as described in previous chapters, may help the nurse to anticipate these needs. Although explaining the reason for a certain procedure may help the patient understand its benefit, a nurse must never attempt to influence or coerce the patient to agree to any procedure. In all cases, the nurse must document which procedures took place and any that were refused.

The physical assessment may be an exhausting experience for a patient who is elderly, debilitated, frail, or suffering from a chronic illness, because the nurse must examine every part of the body and the patient must make frequent changes in position. Consequently, the nurse should consider the patient's age, health status, level of functioning, and severity of illness at all times and adapt the examination accordingly. In addition, the nurse can conserve the patient's energy by moving around the patient during the examination, rather than asking the patient to move, and by carrying out the examination as quickly and efficiently as possible. The techniques and approaches for physical assessment vary for children, pregnant females, and older adults. The chapters in Unit IV discuss health assessment of pregnant women, children, and older adults. ∞

TECHNIQUES AND EQUIPMENT IN ASSESSMENT OF THE OBESE PATIENT Because the prevalence of obesity in the United States continues to remain elevated, nurses must be prepared to address the special needs of the obese patient during a comprehensive assessment (Dambaugh & Ecklund, 2016). This often requires adjustments in the use and selection of equipment and techniques. It is important to note that the nurse should be respectful and sensitive to issues surrounding the need for making these special considerations as this can sometimes generate feelings of embarrassment for the obese patient (McFarlane, 2012).

To ensure both comfort and safety, chairs in the waiting and examination areas and wheelchairs used for transport must be wide and sturdy. Equipment used for assessment must be appropriate for accurate data collection and to ensure patient safety. Extra-large examination gowns should be available. Scales with a capacity of greater than 350 pounds are required. Examination tables should be wide and sturdy with hand bars or footstools to help the patient move onto the table. Examination tables should be bolted to the floor to avoid tipping. If the patient needs helps stepping up or sitting on the exam table, use a gait belt or other assistive device to provide stability and support. If necessary, ask a second person to assist in moving the patient to avoid injury to both the patient and nurse. A large adult-size cuff, a thigh cuff, or special cuffs designed for the obese patient must be considered for accurate measurement of the blood pressure (Dambaugh & Ecklund, 2016).

Because of the weight of the chest wall and fat in the intercostal muscles, respiratory muscles can be exhausted quickly when obese patients are placed in a supine position (Dambaugh & Ecklund, 2016). Nurses should keep the head of the examination table elevated as much as possible during the examination. If the patient's head must be lowered, the nurse should continually monitor the patient's respiratory status, and the head of the bed should be raised as soon as possible after the exam is complete.

Standard Precautions

Throughout the physical assessment, the professional nurse is required to apply the principles of asepsis. The Centers for Disease Control and Prevention (CDC, 2008), Occupational Safety and Health Administration (OSHA, n.d.), and World Health Organization (WHO, 2009) have provided guidelines to protect patients and healthcare workers. Hand washing, use of gloves, use of protective barriers, disposal of sharps, cleaning of equipment after use, handling of specimens, and proper disposal of body wastes are included in the guidelines. Each healthcare agency has created agency policies based on these guidelines. A nurse working at an agency is responsible for knowing the policies and following the guidelines. Refer to Appendix A to review standard precautions.

Hand Hygiene Before beginning the physical assessment, the nurse should wash his or her hands in the presence of the patient. Hand hygiene not only protects the nurse and the patient, but also signals that the nurse is providing for the patient's safety. According to the World Health Organization (WHO, 2009) recommendations, nurses should scrub and rinse hands with soap for 40 to 60 seconds when the hands are visibly soiled, after using the restroom, after removing gloves, and before and after contact with medical equipment. In addition, alcohol-based antiseptic hand rubs in the form of rinses, gels, or foams should be used before and after direct patient contact. Nonsterile examination gloves should be available and used appropriately during the assessment. The bell and diaphragm of the stethoscope should

Evidence-Based Practice:
Assessment Considerations for Obese Patients

- Because of the weight of the chest wall and fat in the intercostal muscles in obese patients, respiratory muscles can be exhausted quickly when obese patients are placed in a supine position. Nurses should keep the head of the examination table elevated as much as possible during the examination. (Dambaugh & Ecklund, 2016)
- A large adult-size cuff, a thigh cuff, or special cuffs designed for the obese patient must be considered for accurate measurement of the blood pressure (Dambaugh & Ecklund, 2016)

be cleaned after the assessment of each patient to prevent the spread of infection.

Healthcare-associated infections (HAIs) are a common cause for prolonged hospital stays and complications of both simple and complex procedures. Using safety precautions to prevent the spread of infections is particularly important for high-risk patients such as patients with compromised immune systems or older patients. Hand washing and the use of antiseptic hand rubs are the most effective ways to prevent transfer of infection from one patient to another in both clinical and hospital settings. Refer to Appendix B for isolation precautions.

Use and Care of Medical Equipment   To decrease the risk of infection transfer between patients, medical staff should ensure the proper cleaning, use, and disposal of medical equipment that is used during the physical assessment. For noncritical surfaces such as bed rails, blood pressure cuffs, stethoscope surfaces, and other equipment that touches the patient's intact skin but not open sores or mucous membranes, a light disinfectant should be used to cleanse the surface between use on different patients (Centers for Disease Control and Prevention, 2008). Equipment that touches non-intact skin or mucous membranes should be cleaned with a high-level disinfectant between all patients. Equipment that enters normally sterile areas or the bloodstream should be cleaned and sterilized between every use. In addition, nurses should use sterile disposable equipment when possible, especially for procedures that require contact with mucous membranes, non-intact skin, or sterile tissues.

When using medical equipment during a physical examination, the nurse should prepare all the needed instruments and tools in a clean area. The clean area should be draped with a sterile cloth or paper liner, and clean or sterile instruments should be placed on the clean surface. After use, the dirty instruments should be placed either directly in a regular or biohazard trash can as appropriate or in a separate area reserved for dirty equipment. Dirty equipment should be separated from clean equipment to prevent potential cross-contamination of infectious agents between different areas of the body.

Patient Hazards   Some situations that arise during a physical assessment pose a potential hazard for the patient. For example, a patient might become light-headed and dizzy from taking deep breaths during a respiratory assessment or fall when asked to touch the toes during a musculoskeletal assessment. A patient who is frail, weak, debilitated, or suffering from a chronic illness is at greatest risk. Throughout the procedure, it is necessary to anticipate potential hazards and modify the assessment to prevent them. In addition, some assessment techniques may injure the patient if used indiscriminately. For example, vigorous, deep palpation of a throbbing mass might lead to a ruptured abdominal aneurysm.

Application Through Critical Thinking

CASE STUDY

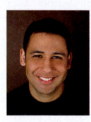

Source: Phase4Studios/ Shutterstock.

As part of a comprehensive health assessment course, *José Espero,* a student nurse, must conduct a physical assessment of an adult patient. José knows that it is important to understand proper techniques and gather the necessary equipment before approaching the patient. Before entering the room, his instructor asks José to review this information with her.

CRITICAL THINKING QUESTIONS

1. What should José include in his explanation of the assessment procedures to the patient?

2. What equipment must José prepare for the physical assessment?

3. What safety and comfort issues must be addressed when conducting the assessment for the patient?

4. Are there any other considerations José should take into account before or during the assessment of the patient?

REFERENCES

Centers for Disease Control and Prevention (CDC). (2008). *Guideline for disinfection and sterilization in healthcare facilities, 2008*. Retrieved from https://www.cdc.gov/infectioncontrol/pdf/guidelines/disinfection-guidelines.pdf

Dambaugh, L. A., & Ecklund, M. M. (2016). Progressive care of obese patients. *Critical Care Nurse, 36*(4), 58–63.

Douglas, C., Booker, C., Fox, R., Windsor, C., Osborne, S., & Gardner, G. (2016). Nursing physical assessment for patient safety in general wards: Reaching consensus on core skills. *Journal of Clinical Nursing, 25*, 1890–1900. doi:10.1111/jocn.13201

Douglas, C., Windsor, C., & Lewis, P. (2015). Too much knowledge for a nurse? Use of physical assessment by final-semester nursing students. *Nursing and Health Sciences, 17*, 492–499. doi:10.1111/nhs.12223

National Institute for Occupational Safety and Health (NIOSH). (1998). *Preventing allergic reactions to natural rubber latex in the workplace*. Retrieved from http://www.cdc.gov/niosh/docs/97-135

Occupational Safety and Health Administration (OSHA). (n.d.). *Healthcare wide hazards (Lack of) universal precautions*. Retrieved from https://www.osha.gov/SLTC/etools/hospital/hazards/univprec/univ.html

World Health Organization. (2009). *WHO guidelines on hand hygiene in health care*. Geneva, Switzerland: WHO Press.

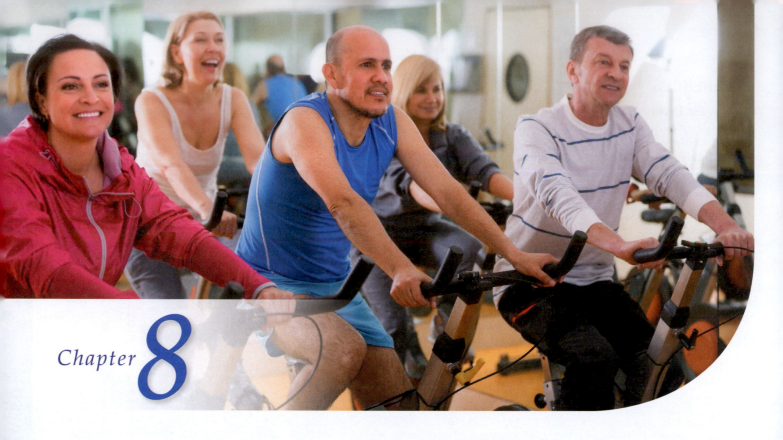

Chapter 8

General Survey and Physical Exam: Objective Data

LEARNING OUTCOMES

Upon completion of this chapter, you will be able to:

1. Identify the components of the general survey.

2. Identify the necessary steps and equipment for measuring height and weight.

3. Determine which techniques will ensure accurate measurement of vital signs.

4. Interpret nurse–patient encounter findings accurately.

KEY TERMS

blood pressure, 101	hyperthermia, 102	pulse, 101	systolic pressure, 106
diastolic pressure, 106	hypothermia, 102	respiratory rate, 101	temperature, 101
functional assessment, 110	oxygen saturation, 105	sinus arrhythmia, 109	vital signs, 101
general survey, 97	pain, 101	sphygmomanometer, 107	

MEDICAL LANGUAGE

a-	Prefix meaning "no," "not," "without"	**dys-**	Prefix meaning "abnormal," "difficult," "painful"
brady-	Prefix meaning "slow"		
cephalo-	Prefix meaning "head"	**tachy-**	Prefix meaning "fast"
		vaso-	Prefix meaning "vessel," "duct"

Introduction

The **general survey** includes objective data about the patient's physical appearance, body structure, mobility, behavior, height, weight, and vital signs. It begins during the interview phase of a comprehensive health assessment (see Figure 8.1 ■). While collecting subjective data during the health history, the nurse starts observing the patient, developing initial impressions about the individual's health and formulating strategies for the physical assessment. The initial impression should include what is seen, heard, or smelled during the initial phase of assessment. The objective data collected during the general survey will guide the nurse later during the assessment of body regions and systems. In addition, this data will help to determine the patient's ability to participate in all aspects of the assessment process. Should assessment reveal urgent or emergent problems, the patient will require treatment before proceeding. For example, the patient having chest pain or difficulty breathing (dyspnea) will need appropriate evaluation and treatment before conducting a full assessment.

Upon completion of the general survey, the nurse will assess height, weight, and vital signs. Information about each of these important phases of comprehensive health assessment is discussed in the following sections.

Components of the General Survey

The general survey is composed of four major categories of objective data: physical appearance, mental status, mobility, and patient behavior. Lifespan considerations also must be taken into account for each patient. The age and developmental stage of the patient will significantly affect the survey, as expected findings will vary. (See Unit IV for detailed information about lifespan considerations.)

Specific observations are required in the general survey. The following sections identify these required observations, which provide objective data. During the general survey, the nurse will determine if the observed behaviors fall within an expected

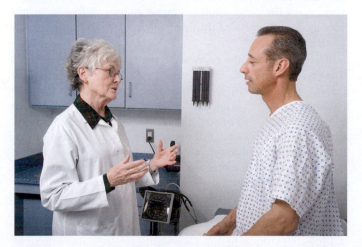

Figure 8.1 The nurse begins the general survey.

range for the patient's sex, age, race or ethnic background, and culture. The nurse must also determine the patient's ability to participate in all aspects of the process before proceeding.

Physical Appearance

The patient's physical appearance provides immediate and important cues to the level of individual wellness. Thus, beginning with the initial meeting, the nurse notes any factors about the patient's physical appearance that are in any way unexpected. For example, the nurse might note that a patient appears undernourished, seems older than his or her stated age, has a frown, is smiling, or has skin color that is pale, flushed, ruddy, or cyanotic.

Body shape and build may indicate the patient's general level of wellness. The patient's height and weight should be within normal ranges for age and body build. Extreme thinness or obesity may indicate an eating disorder. The nurse must consider the patient's lifestyle, socioeconomic level, and environment.

Mental Status

The nurse assesses the patient's mental status while the patient is responding to questions and giving information about health history. The nurse notes the patient's affect, mood, level of anxiety, orientation, and speech. Findings in these areas may be evaluated further during the assessment of the patient's psychosocial status and neurologic system.

The nurse assesses the patient for orientation to person, place, and time. Patients should typically be able to state their name, location, the date, month, season, and time of day. In most cases, the nurse will be able to sense a patient's orientation during the initial interview. If the patient appears confused, the nurse should ask him or her to respond to the following: "Tell me your name." "Where are you now?" "What is today's date?" and "What time is it?" If the patient cannot respond or responds incorrectly, a more detailed assessment of mental status must be performed. (Tools for assessment of mental status in adults are discussed in Chapter 24. ∞)

Mobility

The nurse observes the patient's gait, posture, and range of motion (the complete movement possible for a joint). Normally, the patient walks in a rhythmic, straight, upright position with arms swinging at each side of the body. The shoulders are level and straight. Difficulty with gait and posture, such as stumbling, shuffling, limping, or the inability to stand erect, calls for further evaluation. Range of motion should be fluid and appropriate to the age of the patient. The nurse will observe for deviations from the normal that include weakness, stiffness, involuntary motor activity, or limitations in movement related to trauma, deformity, or those associated with obesity. (See Chapter 23 for information on assessing the musculoskeletal system and range of motion. ∞)

Patient Behavior

An assessment of patient behavior includes objective data about dress and grooming, body odors, facial expression, mood and affect, ability to make eye contact, and level of anxiety. The way in which patients' dress may provide clues to their sense of self-esteem and body image. However, the nurse must consider many factors before drawing conclusions based on a patient's appearance. For example, a patient who wears clothing that is inappropriate for the situation or weather may be blind, mentally ill, experiencing situational grief or anxiety, or mentally fit but unable to buy other clothes because of financial constraints.

The nurse observes the patient for cleanliness and personal hygiene. The patient who is dirty or has a strong body odor or poor dental hygiene may be depressed, have poor self-concept, lack knowledge about personal hygiene practices, or have difficulty managing hygiene because of obesity. The nurse must consider the patient's environment, habits, and cultural background before drawing conclusions. For example, a patient who is dirty may have just come from working on a construction site.

The nurse assesses the patient's emotional state by noting what the patient says, as well as the body language, facial expression, and appropriateness of behavior in relation to the situation and circumstances. The patient should exhibit comfort in talking with the examiner. Giggling when answering questions about bowel movements may simply indicate embarrassment, whereas giggling when describing the death of a loved one may be an example of inappropriate affect.

The nurse also assesses the patient for apprehension, fear, and nervousness. Like affect and mood, the patient's level of anxiety is revealed through speech, body language, and facial expression. During the health assessment, the patient may exhibit anxiety because of embarrassment, fear of pain, or worry about the outcome of the examination. If the patient's anxiety seems to have no cause, the patient must be evaluated further. To obtain a relative impression of the level of anxiety, patients may be asked to rate their feelings of anxiety on a scale of 0 to 10. The nurse uses the patient's response as an indicator of the need for further assessment and as a baseline for future assessment of anxiety levels. (Chapter 11 provides more information about assessment for anxiety. ∞)

The nurse assesses the patient's speech for quantity, volume, content, articulation, and rhythm. The patient should speak easily and fluently to the nurse or to an interpreter. Disorganized speech patterns, silence, or constant talking may indicate normal nervousness or shyness or may signal a speech defect, neurologic deficit, depression, or another disorder.

Lifespan Considerations

For pediatric patients, instead of assessing mental status based on orientation, nursing assessment includes comparing the patient's developmental stage to the expected findings based on age. Just as the brain is not fully mature at birth, all of the major organ systems are immature and develop throughout childhood. The most dramatic development changes occur primarily in infancy and adolescence, although each stage of childhood is marked by unique changes.

Newborns are children between birth and 1 month of age. Infants are children between 1 and 12 months of age. Infancy is characterized by dramatic changes in height and weight and the development of gross physical and social skills. Young children have cephalocaudal physical growth—that is, their development progresses in a head-to-toe fashion. Development and growth begin proximally before developing distally. For example, fine motor skills follow gross motor skills, and the ability to grasp precedes the ability to stand or walk. Toddlers are children who are at least 1 year old but who have not yet reached 3 years of age. Toddlerhood is marked by slower, steadier growth, fine motor skill improvement, and language development. Preschoolers are children between 3 and 5 years of age. The preschool years are characterized by motor and language skill refinement and beginning social skill development. School-age children are between 6 and 10 years old. The major developmental tasks of school-age children involve cognitive and social growth. Adolescence is characterized by periods of rapid growth, sexual maturation, and cognitive refinement. Adolescence is the period between 11 and 21 years of age.

For patients across the lifespan, general appearance can provide very useful assessment data. For example, the appearance of the younger child reveals a great deal of information about the child's parents or caretakers, and the appearance of an older child gives clues about self-care. In other words, a child 3 years of age whose skin and clothes are dirty may be a victim of neglect, whereas a 13-year-old in the same condition may lack knowledge about proper hygiene.

The nurse should note the child's interaction with the parents or caretakers. Their relationship should exhibit mutual warmth and caring. Signs of child abuse include clinging to a parent or strong attachment to a parent because of fear of parental anger; absence of separation anxiety in a child who, because of developmental stage, would ordinarily demonstrate it; avoidance of eye contact between caretaker and child; a caretaker's demonstration of disgust with a child's behavior, illness, odor, or stool; flinching when people move toward the child; and regression to infantile behavior.

Assessment of general appearance also offers insight into the older adult's overall health status. The dress, grooming, and personal hygiene of an older adult may be affected by limitations in mobility from arthritis, cardiovascular disease, and other disorders or by a lack of funds.

The gait of an older adult is often slower and the steps shorter. To maintain balance, older adults may hold their arms away from the body or use a cane. The posture of an older adult may look slightly stooped because of a generalized flexion, which also causes the older adult to appear shorter. A loss in height may also be because of thinning or compression of the intervertebral disks.

The behavior of the older adult may be affected by various disorders common to this age group, such as vascular insufficiency and diabetes. In addition, medications may affect the patient's behavior. Some medications may cause the patient to feel anxious, and others may affect the patient's alertness, orientation, or speech. Older adults are likely to have one or more chronic conditions associated with age, such as arthritis, hypertension, or diabetes. As a result, older adults must consume several prescription medications. Overmedication may occur because older adults seek care from multiple healthcare providers without collaboration regarding treatment. Multiple medications may combine to produce dangerous side effects. Additionally, the schedules for multiple medications may be confusing and result in overmedication, forgotten doses, negative side effects, or ineffectiveness of medication. Therefore, the nurse must conduct a thorough assessment of the patient's medication schedule and history.

Measuring Height and Weight

The nurse measures the patient's height and weight to establish baseline data and to help determine health status. The patient should be asked about height and weight before any measurements are taken. Large discrepancies between the stated height and weight and the actual measurements may provide clues to the patient's self-image. Alternatively, discrepancies in weight may indicate the patient's lack of awareness of a sudden loss or gain in weight that may be caused by illness. The importance of gathering accurate measurements is addressed in the feature Evidence-Based Practice: Accuracy in Height and Weight Measurement.

Height

To measure height, the nurse uses a measuring stick attached to a platform scale or to a wall. The patient should look straight ahead while standing as straight as possible with heels together and shoulders back. When using a platform scale, the nurse raises the height attachment rod above the patient's head, then extends and lowers the right-angled arm until it rests on the crown of the head. The measurement is read from the height attachment rod (see Figure 8.2 ■). When using a measuring stick, the nurse should place an L-shaped level on the crown of the patient's head at a right angle to the measuring stick (see Figure 8.3 ■). To determine the height of a bedridden patient, a disposable measuring tape should be used while the patient is in a lying position. Measure from the top of the patient's head to the bottom of the heel to obtain accurate height data.

Weight

A standard platform scale or digital scale (see Figure 8.4 ■) is used to measure the weight of older children and adults. It is

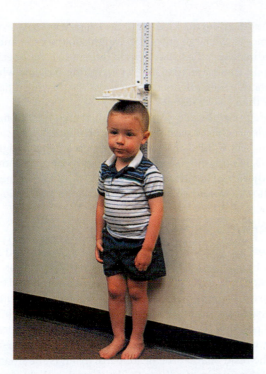
Figure 8.3 Measuring the patient's height with a measuring stick.

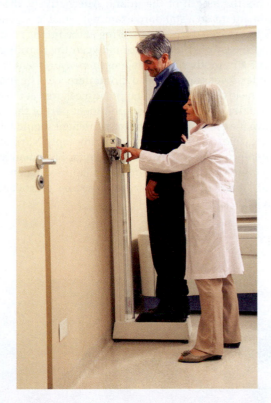
Figure 8.4 Measuring the patient's weight with a standard platform scale.
Source: jovannig/123RF.

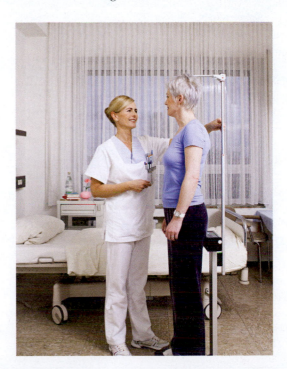
Figure 8.2 Measuring the patient's height with a platform scale.
Source: Joos Mind/Stone/Getty Images.

best to use the same scale at each visit and to weigh the patient at the same time of day in the same kind of clothing (e.g., the examination gown) and without shoes. If using a digital scale, the nurse simply reads the weight from the lighted display panel. Otherwise, the scale is calibrated by moving both weights to 0 (zero) and turning the knob until the balance beam is level. The nurse moves the large and small weights to the right and takes the reading when the balance beam returns to level. Special bed and chair scales are available for weighing patients who cannot stand. Obese patients require scales that have a capacity of greater than 159 kg (350 lb).

Average height and weight for adult men and women are available in charts prepared by governmental agencies and insurers. Table 8.1 illustrates average acceptable weights for adults. The body mass index (BMI) is considered a more reliable indicator of healthy weight. (The BMI and other measures in relation to weight are discussed in Chapter 10. ∞)

Lifespan Considerations

Children who are able to stand on their own at full height should be measured for height in a standing position rather than length in a lying position. However, length should be used to measure infants who are unable to stand independently. To measure an infant's length, the nurse places the child in a supine position on an examining table that is equipped with a ruler, headboard, and adjustable footboard. The nurse positions the head against the headboard, extends the infant's leg nearest the ruler, and adjusts the footboard until it touches the infant's foot. The space between the headboard and footboard represents the length of the infant. Alternatively, the nurse places the infant on a standard examination table, extends the infant's leg, marks the paper covering at the infant's head and foot, and measures the distance between the markings (see Figure 8.5 ■). Another common length measurement for children under 3 years old is head circumference. The infant or toddler's head circumference should be measured at the widest point, usually around the most prominent part of the occiput and above the eyebrows, and the measurement should be taken with a flexible, unstretchable measuring tape. Normal head circumference ranges from 34 to 37 cm (approximately 13 to 14.5 in.) in newborns up to 47 to 51 cm (approximately 18.5 to 20 in.) at 3 years of age (Centers for Disease Control and Prevention [CDC], 2001).

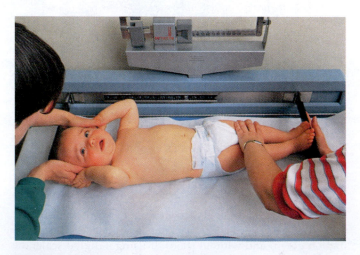

Figure 8.5 Measuring an infant's length.

Evidence-Based Practice
Accuracy in Height and Weight Measurement

Drug dosages, nutritional support, and ventilator settings are just some of the healthcare interventions dependent upon accurate height and weight measurements. Subjective reporting of height and weight has been shown to be inaccurate. Overestimation of weight may lead to inaccurate dosing of critical medication, inappropriate or inadequate nutritional support, and incorrect estimation of tidal volumes for mechanical ventilation potentially resulting in severe lung injury or an inability to wean from the ventilator.

- A study done by Byers, France, and Kuiper (2014) found that nursing staff members incorrectly assumed a physician's order was required to obtain height and weight on a patient.
- They were also unaware that the scales used for weight must be routinely calibrated and zeroed before putting the patient on the scale (Byers et al., 2014).

Table 8.1 Guidelines for Ideal Weight Based on Height

HEIGHT	IDEAL WEIGHT
4′10″	91–115 lb
4′11″	94–119 lb
5′0″	97–123 lb
5′1″	100–127 lb
5′2″	104–131 lb
5′3″	107–135 lb
5′4″	110–140 lb
5′5″	114–144 lbs.
5′6″	118–148 lb
5′7″	121–153 lb
5′8″	125–158 lb
5′9″	128–162 lb
5′10″	132–167 lb
5′11″	136–172 lb
6′0″	140–177 lb
6′1″	144–182 lb
6′2″	148–186 lb
6′3″	152–192 lb
6′4″	156–197 lb

Source: Rush University Medical Center. (n.d.). *What is a healthy weight?* Retrieved from http://www.rush.edu/rumc/page-1108048103230.html

Infants are weighed on a modified platform scale with curved sides to prevent injury. The scale measures weight in grams and in ounces. The nurse places the unclothed baby on the scale on a paper drape and watches the baby to prevent a fall (see Figure 8.6 ■). Measurements are taken to the nearest 10 grams (0.5 oz.).

Children over the age of 2 or 3 years may be weighed on the upright scale or seated on the infant scale. The child's underpants should be left on. To measure height, the nurse uses the platform scale or a measuring stick attached to the wall, as for an adult. By the age of 4, most children enjoy being weighed and measured and finding out how much they have grown.

The height of older adults may decline somewhat as a result of thinning or compression of the intervertebral disks and a general flexion of the hips and knees. Body weight may decrease because of muscle shrinkage. The older patient may appear thinner, even when properly nourished, because of loss of subcutaneous fat deposits from the face, forearms, and lower legs. At the same time, fat deposits on the abdomen and hips may increase.

Measuring Vital Signs

Vital signs include body **temperature**, **pulse**, **respiratory rate**, and **blood pressure**. Measurement of oxygen saturation and pain assessment may be included when taking vital signs (see Box 8.1 Pain—The Fifth Vital Sign?). The nurse measures vital signs to obtain baseline data, to detect or monitor a change in the patient's health status, and to monitor patients at risk for alterations in health.

Measuring Body Temperature

The body's surface temperature—the temperature of the skin, subcutaneous tissues, and fat—fluctuates in response to environmental factors and is, therefore, unreliable for monitoring a patient's health status. Instead, the nurse should measure the patient's core temperature, or the temperature of the deep tissues of the body (e.g., the thorax and abdominal cavity). This temperature remains relatively constant at about 37°C (98.6°F).

Sensors in the hypothalamus regulate the body's core temperature. When these hypothalamic sensors detect heat, they signal the body to decrease heat production and increase heat loss (e.g., by vasodilation and sweating). When sensors in the hypothalamus detect cold, they signal the body to increase heat production and decrease heat loss (e.g., by shivering, vasoconstriction, and inhibition of sweating).

Factors That Influence Body Temperature A variety of factors may influence normal core body temperature, including the following:

- *Age.* The core temperature of infants is highly responsive to changes in the external environment; therefore, infants need extra protection from even mild variations in temperature. Indicators for assessing rectal temperature in children rather than tympanic temperature include recent exposure to extreme temperatures (cold winters or hot summers) and illness, especially otitis media. The core body temperature of children is more stable than that of infants but less so than that of adolescents or adults. However, older adults are more sensitive than middle adults to variations in external environmental temperature. This increased sensitivity may be because of the decreased thermoregulatory control and loss of subcutaneous fat common in older adults, or it may be because of environmental factors such as lack of activity, inadequate diet, or lack of central heating.

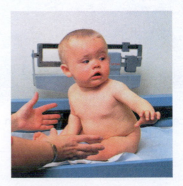

Figure 8.6 Weighing an infant.

> ## Box 8.1 Pain—The Fifth Vital Sign?
>
> Assessment of **pain** is essential in comprehensive health assessment. Pain is an entirely subjective and personal experience. When pain is present, it impacts every aspect of an individual's health and well-being. Pain can be acute and chronic, or severe, or mild, but overall it is an experience unique to the individual. The perception of pain and the ways in which the individual responds to pain vary according to age, sex, culture, and developmental level. When conducting a pain assessment, the nurse must consider all factors influencing the individual's experience with pain.
>
> The phrase "Pain as the Fifth Vital Sign" was originally promoted in the late 1990s to encourage healthcare professionals to have an elevated awareness of pain, pain assessment, and pain treatment in their patients. A determination about the presence of pain, followed by a numerical or facial rating score to indicate the intensity of pain, usually occurred during assessment of the other vital signs. At the time this initiative was launched, postoperative pain and cancer pain were often ignored. Healthcare has moved forward by leaps and bounds, with some thinking the pendulum has swung too far in the other direction. Hospital ratings for quality are now determined in part by how well the patient's pain was controlled. This has led some to believe that the overemphasis on pain assessment and pain control has contributed to the overuse of opioids (Campell, 2016; Greenwell, 2015; Purser, Warfield, & Richardson, 2014). The Joint Commission, an independent agency that accredits thousands of healthcare organizations in the United States, issued a statement in 2016 supporting the need for pain assessment but denounced the notion that they required the use of drugs to manage pain (Baker, 2016). At the 2016 American Medical Association (AMA) meeting, the delegates voted to stop the use of pain as the fifth vital sign because of their concern that the initiative was one factor that has impacted the opioid crisis (Anson, 2016; Scher, Meador, VanCleave, & Reid, 2018). Refer to Chapter 9 for a thorough discussion of pain. ∞

- *Diurnal variations.* Core body temperature is usually highest between 8:00 p.m. and midnight and lowest between 4:00 a.m. and 6:00 a.m. Normal body temperature may vary between these times by as much as 1°C (1.8°F). Some individuals have more than one complete cycle in a day.

- *Exercise.* Strenuous exercise can increase core body temperature by as much as 2°C (5°F).

- *Hormones.* A variety of hormones affect core body temperature. For example, in women, progesterone secretion at the time of ovulation raises core body temperature by about 0.35°C (0.5°F).

- *Stress.* The temperature of a highly stressed patient may be elevated as a result of increased production of epinephrine and norepinephrine, which increase metabolic activity and heat production.

- *Illness.* Illness or a central nervous system disorder may impair the thermostatic function of the hypothalamus. **Hyperthermia**, also called fever, may occur in response to viral or bacterial infections or from tissue breakdown following myocardial infarction, malignancy, surgery, or trauma. **Hypothermia** is usually a response to prolonged exposure to cold.

Routes for Measuring Body Temperature Core body temperature was once typically measured with a mercury-in-glass thermometer. However, because of the toxicity associated with mercury, most glass thermometers now use alcohol and galinstan, and even these are being replaced. Today, nurses are more likely to use an electronic thermometer (see Figure 8.7 ■), which gives a highly accurate reading in only 2 to 60 seconds. These portable, battery-operated devices consist of an electronic display unit, a probe, and disposable probe sheaths. The nurse attaches the appropriate probe to the unit, covers it with a sheath, and inserts it into the body orifice. The probe is left in place until the temperature appears on the liquid crystal display (LCD). There are five routes for measuring core body temperature: oral, rectal, axillary, tympanic, and temporal artery.

ORAL Measuring the oral temperature is the most accessible, accurate, and convenient method. Because of safety concerns, the U.S. Environmental Protection Agency (EPA) is working to phase out the manufacture, sale, and use of mercury thermometers. In several states, the sale of mercury thermometers is prohibited (EPA, 2014). Mercury thermometers are no longer used in the clinical setting because of the possibility of breaking and mercury exposure. (For more information, visit the U.S. Environmental Protection Agency website.)

Oral temperatures may be evaluated by using an electronic or digital probe device. Place the covered probe, usually blue in color, at the base of the tongue in either of the sublingual pockets to the right or left of the frenulum (see Figure 8.8 ■), and instruct the patient to keep the lips tightly closed around the thermometer. The thermometer is left in place until the device beeps or shows indication that the measurement is completed. After removing the thermometer, the nurse either discards the disposable sheath or cleans the device. The temperature reading will appear in the display window.

RECTAL A rectal temperature is taken if the patient is comatose, confused, having seizures, or unable to close the mouth. It is

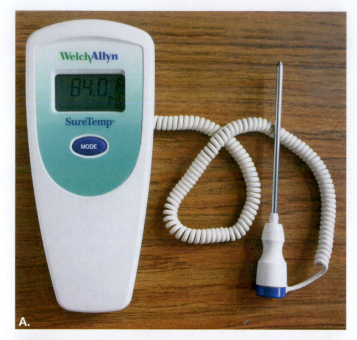

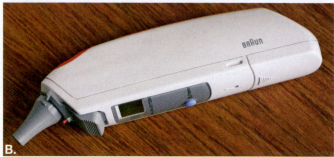

Figure 8.7 Electronic thermometers. A. This device may be used to measure oral, rectal, or axillary temperature. B. This device is used to measure tympanic temperature.

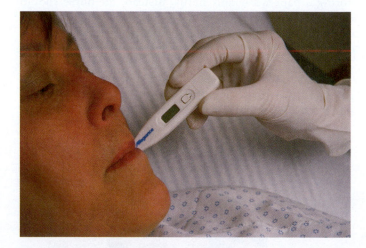

Figure 8.8 Placement of the thermometer for an oral temperature.

important to use pre-lubricated thermometer covers and put on disposable examination gloves. The patient should be in a side-lying position. The nurse then inserts the thermometer into the anus from 1.3 cm to 2.5 cm (approximately 0.5 in. to 1.0 in.) for infants or 2.5 cm to 4 cm (1 in. to 1.5 in) for an adult, being careful not to force insertion of the thermometer. The probe, usually red in color, is left in place until there is a beep or the device indicates that the reading is completed. Remove the probe, dispose of the disposable sheath, and obtain the reading in the display window.

AXILLARY Occasionally, the nurse needs to take an axillary temperature. This is the safest method and is less invasive than the oral or rectal routes, especially for infants and young children. Because of the variability of probe positioning, many authorities consider the axillary route to be least accurate. For an axillary temperature, the nurse places the thermometer in the patient's axilla and assists the patient in placing the arm tightly across the chest to keep the thermometer in place.

TYMPANIC The tympanic temperature can be taken only with an electronic thermometer. Using infrared technology, it measures a patient's core body temperature quickly and accurately. This method is comfortable and noninvasive for the patient. The measuring probe resembles an otoscope. The nurse gently places the covered tip of the probe at the opening of the ear canal, being careful not to force the probe into the ear canal or occlude the canal opening. After about 2 seconds, the patient's temperature reading will appear on the LCD.

TEMPORAL ARTERY The temporal artery thermometer (TAT) is a noninvasive device to measure temperature using an infrared sensor. To measure the temperature, the TAT is placed in the center of the forehead and moved in a straight line toward the temple into the hairline. Without letting up on the scan button, lift the device and place the tip behind the ear lobe. The reading is taken after these steps are completed and appears on an LCD in seconds. This two-step approach is used to improve accuracy by eliminating the possibility of diaphoresis causing an evaporative cooling effect, thus lowering the temperature seen on the TAT. Incorrect technique with the TAT can produce significantly inaccurate readings (Barry et al., 2016).

The accuracy of each method of taking a temperature has long been debated. Numerous studies have examined various factors, such as use of correct technique and the correlation or accuracy of the results for the various types of thermometers, some of which are described in the feature Evidence-Based Practice: Accuracy in Temperature Measurement.

Measuring Pulse Rate

The heart is a muscular pump. The left ventricle of the heart contracts with every beat, forcing blood from the heart into the systemic arteries. The amount of blood pumped from the heart with each heartbeat is called the *stroke volume*. The force of the blood against the walls of the arteries generates a wave of pressure that is felt at various points in the body as a pulse. The ability of the arteries to contract and expand is called *compliance*. When compliance is reduced, the heart must exert more pressure to pump blood throughout the body.

Location of Pulse Points The apical pulse is felt at the apex of the heart. Figure 8.9 ■ illustrates the location of the apical pulse for an adult. The peripheral pulse is the pulse as felt in the body's periphery (e.g., in the neck, wrist, or foot). Figure 8.10 ■ shows eight sites where the peripheral pulse is most easily palpated.

Evidence-Based Practice
Accuracy in Temperature Measurement

- TATs have been found to correlate well with rectal temperatures and are more accurate than tympanic and axillary temperatures in children, thus allowing the use of the TAT in place of the rectal thermometer (Allegaert, Casteels, Gorp, & Bogaert, 2014; Batra & Goyal, 2013; Reynolds et al., 2014). A high correlation was also found in adults (Kemp, 2013).
- Acutely ill patients were studied to determine the most accurate method of temperature collection. Compared with an electronic oral thermometer, the TAT overestimated temperature and the disposable axillary thermometer underestimated temperature. It was concluded that for acutely ill hospitalized trauma patients the TAT and the disposable axillary temperatures were not recommended (Johnstone, 2017).
- A study was done comparing an oral electronic thermometer and a TAT in febrile cancer patients. The TAT was found to be unreliable in detecting fever in this group of cancer patients (Mason et al., 2017).
- Temperatures taken with a tympanic thermometer in each ear were compared in a study using subjects ages 10 to 94 years of age. No significant difference was found between the temperatures taken in the two ears, indicating that checking one ear with a TAT is sufficient practice (Salota et al., 2016).

In a healthy patient, the peripheral pulse rate is equivalent to the heartbeat. Assessment of the peripheral pulse is an important component of a thorough health assessment.

Alterations in the patient's health can weaken the peripheral pulse, making it difficult to detect. In obese patients, the radial pulse is the most accessible and palpable of peripheral pulses. The carotid pulse is difficult to assess due to the short, thick neck in morbidly obese patients. The use of a Doppler device may be required to assess peripheral pulses in obese patients. A Doppler is a noninvasive device that produces a swishing sound if there is blood flow through the blood vessels. The sound is created by bouncing high-frequency sound waves, or ultrasound, off circulating red blood cells. (More detailed information related to assessment of peripheral pulses is located in Chapter 18 and Chapter 19. ∞)

Factors That Influence Pulse Rate A variety of factors may influence the normal pulse rate, including the following:

- *Age.* The average pulse rate of infants and children is higher than that of teens and adults. After age 16, the pulse stabilizes to an average of about 70 beats per minute (beats/min) in males and 75 beats/min in females.
- *Sex.* As noted, the average pulse rate of the adult male is slightly lower than that of the adult female.
- *Exercise.* The pulse rate normally increases with exercise.

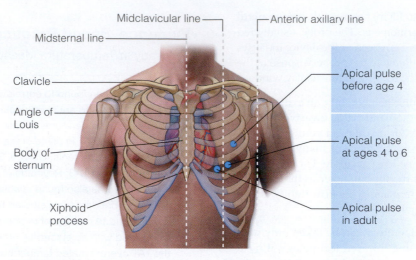

Figure 8.9 Location of the apical pulse in a child under age 4, a child ages 4 to 6, and an adult.

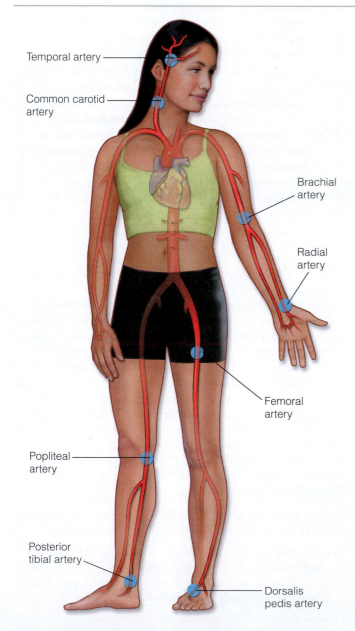

Figure 8.10 Body sites where the peripheral pulse is most easily palpated.

- *Stress.* In response to stress, fear, and anxiety, the heart rate and the force of the heartbeat increase.
- *Fever.* The peripheral vasodilation that accompanies an elevated body temperature lowers systemic blood pressure, in turn causing an increase in pulse rate.
- *Hemorrhage.* Pulse rate increases in response to significant loss of blood from the vascular system.
- *Medications.* A variety of medications may either increase or decrease the heart rate.
- *Position changes.* When patients sit or stand for long periods, blood may pool in the veins, resulting in a temporary decrease in venous blood return to the heart and, consequently, reduced blood pressure and lowered pulse rate.

Palpation of the Radial Pulse The radial pulse is the most commonly measured peripheral, although not as accurate as an EKG. (See the feature Evidence-Based Practice: Accuracy in Pulse Measurement). The radial pulse is palpated by placing the pads of the first two or three fingers on the anterior wrist along the radius bone (see Figure 8.11 ■). If the pulse is regular, the nurse counts the beats for 30 seconds and multiplies by 2 to obtain the total beats per minute. If the pulse is irregular, the nurse counts the beats for a full minute.

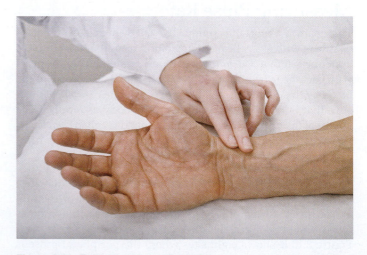

Figure 8.11 Palpating the radial pulse.

Evidence-Based Practice
Accuracy in Pulse Measurement

- Checking the radial pulse for 30 seconds and multiplying by 2 is considered typical practice when used with a heart rate less than 100 beats/min. Hollerbach and Sneed (1990) substantiated this finding along with evidence that counting the pulse for 15 seconds and multiplying by 4 was not consistently as accurate as the 30-second count, especially when the pulse rate was greater than 100 beats/min.
- When a palpated radial pulse rate is compared with an electrocardiograph (ECG) heart rate reading in an acutely ill patient, there is poor correlation between the two rates (Kellett, Li, Rasool, Green, & Seely, 2011; Opio & Kellett, 2017). The ECG rate was shown to be much more accurate than the radial pulse rate in acutely ill patients, especially when the pulse rate exhibited tachycardia (Kellet et al., 2011; Opio & Kellett, 2017).

Four factors are considered when assessing the pulse: rate, rhythm, force, and elasticity. A pulse rate of less than 60 beats/min, called *bradycardia*, may be found in a healthy, well-trained athlete. A pulse rate of more than 100 beats/min, called *tachycardia*, may also be found in the healthy patient who is anxious or has just finished exercising. The pulse of a healthy adult has a relatively constant rhythm—that is, the intervals between beats are regular. (Irregularities in heart rhythm are discussed fully in Chapter 18. ∞)

The nurse assesses the force of a pulse, or its stroke volume, by noting the pressure that must be exerted before the pulse is felt. A full, bounding pulse is difficult to obliterate. It may be caused by fear, anxiety, exercise, or a variety of alterations in health. A weak, thready pulse is easy to obliterate. It also may indicate alterations in health such as hemorrhage. The nurse palpates along the radial artery in a proximal-to-distal direction to assess the elasticity of the artery. A normal artery feels smooth, straight, and resilient.

Measuring Respiratory Rate

The human body continuously exchanges oxygen and carbon dioxide through the act of respiration. Normal respiratory rates are dependent on age. The normal respiratory rate for adults is 12 to 20 breaths per minute.

Assessment of Respiratory Rate Counting the number of respirations per minute assesses respiratory rate. The nurse observes the full respiratory cycle (one inspiration and one expiration) for rate and pattern of breathing. The patient's respiratory rate is assessed by counting the number of breaths for 30 seconds and then multiplying by 2. If the nurse detects irregularities or difficulty breathing, the respirations are counted for one full minute.

Factors That Influence Respiratory Rate Respiratory rate is an indicator of many conditions and must be accurately measured, which is addressed in the feature Evidence-Based Practice: Accuracy in Respiratory Rate Measurement. The respiratory rate may increase in some patients if they become aware that their breaths are being counted. For this reason, while counting breaths per minute, the nurse should maintain the posture of counting the radial pulse.

Other factors that may increase respiratory rate include exercise, stress, increased temperature, and increased altitude. Some medications may either increase or decrease respiratory rate. Obese patients have difficulty with respiration as a result of increased fatty tissue in the chest wall and abdomen. These patients are most comfortable in a sitting position for all assessments. Exertion from moving onto an examination table may cause an increased respiratory rate. Allow time for the patient to adjust to a change in position and to recover from movement before counting respirations. (See Chapter 16 for a more detailed discussion of respiration. ∞)

Oxygen Saturation Level The blood **oxygen saturation** level, or SpO_2, is the percentage of oxygen carried by the hemoglobin and is measured using a pulse oximeter (see Figure 8.12). The pulse oximeter uses a sensor and a photodetector to determine the light sent and absorbed by the hemoglobin. The reported percentage represents the light absorbed by oxygenated and deoxygenated hemoglobin. This noninvasive procedure allows oxygen saturation values to be easily obtained and rapidly updated. The sensor is usually placed on the finger of the patient. In a healthy individual, a value of 97% to 99% is considered normal (Osborn, Wraa, Watson, & Holleran, 2014), and an oxygen saturation of less than 90% should be investigated further. The amount of oxygen dissolved in the plasma of the arterial blood is represented by the abbreviation PaO_2. While the SpO_2 and the PaO_2 are related via the oxyhemoglobin disassociation curve, an SpO_2 of 90% correlates to a PaO_2 of 60 mmHg.

Evidence-Based Practice
Accuracy in Respiratory Rate Measurement

- Cretikos et al. (2008) identified that the respiratory rate is commonly omitted when a set of vital signs is obtained.
- A resting respiratory rate in an adult greater than 20 breaths per minute indicates that a patient is ill, and a rate greater than 24 breaths per minute is of critical concern (Cretikos et al, 2008).
- Pulse oximetry readings from the hand can be inaccurate if the fingers are cold, if there is poor circulation to the site, or if nail polish or artificial nails are in place. Placement of the sensor on the earlobe promotes more accurate findings (Fahy, Lareau, & Sockrider, 2013).
- Pulse oximetry can detect hypoxemia before symptoms such as cyanosis (blue color) of the skin appear. Pulse oximetry readings can be altered by conditions such as low hemoglobin and low body temperature (hypothermia), especially in children (Ross, Newth, & Khemani, 2014).

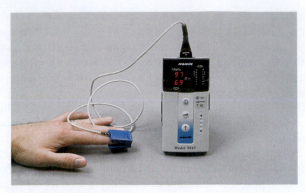

Figure 8.12 Pulse oximeter.

Lifespan Considerations Lung development is complete in healthy full-term newborns; however, there are significant differences between child and adult respiratory tracts. Infants have thinner, less muscular chest walls with a more noticeable xiphoid process. Breath sounds are louder and harsher. Referred sounds from the upper airways are common. The anterior–posterior chest diameter is approximately equal in infants, and the ribs appear more horizontal. Infants are obligate nose breathers until 6 months of age; they cannot breathe through their mouths. The nurse should carefully assess children under the age of 6 months with nasal congestion for signs of respiratory distress. Abdominal breathing is common until age 6 years. Thoracic breathing begins in the school-age years. (For additional discussion of life-span considerations related to the pediatric respiratory system, see Chapter 26. ∞)

Measuring Blood Pressure

Blood ebbs and flows within the systemic arteries in waves, causing two types of pressure. The **systolic pressure** is the pressure of the blood at the height of the wave, when the left ventricle contracts. This is the first (top) number recorded in a blood pressure measurement. The **diastolic pressure** is the pressure between the ventricular contractions, when the heart is at rest. This is the second (bottom) number recorded in a blood pressure measurement.

To measure blood pressure, the bladder of the blood pressure cuff must fit the length and width of the patient's limb. The cuff should cover two-thirds of the upper arm from shoulder to elbow, and the lower edge of the cuff should be positioned approximately 1 inch above the elbow. In addition, the inflatable portion of the cuff should cover 80% of the arm width (James et al., 2014). In adults under 60 years of age or those of any age with diabetes or chronic kidney disease, the ideal blood pressure reading is less than 140/90 mmHg. For adults over 60 years of age without diabetes or chronic kidney disease, the recommended blood pressure level is less than 150/90.

Circulatory Factors That Influence Blood Pressure Factors that influence blood pressure include but are not limited to the following:

- *Cardiac output.* Cardiac output is the amount of blood ejected from the heart. Cardiac output is equal to the stroke volume, or the amount of blood ejected in one heartbeat (measured in milliliters per beat), multiplied by the heart rate (measured in beats per minute). Cardiac output averages about 5.5 liters per minute (L/min).

- *Blood volume.* Blood volume is the total amount of blood circulating within the entire vascular system. Blood volume averages about 5 L in adults. In children, blood volume is approximately 80 mL/kg (London et al., 2014). A sudden drop in blood pressure may signal sudden blood loss, as with internal bleeding.

- *Peripheral vascular resistance.* Peripheral vascular resistance is the resistance the blood encounters as it flows within the vessels. Peripheral resistance is in turn influenced by various factors, such as vessel length and diameter. Two of the most important factors influencing peripheral resistance are blood viscosity and vessel compliance.

- *Blood viscosity.* Blood viscosity is the ratio between the blood cells (the formed elements) and the blood plasma. When the total amount of formed elements is high, the blood is thicker, or more viscous. The molecules pass one another with greater difficulty, and more pressure is required to move the blood.

- *Vessel compliance.* Vessel compliance describes the elasticity of the smooth muscle in the arterial walls. Highly elastic arteries respond readily and fully to each heartbeat. Rigid, hardened arteries, as are found with arteriosclerosis, are less responsive, and greater force is required to move the blood along.

Note that blood in the systemic circulation flows along a pressure gradient from central to peripheral; in other words, pressure is higher in the arterioles than in the capillaries and higher still in the aorta.

Additional Factors Affecting Blood Pressure Additional factors that influence blood pressure include but are not limited to the following:

- *Age.* Systolic blood pressure in newborns averages about 78 mmHg. Blood pressure rates tend to rise with increasing age through age 18 and then tend to stabilize. In older adults, blood pressure rates tend to rise again as elasticity of the arteries decreases.

- *Sex.* After puberty, females tend to have lower blood pressure than males of the same age. Reproductive hormones may influence this difference because blood pressure in women usually increases after menopause.

- *Race.* The prevalence of hypertension in African American adults in the United States is among the highest in the world when compared with Hispanic, non-Hispanic, and Asian males and females (Benjamin et al., 2017).

- *Obesity.* Blood pressure tends to be higher in people who are overweight and obese than it is in people of normal weight and the same age.

- *Physical activity.* Physical activity (including crying in infants and children) increases cardiac output and, therefore, increases blood pressure.

- *Stress.* Stress increases cardiac output and arterial vasoconstriction, resulting in increased blood pressure.

- *Diurnal variations.* Blood pressure is usually lowest in the early morning and rises steadily throughout the day, peaking in the late afternoon or early evening.

- *Medications.* A variety of medications may increase or decrease blood pressure.

Blood pressure is also affected by alterations in health. Any condition that affects the cardiac output, peripheral vascular resistance, blood volume, blood viscosity, or vessel compliance can affect blood pressure.

Assessment of Blood Pressure An accurate measurement of blood pressure is an essential part of any complete health assessment.

PATIENT PREPARATION It is important to reassure the patient that the procedure for taking blood pressure is generally quick and painless. The patient should be at rest for at least 5 minutes before taking a blood pressure measurement and up to 20 minutes if the patient has been engaging in heavy physical activity. Patient anxiety may also cause a temporary elevation of blood pressure.

EQUIPMENT The nurse measures blood pressure with a blood pressure cuff, a sphygmomanometer, and a stethoscope. There are various cuff sizes, as shown in Figure 8.13 ■. The cuff consists of an inflatable bladder, which is covered by cloth and has two tubes attached to it. One of these tubes ends in a rubber bulb with which to inflate the bladder. A small valve on the side of the bulb regulates air in the bladder. When the valve is loosened, air in the bladder is released. After the valve is tightened, pumped air remains in the bladder. The second tube attached to the bladder ends in a **sphygmomanometer**, a device that measures the air pressure in the bladder. Blood pressure is measured with an aneroid sphygmomanometer. The aneroid sphygmomanometer has a small, calibrated dial with a needle. The bladder of the blood pressure cuff must fit the length and width of the patient's limb. If the bladder is too narrow, the blood pressure reading will be falsely high (see Table 8.2). Conversely, if the bladder is too wide the blood pressure reading will be falsely low. The width of the bladder should equal 40% of the circumference of the limb. The length of the bladder should equal 80% of the circumference of the limb. This is important in accurate measurement of blood pressure in obese

Table 8.2 Selected Sources of Error in Blood Pressure Assessment

ERROR	EFFECT
Bladder cuff too narrow	Erroneously high
Bladder cuff too wide	Erroneously low
Arm unsupported	Erroneously high
Insufficient rest before the assessment	Erroneously high
Repeating assessment too quickly	Erroneously high systolic or low diastolic readings
Cuff wrapped too loosely or unevenly	Erroneously high
Deflating cuff too quickly	Erroneously low systolic and high diastolic readings
Deflating cuff too slowly	Erroneously high diastolic reading
Failure to use the same arm consistently	Inconsistent measurements
Arm above level of the heart	Erroneously low
Assessing immediately after a meal or while client smokes or has pain	Erroneously high
Failure to identify auscultatory gap	Erroneously low systolic pressure and erroneously low diastolic pressure

patients, who may require special cuffs. Note that the circumference of the patient's limb, and not the age of the patient, determines the cuff used. Automatic monitors can be used to measure blood pressure. These devices include a cuff attached to an electronic monitor. Application of the cuff is the same as in the manual method. The monitor provides a reading on an LCD of the systolic, diastolic, and mean blood pressures.

THE PROCEDURE Blood pressure measurements are usually taken by placing the cuff on the patient's arm and auscultating, or using the stethoscope to listen to the pulse in the brachial artery. Accuracy can be compromised by many factors (see the feature Evidence-Based Practice: Accuracy in Blood Pressure Measurement). The nurse must use common sense when choosing which arm to use for the measurement. For example, blood pressure should not be measured in an arm on the same side as a mastectomy or in an arm with a shunt. If blood pressure cannot be measured in either arm because of disease or trauma, a thigh blood pressure may be taken, using the popliteal artery, or a calf blood pressure may be taken, using the posterior tibial or dorsalis pedis arteries.

To measure the blood pressure in the patient's arm, the nurse follows these steps:

1. Place the patient in a comfortable position in a quiet room. Instruct the patient to not cross the legs during the procedure.

2. Confirm that the blood pressure cuff is the appropriate size for the patient's arm.

3. Remove any clothing from the patient's arm.

4. Slightly flex the arm and hold it at the level of the heart with the palm upward.

5. Palpate the brachial pulse.

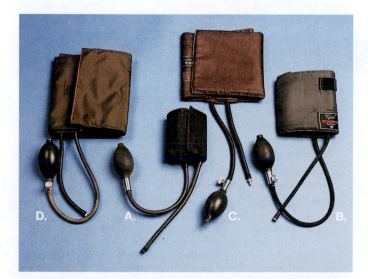

Figure 8.13 A variety of cuff sizes: A. a pediatric small cuff for a child; B. a small adult cuff for a frail adult or large child; C. a normal adult-size cuff; and D. a large cuff for use on the arm of an obese adult or the leg of an average-size adult.

6. Place the cuff on the arm with the lower border 1 inch above the antecubital area, making sure that the cuff is smooth and snug. One finger should fit between the cuff and the patient's arm. Be sure that the center of the bladder is over the brachial artery. Many cuffs have an arrow to indicate the center of the bladder, thus the part of the cuff to be over the artery.

7. Palpate the radial pulse.

8. Close the release valve on the pump.

9. Inflate the cuff until the radial pulse is no longer palpable and note the reading on the sphygmomanometer. Release the valve and rapidly deflate the cuff. Wait 15 to 30 seconds before proceeding to the next step. This is the palpatory systolic blood pressure.

10. Place the diaphragm of the stethoscope over the brachial pulse (see Figure 8.14 ■).

11. Pump up the cuff until the sphygmomanometer registers 30 mmHg above the palpatory systolic blood pressure (the point at which the radial pulse disappeared).

12. Release the valve on the cuff carefully so that the pressure decreases at the rate of 2 to 3 mmHg per second.

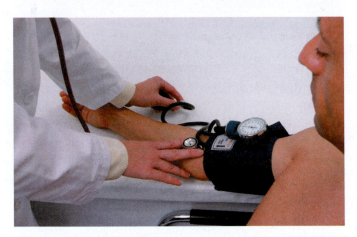

Figure 8.14 Measuring the patient's blood pressure.

13. Note the manometer reading at each of the five Korotkoff phases (see Box 8.2). The first sound is recorded as the systolic blood pressure, and the last sound is recorded as the diastolic blood pressure.

14. Deflate the cuff rapidly and completely.

15. Remove the cuff from the patient's arm.

Lifespan Considerations

The patient's age can impact the methods and equipment used to assess vital signs. The following sections address considerations the nurse should take into account when caring for patients throughout the lifespan. See Table 8.3 for an overview of normal ranges of vital signs based on age.

Temperature   Respirations and pulse rate are assessed before measuring rectal temperature in infants because taking a rectal temperature may cause an infant to cry. While holding the infant in a lateral position with the knees flexed onto the abdomen, or prone on the nurse's lap, the nurse separates the infant's buttocks with the nondominant hand and inserts the thermometer with the dominant gloved hand. The nurse should use a blunt-tipped thermometer, insert it no more than 2.5 cm, or 1 inch, and hold onto the exposed end. To avoid the risk of rectal perforation, an axillary temperature may be taken rather than a rectal temperature in newborns. The nurse also should take the axillary temperature in toddlers and older children whenever possible to eliminate their anxiety over the invasive rectal procedure. An oral route may be used as early as 5 years of age if the child is able to keep his or her mouth closed. Electronic thermometers, which are unbreakable and register quickly, are particularly useful with children.

Body temperature in the older adult may be reduced because of decreased thermoregulatory control and loss of subcutaneous fat. Older adults are more sensitive to environmental changes in temperature, possibly because of lack of physical activity, inadequate diet, or inability to afford adequate heating.

Pulse   The apical site is used for children younger than 2 years of age. In preschool children, the nurse uses the brachial site and

---

Box 8.2 Korotkoff Sounds

When measuring blood pressure, auscultate to identify the following five phases in a series of sounds called Korotkoff sounds, named after the Russian surgeon who first described them:

Phase 1: The period initiated by the first faint, clear, tapping sounds. These sounds gradually increase in intensity. Sounds heard during this phase correspond to appearance of a palpable pulse. To verify that they are not extraneous sounds, identify at least two consecutive tapping sounds.

Phase 2: The period during which the sounds become softer and longer; murmuring or swishing sounds are reflective of turbulent blood flow.

Phase 3: The period during which the sounds are crisper and louder; sounds have a rhythmic pattern.

Phase 4: Rhythmic sounds become muffled and have a soft, blowing quality.

Phase 5: The point at which the sounds disappear. The silence reflects the absence of pressure in the cuff. Normal blood flow is inaudible.

Document the blood pressure measurements as follows:

- The systolic pressure is the point at which the first tapping sound is heard (Phase 1).

- In adults, the diastolic pressure is the point at which the sounds become inaudible (Phase 5).

- In children, the diastolic pressure is the point at which the sounds become muffled (Phase 4).

- Older patients may have a wide pulse pressure. A pulse pressure is calculated by finding the difference between the systolic and diastolic pressures. In older patients with a wide pulse pressure, Korotkoff sounds may become inaudible between systolic and diastolic pressure and reappear as cuff deflation continues. This is known as auscultatory gap. This can often be eliminated by elevating the arm overhead for 30 seconds before inflating the cuff and bringing the arm to the usual position for continued measurement.

Table 8.3 Variations in Normal Ranges of Vital Signs by Age

AGE	PULSE	RESPIRATIONS	BLOOD PRESSURE SYSTOLIC	DIASTOLIC
Newborn	100–205 (awake) 90–160 (asleep)	30–80	60–76	31–45
Infant (1–12 months)	100–180 (awake) 90–160 (asleep)	30–53	72–104	37–56
1–2 years	98–140 (awake) 80–120 (asleep)	22–37	86–106	42–63
3–5 years	98–140 (awake) 80–120 (asleep)	22–34	89–112	46–72
6–12 years	70–120 (awake) 50–90 (asleep)	18–25	97–120	57–80
Adolescent	60–100	12–18	110–135	75–85
Adult	60–100	12–20	Less than 140	Less than 90
Older adult	60–100	15–20	Less than 150	Less than 90

Source: Based on Charbek, E. (2015). Normal vital signs. *Medscape,* updated August 27, 2015. Retrieved from https://emedicine.medscape.com/article/2172054-overview; and James, P. A., Oparil, S., Carter, B. L., Cushman, W. C., Dennison-Himmelfarb, C., Handler, J., . . . E. O. (2014). 2014 Evidence-Based Guideline for the Management of High Blood Pressure in Adults Report From the Panel Members Appointed to the Eighth Joint National Committee (JNC 8) [Abstract]. *JAMA, 311*(5), 507–520. doi:10.1001/jama.2013.284427

counts the pulse for a full minute. It is important to pay attention to any irregularities in rhythm, such as **sinus arrhythmia**, which is not uncommon in children. The pulse rate of the healthy older adult is in a range between 60 and 100 beats/min. The radial artery may feel rigid if there is loss of elasticity in the arterial walls.

Respirations The nurse should count respirations for 1 full minute in infants because the breathing pattern may show considerable variation. Infants have irregular breathing patterns characterized by frequent brief rate accelerations or decelerations. This is a normal variant that disappears during the first few months of life. The respiratory rate in older adults may be increased to accommodate a decrease in vital capacity and inspiratory reserve volume.

Table 8.4 shows the expected blood pressure goals for adults.

Table 8.4 Classification of Blood Pressure Goals for Adults 18 Years and Older

	SYSTOLIC		DIASTOLIC
18–59 years	Less than 140mm/Hg	and	Less than 90mm/Hg
60 YEARS			
Without diabetes, renal disease, or other comorbidities	Less than 150 mmHg	and	Less than 90mm/Hg
With diabetes, renal disease, or other comorbidities	Less than 140 mmHg	and	Less than 90mm/Hg

Sources: Seckel, M. A., Bradley, E. G., & Thompson, H. (2016). Obtaining accurate noninvasive blood pressure measurements in adults. *Critical Care Nurse, 36*(3), E12–E16. http://dx.doi.org/10.4037/ccn2016590; James, P. A., Oparil, S., Carter, B. L., Cushman, W. C., Dennison-Himmelfarb, C., Handler, J., . . . Ortiz, E. (2014). 2014 Evidence-based guideline for the management of high blood pressure in adults: Report from the panel members appointed to the Eighth Joint National Committee (JNC 8) [Abstract]. *Journal of the American Medical Association, 311* (5), 507–520. doi:10.1001/jama.2013.284427; Burton, M. A., & Ludwig, L. J. M. (2014). *Fundamentals of nursing care: Concepts, connections & skills,* 2nd ed.). Philadelphia, PA: F. A. Davis.

The Functional Assessment as Part of the General Survey

Nurses use their observational skills in many situations. When making observations, nurses are continually thinking about the data and using their knowledge of the physical, behavioral, and

Evidence-Based Practice
Accuracy in Blood Pressure Measurement

- The patient's arm position is important to ensure accurate blood pressure measurement. If the arm is above the level of the heart, the blood pressure will be lower than the actual. If the arm is below the heart, the blood pressure will be higher than the actual (Seckel, Bradley, & Thompson, 2016).
- Overall systolic blood pressures tend to be higher in the calf than in the arm; thus, calf blood pressures should be only used if the arm is not accessible (Seckel et al., 2015).
- When the blood pressure is checked while the patient is sitting up or standing, the arm must be supported and held horizontally to the level of the heart to achieve the most accurate blood pressure reading. If the arm is left hanging down or resting on the armrest of the chair, the blood pressure will be up to 10 mmHg higher or, in patients with hypertension, up to 20 mmHg higher (Rauen, Chulay, Bridges, Vollman, & Arbour, 2008).

social sciences to interpret the findings. The findings are interpreted according to the expected norms for patients in relation to age, sex, race, development, and culture.

Functional Assessment During the General Survey

The **functional assessment** is an observation to gather data while the patient is performing common or routine activities. During the general survey of a healthy patient, the nurse will observe the patient while performing the following common activities: walking into the examination room, taking a seat for the interview, and moving the arms and hands to arrange clothing or to shake hands as an introduction. The nurse will also observe the facial expression while these acts occur. From this brief encounter, the nurse applies knowledge to begin to gather and interpret data about the patient's mobility and strength as well as the symmetry of the face and parts of the body.

Critical Thinking

When applying the critical thinking process, the professional nurse uses a variety of skills that culminate in assisting patients to make healthcare decisions.

The following case study and analysis is presented to demonstrate the application of critical thinking in the functional assessment of a patient as part of the general survey.

The nurse conducted a comprehensive health assessment of a 21-year-old African American male who was new to the clinic. The interaction began when the nurse went to the waiting area to bring the patient to the interview area. The following occurred: As the nurse entered the waiting area, all of the patients looked up. The nurse called out "Jason C." and looked about the room. An African American male wearing a local college football jersey said, "That's me." The man rose quickly, pushing himself up with his hands placed on the arms of the chair. Upon standing, he grimaced slightly. The patient demonstrated a slight limp and appeared to be bearing only partial weight on his right leg. As the patient approached, the nurse noted that he had smooth skin on his face and hands. He was approximately 6'2" and muscular. As he moved through the door, he stated, "Just tell me I didn't tear anything in my knee that's going to need surgery."

As stated previously in this chapter, the general survey begins with the initial encounter with the patient and provides cues about the patient. The observations from this brief case study include the following:

- All of the patients looked up when the nurse entered the waiting area.
- When a name was called, a young adult African American male wearing a local college football jersey responded.
- The young man rose quickly.
- The young man used his arms to push himself out of the chair.
- The young man grimaced slightly upon standing.
- The young man had smooth skin on his face and hands.
- The young man was approximately 6'2" tall and was muscular.
- He walked with a slight limp.
- He appeared to be bearing only partial weight on his right leg.

- As he entered the exam area, he stated, "Just tell me I didn't tear anything in my knee that's going to need surgery."

In applying critical thinking, the nurse will begin to sort information and determine an approach to continue data gathering. The nurse considers each of the observations in terms of normal and abnormal findings in relation to the age, sex, race, and culture of the patient. Interpretations of the nurse's observations in this case study are as follows:

- All the patients looked up when the nurse entered the room.
  The patient was aware that someone entered the room; this indicates that his vision and hearing are intact. This is considered a normal finding.
- The patient responded when his name was called.
  This is further indication that hearing is intact. This is a normal finding.
- The patient rose quickly.
  This is an expected finding in a young adult because of good muscle tone and strength.
- The patient used his arms to push himself out of the chair.
  This is an indication of diminished strength or mobility in one or both lower extremities. This is an unexpected finding in a young adult because of increased muscle tone and strength. This requires follow-up to determine the actual muscle strength of the patient.
- The patient grimaced upon standing.
  This indicates discomfort. This is initially interpreted as an abnormal finding. Discomfort is indicative of an underlying problem. In this case, the problem may be musculoskeletal.
- The patient had smooth skin on his face and hands.
  This finding suggests that the patient is in a state of fluid and nutritional balance and that he follows hygiene practices. This has the suggestion of being a normal finding. However, the nurse will consider other factors during the assessment.
- The patient was approximately 6'2" tall and was muscular.
  Increased muscular tone may be a normal finding among young adults. Additionally, the nurse recognizes that the young man is wearing a football jersey from a local college, which suggests he may be a college athlete.
- The patient limped and appeared to be bearing only partial weight on his right leg.
  This is an abnormal finding. The nurse must explore the underlying cause. This is suggestive of a musculoskeletal problem.
- As he entered the exam area, he stated, "Just tell me I didn't tear anything in my knee that's going to need surgery."
  This response indicates the patient's concern regarding an injury. The statements are not unexpected in relation to observations about the movements and gait of the patient. This statement forces the nurse to make a rapid decision about the process of the health assessment. The nurse must quickly gather more data to determine the patient's ability to participate in all aspects of the assessment.

The preceding analyses demonstrate that a great deal of information can be obtained through observation. In this situation much information is missing. As this information is gathered, the nurse will determine the relevance of each piece of data to the overall situation. The nurse applies critical thinking throughout the comprehensive health assessment while working with the patient to meet health-related needs.

CASE STUDY

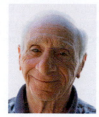

Source: Bloom Productions/ Digital Vision/Getty Images.

It is a Friday morning. You are the nurse who is conducting a physical examination of Joseph Miller, a 73-year-old Caucasian male. You begin with a patient interview during which the following occurs.

The patient enters the room, looks right at you, smiles, and states, "How do you do?" in a clear voice. When you introduce yourself, he gives you a firm handshake, then holds both of your hands in his and comments, "Boy, you sure have cold hands." He walks steadily to the chair you indicate but holds onto the desk while getting seated. You inform the patient of the purpose of the interview. He denies any specific complaints or problems when asked. He then shrugs his shoulders and comments, "I don't think I have anything special going on. I'm here for my three-month check, and I expect to get a clean bill of health." You ask him to sign an admission form. He puts on reading glasses, peruses the form, and signs it.

When asked about current medications, the patient states, "I have them with me, let me show you." He then takes out three medicine bottles. He reads each label and comments as follows about each: "This is Pardivil, it's for my blood pressure; this one is ferrous sulfate, that's iron, I have some anemia; this last one is Digit, I take it every other day for my heart." He frowns and says, "This bottle is nearly empty." After opening the bottle and looking at the contents, he says, "Yup, just as I thought, I only have three pills left, so I'll have to fill it. I'll be out of pills by Thursday, and the drugstore is always packed just before the weekend." You continue the interview and conclude it by telling the patient you are going to check his blood pressure, pulse, temperature, and weight before escorting him to the examination room.

CRITICAL THINKING QUESTIONS

1. What are the findings from the case study for Mr. Miller?

2. How would you interpret the findings in relation to the categories for observation in the general survey?

3. Which findings indicate the need for follow-up in the interview or physical assessment?

4. What factors must be considered when evaluating the vital signs assessment for Mr. Miller?

5. What psychosocial factors (if noted) would indicate further follow-up is needed?

REFERENCES

Allegaert, K., Casteels, K., Gorp, I., & Bogaert, G. (2014). Tympanic, infrared skin, and temporal artery scan thermometers compared with rectal measurement in children: A real-life assessment. *Current Therapeutic Research, 76,* 34–38.

Anson, P. (2016). AMA drops the pain as the fifth vital sign. Retrieved from https://www.painnewsnetwork.org/ stories/2016/6/16/ama-drops-pain-as-vital-sign

Baker, D. (2016). Joint Commission statement on pain management. Retrieved from https://www.jointcommission.org/ joint_commission_statement_on_pain_management

Barry, L., Branco, J., Kargbo, N., Venuto, C., Werfel, E., Barto, D., & Glasofer, A. (2016). The impact of user technique on temporal artery thermometer measurements. *Nursing 2016 Critical Care, 11*(5), 12–14.

Batra, P., & Goyal, S. (2013). Temporal artery thermometers may rival rectal thermometers in ED. *Pediatric Emergency Care, 29,* 63–66.

Benjamin, E., Blaha, M., Chiuve, S., Cushman, M., Das, S., Deo, R., . . . & Muntner, P. (2017). Heart disease and stroke statistics—2017 update: A report from the American Heart Association. *Circulation, 135,* e6–e458. Retrieved from http://circ.ahajournals.org/content/early/2017/01/25/ CIR.0000000000000485.citation

Burton, M. A., & Ludwig, L. J. M. (2014). *Fundamentals of nursing care: Concepts, connections & skills,* 2nd ed. Philadelphia, PA: F. A. Davis

Byers, D., France, N., & Kuiper, B. (2014, June). Measuring height and weight: From research to policy. *Nursing 2014,* 19–21. doi:10.1097/01.NURSE.0000444726.83265.c6

Campbell, J. (2016). The fifth vital sign revisited. *Pain, 157*(1), 3–4.

Centers for Disease Control and Prevention. (2001). Data table of infant head circumference-for-age charts. Retrieved from https://www.cdc.gov/growthcharts/html_charts/hcageinf .htm

Charbek, E. (2015). *Normal vital signs.* Medscape. Retrieved from https://emedicine.medscape.com/article/2172054-overview

Cretikos, M. A., Bellomo, R., Hillman, K., Chen, J., Finfer, S., & Flabouris, A. (2008) Respirator rate: The neglected vital sign. *Medical Journal of Australia, 188*(11): 657–659.

Fahy, B., Lareau, S., & Sockrider, M. (2013) Patient information series: Pulse oximetry. American Thoracic Society. Retrieved from www.thoracic.org/patients/patientresources/ resources/pulse-oximetry.pdf

Greenwell, S. (2015). My pain – the 5th vital sign. *Family Doctor, 3*(3), 28–30.

Hollerbach, A., & Sneed, N. (1990). Accuracy of radial pulse assessment by length of counting interval. *Heart and Lung: Journal of Critical Care, 19*(3), 258–264.

James, P. A., Oparil, S., Carter, B. L., Cushman, W. C., Dennison-Himmelfarb, C., Handler, J., . . . Ortiz, E. (2014). 2014 Evidence-based guideline for the management of high blood pressure in adults: Report from the panel members appointed to the Eighth Joint National Committee (JNC 8) [Abstract]. *Journal of the American Medical Association, 311*(5), 507–520. doi:10.1001/jama.2013.284427

Johnstone, M. (2017). Comparison of level of agreement for 3 temperature-measurement devices and methods. Presented at the AACN National Teaching Institute in Houston, Texas, May 22–25, 2017. 2017 National Teaching Institute Research Abstracts.

Kellett, J., Li, M., Rasool, S., Green, G., & Seely, A. (2011). Comparison of the heart and breathing rate of acutely ill medical patients recorded by nursing staff with those measured over 5 min by a piezoelectric belt and ECG monitor at the time of admission to hospital. *Resuscitation, 82*, (11), 1381–1386.

Kemp, C. (2013). Temporal artery thermometers may rival rectal thermometers in ED. *AAP News, 34*(4), 2.

London, M. L., Ladewig, P. A. W., Davidson, M. R., Ball, J. W., Bindler, R. C., & Cowen, K. J. (2014). *Maternal & child nursing care* (4th ed.). Upper Saddle River, NJ: Pearson.

Mason, T., Boubekri, A., Lalau, J., Patterson, A., Hartranft, S., & Sutton, S. (2017). Equivalence study of two temperature-measurement methods in febrile adult patient with cancer. *Oncology Nursing Forum, 44*(2), E82–E87.

Opio, M., & Kellett, J. (2017). How well are pulses measured? Practice-based evidence from an observational study of acutely ill medical patients during hospital admission. *The American Journal of Medicine, 130*, 863.e13–863.e16.

Osborn K. S., Wraa, C. E., Watson, A., & Holleran, R. S. (2014). *Medical-surgical nursing: Preparation for practice* (2nd ed.). Upper Saddle River, NJ: Pearson.

Purser, L., Warfield, K., & Richardson, C. (2014). Making pain visible: An audit and review of documentation to improve the use of pain assessment by implementing pain as the fifth vital sign. *Pain Management Nursing, 15*(1), 137–142.

Rauen, C., Chulay, M., Bridges, E., Vollman, K., & Arbour, R. (2008). Seven evidence-based habits: Putting some cows out to pasture. *Critical Care Nurse, 28*(2), 98–124.

Reynolds, M., Bonham, L., Gueck, M., Hammond, K., Lowery, J., Redel, C., . . . Craft, M. (2014). Are temporal artery temperatures accurate enough to replace rectal temperature measurement in pediatric ED patients? *Journal of Emergency Nursing, 40*(1), 46–50.

Ross, P., Newth, C., & Khemani, R. (2014). Accuracy of pulse oximetry in children. *Pediatrics 133*(1), 22–29.

Rush University Medical Center. (n.d.). *What is a healthy weight?* Retrieved from http://www.rush.edu/rumc/page-110804810 3230.html

Salota, V., Slovakova, Z., Panes, C., Nundlall, A., & Goonasekera, C. (2016). Is postoperative tympanic membrane temperature measurement effective? *British Journal of Nursing, 25*(9), 490–493.

Scher, C., Meador, L., Van Cleave, J., & Reid, M. (2018, April). Moving beyond pain as the fifth vital sign and patient satisfaction scores to improve pain care in the 21st century. *Pain Management Nursing, 19*(2), 125–129. https://doi.org/10.1016/j.pmn.2017.10.010

Seckel, M. A., Bradley, E. G., & Thompson, H. (2016). Obtaining accurate noninvasive blood pressure measurements in adults. *Critical Care Nurse, 36*(3), E12–E16. Retrieved from http://dx.doi.org/10.4037/ccn2016590

U.S. Environmental Protection Agency (EPA). (2014). *Phase-out of mercury thermometers used in industrial and laboratory settings.* Retrieved from http://www.epa.gov/mercury/thermometer.htm

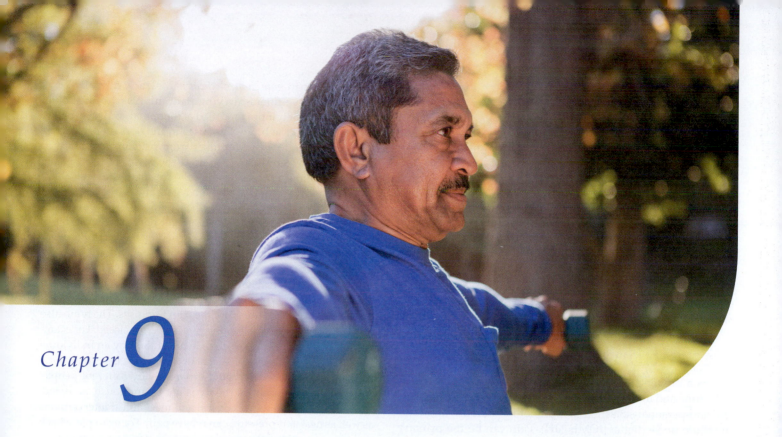

Chapter 9

Pain Assessment

LEARNING OUTCOMES

Upon completion of this chapter, you will be able to:

1. Define pain.

2. Outline the physiologic process involved in the perception of pain.

3. Discuss the nature of pain, including types and other concepts related to pain.

4. Examine factors that influence perception and expression of pain.

5. Demonstrate techniques and tools used for assessment of pain.

KEY TERMS

acute pain, 116
chronic pain, 116
cutaneous pain, 116
deep somatic pain, 116
hyperalgesia, 118

intractable pain, 117
neuropathic pain, 117
nociception, 115
nociceptors, 115
pain, 114

pain rating scales, 122
pain reaction, 118
pain sensation, 118
pain threshold, 118
pain tolerance, 118

phantom pain, 117
radiating pain, 116
referred pain, 117
visceral pain, 116

MEDICAL LANGUAGE

-algesia Suffix meaning "sensitivity to pain"

-algia Suffix meaning "pain"

hyper- Prefix meaning "high," "elevated," "above normal"

neur- Prefix meaning "nerve"

psych Root word meaning "mind"

somat- Prefix meaning "body"

Introduction

Pain comes from the Greek word *poinē* meaning "penalty," implying the person is paying for something. It is a highly unpleasant sensation that affects a person's physical health, emotional health, and well-being. Pain assessment, treatment, and relief present one of the greatest challenges to the nurse and other members of the healthcare team. The nurse has a primary role regarding the collection and analysis of data, the implementation of treatment modalities, and the evaluation of the patient regarding pain experiences.

Pain assessment requires a strong knowledge base regarding the concept of pain and methods used to collect information about the pain experience. Accurate assessment of pain is essential to developing, monitoring, and evaluating the effectiveness of pain relief interventions.

Definition of Pain

Pain is a universal experience, meaning everyone has pain at some time and to some degree. It is a highly subjective, unpleasant, and personal sensation that cannot be shared with others (Institute of Medicine [IOM], 2011). Pain can be the primary problem or be associated with a specific diagnosis, treatment, or procedure. A widely accepted definition of this phenomenon by the International Association for the Study of Pain (IASP) is that **pain** is "an unpleasant sensory and emotional experience associated with actual or potential tissue damage, or described in terms of such damage" (IASP, 1994, p. 210).

No two people experience pain in the same manner. It can occupy all of a person's thinking, force changes in the ability to function on a daily basis, and produce changes in the individual's life. For the patient, it is a difficult concept to describe, thus making pain treatment and relief most difficult. The nurse cannot see or feel the pain being experienced by the patient; however, the effects produced by the pain will be assessed. These changes can be physiologic, psychologic, and behavioral in nature.

Physiology of Pain

Pain is a complex and multidimensional phenomenon that is not clearly understood. Theories have been developed to explain the conceptual and physiologic aspects of pain.

Theories of Pain

Among the theories of pain are the specificity theory, pattern theory, and gate control theory.

The *specificity theory* explains the complexity of pain. This theory contends that pain neurons are as specific and unique as other specific neurons (e.g., taste, smell) in the body. The special pain neurons transport the sensation to the brain for interpretation. The transport occurs in a straight line to the brain, making the pain equal to the injury. This theory does not include a consideration of any psychologic component to pain.

The *pattern theory* maintains that individuals will respond in a different manner to a similar stimulus. This theory implies that the pattern of the stimulus is more important than the specific stimulus. It does not take into consideration the psychosocial component to pain.

According to *gate control theory* (Melzack & Wall, 1965), peripheral nerve fibers carrying pain impulses to the spinal cord can have their input modified at the spinal cord level before transmission to the brain. Synapses in the dorsal horns act as gates that close to keep impulses from reaching the brain or open to permit impulses to ascend to the brain.

In application of the gate control theory, small-diameter nerve fibers carry pain impulses through a gate and, ultimately, to the brain. However, according to this theory, impulses that are simultaneously transmitted by large-diameter nerve fibers can block transmission of the pain impulses carried by the small-diameter nerve fibers—that is, they close the gate (see Figure 9.1 ■). The gate mechanism is thought to be situated in the substantia gelatinosa cells in the dorsal horn of the spinal cord. Because a limited amount of sensory information can reach the brain at any given time, certain cells can interrupt the pain impulses. The brain also appears to influence whether the gate is open or closed. For example, previous experiences with pain affect the way an individual responds to pain. The involvement of the brain helps explain why painful stimuli are interpreted differently by different people. Although the gate control theory is not unanimously accepted, it does help explain why electrical and mechanical interventions as well as heat and pressure can relieve pain. For example, a back massage may stimulate impulses in large nerves, which in turn close the gate to back pain.

Nervous System

The nervous system must receive and interpret a stimulus to allow the individual to recognize the pain process. How pain is transmitted and perceived is not completely understood. Whether pain is perceived and to what degree depends on the interaction between the body's analgesia system and the nervous system's transmission and interpretation of stimuli.

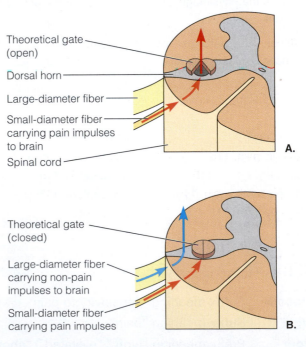

Theoretical gate (open)
Dorsal horn
Large-diameter fiber
Small-diameter fiber carrying pain impulses to brain
Spinal cord

A.

Theoretical gate (closed)
Large-diameter fiber carrying non-pain impulses to brain
Small-diameter fiber carrying pain impulses

B.

Figure 9.1 Gate control theory: A. open gate, B. closed gate.

Nociception The peripheral nervous system includes primary sensory neurons specialized to detect tissue damage and to evoke the sensations of touch, heat, cold, pain, and pressure. The receptors that transmit pain sensation are called **nociceptors**. These pain receptors or nociceptors can be excited by mechanical, thermal, or chemical stimuli (see Table 9.1). The physiologic processes related to pain perception are described as **nociception**. The processes involved in nociception include transduction, transmission, perception, and modulation (Paice, 2002).

TRANSDUCTION During the transduction process, biochemical mediator release is triggered by injury to the tissues. These biochemical mediators—such as prostaglandins, bradykinin, serotonin, histamine, and substance P—sensitize the nociceptors. Painful or noxious stimulation also causes ions to move across cellular membranes, which leads to excitement of the nociceptors. Pain medications, or analgesics, act during the transduction process by inhibiting the synthesis of prostaglandin (e.g., nonsteroidal anti-inflammatory medications, such as ibuprofen) or by decreasing the movement of ions across the cellular membrane (e.g., local anesthetic agents) (Berman & Snyder, 2016).

TRANSMISSION Pain transmission, which is the second process involved in nociception, incorporates three phases (McCaffery & Pasero, 1999). During the first phase, the pain impulse is transmitted from the peripheral nerve fibers to the spinal cord. At this point, substance P functions as a neurotransmitter, promoting the movement of impulses across the nerve synapse from the primary afferent neuron to the second-order neuron in the dorsal horn of the spinal cord (see Figure 9.2 ■). Transmission of the pain impulse to the dorsal horn of the spinal cord involves two types of nociceptive fibers: A-delta fibers, which transmit localized, sharp pain; and C fibers, which transmit dull, aching pain. During phase two of transmission, the pain impulse travels from the spinal cord and ascends via spinothalamic tracts to the brainstem and thalamus (see Figure 9.3 ■). In phase three of transmission, signals are transmitted between the thalamus and the somatic sensory cortex, which is the site of pain perception (Berman & Snyder, 2016).

Pain control can take place during the transmission process. For example, opioids (narcotic analgesics) inhibit the release of certain neurotransmitters, particularly substance P, thus blocking pain at the spinal level.

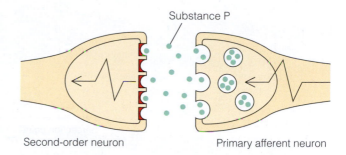

Figure 9.2 Substance P assists the transmission of impulses across the synapse from the primary afferent neuron to a second-order neuron in the spinothalamic tract.

PERCEPTION During perception, which is the third process, the patient becomes aware of the pain. Pain perception is believed to occur in the cortical structures, which allows for different cognitive-behavioral strategies to be applied to reduce the sensory and affective components of pain (McCaffery & Pasero, 1999). For example, nonpharmacologic interventions such as distraction, guided imagery, and music can help direct the patient's attention away from the pain (Berman & Snyder, 2016).

MODULATION The fourth process, modulation, is commonly referred to as the descending system. During modulation, neurons in the brainstem transmit signals back to the dorsal horn of the spinal cord (Paice, 2002). At this point, these descending fibers release substances that can block the ascending painful impulses in the dorsal horn—for example, endogenous opioids, serotonin, and norepinephrine may be released. Because these neurotransmitters undergo reuptake, during which they are taken back by the body, their analgesic effectiveness is limited (McCaffery & Pasero, 1999). Patients with chronic pain may be prescribed tricyclic antidepressants, which inhibit the reuptake of norepinephrine and serotonin. This action increases the modulation phase that helps inhibit painful ascending stimuli (Berman & Snyder, 2016).

Responses to Pain The pain response is complex and incorporates both physiologic and psychosocial aspects. Initially, sympathetic nervous system stimulation triggers the fight-or-flight response. Eventually, as the body adapts to the pain, the

Table 9.1 Types of Pain Stimuli

STIMULUS TYPE	PHYSIOLOGIC BASIS OF PAIN
Mechanical	
1. Trauma to body tissues (e.g., surgery)	Tissue damage; direct irritation of the pain receptors; inflammation
2. Alterations in body tissues (e.g., edema)	Pressure on pain receptors
3. Blockage of a body duct	Distention of the lumen of the duct
4. Tumor	Pressure on pain receptors; irritation of nerve endings
5. Muscle spasm	Stimulation of pain receptors (also see chemical stimuli)
Thermal	
1. Extreme heat (e.g., burns)	Tissue destruction; stimulation of thermosensitive pain receptors
2. Extreme cold (e.g., frostbite)	
Chemical	
1. Tissue ischemia (e.g., blocked coronary artery)	Stimulation of pain receptors because of accumulated lactic acid (and other chemicals, such as bradykinin and enzymes) in tissues
2. Muscle spasm	Tissue ischemia secondary to mechanical stimulation (see above)

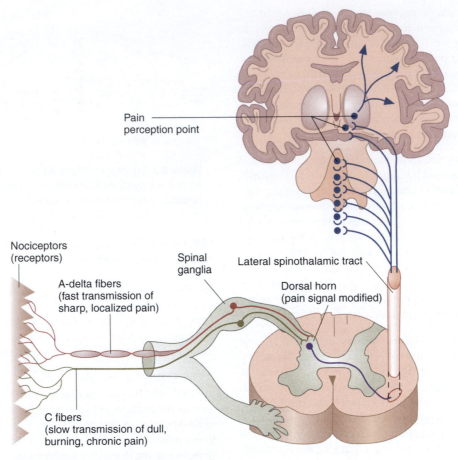

Pain perception point

Nociceptors (receptors)

A-delta fibers (fast transmission of sharp, localized pain)

Spinal ganglia

Lateral spinothalamic tract

Dorsal horn (pain signal modified)

C fibers (slow transmission of dull, burning, chronic pain)

Figure 9.3 Physiology of pain perception.

parasympathetic nervous system takes over, reversing many of the initial physiologic responses. This adaptation to pain occurs after several hours or days of pain. The actual pain receptors adapt very little and continue to transmit the pain message. The person may learn to cope through cognitive and behavioral activities, such as diversions, imagery, and excessive sleeping. The individual may seek out physical interventions to manage the pain, such as analgesics, massage, and exercise.

A proprioceptive reflex also occurs with the stimulation of pain receptors. Impulses travel along sensory pain fibers to the spinal cord. There they synapse with motor neurons, and the impulses travel back via motor fibers to a muscle near the site of the pain (see Figure 9.4 ■). The muscle then contracts in a protective action—for example, when a person touches a hot stove, the hand reflexively draws back from the heat even before the person is aware of the pain.

Nature of Pain

Pain, which is a subjective and personal experience, can be described in many ways. The nurse and other members of the healthcare team may use both the type of pain and the concepts associated with pain to elicit descriptions of pain.

Types of Pain

Pain may be described in terms of duration, location, and etiology. When pain lasts only through the expected recovery period from illness, injury, or surgery, it is described as **acute pain**, whether it has a sudden or slow onset and regardless of the intensity. Depending on the patient's condition, acute pain may last for a few minutes up to several weeks, but usually it does not last longer than 6 months. **Chronic pain** is prolonged, usually recurring or persisting over 6 months or longer, and it interferes with functioning. Chronic pain can be further classified as chronic malignant (or cancer) pain, when associated with cancer or other life-threatening conditions, or as chronic nonmalignant pain, when the etiology is a nonprogressive disorder (American Pain Society, 2016). Such disorders include cluster headaches, low back pain, and myofascial pain dysfunction. Acute pain and chronic pain result in different physiologic and behavioral responses, as shown in Table 9.2.

Pain may be categorized according to its origin as cutaneous, deep somatic, or visceral. **Cutaneous pain** originates in the skin or subcutaneous tissue. A paper cut causing a sharp pain with some burning is an example of cutaneous pain. **Deep somatic pain** arises from ligaments, tendons, bones, blood vessels, and nerves. It is diffuse and tends to last longer than cutaneous pain. An ankle sprain is an example of deep somatic pain. **Visceral pain** results from stimulation of pain receptors in the abdominal cavity, cranium, and thorax. It tends to appear diffuse and often feels like deep somatic pain—that is, burning, aching, or a feeling of pressure. Visceral pain is frequently caused by stretching of the tissues, ischemia, or muscle spasms—for example, an obstructed bowel will result in visceral pain.

Pain may also be described according to where it is experienced in the body. **Radiating pain** is perceived at the source

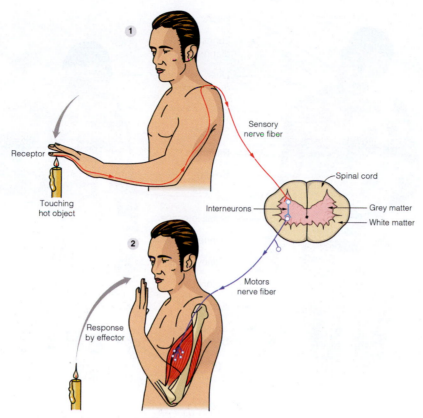

Figure 9.4 Proprioceptive reflex to a pain stimulus.
Source: lukaves/123RF.

Table 9.2 Comparison of Acute and Chronic Pain

ACUTE PAIN	CHRONIC PAIN
Mild to severe	Mild to severe

Sympathetic nervous system responses:
  Increased pulse rate
  Increased respiratory rate
  Elevated blood pressure
  Diaphoresis
  Dilated pupils
	Parasympathetic nervous system responses:
	  Vital signs normal
	
	  Dry, warm skin
	  Pupils normal or dilated

Related to tissue injury; resolves with healing	Continues beyond healing
Patient appears restless and anxious	Patient appears depressed and withdrawn
Patient reports pain	Patient often does not mention pain unless asked
Patient exhibits behavior indicative of pain: crying, rubbing area, holding area	Pain behavior often absent

of the pain and extends to nearby tissues. For example, cardiac pain may be felt not only in the chest but also along the left shoulder and down the arm. **Referred pain** is felt in a part of the body that is considerably removed from the tissues causing the pain. For example, pain from one part of the abdominal viscera may be perceived in an area of the skin remote from the organ causing the pain (see Figure 9.5 ■)

Intractable pain is highly resistant to relief. One example is the pain from an advanced malignancy. When caring for a patient experiencing intractable pain, nurses are challenged to use a number of methods, pharmacologic and nonpharmacologic, to provide pain relief.

Neuropathic pain is the result of current or past damage to the peripheral or central nervous system and may not have a stimulus, such as tissue or nerve damage, for the pain. Neuropathic pain is long lasting, is unpleasant, and can be described as burning, dull, and aching. Episodes of sharp, shooting pain can also be experienced (Sadosky, Hopper, & Parsons, 2014). Examples of this pain include trigeminal neuralgia and peripheral neuropathy.

Phantom pain, which is perceived in a body part that is missing (e.g., an amputated leg) or that is paralyzed by a spinal cord injury, is an example of neuropathic pain. This can be distinguished from phantom sensation—that is, the feeling that

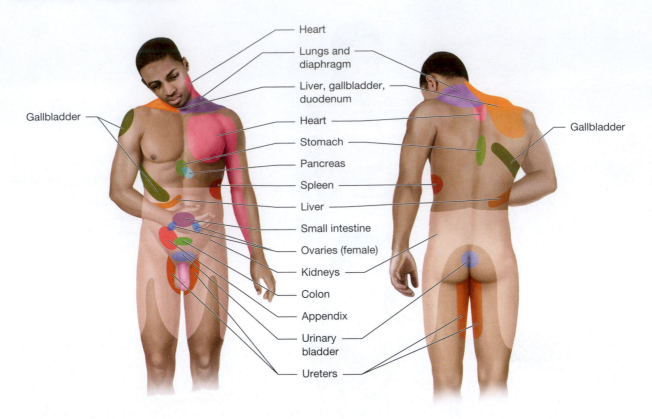

Figure 9.5 Sites of referred pain.

---

the missing body part is still present. The incidence of phantom pain can be reduced when analgesics are administered via epidural catheter before an amputation.

Concepts Associated with Pain

When a person perceives pain from injured tissue, the pain threshold is reached. An individual's **pain threshold** is the amount of pain stimulation the person requires to feel pain. A person's pain threshold is fairly uniform; however, it can change. For example, the same stimuli that once produced mild pain can at another time produce intense pain. Excessive sensitivity to pain is called **hyperalgesia**.

Two additional terms used in the context of pain are *pain sensation* and *pain reaction*. **Pain sensation** can be considered the same as pain threshold; **pain reaction** includes the autonomic nervous system and behavioral responses to pain. The autonomic nervous system response is the automatic reaction that often protects the individual from further harm—for example, the automatic withdrawal of the hand from a hot stove. The behavioral response is a learned response used as a method of coping with pain.

Pain tolerance is the maximum amount and duration of pain that an individual is willing to endure. Some patients are unable to tolerate even the slightest pain, whereas others are willing to endure severe pain rather than be treated for it. Pain tolerance is widely influenced by psychological and sociocultural factors. According to current research, many studies suggest that there are sex differences with pain (Bartley & Fillingim, 2013). Although more research needs to be conducted to determine the extent of the differences, women tend to experience more chronic and clinical pain and demonstrate higher levels of pain

sensitivity when compared with males. According to a National Health Interview Survey, 2010–2011 (Centers for Disease Control and Prevention [CDC], 2013), of all individuals 18 and older who were surveyed, 20.7% of women reported having pain within the last 3 months, whereas only 16.9% of men reported pain during the same period of time. Sex-based cultural influences may also shape an individual's expression of pain.

Factors Influencing Pain

Many factors influence perception of and reaction to pain (IOM, 2011). These factors include lifespan considerations, race, ethnicity, sex, and culture, as well as various aspects of the environment.

Lifespan Considerations

The age and developmental stage of a patient will influence both the reaction to and the expression of pain. (See the Evidence-Based Practice feature, Pain Assessment and Response.) The expression of pain may also be influenced by past experience. Age variations and related nursing interventions are presented in Table 9.3.

The field of pain management for infants and children has grown significantly. It is now accepted that anatomic, physiologic, and biochemical elements necessary for pain transmission are present in newborns, regardless of their gestational age. Harrison, Bueno, & Reszel (2015) recommend that environmental, nonpharmacologic, and pharmacologic interventions be used to prevent, reduce, or eliminate pain in neonates. Physiologic indicators may vary in infants, so behavioral observation is recommended for pain assessment (Ball, Bindler, Cowen, &

Table 9.3 Lifespan Considerations Related to the Pain Experience

AGE GROUP	PAIN PERCEPTION AND BEHAVIOR	SELECTED NURSING INTERVENTIONS
Infant	Perceives pain Responds to pain with increased sensitivity Older infant tries to avoid pain—for example, turns away and physically resists	Give a glucose pacifier. Use tactile stimulation. Play music or tapes of a heartbeat.
Toddler and Preschooler	Develops the ability to describe pain and its intensity and location Often responds with crying and anger because child perceives pain as a threat to security Reasoning with child at this stage not always successful May consider pain a punishment Feels sad May learn there are gender differences in pain expression Tends to hold someone accountable for the pain	Distract the child with toys, books, pictures. Involve the child in blowing bubbles as a way of "blowing away the pain." Appeal to the child's belief in magic by using a "magic" blanket or glove to take away pain. Hold the child to provide comfort. Explore misconceptions about pain.
School-age Child	Tries to be brave when facing pain Rationalizes in an attempt to explain the pain Responsive to explanations Can usually identify the location and describe the pain With persistent pain, may regress to an earlier stage of development	Use imagery to turn off "pain switches." Provide a behavioral rehearsal of what to expect and how it will look and feel. Provide support and nurturing.
Adolescent	May be slow to acknowledge pain Recognizing pain or "giving in" may be considered weakness Wants to appear brave in front of peers and not report pain	Provide opportunities to discuss pain. Provide privacy. Present choices for dealing with pain. Encourage music or TV for distraction.
Adult	May exhibit gender-based behaviors learned as a child May ignore pain because to admit it is perceived as a sign of weakness or failure May not take action because of fear of what the pain may indicate	Deal with any misconceptions about pain. Focus on the patient's control in dealing with the pain. Allay fears and anxiety when possible.
Older Adult	May have multiple conditions presenting with vague symptoms May perceive pain as part of the aging process May have decreased sensations or perceptions of the pain May exhibit such indicators of pain as lethargy, anorexia, and fatigue May withhold complaints of pain because of fear of the treatment, fear of any lifestyle changes that may be involved, or fear of becoming dependent May describe pain differently—that is, as "ache," "hurt," or "discomfort" May consider it unacceptable to admit or show pain	Thorough history and assessment are essential. Spend time with the patient and listen carefully. Clarify misconceptions. Encourage independence whenever possible.

Shaw, 2017). Children may be less able than an adult to articulate their experience or needs related to pain, which may result in their pain being undertreated. When interpreting pediatric complaints, the nurse should take into consideration reports from parents or caregivers, the child's developmental stage, and psychosocial factors, such as the following:

- Small children commonly will complain of a "tummy ache" or "my throat hurts," whereas parents may be concerned about fussiness or altered sleep patterns.
- Preadolescent children will complain of stomach pain when they are gassy, if they are nauseated, or if they actually feel abdominal pain.
- Children with sore throats often present with a history of normal fluid intake but decreased solid food intake.
- Anxious or frightened preschool and school-age children may complain of headache or stomachache.

Older adults constitute a major portion of the individuals within the healthcare system. The prevalence of pain in the older population is generally higher because of both acute and chronic disease conditions. However, pain is often underassessed and undertreated for a variety of reasons, including difficulty accessing care to report pain, misconceptions about the aging process, and patient reluctance to report pain because of the stigma surrounding pain and the treatment of pain (Denny & Guido, 2012). Therefore, it is essential for nurses to ensure adequate assessment of pain and educate patients regarding pain treatment. Although pain threshold does not appear to change with aging, the effect of analgesics may increase because of physiologic changes related to drug metabolism and excretion (Kee, Hayes, & McCuistion, 2012).

Race, Ethnicity, Sex, and Cultural Influences

Race, ethnicity, sex, and cultural influences have long been recognized as influencing pain (Campbell & Edwards, 2012; IOM, 2011; Ostrom et al., 2017). Race and sex are among the most commonly studied demographic factors in relation to pain sensitivity and pain expression (Ostrom et al., 2017). For example,

Ostrom and colleagues (2017) found that women displayed more sensitivity to certain pain sensitivity measures (29 of 34) than men. In regard to race, results showed that African American and Hispanic subjects had greater sensitivity to certain types of pain stimuli (i.e., mechanical cutaneous pain) than non-Hispanic White subjects, although there were no differences among the subjects for other types of stimuli (i.e., pressure pain thresholds).

Behavior related to pain is part of the socialization process. Sociocultural impact on pain is another factor that researchers seek to understand in order to know more about pain experiences, coping, and improve pain management (Pillay, van Zyl, & Blackbeard, 2014). For example, findings from an extensive systematic literature review by Pillay and colleagues (2014) indicate cultural differences in pain expression: Certain groups of individuals were more likely to communicate with providers about their pain experience, whereas others took a more stoic approach and chose to endure pain without reporting. Gender-role expectations within cultures were significant as well.

The culture of healthcare also influences the healthcare provider's perception of the patient's pain. Some studies support the notion that factors such as race and ethnicity, age, and sex may play a part in how providers across disciplines view pain

in certain groups of individuals based on these factors (IOM, 2011; Wadner, Scipio, Hirsh, Torres, & Robinson, 2012). Nurses may have their own attitudes and expectations about pain (Jarrett, Church, Fancher-Gonzalez, Shackelford, & Lofton, 2013). For example, nurses may place a higher value on silent suffering or self-control in response to pain (Jarrett et al., 2015). They may expect patients to be objective about pain and to be able to provide a detailed description of their pain. Nurses may deny or minimize the pain they observe in others. Because nurses serve a more diverse population in terms of ethnicity and cultural responses to pain than they once did, nurses must identify their own personal attitudes about pain in order to provide culturally competent care for patients in pain.

Environmental Considerations

Environmental factors will influence a person's ability to identify and seek relief for pain. The external environment includes a variety of stimuli for pain. Objects that may contribute to pain include restrictive clothing, ill-fitting shoes, or furniture and other objects in the work and home environments that cause pressure, strain, discomfort, or pain in healthy or already painful areas of the body. The ability to move freely influences the person's ability to avoid or control painful stimuli.

Family members and support systems, including members of the healthcare team, are factors in the external environment that must be considered. A strange environment such as a hospital, with its noises, lights, and activity, can compound pain. The lonely person who is without a support network may perceive pain as severe, whereas the person who has supportive people around may perceive less pain. Some people prefer to withdraw when they are in pain; others prefer the distraction of people and activity around them. Family caregivers can be a significant support for a person in pain. With the increase in outpatient and home care, families are assuming an increased responsibility for pain management. Education related to the assessment and management of pain can positively affect the perceived quality of life for both patients and their caregivers (McCaffery & Pasero, 1999).

Expectations of significant others can affect a person's perceptions of and responses to pain. In some situations, girls may be permitted to express pain more openly than boys. Family role can also affect how a person perceives or responds to pain. For instance, a single mother supporting three children may ignore pain because of her need to stay on the job. The presence of support people often changes a patient's reaction to pain. For example, toddlers often tolerate pain more readily when supportive parents or nurses are nearby.

The internal environment includes individual perceptions and experiences related to pain. Previous pain experiences alter a patient's sensitivity to pain. People who have experienced pain, or who have been exposed to the suffering of someone close who experienced pain, are often more threatened by anticipated pain than people without a pain experience. The success or lack of success of pain relief measures influences a person's expectations for relief. For example, a person who has tried several pain relief measures without success may have little hope about the helpfulness of nursing interventions.

Some patients may accept pain more readily than others, depending on the circumstances. A patient who associates the pain with a positive outcome may withstand the pain amazingly

---

Evidence Based Practice:

Pain Assessment and Response

- Differences exist in reporting of pain among certain groups of individuals.

  ○ Women tend to report pain more frequently than men (Bartley & Fillingim, 2013; CDC, 2013).

  ○ Women displayed more sensitivity to certain pain sensitivity measures (29 of 34) than men (Ostrom et al., 2017).

  ○ Because of variations in physiologic indicators in infants, behavioral observation is recommended for pain assessment (Ball et al., 2017).

  ○ The prevalence of pain in the older population is generally higher because of both acute and chronic disease conditions, but it is often underassessed and undertreated (Denny & Guido, 2012).

  ○ African American and Hispanic subjects tend to have greater sensitivity to certain types of pain stimuli (i.e., mechanical cutaneous pain) than non-Hispanic White subjects (Ostrom et al., 2017).

- Negative emotions such as anxiety, depression, and anger have been found to influence and intensify the pain experience in several studies. Fatigue also reduces a person's ability to cope, thereby increasing pain perception (IOM, 2011).

- There is increasing evidence to support a shift from the use of unidimensional pain assessment tools to multidimensional tools (Scher, Meador, Cleave, & Reid, 2017)

well. For example, a woman giving birth to a child or an athlete undergoing knee surgery to prolong his career may tolerate pain better because of the benefit associated with it. These patients may view the pain as a temporary inconvenience rather than a potential threat or disruption to daily life.

In contrast, patients with unrelenting chronic pain may suffer more intensely (IOM, 2011). They may respond with despair, anxiety, and depression because they cannot attach a positive significance or purpose to the pain. In this situation, the pain may be looked upon as a threat to body image or lifestyle and as a sign of possible impending death.

The threat of the unknown and the inability to control the pain or the events surrounding it often augment the pain perception. Negative emotions such as anxiety, depression, and anger have been found to influence and intensify the pain experience in several studies (IOM, 2011). Fatigue also reduces a person's ability to cope, thereby increasing pain perception. When pain interferes with sleep, fatigue and muscle tension often result and increase the pain; thus a cycle of pain–fatigue–pain develops. People who believe that they have control of their pain have decreased fear and anxiety, which decreases their pain perception. A perception of lacking control or a sense of helplessness tends to increase pain perception. Patients who are able to express pain to an attentive listener and participate in pain management decisions can increase their sense of control and decrease pain perception.

Assessment of Pain

Accurate and timely patient assessment is imperative for effective pain management. Poorly managed or untreated pain will influence every aspect of an individual's health and well-being. Because pain is subjective and experienced uniquely by each person, nurses need to assess all factors affecting the pain experience—physiologic, psychologic, behavioral, emotional, and sociocultural. Healthcare professionals may include pain as a component of vital signs assessment and consider it to be the fifth vital sign. However, the growing opioid epidemic has many healthcare professionals calling for removal of this label (Ault, 2017; Scher et al., 2017). In addition, there is evidence to support the determination that current methods of pain assessment within clinical settings are not resolving the issue of undertreatment of pain in certain individuals, as well as that there may be a link to the opioid crisis (Scher et al, 2017). The American Medical Association (AMA) and American Academy of Family Physicians (AAFP) have already voted to eliminate pain as the fifth vital sign. Many physicians and nurses feel that assessment of pain should be more comprehensive, including more than just assessment by a pain scale (Ault, 2017; Scher et al, 2017). They indicate that other factors, such as functional assessment and collaboration of an interprofessional team using multidimensional assessment tools, should be included. Because of the currency of this call for change, new standards and protocols have not been established and more details will likely be forthcoming in the near future.

The extent and frequency of the pain assessment vary according to the situation. For patients experiencing acute or severe pain, the nurse may focus only on location, quality, severity, and early intervention. Patients with less severe or chronic pain can usually provide a more detailed description of the experience. Frequency of pain assessment usually depends on the pain

control measures being used and the clinical circumstances. For example, in the initial postoperative period, pain is often assessed whenever vital signs are taken, which may be as often as every 15 minutes and then extended to every 2 to 4 hours. Following pain management interventions, pain intensity should be reassessed at an interval appropriate for the intervention. For example, following the intravenous administration of morphine, the severity of pain should be reassessed in 20 to 30 minutes.

Because many people will not voice their pain unless asked about it, pain assessments must be initiated by the nurse. It is also essential that nurses listen to and rely on the patient's perceptions of pain. Believing the patient who is experiencing and conveying the perceptions is crucial in establishing a sense of trust.

Pain assessments consist of two major components, or phases: (a) a pain history to obtain facts from the patient and (b) direct observation of behavioral and physiologic responses to pain by the patient. The goal of assessment is to gain an objective understanding of a subjective experience. The nurse typically initiates pain assessment because many individuals do not discuss their pain until asked about it.

Pain History

A detailed history to obtain subjective data from the patient is essential for successful treatment and relief from pain. During the history taking and focused interview, the nurse provides patients an opportunity to express in their own words how they view pain. It also gives the nurse an opportunity to observe the body language or nonverbal communication of the patient. The responses made by the patient will help the nurse understand the meaning of pain to the patient and the coping strategies being used. Each person's pain experience is unique, and the patient is the best interpreter of the pain experience.

A pain history includes collection of data about the onset, location, duration, characteristics (including intensity, quality, and pattern of pain); precipitating factors; actions aimed at relief of pain; impact on activities of daily living (ADLs); coping strategies; and emotional responses. A suggested method for assessment of physical complaints, including pain, is the acronym OLDCART & ICE. Figure 9.6 ■ describes the meanings of the letters in the OLDCART and ICE acronym. (Also see Chapter 5, Interviewing and Health History: Subjective Data. ∞) The following subsections present the factors related to each aspect of pain assessment.

OLDCART & ICE Acronym
O = Onset
L = Location
D = Duration
C = Characteristics
A = Aggravating Factors
R = Relieving Factors
T = Treatment
&
I = Impact on ADLs
C = Coping Strategies
E = Emotional Response

Figure 9.6 OLDCART and ICE acronym.

Onset The nurse asks the patient to discuss and describe when the pain began.

Location The nurse should ask the patient to point to the specific location of pain. Charts in which body outlines are depicted are a useful method for children and adults to accurately identify the site of pain. When recording the location, the body outline charts may be used. The nurse is also expected to record locations, using appropriate terminology in relation to the proximity or distance from known landmarks (e.g., "pain in substernal area 3 cm [1.18 in.] below the xiphoid process").

Duration The patient is asked to describe the length of time the pain lasts. Included would be a determination of the pain as constant or intermittent. If the pain is intermittent, the nurse must assess the length of time without pain or between episodes of pain.

Characteristics The characteristics of the pain are assessed by asking the patient to apply an adjective to the pain. For example, pain may be experienced as burning, stabbing, piercing, or throbbing. Children may have difficulty describing pain; therefore, it is important to use familiar terminology, such as "boo-boo," "feel funny," or "hurt." The nurse must use quotation marks to record the description of the pain in the exact words spoken by the patient.

The intensity of pain is most accurately assessed through the use of **pain rating scales** (see Figure 9.7 ■). Most scales use a numerical rating of 0 to 5 or 0 to 10, with 0 indicating the absence of pain. Descriptors accompany the number ratings in many scales. The descriptors assist the patient to "quantify" the intensity of the pain. For children and adults who cannot read or are unable to numerically rate their pain, self-report measures may include using drawings that depict facial expressions or visual analog scale (VAS) tools. Several variations of VAS tools are available, with one of the earliest and best-known being the Faces Pain Scale (Bieri, Reeve, Champion, Addicoat, & Ziegler, 1990). Numbers accompany each facial expression so that pain intensity can be identified.

Aggravating Factors A variety of factors can precipitate pain. These aggravating factors include activity, exercise, turning, breathing, swallowing, urinating, and temperature or other climactic changes. Fear, anxiety, and stress can also aggravate pain.

Relieving Factors Assessment of pain includes gathering data about the measures taken by the patient to relieve or alleviate the pain. The nurse will inquire about the use of medications,

home and folk remedies, and alternative or complementary therapies such as acupuncture, massage, and imagery. The nurse must also gather data about the effectiveness of the measures.

Treatment This assessment includes gathering data about pharmacologic and nonpharmacologic treatments for pain.

Impact on Activities of Daily Living (ADLs) Assessment of the impact of pain on ADLs enables the nurse to understand the severity of the pain and the impact of the pain on the patient's quality of life. ADLs include work, school, household and family management, mobility and transportation, leisure activities, and marital and family relationships. The nurse may ask the patient to rate the impact of the pain on each of the ADLs.

Coping Strategies Individuals cope with pain in a variety of ways. Various coping strategies include but are not limited to prayer, yoga, tai chi, chi quong (also known as chi gung, chi kung, or qi gong), support groups, distraction, relaxation techniques, or withdrawal. The strategies are often unique to the individual or reflect cultural values and beliefs. The nurse attempts to identify coping strategies employed by the patient and to determine if they are effective in pain management.

Emotional Responses An assessment of the patient's emotional response to pain is important. Pain, especially chronic or debilitating pain, can result in depression, anxiety, and physical and emotional exhaustion. The emotional response to pain is often related to the type, intensity, and duration of pain.

Behavior and Physiologic Reponses to Pain

The observation phase of the pain assessment includes the direct observation of the patient's behavior and physiologic responses. During observation, the nurse should remember that cultural factors may significantly affect the patient's behavioral responses to pain.

Behavior A variety of behaviors indicate the presence of pain. Many of these behaviors are nonverbal or consist of vocalizations. Behaviors indicative of pain include facial grimacing, moaning, crying or screaming, guarding or immobilization of a body part, tossing and turning, and rhythmic movements.

Physiologic Responses The site of the pain and the duration of the pain influence physiologic responses to pain. The sympathetic nervous system is stimulated in the early stage of acute pain. The response is demonstrated in elevation of blood pressure and pulse and respiratory rates, pallor, and diaphoresis. Parasympathetic stimulation often accompanies visceral pain. This results in lowered blood pressure and pulse rate and warm, dry skin.

Focused Interview

During the focused interview, information regarding pain will be collected. The subjective data will include the factors under consideration when using the OLDCART & ICE acronyms described earlier in this chapter. These factors include onset, location, duration, and characteristics of the pain. Information regarding the intensity of the pain will be obtained as a part of the interview. Further questions address aggravating and relieving factors, treatments, impact on activities of daily

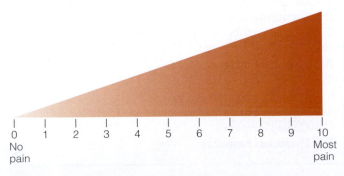

Figure 9.7 Pain rating intensity scale.

```
|   |   |   |   |   |   |   |   |   |   |   |
0   1   2   3   4   5   6   7   8   9   10
No                                     Most
pain                                   pain
```

living (ADLs), coping strategies, and emotional responses. These subjective data will be obtained using open-ended and closed questions. Follow-up questions may be needed for greater clarification regarding the pain experience. Sample questions are provided for the nurse to use to obtain the subjective data. This list of questions is not all-inclusive but does represent the types of questions required in a comprehensive focused interview. Additional questions specific to a body system are found in the assessment chapters in Unit III of this text. ∞

Questions Regarding Onset

1. When did the pain begin?
2. Can you describe any circumstances associated with the onset of pain?

   Questions 1 and 2 allow the patient to describe the time frame and circumstances, both physical and emotional, that accompanied the start of the pain experience.

Questions Regarding Location

1. Where is your pain?
2. Does the pain move, or is it just in one place?
3. Are you able to point to or put your finger on the painful area?

   Questions 1 to 3 give patients the opportunity to specifically locate the pain and identify the body parts involved. An alternative method would be to give patients a picture of the body and ask them to color the areas of the body affected by the pain.

Questions Regarding Duration

1. Do you have pain now?
2. Is the pain constant or intermittent?
3. How long does the pain last?

   Questions 1 to 3 give the patient the opportunity to explain a pattern associated with pain.

Questions Regarding Characteristics of the Pain

1. How bad is the pain now?
2. Using a scale of 0 to 10, with 0 being no pain and 10 being the worst possible pain, how would you rate your present pain level?

   Questions 1 and 2 give the patient the opportunity to describe the level or intensity of the pain being experienced at the present time.

3. An alternative method would be to give the patient a pain-intensity scale (refer to Figure 9.7) and ask the patient to place a mark to correspond to the pain being experienced. The nurse should be sure to use a tool appropriate for the patient. Rating scales include use of numbers and pictures, and they are language specific.
4. What does the pain feel like?
5. Describe your pain.

   Questions 4 and 5 give patients the opportunity to describe the pain using their own words.

6. An alternative method would be to list the possible descriptive terms and ask the patient to respond "yes" or "no" to each descriptor, such as these: *deep, superficial, burning, aching, pressure-like, dull, sharp, shooting, stabbing, piercing, crushing,* or *tingling.*

This is a comprehensive and easy way to elicit information regarding the quality of the pain.

Questions Regarding Aggravating Factors

1. What do you think started the pain?

   This question elicits patient perceptions about the cause of pain.

2. What were you doing just before the pain started?

   This question is intended to identify triggers or factors related to the onset of pain.

3. Have you been under a great deal of stress lately?

   This is an attempt to determine a link to psychosocial factors or psychogenic sources of pain.

4. An added method to determine aggravating factors is to list common factors and ask the patient to respond "yes" or "no" when the list is read. The factors would include but are not limited to moving, walking, turning, breathing, swallowing, and urinating.

   This permits the patient to provide specific information regarding the pain.

Questions Regarding Relieving Factors

1. What have you done to relieve the pain?
2. Did it work?
3. Have you used this before? When?
4. Why do you think it worked (or did not work) this time?

   Questions 1 to 4 provide the patient the opportunity to discuss what actions have been taken to help decrease or eliminate the pain.

Questions Regarding Treatment

1. Do you take a prescribed pain pill?
2. Do you take an over-the-counter medicine for the pain?
3. Do you change your diet in any way when you have pain?
4. Do you use an ice pack or heating pad on the pain?
5. Do you use prayer?
6. Do you or a family member perform some type of ritual?
7. Do you rest when you have the pain?
8. Do you do anything that has not been mentioned?

   When the patient responds "yes" to any of these questions, the nurse must then determine the effectiveness of the strategy.

Questions Regarding Impact on Activities of Daily Living

1. Describe your daily activities.
2. How well are you able to perform these activities?
3. Does the pain in any way hinder your ability to function?

   Questions 1 to 3 encourage the patient to describe the ability to function independently on a daily basis.

4. An alternative method would be to list possible daily activities and ask the patient to respond with a "yes" or "no" if the pain hinders the ability to perform the actions.

   Examples include the following:
      Do you have difficulty sleeping?
      Has your appetite changed?
      Are you able to get out of bed without help?

Do you have difficulty walking, standing, sitting, or climbing stairs?

Are you able to perform your work activities?

Are you able to concentrate at school, work, or home?

Are you able to drive? To ride in a car?

Do you have mood swings?

Do you find yourself being short with family members and friends?

Questions Related to Coping Strategies

1. Describe how you deal or cope with the pain.

2. Are you in a support group for pain?

3. What do you do to decrease the pain so you can function and feel better?

   Questions 1 to 3 enable the patient to share his or her coping strategies. These may be unique to the individual and may reflect family values and cultural beliefs.

Questions Related to Emotional Responses

1. Emotionally, how does the pain make you feel?

2. Does your pain make you feel depressed?

3. Does your pain ever make you feel anxious, tired, or exhausted?

   Questions 1 to 3 give the nurse an opportunity to explore emotional feelings related to pain with the patient.

Physiologic Responses

Assessment of patient behaviors will include the collection of objective data. There are wide variations in nonverbal responses to pain. For patients who are very young, aphasic, confused, or disoriented, nonverbal expressions may be the only means of communicating pain. Facial expression is often the first indication of pain, and it may be the only one. Clenched teeth, tightly shut eyes, open somber eyes, biting of the lower lip, and other facial grimaces may be indicative of pain. Vocalizations like moaning and groaning or crying and screaming are sometimes associated with pain.

Immobilization of the body or a part of the body may also indicate pain. The patient with chest pain often holds the left arm across the chest. A person with abdominal pain may assume the position of greatest comfort, often with the knees and hips flexed, and may move reluctantly.

Purposeless body movements can also indicate pain—for example, tossing and turning in bed or flinging the arms about. Involuntary movements such as a reflexive jerking away from a needle inserted through the skin indicate pain. An adult may be able to control this reflex; however, a child may be unable or unwilling to do so.

Rhythmic body movements or rubbing may indicate pain. An adult or child may assume a fetal position and rock back and forth when experiencing abdominal pain. During labor a woman may massage her abdomen rhythmically with her hands. Because behavioral responses can be controlled, they may not be very revealing. When pain is chronic, there are rarely overt behavioral responses because the individual develops personal coping styles for dealing with pain, discomfort, or suffering.

Physiologic responses vary with the origin and duration of the pain. Early during the onset of acute pain, the sympathetic nervous system is stimulated, resulting in increased blood pressure, increased pulse rate, increased respiratory rate, pallor, diaphoresis, and pupil dilation. The body does not sustain the increased sympathetic function over a prolonged period. Therefore, the sympathetic nervous system adapts, making the physiologic responses less evident or even absent. Physiologic responses are most likely to be absent in people with chronic pain because of central nervous system adaptation. Thus, it is important that the nurse assess more than the physiologic responses because they may be poor indicators of pain.

Assessment Tools

Assessment tools employed by the nurse help patients describe their pain, and numeric scales and surveys assist the nurse in quantifying their pain. The chosen tools will help the nurse obtain precise data needed to implement treatment modalities and evaluate pain relief. The holistic approach to nursing assessment of pain permits the assessment plan to reflect the individual beliefs, needs, and wishes of the patient. Establishing a caring relationship, listening to the patient, and using comprehensive interview techniques are essential in the assessment of pain.

The chosen assessment tool should be easy to use, tabulate, and score. It should be in the language of the patient, and it should be used consistently. The nurse must teach the patient, family members, and other members of the healthcare team the correct use of the tool. All tools have advantages and disadvantages. It is the responsibility of the nurse to identify these factors before implementation of the appropriate tool. Tools used for pain assessment are designed and classified as unidimensional or multidimensional.

Successful management of pain is dependent on an accurate assessment of the type and degree of pain the patient is experiencing as well as the identification of underlying causes. The assessment data are used by the nurse in interaction with the patient and other health professionals to develop a plan for pain management.

Unidimensional Assessment Tools   Unidimensional tools are used to help determine the patient's level of acute pain. The tool is called unidimensional because it assesses one aspect of pain. Many times this single element relates to the intensity of pain. Numeric rating scales, visual analog scales, the Oucher Scale, and the Poker Chip Scale are examples of unidimensional tools (Partners Against Pain, 2013)

Unidimensional tools can be used in any clinical setting across the age span. It is important for the nurse to use the tool consistently throughout the assessment, treatment, and reassessment of the patient. Because they measure just one element of the pain experience, unidimensional tools can lead to inadequate use of treatment modalities; therefore, nurses and other members of the healthcare team should not use these tools in isolation to make decisions about treating pain (Scher et al., 2017).

The Numeric Rating Scale asks the patient to describe pain intensity with a number. The selected number then equates to pain severity. The Simple Verbal Descriptive Scale is another unidimensional tool. The individual is presented with six descriptive words and is asked to select one that corresponds to the present level of intensity.

The Body Diagram tool presents an outline of the body. The individual is asked to mark the picture showing the location of the pain. Shading of the body parts by the patient will describe the intensity of the pain.

As previously discussed, visual methods of rating pain have been developed that use illustrations of faces ranging from neutral to distressed. Examples of the most commonly used faces-type pain rating scales include the following:

- Faces Pain Scale (FPS) (scored 0–6)
- Faces Pain Scale–Revised (FPS-R) (scored 0–10)
- Oucher Pain Scale (scored 0–10)
- Wong-Baker FACES Pain Rating Scale (WBFPRS) (scored 0–10)

Research suggests that children tend to prefer the WBFPRS; however, all of the scales have proven useful in the clinical setting (Tomlinson, von Baeyer, Stinson, & Sung, 2010).

Multidimensional Assessment Tools   The multidimensional assessment tools assess two or more elements of pain. These tools go beyond pain intensity and include affective and sensory elements. The McGill Pain Questionnaire, short and long form, is an example of a multidimensional assessment tool.

Multidimensional assessment tools assess the nature and location of pain, the patient's mood, and the impact of pain regarding ADLs. The McGill Pain Questionnaire is available in a long and short form and is used when pain is prolonged. The long form measures intensity, location, pattern, sensory dimensions, and affective dimensions of pain. The short form measures intensity, sensory dimensions, and affective dimensions of pain.

The Brief Pain Inventory is another multidimensional scale used for assessment of pain. This tool provides information on pain and how pain interferes with the person's ability to function. Questions on this tool address medications, relief, individual beliefs, and quality of life.

Tool Selection   Many tools are available to assist the patient and nurse to assess, treat, and evaluate pain and to measure the effectiveness of the treatment modalities. Tools must be appropriate for the age, culture, language, and cognitive abilities of the individual. Additional information about pain rating scales and tools to assess pain are available through authoritative online references.

Application Through Critical Thinking

CASE STUDY

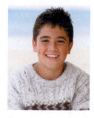

Source:
Oliveromg/
Shutterstock.

A car hit John Taylor, age 12, while he was riding his bicycle. He has several injuries and is brought to the emergency department at the local community hospital. The emergency technician informs the staff that John's right leg was splinted at the scene, right pedal pulse was 56, and left pedal pulse was 76. John has a cut above his right eye that is bleeding, and his right eye is swollen and partially closed. John has had no loss of consciousness; however, his respirations are 32 and shallow. He is crying and tells the nurse he has a lot of pain in his right leg, his head hurts, and he cannot seem to catch his breath. His father is at the bedside and tells him that big boys don't cry. His mom is hysterical and keeps telling John that it's okay to cry.

The emergency department physician asks for a chest x-ray immediately, starts supportive oxygen therapy, and gives direction for administration of pain medication.

CRITICAL THINKING QUESTIONS

1. How and when should the nurse assess the pain in this patient?
2. What pain-scale tool, if any, would be appropriate to use?
3. What additional information regarding pain is needed?
4. What role will the parents have at this time?
5. How do cultural values and belief systems impact the perception and management of pain?

REFERENCES

American Pain Society. (2016). *Principles of analgesic use in the treatment of acute pain and cancer pain* (7th ed.). Glenview, IL: Author.

Ault, A. (2017, February 21). Many physicians, nurses want pain removed as fifth vital sign. *Medscape*. Retrieved from https://www.medscape.com/viewarticle/875980

Ball, J. W., Bindler, R. C., Cowen, K., & M. R. Shaw. (2017). *Pediatric nursing: Caring for children* (7th ed.). Hoboken, NJ: Prentice Hall.

Bartley, E. J., & Fillingim, R. B. (2013). Sex differences in pain: A brief review of clinical and experimental findings. *British Journal of Anaesthesia, 111*(1), 52–58. doi:10.1093/bja/aet127

Berman, A. J., & Snyder, S. (2016). *Kozier and Erb's fundamentals of nursing: Concepts, process, and practice* (10th ed.). Hoboken, NJ: Prentice Hall.

Bieri, D., Reeve, R., Champion, G., Addicoat, L., & Ziegler, J. B. (1990). The Faces Pain Scale for the assessment of the severity of pain experienced by children: Development, initial validation, and preliminary investigation for ratio scale properties. *Pain, 41*(2), 139–150.

Campbell, C. M., & Edwards, R. R. (2012). Ethnic differences in pain and pain management. *Pain Management, 2*(3), 219–230. doi:10.2217/pmt.12.7

Centers for Disease Control and Prevention (CDC). (2013). QuickStats: Percentage of adults aged ≥18 years who often had pain in the past 3 months, by sex and age group — National Health Interview Survey, United States, 2010–2011. Retrieved from https://www.cdc.gov/mmwr/preview/mmwrhtml/mm6217a10.htm

Denny, D. L., & Guido, G. W. (2012). Undertreatment of pain in older adults: An application of beneficence. *Nursing Ethics, 19*(6), 800–809. doi:10.1177/0969733012447015

Harrison, D., Bueno, M., & Reszel, J. (2015). Prevention and management of pain and stress in the neonate. *Research and Reports in Neonatology, 5*, 9–16. doi:10.2147/RRN.S52378

Institute of Medicine (IOM). (2011). *Relieving pain in America: A blueprint for transforming prevention, care, education, and research.* Washington, DC: The National Academies Press. Retrieved from https://www.nap.edu/read/13172/chapter/1

International Association for the Study of Pain (IASP). (1994). Part III: Pain terms, a current list with definitions and notes on usage. In H. Merskey & N. Bogduk (Eds.), *Classification of chronic pain* (2nd ed., pp. 209–214). Seattle, WA: IASP Press. Retrieved from http://www.iasp-pain.org/files/Content/ContentFolders/Publications2/FreeBooks/Classification-of-Chronic-Pain.pdf

Jarrett, A., Church, T., Fancher-Gonzalez, K., Shackelford, J., & Lofton, A. (2013). Nurses' knowledge and attitudes about pain in hospitalized patients. *Clinical Nurse Specialist, 27*(2), 81–87. doi:10.1097/NUR.0b013e3182819133

Kee, J., Hayes, E., & McCuistion, L. (2012). *Pharmacology: A nursing process approach* (7th ed.). St. Louis, MO: Mosby.

McCaffery, M., & Pasero, C. (1999). *Pain: Clinical manual* (2nd ed.). St. Louis, MO: Mosby.

Melzack, R., & Wall, P. D. (1965). Pain mechanisms: A new theory. *Science, 150*, 971–979.

Ostrom, C., Bair, E., Maixner, W., Dubner, R., Fillingim, R. B., Ohrbach, R., . . . Greenspan, J. D. (2017). Demographic predictors of pain sensitivity: Results from the OPERRA study. *The Journal of Pain, 18*(3), 295–307. doi:10.1016/j.jpain.2016.10.018

Paice, J. A. (2002). Understanding nociceptive pain. *Nursing, 32*(3), 74–75.

Partners Against Pain. (2013). *Pain assessment scales.* Stanford, CT: Purdue Pharma LP. Retrieved from http://www.partnersagainstpain.com/measuring-pain/assessment-tool.aspx

Pillay, T., van Zyl, H. A., & Blackbeard, D. (2014). Chronic pain perception and cultural experience. *Procedia - Social and Behavioral Sciences, 113*(7), 151–160. doi:10.1016/j.sbspro.2014.01.022

Sadosky, A., Hopper, J., & Parsons, B. (2014). Painful diabetic peripheral neuropathy: Results of a survey characterizing the perspectives and misperceptions of patients and healthcare practitioners. *The Patient - Patient-Centered Outcomes Research, 7*(1), 107–114.

Scher, C., Meador, L., Cleave, J. H., & Reid, M. C. (2017). Moving beyond pain as the fifth vital sign and patient satisfaction scores to improve pain care in the 21st century. *Pain Management Nursing*, Advance online publication. doi:10.1016/j.pmn.2017.10.010

Tomlinson, D., von Baeyer, C. L., Stinson, J. N., & Sung, L. (2010). A systematic review of faces scales for the self-report of pain intensity in children. *Pediatrics, 126*(5), e1168–e1198.

Wadner, L. D., Scipio, C. D., Hirsh, A. T., Torres, C. A., & Robinson, M. E. (2012). The perception of pain in others: How gender, race, and age influence pain expectations. *Journal of Pain, 13*(3), 220–227. doi:10.1016/j.jpain.2011.10.014

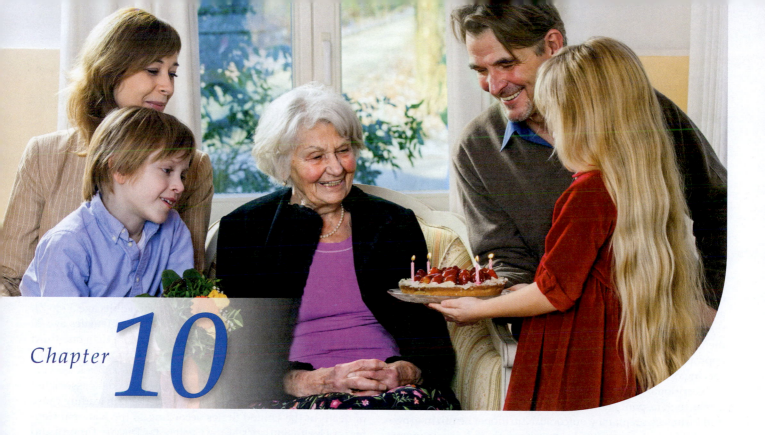

Chapter 10

Nutritional Assessment

LEARNING OUTCOMES

Upon completion of this chapter, you will be able to:

1. Define nutritional health.

2. Identify factors that affect or influence a nutritional assessment of an adult.

3. Describe the components and tools used to obtain a nutritional history.

4. Describe the components and tools of a physical assessment as they pertain to nutrition.

5. Identify the laboratory parameters used in a nutritional assessment.

6. Identify the most commonly used nutritional screening and assessment tools.

KEY TERMS

alopecia, 140
angular stomatitis, 140
anthropometric, 133
ascites, 142
atrophic papillae, 141
cheilosis, 140
diet recall, 131
flag sign, 140
follicular hyperkeratosis, 142

food deserts, 128
food frequency
   questionnaire, 132
food security, 131
glossitis, 141
immunocompetence, 143
koilonychia, 141
malnutrition, 128
nutritional health, 128

obesity, 128
obesity paradox, 128
overnutrition, 128
overweight, 128
pellagra, 142
petechiae, 142
pica, 131
protein-calorie
   malnutrition, 128

purpura, 142
rickets, 142
somatic protein, 138
undernutrition, 128
xanthelasma, 140
xerophthalmia, 140

MEDICAL LANGUAGE

-graphy Suffix meaning "process of recording"

hyper- Prefix meaning "high," "elevated," "above normal"

hypo- Prefix meaning "below," "deficient"

-itis Suffix meaning "inflammation"

-osis Suffix meaning "condition, usually abnormal"

-pathy Suffix meaning "disease," "emotion"

somat- Prefix meaning "body"

Introduction

The determination of an individual's nutritional status is based on the foundation of a thorough nutritional assessment. The assessment portion of the nursing care process incorporates the gathering and interpretation of data for a nutritional assessment. These data then create the base for later development of appropriate nursing and nutritional interventions aimed at preserving or improving nutritional health.

Nutritional health is a crucial component of overall health across the lifespan. The nutritional health of a pregnant female will influence pregnancy outcome. Nutritional health in growing children plays a central role in growth and development. In adults and older adults, nutritional health can be associated with the prevention or development of chronic disease. Aspects of nutritional health in individuals within these special populations are addressed in more detail in Unit IV. Religious and cultural influences on health, nutrition beliefs, and food habits vary among and within ethnic groups, as well. Refer to Chapter 3 for more detail. ∞

Defining Nutritional Health

Nutritional health can be defined as the physical result of the balance between nutrient intake and nutritional requirements. A patient who consumes adequate nutrition to meet individual needs and avoids habitual excesses and insufficiencies would be considered to be in good nutritional health. **Undernutrition**, also called **malnutrition**, describes the condition of insufficient nutrient intake or poor nutrient stores, both of which cause adverse health effects. For example, a pregnant female who consumes less than the required amounts of folic acid may place her unborn child at risk for certain birth defects, such as neural tube defects, and could be considered in poor nutritional health because of undernutrition. **Overnutrition** results from excesses in nutrient intake or stores. For example, an individual who consumes excess saturated fat may be at risk for elevated blood cholesterol and cardiovascular disease. This person may, therefore, be considered to have poor nutritional health because of overnutrition.

Many factors can influence nutritional health. When gathering data for a nutritional assessment, it is important to realize common risk factors for a poor nutritional status. Overnutrition in the form of excess dietary intake of fat, especially saturated fat, has been associated with an increased risk of atherosclerosis. **Overweight** and **obesity** are linked with increased risk

of hypertension, cardiovascular disease, type 2 diabetes, some cancers, degenerative joint disease, and other conditions. In addition, excess body weight has been shown to increase the risk of mortality from cardiovascular disease, diabetes mellitus, kidney disease, and certain cancers in adults age 30 to 74. In the United States, almost 70% of males and females age 20 to 74 are considered overweight or obese. More than one-third of adults are obese, a statistic that has not improved over the last decade. More than one-third of children and adolescents are overweight or obese. Excess alcohol intake is associated with chronic liver disease and cirrhosis, the 12th leading cause of death in the United States according to the National Center for Health Statistics at the Centers for Disease Control and Prevention (CDC, 2009).

Undernutrition is less common than overnutrition in the United States, but it can have devastating physical health consequences when **protein-calorie malnutrition** or other nutrient deficiencies develop. Undernutrition can lead to faltering growth, compromised immune status, poor wound healing, muscle loss, physical and functional decline, and lack of proper development. Generally, individuals at risk for undernutrition include those who have a chronic illness; are poor, elderly, or hospitalized; are restrictive eaters (from chronic dieting or disordered eating); or are alcoholics. An individual can have both overnutrition and undernutrition, such as an overweight child who consumes no fruits or vegetables. The **obesity paradox** is a term used to denote the joint presence of obesity and nutritional deficiency (Koh, Hoy, O'Connell, & Montgomery, 2012). **Food deserts** contribute to the obesity paradox. Food deserts are low-income, urban or rural areas that lack access to healthy, affordable food. When food is available in a food desert, it is generally high-calorie food of poor nutritional quality, such as food that is found in fast-food restaurants and convenience stores (Ver Ploeg & Rahkovsky, 2016). Box 10.1 outlines additional risk factors for overnutrition and undernutrition to consider when conducting a nutrition assessment.

Health Promotion

The U.S. Department of Health and Human Services, Office of Disease Prevention and Health Promotion, has established a collaborative public health initiative called *Healthy People 2020* aimed at both increasing the quality and years of healthy life in the U.S. population and reducing health disparities. Overarching goals of *Healthy People 2020* are to promote health and prevent disease. The *Healthy People 2020* objectives are important reminders to the clinician of the central role nutrition plays

Box 10.1 Risk Factors for Poor Nutritional Health

Undernutrition

- Chronic disease, acute illness, wounds, or injury—including symptoms and treatment
- Multiple medications and medication side effects that reduce intake or alter nutrient metabolism
- Food insecurity—lack of money or access to adequate and safe food, including food deserts
- Restrictive eating because of medical conditions requiring altered diet that reduces intake of food groups or nutrients—for example, a very low-fat diet with fat malabsorption, a gluten-free diet with celiac disease, or a low potassium and protein modified diet with renal failure
- Food allergies and intolerances (Multiple food allergies further increase risk because of broader avoidance of food groups.)
- Self-diagnosed or self-prescribed diets (Avoidance of foods or food groups without demonstrated medical need leads to unnecessary elimination of foods, food groups, and accompanying nutrients—for example, eliminating gluten without celiac disease or diagnosed gluten intolerance.)
- Restrictive eating because of chronic dieting, disordered eating, or food faddism such as trendy diets, cleanses, or nutritional beliefs—for example, following a vegan diet and not ensuring adequate supplemental sources of vitamins B_{12} and D, which are lacking in a plants-only diet

- Alcohol abuse, which may cause both reduced intake and altered nutrient metabolism
- Depression, bereavement, loneliness, social isolation
- Poor dental health
- Chewing and swallowing difficulties, including those from altered dental/oral health, decreased saliva production, medication side effects, or a medical diagnosis
- Alterations in sensory perception such as decreased vision, hearing, taste and smell, touch
- Decreased functional status—for example, dependency on others, cognitive changes
- Decreased knowledge or skills about food preparation and recommendations
- Extreme age—premature infants or adults over age 80

Overnutrition

- Excess intake of solid fats, added sugars, or calories
- Excess intake of any nutrient from foods, fortified foods, or dietary supplements
- Alcohol abuse
- Sedentary lifestyle
- Decreased knowledge or skills about food preparation and recommendations

in overall health across the life lifespan. Issues related to overweight and obesity are considered to be among the areas monitored to track progress toward achievement of overall goals. The *Healthy People 2020* goals related to nutrition and weight status (NWS) and Maternal, Infant, and Child Health (MICH) are presented in Table 10.1.

The increasing prevalence of overweight and obesity in the United States, as well as the statistics on nutritional health disparities, illustrate the importance of nutritional screening and assessment as the first step toward reaching these important goals. Box 10.2 outlines the cultural and socioeconomic influences that may affect nutritional health.

Box 10.2 Cultural and Socioeconomic Influences on Nutritional Health

Overweight and Obesity

- Almost 70% of adults age 20 to 74 are overweight or obese. Almost 35% of adults are obese, a statistic that has not improved in the last decade.
- Over 17% of children age 2 to 19 are obese.
- Prevalence of obesity in males is highest among Hispanic males.
- Prevalence of obesity in females is highest among Black females.
- Hypertension, a comorbidity of overweight and obesity, affects 55.1% of adults in the United States.
- Prevalence of hypertension is highest among Mexican American and Black males.
- Adults of low socioeconomic status have almost double the rate of overweight or obesity compared with those of medium and high socioeconomic status.

Undernutrition

- Up to 60% of older adults in dependent care or hospitals are malnourished.
- Adequate folic acid and iron status are important for healthy outcomes during pregnancy. Pregnant Mexican American and Black females are more likely than other ethnic groups to have iron deficiency and low folic acid levels. Females of lower economic status and those with less education are also more likely to have inadequate folic acid or iron status.
- Black women and adolescents under age 15 are more likely to have insufficient gestational weight gain and are more likely to deliver low–birth weight babies than other populations.

Poverty and Food Insecurity

- Among Americans, the prevalence of poverty is 15%.
- Children under age 18 experience a 21.8% poverty rate.
- Prevalence of poverty is highest among Blacks (27.2%) and Hispanics (25.6%).

Sources: Centers for Disease Control and Prevention (CDC; 2014); Ogden, Carroll, Kit, & Flegal (2014); U.S. Census Bureau (2013); U.S. Department of Health and Human Services (2013).

Table 10.1 Examples of *Healthy People 2020* Objectives Related to Nutrition and Weight Status (NWS) and Maternal, Infant, and Child Health (MICH)

OBJECTIVE NUMBER	DESCRIPTION
NWS-1/2	Increase the number of States with nutrition standards for foods and beverages provided to preschool-aged children in child care. Increase the proportion of schools that offer nutritious foods and beverages outside of school meals.
NWS-3	Increase the number of States that have State-level policies that incentivize food retail outlets to provide foods that are encouraged by the Dietary Guidelines for Americans.
NWS-4	(Developmental) Increase the proportion of Americans who have access to a food retail outlet that sells a variety of foods that are encouraged by the Dietary Guidelines for Americans.
NWS-5	Increase the proportion of primary care physicians who regularly measure the body mass index of their patients.
NWS-6	Increase the proportion of physician office visits that include counseling or education related to nutrition or weight.
NWS-7	(Developmental) Increase the proportion of worksites that offer nutrition or weight management classes or counseling.
NWS-8/9/10/11	Increase the proportion of adults who are at a healthy weight. Reduce the proportion of adults who are obese. Reduce the proportion of children and adolescents who are considered obese. Prevent inappropriate weight gain in youth and adults.
NWS-12/13	Eliminate very low food security among children. Reduce household food insecurity and in doing so reduce hunger.

NWS-14/15/16/17/18/19/20	In the diet of the population aged 2 years and older:
	  Increase the variety and contribution of vegetables.
	  Increase the contribution of whole grains.
	  Reduce the consumption of calories from solid fats and added sugars.
	  Reduce consumption of saturated fat.
	  Reduce consumption of sodium.
	  Increase consumption of calcium.

NWS-21/22	Reduce iron deficiency among young children and females of childbearing age. Reduce iron deficiency among pregnant females.
MICH-8	Reduce low birth weight (LBW) and very low birth weight (VLBW).
MICH-14	Increase the proportion of women of childbearing potential with intake of at least 400 mcg of folic acid from fortified foods or dietary supplements.

Source: U.S. Department of Health and Human Services, Office of Disease Prevention and Health Promotion (2014).

Source: United States Department of Health and Human Services. (2014). Healthy People 2020. Retrieved from http://www.healthypeople.gov/2020/topicsobjectives2020/default.aspx

Nutritional Assessment Factors

A nutritional assessment is the foundation on which nursing diagnoses are developed and on which the implementation of goals and objectives in the nursing care process are later created. The prevention or treatment of malnutrition and overnutrition first requires a nutritional assessment. Determination of an individual's nutritional status should be accomplished while gathering data for a nursing assessment. The components used in a nutritional assessment include the nutritional history, physical assessment, and laboratory values.

Nutritional assessment techniques and tools vary in their level of sophistication and depth. No one piece of data can give a complete nutritional assessment. Many parameters used to assess nutritional status can be affected by nonnutritional influences such as disease, medication, or environment. This illustrates the need to gather data from varying resources. Generally, an assessment done using multiple variables will be more valuable than an assessment made with limited data. In some healthcare situations, not all parameters or data are available. The nurse must rely on available information and sharp clinical judgment when making an assessment.

Varying medical diagnoses or issues specific to the lifespan will also influence pertinent parameters and techniques used in assessing a patient's nutritional status, which will be addressed in more detail within chapters for special populations. For example, measuring waist circumference may be of use when assessing potential overnutrition in some adults, but it would be of little nutritional use when assessing either a patient with ascites or a pregnant female.

Nutritional assessment of the adult focuses on evaluating the issues of both overnutrition and undernutrition. Overnutrition and undernutrition are not mutually exclusive conditions. For example, an obese individual can have nutrient deficiencies from consuming poor-quality food that contains excess calories. Good food habits developed early in life and maintained later may help to promote good health well into adulthood and older adulthood.

The presence of a chronic disease or condition may become a significant factor affecting nutritional health. Medications can have nutritional health implications. In addition to dietary habits, nutrition status can be affected by lifestyle choices, socioeconomic status, education, and cultural influences. Box 10.3 outlines pertinent nutritional history data to obtain when assessing the adult.

A registered dietitian (RD) is generally responsible for completing a comprehensive nutritional assessment in most acute or long-term care settings; a nurse may do this as well and is most often the frontline clinician who obtains the data needed for a nutritional assessment. A nurse is ideally situated to identify nutritionally at-risk patients who need further intervention targeting nutritional health. Along with identification, nurses should recognize their role as part of the interprofessional care team in partnering with the RD in preventing and treating malnutrition (Guenter, Malone, & DiMaria-Ghalili, 2015).

Cultural Considerations for Nutritional Assessment

Religious and cultural influences on health, beliefs about nutrition, and food habits vary among and within ethnic groups. It is important to ask specific questions about these influences to understand how they affect or are interpreted by the individual patient. Assumptions and generalizations based on the patient's association with a cultural or ethnic population will not provide the nurse with accurate personal information about the patient.

During the physical assessment and anthropometric portion of the assessment, careful and sensitive questioning of the patient—in some cases with the help of a translator—is needed to determine whether issues exist that may interfere with the gathering of data. Removal of certain garments may be prohibited; this can interfere with obtaining accurate weight, determining body measurements, or assessing clinical signs and symptoms. Examination or touching by a member of the opposite sex may be taboo. The nurse should engage in decision making with the patient on how best to proceed when such issues are present. Chapter 3 provides sample questions for such an assessment. ∞

Nutritional History

A careful nutritional history is part of a comprehensive nutritional assessment and is best accomplished using more than one tool. A diet recall, a food frequency questionnaire, and a food record are components of a nutritional history that can be complemented with a focused interview for more specific information.

Diet Recall

A **diet recall**, also called a 24-hour recall, can be done quickly in most settings to obtain a snapshot assessment of dietary intake. A patient is asked to verbally recall all food, beverages, and nutritional supplements or products consumed in a set 24-hour period. Obtaining a recall for both a weekday and one weekend day will strengthen the data obtained by showing examples of more than one type of typical day. In order to appear nonjudgmental and not hint at "correct" answers to questions, the nurse should ask primarily open-ended questions. The nurse should begin the diet recall by asking "Tell me what you ate yesterday (or on a specific day). When was the first time you had something to eat or drink during the day?" This type of questioning avoids asking the assuming question "What did you have for breakfast?" Patients may feel judged if they admit they skip breakfast or feel too embarrassed to admit missing a meal. The result may

---

Box 10.3 Nutritional History Data

Food

- All meals and snacks—note timing to assess for large gaps or missed meals
- All liquids, including water, alcohol, and sweetened and caffeinated beverages
- Use of fortified foods
- Preparation methods, including whether food was fresh, frozen, canned, packaged, or premade
- Portion sizes
- Grocery habits

Beliefs and Practices

- Adherence to a therapeutic diet for medical reasons or because of food allergy or food intolerance
- Cultural or religious influences on food choices and practices
- Faddism—trendy food and nutrition beliefs
- Lifestyle diet choices—vegetarianism, vegan diet, avoidance of certain foods or food groups
- **Pica**—if craving for nonfood substances present: types of substances eaten, source, and amounts

- Meal patterns—number and frequency of meals and snacks, missed meals, location of meals

Supplement and Medication Use

- Vitamin and mineral use—dose, frequency, and constituents
- Herbal use—dose, frequency, and constituents
- Over-the-counter weight loss or sports supplements—dose, frequency, and ingredients
- Over-the-counter and prescription medications to assess for drug–nutrient interactions or drug–herb interactions

Socioeconomic and Educational Influences

- Education and literacy level
- Knowledge and skills related to food and nutrition
- Social environment—assess for isolation and social support system
- General economic status and access to adequate food (**food security**)
- Functional capacity related to activities of daily living (ADL) and instrumental activities of daily living (IADL), such as shopping, meal preparation, self-feeding
- Activity level

be an inaccurate recall in which patients contrive answers they feel the nurse is seeking. Gentle prompting to obtain complete information is often needed. The nurse should ask about all food from meals and snacks; all liquids, including alcohol; and any use of nutritional supplements such as herbs, vitamins, minerals, and diet and sports nutritional products. In order to assess nutrient intake accurately, one must determine whether fortified versions of common foods are consumed. Many foods are now fortified and should not be overlooked as significant sources of vitamins and minerals. Cereals and juices are examples of fortified foods to which nutrients not normally found in the product, such as calcium, have been added. The nurse can prompt the patient to share information regarding modifications in the diet by asking "Have you ever followed a special diet for any reason, such as to change your weight, treat a condition, or alter your nutritional health?" If an affirmative answer is given, the nurse can continue with "Please tell me more about that." Notice that the question uses the phrase "change your weight" and does not specifically ask about weight loss or gain so as to not appear judgmental. A family member may participate in the interview with the permission of the patient or if the patient is unable to recall for any reason, as in the case of an adult with communication difficulties or a child. Accuracy of a secondhand recall, even from a family member, has been found to be variable.

A best estimate of portion sizes will improve the accuracy of a recall. It is easy to over- and underestimate portion sizes of foods and liquids without a visual comparison. Life-size, culturally appropriate food models are available. Digital photographs are less cumbersome and are easily available. It is not always convenient to carry facsimiles to different settings where the nurse may be interviewing a patient. In such cases, use of the food analogies in Figure 10.1 ■ can be helpful.

There are drawbacks to the exclusive use of diet recall for obtaining a patient's nutritional history. A 24-hour recall is simply a 1-day example of intake and may not be indicative of normal habits. Other types and amounts of intake may occur on different days that were not assessed. Patients may have significant food habits that occur occasionally but not on the day recalled. The use of dietary supplements or alcohol often does not occur in the same fashion each day, yet it is crucial information to assess. Many other important data related to diet could be overlooked by relying on the recall alone. The accuracy of the recall relies heavily on the memory of the patient and the good interviewing skills of the nurse. Repeated diet recalls taken during subsequent healthcare visits can be used for comparison purposes and validation of intake.

Underreporting bias can occur with all parts of a nutritional history and may become apparent during the recall. Patients seeking the social approval of the nurse or wanting to avoid disapproval for their habits may underreport. Underreporting occurs for all ages and is seen more often in smokers, the obese, and individuals with lower educational and socioeconomic levels. In addition, alcohol and drug use are frequently underreported. A nonjudgmental approach during the nutritional history will provide an environment conducive to full answers by the patient. In addition to asking open-ended questions, using a neutral tone of voice and maintaining facial expressions that do not hint at approval or disapproval are key to appearing nonjudgmental. Combining the recall with a food frequency assessment and a focused interview will yield the best information on which to base an assessment.

Small potato or piece of fruit: computer mouse

3 oz animal protein: deck of cards

1 oz cheese: small box of wooden matches

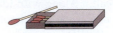

2 tbsp: golf ball

4 tbsp: four thumbs

1 cup dry measure: tightly clenched small woman's fist

Figure 10.1 Analogies for estimating portion size.

Food Frequency Questionnaire

A **food frequency questionnaire** assesses intake of a variety of food groups on a daily, weekly, or longer basis. This questionnaire helps to fill in some of the missing data not captured by a 24-hour recall and helps to provide a more balanced assessment of intake. For example, in a 24-hour recall a patient may indicate no fruit intake, whereas during a food frequency assessment, two servings of fruit and one serving of juice are reported as a daily average. When an entire category of food seems missing, the nurse can ask further questions to ascertain the reason. In this way, using both the recall and the food frequency questionnaire can uncover information that might not otherwise have surfaced in the conversation. Food intolerances, allergies, dieting, and food faddism are examples. Food frequency questionnaires can be formal instruments composed of a checklist of food groups and foods or shorter questionnaires aimed at gathering general information. All food, beverage, and supplement groups should be included. Patients can fill out longer checklists before or after an interview but may find such tools cumbersome. Shorter questionnaires can be administered verbally and

Table 10.2 Completed Food Frequency Questionnaire

FOOD	VARIETY	TYPE	AMOUNT PER DAY	AMOUNT PER WEEK	LESS THAN ONCE PER WEEK (LIST)
Fruit	Juice Fresh Canned/frozen	Apple Melon None	12 oz	1 cup	
Vegetables	Green Other	Varied Squash		1–2× 1×	
Dairy	Milk Cheese Yogurt	Low fat Never	2 cups		1× month
Protein	Animal/Plant	Poultry or fish Soyburger or tofu	Each night	 1–2×	
Fats	Saturated Unsaturated	Butter Olive oil	1–2 pats	 1 tbsp	
Fluids	General Caffeine Alcohol	Water Tea Wine	4 oz 4× with meds Each a.m.	 3×	
Sweets and Sugars		Cookies	2×		
Supplements	Vitamin/mineral Herbal Other:	Multivitamin Echinacea Over-the-counter weight-loss product (cannot recall ingredients)	one		4–5× year for cold Tried once and stopped, because of dizziness

are more practical. Table 10.2 is an example of a basic food frequency questionnaire.

Food Record

Keeping a food record or diary for up to 3 days can provide supplemental information for a nutritional history. Recording 2 sequential weekdays and 1 weekend day works well. Food diaries longer than 3 days in length tend to be recorded retrospectively with a loss of accuracy. Underreporting bias should also be considered when evaluating a food diary (Lopes et al., 2016). Food records are generally thought of as the gold standard for establishing nutritional habits, but it is worth noting that the act itself of maintaining a food record can directly influence a person's consumption. This phenomenon is attributed to the patient's concern that consumption habits may be met with judgment by the healthcare practitioner, causing the patient to alter food selections during the recording period. Instructing the individual not to alter food habits while recording may alleviate this.

Focused Nutritional History Interview

A diet recall, food frequency questionnaire, or food diary can be used individually or in combination as parameters in a quick nutritional assessment. Conducting a more focused interview along with these tools, either as part of a nursing assessment or just concerning nutrition, will give the clearest picture of nutritional status.

A nutrition-focused interview can easily occur at the same time as a diet recall. As the recall is conducted, pertinent ancillary questions can be asked. For example, a patient may report drinking cranberry juice at breakfast because of intolerance to citrus fruits. The nurse could then use that cue to ask if there are other intolerances or food allergies before getting back on track to the recall. The remainder of the needed nutrition history data can be gathered from the patient and the medical chart after the recall portion of the interview. This more extensive form of a nutritional history assesses current habits but also can assess former habits. Past chronic dieting, supplement use, and therapeutic diets are examples of important historic data to gather. Box 10.3 outlines data topics to gather during the focused interview in addition to diet recall data. Box 10.4 is an example of a nutrition assessment form combining diet recall, food frequency, and focused interview data.

Physical Assessment

The physical assessment portion of a nutritional assessment consists of two parts: anthropometric measurements and a head-to-toe physical assessment of a patient.

Anthropometric Measurements

Anthropometric measurements include any scientific measurement of the body. Pertinent data from the medical history and examination should be considered during this portion of a nutritional assessment. The healthcare setting and the patient's needs dictate the depth of data gathered. Height, weight, and measurements of body fat and muscle composition are

Box 10.4 Nutrition Assessment Form

NUTRITION VALUATION

Name: _____   Date: _____

Home Address: _____   Referred By: _____

_____   _____

Phone: _____   Signed Consent/Date: _____

Age: _____

Height (Ht)	Weight (Wt)	Recent wt change	Max/Min wts	Patient goal
Body fat	Wt Hx	Exercise	Ex. freq/duration	Other activities
Medical Hx/Dx	Rx and OTC meds	Vits/minerals	Supplements	Herbs
Previous diets	Food allergies/intolerances	Food prep/refrig	Restrictive?	Living with
Binge?	Purge?	Laxatives?	Other?	

Diet Hx:

M–F   Weekends

FOOD FREQUENCY

Fruit (indicate day/week/other)

vit C _____

other _____

Dairy (indicate day/week/other)

milk/yogurt _____

cheese _____

other _____

Fats (indicate day/week/other)

saturated _____

polyunsaturated _____

monounsaturated _____

Vegetables

green _____

other _____

Animal Protein

_____

_____

Sugars/Sweets

_____

_____

Grains/Starch

whole grain _____

other _____

Plant Protein

_____

_____

Fluids/Water

caffeinated _____

alcohol _____

other _____

Source: Provided courtesy of Sheila Tucker, MA, RD, CSSD, LDN.

Box 10.5 Calculating Weight Loss Percentage

A community health nurse is visiting the senior center for a seasonal flu shot clinic. Miss M., an 80-year-old female, complains that she needs to sew new elastic into her skirt as the old elastic is not working to keep the skirt snug at her waistline. The nurse wonders if Miss M. has lost some weight since the last visit and weighs her. She weighs 108 lb, down from 120 lb 6 months ago.

(120 lb prior weight - 108 lb current weight)/120 lb prior weight

= 12 lb weight loss / 120 lb prior weight = 0.10

0.10 × 100 = 10% weight loss in 6 months

---

anthropometric measurements. At times, estimated measurements and alternative techniques for obtaining anthropometric data may be necessary because of specific circumstances that make standard measurement difficult or impossible.

Height Measurement of height is needed in adults to make an accurate assessment of weight status. In children, height is monitored on a continuum to assess growth and, indirectly, nutritional status. See Chapter 8 for accurate height assessment methods. ∞

Alternative methods of height measurement (e.g., fingertip-to-fingertip length, sternum-to-fingertip doubled, knee height) may be used when the standard method of measurement is not possible. When no means of obtaining measured height is feasible, self-reported height may be used. Every effort should be made to obtain a current measured height, but this is not always possible. The accuracy of self-reported heights can be questionable (Sagna, Schopflocher, Raine, Nykiforuk, & Plotnikoff, 2013). Men, women, and adolescents have been reported to overstate self-reported height by up to 2 cm (.787 in.). Adults over age 60 have been reported to overstate height by approximately 2.5 cm (.984 in.). Whichever method of measurement is used (including self-report), it should be noted in the documentation to decrease the chance of subsequent disparities in measurement using alternative methods.

Weight Current body weight and weight history are essential components of a nutritional assessment. Every effort should be made to obtain actual weight because self-reported weights are often underreported in men and women (Sagna et al., 2013). In the individual with undetected weight loss, self-reported weight could delay proper nutritional intervention by masking the clinical change. See Chapter 8 for accurate methods to determine the patient's weight. ∞

Weight history is crucial for determining the presence of any intentional or unplanned weight losses. Weight history is also followed in children and pregnant females to monitor growth and development. Weight guidelines for children and pregnant females are outlined in Chapter 25 and Chapter 26. ∞ When obtaining a weight history, the nurse should look for prior documentation of actual weight, if available. Otherwise, open-ended questions can be asked, such as "When was the last time you were weighed?" followed by "What did you weigh then?" The nurse may also ask for weights at specific points in time as a cross-check: "What did you weigh this past summer before coming to college?" The nurse should not simply ask "Has your weight changed recently?" because the patient may not have an accurate answer or may not want to divulge any known gain or loss. The nurse can discern whether weight change has occurred by asking for specific weight information and calculating any noted differences.

It is important to note increases as well as decreases in weight. A weight *gain* of 3 pounds or more in a 1-week period is a useful marker in determining issues related to fluid retention, edema, or dehydration, which may indicate conditions such as congestive heart failure or renal disease. In contrast, unintentional weight *loss* of 5% or more of body weight over a month or 10% or more over 6 months is considered clinically significant and warrants attention. Weight change is calculated using the following formula:

([prior weight − current weight]/prior weight) ×100 = % weight change

Box 10.5 outlines an example of calculations used to determine percent weight change.

Body Mass Index Body mass index (BMI) is widely used to assess appropriate weight for height using the following formula: BMI = weight (kg)/height^2 (meters). Parameters have been established to delineate underweight, healthy weight, and overweight standards in adults based on current scientific findings of morbidity and mortality prevalence associated with various BMI values. The U.S. Department of Health and Human Services, National Heart, Lung, and Blood Institute (NHLBI; n.d.), along with the World Health Organization (WHO; 2014), have established internationally used classifications for BMI, which are outlined in Table 10.3. Many charts, tables, and nomograms exist to make BMI calculations quick and easy for clinical application.

Exclusive use of BMI as an indicator of weight status makes the assumption that all individuals have equal body composition at each given weight—that every person of the same weight has the same amount of muscle mass, body fat, and bone mineral content. This generalization has not been found to be true and, therefore, represents a clinical limitation to the use of BMI alone when

Table 10.3 Classification of Body Mass Index in Adults

BODY MASS INDEX (BMI)	CLASSIFICATION
<16	Severe underweight
16–16.99	Moderate underweight
17–18.49	Mild underweight
18.5–24.9	Normal
25–29.9	Overweight
30–34.9	Obese class 1
35–39.9	Obese class 2
≥ 40	Obese class 3

Sources: U.S. Department of Health and Human Services, National Heart, Lung, and Blood Institute. (n.d.); World Health Organization (2014).

assessing weight. Athletic people with little body fat and ample muscle mass can be classified as overweight using BMI despite a visual assessment that reveals a high level of fitness. Likewise, an individual's BMI may fall within the classification of healthy, yet the person may have little muscle mass and excess body fat.

BMI classifications exist as generic standards of height–weight comparisons for the general population. Racial differences have been observed in body composition. Asian adults have been reported to have a higher proportion of body fat mass at a given BMI than Caucasians have. African American adults have greater muscle mass and bone mineral density at a given BMI than Caucasians have. In addition, ethnic differences within race categories have been observed (Harvard School of Public Health, 2014). For example, Chinese adults have been observed to have proportionately higher body fat mass at a given BMI than Polynesians. Despite these variances, different standards for BMI do not exist for any ethnic populations. These drawbacks indicate the problem of using BMI as a sole indicator of weight status or nutritional health and are an excellent example of the need to use multiple parameters when conducting an assessment. In particular, it is recommended that BMI be used in conjunction with waist circumference when assessing the adult for health risks associated with overweight or obesity (Cerhan et al., 2014).

Height–Weight Tables Height–weight tables have been used in the past to assess body weight in adults but are no longer a standard. Such tables outlined reference weights for given heights for both males and females or were gender specific. Table 10.4 is an example of a current height–weight table based on BMI calculations presented in an easy-to-use form.

Use of such height–weight tables has the same limitations as does use of BMI as a sole indicator of weight status. Differences in body composition go largely unaccounted for, and the clinician must remember to assess each person for these individual differences.

Waist Circumference Excess, centrally located abdominal fat deposition is considered to be an independent risk factor for cardiovascular disease in adults. Measurement of waist circumference can be included in a comprehensive nutritional assessment, especially when risk factors for cardiovascular disease exist. The NHLBI considers waist circumference greater than 102 cm (40.16 in.) in males and greater than 88 cm (34.65 in.) in females indicative of risk.

Waist circumference should be measured with a spring-loaded measuring tape to ensure reliable tension is applied with each measurement. Use of the bony landmark on the lateral border of the ilium is recommended when marking a site guide for the measurement. Figure 10.2 ■ depicts the location of this landmark. Standing behind the patient and palpating the right hip can locate the lateral ilium. A line should be drawn at the uppermost lateral line of the ilium at the midaxillary point. Other references suggest measuring waist circumference just below the umbilicus, but this can be unreliable because an obese state can change the position of the umbilicus. Waist circumference should be measured at the marked midaxillary line while keeping the measuring tape parallel to the floor. Measurement should be done directly on the surface of the skin and not over clothing. It has been suggested that taking measurements with the patient in front of a mirror is helpful to ensure a true horizontal extension of the measuring tape, especially in those who are obese or have wider hips than waist. The spring-loaded measuring tape should be pulled taut but should not compress the skin. Uneven tension on the measure between sequential measurements will alter reliability of waist circumference measurements.

Waist circumference validity can be limited by obesity when increases in abdominal fat mass become pendulous because of the effects of gravity and no longer are situated along the waistline. Increases in abdominal subcutaneous fat and increases in body weight may not always be reflected by increases in waist circumference. In addition, waist circumference is not a valid nutritional tool for use in adults with ascites, for pregnant females, or for those with other medical conditions associated with increases in fat-free abdominal girth, such as polycystic kidney disease.

Body Composition Measurement More specific assessment of body fat and muscle mass than weight alone can be made

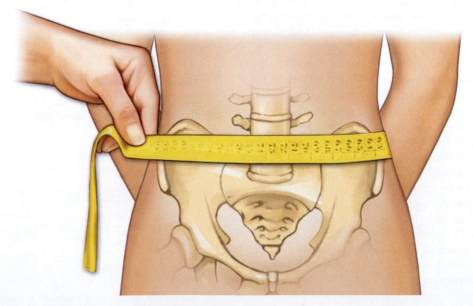

Figure 10.2 Landmarks for waist circumference.

Table 10.4 Height–Weight Table with BMI Calculation

Locate the height of interest in the leftmost column, then read across the row for that height to the weight of interest. Follow the column of the weight up to the top row that lists the BMI. BMI of 19–24 is the healthy weight range, BMI of 25–29 is the overweight range, BMI of 30–39 is the obese range, and BMI of 40 and above is in the extreme obesity range.

Body Mass Index Table

	NORMAL						OVERWEIGHT					OBESE										EXTREME OBESITY															
BMI	19	20	21	22	23	24	25	26	27	28	29	30	31	32	33	34	35	36	37	38	39	40	41	42	43	44	45	46	47	48	49	50	51	52	53	54
Height (inches)																																				
58	91	96	100	105	110	115	119	124	129	134	138	143	148	153	158	162	167	172	177	181	186	191	196	201	205	210	215	220	224	229	234	239	244	248	253	258
59	94	99	104	109	114	119	124	128	133	138	143	148	153	158	163	168	173	178	183	188	193	198	203	208	212	217	222	227	232	237	242	247	252	257	262	267
60	97	102	107	112	118	123	128	133	138	143	148	153	158	163	168	174	179	184	189	194	199	204	209	215	220	225	230	235	240	245	250	255	261	266	271	276
61	100	106	111	116	122	127	132	137	143	148	153	158	164	169	174	180	185	190	195	201	206	211	217	222	227	232	238	243	248	254	259	264	269	275	280	285
62	104	109	115	120	126	131	136	142	147	153	158	164	169	175	180	186	191	196	202	207	213	218	224	229	235	240	246	251	256	262	267	273	278	284	289	295
63	107	113	118	124	130	135	141	146	152	158	163	169	175	180	186	191	197	203	208	214	220	225	231	237	242	248	254	259	265	270	278	282	287	293	299	304
64	110	116	122	128	134	140	145	151	157	163	169	174	180	186	192	197	204	209	215	221	227	232	238	244	250	256	262	267	273	279	285	291	296	302	308	314
65	114	120	126	132	138	144	150	156	162	168	174	180	186	192	198	204	210	216	222	228	234	240	246	252	258	264	270	276	282	288	294	300	306	312	318	324
66	118	124	130	136	142	148	155	161	167	173	179	186	192	198	204	210	216	223	229	235	241	247	253	260	266	272	278	284	291	297	303	309	315	322	328	334
67	121	127	134	140	146	153	159	166	172	178	185	191	198	204	211	217	223	230	236	242	249	255	261	268	274	280	287	293	299	306	312	319	325	331	338	344
68	125	131	138	144	151	158	164	171	177	184	190	197	203	210	216	223	230	236	243	249	256	262	269	276	282	289	295	302	308	315	322	328	335	341	348	354
69	128	135	142	149	155	162	169	176	182	189	196	203	209	216	223	230	236	243	250	257	263	270	277	284	291	297	304	311	318	324	331	338	345	351	358	365
70	132	139	146	153	160	167	174	181	188	195	202	209	216	222	229	236	243	250	257	264	271	278	285	292	299	306	313	320	327	334	341	348	355	362	369	376
71	136	143	150	157	165	172	179	186	193	200	208	215	222	229	236	243	250	257	265	272	279	286	293	301	308	315	322	329	338	343	351	358	365	372	379	386
72	140	147	154	162	169	177	184	191	199	206	213	221	228	235	242	250	258	265	272	279	287	294	302	309	316	324	331	338	346	353	361	368	375	383	390	397
73	144	151	159	166	174	182	189	197	204	212	219	227	235	242	250	257	265	272	280	288	295	302	310	318	325	333	340	348	355	363	371	378	386	393	401	408
74	148	155	163	171	179	186	194	202	210	218	225	233	241	249	256	264	272	280	287	295	303	311	319	326	334	342	350	358	365	373	381	389	396	404	412	420
75	152	160	168	176	184	192	200	208	216	224	232	240	248	256	264	272	279	287	295	303	311	319	327	335	343	351	359	367	375	383	391	399	407	415	423	431
76	156	164	172	180	189	197	205	213	221	230	238	246	254	263	271	279	287	295	304	312	320	328	336	344	353	361	369	377	385	394	402	410	418	426	435	443

Body Weight (pounds)

Source: Adapted from Clinical Guidelines on the Identification, Evaluation, and Treatment of Overweight and Obesity in Adults: The Evidence Report.

using skinfold measurements or technologic instruments. Muscle mass is also referred to as **somatic protein** stores or skeletal muscle. This second tier of anthropometric measurements can assess body composition either in just two components, fat and fat-free mass, or in multicomponents, which can include more precise analysis of fat-free mass for muscle, bone, and fluid components. Increasing levels of technology and updating of older reference values to include multicomponent analysis will allow more valid assessment of body composition in the future.

SKINFOLD MEASUREMENTS Skinfold thickness measurements can estimate subcutaneous body fat stores. Measurements taken at up to eight sites on the body are believed to be predictive of overall body fat composition. Sites include the triceps; the chest; the subscapular, midaxillary, and suprailiac regions; the abdomen; and the upper thigh.

The tricep skinfold (TSF) is the site most often used to estimate subcutaneous fat because of easy access to this measurement in most situations. Tricep measurements are done at the midpoint of the arm equidistant from the uppermost posterior edge of the acromion process of the scapula and the olecranon process of the elbow. A measuring tape should be used to determine this midpoint on the back of the upper arm, and the site should be marked for reference. It is helpful to have the patient flex the arm at a 90-degree angle while locating the bony landmarks and measuring the midpoint. However, the arm should hang freely during the skinfold measurement itself. Figure 10.3 ■ illustrates the location of the TSF measurement.

Skinfold measurements are made using professional grade calipers and a flexible measuring tape. Plastic calipers should not be used because they become bent or warped with use and then measurements are inaccurate. The technique for properly grasping the skinfold layers and subcutaneous fat takes practice before reliable measurements can be made. Both skinfold layers and subcutaneous fat are pinched and then held gently between the thumb and forefinger with care taken not to grasp underlying muscle. The fold is then measured between the calipers for each marked site on the body. Body composition results will not be representative if a distinct separation of subcutaneous fat and muscle cannot be accomplished when grasping the skinfold. To allow for even compression before the reading is taken, the caliper jaws should be placed perpendicular to the fold and left in place for several seconds after tension is released. Three measurements should be taken at each site and then averaged. For consistency purposes, skinfold measurements should be taken on the right side of the body.

Measurement values for each skinfold site can be evaluated in two ways. First, they may be used to monitor a patient over time, comparing measurements at intervals for changes in body composition. Second, they may be compared with reference values that are specific for gender, age, race, and fitness level. Reference values are simply descriptions of body composition compiled from subjects in population studies and should not be

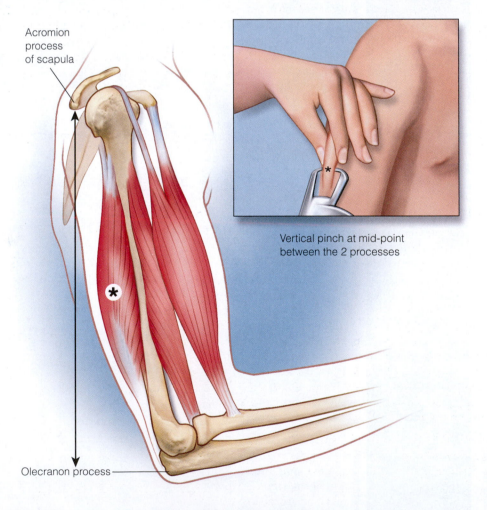

Acromion process of scapula

Olecranon process

Vertical pinch at mid-point between the 2 processes

Figure 10.3 Landmarks for triceps skinfold measurement.

considered the same as a standard. Reference values allow the clinician to assess an individual's measurements compared with others in a similar, well-defined population group. Standards, however, are values that are known to be desirable targets for health regardless of population norms.

Commonly used reference values to assess skinfold measurements in some populations are more than 20 years old. Another problem is that these older references were not obtained from diverse population groups, which makes them difficult to apply to the wider population that exists today. Newer reference standards are constantly being published and are becoming more population specific, but no widely used single reference exists. Therefore, the nature of human diversity requires even more research to be done in this area to appreciate the variety of reference values needed for racial, ethnic, age, fitness, and gender categories. Age-related differences in body fat distribution necessitate use of the specific skinfold references established for older adults because the relationship between specific-site subcutaneous fat measurements and total body fat is different than in younger adults. Changes in skin elasticity and connective tissue also affect skinfold accuracy with age.

MIDARM MUSCLE CIRCUMFERENCE AND CALF CIRCUMFERENCE Circumference measurements of limbs can be used alone or in conjunction with skinfold measurements to provide additional or confirmational body composition information. Midarm muscle circumference (MAMC) is obtained by measuring the midarm circumference (MAC) at the same site as the tricep skinfold. A spring-loaded flexible measuring tape is used to provide tension without compressing the skin. Calf circumference is measured at the site of maximum calf width, which can be determined by placing the measure around the calf and sliding it along the calf until a maximum value is noted. Limb circumferences are measured in centimeters in adults.

BIOELECTRICAL IMPEDANCE ANALYSIS Bioelectrical impedance analysis (BIA) is a noninvasive tool for assessing body composition employing principles of electroconduction through water, muscle, and fat. In traditional BIA, electrodes are placed on the dorsal surfaces of the right foot and hand with the patient in the supine position on a nonconductive surface. Calculations are based on the knowledge that muscle and fluids have a higher electrolyte and water content than does fat, and thus they conduct electric current differently. Altered hydration and altered skin temperature will cause measurement error by altering electric current flow. Patients should be well hydrated when employing BIA technology, or dehydration will slow conductivity and give a falsely high body fat measurement. Equations used to predict body fat composition with BIA must be population specific. Standard error for BIA measurements approximates that of skinfold measurements at 3% to 4%, provided correct equations are used and the patient is hydrated. Handheld BIA devices are being manufactured for easier clinical use (see Figure 10.4 ■). This version of the device measures segmental electric impedance from arm to arm rather than the traditional whole-body method.

NEAR-INFRARED INTERACTANCE Near-infrared interactance devices measure body fat at specific sites by passing infrared light through tissue and measuring reflected light. Predictive equations estimate body fat composition at the site. Gender, body weight, height, frame size, and fitness level are included in the calculation to determine total body fat percentage. Generally this measurement is performed on the bicep. Small, handheld

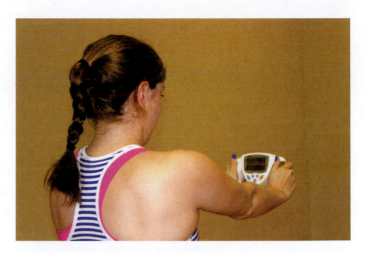

Figure 10.4 Handheld BIA device.
Source: Sheila Tucker.

near-infrared devices are available for clinical use. Standard error for near-infrared measurement exceeds 3.5% and can be as high as 5.5%; error is greater with increased body fat.

LABORATORY BODY COMPOSITION Several other more sophisticated and expensive tools exist for measuring body composition. These are primarily used in laboratory research and not in clinical situations. Underwater weighing, dual energy x-ray absorptiometry (DEXA), and body plethysmography are examples of research tools. Underwater weighing requires the patient to be completely submersed underwater to measure water displacement by the body. Regression equations calculate body fat based on known density of fat-free and fat tissue. Underwater weighing has long been called the gold standard for body composition although it uses only a two-component model and does not measure bone mineral content or total body water. DEXA takes advantage of x-ray technology to measure a multicomponent model of body composition and is quickly becoming the research tool of choice. *Plethysmography* measures air volume displacement by the body using similar methodology to underwater weighing.

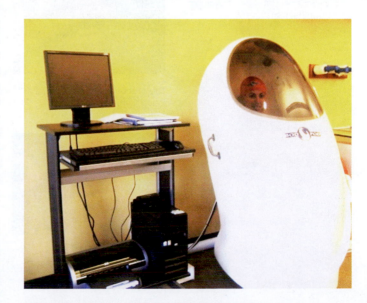

Figure 10.5 BOD POD Body Composition Tracking System.

Patients are measured in a small chamber called a BOD POD Body Composition Tracking System (see Figure 10.5 ■).

Body Fat References or Standards Standards of body fat percentage that are associated with health or morbidity and mortality have not been established. Many sources agree that a minimum essential body fat percentage exists. A minimum of 3% body fat in men and 12% in women is considered essential. These minimums are the lowest value compatible with health, but optimal body fat is higher and should be determined on an individual basis. It is recommended that a range of body fat be given rather than a specific target because of the errors associated with predicting specific values. A range of 12% to 20% body fat in men and 20% to 30% in women has been suggested for health, but more research is necessary to develop population-specific recommendations. Research aimed at the development of future standards and references for body fat percentage is needed. Research specifically addressing the relationship between BMI and body fat percentage will allow the nurse a clearer assessment of body composition traits associated with health risks. Age-specific recommendations are also needed.

Head-to-Toe Physical Assessment

A visual head-to-toe physical assessment can yield findings that may be indicative of normal or abnormal nutritional status. Like all other components of a nutritional assessment, the physical assessment is most useful when used in conjunction with other nutritional assessment parameters. Table 10.5 outlines physical findings associated with poor nutritional health.

Table 10.5 Clinical Findings Associated with Poor Nutritional Health

FINDING	POTENTIAL DEFICIENT NUTRIENT	FINDING	POTENTIAL DEFICIENT NUTRIENT
Hair Dull, sparse, brittle hair Dyspigmentation (**flag sign**) Hair loss (**alopecia**)	Protein Protein, biotin, or zinc Protein, iron, or biotin **Flag sign** *Source:* Centers for Disease Control and Prevention.	*Face* Moon face Pallor	Protein Iron **Pallor** *Source:* Dmytro Zinkevych/123RF.
Eyes Dry mucosa (**xerophthalmia**), blindness and night blindness, Bitot's spot Pale conjunctiva Yellow subdermal fat deposits around lids (**xanthelasma**)	Vitamin A **Dry mucosa** Iron High cholesterol **Xanthelasma** *Source:* Centers for Disease Control and Prevention.	*Lips* Cracks at corners (**angular stomatitis**); inflammation (**cheilosis**)	Riboflavin **Angular stomatitis** *Source:* Centers for Disease Control and Prevention.

(continued)

Table 10.5 Clinical Findings Associated with Poor Nutritional Health (continued)

FINDING	POTENTIAL DEFICIENT NUTRIENT	FINDING	POTENTIAL DEFICIENT NUTRIENT
Tongue Smooth, beefy red or magenta (**glossitis**)	Niacin, pyridoxine (B_6), riboflavin **Glossitis** *Source:* Iryna Timonina/123RF.	**Teeth** Delayed eruption Caries in a baby Mottled enamel	Vitamin D May indicate baby-bottle tooth decay **Baby bottle caries** Excess fluoride *Source:* Levent Konuk/123RF.
Atrophic papillae Diminished taste (hypogeusia)	Iron Zinc **Atrophic papillae** *Source:* Centers for Disease Control and Prevention.	**Glands** Increased parotid size Increased thyroid (goiter)	Protein-calorie malnutrition (PCM) or bulimia Iodine **Goiter, neck** *Source:* Karan Bunjean/Shutterstock.
Gums Spongy, bleeding (scorbutic)	Vitamin C **Scorbutic gums** *Source:* Centers for Disease Control and Prevention.	**Nails** Spoon-shaped (**koilonychia**) ridges	Iron **Koilonychia** *Source:* Mediscan/Alamy Stock Photo. *(continued)*

Table 10.5 Clinical Findings Associated with Poor Nutritional Health (continued)

FINDING	POTENTIAL DEFICIENT NUTRIENT	FINDING	POTENTIAL DEFICIENT NUTRIENT
Skin Poor wound healing/decubitus ulcer Goose bump flesh (**follicular hyperkeratosis**) Dry, scaly Photosensitive symmetric rash (**pellagra**) Bruising (**purpura**) Pinpoint hemorrhages (**petechiae**)	Protein, calories, essential fatty acids Vitamin A Vitamin C Vitamin K Niacin Zinc	**Skeleton/Trunk** Stunted growth Fluid-filled abdomen (**ascites**) Beading on ribs (rachitic rosary), bowed legs (**rickets**), widened epiphysis, narrow chest (pigeon breast) Loss of fat, muscle wasting	PCM, zinc Protein Vitamin D Protein, calories

Skin in pellagra (vitamin B3 deficiency)
Source: Dr. M. A. Ansary/Science Source.

Rickets
Source: Jeff Rotman/Alamy Stock Photo.

FINDING	POTENTIAL DEFICIENT NUTRIENT	FINDING	POTENTIAL DEFICIENT NUTRIENT
Genitalia Delayed sexual maturation (hypogonadism)	Zinc	**Limbs** Loss of fat, muscle wasting Pitting edema	PCM Protein

Hypogonadism
Source: Clinical Photography, Central Manchester University Hospitals NHS Foundation Trust, UK/Science Source.

Pitting edema
Source: Akkalak Aiempradit/ Shutterstock.

FINDING	POTENTIAL DEFICIENT NUTRIENT	FINDING	POTENTIAL DEFICIENT NUTRIENT
Cardiovascular System Arrhythmia	Potassium, magnesium	**Nervous System** Hyporeflexia, confabulation Dementia, confusion, ataxia Neuropathy Tetany	Thiamine Vitamin B_{12} Excess vitamin B_6 Calcium, magnesium

Data that are gathered as part of the physical assessment are also pertinent to the nutritional assessment. Existing medical diagnoses and treatment such as medication or surgical plans are important when evaluating nutritional status. Physical findings such as poor dental health, problems with chewing or swallowing, gastrointestinal complaints, functional decline in physical or mental status, and declining vision, taste, or smell all have negative effects on nutritional health.

Biochemical Assessment— Laboratory Measurements

Several biochemical parameters are commonly used in a nutritional assessment. No one laboratory value is unique in its sensitivity to predict nutritional status because each has confounding reasons for abnormal values. As in the case of physical findings of malnutrition, laboratory values may not reflect current known nutrition status because half-lives and body pools of plasma components vary.

The biochemical assessment and laboratory measurements along with their significance, values, and findings are summarized in Table 10.6.

Nutritional Screening and Assessment Tools

Nutritional assessment data can be gathered and evaluated in a comprehensive fashion, or a more formal validated tool can be used to streamline the process. Numerous nutritional screening and assessment tools exist, but none is considered the gold standard for use in most populations. Until aconsensus is reached defining malnutrition, a variety of nutritional screening and assessment tools will continue to be published.

Nutritional screening tools are used for quick assessment of risk factors for poor nutritional health. Screening tools are not meant for diagnostic purposes and are instead used to triage patients who may require further assessment or intervention. Screening tools give a rough estimate of nutrition risk or status. Nutritional assessment tools are generally more comprehensive than screening tools for the goal of identifying or diagnosing malnutrition. Not all assessment or screening tools are validated for use in the populations where they are being used. The nurse should be aware that use of a screening tool that has not

Table 10.6 Biochemical Assessment Laboratory Measurements

LABORATORY MEASUREMENT	SIGNIFICANCE	VALUES AND FINDINGS
Albumin	Low albumin levels can be indicative of depleted visceral protein status and malnutrition. Dehydration or overhydration will lead to false levels because of hemoconcentration or dilution. Liver disease, infection, and inflammation can alter albumin unrelated to nutrition.	Expected 3.5 g/L to 5 g/L Half-life in days 14 to 20 Mild malnutrition 2.8 g/L to 3.4 g/L Moderate malnutrition 2.1 g/L to 3.4 g/L Severe malnutrition < 2.1 g/L
Prealbumin	Also called thyroxine-binding prealbumin, has a shorter half-life and is therefore felt to provide a more current picture of protein status than does albumin. Prealbumin is an acute-phase reactant protein and is affected by inflammation and infection. Hemoconcentration or dilution will cause false values.	Expected 150 mg/L to 350 mg/L Half-life in days 2 to 3 Mild malnutrition 110 mg/L to 150 mg/L Moderate malnutrition 50 mg/L to 109 mg/L Severe malnutrition < 50 mg/L
Transferrin	Responsible for iron binding and transport. Inflammation, infection, or iron deficiency can alter transferrin value.	Expected > 200 mg/dL Half-life in days 8 to 10 Mild malnutrition 180 mg/L to 200 mg/L Moderate malnutrition 160 mg/L to 180 mg/L Severe malnutrition < 160 mg/L
Total Lymphocyte Count (TLC)	Decreased value can indicate poor immunocompetence from malnutrition. Confounding medical conditions such as cancer or immunosuppressive drugs interfere with TLC usefulness in nutritional assessment.	Expected TLC is 2,000 cells/mm^3 to 3,500 cells/mm^3. Plasma level below 1,500 cells/mm^3 may indicate malnutrition and poor immunocompetence.
Delayed Skin Hypersensitivity Testing	A delayed response to intradermal injection of foreign substances such as *Streptococcus* or *Candida.*	Delayed or no response may indicate malnutrition, poor immune system, or no previous exposure.
Cholesterol	High cholesterol may indicate overnutrition or undernutrition. Low cholesterol because of drug treatment is not a risk factor for malnutrition.	≥ 200 mg/dL is associated with cardiovascular disease. ≤ 160 mg/dL may indicate malnutrition.
Nutritional Anemia Assessment	Poor nutrition may be evidenced by low stores of iron, folic acid, vitamin B_{12}.	*Macrocytic anemia* as evidenced by increased red blood cell volume and deficient folic acid or vitamin B_{12} level. *Microcytic anemia* as evidenced by decreased red blood cell volume and iron indices. *Iron deficiency anemia* as evidenced by low plasma hemoglobin, hematocrit, ferritin, iron.
Nitrogen Balance	Measured to estimate adequacy of dietary protein intake in relation to protein losses. Nitrogen is used as the marker to measure protein losses.	*Nitrogen balance* as evidenced by nitrogen intake equals nitrogen loss. *Catabolism* occurs when there is a negative nitrogen balance because losses exceed intake. *Anabolism* occurs when the intake of protein and calories exceeds the nitrogen loss.
Plasma Proteins	Albumin, prealbumin, and transferrin are each used to assess visceral protein status.	
Immunocompetence	A depressed immune status can result from malnutrition, disease, medication, or other disease treatments.	

been validated through in-depth research may lead to frequent missed diagnoses or incorrect diagnoses of poor nutritional health. Sharp clinical judgment by the nurse is a necessary adjunct to any tool. Any risk of malnutrition identified within a screen warrants a referral to a registered dietitian.

ChooseMyPlate

Dietary Guidelines for Americans is published jointly by the U.S. Department of Health and Human Services (USDHHS) and the U.S. Department of Agriculture (USDA). The *Guidelines* (USDA, n.d.) provide authoritative advice for people age 2 and older about how good dietary habits can promote health and reduce risk for major chronic diseases. The most recent guidelines provide an accompanying food guide icon called MyPlate and an interactive website that may be used for individual food guide planning and diet analysis (see Figure 10.6 ■). This site is located at *www.choosemyplate.gov*. The nurse can compare the diet recall or nutrition history data with the distribution of food groups recommended on MyPlate and make a general assessment of diet adequacy. The number and size of food servings included in MyPlate are generic and should be adjusted for more active or less active individuals. The comprehensive website has tools for calculating and tracking individual nutritional needs for calories, major nutrients, and food groups. The benefit of the new icon is that it presents an easily understood image of what an individual meal looks like that would meet current guidelines for health and therefore can be used with all levels of knowledge and literacy skills. The accompanying website has more in-depth information for use with a variety of learning levels.

Other Screening and Assessment Tools

In addition to dietary guideline resources such as *www.choosemyplate.gov,* there are specialized screening and assessment tools that many clinicians have found helpful.

The DETERMINE Checklist DETERMINE is an acronym standing for **D**isease, **E**ating poorly, **T**ooth loss/mouth pain, **E**conomic hardship, **R**educed social contact, **M**ultiple medicines, **I**nvoluntary weight loss/gain, **N**eeds assistance in self-care, and **E**lder years above 80 years.

The DETERMINE checklist may be used to screen the nutritional status of the older adult. The mnemonic scores the nine warning signs of poor nutrition in the older adult. The scoring of the tool provides a stratified nutritional risk score. This tool has been validated for use with community-based older adults (Sinnett et al., 2010).

The Minimum Data Set The Minimum Data Set (MDS) is a component of the Residential Assessment Instrument mandated for all patients in Medicare-certified long-term healthcare facilities (Centers for Medicare and Medicaid Services, 2013). MDS nutritional components are to be included in admission assessments for all residents, as well as in quarterly and annual updates. Any changes in patient status that involve a nutritional component of the MDS require a complete reassessment of nutritional status.

Mini Nutritional Assessment and Subjective Global Assessment The Mini Nutritional Assessment (MNA) and Subjective Global Assessment (SGA) have both been validated for use in the nutritional assessment of older adults. The SGA has also been used in the assessment of other populations since its development more than 20 years ago (Subjective Global Assessment, 2012). The MNA is a newer tool with extensive data validating its use with older adults (Diekmann et al., 2013; Mini Nutritional Assessment, n.d.). The MNA can be included as a routine component of a physical examination or as a quick bedside tool and is available in an online version and as a mobile application.

Malnutrition Universal Screening Tool The Malnutrition Universal Screening Tool (MUST) is a five-step tool that is validated for use with adults in all healthcare settings (BAPEN, 2011) (see Figure 10.7 ■). BMI, unplanned weight loss, and any acute illness factor into this quick-scoring tool that helps triage the patient to further assessment, if indicated. Both online and mobile applications of this tool are available.

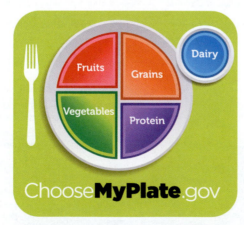

Balancing Calories
- Enjoy your food, but eat less.
- Avoid oversized portions.

Foods to Increase
- Make half your plate fruits and vegetables.
- Make at least half your grains whole grains.
- Switch to fat-free or low-fat (1%) milk.

Foods to Reduce
- Compare sodium in foods like soup, bread, and frozen meals—and choose the foods with lower numbers.
- Drink water instead of sugary drinks.

Figure 10.6 MyPlate.
Source: U.S. Department of Agriculture.

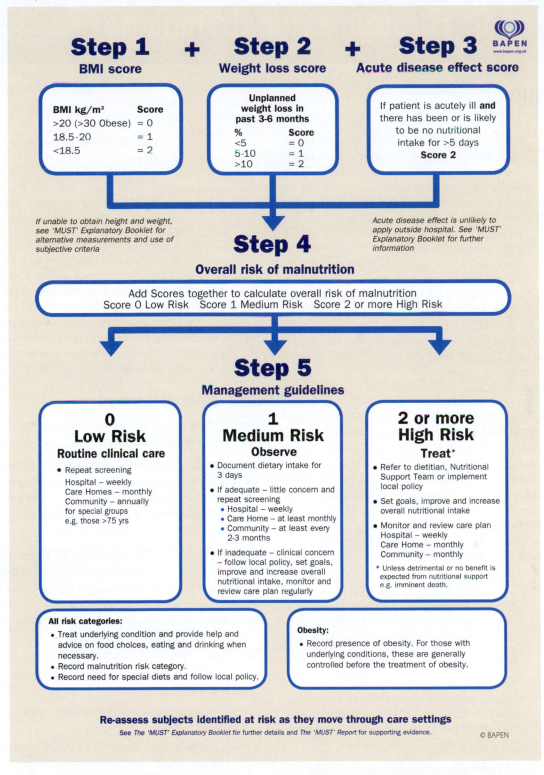

Figure 10.7 MUST is a five-step screening tool to identify adults who are malnourished, at risk of malnutrition (undernutrition), or obese. It also includes management guidelines that can be used to develop a care plan.

Source: © BAPEN. First published May 2003 by MAG, the Malnutrition Advisory Group, a Standing Committee of BAPEN. Reviewed and reprinted with minor changes March 2008, September 2010, and August 2011. MUST is supported by the British Dietetic Association, the Royal College of Nursing, and the Registered Nursing Home Association.

Application Through Critical Thinking

CASE STUDY

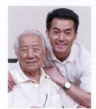

Source: imtmphoto/ Shutterstock.

Harry Chien is a 72-year-old brought to the clinic by his wife and son, who are concerned about his diminished dietary intake. His past medical history is significant for mild hypertension, which is treated with a diuretic and a 2-g sodium therapeutic diet. Physical assessment reveals blood pressure of 110/75 and pulse of 72. Height is 5'8', and weight is 156 lb. Weight 6 months prior was 175 lb. Significant laboratory measures: albumin 3.0 mg/dL. Urinalysis sent: sample dark and scant volume. His skin appears dry with dry axillae and petechiae on the trunk and arms. His eyes are sunken. Temporal wasting is noted, as well as diminished subcutaneous fat stores on the limbs. The assessment of the oral cavity reveals poorly fitting dentures, spongy gums, and deep tongue furrows.

Upon talking to Mr. Chien, the nurse learns that food does not taste the same to him anymore. He blames this on his low-sodium diet. His wife reports that she tries to provide him with good meals each day, but he often doesn't want to eat. She tells the nurse that her husband is a retired professional chef and used to love to cook until the last few months. He has resorted to heating food in the microwave and often overcooks it. Mr. Chien states he overheats the food because the microwave is unpredictable. His wife is reading her concerns from a list she has made and passes the list to him for further comment. The nurse notices he squints at the list and then says he has nothing to add.

The nurse conducts a diet recall that reveals:

Breakfast	Large mug black coffee
	Either cold cereal (flake type, not fortified) and whole milk or 2 pieces of toast or 1 English muffin with butter and jelly
	6 oz apple juice or cider, unfortified
Midday meal	Sandwich on white bread—such as tuna salad, peanut butter and jelly, or sliced turkey with mayonnaise and iceberg lettuce. Used to add tomato to sandwich but "can't be bothered cutting up one."
	Occasionally heats leftovers from restaurant meal with wife; usually has enough for two or three reheated meals during week. Pasta or meat and potato- or rice-type meals. No vegetables. Overheats and discards often.
	Cookie
	Cup of tea with whole milk and 2 tsp sugar
Evening	6 oz ready-to-eat pudding
	4 oz milk with comment "no liquids after 7 p.m. or I have to get up all night"

Mr. Chien takes no nutritional supplements of any kind. The nurse asks further questions about the lack of fruit and vegetables and learns that it has been almost 6 months since Mr. Chien had fruit other than applesauce or apple juice. He also has stopped eating vegetables in the same time frame. He states that he cannot be bothered preparing either type of food, but on further questioning admits that he is having difficulty chewing some foods and has some vision problems that make food preparation difficult or unsafe.

SAMPLE DOCUMENTATION

The following is a sample documentation from the nutrition assessment of Harry Chien.

SUBJECTIVE DATA Brought by wife who notes diminished intake. c/o low Na+ rx causing hypogeusia with secondary anorexia. Also c/o difficulty chewing, vision changes. Diet recall 2-meal/day pattern with no liquids after 7 p.m. Liquid intake, 32 oz/day (only 10 oz noncaffeine). No fruit/vegetable 3–6 mos.

OBJECTIVE DATA VS: BP 110/75—Pulse 72. Height 5'8', weight 156 lb. BMI 23.5. Weight 6 months ago 175 lb. Albumin 3.0 mg/dL. UA: sample dark and scant. Skin and axillae dry/petechiae present. Temp/limb wasting noted. Eyes sunken. Oral cavity: spongy gums, poorly fitting dentures, tongue furrows. Medications: hydrochlorthiazide.

CRITICAL THINKING QUESTIONS

1. How would the data from the case study be clustered to identify the problem areas?

2. How should the nurse interpret the data related to Mr. Chien's fruit and vegetable intake?

3. What additional data would the nurse require to develop a plan of care for Mr. Chien?

4. What additional information should the nurse gather to determine why Mr. Chien is experiencing an alteration in the way food tastes to him?

5. How would the nurse address the signs and symptoms of dehydration in Mr. Chien?

REFERENCES

BAPEN. (2011). Malnutrition Universal Screening Tool (MUST). Retrieved from http://www.bapen.org.uk/pdfs/must/must_full.pdf

Centers for Disease Control and Prevention (CDC), National Center for Health Statistics. (2009). *Anthropometry procedures manual.* Retrieved from http://www.cdc.gov/nchs/data/nhanes/nhanes_09_10/BodyMeasures_09

Centers for Disease Control and Prevention (CDC). (2014). *Health, United States, 2012.* Retrieved from http://www.cdc.gov/nchs/hus.htm

Centers for Medicare and Medicaid Services (CMS). (2013). *Minimum data set manual version 3.0 for nursing homes, October 2013 update.* Retrieved from http://www.cms.gov/Medicare/Quality-Initiatives-Patient-Assessment-Instruments/Nursing-HomeQualityInits/MDS30RAIManual.html

Cerhan, J. R., Moore, S. C., Jacobs, E. J., Kitahara, C. M., Rosenberg, P. S., Adami, H. O., … Berrington de Gonzalez, A. (2014). A pooled analysis of waist circumference and mortality in 650,000 adults. *Mayo Clinic Proceedings, 89,* 335–345.

Diekmann, R., Winning, K., Uter, W., Kaiser, M. J., Sieber, C. C., Volkert, D., & Bauer, J. M. (2013). Screening for malnutrition among nursing home residents: A comparative analysis of the mini nutritional assessment, the nutritional risk screening, and the malnutrition universal screening tool. *The Journal of Nutrition, Health, and Aging, 17*(4), 326–331.

Guenter, P., Malone, A., & DiMaria-Ghalili, R. A. (2015). Six steps to optimal nutrition care. *American Nurse Today, 10*(11). Retrieved from https://www.americannursetoday.com/essence-nutrition

Harvard School of Public Health. (2014). *Ethnic differences in BMI and disease risk.* Retrieved from http://www.hsph.harvard.edu/obesity-prevention-source/ethnic-differences-in-bmi-and-disease-risk

Koh, K. A., Hoy, J. S., O'Connell, J. J., & Montgomery, P. (2012). The hunger-obesity paradox: Obesity in the homeless. *Journal of Urban Health, 89,* 952–964.

Lopes, T. S., Luiz, R. R., Hoffman, D. J., Ferriolli, E., Pfrimer, K., Moura, A. S., … Periera, R. A. (2016). Misreport of energy intake assessed with food records and 24-h recalls compared with total energy expenditure estimated with DLW. *European Journal of Clinical Nutrition, 70,* 1259–1264. doi:10.1038/ejcn.2016.85

Mini Nutritional Assessment. (n.d.). *Overview.* Retrieved from http://www.mna-elderly.com

National Institutes of Health Heart, Lung, and Blood Institute. (n.d.). Body mass index table. Retrieved from https://www.nhlbi.nih.gov/health/educational/lose_wt/BMI/bmi_tbl.pdf

Ogden, C. L., Carroll, M. D., Kit, B. K., & Flegal, K. M. (2014). Prevalence of childhood and adult obesity in the United States, 2011–2012. *Journal of the American Medical Association, 311,* 806–814.

Sagna, M. L., Schopflocher, D., Raine, K., Nykiforuk, C., & Plotnikoff, R. (2013). Adjusting divergences between self-reported and measured height and weight in an adult Canadian population. *American Journal of Health Behavior, 37,* 841–850.

Sinnett, S., Bengle, R., Brown, A., Glass, A. P., Johnson, M. A., & Lee, J. S. (2010). The validity of Nutrition Screening Initiative DETERMINE Checklist responses in older Georgians. *Journal of Nutrition for the Elderly, 29,* 393–409.

Subjective Global Assessment. (2012). *Home.* Retrieved from http://subjectiveglobalassessment.com

U.S. Census Bureau. (2013). *Current Population Survey Annual Social and Economic Supplement (CPS ASEC): Income, poverty, and health insurance coverage in the United States, 2012.* Retrieved from https://www.census.gov/content/dam/Census/library/publications/2013/demo/p60-245.pdf

U.S. Department of Agriculture (USDA). (n.d.). *ChooseMyPlate.gov.* Retrieved from http://www.choosemyplate.gov

U.S. Department of Health and Human Services, National Heart, Lung, and Blood Institute. (n.d.). *Classification of overweight and obesity by BMI, waist circumference, and associated disease risks.* Retrieved from http://www.nhlbi.nih.gov/health/public/heart/obesity/lose_wt/bmi_dis.htm

U.S. Department of Health and Human Services, Office of Disease Prevention and Health Promotion. (2013). *Nutrition and weight status.* Retrieved from https://www.healthypeople.gov/2020/topics-objectives/topic/nutrition-and-weight-status

U.S. Department of Health and Human Services, Office of Disease Prevention and Health Promotion. (2014). *Healthy people 2020.* Retrieved from http://www.healthypeople.gov/2020/topicsobjectives2020/default.aspx

Ver Ploeg, M., & Rahkovsky, I. (2016). *Recent evidence on the effects of food store access on food choice and diet quality.* Retrieved from https://www.ers.usda.gov/amber-waves/2016/may/recent-evidence-on-the-effects-of-food-store-access-on-food-choice-and-diet-quality/

World Health Organization. (2014). *BMI classification.* Retrieved from http://apps.who.int/bmi/index.jsp?introPage=intro_3.html

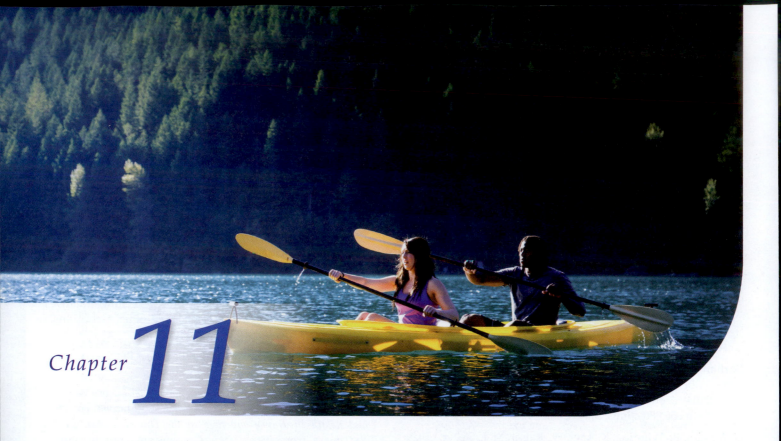

Chapter 11

Psychosocial Health, Substance Abuse, and Intimate Partner Violence

LEARNING OUTCOMES

Upon completion of the chapter, you will be able to:

1. Understand the major components of psychosocial health and apply to overall health and wellness.

2. Analyze the health and other impacts of substance abuse and substance use disorder.

3. Synthesize the importance of intimate partner violence (IPV) screening and violence identification in holistic patient care.

4. Describe application of the nursing process in the assessment of psychosocial health for patients across the lifespan.

KEY TERMS

anorexia nervosa, 152
binge eating disorder (BED), 152
bulimia nervosa, 152
gender identity, 154
interdependent relationships, 154

intimate partner violence (IPV), 152
nonsuicidal self-injury (NSSI), 164
psychosocial functioning, 149
psychosocial health, 149

role development, 153
self-concept, 152
sexual orientation, 154
sexual orientation label, 154
stress, 150

substance use disorder (SUD), 151
suicidal ideation, 164
transgender, 154

MEDICAL LANGUAGE

dys- Prefix meaning "abnormal," "difficult," "painful"

neur- Prefix meaning "nerve"

psych Root word meaning "mind"

Introduction

When performing an assessment, it is important for the nurse to consider the entirety of the individual's body, mind, and spirit and how they interact, rather than considering them as separate body systems. When one part is missing or dysfunctional, all other parts of the individual are affected. Illness, developmental changes, or trauma may bring about changes in psychosocial functioning. The patient may become stressed, may lose self-esteem, or may experience positive changes such as greater closeness with family. Changes in psychosocial functioning may, in turn, affect the patient's physical health or response to treatment. For example, a patient who is extremely stressed may not be able to understand or remember instructions for self-care, and a patient who is socially isolated may not be able to get needed help at home. There is increasing evidence supporting the theory that mind–body interactions play a key role in both health and illness. Nurses need to be aware that physical health problems and mental health problems often coexist (Doherty & Gaughran, 2014). No matter what the source of the patient's concern, a psychosocial assessment can provide significant insights to provide comprehensive and individualized patient care.

Psychosocial Health

Psychosocial health can be defined as being mentally, emotionally, socially, and spiritually well (see Figure 11.1 ■). Psychosocial health includes mental, emotional, social, and spiritual dimensions. The mental dimension refers to an individual's ability to reason, to find meaning in and make judgments from information, to demonstrate rational thinking, and to perceive realistically. The emotional dimension is subjective and includes one's feelings. Social functioning refers to the individual's ability to form relationships with others. Included in the spiritual dimension are beliefs and values that give meaning to life.

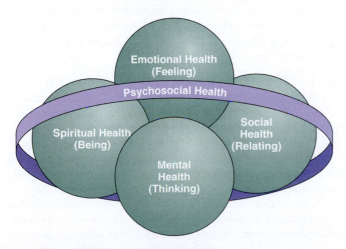

Figure 11.1 Psychosocial health.

Psychosocial functioning includes the way a person thinks, feels, acts, and relates to self and others. Involving aspects of both social interaction and psychological ability to cope and tolerate stress, the individual's level of psychosocial functioning includes the capacity for developing a value and belief system. Some psychosocial factors include socioeconomic status, emotional factors, stressful events, and family and relationship factors. These and others influence the health and well-being in a variety of ways. (Pulkki-Raback et al., 2015). Psychosocial health and functioning are influenced by internal and external factors. Internal factors consist of a person's genetic makeup, physical health, and physical fitness. External factors include the influence of those responsible for one's upbringing and experiences in the social environment, in which culture, geography, and economic status are contributory aspects. Additional factors to consider when assessing a patient's psychosocial health are substance use, exposure to violence, self-concept, role development, interdependent relationships, and the abilities to manage stress, to cope with and adapt to change, and to develop a belief and values system.

Internal Factors That Influence Psychosocial Health

Internal factors that affect psychosocial health include hereditary characteristics or those related to genetic makeup. In addition, the individual's physical health, developmental stage, and level of fitness influence psychosocial health.

Genetics The majority of health disorders have a basis in genetics (National Human Genome Research Institute, 2015). With the completion of the Human Genome Project, gene-based testing and treatment are expected to be incorporated into healthcare with the goal of promoting public health. The Office of Public Health Genomics (OPHG), which is a division of the Centers for Disease Control and Prevention (CDC), is evaluating strategies for responsibly incorporating genomic advances into public health programs (Office of Public Health Genomics [OPHG], 2013).

An individual's genetic makeup influences physical and psychosocial health throughout life. For example, children whose parents or siblings have bipolar disorder have an increased risk for diagnosis of the condition (Shinozaki & Potash, 2014).

Parents with attention-deficit/hyperactivity disorder (ADHD) have an increased likelihood of having offspring with the disorder, and there appears to be a genetic link to conditions such as obesity, alcoholism, and depressive disorders (Shinozaki & Potash, 2014). Some studies of identical twins reveal that they often have the same habits, mannerisms, and perceptions of anxiety, even when raised separately (Byrne et al., 2013).

Hereditary differences impact one's development in two ways: First, experiences impact a hereditary predisposition for certain health problems. For example, an individual with a genetic predisposition to develop schizophrenia would likely develop the disease in a particular environment. Second, genetic characteristics result in reactions from others that can have an impact on the developing personality. Consider the fact that body structure, appearance, and overall physical attractiveness are inherited. Most people respond more positively to children who are physically attractive than to those who are not. Repeated responses of a positive or negative nature can impact one's developing self-concept and self-esteem as well as one's overall behavior and interaction with others. Positive responses result in feelings of self-worth and confidence. Negative responses lead to low self-concept and may result in unmanageable levels of stress, which could trigger unacceptable behavior or mental illness. Furthermore, cognitive processes, including the abilities to think, perceive, remember, and make judgments, are dependent on one's innate or inherited capacity and are enhanced or diminished in response to environmental and educational factors.

Physical Health
Physical health is associated with satisfaction of basic needs, quality of life, and psychosocial well-being, often referred to as the mind–body–spirit connection. Physical health enables an individual to respond to stressors and, therefore, to adapt, cope with change, and grow as a functioning individual capable of personal and social interaction. Conversely, problems with health, particularly chronic illness, can negatively impact coping, adaptation, and personal and emotional fulfillment.

The mind–body–spirit connection can be further explained as the body's response to thoughts and feelings. Positive and negative stress and anxiety may result in physical symptoms. Situations of positive and negative stress include marriage, childbirth, success in school or job performance, financial difficulties, the death of a friend or family member, or loss of a job. Physical symptoms that indicate a problem related to emotional stress or distress include the following:

- Back pain
- Chest pain
- Difficulty breathing
- Constipation
- Fatigue
- Hypertension
- Palpitations
- Dry mouth
- Nausea
- Weight loss or gain

Emotional **stress** affects health in several ways. First, stress affects the immune system, resulting in increased susceptibility to infection. Second, during periods of stress or change, individuals are less likely to attend to habits that promote health, such as eating nutritious meals or following an exercise routine. Third, research points to a molecular link between prolonged stress and obesity. Researchers have found that the neurobiology of stress overlaps with that of appetite regulation. High levels of stress have the ability to influence a person's eating patterns and increase the consumption of highly palatable or comfort foods (Sinha & Jastreboff, 2013) In addition, some individuals use alcohol, tobacco, or drugs in order to self-medicate and "feel better."

Measures to deal with stress and reduce the negative impact on physical and emotional health include talking openly about feelings; thinking about positive aspects of life; using relaxation techniques such as meditation, yoga, prayer, or positive imagery;

and following a regimen to promote health that includes healthy eating, exercise, and sleep.

Developmental Stage
The patient's developmental stage greatly influences psychosocial health. For example, even at the most basic level, children and adults have different understandings of health and illness.

CHILDREN It is common for children to believe they are ill because of bad thoughts or behaviors. The belief that illness is a punishment for wrongdoing is common. Young children cannot identify or modify health risks. Children do not have the cognitive ability to understand cause-and-effect relationships until preadolescence or early adolescence. Parents and guardians function as proxies for their children in most healthcare decisions.

Nurses should use a caring and supportive yet firm approach with children. Whenever possible, play should be incorporated into nursing procedures. It is helpful to allow children to touch and manipulate equipment when safe. Adhesive bandages or empty syringes can be provided for playacting with teddy bears or dolls. The nurse should encourage children to talk about their fears and concerns. Painful procedures should not be performed in a child's bed or while a child is seated on a parent's lap. Children need to know they are safe from painful experiences when they are with their parents. When possible, give the child choices and incorporate the child's caregivers in the nursing plan of care. Chapter 26 provides more information on assessing infants, children, and adolescents. ∞

OLDER ADULTS Unique developmental and lifespan considerations also significantly affect the older adult's psychosocial health. For the older adult, psychosocial assessment should include functional ability, cognition, and lifestyle changes.

Functional ability refers to the ability to perform tasks required for independent living. These activities include eating, bathing, dressing, cooking, shopping, and management of finances. Strength and mobility are essential factors related to functional ability. They require the objective assessment of test administrators in observations of tasks or movements. Performance tests measure upper and lower body strength, range of motion, balance, or speed of gait. Tests of the upper body include dexterity and strength.

The maintenance and improvement of learning, memory, decision making, and planning are skills associated with cognitive health. Cognitive changes do occur with aging; however, forgetting or becoming senile (cognitive decline) is not a normal part of aging. Chapter 27 provides more information on these assessments. ∞

Physical Fitness
Physical fitness can be described as a condition that helps individuals to feel, appear, and perform at an optimal level. The President's Council on Physical Fitness, Sports & Nutrition (2017) describes its mission as to educate and empower a healthy lifestyle for Americans, which includes regular physical activity and good nutrition. Included among the physical fitness components are cardiovascular fitness, body composition, muscular endurance, strength, and flexibility.

Physical health can affect emotional and psychosocial well-being. Maintaining fitness requires fulfilling needs related to exercise, nutrition, rest, and relaxation, as well as adopting practices that promote and preserve health. Physical activity and healthy nutrition are factors in the prevention of overweight and obesity. In the United States, obesity is an epidemic across all age groups.

External Factors That Influence Psychosocial Health

An individual's personality, sense of self, and role as a member of a larger society are influenced by a number of external factors. The manner and conditions in which a child is raised are an important influence. In addition, the experiences during childhood and throughout life that are framed by culture, geography, and economic status contribute in great part to psychosocial well-being.

Family It is widely accepted that children who experience consistent love, attention, and security grow into adults who are able to adapt to change and stress. Child-rearing or caregiving generally occurs within a family unit. Families are considered social units of individuals who are related or live together over a period of time. Individual members in families have ongoing contact with each other; share goals, values, and concerns; and develop practices common to that specific group. Today, families involved in child rearing can be two-parent families, single-parent families, heterosexual or homosexual domestic partnerships, blended or stepfamilies, adoptive families, or families in which grandparents, members of the extended family, or others provide child care in the absence of parents (Masten & Monn, 2015).

Families influence psychosocial health because they are expected to provide for physical safety and economic needs; to help members develop physically, emotionally, and spiritually; and to help each individual develop an identity as self and member of the family. Families foster the development of social skills, spiritual beliefs, and a value system. Families promote adaptive and coping skills and assist members to become part of the greater society. The ability to provide these basic needs is dependent on the maturity of the caregivers and the support system available to them from the family, community, and society.

Culture Culture is a complex system that includes knowledge, beliefs, morals, and customs that provide a pattern for living. Cultures may be composed of individuals from the same ethnic or racial group or background, in the same socioeconomic group, from the same geographic region, who practice a certain religion, or who share common values and beliefs. Culture influences the roles and relationships within families and groups that may be gender specific or determined by age. A person's culture may influence child rearing and health practices. The cultural norms affect physical, social, and mental well-being. An individual's experience and the ways in which one responds to stress, coping, and life situations are determined in great part by culture. Recall the details about the relationship of cultures and health described in Chapter 3. ∞

Geography Geography refers to the country, region, community, or neighborhood in which one was born and raised or in which one currently resides or works. The geography of an area affects family life and the development of individuals within families. Psychosocial health is influenced by the climate, terrain, resources, and aesthetics in varied locations. Community resources including schools, churches, healthcare facilities, transportation systems, support services, and safety systems affect the social development and emotional well-being of individuals within the community. Individuals in urban areas may be subjected to stressors associated with crowded conditions, congestion, and crime rates higher than in other areas. Residents of rural areas may experience the stressors of limited resources and isolation.

In addition, in the United States one must consider the geographic impacts on psychosocial health that accompany regional characteristics, immigration, and the increased mobility of individuals and families. Some regions in the United States have a highly ethnic character. This character shapes the individual's self-concept and the ways one appraises, is appraised, and interacts with others from within and outside the regional/ethnic norm. Immigrants face the stress of adapting to new geographic characteristics and cultural norms. Communities into which immigrants settle and the individuals within them must adapt to the differences in language, customs, morals, values, and roles of the immigrant population. Children of immigrants face the difficulty of being raised in a family with the previous culture's values and norms, while growing and developing as members of their adopted community and culture. Because of economic demand or opportunity, families tend to move more frequently today than in the past. Adults and children then must adjust to the culture of the new location, the loss of the familiar, and the stress of separation from family and friends.

In addition, geography, or one's local environment, influences health-related habits including access to healthy foods and places to walk and exercise. It has been suggested that the increase in obesity in the United States is a result of increasing numbers of people living where driving to work is required; residing in neighborhoods that are unsafe for walking or exercise; and eating convenient, readily available, high-fat "fast foods" rather than healthy foods.

Economic Status Economic status affects the formation of values and attitudes. Values and role expectations related to marriage, gender roles, family roles, sex, parenting, education, housing, leisure activities, clothing, occupation, and religious practice are influenced by the economic status of individuals and families. In the United States, the higher the income the more likely it is that individuals and families will have achieved higher levels of education or provide for higher levels of education for their children. Higher education leads to greater occupational opportunity, improved housing, and the ability to participate in a greater variety of leisure activities. Economic advantages may contribute to the development of increased self-esteem, which can improve an individual's ability to adapt and cope with life changes. Those in lower socioeconomic groups or living in poverty may need to focus on their immediate survival needs of food, clothing, and shelter. Continual confrontation with the results of poverty may result in anger, frustration, difficulty in coping, family disturbances, abnormal behaviors, and mental illness. Access to the healthcare delivery system may be impacted by an individual's or family's socioeconomic status.

Additional Factors in Psychosocial Health

Additional factors to consider when addressing a patient's psychosocial health include substance use and exposure to violence, self-concept, role development, sexuality, interdependent relationships, and the abilities to manage stress, to cope and adapt to change, and to develop a belief and value system.

Substance Use Disorders **Substance use disorders (SUDs),** including abuse of alcohol and prescription medications, are prevalent in the United States with almost 22 million individuals ages 12 and older identifying as having an SUD (Substance Abuse and Mental health Services Administration [SAMHSA], 2015). Substance abuse leads to physical health deterioration and impairs daily functioning. Interpersonal relationships are often neglected when a partner is abusing substances. In addition, substance abuse is a risk factor for negative health impacts and diseases, such as cirrhosis, cancer, infertility, and malnutrition. Substance abuse assessment is presented later in this chapter.

Intimate Partner Violence

Intimate partner violence (IPV) is a serious public health issue affecting millions of women and men across their lifespan (Centers for Disease Control and Prevention [CDC], 2017a). IPV may include neglect, physical abuse, emotional intimidation, and sexual assault. Many individuals who are exposed to IPV are financially or emotionally dependent on their abusive partner. IPV remains a silent health epidemic as it is often undetected (Niolon et al., 2017). Women exposed to IPV display an array of health consequences, including acute physical injury, depression, anxiety, and chronic pain (Paterno & Draughon, 2016). Screening for IPV in healthcare settings has the ability to identify a higher number of individuals who are exposed to violence. The nurse has the ability to promote health and safety through routine screening of IPV. More information on IPV is located later in this chapter.

Self-concept

Self-concept refers to the beliefs and feelings one holds about oneself. A positive self-concept is essential to a person's mental and physical health. Individuals with a positive self-concept are better able to develop and maintain interpersonal relationships and resist psychologic and physical illness.

Self-concept develops over time as a person reacts to and learns from interactions with others. As an individual develops across the lifespan, the interactions move from the immediacy of contact as children with caregivers to contact with individuals in the greater environment.

Body image and self-esteem are components of self-concept. Body image is the way one thinks about physical appearance, size, and body functioning. Self-esteem refers to the sense of worth or self-respect of an individual. All aspects of self-concept affect psychosocial health. Psychosocially healthy people have a realistic sense of self, adapt to change, develop ways to cope with problems, and form relationships that promote growth and development. In contrast, psychosocially unhealthy individuals often have problems with self-concept, which manifest as pessimism, social isolation, feelings of worthlessness, neglect of physical health, depression, anxiety, substance abuse, or suicidal thoughts (see Figure 11.2 ■).

Body image is affected by a variety of factors, including the individual's size and weight. Among children and adolescents, being overweight or obese can result in physical problems later in life. For example, overweight and obesity in childhood are linked to an increased risk for illness and premature death in adulthood (Li, Eriksson, He, Hall, & Czene, 2017).

Likewise, overweight children are subject to bias and stereotyping from peers, teachers, and even parents. Overweight and obese children are prone to low self-esteem, depression, and anxiety. The long-term effects of obesity in childhood and adolescence include an increased risk of metabolic disorders, such as diabetes, cancer, and cardiovascular disease (Wang et al., 2015). The incidence of overweight and obesity is more prevalent in people of low economic status. Causative factors include the use of less expensive, high-calorie, processed foods;

unsafe conditions for exercise; and differing perceptions about body weight in relation to health.

EATING DISORDERS   An eating disorder is a condition in which a person's current intake of food differs significantly from that person's normal intake. Eating disorders can result from an attempt to lose weight; however, the attempt to lose weight may be a misguided response to psychosocial problems.

Anorexia nervosa is a complex psychosocial problem characterized by a severely restricted intake of nutrients and a low body weight. Subjective findings associated with anorexia nervosa include the following:

- Intense fear of gaining weight or becoming fat
- Perception of being overweight even when in an emaciated state
- Refusal to maintain body weight over a minimal normal weight for age and height
- Constipation and gastrointestinal bloating
- Abdominal pain

Objective manifestations associated with anorexia nervosa may include the following:

- Emaciation or extreme weight loss
- Refusal to consume food or nutritional supplements
- Electrolyte imbalances due to fluid loss through vomiting or abuse of laxatives
- Damage to teeth enamel due to overexposure to gastric acid if purging behaviors include vomiting
- Esophageal and stomach injury if purging behaviors include vomiting
- Irregular or absent menses (National Alliance on Mental Illness [NAMI], 2013a)

Bulimia nervosa is an eating disorder characterized by binge eating and purging or another compensatory mechanism to prevent weight gain. Typically, the bulimic consumes large portions of high-calorie food, typically up to 4,000 calories at one time. The individual then tries to force the food out of the body by vomiting or using laxatives, enemas, diuretics, or diet pills. Subjective manifestations associated with bulimia nervosa may include the following:

- Obsession with physical appearance
- Periods of excessive food consumption followed by purging activities (e.g., vomiting, diuretic or laxative abuse, or extreme exercise)

Objective manifestations associated with bulimia nervosa may include the following:

- Normal weight or slightly overweight
- Electrolyte imbalances due to fluid loss through vomiting or abuse of laxatives
- Esophageal and stomach injury
- Damage to teeth enamel due to overexposure to gastric acid if purging through vomiting (National Alliance on Mental Illness [NAMI], 2013b)

Binge eating disorder (BED) is characterized by an individual's maladaptive behavior of recurrent binge eating (Myers

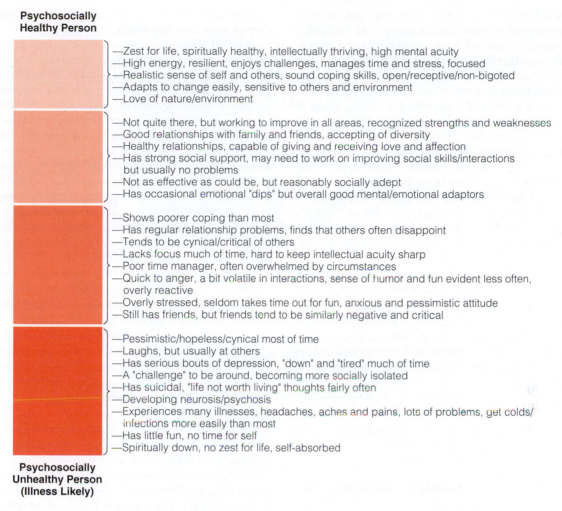

Figure 11.2 Psychosocially healthy person versus psychosocially unhealthy person.

& Wiman, 2014). The disorder is linked to obesity and morbid obesity as it does not include calorie-limiting behaviors such as vomiting, laxative use, or excessive exercise. BED is commonly accompanied by feelings of loss of control and distress. As with other eating disorders, research demonstrates BED can co-occur with other psychiatric disorders, including mood disorders and bipolar disorder, SUD, and anxiety disorders (Myers & Wiman, 2014). Screening, early identification, and specialized treatment of BED assists the healthcare team to promote optimal patient outcomes. Subjective manifestations of BED include the following:

- Recurrent episodes of binge eating

- Binge eating episodes associated with three (or more) of the following: eating faster than normal, eating until feeling uncomfortably full, eating large amounts of food when not hungry, eating alone due to embarrassment associated with eating, feeling disgusted or depressed or guilty after eating

- Marked distress regarding eating habits

- Episodes occur at least once a week for 3 months

- Does not occur with vomiting, laxative use, or excessive exercise (Myers & Wiman, 2014)

Role Development **Role development** refers to the individual's capacity to identify and fulfill the social expectations related to the variety of roles assumed in a lifetime. Roles are reciprocal relationships in which expectations exist for each participant. Examples of reciprocal roles are child–parent, student–teacher, and employee–employer, as well as the reciprocal roles of spouse, sibling, friend, and neighbor. Roles are learned through socialization. The earliest learning generally occurs within the family when children observe and model adult behavior. When role development is healthy and occurs in a supportive environment, self-concept and psychosocial well-being are enhanced as the individual gains confidence in the ability to interact with others according to societal norms. However, unsupportive, violent, or abusive family relationships are stressful and can lead to unsuccessful role relationships. Individuals who receive support and understand role expectations are able to meet the challenges of changing roles as they develop and mature. Individuals who have experienced family stress have conflicting views of role expectations or are unclear regarding social norms. They often experience frustration or a sense of inadequacy associated with fear or negative judgment from others if their performance is not in accordance with expectations for new or changing roles.

Sexuality Sexuality and sexual development also greatly influence an individual's health, both physically and psychosocially. Key components of sexuality include gender identity, sexual orientation, and sexual orientation label.

Gender identity is self-assigned and comprises the most significant aspects of an individual's sexual life, including sexual attractions, behaviors, and desires (Wood & Eagly, 2015). **Sexual orientation** refers to an individual's innate predisposition toward affiliation, affection, bonding, and thoughts in relationship to members of the same sex, the other sex, both sexes, or neither sex (Sornberger, Smith, Toste, & Heath, 2013). A **sexual orientation label** is sometimes used to simplify and describe an individual's sexual orientation. Examples of sexual orientation labels include straight (or heterosexual), gay, lesbian, and bisexual (Sornberger et al., 2013). **Transgender** individuals identify themselves as the gender that is different from their biologically assigned gender. Transgender identity is not associated with any specific sexual orientation label. As such, an individual who is transgender may be heterosexual, gay, lesbian, or bisexual (Morrow & Messinger, 2013).

Historically and at present, members of the lesbian, gay, bisexual, and transgender (LGBT) community have been subject to discrimination, intolerance, and violence. Greater levels of stress have been found in individuals who identify as LGBT (Sornberger et al., 2013). When caring for lesbian, gay, bisexual, and transgender individuals, the nurse needs to be aware of the patient's potential fear of being stereotyped, judged, or discriminated against due to sexuality-related issues. As with all patients, respectful, compassionate care helps build trust, which is the foundation of the nurse–patient relationship. Once trust is established, if the patient so desires, the nursing assessment should include a professional and sensitive discussion about health-related aspects of the patient's sexuality.

Interdependent Relationships

Interdependent relationships are those in which the individual establishes bonds with others based on trust. Interdependent relationships are characterized by mutual reliance and support. According to Roy and Andrews (1999), these relationships are based on the human needs of love, respect, and value for another. These important relationships include the individuals one identifies as the significant other and one's support system. The ability to form, maintain, and adapt to changes in interdependent relationships is impacted by the individual's self-esteem. Individuals generally choose loving and close relationships with those who have similar levels of self-esteem. For example, when two people with high self-esteem form a loving and caring relationship, the high self-esteem is reinforced. Conversely, individuals with low self-esteem choose relationships with others with low self-esteem. As a result, feelings of negative self-worth are reinforced. Positive self-esteem enhances psychosocial health and enables the individual to grow and develop, adapt to change, solve problems, make decisions, maintain physical well-being, and seek help when needed for physical or emotional difficulties. Further, quality of life and length of life, which are measures of psychosocial health, have been linked to positive interdependent relationships.

Maltreatment

Maltreatment or abuse can occur in all age groups and has been identified as physical, sexual, or psychologic abuse, neglect, acts of omission, discriminatory behavior, and financial abuse. The nurse is a "mandated reporter" and must report to the state any suspicion of maltreatment of children and older adult patients.

Physical abuse may present in a variety of ways, including hitting, punching, slapping, burning, choking, shaking, or otherwise harming another person. Patients of all ages can present with signs and symptoms such as bruising at different stages of healing, unexplained injuries, fractures, malnourishment, and marks associated with physical restraint. It is important to note that some cultural practices use treatments that may cause petechiae that imitate physical signs of child abuse. Coining (rubbing the skin with a coin in a symmetric pattern) and cupping (placing heated cups on the skin to create a vacuum) are cultural practices used to treat illness by bringing a source of illness to the surface of the skin. Healthcare providers' knowledge of these cultural practices along with its incidence history can prevent accusations of physical abuse (Spector, 2017).

Sexual abuse may present as rape, sexual assault, molestation, or sexual contact to which the individual has not consented. It also includes incest, sexual exploitation, and prostitution. Research indicates that sexual abuse is underreported and underidentified in part because of societal taboos and perceptions about the gender roles of the offenders and victims. The unfortunate behavioral and psychologic effects of sexual abuse such as stigmatization, betrayal, and powerlessness may enhance the victim's increasing vulnerability to health problems, illness, disease, and socioeconomic challenges.

Psychologic or emotional abuse can result from humiliation, intimidation, and forced isolation. This type of abuse can be manifested by delays in physical or emotional development, lack of attachment, suicide attempts, low self-esteem, and changes in personality or extremes in behavior (Basu, McLaughlin, Misra, & Koenen, 2017). Neglect refers to the failure or refusal to provide food, shelter, protection, or healthcare for a child or older adult. Self-neglect refers to behaviors of adults that threaten their own health and safety.

Discriminatory abuse related to a person's disability, age, gender, race, sexuality, religion, or cultural background can be difficult for the nurse to identify. In addition, financial abuse is related to theft, fraud, exploitation of inheritance, unexplained bank account withdrawals and unusual bank account activities, and loss of valuables. Financial abuse is often a serious issue for older adult patients who may be dependent on caregivers or others for assistance with bill-paying or other financial matters.

Stress and Coping

Stress and coping are the individual's physical and emotional responses to psychosocial or physical threats, called stressors. An automobile accident, a failing grade, an illness, obesity, and loss of a job are examples of stressors. However, stress is not the event itself but, rather, the individual's response to it. Events that are highly stressful for one individual may not be stressful for another. The stress response may include familiar physical symptoms such as sweaty palms or a pounding heart. The immediate physical reaction to stress is also referred to as the *fight, flight, or freeze* response. Physical response to long-term stress may include symptoms such as chronically cold hands or suppression of immune function. The emotional reactions to stress may include difficulty sleeping, inability to concentrate, or anxiety. Positive as well as negative events may produce stress. The physical signs of stress include the following:

- Increased heart rate
- Decreased blood clotting time
- Increased rate and depth of respirations
- Dilated pupils
- Elevated glucose levels
- Dilated skeletal blood vessels
- Elevated blood pressure
- Dilated bronchi
- Increased blood volume
- Contraction of the spleen
- Increased blood supply to vital organs
- Release of T lymphocytes

Stress, in itself, is not bad. In fact, stress can sometimes motivate or enhance performance. Coping mechanisms are what an individual uses to deal with threats to physical and mental well-being. Like other patterns of behavior, patterns of coping with stress stem from early development when the child models the ways significant people in his or her life have coped with and dealt with stress.

Spiritual and Belief Patterns Spiritual and belief patterns reflect an individual's relationship with a higher power or with something, such as an ideal, a group, or humanity itself, that the person sees as larger than self and that gives meaning to life. The outward demonstration of spirituality may be reflected in religious practice, lifestyle, or relationships with others. A moral code is often included in one's belief patterns. A moral code is the internalized values, virtues, and rules one learns from significant others. It is developed by the individual to distinguish right from wrong. An individual's spiritual beliefs and moral code are affected by culture and ethnic background. See Chapter 3 for more on spirituality. ∞

Substance Abuse

Substance use disorders (SUDs) in the United States are substantial and on the rise. In 2014, approximately 21.5 million (8.1%) Americans above age 12 were reported to have struggled with an SUD within the past year (SAMHSA, 2015). According to the National Institute on Drug Abuse (NIDA; 2015), substance use is reported to be the highest among individuals in their late teens (age 18) to early twenties. Alcohol has the highest rate of abuse among all substances, followed by marijuana. In 2013, 17.3 million Americans were found to be dependent or had problems with alcohol, and 4.2 million Americans met the criteria for marijuana abuse or dependence (NIDA, 2015). In the United States, there is a "large treatment gap" for SUDs, with 22.7 million people meeting the criteria for substance abuse treatment and only 2.5 million people receiving addiction treatment services in 2013 (NIDA, 2015).

SUDs occur when there is recurrent use of drugs and/or alcohol that causes a significant life impairment, which results in a person's failure to meet work, school, or family obligations. SAMHSA (2015) categorizes the most common SUDs as the following: Alcohol Use Disorder, Tobacco Use Disorder, Cannabis Use Disorder, Stimulant Use Disorder, Hallucinogen Use Disorder, and Opioid Use Disorder. In the United States, SUDs are significant and continue to be a major public health issue. Although SUDs are classified by severity (mild, moderate, or severe), all SUDs are chronic and negatively impact an individual's health and wellbeing (Ladegast, 2016).

In 2017, the opioid crisis was declared a national public health emergency by the President of the United States (Kerns, 2018). Nationally, the average rates per year of drug overdose deaths have been steadily increasing since 1999. In the years 2014 to 2016, rates of preventable drug overdose jumped to 18% per year (Kerns, 2018). The opioid crisis was fueled in 2000 to 2010 by a dramatic increase in opioid prescribing by healthcare providers in order to address the surge of patients with chronic pain. Opioid misuse and overdose has led to a significant public health problem and evolution of opioid use disorders. The CDC added opioid overdose prevention as one of its five public health challenges in 2014 (Krashin, Murinova, & Sullivan, 2016).

The increasing use of synthetic cannabinoids (SCBs), also referred to as "Spice," K2," "herbal essence," "Mojo," and "Cloud 9," has become a significant public health concern because of their abuse potential and unpredictable toxicity (Mills, Yepes, & Nugent, 2015). SCBs are relatively low cost and cannot be detected by routine drug screenings. SCB use results in higher rates of toxicity and hospital admissions when compared to natural cannabis (Mills et al., 2015). This is likely a result of SCBs having a higher affinity and binding capacity to cannabinoid receptors. The clinical effects of SCB toxicity are tachycardia, lethargy, agitation or irritability, confusion, hypertension, chest pain, vertigo, nausea and vomiting (Mills et al., 2015). No antidote exists for SCB toxicity; thus, treatment for acute toxicity includes supportive care and observation.

It is vital for the nurse to understand that the overall impact of SUDs are multifactorial. The negative impacts include many health consequences as well as emotional, social, and cognitive impairment. Excessive alcohol intake damages the brain, neurological system, pancreas, liver, and intestines (Mehta, 2016). Consuming alcohol while pregnant can lead to fetal alcohol syndrome in newborns. Mothers with SUDs may have newborns who are impacted. Substance-exposed newborns are at a higher risk for respiratory distress, birth defects, drug withdrawal, and behavior abnormalities. In the area of public safety, alcohol is implicated in almost half of all motor vehicle accidents, injuries, and falls. In addition, SUDs can cause family crises and criminal justice problems (Patestos, Patterson, & Fitzsimons, 2014). Screening for SUDs is the nurse's first step to identifying individuals needing substance use intervention and long-term care.

Predisposing factors that increase a person's risk of acquiring a SUD include biological and sociocultural influences. No single theory has been found to explain the etiology of substance-related disorders. A complex interaction of various elements is thought to influence an individual's susceptibility to substance use and abuse (Jordan & Andersen, 2017).

Biological Risk Factors

Biological risk factors cannot be changed. Identification of these causes is, nevertheless, important in a health assessment.

Biochemistry A person's biochemistry has the potential to influence the risk of addiction. Substance addiction is a chronic disease in which a dysfunction in the brain circuitry exists. The areas of the brain affected by the substance include reward, memory, motivation, and other related functions. An individual does not think the same when the neurological system is influenced by a substance. Neurotransmitters that are thought to be involved in SUDs include dopamine, norepinephrine, serotonin, and gamma-aminobutyric acid (GABA). Neuronal pathways in the brain are believed to be altered with substance addiction in the areas that sense pleasure and reward. When an individual chronically uses substances over time, the brain adapts to the excessive activation of the neurons. This results in a person having the symptoms of physical discomfort associated with the drug's withdrawal. Withdrawal symptoms have been found with the chronic use of substances, including cannabis. Thus, neurotransmitters and other biochemical factors influence a person's risk for developing and suffering from a substance-related disorder (Volkow, Wise, & Baler, 2017).

Genetics Genetic factors are likely involved in a person's development of an SUD. A genetic link for alcoholism is well established in families, with children of alcoholics at a much higher risk to develop alcoholism when compared with other children. It is estimated that hereditary factors in addiction account for 40% to 60% of an individual's susceptibility to the disease (National Institute on Drug Abuse [NIDA], 2016). Although genetic factors contribute to addiction, it is important to note the interaction of an individual's genetics and environment in SUDs. A person's environment has the potential to enhance his risk or protection. For example, providing healthy after-school activities, such as basketball, has been shown to reduce a person's vulnerability to addiction. Addiction is a complex disease that researchers continue to investigate. Genetics have been identified as a biologic risk factor for an SUD (NIDA, 2016).

Sociological Risk Factors

To complete an accurate and comprehensive assessment of the addicted individual, it is important for the nurse to understand the social influences and ethnic and cultural influence in substance-related disorders.

Social Learning and Conditioning Social learning and conditioning are predisposing factors to SUDs. A person's family and friends influence one's perspective on substance use. If parents or caregivers provide a model of drug or alcohol use, children and adolescents have a higher rate of using substances. Modeling and imitation of parental behaviors is seen from early childhood to adolescence. In the child and adolescent, peer influence is a significant factor in the development of SUDs. In addition, modeling and peer influence continue to be factors in substance abuse in adulthood. This is mostly related to a person's social network and workforce culture. For example, a patient binges on alcohol approximately 10 times a month with coworkers and states that drinking with coworkers is viewed as a way to express group cohesiveness.

SUDs include a learned response from a substance, or multiple substances, in an environment. The term *conditioning* refers to this learned response, which is elicited after a person has repeated exposure to a stimulus. The euphoria experienced secondary to the substance itself encourages a person to repeat it. Also, the environment appears to contribute to the reinforcement of a person's substance use. A more pleasurable environment for the substance user is related to an increase of substance use in that environment.

Cultural Influences A person's culture may impact the development of an SUD. Patterns of consumption and attitudes and acceptance of a substance within an individual's culture influence an individual's substance use. In addition, a culture that has a high rate of consumption of a substance will likely have an increased availability of a substance for its community members.

Substance Abuse Screening

Abuse of alcohol, methamphetamines, opioids, and other substances ranks among the leading causes of preventable disease and death in the United States (McNeely et al., 2017). Healthcare settings offer an opportunity for substance abuse screening in order to identify substance problems, provide intervention, and link patients to treatment services. Many individuals who need substance abuse treatment are overlooked in healthcare settings. In order to detect SUDs, screening in healthcare settings is recommended for all adolescents and adults.

Screening is a simple and fast way for the nurse to recognize patients who need further assessment. Screening, brief intervention, and referral to treatment (SBIRT) make up an approach that can be used for the nursing management of substance use (Ladegast, 2016). The three components include (1) assessment for substance use concerns by using a standardized screen, such as the TAPS or CAGE screening tools, or other format, such as the single and two-question screening tests; (2) a brief intervention by the nurse; and (3) referring patients who screen positive for treatment services. In addition, screening for SUDs supports the nurse's aim of providing holistic patient care.

Early detection coupled with referral for treatment and long-term care has the potential to positively influence the individual with the disorder (Ladegast, 2016). A gap in SUD treatment exists with an estimated 17 million Americans undertreated for substance abuse (Wu et al., 2016). Routine screening for SUDs in healthcare settings is recommended to address this healthcare gap in treatment services. SUD screening supports substance abuse identification, informs healthcare plans, has the ability to increase referrals, and improves patient access to recovery services.

Substance Abuse Assessment Tools

The nurse has the ability to intervene in the patient's SUD progression through routine screening, early identification, and treatment referrals (Ladegast, 2016). Brief and accurate screening tools in clinical settings allow for informed medical decision making. Examples of clinically relevant SUD screening tools are the CAGE tool for alcohol use and the TAPS tool (Wu et al., 2016). The TAPS tool is a validated, two-step screening and assessment tool that identifies patient use of tobacco, alcohol, illicit drugs, and nonmedical use of prescription drugs (see Figure 11.3 ■). The first step is a four-item screen completed by the patient. If a person is found to be at risk in any of these four areas (tobacco, alcohol, drugs, prescription medications), a further screening is warranted with the ASSIST-Lite (McNeely et al., 2017). The ASSIST-Lite is an in-depth screening that provides a more detailed view of the patient's substance use, including questions on marijuana (hash, weed), cocaine, crystal meth, heroin, anxiety medication, and more (Wu et al., 2016). Patients who are identified as at risk for an SUD must be referred to addiction treatment services.

Substance Use Screening Questions Single-question screenings or tests provide a quick way to screen for patient substance use in healthcare settings. To screen for alcohol, the nurse can ask the patient "How often in the past year have you had four or five drinks in a day?" This allows the nurse to assess for binge drinking and high amounts of alcohol intake. A question that can be used when the nurse screens for patient drug use is "How often in the past year have you used illicit or prescription medications for nonmedical reasons?" Asking questions or screening in healthcare settings is the first step to using the SBIRT approach for substance-related disorders.

CAGE Tool The CAGE Substance Abuse Screening Tool assesses for alcohol problems and has an adapted version for drug problems. Developed in 1974, the four-question CAGE tool, which is shown in Box 11.1, is easy to use and is widely administered in healthcare settings, including psychiatric settings. A patient response of "yes" on two or more of the questions strongly indicates an alcohol problem.

Box 11.1 The CAGE Questionnaire

1. Have you ever felt you should **C**ut down on your drinking or drug use?
2. Have people **A**nnoyed you by criticizing your drinking or drug use?
3. Have you ever felt bad or **G**uilty about your drinking or drug use?
4. Have you ever had a drink or used drugs first thing in the morning to steady your nerves or get rid of a hangover (**E**ye-opener)?

Intimate Partner Violence

In the United States, intimate partner violence (IPV) is a preventable public health issue that affects millions of individuals (Niolon et al., 2017). IPV by definition includes physical violence, sexual violence, stalking, and psychologic aggression that is perpetrated by a current or past intimate partner (CDC, 2017a).

TAPS Tool Part 1

Web Version: 2.0; 4.00; 09-19-17

General instructions:
The TAPS Tool Part 1 is a 4-item screening for tobacco use, alcohol use, prescription medication misuse, and illicit substance use in the past year. Question 2 should be answered only by males and Question 3 only be females. Each of the four multiple-choice items has five possible responses to choose from. Check the box to select your answer.

Segment:
Visit number:

1. In the PAST 12 MONTHS, how often have you used any tobacco product (for example, cigarettes, e-cigarettes, cigars, pipes, or smokeless tobacco)?

   ☐ Daily or Almost Daily ☐ Weekly ☐ Monthly
   ☐ Less Than Monthly ☐ Never

2. In the PAST 12 MONTHS, how often have you had 5 or more drinks containing alcohol in one day? One standard drink is about 1 small glass of wine (5 oz), 1 beer (12 oz), or 1 single shot of liquor. (Note: This question should only be answered by males).

   ☐ Daily or Almost Daily ☐ Weekly ☐ Monthly
   ☐ Less Than Monthly ☐ Never

3. In the PAST 12 MONTHS, how often have you had 4 or more drinks containing alcohol in one day? One standard drink is about 1 small glass of wine (5 oz), 1 beer (12 oz), or 1 single shot of liquor. (Note: This question should only be answered by females).

   ☐ Daily or Almost Daily ☐ Weekly ☐ Monthly
   ☐ Less Than Monthly ☐ Never

4. In the PAST 12 MONTHS, how often have you used any drugs including marijuana, cocaine or crack, heroin, methamphetamine (crystal meth), hallucinogens, ecstasy/MDMA?

   ☐ Daily or Almost Daily ☐ Weekly ☐ Monthly
   ☐ Less Than Monthly ☐ Never

5. In the PAST 12 MONTHS, how often have you used any prescription medications just for the feeling, more than prescribed or that were not prescribed for you? Prescription medications that may be used this way include: opiate pain relievers (for example, OxyContin, Vicodin, Percocet, Methadone); medications for anxiety or sleeping (for example, Xanax, Ativan, Klonopin); medications for ADHD (for example, Adderall or Ritalin).

   ☐ Daily or Almost Daily ☐ Weekly ☐ Monthly
   ☐ Less Than Monthly ☐ Never

Figure 11.3 TAPS Tool.

According to the CDC (2017a), approximately 27% of women and 11% of men reported an experience of partner rape, violence, and/or stalking by an intimate partner. Over the course of their lifetime, 23% of women and 14% of men report experiencing severe physical violence (e.g., being beaten, choked, burned) by an intimate partner (CDC, 2017a). Almost half of women in the United States say they have experienced psychologic aggression by an intimate partner at some point during their life (Dagher, Garza, & Backes Kozhimannil, 2014). Further, IPV is a serious concern in pregnant women with high morbidity and many adverse outcomes.

IPV impacts patients, family health, and safety. Women who are between the ages of 30 to 49 experience the highest rate of intimate homicide, whereas younger women, ages 19 to 25, experience the highest rate of nonfatal IPV (Smith et al., 2017). For some women, IPV can worsen in severity or begin during pregnancy (Paterno & Draughon, 2016). The CDC (2017a) estimates that 15 million children in the United States are exposed to violence in the home annually. This demonstrates the prevalence of IPV among American families and the significance of IPV as a public health concern.

It is important for the nurse to understand that there are short- and long-term health consequences of IPV. Adults exposed to IPV experience a range of adverse physical health effects, such as serious injuries, death, and chronic medical and mental health conditions (Dagher et al., 2014). Physiologic adverse health effects include chronic pain, gastrointestinal disorders, hypertension, chest pain, and sexually transmitted infections (Dagher et al., 2014). The most common psychological health effects on the victim include depression, post-traumatic stress disorder (PTSD), substance abuse, and attempted or completed suicide. Children who are chronically exposed to IPV experience difficulties in emotional regulation as well as sleep and appetite dysregulation (Cruz & Bair-Merritt, 2013). The impact of IPV on individuals and families in the United States is profound.

Cycle of Abuse

The cycle of abuse or battering was identified by Walker in 1979 and includes repeated actions with predictable behaviors over time (Walker, 1979). There are three phases in the cycle: Phase I. The Tension Building Phase; Phase II. The Acute Abuse or Battering Incident; and Phase III. The Calm, Loving, Respite Phase. During the third phase, often referred to as the "honeymoon phase," the perpetrator becomes loving, kind, and often remorseful. Promises of cessation of the abuse and begging for forgiveness are common perpetrator actions in the cycle. As the abuse progresses, fear and intimidation are often used by the perpetrator to maintain power and control. With a sense of powerlessness, many victims of violence cannot see a way out.

Common responses from women regarding why they stayed in an abusive relationship include the following:

- Fear of retaliation—fear for their life and/or for the lives of their children
- Fear of losing children—loss of custody
- Financial dependence
- Religious or cultural reasons
- Hopefulness that the behavior will change

- Lack of a support system
- Lack of concern or attention to the threat of interpersonal violence

Victim Characteristics It is important to note that partner violence crosses all populations. Women and men of all ages, races, religions, cultures, and socioeconomic groups are exposed to IPV. Partners may be married or single, stay-at-home caregivers, or executives in business. Two common characteristics identified by women who have been abused are low self-esteem and willingness to accept the blame for another person's actions. Further, people who grew up in homes with violent relationships are more likely to have or be an abusive partner (Islam et al., 2017). Victims who are chronically exposed to violence can develop a "learned helplessness" due to lack of control over the situation and the inability to change the circumstances.

Perpetrator Characteristics The victimizer or perpetrator of violence often displays a sense of low self-esteem and a need to maintain control. Pathologic jealousy and a limited ability to cope are common traits of a perpetrator. Perpetrators often display possessive behavior and become threatened when a partner is independent. A "dual personality" can be presented as controlling and jealous behavior shown to the partner, whereas calm and charming behavior is presented to the rest of society. The perpetrator seeks power through intimidation and seeks to isolate the victim. In addition, the perpetrator may use threats of suicide or homicide (against the victim, children, family member, and pets) as a tactic of emotional abuse. Such tactics have the potential to keep the victim fearful, and they can impact the victim's ability to leave the dangerous situation.

IPV Screening

IPV can have a lasting harmful effect on individuals, families, and communities. The goal is to stop it from happening in the first place by using prevention efforts including promoting healthy, respectful, nonviolent relationships to reduce known risk factors (CDC, 2017a). The U.S. Preventive Services Task Force (2013) issued recommendations to screen women ages 18 to 46 for IPV, with referral to appropriate intervention services. The assessment should be routinely conducted on all adolescent and adult women at each patient encounter. The assessment should take place in private, as part of routine practice, using neutral terms such as *hit* or *forced to have sex*, rather than *abuse* or *rape*. Ask questions such as "Tell me about your relationship with your partner," or ask "Has your partner ever hit, slapped, kicked, or otherwise hurt you?" These are initial questions that are broad and nonthreatening and help to progress toward more sensitive questions if IPV is disclosed.

IPV screening also includes an observational assessment for possible IPV-related injuries. Once IPV is disclosed, the nurse's validation that no one deserves to be hurt is followed by assessment of the patient's immediate safety, such as asking "Is it safe for you to go home?" or "Is your partner here with you now?" The emphasis should be on appropriate concern for safety and on offering information that would include appropriate resources and referrals (Davila, Mendias, & Juneau, 2013).

When screening for IPV is routinely performed, it has been found to identify an increased number of individuals and children who are exposed to violence. IPV screening is recommended by most medical and nursing organizations, including the American College of Obstetricians and Gynecologists and the American Academy of Pediatrics (Cruz & Bair-Merritt, 2013). In healthcare settings, IPV is the primary cause of injury for women between the ages of 16 and 44. Up to 19% of women screened in emergency departments reported experiencing IPV in the previous year (Dagher et al., 2014). The first step to IPV intervention is identifying individuals who are exposed to violence through screening.

IPV screening in healthcare settings promotes IPV identification in order to provide resources and mitigate the potential health impacts of partner violence. Screening and treatment reduced IPV and improved health outcomes for women, which varied by population group. Improved outcomes of IPV intervention include women reporting increased safety planning, increased community connections, increased quality of life, and decreased exposure to violence (Nelson, Bougatsos, & Blazina, 2012). Increased identification of IPV allows for the nurse to assess safety and to ensure the delivery of resources. Referral pathways or IPV care guidelines need to be established and used for IPV screening. This allows for evidence-based intervention and standardization of referrals and resources when IPV is identified (Bradbury-Jones & Taylor, 2013).

IPV Best Practice

Best practices for IPV screening in healthcare settings have been well established in the research. Best clinical practices for IPV screening include being systematic with the implementation of an IPV screening protocol or guideline for healthcare personnel to follow, training healthcare workers who are to complete the screening, using a validated IPV screening tool, and being

---

Box 11.2 IPV Screening Script Example

- Use an opener—for example, "At this facility we routinely screen for safety" or "We ask all of our patients about partner violence."

- Follow up with IPV screening questions or tool—for example, the HITS (see Box 11.3) or ABUSE tools.

- Respond when an IPV screen is negative (no violence)—for example, "Thank you for answering as some topics can be difficult to talk about" or "If you or a friend is ever in an unsafe relationship, there are people and resources to help."

- Respond when IPV screening is positive—for example, "Everyone deserves to be treated with respect" or "No one deserves to be hurt by a partner."

---

prepared to provide community resources to patients and families (Paterno & Draughon, 2016). It is imperative for nurses to routinely screen for IPV in a private manner, with absolutely no children or others present during the screening.

Before implementation of routine IPV screening, healthcare personnel training, including responses and resources, is needed in order to optimize patient care. It is important to train and support IPV screeners, including the contact information for referral and community resources when partner violence is disclosed. The development of a "what to say" or a screening script was found to be beneficial for the screener (see Box 11.2). When partner violence is identified, the screener may need to report the incident and must understand the mandatory reporting requirements for IPV, which vary by state (Paterno & Draughon, 2016). Some states require the nurse to report partner violence only if there is "material injury." Also, nurses need to know the policy of their healthcare organization on IPV screening. Survivors of partner violence report that calling

---

Box 11.3 HITS Screening Tool

"HITS" A domestic violence screening tool for use in the community

HITS Tool for Intimate Partner Violence Screening: Please read each of the following activities and fill in the circle that best indicates the frequency with which your partner acts in the way depicted.

How often does your partner:	Never	Rarely	Sometimes	Fairly often	Frequently
1. physically hurt you?	O	O	O	O	O
2. insult or talk down to you?	O	O	O	O	O
3. threaten you with harm?	O	O	O	O	O
4. scream or curse at you?	O	O	O	O	O
	1	2	3	4	5

Each item is scored from 1–5. Thus, scores for this inventory range from 4–20. A score of greater than 10 is considered positive.

Clinical Research and Methods
(Fam Med 1998;30(7):508-12.)

HITS is copyrighted in 2003 by Kevin Sherin MD, MPH; For permission to use HITS, Email kevin_sherin@doh.state.fl.us; *HITS is used globally in multiple languages 2006

Box 11.4 Abuse Assessment Screen

Instructions: Circle Yes or No for each question

1. Have you ever been emotionally or physically abused by your partner or someone important to you?   YES   NO

2. Within the last year, have you been hit, slapped, kicked, or otherwise physically hurt by someone?   YES   NO

   If YES, who? (Circle all that apply)

   Husband   Ex-Husband   Boyfriend   Stranger   Other   Multiple

   Total no. of times _____

3. Since you've been pregnant, have you been slapped, kicked, or otherwise physically hurt by someone?   YES   NO

   If YES, who? (Circle all that apply)

   Husband   Ex-Husband   Boyfriend   Stranger   Other   Multiple

   Total no. of times_____

Mark the area of injury on the body map.

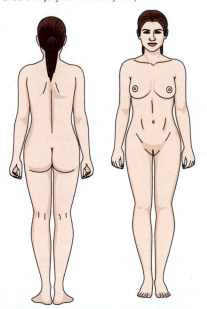

Score each incident according to the following scale:

   1 = Threats of abuse including use of weapon _____

   2 = Slapping, pushing; no injuries and/or lasting pain _____

   3 = Punching, kicking, bruises, cuts, and/or continuing pain _____

   4 = Beating up, severe contusions, burns, broken bones _____

   5 = Head injury, internal injury, permanent injury _____

   6 = Use of weapon; wound from weapon _____

4. Within the last year, has anyone forced you to have sexual activities?   YES   NO

   If YES, who? (Circle all that apply)

   Husband   Ex-Husband   Boyfriend   Stranger   Other   Multiple

   Total no. of times _____

5. Are you afraid of your partner or anyone you listed above?   YES   NO

Source: Copyright (c) 1992, American Medical Association. All rights reserved.

Journal of the American Medical Association, 1992, 267, 3176–3178.

Developer: Judith McFarlane, Barbara Parker, Karen Soeken, and Linda Bullock.

the police with every occurrence is well intended but not helpful (Paterno & Draughon, 2016). Partnering with the patient is necessary to individualize the plan of care and increase safety. The nurse's role when IPV is discovered is to provide empathy, assess the patient's situation, offer assistance and referral choices, and encourage safety planning.

IPV Assessment Tools

If a patient has a positive IPV screen, the nurse needs to act immediately. The nurse must gather more patient information in order to assess for adequate patient safety and to formulate a plan of care. A referral should be made to a community domestic violence agency (when available). This allows for increased support and often provides the patient with an advocate (Miller, McCaw, Humphreys, & Mitchell, 2015).

See Box 11.3 and Box 11.4 for examples of IPV assessment tools.

The Nursing Process in Psychosocial Assessment

The professional nurse uses knowledge, effective communication skills, and critical thinking in applying the nursing process in psychosocial assessment. In conducting psychosocial assessment, the professional nurse uses a holistic approach in assessing the patient's responses to life experiences and the environment. The information is used to formulate nursing diagnoses and to plan care for the patient.

Assessment

When assessing psychosocial health, the nurse gathers data related to several important areas. These include psychosocial concerns, self-concept and beliefs, stress and coping mechanisms, and reasoning ability.

Psychosocial assessment begins before the initial interview when the nurse gathers information from the medical record relating to past emotional or psychiatric problems as well as physiologic illnesses that may have affected the patient's psychologic or social functioning. For example, psychosocial problems may be related to brain tumors, multiple sclerosis, or bipolar disorder.

During the initial interview, the nurse gathers more information about the patient's social history (e.g., marital status and occupation), history of growth and development, past emotional problems, response to crises and illnesses, and family history of emotional or psychiatric illness. If an area of heightened concern is discovered, the nurse may focus on that area during the initial interview and may also conduct a focused interview at a later time during the course of the patient's care. During the focused interview, the nurse uses information obtained from the medical history, the initial interview, and subsequent patient interactions to help the patient conduct a careful inventory of past and current psychosocial health status.

Psychosocial Well-Being The nurse conducts an interview focused on psychosocial well-being in the following situations:

- The patient presents with multiple complaints.

- The information collected during the health history indicates psychosocial dysfunction.

- The patient's behavior during the initial interview is anxious, depressed, erratic, or bizarre.

- More information is needed to determine if any relationships exist between past disease processes and potential emotional or psychiatric concerns.

In some situations, a psychosocial concern is not apparent at the time of the initial interview but becomes apparent at a later time, such as when a patient learns of a negative prognosis or undergoes disfiguring surgical procedures. In such cases, the nurse should seek a focused psychosocial interview whenever the emotional problem becomes apparent. The case study that follows describes a situation in which anxiety and fear impeded a patient's recovery from a physical illness.

Mrs. Ada Sweeney, a 54-year-old grandmother, was admitted to intensive care with gastrointestinal bleeding. Over the next few days, Mrs. Sweeney was diagnosed with severe ulcerative colitis, anemia, and dehydration. Although the physician initiated an aggressive therapeutic medical regimen, Mrs. Sweeney failed to respond to therapy and continued to experience diarrhea accompanied by gastrointestinal bleeding, elevated temperatures, and severe abdominal pain. Indira Singh, the nurse on duty one night, discovered Mrs. Sweeney crying in her room. Ms. Singh then used a focused interview to gather information regarding the behavior Mrs. Sweeney was demonstrating. "I'm worried about my grandson," Mrs. Sweeney told the nurse. "I'm raising him and his sisters until their mother is able to come back for them." Mrs. Sweeney went on to tell Ms. Singh that her daughter had been sent to prison on drug charges and no one else was available to care for her four children. "I do the best I can, but there's never enough money to go around, and I'm terrified the authorities will take the children away from me." Ms. Singh questioned Mrs. Sweeney about her immediate and extended family, income, job, and available support systems. After Ms. Singh reviewed the data she gathered during the focused interview, it became clear that Mrs. Sweeney's anxiety and fear over the future of her grandchildren were interfering with her recovery.

Within the next few days the social service department at the hospital found a state program that provided a homemaker for the children until their grandmother recovered, assisted the family in obtaining food stamps, and began a search for better housing. Mrs. Sweeney immediately began to show a response to her nursing and medical treatment and was able to leave the hospital within 2 weeks.

Only after the nurse focused on the emotional impact of the illness was the patient able to respond to therapy.

In some situations, the patient's primary health concern is psychosocial in nature. Patients with substance abuse, depression, neurosis, or psychosis fall into this category. In these situations, the nurse should integrate the questions outlined here into the initial focused interview during the first contact with the patient, family, or friends.

The focused interview should be structured to obtain the most information with the fewest questions. Patients may feel uncomfortable answering questions about themselves, making it difficult for the nurse to gather accurate and detailed data regarding the psychosocial aspects of the patient's life.

Physical Observation During the initial or focused interview, the nurse should also observe the patient's general appearance, speech patterns, posture, gait, and body language.

The patient's *general appearance* includes the manner of dress, personal hygiene, and grooming.

- The patient should be clean and well groomed. The clothes should be clean, worn properly, and appropriate for the patient's age and the time and place. The nurse must be careful not to impose his own standards when judging the dress of another.

- The patient who is dirty, disheveled, or unshaven or who has a body odor may have an altered body image caused by low self-esteem. The nurse should further assess the patient for changes in skin integrity due to unclean conditions and should look for signs of ringworm, pediculosis, or other skin problems (see Chapter 12 ∞).

The *speech patterns* of the patient are also important for the nurse to assess during the initial interview. The content, tone, pace, and volume of the speech should be appropriate for the situation.

- Abnormal speech patterns may indicate anxiety, fear, or altered thought processes (see Box 11.5). The nurse should observe the coherence and organization of the patient's speech. The patient's speech should be logical and sequential.

- Patients talking to themselves (auditory hallucinations); reacting to objects, noises, or other people in strange ways (illusions); manifesting erratic beliefs (delusions); or appearing aphasic or incoherent may be experiencing altered communication, altered thought processes, and ineffective coping.

The nurse should next observe the patient's *posture, gait, and general body language.*

- The patient's posture should be erect and relaxed.

- The body language should be open with direct eye contact unless inappropriate for the patient's cultural heritage.

- Movements should be fluid, relaxed, and spontaneous. A closed, guarded posture with poor eye contact may indicate fear, anxiety, or defense mechanisms.

- The patient who paces, wrings hands, appears restless, or exhibits tics (involuntary movements) may also be experiencing anxiety.

- A slow, shuffling gait may indicate depression or poor contact with reality.

The nurse must also observe the *facial expression and affect.* The expression and affect should be appropriate for the conversation and circumstances.

- An unusually sad (depressed) or extremely happy (euphoric) demeanor that is inappropriate for the circumstances, labile (rapid) mood swings, or flat affect (absence of emotional expression) may indicate difficulty coping.

Box 11.5 Abnormal Speech Patterns Associated with Altered Thought Processes

- Loud, rapid, pressured, and high-pitched
- Circumlocution (inability to communicate an idea due to numerous digressions)
- Flight of ideas (jumping from one subject to another)
- Word salad (a conglomeration of multiple words without apparent meaning)
- Neologisms (coining new words that have symbolic meaning to the patient)
- Clanging (rhyming conversation)
- Echolalia (constant repetition of words or phrases that the patient hears others say)

Sensory Perception and Cognition Patients who are out of contact with reality may display illusional, delusional, and hallucinatory speech and behaviors, such as talking to themselves (auditory hallucinations); reacting to objects, noises, or other people in strange ways (illusions); or discussing false beliefs (delusions). Direct questioning may increase the patient's anxiety and escalate abnormal behavior or cause confusion; thus, its use must be limited to patients who appear to be in touch with reality

If the patient does appear to be in control and in touch with reality, the following questions are helpful for gathering additional information. The nurse should preface these questions by first explaining to the patient that some of the questions may seem silly or unimportant, but they are helpful in assessing memory.

1. What is your name?

2. How old are you?

3. Where were you born?

4. Where are you right now?

5. What day of the week is it? What is the date?

   Questions 1 through 5 determine whether the patient is oriented to person, place, and time.

6. What would you take with you if a fire broke out?

   The patient's ability to make a judgment is tested here.

7. Count backward from 10 to 1.

   Tests cognitive function.

8. What did you have for breakfast?

   Tests recent memory.

9. Who were the last two presidents?

   Tests remote memory.

10. Describe what the following statement means: People who live in glass houses should not throw stones.

    Tests the patient's ability to do abstract or symbolic thinking.

11. Are you having any problems thinking? If so, describe what happens.

    The patient may not be able to answer this question if a thought disorder is present. Patients with bipolar disorders and who are manic describe their thoughts as "racing."

12. Do you have trouble making decisions? Describe what happens when you have to make a decision.

    The inability to make decisions may indicate depression or low self-esteem.

13. Do you ever hear voices, see objects, or experience other sensations that do not make sense? If so, describe your experiences.

    The patient who is out of touch with reality may experience auditory, visual, gustatory, somatic, and olfactory hallucinations (hearing, seeing, tasting, feeling, and smelling stimuli that are not real). Discussing hallucinatory experiences in detail may reinforce them for the patient; therefore, it is important not to dwell on these symptoms with the patient.

14. If you hear voices, do they tell you what you must do?

    The nurse asks this question to determine if the patient is experiencing command hallucinations. These are dangerous hallucinations that may lead the patient to self-destructive behavior or to harm others.

15. Do you ever misinterpret objects, sounds, or smells? If so, please describe.

    Patients who are very anxious or out of contact with reality may experience illusions (misinterpretation of environmental stimuli).

In order to provide for the patient's safety and the safety of others, it is important to assess the content of a patient's hallucinations and delusions. Command hallucinations tell patients to carry out acts against themselves or others that are usually harmful. The command hallucinations may be part of an elaborate delusional system in which patients feel persecuted or in danger. In some cases, patients are disturbed by these thoughts and share them with others. In other situations, however, patients keep their thoughts to themselves, and these thoughts do not become apparent until they commit some violent act. A patient who demonstrates these symptoms should be referred to a psychiatric/mental health nurse or clinical specialist who has the skill and expertise needed to uncover hallucinatory and delusional thinking without exacerbating the symptoms.

History of Psychosocial Concerns Some psychosocial concerns begin early in life and reappear whenever a patient faces a major stressor or life crisis. The way the patient coped with problems and treatment modalities in the past can be useful information for planning for the patient's current problems. The following questions are helpful in eliciting this information:

1. Describe any emotions you find yourself frequently experiencing both currently and in the past.

   When the nurse assesses patients, a complete psychosocial history is helpful in determining whether the current health problem is related to previous psychosocial dysfunction.

2. If you had an emotional problem in the past, were you treated for it? What kind of treatment did you have? Was the treatment successful? Who gave you the treatment? When? Do you still have the problem?

   This information is helpful in developing the current nursing care plan if previous methods of treatment were successful.

3. Do you use alcohol or drugs? If so, what do you use, how much, and how often? Have you had any treatment for substance abuse? What kind of treatment? Where?

   Substance abuse may be the underlying cause of physiologic or psychosocial health problems or may be the result of some other underlying problem.

4. Have you had any eating problems, such as anorexia, bulimia, or binge eating? Were you treated? How? By whom? When?

   A patient who has an eating disorder may be in denial and unable to give accurate information on this question. If an eating disorder is suspected, the nurse should look for the diagnostic cues during the physical assessment.

History of Physiologic Alterations or Diseases During treatment for medical–surgical conditions, patients and their families may be unaware that the physical problems may be related to or caused by an underlying psychosocial problem. An understanding of the mind–body interaction, both positive and negative, can help nurses and patients realize when covert cognitive, perceptual, or affective problems are related to the overt signs and symptoms. Sometimes the underlying problem does not surface immediately but becomes apparent only after several days of nursing care.

The following questions are helpful for uncovering additional information:

1. Describe any chronic illnesses you have had.

   Patients with recent onset of a chronic illness often have problems complying with treatment or adjusting to living with the condition.

2. How has your illness changed your mood or feelings? When you are nervous or anxious, how does your body feel?

   A physiologic condition may be an underlying cause of anxiety, nervousness, or other abnormal behavior. Conversely, abnormal psychosocial behavior may aggravate or cause a physiologic condition.

3. Have you had any of the following health problems: arthritis? asthma? bowel disorders? heart problems? glandular problems? headaches? stomach ulcer? skin disorders? If so, describe how the condition has affected your life.

   These conditions sometimes have both a psychologic and physiologic component. The presence of the condition may signal an underlying psychosocial disturbance.

Family History   The nurse should explore this area more fully if the health history indicates a family history of psychosocial dysfunction. Although no member of the family may have been diagnosed as being mentally ill, the nurse should explore individual as well as family dysfunction.

The nurse should ask the following questions in relation to the patient's parents, siblings, and extended family in the case of a child, as well as in relation to the patient's current family if an adult.

1. Describe any problems your family members may have had with mental disorders.

   Some mental disorders, such as schizophrenia, are familial—that is, the illness recurs in the same family over several generations.

2. Describe your relationships with your parents and extended family.

   As the patient describes his or her family life, the nurse should look for family dysfunction problems such as schisms (families in chronic controversy), disengagement (detached relationships), or enmeshment (family interactions that are intense and focus on power conflicts rather than affections).

3. Describe your relationship with your siblings growing up at home. Did you and your siblings have problems getting along? If so, how did you solve them?

   The way a patient learned to handle stress and conflict with siblings as a child influences the way the patient handles these issues throughout life.

4. Did you have death or losses in your family as you grew up? How did your parents teach you to cope with the loss? How did they cope with the loss?

   Patients who are depressed may not have learned how to deal with loss as a child and may have difficulty dealing with the loss of a loved one or with their own or a significant other's declining health status.

5. Describe how your parents raised you. How did it affect you?

   Patients who were raised by parents who had serious emotional problems, or who were abused by their parents, are more likely to have emotional problems as adults.

6. How did your family deal with adversity and conflict?

   Patients learn to deal with problems from their family. Knowing how the patient learned to deal with problems as a child helps the nurse understand how the patient might deal with the present health problem.

7. When disagreement arose in your family, how was it solved? Who sided with whom?

   In dysfunctional families, schisms result, causing family members to align themselves into coalitions against other family members, such as parents against children, father and sons against mother and daughters, and sisters against brothers.

Self-concept   It is difficult to gather significant data about self-concept because most patients find it embarrassing to answer questions about themselves. Patients feel more comfortable divulging this information after a positive nurse–patient relationship has been established and when the nurse integrates questions into general conversation.

The following questions are helpful in obtaining additional information about self-concept:

1. How would you describe yourself to others?

   Asking patients to describe themselves is an excellent technique for determining how they perceive themselves.

2. What are your best characteristics? What do you like about yourself?

3. What would you change about yourself if you could?

   This is a positive way of asking a patient to talk about negative self-perceptions.

4. Have your feelings about your appearance changed? If so, how?

   Self-image may change if the illness or treatment has caused a change in appearance.

5. Do you like to be alone?

   Patients with positive self-concept enjoy spending time by themselves, but those who indicate that they would rather be alone most of the time may be experiencing emotional problems.

6. Describe your social life. What do you do for fun?

   Patients who are unable to answer this question may be depressed or out of touch with reality.

7. Are you comfortable with your sexual preference? If not, why not?

   Patients who are homosexual and have not learned to accept their sexuality may experience a self-image problem.

Other Roles and Relationships   It is also important for the nurse to ask questions about other roles and relationships in the patient's life.

1. Describe your relationships with your friends, neighbors, and coworkers.

2. Do you belong to any social groups? Community groups?

3. Who is your closest friend? How do you maintain your friendship?

   An individual's ability to form close relationships indicates a healthy self-concept. An individual who consistently fails to form close relationships may have a self-concept problem.

4. Is your closest friend the most important person in your life? If not, who is the most important person in your life? Explain why.

Stress and Coping

A person learns coping mechanisms from significant others during early childhood and throughout life. The ability to cope is also greatly affected by the number and severity of stressors that have occurred in a person's life. One method for assessing stress in a patient's life is to administer the Holmes Social Readjustment Rating Scale (SRRS). Developed by psychiatrists Thomas Holmes and Richard Rahe in 1967, the SRRS—and modifications of this tool—are still used today. The SRRS lists a series of life stressors that require the individual to change established norms and patterns, along with an assigned point value for each stressor (Holmes & Rahe, 1967). Because stress is a response to events—not the events themselves—not all people are equally stressed by these events. However, on average, the higher the patient's score, the more likely it is that the individual has responded with stress. As a result, the individual is more likely to experience stress-related disorders (e.g., headaches, asthma, skin rashes, back pain, frequent colds, anxiety). Because positive life events also evoke a stress response, they also should be part of a psychosocial assessment. For example, the death of a spouse has a relative point value of 100, marriage has a relative point value of 50, and a vacation has a relative point value of 13 (Holmes & Rahe, 1967). The complete SRRS is available at the American Institute of Stress website: http://www.stress.org.

As a baseline assessment, the following questions are helpful to gather additional information about the patient's stress and coping mechanisms:

1. What is your greatest source of comfort when you are feeling upset?

   This question identifies the patient's coping mechanisms.

2. Who do you call when you need help?

   This question identifies important persons in the patient's support system.

3. What is the greatest source of stress in your life at the present time? How have you coped with similar situations in the past?

   A person who has successfully coped with stress in the past may be able to call upon these coping skills to deal with current problems.

4. Describe how you are dealing with your illness. Have you had difficulty adjusting to changes in your appearance, your ability to carry out activities of daily living, or your relationships? If so, describe how you feel.

   Patients who have undergone severe, sudden changes that are apparent to others frequently have difficulty adjusting to these changes.

5. Do you take any drugs, medications, or alcohol to cope with your stress? If so, describe what you are taking.

   Patients who are experiencing stress are at risk for becoming addicted to these substances, especially if there is a family history of drug or alcohol abuse.

6. Do you use comfort foods, or do you overeat when you are feeling stressed?

   A link between prolonged stress, eating comfort foods, and obesity has been described.

Self-Directed Violence Ineffective coping may lead to a variety of maladaptive behaviors, including self-directed violence (SDV). **Nonsuicidal self-injury (NSSI)** is characterized by behaviors committed by and aimed at oneself that result in deliberate actual or potential self-harm (Sornberger et al., 2013). NSSI is identified as a maladaptive coping mechanism. **Suicidal ideation** is considering, planning, or thinking about committing suicide (Valois, Zullig, & Hunter, 2015). Associations found with completed adolescent suicide include drug or alcohol use, access to lethal opportunity, and precipitation of an acute event, such as a parental divorce or breakup.

Suicide is the 10th leading cause of death in the United States and remains a major health concern (Steele, Thrower, Noroian, & Saleh, 2018). In 2009, the number of suicide-related deaths exceeded the number of deaths due to motor vehicle crashes (Centers for Disease Control and Prevention [CDC], 2013). In the United States in 2014, 43,773 suicides were reported. This demonstrates an upward trend in completed suicides (Steele et al., 2018). Although traditional suicide prevention efforts have focused on adolescents and older adults, current research suggests that individuals of all ages are at risk for suicide (CDC, 2013).

For the nurse, awareness of the widespread problem of suicide and knowledge of the factors that may increase an individual's risk for NSSI, including one or more previous suicide attempts, are keys to identifying at-risk patients. (See Box 11.6 for an overview of factors associated with an increased risk for attempting suicide.)

In addition to being familiar with risk factors for suicide, the nurse also should be aware of the warning signs of an impending potential suicide attempt. Warning signs of an impending suicide attempt vary among individuals. However, certain behaviors—such as researching methods of suicide or giving away prized personal belongings—are critical indicators that should be immediately reported to the patient's primary care provider. (See Box 11.7 for examples of warning signs that may

---

Box 11.6 Factors That Increase an Individual's Risk for Attempting Suicide

- History of suicide attempt(s)
- Family history of attempted or completed suicide
- Age (with highest risk among older adults)
- Lower socioeconomic status
- Limited education
- Single/unmarried status
- Lesbian, gay, bisexual, transgender (LGBT) sexual orientation
- Unemployment
- History of drug or alcohol abuse
- History of substance use disorder (SUD)
- History of childhood trauma (including physical or sexual abuse, neglect or exposure to intimate partner violence)
- History of mental illness/psychiatric disorder
- Physiologic disorders, such as cancer, HIV, or a terminal illness
- Recent legal/criminal problems
- Chaotic or troubled interpersonal relationships

Sources: Adapted from Borges, et al., 2010; Haw, Hawton, Niedzwiedz, & Platt (2013); and Steele, Thrower, Noroian, & Saleh (2018).

Box 11.7   Potential Warning Signs of an Impending Suicide Attempt

- Reckless behavior
- Increased incidence of alcohol and/or drug abuse
- Seeking out information on suicide methods
- Purchasing a weapon
- Changes in sleep patterns, insomnia
- Sudden change in mood
- Depression, panic attacks, anxiety, or agitation
- Giving away treasured personal belongings
- Expression of feelings of hopelessness or burdensomeness
- Contacting people to say good-bye
- Social withdrawal
- Nonsuicidal self-injury

Sources: Adapted from American Foundation for Suicide Prevention (n.d.); and Steele, Thrower, Noroian, & Saleh (2018).

Box 11.8   Healthy Days Measures

The CDC uses a set of questions called the "Healthy Days Measures." These questions include the following:

1. Would you say that in general your health is

   A. Excellent
   B. Very good
   C. Good
   D. Fair
   E. Poor

2. Now thinking about your physical health, which includes physical illness and injury, for how many days during the past 30 days was your physical health not good?

3. Now thinking about your mental health, which includes stress, depression, and problems with emotions, for how many days during the past 30 days was your mental health not good?

4. During the past 30 days, for about how many days did poor physical or mental health keep you from doing your usual activities, such as self-care, work, or recreation?

Source: Adapted from Centers for Disease Control and Prevention (2017b).

---

signal an impending suicide attempt.) Questions for the nurse to ask to further assess for depression and suicidal ideation include the following:

1. Are you experiencing any of the following: sadness? crying spells? insomnia? lack of appetite? weight loss? weight gain? loss of sex drive? constipation? fatigue? hopelessness? irritability? indecisiveness? confusion? pounding heart or pulse? trouble concentrating?

   These may indicate a high level of stress or major depression.

2. Have you ever considered taking your life? If so, describe what you would do.

   Patients who are suicidal often admit their intentions if questioned directly. Patients are at high risk for suicide if they can describe a method for committing the suicide and have the necessary means at their disposal.

Should analysis of nursing assessment data suggest that a patient is at risk for attempting suicide or committing any other form of NSSI, the nurse should immediately notify the patient's primary care provider. Patients who are known or believed to be at risk for NSSI should be continually monitored, and care of these patients should include immediate implementation of the hospital or organization's safety protocols.

Measures, scales, and instruments are available to assess particular aspects of psychosocial health, including quality of life, social support, stress, and psychosocial well-being. For example, the CDC uses "Healthy Days Measures" to assess quality of life in populations (Centers for Disease Control and Prevention [CDC], 2017b). Box 11.8 includes questions used in Healthy Days Measures.

Organizing the Data

Once the nurse has collected the data from all of the various sources, the information is sorted, grouped, and categorized. Each diagnostic cue falls under one of the psychosocial functioning groups mentioned earlier in this chapter: substance use, exposure to violence, self-concept, roles and relationships, stress and coping, the senses and cognition, and spiritual and belief systems. After the diagnostic cues have been grouped and clustered under one of the psychosocial groups, the nurse determines the final nursing diagnoses.

The following example demonstrates how diagnostic cues obtained during the assessment lead to nursing diagnoses related to psychosocial well-being and function.

Mr. Abe Johnson, a veteran of the Iraq War, was admitted to the local hospital emergency department after being arrested for loitering. The guards at the jail brought him to the hospital after they found heroin in his pocket and were unable to arouse him. When approached by the admitting nurse, Jim, Mr. Johnson shouted, "Don't come near me with that gas machine! The High Lord has told me that I control the secret of life and death, and if you touch me you must die!" Jim recognized that Mr. Johnson presented as delusional, having seen Jim's stethoscope as a "gas machine." After observing Mr. Johnson's manner and tone for a few minutes, Jim noted that he was hearing voices. He knew that Mr. Johnson's behavior could become violent if he continued to experience command hallucinations. To address his concern, Jim removed his stethoscope and showed it to Mr. Johnson. He said, speaking in a quiet calm voice, "This is the stethoscope that I use to listen to a patient's heart. Sometimes I use it to take blood pressures." This seemed to settle Mr. Johnson, who became quiet and withdrawn. After a few minutes Jim said, "You've been brought to the hospital, Mr. Johnson. I'm Jim, your nurse, and I'm here to take care of you."

Discussion: In this clinical situation, the nurse showed Mr. Johnson respect and concern for his feelings and well-being. He did not, however, validate his perceptions about the stethoscope or acknowledge the voices he heard.

The nurse then clustered the information gained from the assessment and identified the significant cues demonstrated by Mr. Johnson:

- Hallucinations
- Delusions
- Illusions
- Fearful thoughts
- Irritability
- Inaccurate interpretation of environment

The nurse reviewed all the data and saw the following factors as contributing to Mr. Johnson's problems:

- Substance use
- Possible homelessness
- Possible post-traumatic stress disorder (PTSD)

Then, after reviewing the assessment data, identifying contributing factors, and clustering the information, the nurse formulated diagnoses and a plan of care.

The holistic approach to nursing holds that the individual must be viewed as a total being, with body, mind, and spirit continuously interacting with self and with the environment. The psychosocial assessment is a key component that must be integrated into the nurse's holistic approach to data collection. This assessment guides the nurse toward a true and accurate picture of the patient as a total human being.

Application Through Critical Thinking

CASE STUDY

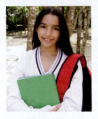

Source: Tono Balaguer/ Shutterstock.

Crystal is a 15-year-old Hispanic female who has come to the women's clinic for birth control. During her interview you find out she has been abusing prescription drugs for the past 3 years. This began shortly after her father passed away from a long battle with colon cancer. She was very close to her father, and when he died she was feeling very sad and took some of his pain medication to help her sleep. She began to use the drugs and eventually became addicted. Her father was the main support in the home, and when he was alive he kept the family together. He worked in the restaurant industry and did not have any death benefits other than Social Security and a small life insurance policy. Crystal's mother suffers from depression and has been unable to work since her father died, and she has times when she is so depressed she is unable to get out of bed. She refuses to get any help. Crystal is left to care for herself and her mom and says she

uses drugs just to escape from her life. She does not attend school regularly and has poor grades. She has a part-time job at a restaurant to pay for her drugs and to buy food. She and her mom have been living in an apartment in a low-income housing area since they lost their home due to foreclosure. Crystal shares with you that she is sexually active and does not want to become pregnant.

CRITICAL THINKING QUESTIONS

1. What external/internal factors contributed to Crystal's current situation?
2. What additional factors are applicable in psychosocial health?
3. What questions might you ask to understand Crystal's self-concept?
4. What questions might you ask to find out more information about Crystal's relationship with her mother?
5. What suicide risk factors does Crystal have?

REFERENCES

American Foundation for Suicide Prevention. (n.d.). *Risk factors and warning signs.* Retrieved from http://www.afsp .org/understanding-suicide/risk-factors-and-warning -signs

Basu, A., McLaughlin, K. A., Misra, S., & Koenen, K. C. (2017). Childhood maltreatment and health impact: The examples of cardiovascular disease and type 2 diabetes mellitus in adults. *Clinical Psychology Science and Practice, 24*(2), 125-139. doi: 10.1111/cpsp.12191

Borges, G., Nock, M. K., Haro, J. M., Hwang, I., Sampson, N. A., Alonso, J., . . . Kessler, R. C. (2010). Twelve-month prevalence of and risk factors for suicide attempts in the World Health Organization mental health surveys. *Journal of Clinical Psychiatry, 71*(12), 1617–1628. doi:10.4088/JCP.08m04967blu

Bradbury-Jones, C., & Taylor, J. (2013). Establishing a domestic abuse care pathway: Guidance for practice. *Nursing Standard, 27*, 42–47. Retrieved from http://www.nursing-standard.co .uk/

Byrne, E., Gehrman, P., Medland, S. Nyholt, D., Heath, A., Madden, P., . . . The Chrongen Consortium. (2013). A genome-wide association of sleep habits and insomnia. *American Journal of Medical Genetics, 162*(5), 439-451. doi:10.1002/ajmg.b.32168

Centers for Disease Control and Prevention (CDC). (2013). Suicide among adults aged 35–64 years—United States, 1999–2010. *Morbidity and Mortality Weekly Report (MMWR), 62*(17), 321–325. Retrieved from https://www.cdc.gov/mmwr/preview/mmwrhtml/mm6217a1.htm?s_cid=mm6217a1_w"

Centers for Disease Control and Prevention (CDC). (2017a). *Intimate partner violence.* Retrieved from https://www.cdc.gov/violenceprevention/intimatepartnerviolence/index.html

Centers for Disease Control and Prevention (CDC). (2017b) *Health-related quality of life (HRQOL): CDC HRQOL–14 "Healthy Days Measure."* Retrieved from http://www.cdc.gov/hrqol/hrqol14_measure.htm

Cruz, M., & Bair-Merritt, M. H. (2013). Screening and intervention of intimate partner violence. *Contemporary Pediatrics, 30*(5), 12–25. Retrieved from http://www.advanstar.com/healthcare

Dagher, R. K., Garza, M. A., & Backes Kozhimannil, K. (2014). Policymaking under uncertainty: Routine screening for intimate partner violence. *Violence Against Women, 20*(6), 730–749. doi:10.1177/1077801214540540

Davila, Y. R., Mendias, E. P., & Juneau, C. (2013). Under the RADAR: Assessing and intervening for intimate partner violence. *Journal of Nurse Practitioners, 9*(9), 594–599.

Doherty, A., & Gaughran, F. (2014). The interface of physical and mental health. *Social Psychiatry & Psychiatric Epidemiology, 49*(5), 673–682. doi:10.1007/s00127-014-0847-7

Haw, C., Hawton, K., Niedzwiedz, C., & Platt, S. (2013). Suicide clusters: A review of risk factors and mechanisms. *Suicide and Life-Threatening Behavior, 43*(1), 97–108.

Holmes, T., & Rahe, R. J. (1967). Social Readjustment Rating Scale. *Journal of Psychosomatic Research, 11*(2), 213–218.

Islam, M. J., Rahman, M., Broidy, L., Haque, S. E., Yu Mon, S., Nguyen Huu Chau, D., . . . Duc, N. C. (2017). Assessing the link between witnessing inter-parental violence and the perpetration of intimate partner violence in Bangladesh. *BMC Public Health, 17*(1), 1–10. doi:10.1186/s12889-017-4067-4

Jordan, C. J., & Andersen, S. L. (2017). Sensitive periods of substance abuse: Early risk for the transition to dependence. *Developmental Cognitive Neuroscience, 25*, 29-44. doi:10.1016/j.dcn.2016.10.004

Kerns, T. L. (2018). The opioid crisis. *Nevada RNFormation, 27*(2), 12.

Krashin, D., Murinova, N., & Sullivan, M. (2016). Challenges to treatment of chronic pain and addiction during the "opioid crisis." *Current Pain Headache Reports. 20*: 65. doi:10.1007/s11916-016-0595-2

Ladegast, S. (2016). The use of SBIRT in substance abuse screening. *The Nurse Practitioner, 41*(10), 1–3. doi:10.1097/01NPR.0000497009.2998.6c

Li, J., Eriksson, M., He, W., Hall, P., & Czene, K. (2017). Associations between childhood body size and seventeen adverse outcomes: Analysis of 65,057 European women. *Scientific Reports, 7*(1), Article number: 16917. http://doi.org/10.1038/s41598-017-17258-5

Masten, A. S., & Monn, A. R. (2015). Child and family resilience: A call for integrated science, practice, and professional training. *Family Relations: Interdisciplinary Journal of Applied Family Science, 64*(1), 5-21. doi:10.1111/fare.12103

McNeely, J., Wu, L.-T., Subramaniam, G., Sharma, G., Cathers, L. A., Svikis, D., . . . Schwartz, R. P. (2017). Performance of the Tobacco, Alcohol, Prescription Medication, and Other Substance Use (TAPS) Tool for substance use screening in primary care patients. *Annals of Internal Medicine, 165*(10), 690–699. http://doi.org/10.7326/M16-0317

Mehta, A. J. (2016). Alcoholism and critical illness: A review. *World Journal of Critical Care Medicine, 5*(1), 27-35. doi:10.5492/wjccm.v5.i1.27

Miller, E., McCaw, B., Humphreys, B. L., & Mitchell, C. (2015). Integrating intimate partner violence assessment and intervention into healthcare in the United States: A systems approach. *Journal of Women's Health, 24*(1), 92-99. doi:10.1089/jwh.2014.4870

Morrow, D. F., & Messinger, L. (Eds.). (2013). *Sexual orientation and gender expression in social work practice: Working with gay, lesbian, bisexual, and transgender people.* New York, NY: Columbia University Press.

Myers, L. L., & Wiman, A. M. (2014). Binge eating disorder: A review of a new "DSM" diagnosis. *Research on Social Work Practice, 24*(1), 86–95. doi:10.177/1049735153507755

National Alliance on Mental Illness (NAMI). (2013a). *Anorexia nervosa.* Retrieved from http://www.nami.org/Template.cfm?Section=By_Illness&Template=/ContentManagement/ContentDisplay.cfm&ContentID=149438

National Alliance on Mental Illness (NAMI). (2013b). *Bulimia nervosa.* Retrieved from http://www.nami.org/Content/ContentGroups/Helpline1/Bulimia.htm

National Human Genome Research Institute. (2015). *Frequently asked questions about genetic disorders: What are genetic disorders?* Retrieved from https://www.genome.gov/19016930

National Institute on Drug Abuse (NIDA). (2015). *Advancing addiction science: Nationwide trends.* Retrieved from https://www.drugabuse.gov/publications/drugfacts/nationwide-trends

National Institute on Drug Abuse (NIDA) (2016). *Genetics and epigenetics of addiction.* Retrieved from https://www.drugabuse.gov/publications/drugfacts/genetics-epigenetics-addiction

Nelson, H. D., Bougatsos, C., & Blazina, I. (2012). Screening women for intimate partner violence: A systematic review to update the U.S. Preventive Services Task Force (USPSTF) recommendation. *Annals of Internal Medicine, 156,* 796–808.

Niolon, P. H., Kearns, M., Dills, J., Rambo, K., Irving, S., Armstead, T. L., & Gilbert, L. (2017). *Preventing intimate partner violence across the lifespan: A technical package of programs, policies, and practices.* Atlanta, GA: National Center for Injury Prevention and Control Centers for Disease Control and Prevention.

Office of Public Health and Genomics (OPHG). (2013). *Identifying opportunities to improve health and transform healthcare.* Retrieved from http://www.genome.gov/Pages/Health/PatientsPublicInfo/GeneticTestingWhatItMeansForYourHealth.pdf

Paterno, M. T., & Draughon, J. E. (2016). Screening for intimate partner violence. *Journal of Midwifery & Women's Health, 61,* 370–375. doi:10.1111/jmwh.12443

Patestos, C., Patterson, K., & Fitzsimons, V. (2014). Substance abuse prevention. *NASN School Nurse, 29*(6), 310–314.

President's Council on Physical Fitness, Sports & Nutrition. (2017). *About PCPFSN.* Washington, DC: U.S. Department of Health and Human Services. Retrieved from https://www.hhs.gov/fitness

Pulkki-Raback, L., Elovainio, M., Hakulinen, C., Lipsanen, J., Hintsanen, M., Jokela, M., . . . Keltikangas-Jarvinen, L. (2015). Cumulative effect of psychosocial factors in youth on ideal cardiovascular health in adulthood: The cardiovascular risk in young Finns study. *Circulation, 131*(3), 245–253. doi:10.1161/CIRCULATIONAHA.113.007104

Roy, C., & Andrews, H. (1999). *The Roy adaptation model* (2nd ed.). Stamford, CT: Appleton & Lange.

Shinozaki, G., & Potash, J. B. (2014). New developments in the genetics of bipolar disorder. *Current Psychiatry Reports, 16*:493, 1–10. doi:10.1007/s11920-014-0493-5

Sinha, R., & Jastreboff, A. M. (2013). Stress as a common risk factor for obesity and addiction. *Biological Psychiatry, 73*(9), 827–835.

Smith, S. G., Chen, J., Basile, K. C., Gilbert, L. K., Merrick, M. T., Patel, N., . . . Jain, A. (2017). *The National Intimate Partner and Sexual Violence Survey (NISVS): 2010–2012 State report.* Atlanta, GA: National Center for Injury Prevention and Control, Centers for Disease Control and Prevention. Retrieved from https://stacks.cdc.gov/view/cdc/46305

Sornberger, M. J., Smith, N. G., Toste, J. R., & Heath, N. L. (2013). Nonsuicidal self-injury, coping strategies, and sexual orientation. *Journal of Clinical Psychology, 69,* 571–583. doi:10.1002/jclp.21947

Spector, R. (2017). *Cultural diversity in health and illness.* New York, NY: Pearson.

Steele, I. H., Thrower, N., Noroian, P., & Saleh, F. M. (2018). Understanding suicide across the lifespan: A United States perspective of suicide risk factors, assessment & management. *Journal of Forensic Science, 63,* 162–171. doi:10.1111/1556-4029.13519

Substance Abuse and Mental Health Services Administration [SAMHSA]. (2015). *Mental and substance use disorders.* Retrieved from https://www.samhsa.gov/disorders

U.S. Preventive Services Task Force. (2018.) *Draft recommendation statement: Intimate partner violence, elder abuse, and abuse of vulnerable adults: Screening.* Retrieved from: https://www.uspreventiveservicestaskforce.org/Page/Document/draft-recommendation-statement/intimate-partner-violence-and-abuse-of-elderly-and-vulnerable-adults-screening1

Valois, R., Zullig, K., & Hunter, A. (2015). Association between adolescent suicide ideation, suicide attempts and emotional self-efficacy. *Journal of Child & Family Studies, 24*(2), 237–248. doi:10.1007/s10826-013-9829-8

Volkow, N. D., Wise, R. A., & Baler, R. (2017). The dopamine motive system: Implication for drug and food addiction. *Nature Reviews Neuroscience, 18,* 741–752. doi:10.1038/nrn.2017.130

Walker, L. E. 1979. *Battered woman.* New York, NY: Harper and Row.

Wang, J., Freire, D., Knable, L., Zhao, W., Gong, B., Mazzola, P., . . . Pasinetti, G. M. (2015). Childhood and adolescent obesity and long-term cognitive consequences during aging. *Journal of Comparative Neurology, 523,* 757–768. doi:10.1002/cne.23708

Wood, W., & Eagly, A. (2015). Two traditions of research on gender identity. *Sex Roles, 73*(11–12), 461–473. doi:10.1007/s11199-015-0480-2

Wu, L., McNeely, J., Subramaniam, G. A., Sharma, G., Vanveldhuisen, P., & Schwartz, R. P. (2016). Design of the NIDA clinical trials network validation study of Tobacco, Alcohol, Prescription Medications, and Substance Use/Misuse (TAPS) tool. *Contemporary Clinical Trials, 19*(50), 90–97. doi:10.1016/j.cct2016.07.013

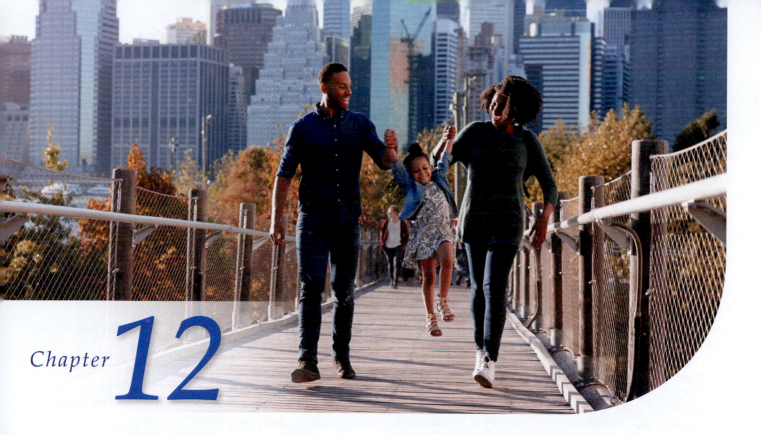

Chapter 12

Skin, Hair, and Nails

LEARNING OUTCOMES

Upon completion of this chapter, you will be able to:

1. Describe the anatomy and physiology of the skin, hair, and nails.

2. Identify the anatomic, physiologic, developmental, psychosocial, and cultural variations that guide assessment of the skin, hair, and nails.

3. Determine which questions about the skin, hair, and nails to ask for the focused interview.

4. Outline the techniques for assessment of the skin, hair, and nails.

5. Generate the appropriate documentation to describe the assessment of the skin, hair, and nails.

6. Identify abnormal findings in the physical assessment of the skin, hair, and nails.

KEY TERMS

alopecia areata, 177
apocrine glands, 171
cuticle, 172
dandruff, 177
dermis, 170
diaphoresis, 174
ecchymosis, 185
eccrine glands, 171

edema, 184
epidermis, 170
hair, 171
hirsutism, 178
hypodermis, 171
integumentary system, 170
keratin, 170
lunula, 172

melanin, 170
Mongolian spots, 191
nails, 172
onycholysis, 203
paronychia, 203
pediculosis capitis, 188
pressure ulcers, 185
primary lesions, 190

sebaceous glands, 171
secondary lesions, 185
terminal hair, 172
trichotillomania, 172
vellus hair, 172
vitiligo, 180

MEDICAL LANGUAGE

-cyte	Suffix meaning "cell"	**-lysis**	Suffix meaning "breakdown," "separation," "destruction"
-emia	Suffix meaning "blood condition"		
epi-	Prefix meaning "above," "upon," "on"	**-oma**	Suffix meaning "tumor," "mass," "fluid collection"
-itis	Suffix meaning "inflammation"	**onycho-**	Prefix meaning "nail"

Introduction

A thorough assessment of the skin, hair, and nails is one of the first steps in learning about a patient's overall health status. The skin, hair, and nails make up the **integumentary system**. A patient's activities of daily living, habits and behaviors, beliefs, and physical environment, both at home and at work, can greatly influence integumentary health and are an integral part of the assessment data. The nurse must have a thorough knowledge base regarding the anatomy, physiology, and health assessment techniques for the integumentary system.

Information from the history and physical assessment can reveal the status of a patient's hydration, nutrition, airway clearance, thermoregulation, and tissue perfusion, all of which directly impact the skin, hair, and nails. Alterations in the skin, hair, and nails can also reveal the health status in relation to activity, sleep and rest, level of stress, and self-care ability.

Anatomy and Physiology Review

The skin and the accessory structures, the sweat and oil glands, hair, and nails are the major components of the integumentary system. The largest of these is the skin, a cutaneous membrane; the skin is made up of two primary layers, and this complex shield protects the body against heat, ultraviolet rays, trauma, and invasion by bacteria. In addition, the skin works with other body systems to regulate body temperature, synthesize vitamin D, store blood and fats, excrete body wastes, and help humans sense the world around them (Marieb & Keller, 2018).

The skin is composed of the epidermal, dermal, and subcutaneous layers. The cutaneous glands, which are located in the dermal layer, release secretions to lubricate the skin and to assist in temperature regulation. The hair and nails are composed of keratinized (hardened) cells and serve to protect the skin and the ends of the fingers and toes. Each of these anatomic structures is described in the following sections.

Skin and Glands

The skin is composed of two distinct layers. The outer layer, called the **epidermis**, is firmly attached to an underlying layer called the **dermis**. Deep in the dermis is a layer of subcutaneous tissue that anchors the skin to the underlying body structures. The major functions of the skin are the following:

- Perceiving touch, pressure, temperature, and pain via the nerve endings
- Protecting against mechanical, chemical, thermal, and solar damage
- Protecting against loss of water and electrolytes
- Regulating body temperature
- Repairing surface wounds through cellular replacement
- Synthesizing vitamin D
- Allowing identification through uniqueness of facial contours, skin and hair color, and fingerprints

Epidermis The epidermis is a layer of epithelial tissue that comprises the outermost portion of the skin. Where exposure to friction is greatest, such as on the fingertips, palms, and soles of the feet, the epidermis consists of five layers (or strata), as shown in Figure 12.1 ■. These five layers, from deep to superficial, are the stratum basale, stratum spinosum, stratum granulosum, stratum lucidum, and stratum corneum.

New skin cells are formed in the stratum basale, or basal layer, which is also known as the stratum germinativum (germinating layer). These new skin cells consist mostly of a fibrous protein called **keratin**, which gives the epidermis its tough, protective qualities. About 25% of the cells in the stratum basale are *melanocytes*, which produce the skin pigment called **melanin**. All humans have the same relative number of melanocytes, but the amount of melanin they produce varies according to genetic, hormonal, and environmental factors.

Cells produced in the stratum basale gradually move through the layers of the epidermis toward the stratum corneum, where they are sloughed off. The abundance of keratin in this tough "horny layer" protects against abrasion and trauma, repels water, resists water loss, and renders the body insensitive to a variety of environmental toxins.

Dermis The dermis is a layer of connective tissue that lies just below the epidermis. The dermis consists mainly of two types of fibers: collagen, which gives the skin its toughness and enables it to resist tearing, and elastic fibers, which give the skin its elasticity. The dermis is richly supplied with nerves, blood vessels, and lymphatic vessels; and it is embedded with hair follicles, sweat glands, oil glands, and sensory receptors.

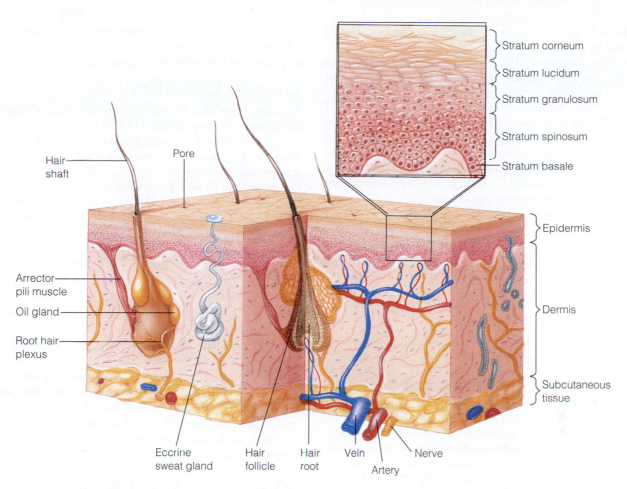

Figure 12.1 Skin structure. Three-dimensional view of the skin, subcutaneous tissue, glands, and hairs.

Subcutaneous Tissue The subcutaneous tissue (or **hypodermis**) is a loose connective tissue that stores approximately half the body's fat cells. Thus, it cushions the body against trauma, insulates the body from heat loss, and stores fat for energy.

Cutaneous Glands The cutaneous glands are formed in the stratum basale and push deep into the dermis. They release their secretions through ducts onto the skin surface. The major functions of the cutaneous glands are the following:

- Excreting uric acid, urea, ammonia, sodium, potassium, and other metabolic wastes
- Regulating temperature through evaporation of perspiration on the skin surface
- Protecting against bacterial growth on the skin surface
- Softening, lubricating, and waterproofing skin and hair
- Resisting water loss from the skin surface in low-humidity environments
- Protecting deeper skin regions from bacteria on the skin surface

There are two types of sweat (or sudoriferous) glands: eccrine and apocrine. **Eccrine glands** are more numerous and more widely distributed. They produce a clear perspiration

mostly made up of water and salts, which they release into funnel-shaped pores at the skin surface. **Apocrine glands** are found primarily in the axillary and anogenital regions. They are dormant until the onset of puberty. Apocrine glands produce a secretion made up of water, salts, fatty acids, and proteins, which is released into hair follicles. When apocrine sweat mixes with bacteria on the skin surface, it assumes a musky odor.

Oil Glands Oil glands, or **sebaceous glands**, are distributed over most of the body except the palms of the hands and soles of the feet. They produce *sebum*, an oily secretion composed of fat and keratin that is usually released into hair follicles.

Hair

A **hair** is a thin, flexible, elongated fiber composed of dead, keratinized cells that grow out in a columnar fashion (see Figure 12.1). Each hair shaft arises from a follicle. Nerve endings in the follicle are sensitive to the slightest movement of the hair. Each hair follicle also has an *arrector pili* muscle that causes the hair to contract and stand upright when a person is under stress or exposed to cold.

The deep end of each follicle expands to form a hair bulb, where new cells are produced. Hair growth is cyclic, and scalp hair typically has an active phase of about 4 years and a resting phase of a few months. Because these phases are not synchronous, only a small percentage of a person's hair follicles shed their hair at any given time.

Hair color is determined by the amount of melanin produced in the hair follicle. Black or brown hair contains the greatest amount of melanin.

The type and distribution of hair vary in different parts of the body. **Vellus hair**, a pale, fine, short strand, grows over the entire body except for the margins of the lips, the nipples, the palms of the hands, the soles of the feet, and parts of the external genitals. The **terminal hair** of the eyebrows and scalp is usually darker, coarser, and longer. At puberty, hormones signal the growth of terminal hair in the axillae, in the pubic region, and on the legs of both sexes, as well as on the face and chest of most males.

The major functions of the hair are to insulate against heat and cold, protect against ultraviolet and infrared rays, perceive movement or touch, protect the eyes from sweat, and protect the nasal passages from foreign particles.

Nails

Nails are thin plates of keratinized epidermal cells that shield the distal ends of the fingers and toes (see Figure 12.2 ■). Nail growth occurs at the nail matrix because new cells arise from the basal layer of the epidermis. As the nail cells grow out from the matrix, they form a transparent layer, called the body of the nail, which extends over the nail bed. The nail body appears pink because of the blood supply in the underlying dermis. A moon-shaped crescent called a **lunula** appears on the nail body over the thickened nail matrix. A fold of epidermal skin called a **cuticle** protects the root and sides of each nail. The major functions of the nails are to protect the tips of the fingers and toes and aid in picking up small objects, grasping, and scratching.

Special Considerations

Throughout the assessment process, the nurse gathers subjective and objective data reflecting the patient's state of health. Using critical thinking and the nursing process, the nurse identifies many factors to be considered when collecting the data. Some of these factors include but are not limited to age, developmental level, race, ethnicity, work history, living conditions, social situation, and emotional well-being.

Lifespan Considerations

A patient's age and developmental stage have a tremendous influence on the appearance and functioning of all parts of the integumentary system. Growth and development are dynamic processes that describe change over time. Data collection and interpretation of these findings in relation to expected values are important. Details about differences in the assessment of the skin, hair, and nails of the pregnant female are located in Chapter 25; in infants, children, and adolescents in Chapter 26; and in older adults in Chapter 27.

Psychosocial Considerations

The appearance of the skin, hair, and nails impacts the self-concept of the individual. Skin disorders may interfere with social relationships, roles, and sexuality. Although stress may exacerbate certain skin conditions, such as rashes or acne, a visible skin disorder may trigger psychosocial health problems leading to social isolation, a body image disturbance, or a self-esteem disturbance. Stress may also be a factor in compulsive behaviors such as hair twisting or plucking (**trichotillomania**) and nail biting, signaled by nails that have no visible free edge or that have short, jagged edges. A lack of cleanliness of the skin, hair, or nails also may result from emotional distress, poor self-esteem, or a disturbed body image.

Social and Environmental Considerations

A patient's living situation, including socioeconomic status, home environment, and type of employment or daily activities, may affect the health of the skin, hair, and nails. In addition, the daily habits of bathing, moisturizing, and other skin, hair, and nail care will be learned through the assessment and physical examination of this system. The nurse must take care to consider all of these factors during the assessment.

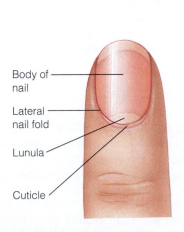
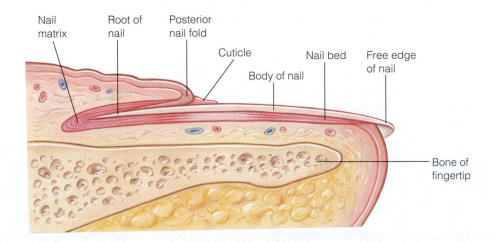

Figure 12.2 Structure of a nail.

The type of soap and other products used as part of the cleansing routine may contribute to the overall health and condition of the skin, hair, and nails. Skin and hair may become dry, oily, or itchy depending on the choices of product and habits. Hairstyling methods, use of hair products, chemical curling, or bleaching may be factors in damage, breakage, or loss of hair.

Depending on skin color, texture, and age, the assessment may reveal skin that is dry or oily. Understanding that skin care and use of products may influence this, the nurse must not make conclusions without taking all these factors into consideration.

Environmental influences on the skin, hair, and nails include sunlight, temperature, and work with the hands. The skin's response to stressors such as ultraviolet radiation is similar in all races. Dark-skinned and light-skinned patients alike will experience the damaging effects from overexposure to the sun. Therefore, assessment of color, texture, moles, and other lesions should be thorough for all patients. Individuals who work with their hands may experience a circumscribed, painless thickening of the epidermis, called a callus. These tend to form on parts of the body that are regularly exposed to pressure, weight bearing, or friction. Common sites of calluses include the fingers, palms, toes, and soles of the feet.

Cleanliness may be influenced by what the patient does for work or play and may make it difficult to keep the fingers and nails unstained. Chemicals used in certain occupations and smoking tobacco may stain the nails. The patient's occupation may require frequent or prolonged immersion of the hands in water, which may lead to paronychia.

Subjective Data—Health History

Assessment of the integumentary system includes gathering subjective and objective data about the skin, hair, and nails. Subjective data collection occurs during the interview, before the actual physical assessment. The nurse will use a variety of communication techniques to elicit general and specific information about the condition of the patient's skin, hair, and nails. The questions in the focused interview form part of the subjective database. Health records and the results of laboratory tests are important secondary sources to be reviewed and included in the data-gathering process See Table 12.1 for more on potential secondary sources of patient data.

Table 12.1 Potential Secondary Sources for Patient Data Related to the Skin, Hair, and Nails

LABORATORY TESTS—SKIN	
Eosinophils	Normal Value 1–4%
IgE	Normal Value < 0.35 kU/L
DIAGNOSTIC TESTS—SKIN	
Gram stain and culture	
Immunostaining	
Patch tests	
Skin biopsy	
Skin scraping	
Tzanck test	
DIAGNOSTIC TESTS—HAIR	
Trichogram–alopecia	
DIAGNOSTIC TESTS—NAILS	
Biopsy	

Focused Interview

The focused interview for the integumentary system concerns data related to the structures and functions of that system. Subjective data related to the condition of the skin, hair, and nails are gathered during the focused interview. The nurse must be prepared to observe the patient and listen for cues related to the integumentary system. The nurse may use open-ended and closed questions to obtain information. A number of follow-up questions or requests for descriptions may be required to clarify data or gather missing information. Follow-up questions are used to identify the source of problems, determine the duration of difficulties, identify measures to alleviate problems, and provide clues about the patient's knowledge of his or her own health. One approach to focused questioning about symptoms would be the OLDCART and ICE method., described in detail in Chapter 5. ∞

The focused interview guides the physical assessment of the integumentary system. The information is always considered in relation to norms and expectations about the function of the integument. Therefore, the nurse must consider age, gender, race, culture, environment, health practices, and past and current problems and therapies when forming questions and using techniques to elicit information. In order to address all of the factors when conducting a focused interview, categories of questions related to the status and function of each part of the integumentary system have been developed. These categories include general questions that are asked of all patients; those addressing illness and infection; questions related to symptoms, pain, and behaviors; those related to habits or practices; and questions that address social or environmental concerns. Questions that are specific to patients according to age and pregnancy are found in Chapter 25, Chapter 26, and Chapter 27. ∞

To conduct the interview about the integumentary system, the nurse must consider the patient's ability and willingness to participate in the focused interview. Further, the nurse must consider that because the appearance of the skin has an impact on self-image, patients with changes in the skin from disease or even the normal aging process may be anxious about the way they appear to others. Patients with visible skin disorders are often sensitive about the condition and their appearance. The nurse must select communication techniques that demonstrate caring and preserve the dignity of the patient.

Focused Interview Questions	Rationales and Evidence

The following sections provide sample questions and bulleted follow-up questions in each of the categories for the integumentary system components. A rationale for each of the questions is provided. The list of questions is not all-inclusive but represents the types of questions required in a comprehensive focused interview related to the integumentary system.

Skin
General Questions

1. **Describe your skin today.**
   - How does it compare to 2 months ago? How does it compare to 2 years ago?

   ▶ This question gives patients the opportunity to provide their own perceptions about the skin.

2. **Do you ever have trouble controlling body odor? If so, at what times?**

   ▶ Body odor becomes stronger during heavy activity because of increased excretion of uric acid. Body odor may also be related to diet. A change in body odor may indicate the presence of a systemic disorder or developmental changes (Mayo Clinic, 2014a).

3. **How much and how easily do you sweat?**

   ▶ **Diaphoresis** (profuse sweating) is a significant avenue for sodium chloride loss and may indicate the presence of a systemic disorder, including infectious disease with a fever. Increased sweating is a side effect of some medications (Shields, Fox, & Liebrecht, 2018). Decreased sweating increases the risk of heat stroke and may be a side effect of medications.

4. **Have you had episodes of increased sweating that occur at certain times, especially at night?**

   ▶ Such episodes can suggest the presence of an infectious process (Mayo Clinic, 2014a).

5. **Have you noticed any changes in the color of your skin?**
   - If so, did the change occur over your entire body or only in one area?

   ▶ Color changes to the skin may result from internal diseases. For example, yellowing of the skin may indicate liver disease (Polley et al., 2015), darkening of the skin may indicate adrenal disease, and a blue tint to the skin (cyanosis) may indicate heart or respiratory diseases.

6. **Has your skin become either oilier or drier recently?**
   - Have you noticed other changes in the way your skin feels?

   ▶ Metabolic disorders or simple age-related changes in the production of sebum may produce changes in the texture of the skin (Cleveland Clinic, 2015).

7. **Is there a history of allergies, rashes, or other skin problems in your family?**

   ▶ Some allergies and skin disorders are inherited or familial (Nutten, 2015). Follow-up is required to obtain details about specific problems, their occurrence, treatments, and outcomes.

Questions Related to Illness or Infection

1. **Have you ever had a skin problem?**
   - When were you diagnosed with the problem?
   - What treatment was prescribed for the problem?
   - Was the treatment helpful?
   - What kinds of things did you do to help with the problem?
   - Has the problem ever recurred (acute)?
   - How are you managing the disease now (chronic)?

   ▶ The patient has an opportunity to provide information about specific skin problems or illnesses. If a diagnosed illness is identified, follow-up about the date of diagnosis, treatment, and outcomes is required. Data about each illness identified by the patient are essential to an accurate health assessment. Illnesses can be classified as acute or chronic, and follow-up regarding each classification will differ.

2. *Alternative to question 1:* **List possible skin problems or illnesses, such as lupus, psoriasis, lesions, burns, and trauma, and ask the patient to respond "yes" or "no" as each is stated.**

   ▶ This is a comprehensive and easy way to elicit information about all skin disorders. Follow-up would be carried out for each identified diagnosis, as in question 1.

3. **Have you had any illnesses recently? If so, please describe them.**

   ▶ Some skin disorders are manifestations of systemic illness (American Academy of Dermatology [AAD], 2013).

4. **Do you have or have you had a skin infection?**
   - When were you diagnosed with the infection?
   - What treatment was prescribed for the problem?
   - Was the treatment helpful? What kinds of things have you done in the past or are you doing now to help with the problem?
   - Has the problem ever recurred (acute)?
   - How are you managing the infection now (chronic)?

   ▶ If an infection is identified, follow-up about the date of infection, treatment, and outcomes is required. Data about each infection identified by the patient are essential to an accurate health assessment. Infections can be classified as acute or chronic, and follow-up regarding each classification will differ.

5. *Alternative to question 4:* **List possible skin infections, such as warts, herpes simplex, herpes zoster, candida, and acne, and ask the patient to respond "yes" or "no" as each is stated.**

   ▶ This is a comprehensive and easy way to elicit information about all skin infections. Follow-up would be carried out for each identified infection.

Questions Related to Symptoms, Pain, and Behaviors

When gathering information about symptoms, many questions are required to elicit details and descriptions that assist in the analysis of the data. Discrimination is made in relation to the significance of a symptom, in relation to specific diseases or problems, and in relation to potential follow-up examination or referral. One rationale may be provided for a group of questions in this category.

Focused Interview Questions	Rationales and Evidence

The following questions refer to specific symptoms and behaviors associated with the skin. For each symptom, questions and follow-up are required. The details to be elicited are the characteristics of the symptom; the onset, duration, and frequency of the symptom; the treatment or remedy for the symptom, including over-the-counter and home remedies; the determination if diagnosis has been sought; the effect of treatments; and family history associated with a symptom or illness.

Questions Related to Symptoms

1. **Do you have any sores or ulcers on your body that are slow in healing?**
   - Where are these?
   - Do you have frequent boils or skin infections?

   ▶ Delayed healing or frequent skin infections may be a sign of diabetes mellitus or inadequate nutrition (American Diabetes Association [ADA], 2015).

2. **Does your skin itch? If so, where?**
   - How severe is it?
   - When does it occur?

   ▶ These questions may help in determining if the itching is because of an allergic reaction or eczema.

3. **Have you noticed any rashes on your body? If so, please describe.**
   - Where on your body did the rash start? Where did it spread?
   - When did you first notice it?
   - Did the rash happen at the same time as any other symptoms, such as fever or chills?
   - Have you made a recent change in any skin care products or laundry detergents that might have contributed to the rash?

   ▶ These factors may help in determining the cause of the rash.

4. **If you have a rash, do you notice it more after wearing certain clothes or jewelry?**
   - After using certain skin products?
   - Did it occur soon after starting a new medication?
   - Does the rash happen during or after any other activities, such as gardening or washing dishes?

   ▶ Rashes related to clothing, jewelry, or cosmetics may be because of contact dermatitis, a type of allergy. Many medications cause allergic skin reactions. A drug reaction can occur even after the patient has taken the drug a long time. Aspirin, antibiotics, and barbiturates are a few of the drugs that fall into this category (Shields et al., 2018).

5. **Have you noticed a change in the size, color, shape, or appearance of any moles or birthmarks?**
   - When did you first notice this?
   - Describe the change.
   - Are they painful? Do they itch? Bleed?

   ▶ Any changes in a mole or birthmark may signal a skin cancer (American Cancer Society, 2013).

6. **Have you noticed any other lesions, lumps, bumps, tender spots, or painful areas on your body?**
   - If so, when did you first notice them? Where?
   - Have they spread? If so, please describe how they spread and where they are now located.

   ▶ The time of onset and pattern of development may help determine the source of the problem. For instance, certain patterns of bruises may signal frequent falls or physical abuse (Clarysse, Kivlahan, Beyer, & Gutermuth, 2017).

7. **Have you noticed any drainage from any skin region?**
   - If so, where does the drainage come from? What does it look like? Does it have an odor?
   - Is the drainage accompanied by any other symptoms? If so, please describe.

   ▶ Diagnostic cues such as pain, chills, or fever may aid in identifying the source of the problem.

8. **Please describe anything you have done to treat your skin condition.**
   - When did you begin this treatment? How has your skin responded to the treatment?

Questions Related to Pain

1. **Please describe any skin pain or discomfort.**

2. **Have you experienced any pain or discomfort in any skin folds—for example, between the toes, under the breasts, between the buttocks, or in the perianal area?**

   ▶ Note that the warm, dark, moist environment in skin folds may breed bacterial and fungal infections (Berman, Snyder, & Frandsen, 2016).

3. **Where is the pain?**

   ▶ Questions 3 through 8 are standard questions associated with pain to determine the location, frequency, duration, and intensity of the pain.

4. **How often do you experience the pain?**

5. **How long does the pain last?**

6. **How long have you had the pain?**

7. **How would you rate the pain on a scale of 0 to 10?**

8. **Is there a trigger for the pain?**

9. **What do you do to relieve the pain?**

   ▶ Questions 9 and 10 are intended to determine if the patient has selected a treatment based on past experience, knowledge of skin disorders, or use of complementary and alternative care and its effectiveness.

10. **Is this treatment effective?**

(continued)

Focused Interview Questions	Rationales and Evidence

Questions Related to Age and Pregnancy

The focused interview must reflect the anatomic and physiologic differences in the skin that exist along the age span as well as during pregnancy. Specific questions related to the integumentary system for each of these groups are provided in Chapter 25, Chapter 26, and Chapter 27. ∞

Questions for the Menstruating Female

1. Are you pregnant? If not, are you menstruating regularly? Describe your menstrual cycle.

▶ The skin may be affected by changes in hormonal balance.

Questions Related to Behaviors

1. Do you spend time in the sun exercising or playing sports?

2. Do you sunbathe, either outdoors or in a tanning bed?

3. Have you ever sunbathed?

4. Do you spend time in the sun exercising or playing sports?

5. Do you work outdoors?

▶ Excessive exposure to the ultraviolet radiation of the sun thickens and damages the skin, depresses the immune system, and alters the deoxyribonucleic acid (DNA) in skin cells, predisposing an individual to cancer (Berman et al., 2016).

6. How does your skin react to sun exposure?
   - Do you use a daily lotion with sun protection factor (SPF)?
   - What SPF lotion do you use? Do you reapply the lotion after several hours outside or after swimming?

▶ The ultraviolet radiation that accompanies sunburn is capable of disabling cells that initiate the normal immune response (World Health Organization, 2014). Individuals who burn easily or have a history of serious sunburns may have a greater risk for developing skin cancer (Mayo Clinic, 2014b). These questions determine if the patient follows recommendations by the American Cancer Society regarding skin exposure.

7. Do you remember having a sunburn that left blisters?

▶ A history of blistering sunburn increases the risk for skin cancer, especially if it occurred in childhood (Mayo Clinic, 2014b).

8. How do you care for your skin?
   - What kind of soap, cleansers, toners, or other treatments do you use?
   - How do you clean your clothes?
   - What kind of detergent do you use?
   - How often do you bathe or shower?

▶ Some skin products and laundry detergents may affect the skin of some patients. Infrequent cleansing of the skin increases the likelihood of skin infections, whereas excessive bathing decreases protective skin oils.

9. Do you now have or have you ever had a tattoo(s)?
   - How long have you had the tattoo(s)?
   - Have you had any problems with that area of the skin?
   - Further follow-up would include questions related to treatment and outcomes if skin problems accompanied tattoos.

▶ Tattoos can cause skin irritation and in some cases infection (Centers for Disease Control and Prevention [CDC], 2012).

10. Do you now have or have you ever had piercing of any part of your body?
    - Where are the sites of piercing?
    - How long have you had the piercing?
    - Have any piercing sites closed?
    - Have you ever had a problem at the piercing site?
    - What was the problem?
    - Did you seek treatment for the problem?
    - What was the outcome of the treatment?
    - What is the current condition of piercing site(s)?

▶ Piercing of any body part puts an individual at risk for infection and hepatitis C and can result in the development of scar tissue at the site (Van Hoover, Rademayer, & Farley, 2017)

Questions Related to the Environment

Environment refers to both the internal and external environments. Questions related to the internal environment include all of the previous questions and those associated with internal or physiologic responses. Questions regarding the external environment include those related to home, work, or social environments.

Internal Environment

1. How would you describe your level of stress? Has it changed in the past few weeks? Few months? Describe.

▶ Emotional stress may aggravate skin disorders (Alexopoulos & Chrousos, 2016).

2. Are you now experiencing, or have you ever experienced, intermittent or prolonged anxiety or emotional upset?
   - Describe the situation.
   - Can you determine precipitating factors?
   - Have you sought care or treatment for the problem?
   - What do you do when the problem arises?

Focused Interview Questions	Rationales and Evidence
3. Are you taking any prescription or over-the-counter medications?	▶ Patients may experience rashes or other skin eruptions in response to various drugs. Some drugs, such as antibiotics, antihistamines, antipsychotics, oral hypoglycemic agents, and oral contraceptives, can cause an adverse effect if the patient is exposed to the sun (Shields et al., 2018).
4. Have you changed your diet recently? Have you recently tried any unfamiliar types of food? Please describe.	▶ Changes in diet or eating new foods may cause rashes and other skin reactions.
5. Has the condition of your skin affected your social relationships in any way? Has it limited you in any way? If so, how?	▶ Skin problems may affect a person's self-concept and body image, interfering with social relationships, roles, and sexuality. This is especially true for adolescents and young adults (Dalgard et al., 2015). Serious skin problems may also affect a person's ability to function and maintain a job.

External Environment

The following questions deal with substances and irritants found in the physical environment of the patient. The physical environment includes the indoor and outdoor environments of the home and the workplace, those encountered for social engagements, and any encountered during travel.

1. Have you been exposed recently to extremes in temperature? • If so, when? How long was the exposure? Where did this occur? • Describe the temperature of your home environment and of your work environment.	▶ Extremes in environmental temperature may exacerbate skin disorders.
2. Do you work in an environment where radioisotopes or x-rays are used? • If so, are you vigilant about following precautions and using protective gear?	▶ Excessive exposure to x-rays or radioisotopes may predispose a patient to skin cancer (Mayo Clinic, 2014b).
3. Do you wear gloves for work? If so, what types of gloves? Do you have any signs of allergy related to wearing these gloves?	▶ Certain types of gloves, especially latex, can cause mild to severe allergic skin reactions.
4. How often do you travel? • Have you traveled recently? • If so, where? • Have you come into contact with anyone who has a similar rash or skin problem?	▶ The nurse should suspect unfamiliar foods, water, plants, or insects as potential causes of rashes and other skin problems if the patient has traveled recently. In addition, some rashes, such as measles and impetigo, are contagious (Eldridge & Cohen, 2014).
5. Does your job or hobby require you to perform repetitive tasks? • Does your job or hobby require you to work with any chemicals? • Does your job or hobby require you to wear a specific type of helmet, hat, goggles, gloves, or shoes?	▶ Regular work with certain tools or regular wear of ill-fitting helmets, hats, goggles, or shoes may cause skin abrasions. In addition, the skin absorbs certain organic solvents used in industry, such as acetone, dry-cleaning fluid, dyes, formaldehyde, and paint thinner. Excessive exposure to these and other types of irritants may contribute to rashes, skin cancers, or other skin reactions (CDC, 2013).

Hair

General Questions

1. Describe your hair now. • How does it compare to 2 months ago? How does it compare to 2 years ago? • Have you ever had problems with your hair? If so, please describe the problem, including any treatment and resolution.	
2. How often do you wash your hair? • What kinds of shampoos do you use? • Do you have excessive dandruff? • If so, do you do anything to control it?	▶ Shampooing too frequently or using too many styling products can irritate or dry out the scalp, increasing the presence of dry flakes of skin called **dandruff**; not shampooing frequently enough can also cause dandruff because of a buildup of dead skin cells and oil. Other skin conditions, such as seborrheic dermatitis, eczema, psoriasis, and *Malassezia* infection, can also contribute to dandruff (Mayo Clinic, 2016a).
3. Have you noticed a recent increase in hair loss? • If so, describe how the hair fell out. • Was it a gradual or sudden onset? • It is symmetric? Are there bald or patchy areas without hair? • Have you been ill in the last few months?	▶ The scalp typically sheds about 50 to 90 hairs each day, and thus some hair loss is normal. Progressive diffuse hair loss is natural in some men (Mayo Clinic, 2016b). Hair loss in women that follows a male pattern may be because of an imbalance of adrenal hormones, such as that which occurs in polycystic ovarian syndrome (Setji & Brown, 2014). When patches of hair fall out, the nurse should suspect trauma to the scalp because of chemicals, infections, or blows to the head. Some chemotherapeutic agents cause hair loss. Also, some people with nervous disorders pull or twist their hair, causing it to fall out (trichotillomania). If hair loss is distributed over the entire head, it may be caused by a systemic disease or fungal infection. Abnormal hair loss sometimes follows a feverish illness. Hair loss may also be the result of an autoimmune disorder called **alopecia areata** (Mayo Clinic, 2016b). Thinning or shedding of the hair on the scalp (telogen effluvium) may occur in pregnancy (Gizlenti & Ekmekci, 2013). Hair shedding may last for several months and continue for up to 15 months after childbirth.

(continued)

Focused Interview Questions	Rationales and Evidence
4. Have you noticed a recent increase in hair growth? • What it a gradual or sudden onset? • Is it symmetric? Are there bald or patchy areas without hair?	▶ **Hirsutism** is shaggy or excessive hair. It is often associated with polycystic ovarian syndrome, Cushing's syndrome, congenital adrenal hyperplasia, androgen-secreting tumors, and some medications (Khomami, Tehrani, Hashemi, Farahmand, & Azizi, 2015).
5. Are you taking any prescription or over-the-counter medications?	▶ Certain medications can change the texture of the hair or lead to hair loss. For instance, oral contraceptives may change the hair texture or rate of hair growth in some women, and drugs used in the treatment of circulatory disorders and cancer may result in a temporary generalized hair loss over the entire body (Patel, Harrison, & Sinclair, 2013).
6. How do you style your hair?	▶ Use of styling products can dry or damage hair, as can use of hair dryers, curling irons, and heated rollers. Some methods of setting hair, as well as sleeping in hair rollers, may cause breakage and lead to patchy hair loss. Repeated tight braiding may damage hair and lead to patchy hair loss.
7. Do you bleach, color, perm, or chemically straighten your hair? • If so, how often? When was the last time?	▶ These chemical processes may damage the scalp and hair and may cause hair loss.
8. Do you remove your eyebrows or facial hair? What method do you use? • Do you shave the hair on your face, on your legs, or under your arms? • Do you use chemical hair removers, wax, or electrolysis?	▶ Each of these hair removal methods can cause trauma to the skin. Use of unclean equipment can contaminate the skin. Plucking leaves an open portal for bacteria and may lead to infection if aseptic technique is not used (Elmann et al., 2012).
9. Do you swim regularly? How often? For how long? Where?	▶ Swimming regularly in salt water or chlorinated pools can dry the scalp and hair and may cause increased dandruff.

Nails

General Questions

1. Describe your nails now. • How do they compare to 2 months ago? How do they compare to 2 years ago? • Have you ever had problems with your nails? • If so, please describe the problem, including any treatment and resolution.	▶ Ridged, brittle, split, or peeling fingernails may be caused by protein or vitamin B deficiencies. Changes in circulation may affect the nails. Newly acquired dark longitudinal lines may signal a nevus or melanoma in the nail root. Dark lines may be normal, especially in dark-skinned patients, or associated with some medications, including antiretrovirals (Shields et al., 2018).
2. Have you noticed any pain, swelling, or drainage around your cuticles? • If so, when did you first notice this? • What do you think might have caused it?	▶ Infection of the cuticles is often because of chronic trauma in a wet environment, such as occurs with nail biters or dishwashers (Tully, Trayes, & Studdiford, 2012).
3. Have you been ill recently?	▶ Cancer, heart disease, liver disease, anemia, and other illnesses can cause various changes in the nails, such as grooves, ridges, or discoloration.
4. Have you been taking any prescription or over-the-counter medications?	▶ Some medications may cause nail changes in some patients. For example, patients who have been treated with the antiviral drug zidovudine (Retrovir, AZT) can develop dark, longitudinal lines on all of their fingernails (Shields et al., 2018).
5. Do you wear nail enamel? Do you wear artificial fingernails, tips, or wraps?	▶ Prolonged use of nail polish may dry or discolor the nails. In addition, some patients may have an allergic reaction to nail polish. Use of artificial nails may encourage growth of fungi or damage the nail plate.
6. Do you spend a great deal of time at work or at home with your hands in water?	▶ Bacterial and fungal infections of the cuticles may occur in people who submerge their hands in water for long periods (Tully et al., 2012).

Patient-Centered Interaction

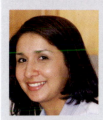

Ms. Tanish Thalia, age 32, reports to the Medi-Center with a chief complaint of pain, swelling, and redness at the nails of two fingers on her left hand. The following is an excerpt of the focused interview.

Source: SW Productions / Getty Images.

Interview

Nurse: Good morning. Ms. Thalia. I see from your information sheet that you have a problem with the fingernails of your left hand.

Ms. Thalia: Yes, I think it's my nails, but I'm not sure.

Nurse: The problem involves two fingers of the left hand.

Ms. Thalia: Yes, the thumb and index finger are the only two. The other three seem to be okay.

Nurse: Looking at your nails, I see they are highly polished.

Ms. Thalia: Yes, I have them done professionally every seven to ten days. They were done five days ago.

Nurse: Are these your natural nails?

Ms. Thalia: Yes, I have silk wraps on all my nails to help make them stronger.

Nurse: Does the manicurist push and cut your cuticles?

Ms. Thalia: Yes, she does both. Do you think this is from having the manicure?

Nurse: It could be. I'm not sure. I need more information. When did you first notice the pain and swelling?

Ms. Thalia: It started several days after I had my nails done, and now it seems to be getting worse. What is causing this?

Nurse: Is this the first time the manicurist did your nails?

Ms. Thalia: Oh no. Sally has been doing my nails for three years. This is the first time I have had anything like this.

Nurse: How much time are your hands and nails in water?

Ms. Thalia: Not much. I use gloves when I do the dishes.

Analysis

The nurse uses closed questions to obtain the necessary information from Ms. Thalia. The nurse seeks clarification regarding the fingers involved and also confirms the condition of the nails, the frequency of care, and the type of care regarding cutting of the cuticles. When asked, Ms. Thalia is able to provide specific information regarding date of last manicure, symptoms involved, and the relationship between these two factors. The nurse does not make a judgment and indicates that more information is needed.

Objective Data—Physical Assessment

Assessment Techniques and Findings

Physical assessment of the skin, hair, and nails requires the use of inspection and palpation. Inspection includes looking at the skin, hair, and nails to determine color, consistency, shape, and hygiene-related factors. Knowledge of norms or expected findings is essential in determining the meaning of the data as the nurse performs the physical assessment.

EQUIPMENT

- Examination gown and drape
- Examination light
- Examination gloves, clean and nonsterile
- Centimeter ruler
- Magnifying glass
- Penlight

HELPFUL HINTS

- Provide a warm, private environment that will reduce patient anxiety.
- Provide special instructions and explain the purpose for removal of clothing, jewelry, hairpieces, and nail enamel.
- Maintain the patient's dignity by using draping techniques.
- Monitor one's verbal responses to skin conditions that already threaten the patient's self-image.
- Be sensitive to a patient's individual needs. Ask permission before touching or examining.
- Because covering the head, hair, face, or skin may be part of religious or cultural beliefs, provide careful explanations regarding the need to expose these areas for assessment.
- Direct sunlight is best for assessment of the skin, so if it is not available, the lighting still must be strong and direct. Tangential lighting may be helpful in assessment of dark-skinned patients.
- Use standard precautions throughout the assessment.

Healthy skin should be clean, free from odor, and consistent in color. It should feel warm and moist and have a smooth texture. The skin should be mobile, with blood vessels visible beneath the surfaces of the abdomen and eyelids. It should be free of lesions other than findings of freckles, birthmarks, and normal age variations. The skin should be sensitive to touch and temperature.

The scalp and hair in the adult should be clean. Hair color is determined by the amount of melanin. Gray hair can occur as a result of decreased melanin, genetics, or aging. Hair texture may be coarse or thin. Hair is expected to be evenly distributed over the scalp. Male pattern baldness is a normal finding. Fine hair is distributed over the body with coarser, darker, longer hair in the axillae and pubic regions in adults. The nails should have a pink undertone and lie flat or form a convex curve on the nail bed.

Physical assessment of the skin, hair, and nails follows an organized pattern. It begins with a survey and inspection, followed by palpation, of the skin. Inspection and palpation of the hair and nails are then carried out. When lesions are present, measurements are used to identify the size of the lesions and the location in relation to accepted landmarks.

The first step in the physical assessment is to visually inspect the skin. Assessment of the skin color gives the nurse information about the overall health of the patient. Variations in skin color from light to dark must be taken into account when describing the findings. See Table 12.2 for how to assess for changes in skin appearance based on skin tone. Changes in skin color may be difficult to evaluate in patients with dark skin. It is helpful to inspect areas of the body with less pigmentation, such as the lips, oral mucosa, sclerae, palms of the hands, and conjunctivae of the inner eyelids. The nurse must be careful not to mistake the normal deposition of melanin in the lips of some olive to dark-skinned people for cyanosis. Some individuals with dark skin have increased pigmentation in the creases of the palms and soles, as well as yellow or brown-tinged sclerae. These are normal findings (see Table 12.2 for evaluating color variations in light and dark skin).

Table 12.2 Color Variations in Light and Dark Skin

COLOR VARIATION/LOCALIZATION	POSSIBLE CAUSES	APPEARANCE IN LIGHT SKIN	APPEARANCE IN DARK SKIN
Pallor *Loss of color in skin because of the absence of oxygenated hemoglobin.* Widespread, but most apparent in face, mouth, conjunctivae, and nails.	May be caused by sympathetic nervous stimulation resulting in peripheral vasoconstriction because of smoking, a cold environment, or stress. May also be caused by decreased tissue perfusion because of cardiopulmonary disease, shock and hypotension, lack of oxygen, or prolonged elevation of a body part. May also be caused by anemia.	White skin loses its rosy tones. Skin with natural yellow tones appears more yellow; may be mistaken for mild jaundice.	Black skin loses its red undertones and appears ash-gray. Brown skin becomes yellow tinged. Skin looks dull.
Absence of Color *Congenital or acquired loss of melanin pigment.* Congenital loss is typically generalized, and acquired loss is typically patchy.	Generalized depigmentation may be caused by albinism. Localized depigmentation may be because of **vitiligo** or *tinea versicolor*, a common fungal infection.	Albinism appears as white skin, white or pale blond hair, and pink irises. Vitiligo is very noticeable as patchy milk-white areas. *Tinea versicolor* appears as patchy areas paler than the surrounding skin.	Albinism appears as white skin, white or pale blond hair, and pink irises. Vitiligo appears as patchy milk-white areas, especially around the mouth. *Tinea versicolor* appears as patchy areas paler than the surrounding skin.
Cyanosis *Mottled blue color in skin and its appendages because of inadequate tissue perfusion with oxygenated blood.* Most apparent in the nails, lips, oral mucosa, and tongue.	Systemic or central cyanosis is because of cardiac disease, pulmonary disease, heart malformations, and low hemoglobin levels. Localized or peripheral cyanosis is because of vasoconstriction, exposure to cold, and emotional stress.	The skin, lips, and mucous membranes look blue tinged. The conjunctivae and nail beds are blue.	The skin may appear a shade darker. Cyanosis may be undetectable except for the lips, tongue, oral mucous membranes, nail beds, and conjunctivae, which appear pale or blue tinged.
Reddish Blue Tone *Ruddy tone because of an increase in hemoglobin and stasis of blood in capillaries.* Most apparent in the face, mouth, hands, feet, and conjunctivae.	Polycythemia vera, an overproduction of red blood cells, granulocytes, and platelets.	Reddish purple hue.	Difficult to detect. The normal skin color may appear darker in some patients. Check lips for redness.
Erythema *Redness of the skin because of increased visibility of normal oxyhemoglobin.* Generalized, or on face and upper chest, or localized to area of inflammation or exposure.	Hyperemia, congestion of blood and accompanying dilatation in superficial arteries. Because of fever, warm environment, local inflammation, allergy, emotions (blushing or embarrassment), exposure to extreme cold, consumption of alcohol, or dependent position of body extremity.	Readily identifiable over entire body or in localized areas. Local inflammation and redness are accompanied by higher temperature at the site.	Generalized redness may be difficult to detect. Localized areas of inflammation appear purple or darker than surrounding skin. May be accompanied by higher temperature, hardness, swelling.
Jaundice *Yellow undertone because of increased bilirubin in the blood.* Generalized, but most apparent in the conjunctivae and mucous membranes.	Increased bilirubin may be because of liver disease, biliary obstruction, or hemolytic disease following infection or severe burns, or resulting from sickle cell anemia or pernicious anemia.	Generalized. Also visible in sclerae, oral mucosa, hard palate, fingernails, palms of hands, and soles of the feet.	Visible in the sclerae, oral mucosa, junction of hard and soft palate, palms of the hands, and soles of the feet.

COLOR VARIATION/LOCALIZATION	POSSIBLE CAUSES	APPEARANCE IN LIGHT SKIN	APPEARANCE IN DARK SKIN
Carotenemia *Yellow-orange tinge caused by increased levels of carotene in the blood and skin.* Most apparent in the face, palms of the hands, and soles of the feet.	Excess carotene because of ingestion of foods high in carotene, such as carrots, egg yolks, sweet potatoes, milk, and fats. Also may be seen in patients with anorexia nervosa or endocrine disorders, such as diabetes mellitus, myxedema, and hypopituitarism.	Yellow-orange tinge most visible in palms of the hands and soles of the feet. No yellowing of sclerae or mucous membranes.	Yellow-orange tinge seen in forehead, palms, soles. No yellowing of sclerae or mucous membranes.
Uremia *Pale yellow tone because of retention of urinary chromogens in the blood.* Generalized, if perceptible.	Chronic renal disease, in which blood levels of nitrogenous wastes increase. Increased melanin may also contribute, and anemia is usually present as well.	Generalized pallor and yellow tinge, but does not affect the conjunctivae or mucous membranes. Skin may show bruising.	Very difficult to discern because the yellow tinge is very pale and does not affect the conjunctivae or mucous membranes. Rely on laboratory and other data.
Brown *An increase in the production and deposition of melanin.* Generalized or localized.	May be because of Addison disease or a pituitary tumor. Localized increase in facial pigmentation may be caused by hormonal changes during pregnancy or the use of birth control pills. More commonly because of exposure to ultraviolet radiation from the sun or from tanning booths.	With endocrine disorders, general bronzed skin. Hyperpigmentation in nipples, palmar creases, genitals, and pressure points. Sun exposure causes red tinge in pale skin, and olive-toned skin tans with little or no reddening.	With endocrine disorders, general deepening of skin tone. Hyperpigmentation in nipples, genitals, and pressure points. Sun exposure leads to tanning in various degrees from brown to black.

Techniques and Normal Findings

Abnormal Findings and Special Considerations

Survey

A quick survey enables the nurse to identify any immediate problem and the patient's ability to participate in the assessment. The nurse inspects the overall appearance of the patient, notes hygiene and odor, and observes for signs of anxiety.

▶ Patients experiencing pain or discomfort may not be able to participate in the assessment. Severe pain or distress warrants evaluation by a primary care provider.

▶ Patients experiencing anxiety may demonstrate pallor and diaphoresis. Acknowledgment of the problem and discussion of the procedures often provide relief.

ALERT! *The nurse must be alert for the possibility of impending shock if the patient has pallor accompanied with a drop in blood pressure, increased pulse and respirations, and marked anxiety. If these cues are present, a physician should be consulted immediately.*

Inspection of the Skin

1. **Position the patient.**
   - The patient should be in a sitting position with all clothing removed except the examination gown (see Figure 12.3 ■).

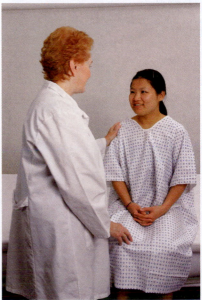

Figure 12.3 Positioning of patient.

(continued)

Techniques and Normal Findings	Abnormal Findings and Special Considerations

2. Instruct the patient.
- Explain that you will be looking carefully at the patient's skin.

3. Observe for cleanliness, perspiration, or sheen on the skin and use the sense of smell to determine body odor.
- Some perspiration is normal and results in a sheen on the skin in healthy individuals. Body odor is produced when bacterial waste products mix with perspiration on the skin surface. During heavy physical activity, body odor increases. Amounts of urea and ammonia are excreted in perspiration.

▶ Urea and ammonia salts may be found on the skin of patients with advanced kidney disease.

4. Observe the patient's skin tone.
- Evaluate any widespread color changes such as cyanosis, pallor, erythema, or jaundice. For example, always assess patients with cyanosis for vital signs and level of consciousness. Use Table 12.2 to evaluate color variations in light and dark skin.
- The amount of melanin and carotene pigments, the oxygen content of the blood, and the level of exposure to the sun influence skin color. Dark skin contains large amounts of melanin, whereas fair skin has small amounts. The skin of most Asians contains a large amount of carotene, which causes a yellow cast.

▶ Cyanosis or pallor indicates abnormally low plasma oxygen, placing the patient at risk for altered tissue perfusion. Pallor is seen in anemia.

5. Inspect the skin for even pigmentation over the body.
- In most cases, increased or decreased pigmentation is caused by differences in the distribution of melanin throughout the body. These are normal variations. For example, the margins of the lips, areolae, nipples, and external genitalia are more darkly pigmented. Freckles (see Figure 12.4 ■) and certain *nevi* (congenital marks [see Figure 12.5 ■]) occur in people of all skin colors in varying degrees.

▶ For unknown reasons, some people develop patchy and depigmented areas over the face, neck, hands, feet, and skin folds. This condition is called **vitiligo** (see Figure 12.6 ■). Skin is otherwise normal. Vitiligo occurs in all races in all parts of the world, but it seems to affect dark-skinned people more severely. Patients with vitiligo may suffer a severe disturbance in body image.

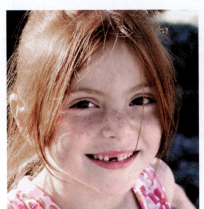

Figure 12.4 Freckles.
Source: Margot Petrowski/Shutterstock.

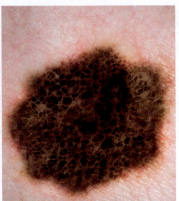

Figure 12.5 Nevus.
Source: Australis Photography/Shutterstock.

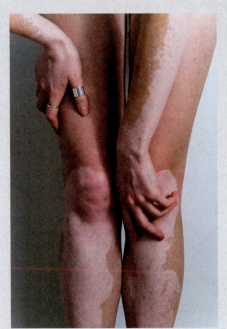

Figure 12.6 Vitiligo.
Source: Olena Gorbenko/Shutterstock.

6. Inspect the skin for superficial arteries and veins.
- A fine network of veins or a few dilated blood vessels visible just beneath the surface of the skin are normal findings in areas of the body where skin is thin (e.g., the abdomen and eyelids).

Techniques and Normal Findings	Abnormal Findings and Special Considerations

Palpation of the Skin

1. Instruct the patient.
- Explain that you will be touching the patient in various areas with different parts of your hand.

2. Determine the patient's skin temperature.
- Use the dorsal surface of your fingers, which is most sensitive to temperature. Palpate the forehead or face first. Continue to palpate inferiorly, including the hands and feet, comparing the temperature on the right and left side of the body (see Figure 12.7 ■).

▶ The temperature of the skin is higher than normal in the presence of a systemic infection or metabolic disorder such as hyperthyroidism, after vigorous activity, and when the external environment is warm.

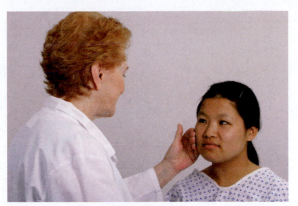

Figure 12.7 Palpating skin temperature.

- Local skin temperature is controlled by the amount and rate of blood circulating through a body region. Normal temperatures range from mildly cool to slightly warm.

▶ The temperature of the skin is lower than normal in the presence of metabolic disorders such as hypothyroidism or when the external environment is cool. Localized coolness results from decreased circulation because of vasoconstriction or occlusion, which may occur from peripheral arterial insufficiency.

- The skin on both sides of the body is warm when tissue is perfused. Sometimes the hands and feet are cooler than the rest of the body, but the temperature is normally similar on both sides.

▶ A difference in temperature *unilaterally* may indicate an interruption in or lack of circulation on the cool side because of compression, immobilization, or elevation. If one side is warmer than normal, inflammation may be present on that side.

3. Assess the amount of moisture on the skin surface.
- Inspect and palpate the face, skin folds, axillae, palms, and soles of the feet, where perspiration is most easily detected.

▶ Diaphoresis occurs during exertion, fever, pain, and emotional stress and in the presence of some metabolic disorders such as hyperthyroidism. It may also indicate an impending medical crisis such as a myocardial infarction.

- A fine sheen of perspiration or oil is not an abnormal finding, nor is moderately dry skin, especially in cold or dry climates.

▶ Severely dry skin typically is dark, weathered, and fissured. Pruritus frequently accompanies dry skin and, if prolonged, may lead to abrasion and thickening. Generalized dryness may occur in an individual who is dehydrated or has a systemic disorder such as hypothyroidism.

▶ Dry, parched lips and mucous membranes of the mouth are clear indicators of systemic dehydration. These areas should be checked if dehydration is suspected. Dry skin over the lower legs may be because of vascular insufficiency. Localized itching may indicate a skin allergy.

4. Palpate the skin for texture.
- Use the palmar surface of fingers and finger pads when palpating for texture. Normal skin feels smooth, firm, and even.

5. Palpate the skin to determine its thickness.
- The outer layer of the skin is thin and firm over most parts of the body except the palms, soles of the feet, elbows, and knees, where it is thicker. Normally, the skin over the eyelids and lips is thinner.

▶ The skin may become excessively smooth and velvety in patients with hyperthyroidism, whereas patients with hypothyroidism may have rough, scaly skin.

▶ Very thin, shiny skin may signal impaired circulation.

(continued)

Techniques and Normal Findings	Abnormal Findings and Special Considerations

6. Palpate the skin for elasticity.

- Elasticity is a combination of turgor (resiliency, or the skin's ability to return to its normal position and shape) and mobility (the skin's ability to be lifted).

  Using the forefinger and thumb, grasp a fold of skin beneath the clavicle (see Figure 12.8 ■).

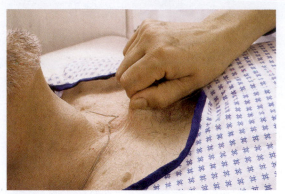

Figure 12.8 Palpating for skin elasticity.

- Notice the reaction of the skin both as you grasp and as you release. Healthy skin is mobile and returns rapidly to its previous shape and position.
- Finally, palpate the feet, ankles, and sacrum. Edema is present if your palpation leaves a dent in the skin.
- Grade edema on a four-point scale: +1 indicates mild edema, and +4 indicates deep edema (see Figure 12.9 ■).
- Note that because the fluid of edema lies above the pigmented and vascular layers of the skin, skin tone in the patient with edema is obscured.

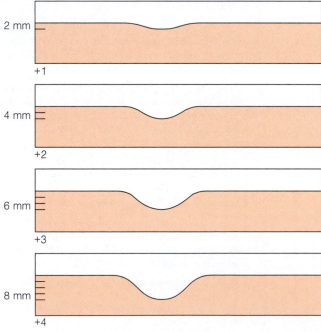

Figure 12.9 Four-point scale for grading edema.

▶ When skin turgor is decreased, the skinfold "tents" (holds its pinched formation) and slowly returns to the former position (see Figure 12.8). Decreased turgor occurs when the patient is dehydrated or has lost large amounts of weight.

Increased skin turgor may be caused by *scleroderma*, literally "hard skin," a condition in which the underlying connective tissue becomes scarred and immobile.

▶ **Edema** is a decrease in skin mobility caused by an accumulation of fluid in the intercellular spaces. Edema makes the skin look puffy, pitted, and tight. It may be most noticeable in the skin of the hands, feet, ankles, and sacral area (see Figure 12.10 ■).

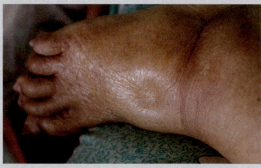

Figure 12.10 Pitting edema.
Source: Akkalak Aiempradit/Shutterstock.

Techniques and Normal Findings	**Abnormal Findings and Special Considerations**

7. Inspect and palpate the skin for lesions.

- Lesions of the skin are changes in normal skin structure. Primary lesions develop on previously unaltered skin. Lesions that change over time or because of scratching, abrasion, or infection are called **secondary lesions** (refer to Table 12.3 and Table 12.4 for more details).
- One specific type of secondary lesion is a **pressure ulcer,** which is a localized region of damaged or necrotic tissue that is caused by the exertion of pressure over a bony prominence. Previously called decubitus ulcers, bedsores, and pressure sores, the current terminology was adopted to avoid implying that only nonambulatory, bed-bound patients are at risk for developing pressure ulcers. Although reduced mobility is a significant risk factor for this condition, ambulatory patients also are at risk for developing pressure ulcers (Qaseem, Mir, Starkey, & Denberg, 2015). Therefore, all patients should have their skin inspected for pressure ulcers at every assessment.
- Pressure ulcers are staged based on their depth (see Box 12.1).

▶ The periumbilical and flank areas of the body should be observed for the presence of **ecchymosis** (bruising). Ecchymoses in the periumbilical area may signal bleeding somewhere in the abdomen (Cullen's sign). Ecchymoses in the flank area are associated with pancreatitis or bleeding in the peritoneum (Grey Turner's sign).

▶ Certain systemic disorders may produce characteristic patterns of lesions on particular body regions. Widespread lesions may indicate systemic or genetic disorders or allergic reactions. Localized lesions may indicate physical trauma, chemical irritants, or allergic dermatitis. The nurse may wish to photograph the patient's skin to document the presence, pattern, or spread of certain lesions.

ALERT! *Physical abuse should be suspected if the patient has any of the following: bruises or welts that appear in a pattern suggesting the use of a belt or stick; burns with sharply demarcated edges suggesting injury from cigarettes, irons, or immersion of a hand in boiling water; additional injuries such as fractures or dislocations; or multiple injuries in various stages of healing. A nurse must be especially sensitive if the patient is fearful of family members, is reluctant to return home, and has a history of previous injuries. When any of these diagnostic cues are evident, it is important to obtain medical assistance and follow the state's legal requirements to notify the police or local protective agency.*

Box 12.1   Pressure Ulcer Staging

Pressure ulcers are staged based on their depth.

- Stage I pressure ulcers demonstrate intact skin with no involvement of the underlying tissues or structures.
- Stage II pressure ulcers involve the epidermal skin layer and also may extend into the dermis.
- Stage III pressure ulcers extend into the subcutaneous tissue; however, whereas underlying muscle, fascia, and bone may be visible, the ulcer is not directly involved with these structures.
- Stage IV pressure ulcers involve muscle and bone (Qaseem et al., 2015).

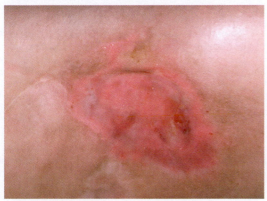

(A) Stage I Pressure Ulcer

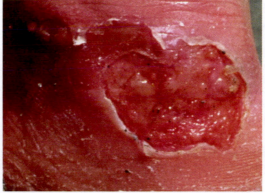

(B) Stage II Pressure Ulcer

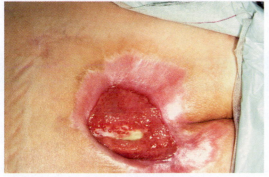

(C) Stage III Pressure Ulcer

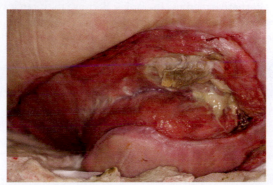

(D) Stage IV Pressure Ulcer

Figure 12.11 The four stages of pressure ulcers.
Source: (A) Mediscan/Alamy Stock Photo. (B) David Nunuk/Science Source. (C) Tierbild Okapia/Science Source. (D) Roberto A. Penne-Casanova/Science Source.

(continued)

Techniques and Normal Findings	Abnormal Findings and Special Considerations

- Carefully inspect the patient's body, including skin folds and crevices, using a good source of light.
- In the obese patient this requires lifting the breasts and carefully examining the skin under folds in the abdomen, back, and perineal areas. Pressure on the bladder and bowel from the weight of the abdomen and from reduced mobility contribute to the increased incidence of incontinence in obese patients. In addition, abdominal girth and reduced mobility contribute to difficulties with hygiene in the perineal and other areas. As a result, the obese patient is at risk for rashes and skin breakdown.
- When lesions are observed, palpate lesions between the thumb and index finger. Measure all lesion dimensions (including height, if possible) with a small, clear, flexible ruler.
- Document lesion size in centimeters. If necessary, use a magnifying glass or a penlight for closer inspection (see Figure 12.12 ■).

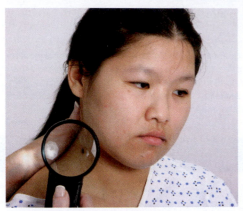

Figure 12.12 Using a magnifying glass.

- Assess any drainage for color, odor, consistency, amount, and location. If indicated, obtain a specimen of the drainage for culture and sensitivity.
- Healthy skin is typically smooth and free of lesions; however, some lesions, such as freckles, insect bites, healed scars, and certain birthmarks, are expected findings.

8. **Palpate the skin for sensitivity.**
   - Palpate the skin in various regions of the body and ask the patient to describe the sensations.
   - Give special attention to any pain or discomfort that the patient reports, especially when palpating skin lesions.
   - Ask the patient to describe the sensation as closely as possible, and document the findings.
   - The patient should not report any discomfort from your touch.

▶ The injection of drugs into the veins of the arms or other parts of the body results in a series of small scars called *track marks* along the course of the blood vessel. A nurse who sees track marks and suspects substance abuse should refer the patient to a mental health or substance abuse professional.

ALERT! *Localized hot, red, swollen painful areas indicate the presence of inflammation and possible infection. These areas should not be palpated, because the slightest disturbance may spread the infection deeper into skin layers.*

Some cultures use therapies such as coining and cupping. These are used in treatment for a variety of illnesses and are among complementary and alternative medical therapies. Because they can leave visible welts and bruising on the skin, the nurse should ask if therapies using coins, cups, or pinching have been recently employed. The nurse should be aware of alternative medical practices and include questions about them in the interview. Box 12.2 describes these therapies.

Box 12.2 Coining, Cupping, Pinching

These treatments stimulate circulation and are thought to restore balance in children and adults with a variety of ailments.

Coining	Coining refers to rubbing the skin of the back, upper chest, neck, and arms with a coin in symmetric patterns which may result in skin bruising.
Cupping	Cupping is conducted by creating a vacuum in a small glass cup by using heat or burning, then placing the cup or glass upside down on the patient's skin. The vacuum created draws blood and lymph to the skin surface. The cup is left in place for a short time and when removed leaves a circular red or dark lesion (Spector, 2017).
Pinching	When pinching, the first and second fingers pull upward on the skin of the neck, back, and chest and between the eyebrows. The pinching produces bruises.

Additional Assessment: Assessment for Cancerous Lesions

According to the American Cancer Society (2014), more than one million cases of basal or squamous cell carcinomas go unreported each year. The number of cases of melanoma has been rising for the past 30 years. Melanoma occurs primarily in Caucasians, with rates 10 times higher than those for African Americans.

Risk factors for skin cancer include sun sensitivity, difficulty tanning, history of prolonged sun exposure, use of tanning booths, diseases in which immunosuppression occurs, a history of skin cancer, or occupational exposure to some chemicals such as coal tar and radiation. Melanoma risks include personal or family history of melanoma, the presence of moles that are atypical in growth or appearance, and the presence of more than 50 moles. Early detection of skin cancer can result in appropriate treatment and cure.

Comprehensive health assessment includes the patient interview and physical examination. Careful attention to detail during the health history interview enables the examiner to elicit information about risks for skin cancer, including family history, sun exposure, and occupational hazards. Physical assessment for skin cancer includes total body skin examination, especially in those who are at high risk for development of skin cancer. The

National Cancer Institute (2017) describes the characteristics of common moles and the signs that a mole may be cancerous. A commonly used tool for screening for melanoma includes the ABCDE appraisal of pigmented lesions (see Figure 12.13 ■).

A = Asymmetry
B = Border Irregularity
C = Color Variegation
D = Diameter Greater than 6 mm
E = Evolving Changes*

*Evolving changes include changes in size, shape, symptoms (itching, tenderness), surface (bleeding), and shades of color.

Figure 12.13 ABCDE Criteria for Melanoma Assessment.

The ABCDE criteria refer to size, shape, color, diameter, and change in lesions. This approach is recommended for both healthcare providers and the public to screen for melanoma. This method improves the rates of identification, diagnosis, and treatment of melanomas (Crowson, Magro, & Mihm, 2014).

Techniques and Normal Findings	Abnormal Findings and Special Considerations

Inspection of the Scalp and Hair

1. **Instruct the patient.**
   - Explain that you will be looking at the patient's scalp and hair. Tell the patient you will be parting the hair to observe the scalp.
2. **Observe for cleanliness.**
   - Ask the patient to remove any hairpins, hair ties, barrettes, wigs, or hairpieces and to undo braids. If the patient is unwilling to do this, examine any strands of hair that are loose or undone.
   - Part and divide the hair at 1-in. intervals and observe (see Figure 12.14 ■).

▶ Lesions, including cancerous lesions, may occur on the scalp.
▶ Apply the ABCDE method (see Figure 12.13) in assessment of lesions.

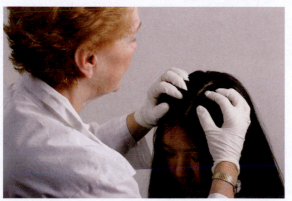

Figure 12.14 Inspecting the hair and scalp.

- A small amount of dandruff (dead, scaly flakes of epidermal cells) may be present.

▶ Excessive dandruff occurs on the scalp of patients with certain skin disorders, such as psoriasis or seborrheic dermatitis, in which large amounts of the epidermis slough away. Dandruff should be distinguished from head lice.
▶ Graying of the hair in patches may indicate a nutritional deficiency, commonly of protein or copper.

3. **Observe the patient's hair color.**
   - Like skin color, hair color varies according to the level of melanin production. Graying is influenced by genetics and may begin as early as the late teens in some patients.

(continued)

Techniques and Normal Findings	Abnormal Findings and Special Considerations

Techniques and Normal Findings

4. **Assess the texture of the hair.**
   - Roll a few strands of hair between your thumb and forefinger.
   - Hold a few strands of hair taut with one hand while you slide the thumb and forefinger of your other hand along the length of the strand.
   - Hair may be thick or fine and may appear straight, wavy, or curly.
5. **Observe the amount and distribution of the hair throughout the scalp.**
   - The amount of hair varies with age, gender, and overall health. Healthy hair is evenly distributed throughout the scalp.
   - In most men and women, atrophy of the hair follicles causes hair growth to decline by the age of 50. Male pattern baldness (see Figure 12.15 ■), a genetically determined progressive loss of hair beginning at the anterior hairline, has no clinical significance. It is the most frequent reason for hair loss in men.

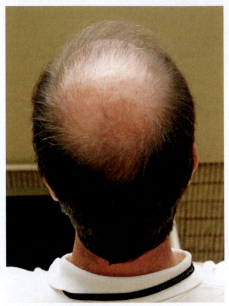

Figure 12.15 Male pattern baldness.

   - Remember to assess the amount, texture, and distribution of body hair. Some practitioners prefer to perform this assessment with the regions of the body.
6. **Inspect the scalp for lesions.**
   - The healthy scalp is free from lesions.

Assessment of the Nails

1. **Instruct the patient.**
   - Explain that you will be looking at and touching the patient's nails and that you will ask the patient to hold the hands and fingers in certain positions while you are inspecting the fingernails.
2. **Assess for hygiene.**
   - Confirm that the nails are clean and well groomed.
3. **Inspect the nails for an even, pink undertone.**
   - Small, white markings in the nail are normal findings and indicate minor trauma.

4. **Assess capillary refill.**
   - Depress the nail edge briefly to blanch, and then release. Color returns to healthy nails instantly upon release.

Abnormal Findings and Special Considerations

▶ Hypothyroidism and other metabolic disorders, as well as nutritional deficiencies, may cause the hair to be dull, dry, brittle, and coarse.

▶ When hair loss occurs in women, it is thought to be caused by an imbalance in adrenal hormones.

▶ Widespread hair loss may also be caused by illness, infections, metabolic disorders, nutritional deficiencies, and chemotherapy. Patchy hair loss (*alopecia areata*) may be because of infection.

▶ Gray, scaly patches with broken hair may indicate the presence of a fungal infection such as ringworm.
▶ Infestation by **pediculosis capitis** (head lice) is signaled by tiny, white, oval eggs (nits) that adhere to the hair shaft. Head lice usually cause intense itching. The scalp should be checked for excoriation from scratching.

▶ Dirty fingernails may indicate a self-care deficit but could also be related to a person's occupation.
▶ The nails appear pale and colorless in patients with peripheral arteriosclerosis or anemia. The nails appear yellow in patients with jaundice, and dark red in patients with *polycythemia,* a pathologic increase in production of red blood cells. Fungal infections may cause the nails to discolor. Horizontal white bands may occur in chronic hepatic or renal disease. A darkly pigmented band in a single nail may be a sign of a melanoma in the nail matrix and should be referred to a physician for further evaluation.
▶ The nail beds appear blue, and color return is sluggish in patients with cardiovascular or respiratory disorders.

Techniques and Normal Findings	Abnormal Findings and Special Considerations

5. Inspect and palpate the nails for shape and contour.
- Perform the Schamroth technique to assess clubbing. Ask the patient to bring together the dorsal aspect of the corresponding fingers, creating a mirror image.
- Look at the distal phalanx and observe the diamond-shaped opening created by nails. When clubbing is present, the diamond is not formed and the distance increases at the fingertip (see Figure 12.16 ■).

▶ *Clubbing of the fingernails* occurs when there is hypoxia or impaired peripheral tissue perfusion over a long time. It may also occur with cirrhosis, colitis, thyroid disease, or long-term tobacco smoking. The ends of the fingers become enlarged, soft, and spongy, and the angle between the skin and the nail base is greater than 160 degrees.

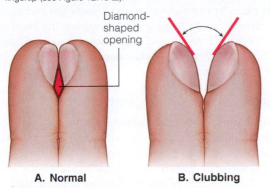

Diamond-shaped opening

A. Normal   **B. Clubbing**

Figure 12.16 Schamroth technique. A. Healthy nail. B. Clubbing.

- The nails normally form a slightly convex curve or lie flat on the nail bed. When viewed laterally, the angle between the skin and the nail base should be approximately 160 degrees (see Figure 12.17 ■).

▶ *Spoon nails* form a concave curve rather than a convex curve.

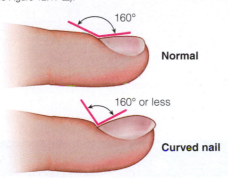

160°

Normal

160° or less

Curved nail

Figure 12.17 Angle of fingernail.

6. Palpate the nails to determine their thickness, regularity, and attachment to the nail bed.
- Healthy nails are smooth, strong, and regular and are firmly attached to the nail bed with only a slight degree of mobility.

▶ Nails may be thickened in patients with circulatory disorders. Onycholysis occurs with trauma, infection, or skin lesions.

7. Inspect and palpate the cuticles.
- The cuticles are smooth and flat in healthy nails.

▶ *Hangnails* are jagged tears in the lateral skin folds around the nail. An untreated hangnail may become inflamed and lead to a *paronychia*, an infection of the cuticle.

Self-Assessment of the Skin

Teach all patients how to examine their skin (see Box 12.3).

Box 12.3 Self-Examination of the Skin

1. Use a room that is well lit and has a full-length mirror. Have a handheld mirror and chair available. Remove all of your clothes.
2. Examine all of your skin surface, front and back. Begin with your hands, including the spaces between your fingers. Continue with your arms, chest, abdomen, pubic area, thighs, lower legs, and toes. Next examine your face and neck. Make sure you inspect your underarms, the sides of your trunk, the back of your neck, the buttocks, and the soles of your feet.
3. Next, sit down with one leg elevated. Use the handheld mirror to examine the inside of the elevated leg, from the groin area to the foot. Repeat on the other leg.
4. Use the handheld mirror to inspect your scalp.
5. Consult your physician promptly if you see any newly pigmented area or if any existing mole has changed in color, size, shape, or elevation. Also report sores that do not heal; redness or swelling around a growth or lesion; any change in sensation such as itching, pain, tenderness, or numbness in a lesion or the skin around it; and any change in the texture or consistency of the skin.

Documenting Your Findings

Documentation of assessment data—subjective and objective—must be accurate, professional, complete, and confidential. When documenting the information from the focused assessment of each body system, the nurse should use measurements where appropriate to ensure accuracy, use medical terminology rather than jargon, include all pertinent information, and avoid language that could identify the patient. The information in the documentation should make it clear what questions were asked and should use language to indicate whether it is the patient's response or the nurse's findings. For patient responses, the documentation will say "denies," "states," or "reports," whereas the nurse's findings will simply list the findings as fact, or say "no" along with the condition—for example, patient "denies itching or rash" and the nurse found "two 5 mm hyperpigmented macules on dorsal aspect of R forearm." See an example of normal results for the integumentary system below.

Sample Documentation: Skin, Hair, and Nails Assessment

Focused History (Subjective Data)

This is information from the Review of Systems (ROS) and other pertinent history information that is or could be related to the patient's integumentary system.

Denies rash, itching, hair loss, and changes in skin or nails since last visit. Denies history of eczema or psoriasis. Reports allergy to nickel, which causes itchy rash where it touches skin. Denies history of tanning bed use or sunburn with blistering. Full body exam by dermatologist was 2 years ago and negative. Immunizations are up to date. Pt. reports having colored her hair for the past 3 years, and wears acrylic nails. States she washes her hair every other day, uses a moisturizing lotion with SPF 30 on her face daily.

Physical Assessment (Objective Data)

Skin is light pink, Caucasian, evenly pigmented, and consistently warm on upper and lower extremities. Skin is smooth, dry, elastic. Two 5 mm hyperpigmented macules on dorsal aspect of R forearm. Eyebrows and lashes are evenly distributed. Facial skin is free of lesions, lips are smooth, dark pink, moist. Hair is fine textured, light blonde, evenly distributed, and scalp is free of lesions or infestations. Nails are pink, rounded with no clubbing. Capillary refill is < 3 sec on upper and lower extremities. Cuticles are smooth and well attached to nail bed.

Abnormal Findings

Abnormal findings of the integumentary system include alterations in the skin, hair, or nails. Skin abnormalities include **primary lesions** (see Table 12.3), secondary lesions (see Table 12.4), and vascular lesions (see Table 12.5). Skin abnormalities also are classified based on configuration and shape (see Table 12.6). Abnormalities of the hair and nails are described at the conclusion of this chapter.

Table 12.3 Primary Lesions

Macule and Patch

Flat, nonpalpable change in the skin color.

Macules are smaller than 1 cm with a circumscribed border.

Examples: freckles, measles, petechiae

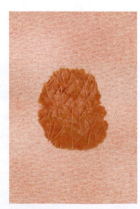

Macule.

Papule and Plaque

Elevated, solid palpable masses with a circumscribed border.

Papules: smaller than 0.5 cm.

Examples: elevated moles, warts, lichen planus

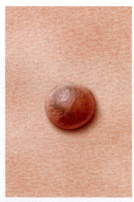

Papule.

Patches are larger than 1 cm and may have an irregular border.

***Examples:* Mongolian spots**, port-wine stains, vitiligo, and chloasma

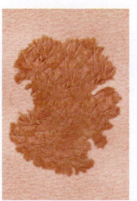

Patch.

Plaques: groups of papules that form lesions larger than 0.5 cm.

Examples: psoriasis, actinic keratosis, lichen planus

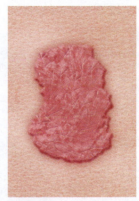

Plaque.

Nodule and Tumor

Elevated, solid, hard or soft palpable mass extending deeper into the dermis.

Nodules are smaller than 2 cm and have circumscribed borders.

Examples: small lipoma, squamous cell carcinoma, fibroma, and intradermal nevi

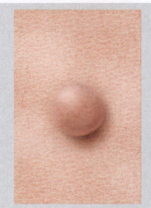

Nodule.

Vesicle and Bulla

Elevated, fluid-filled, round or oval-shaped, palpable masses with thin, translucent walls and circumscribed borders.

Vesicles are smaller than 0.5 cm.

Examples: herpes simplex/zoster, early chickenpox, poison ivy, and small burn blisters

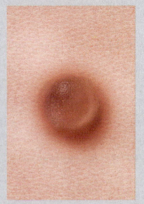

Vesicle.

Tumors may have irregular borders and are larger than 2 cm.

Examples: large lipoma, carcinoma, and hemangioma

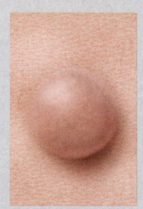

Tumor.

Bullae are larger than 0.5 cm.

Examples: contact dermatitis, friction blisters, and large burn blisters

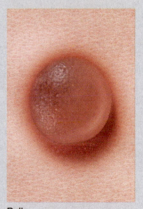

Bulla.

Pustule

An elevated, pus-filled vesicle or bulla with a circumscribed border. Size varies.

Examples: acne, impetigo, and carbuncles (large boils)

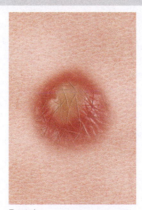

Pustule.

Wheal

An elevated, often reddish area with an irregular border caused by diffuse fluid in tissues. Size varies.

Examples: insect bites, hives (extensive wheals)

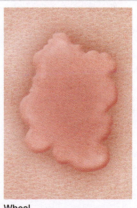

Wheal.

(continued)

Table 12.3 Primary Lesions (continued)

Cyst

Elevated, encapsulated, fluid-filled or semisolid mass originating in subcutaneous tissue or dermis, usually 1 cm or larger.

Examples: sebaceous cysts and epidermoid cysts

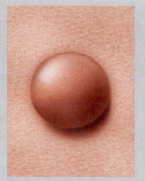

Cyst.

Table 12.4 Secondary Lesions

Atrophy

A translucent, dry, paperlike, sometimes wrinkled skin surface resulting from thinning or wasting of the skin because of loss of collagen and elastin.

Examples: striae, aged skin

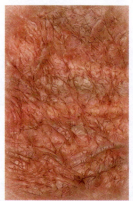

Atrophy.

Crust

Dry blood, serum, or pus on the skin surface from burst vesicles or pustules. It can be red-brown, orange, or yellow. Large crusts are called scabs.

Examples: eczema, impetigo, herpes, or scabs following abrasion

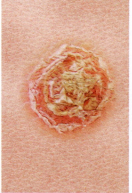

Crust.

Erosion

Wearing away of the superficial epidermis causing a moist, shallow depression. Usually heal without scarring.

Examples: scratch marks, ruptured vesicles

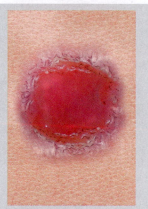

Erosion.

Fissure

A linear crack with sharp edges extending into the dermis.

Examples: cracks at the corners of the mouth or in the hands, athlete's foot

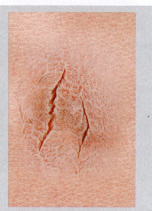

Fissure.

Keloid

An elevated, irregular, darkened area of excess scar tissue caused by excessive collagen formation during healing that extends beyond the site of the original injury.

Example: keloid from ear piercing or surgery

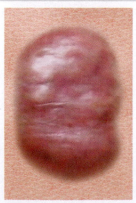

Keloid.

Lichenification

A rough, thickened, hardened area of epidermis resulting from chronic irritation such as scratching or rubbing.

Example: chronic dermatitis

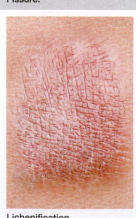

Lichenification.

Scales

Shedding flakes of greasy, keratinized skin tissue. Color may be white, gray, or silver. Texture may vary from fine to thick.

Examples: dry skin, dandruff, psoriasis, and eczema

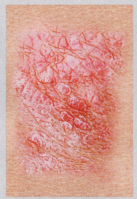

Scales.

Scar

A flat, irregular area of connective tissue left after a lesion or wound has healed. New scars may be red or purple; older scars may be silvery or white.

Examples: healed surgical wound or injury, healed acne

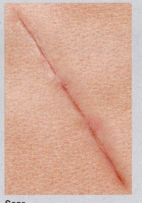

Scar.

Ulcer

A deep, irregularly shaped area of skin loss extending into the dermis or subcutaneous tissue. May be caused by venous hypertension, arterial insufficiency, neuropathy, or lymphedema. Ulcerated skin may bleed or leave a scar.

Examples: stasis ulcers, chancres

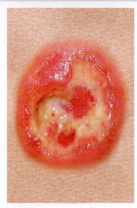

Ulcer.

Table 12.5 Vascular Lesions

NAME/DESCRIPTION	CAUSES	LOCALIZATION/DISTRIBUTION
Ecchymosis Flat, irregularly shaped lesion of varying size with no pulsation; does not blanch with pressure. • In light skin, it begins as a bluish purple mark that changes to greenish yellow. • In brown skin, it varies from blue to deep purple. • In black skin, it appears as a darkened area.	Release of blood from superficial vessels into surrounding tissue because of trauma, hemophilia, liver disease, or deficiency of vitamins C or K.	May occur anywhere on the body at the site of trauma or pressure. 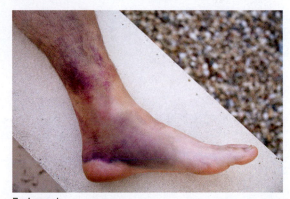 Ecchymosis. *Source:* Paul Cox/Alamy Stock Photo.

(continued)

Table 12.5 Vascular Lesions (continued)

NAME/DESCRIPTION	CAUSES	LOCALIZATION/DISTRIBUTION
Hemangioma A bright red, raised lesion about 2–10 cm in diameter that does not blanch with pressure and is usually present at birth or within a few months of birth. Typically, it disappears by age 10.	A cluster of immature capillaries. Cause is unknown; may be hereditary.	May appear on any part of the body. 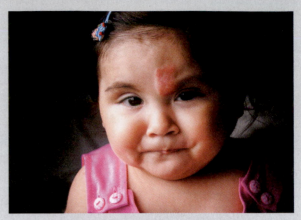 Hemangioma. *Source*: Ruslana Iurchenko/Shutterstock.
Hematoma A raised, irregularly shaped lesion similar to an ecchymosis except that it elevates the skin and looks like a swelling.	A leakage of blood into the skin and subcutaneous tissue as a result of trauma or surgical incision.	May occur anywhere on the body at the site of trauma, pressure, or surgical incision. 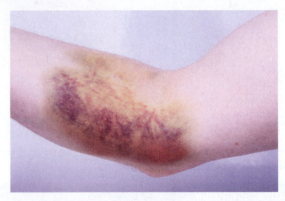 Hematoma. *Source*: Powered by Light/Alan Spencer/Alamy Stock Photo.
Petechiae Flat, red or purple rounded "freckles" approximately 1–3 mm in diameter. They are difficult to detect in dark skin and do not blanch.	Minute hemorrhages resulting from fragile capillaries that are caused by septicemias, liver disease, vitamins C or K deficiency, or anticoagulant therapy.	Most commonly appear on body's dependent surfaces (back, buttocks) but may occur in oral mucosa and conjunctivae. 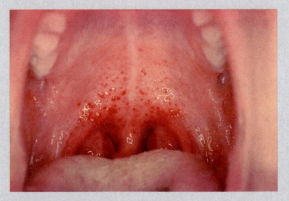 Petechiae on palate. *Source*: Heinz F. Eichenwald/Centers for Disease Control and Prevention (CDC).

NAME/DESCRIPTION	CAUSES	LOCALIZATION/DISTRIBUTION
Port-Wine Stain A flat, irregularly shaped lesion ranging from pale red to deep purple-red. Color deepens with exertion, emotional response, or exposure to extremes of temperature. Present at birth and typically does not fade.	A large, flat mass of blood vessels on the skin surface that is likely caused by a genetic mutation (Shirley et al., 2013).	Most commonly appears on the face and head but may occur at other sites. 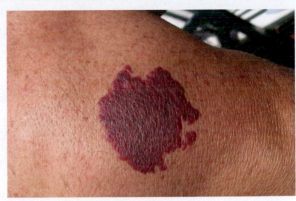 **Port-wine stain (nevus flammeus).** *Source:* guentermanaus/Shutterstock.
Purpura Flat, reddish-blue, irregularly shaped extensive patches of varying size.	Bleeding disorders, scurvy, and capillary fragility in the older adult (senile purpura).	May appear anywhere on the body but are most noticeable on the legs, arms, and backs of hands. 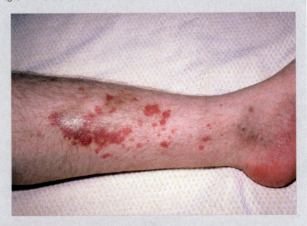 **Purpura.** *Source:* Mediscan/Alamy Stock Photo.
Spider Angioma A flat, bright red dot with tiny radiating blood vessels ranging in size from a pinpoint to 2 cm. It blanches with pressure.	A type of telangiectasis (vascular dilatation) caused by elevated estrogen levels, pregnancy, estrogen therapy, vitamin B deficiency, or liver disease, or it may not be pathologic.	Most commonly appears on the upper half of the body. 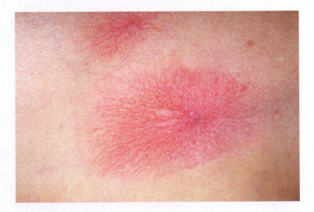 **Spider (star) angioma.** *Source:* Mediscan/Alamy Stock Photo.

(continued)

Table 12.5 Vascular Lesions (continued)

NAME/DESCRIPTION	CAUSES	LOCALIZATION/DISTRIBUTION
Venous Lake A soft, compressible, slightly elevated vascular lesion. Color typically ranges from dark blue to purple.	Venule dilation; most commonly occurs in individuals who are over age 50 and have a history of sun exposure.	Most commonly found on sun-exposed areas, including the lips, ears, neck, face, and posterior hand.

Venous lake.
Source: Science Photo Library/Science Source.

Table 12.6 Configurations and Shapes of Lesions

NAME	EXAMPLE	NAME	EXAMPLE
Annular Lesions with a circular shape. ***Examples:*** Tinea corporis, pityriasis rosea		**Confluent** Lesions that run together. ***Example:*** Urticaria	

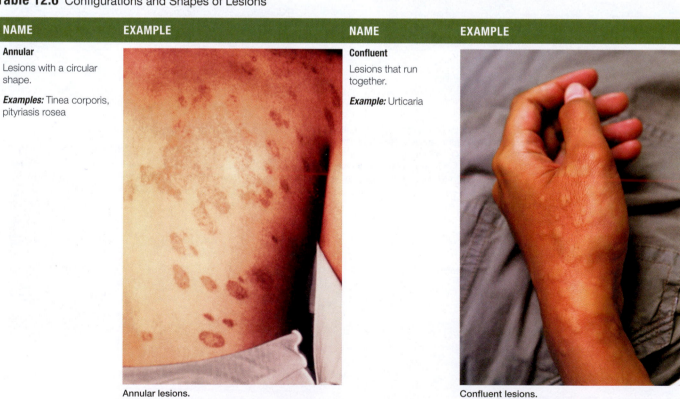

Annular lesions.
Source: Dr. Lucille K. Georg/Centers for Disease Control and Prevention (CDC).

Confluent lesions.
Source: Konmesa/Shutterstock.

NAME	EXAMPLE	NAME	EXAMPLE

Discrete

Lesions that are separate and discrete.

Example: Molluscum.

Grouped

Lesions that appear in clusters.

Example: Purpural lesion

Discrete lesions.
Source: Jodi Jacobson/Getty Images.

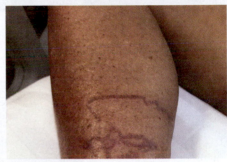

Grouped lesions.
Source: CLS Digital Arts/Shutterstock.

Target

Lesions with concentric circles of color.

Example: Erythema multiforme

Linear

Lesions that appear as a line.

Example: Scratches

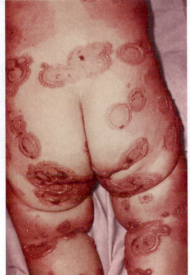

Target lesions.
Source: Arthur E. Kaye/Centers for Disease Control and Prevention (CDC).

Linear lesions.
Source: TisforThan/Shutterstock.

Polycyclic

Polycyclic lesions are lesions that are circular but united.

Example: Psoriasis

Zosteriform

Lesions arranged in a linear manner along a nerve route.

Example: Herpes zoster (shingles)

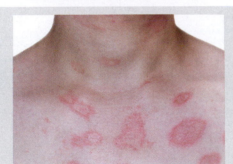

Polycyclic lesions.
Source: Mario Studio/Shutterstock.

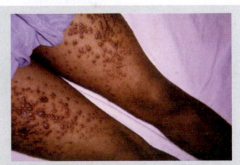

Zosteriform lesions.
Source: John Noble, Jr., MD/Centers for Disease Control and Prevention (CDC).

Overview of Skin Lesions

Skin lesions may have a variety of causes, or etiologies. For example, the etiology of a skin lesion may be an infectious disease, an allergic or inflammatory disorder, or a cancerous condition (malignancy). The following sections provide an overview of these categories of skin lesions.

Infectious Skin Lesions

Skin lesions may be caused by infectious organisms, such as viruses, bacteria, and fungi. In some cases, the lesions may be caused by a combination of organisms. Examples of infectious skin lesions include tinea, measles (rubeola), German measles (rubella), chickenpox (varicella), herpes simplex, and herpes zoster (shingles) (see Table 12.7).

Table 12.7 Common Infectious Skin Lesions

NAME	EXAMPLE	NAME	EXAMPLE

Tinea

Fungal infection affecting the body (tinea corporis); scalp (tinea capitis); or feet (tinea pedis, athlete's foot). Secondary bacterial infection may also be present. Appearance of tinea lesions varies.

Rubeola (measles)

A highly contagious viral disease that causes a rash of red to purple macules or papules that begins on the face and then progresses over the neck, trunk, arms, and legs. Lesions do not blanch. Oral mucosa may demonstrate tiny, white spots that look like grains of salt (Koplik's spots).

Rubeola (measles).
Source: Anukul/Shutterstock.

Tinea corporis.
Source: K. Mae Lennon/Centers for Disease Control and Prevention (CDC).

Rubella (German measles)

A highly contagious disease caused by the rubella virus. Typically it begins as a pink, papular rash that is similar to measles but paler. Skin lesions begin on the face and then spread over the body.

Unlike measles, German measles may be accompanied by swollen glands but not by Koplik's spots. Most common in children.

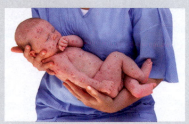

Rubella (German measles).
Source: andriano/123RF.

Vericella (chickenbox)

A mild infectious disease caused by a primary infection with the varicella zoster virus that begins as groups of small, red, fluid-filled vesicles usually on the trunk from which the rash progresses to the face, arms, and legs. Vesicles erupt over several days, forming pustules, then crusts; may cause intense itching. Most common in children.

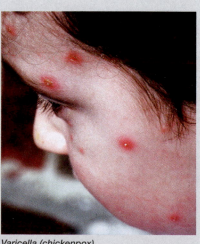

Varicella (chickenpox).

NAME	EXAMPLE	NAME	EXAMPLE

Herpes simplex

A chronic viral infection. Lesions progress from vesicles to pustules and then crusts. The two different types of herpes simplex are oral (HSV-1) and genital (HSV-2). HSV-1 causes lesions on the lips and oral mucosa. HSV-2 causes lesions on the penis, vagina, buttocks, or anus. Although lesions are often confined to the oral mucosa or genitals, lesions from both types of herpes can appear anywhere on the body.

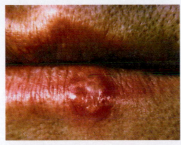

Oral herpes simplex.
Source: National Archives Record Group 11

Herpes zoster (shingles)

A reactivation of the dormant varicella zoster virus, which typically has invaded the body during an attack of chickenpox. Clusters of small vesicles form on the skin along the route of sensory nerves. Vesicles progress to pustules and then crusts and cause intense pain and itching. More common and more severe among older adults.

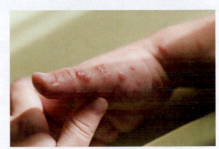

Herpes zoster (shingles).
Source: Angel Simon/Shutterstock.

Impetigo

A contagious bacterial skin infection that usually appears on the skin around the nose and mouth. Lesions may begin as a barely perceptible patch of blisters that breaks, exposing red, weeping area beneath. Tan crust soon forms over this area, and the infection may spread out of the edges. Common in children.

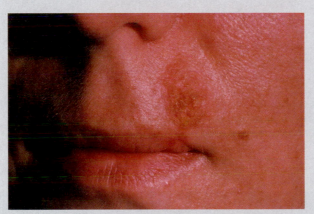

Impetigo
Source: DR ZARA/BSIP SA/Alamy Stock Photo.

Allergic or Inflammatory Skin Lesions

Allergies and inflammatory responses also may cause skin lesions to develop. For example, contact dermatitis is caused by an allergic reaction, whereas eczema and psoriasis are caused by inflammatory responses (see Table 12.8).

Table 12.8 Common Allergic or Inflammatory Skin Lesions

NAME	EXAMPLE	NAME	EXAMPLE

Contact dermatitis

Inflammation of the skin because of an allergy to a substance that comes into contact with the skin, such as clothing, jewelry, plants, chemicals, or cosmetics. Lesion location may help identify the allergen. May progress from redness to hives, vesicles, or scales; usually accompanied by intense itching.

Contact dermatitis.
Source: blickwinkel/Czepluch/Alamy Stock Photo.

Eczema

Internally provoked inflammation of the skin causing reddened papules and vesicles that ooze and weep and possible crust formation. Lesions usually located on the scalp, face, elbows, knees, forearms, torso, and wrists; usually accompanied by intense itching.

Eczema (atopic dermatitis).
Source: Sergio Azenha/Alamy Stock Photo.

(continued)

Table 12.8 Common Allergic or Inflammatory Skin Lesions (continued)

NAME	EXAMPLE
Psoriasis	
Thickening of the skin in dry, silvery, scaly patches that occurs with overproduction of skin cells, resulting in buildup of cells faster than they can be shed. May be triggered by emotional stress or generally poor health. Lesions may form on the scalp, elbows and knees, lower back, and perianal area.	Psoriasis. *Source:* olavs/Shutterstock.

Malignant Skin Lesions

Certain forms of skin lesions are malignant, or cancerous. Examples of malignant skin lesions include basal cell carcinoma, squamous cell carcinoma, malignant melanoma, and Kaposi's sarcoma (see Table 12.9).

Table 12.9 Malignant Skin Lesions

NAME	EXAMPLE	NAME	EXAMPLE
Basal cell carcinoma		**Squamous cell carcinoma**	
The most common but least malignant type of skin cancer. A proliferation of the cells of the stratum basale into the dermis and subcutaneous tissue. Lesions begin as shiny papules that develop central ulcers with rounded, pearly edges and occur most often on regions regularly exposed to the sun.	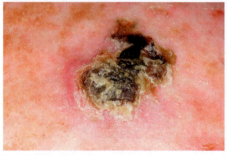Basal cell carcinoma. *Source:* DR P. MARAZZI/SCIENCE PHOTO LIBRARY/Alamy Stock Photo.	Arises from the cells of the stratum spinosum, and begins as a reddened, scaly papule that then forms a shallow ulcer with a clearly delineated, elevated border. Commonly appears on the scalp, ears, back of the hand, and lower lip. Believed to be caused by sun exposure; grows rapidly.	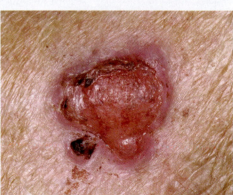Squamous cell carcinoma. *Source:* Dr P. Marazzi/Science Source.

NAME	EXAMPLE	NAME	EXAMPLE

Malignant melanoma

The least common but most serious type of skin cancer because it spreads rapidly to lymph and blood vessels. Lesion contains areas of varied pigmentation and may be black, brown, blue, or red, often with irregular edges with notched borders; diameter is greater than 6 mm.

Malignant melanoma.
Source: Mediscan/Alamy Stock Photo.

Kaposi's sarcoma

Malignant tumor of the epidermis and internal epithelial tissues. Painless lesions are typically soft, blue to purple; other characteristics are variable. Lesions may be macular or papular and may resemble keloids or bruises. Most commonly occurs in people who are HIV positive.

Kaposi's sarcoma.
Source: Steve Kraus/Centers for Disease Control and Prevention (CDC).

Overview of Hair and Scalp Abnormalities

Certain disorders of the integumentary system tend to affect the hair, the scalp, or a combination of these two regions (see Table 12.10).

Table 12.10 Hair and Scalp Abnormalities

NAME	EXAMPLE	NAME	EXAMPLE

Seborrheic dermatitis

Yellow-white greasy scales on the scalp and forehead, similar to eczema but without the significant itching or discomfort characteristic of eczema). Common in infants. Also called cradle cap.

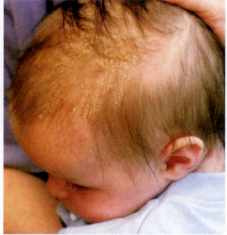

Seborrheic dermatitis (cradle cap).

Tinea capitis

Highly contagious fungal disease (Mayo Clinic, 2014c) that causes patchy hair loss on the head with skin pustules. Transmitted from the soil, from animals, or from person to person. Most common among toddlers and school-age children. Also called scalp ringworm.

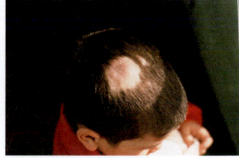

Tinea capitis (scalp ringworm).
Source: PR BOUREE/BSIP SA/Alamy Stock Photo.

(continued)

Table 12.10 Hair and Scalp Abnormalities (continued)

NAME	EXAMPLE	NAME	EXAMPLE
Alopecia Areata There is no known cause for this condition, which produces a sudden loss of hair in a round balding patch on the scalp.	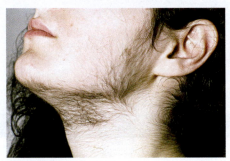 Alopecia areata. *Source:* Fresnel/Shutterstock.	**Folliculitis** Infections of hair follicles, appears as pustules with underlying erythema.	Folliculitis. *Source:* ocskaymark/123RF.
Hirsutism Excess body hair in females on the face, chest, abdomen, arms, and legs, following the male pattern that is typically because of endocrine or metabolic dysfunction. Also may be idiopathic or of unknown origin.	Hirsutism. *Source:* John Radcliffe Hospital/Science Source.	**Furuncle/abscess** Infected hair follicles give rise to *furuncles*, which are hard, erythematous, pus-filled lesions. *Abscesses* are caused by bacteria entering the skin. These are larger lesions than furuncles.	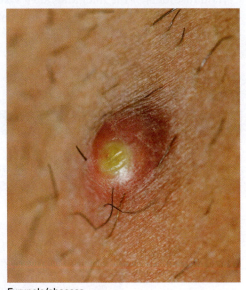 Furuncle/abscess. *Source:* FCG/Shutterstock.

Overview of Nail Abnormalities

Abnormalities of the nails can stem from numerous etiologies, including genetic factors, infectious disease processes, and traumatic injuries. Nail abnormalities also can provide clues to the presence of underlying disease processes involving other body systems. Examples of nail abnormalities include spoon nails, paronychia, Beau's line, splinter hemorrhage, clubbing, and onycholysis (see Table 12.11).

Table 12.11 Nail Abnormalities

NAME	EXAMPLE	NAME	EXAMPLE
Koilonychia Concavity and thinning of the nails, commonly a congenital condition or result from an iron deficiency. Also known as spoon nails.	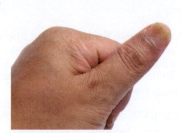 Koilonychia (spoon nails). *Source:* kenary820/shutterstock.	**Paronychia** **Paronychia** is an infection of the skin adjacent to the nail, usually caused by bacteria or fungi. Affected area becomes red, swollen, and painful; pus may ooze from affected area.	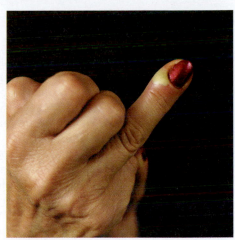 Paronychia. *Source:* Marcel Jancovic/Shutterstock.
Beau's Lines Occur because of trauma or illness affecting nail formation. A linear depression develops at the base and moves distally as the nail grows.	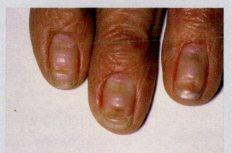 Beau's Line. *Source:* Dr. P. Marazzi/Science Source.	**Splinter hemorrhage** Can occur as a result of trauma or in endocarditis. These appear as reddish-brown spots in the nail.	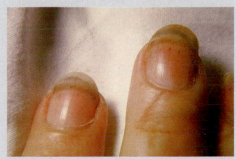 Splinter hemorrhages. *Source:* CDC/Dr. Thomas F. Sellers/Emory University.
Clubbing The nail appears more convex and wide; the nail angle is greater than 160 degrees. Occurs in chronic respiratory and cardiac conditions in which oxygenation is compromised (lung disease, lung cancer, bronchiectasis, cystic fibrosis) (van Manen et al., 2017). Additional causes may include liver disease, congenital heart disease, hypertrophic osteoarthropathy, and HIV.	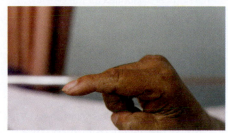 Clubbing of fingernails. *Source:* Casa nayafana/shutterstock.	**Onycholysis** A fungal nail infection that causes the nails to thicken and lift off the nail bed and appear white, yellow, or opaque. Most commonly occurs on toenails; more common in adults. Also called tinea unguium.	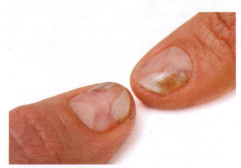 Onycholysis. *Source:* Sergey Kolesnikov/123rf.

CASE STUDY

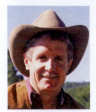

Source: Jess Alford/
Getty Images

Mr. Shelley is a 54-year-old groundskeeper for a large corporation in the Southwest. Today, he visits the company's health and wellness office and says, "My wife told me to have someone check my leathery skin."

Julieta Cardenas, RN, asks Mr. Shelley how much time he spends outdoors. He reveals that he is outside from about 8:00 a.m. until 4:00 p.m. each day, except for his lunch break, which he usually takes in the cafeteria. He reports that he does not use sunscreen. In the summertime, he works in a short-sleeved shirt, shorts, and a hat. He doesn't recall ever having had a bad sunburn. He states that he has a mole on his left thigh that has been present since birth, but to his knowledge it has not changed. He is not aware of any other birthmarks or skin lesions. He has never performed a skin self-assessment. He reports no family history of skin cancer. He states that he never sunbathes or swims and that he plays outdoor baseball only at the annual family picnic. He showers each day before going home and uses deodorant soap. He admits that his skin is often quite dry but said he feels that sunscreens and lotions "are for women."

The nursing assessment of Mr. Shelley's skin reveals the following data: His skin is clean. It is a ruddy brown color where frequently exposed to the sun and a pinkish tan elsewhere. His temperature is warm bilaterally, and he has a mild sheen of perspiration on his face, neck, and upper trunk. Where exposed to the sun, his skin is thick with decreased elasticity. There are no unexpected visible blood vessels or vascular lesions. There is a hyperpigmented papule approximately 0.5 cm by 0.5 cm on the anterior surface of his left thigh. No drainage is noted. Mr. Shelley's scalp and hair are dry but clean and free of lesions. Soil is embedded beneath the free edge of his nails. He states that he had been transplanting cuttings.

Sample Documentation The following information is summarized from the case study.

SUBJECTIVE DATA Seeks checkup for "leathery skin." Works as groundskeeper. Outdoors 7 hours a day. No sunscreen, little protective clothing. No recall of sunburn. "Mole" left thigh since birth, reports unchanged. No other lesions. No self-skin assessment. No family history of skin cancer. Denies sunbathing or swimming. Occasional outdoor baseball. Showers daily with deodorant soap. Feels skin is "dry." "Sunscreens and lotions are for women."

OBJECTIVE DATA Skin clean, ruddy brown where exposed, pinkish tan in unexposed areas. Temperature warm, bilaterally. Mild perspiration on face, neck, upper trunk. Exposed skin thick, decreased elasticity. No unexpected vessels, vascular lesions. Hyperpigmented papule 0.5 cm by 0.5 cm anterior (L) thigh, no drainage. Scalp and hair, no lesions. Nails, soil embedded beneath free edge.

CRITICAL THINKING QUESTIONS

1. Describe the findings from the case study.
2. Identify the findings as normal or abnormal.
3. Determine the categories that emerge from clustering of the data.
4. Analyze the categories to identify the physical and psychosocial nursing care priorities for Mr. Shelley.
5. What might the nurse do to help Mr. Shelley understand the risks of not using sunscreen?

REFERENCES

Alexopoulos, A., & Chrousos, G. P. (2016). Stress-related skin disorders. *Reviews in Endocrine and Metabolic Disorders, 17*(3), 295–304. doi:10.1007/s11154-016-9367-y

American Academy of Dermatology (ADD). (2013). *Skin can show first sign of some internal diseases.* Retrieved from http://www.aad.org/stories-and-news/news-releases/skin-can-show-first-signs-of-some-internal-diseases

American Cancer Society. (2013). *Signs and symptoms of melanoma skin cancer.* Retrieved from http://www.cancer.org/cancer/skincancer-melanoma/detailedguide/melanoma-skin-cancer-signs-and-symptoms

American Cancer Society. (2014). *Cancer facts and statistics.* Retrieved from http://www.cancer.org/research/cancerfactsstatistics/index

American Diabetes Association (ADA). (2015). Diabetes symptoms. Retrieved from http://www.diabetes.org/diabetes-basics/symptoms/?loc=db-slabnav

Berman, A., Snyder, S. J., & Frandsen, G. (2016). *Kozier & Erb's fundamentals of nursing: Concepts, process, and practice* (10th ed.). Hoboken, NJ: Pearson.

Centers for Disease Control and Prevention (CDC). (2012). *The hidden dangers of getting inked.* Retrieved from https://blogs.cdc.gov/publichealthmatters/2012/08/the-hidden-dangers-of-getting-inked

Centers for Disease Control and Prevention (CDC). (2013). *Workplace safety and health topics: Skin exposures & effects.* Retrieved from http://www.cdc.gov/niosh/topics/skin

Clarysse, K., Kivlahan, C., Beyer, I., & Gutermuth, J. (2017). Signs of physical abuse and neglect in the mature patient. *Clinics in Dermatology,* Epub 2017. doi:10.1016/j.clindermatol.2017.10.018

Cleveland Clinic. (2015). *Diseases and conditions: Metabolic syndrome.* Retrieved from http://my.clevelandclinic.org/disorders/metabolic_syndrome/hic_metabolic_syndrome.aspx

Crowson, A. N., Magro, C. M., & Mihm, M. C. (2014). *The melanocytic proliferations: A comprehensive textbook of pigmented lesions.* Hoboken, NJ: John Wiley & Sons.

Dalgard, F. J., Gieler, U., Tomas-Aragones, L., Lien, L., Poot, F., Jemec, G. B . . . . Kupfer, J. (2015). The psychological burden of skin diseases: A cross-sectional multicenter study among dermatological outpatients in 13 European countries. *Journal of Investigative Dermatology, 135*(4), 984–991. doi:10.1038/jid.2014.530

Eldridge, M., & Cohen, S. H. (2014). Cutaneous manifestations of infection in returning travelers. *Current Infectious Disease Reports, 16*(426), 1–8. doi:10.1007/s11908-014-0426-9

Elmann, S., Pointdujour, R., Blaydon, S., Nakra, T., Connor, M., Mukhopadhyay, C., . . . Shinder, R. (2012). Periocular abscesses following brow epilation. *Ophthalmic Plastic & Reconstructive Surgery, 28*(6), 434–437. doi:10.1097/IOP.0b013e3182696552

Gizlenti, S., & Ekmekci, T. R. (2013). The changes in the hair cycle during gestation and the post-partum period. *Journal of the European Academy of Dermatology and Venereology, 28,* 878–881. doi:10.1111/jdv.12188

Khomami, M. B., Tehrani, F. R., Hashemi, S., Farahmand, M., & Azizi, F. (2015). Of PCOS symptoms, hirsutism has the most significant impact on quality of life of Iranian women. *PlosOne, 10*(4), e0123608. doi:10.1371/journal.pone.0123608

Marieb, E., & Keller, S. (2018). *Essentials of human anatomy and physiology* (12th ed.). New York, NY: Pearson

Mayo Clinic. (2014a). *Diseases and conditions: Sweating and body odor.* Retrieved from http://www.mayoclinic.org/diseases-conditions/sweating-and-body-odor/basics/definition/con-20014438

Mayo Clinic. (2014b). *Diseases and conditions: Skin cancer.* Retrieved from http://www.mayoclinic.org/diseases-conditions/skin-cancer/basics/risk-factors/con-20031606

Mayo Clinic. (2014c). *Diseases and conditions: Ringworm (scalp).* Retrieved from http://www.mayoclinic.org/diseases-conditions/ringworm/basics/definition/con-20029923

Mayo Clinic. (2016a). *Diseases and conditions: Dandruff.* Retrieved from http://www.mayoclinic.org/diseases-conditions/dandruff/basics/definition/con-20023690

Mayo Clinic. (2016b). *Diseases and conditions: Hair loss.* Retrieved from http://www.mayoclinic.org/diseases-conditions/hair-loss/basics/definition/con-20027666

National Cancer Institute (NCI). (2017). *Common moles, dysplastic nevi, and risk of melanoma.* Retrieved from https://www.cancer.gov/types/skin/moles-fact-sheet

Nutten, S. (2015). Atopic dermatitis: Global epidemiology and risk factors. *Annals of Nutrition & Metabolism, 66*(suppl. 1), 8–16. doi:10.1159/000370220

Patel, M., Harrison, S., & Sinclair, R. (2013). Drugs and hair loss. *Dermatologic Clinics, 31*(1), 67–73.

Polley, N., Srimoyee, S., Singh, S., Adhikari, A., Das, S., Choudhury, B. R., & Pal, S. K. (2015). Development and optimization of a noncontact optical device for online monitoring of jaundice in human subjects. *Journal of Biomedical Optics, 20*(6), 067001. doi:10.1117/1.JBO.20.6.067001

Qaseem, A., Mir, T. P., Starkey, M., & Denberg, T. D. (2015). Risk assessment and prevention of pressure ulcers: A clinical practice guideline from the American College of Physicians. *Annals of Internal Medicine, 162*(5), 359–369. doi:10.7326/M14-1567

Setji, T. L., & Brown, A. J. (2014). Polycystic ovarian syndrome: Update on diagnosis and treatment. *American Journal of Medicine, 127*(10), 912–919. doi:10.1016/j.amjmed.2014.04.017

Shields, K. M., Fox, K. L., & Liebrecht, C. (2018). *Pearson nurse's drug guide.* Hoboken, NJ: Pearson.

Shirley, M. D., Tang, H., Gallione, C. J., Baugher, J. D., Frelin, L. P., Cohen, B., . . . Pevsner, J. (2013). Sturge-Weber syndrome and port-wine stains caused by somatic mutation in GNAQ. *New England Journal of Medicine, 368*(21), 1971–1979.

Spector, R. (2017). *Cultural diversity in health and illness.* New York, NY: Pearson.

Tully, A. S., Trayes, K. P., & Studdiford, J. S. (2012). Evaluation of nail abnormalities. *American Family Physician, 85*(8), 779–787.

Van Hoover, C., Rademayer, C., & Farley, C. L. (2017). Body piercing: Motivations and implications for health. *Journal of Midwifery & Women's Health, 62*(5), 521–530. doi:10.1111/jmwh.12630

van Manen, M. J. G., Vermeer, L. C., Moor, C. C., Vrijenhoeff, R., Grutters, J. C., Veltkamp, M., & Wijsnebeek, M. S. (2017). Clubbing in patients with fibrotic interstitial lung diseases. *Respiratory Medicine, 132,* 226–231. doi:10.1016/j.rmed.2017.10.021

World Health Organization (WHO). (2014). *Health effects of UV radiation: UV health effects on the immune system.* Retrieved from http://www.who.int/uv/health/uv_health2/en/index3.html

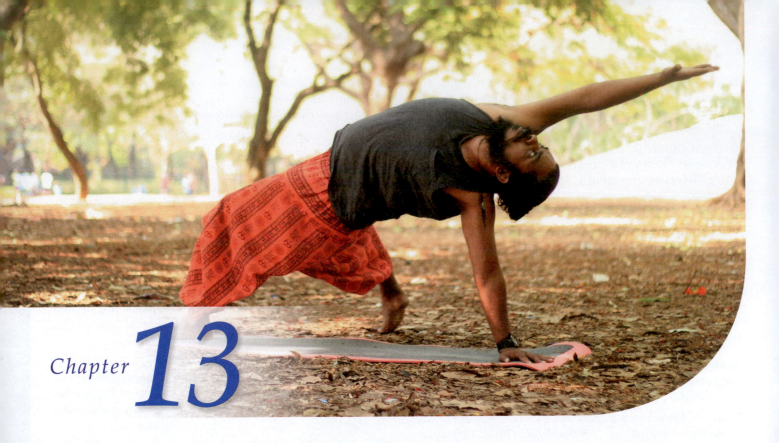

Chapter 13

Head, Neck, and Related Lymphatics

LEARNING OUTCOMES

Upon completion of this chapter, you will be able to:

1. Describe the anatomy and physiology of the head, neck, and related lymphatics.

2. Identify the anatomic, physiologic, developmental, psychosocial, and cultural variations that guide assessment of the head, neck, and related lymphatics.

3. Determine which questions about the head, neck, and related lymphatics to use for the focused interview.

4. Outline the techniques for assessment of the head, neck, and related lymphatics.

5. Generate the appropriate documentation to describe the assessment of the head, neck, and related lymphatics.

6. Identify abnormal findings in the physical assessment of the head, neck, and related lymphatics.

KEY TERMS

acromegaly, 224
anterior triangle, 208
atlas, 207
axis, 207
Bell's palsy, 224
cerebrovascular accident, 225
craniosynostosis, 225
crepitation, 218
Cushing's syndrome, 225
Down syndrome, 225
fetal alcohol syndrome, 226
goiter, 212
hydrocephalus, 226
hyoid, 208
hyperthyroidism, 220
hypothyroidism, 220
lymphadenopathy, 221
Parkinson disease, 226
posterior triangle, 208
sutures, 207
thyroid gland, 210
torticollis, 226

MEDICAL LANGUAGE

-itis   Suffix meaning "inflammation"

-megaly   Suffix meaning "enlargement"

post-   Prefix meaning "after," "behind"

retro-   Prefix meaning "behind," "back," "backward"

supra-   Prefix meaning "above," "upper"

vaso-   Prefix meaning "vessel," "duct"

Introduction

The head and neck region is made up of integrated components of several body systems making assessment of this area complex. The integumentary, musculoskeletal, gastrointestinal, respiratory, cardiovascular, endocrine, and neurological systems are present in this region. The nurse must be aware of the interconnectedness of these systems; the details of each are covered in subsequent chapters.

The interconnected body systems in the head and neck region are assessed at the same time. For example, the integumentary system provides covering and protection, and the musculoskeletal system permits movement of the neck and face and protects the brain, spinal cord, and eyes. Food is taken in through the mouth, which is the beginning of the gastrointestinal system, and air enters the lungs through the nose, mouth, and trachea, which make up the upper respiratory system. The cardiovascular system carries oxygen and other nutrients to the region and transports wastes. The nurse must consider this close interrelationship of systems when assessing the patient's head and neck to obtain data about the patient's nutritional status, airway clearance, tissue perfusion, metabolism, level of activity, sleep and rest, level of stress, and self-care ability.

When performing an assessment of the head and neck, the nurse must be aware of psychosocial, cultural, and environmental factors that may influence the health of this body area. A patient's level of stress, behaviors, and activities influence overall health, and the effects may be apparent in the structure and functioning of the components of the head and neck region. It is also important for the nurse to consider the influence of patient's beliefs, values, and knowledge base related to activities of daily living and self-care practices. For example, many patients spend a great deal of time caring for this area of the body, and alterations in health may affect their ability to provide this care. A patient's ancestry, cultural practices, socioeconomic status, and physical environment both at home and at work can greatly influence the health of the head and neck and are an integral part of the assessment data. In addition, a patient's developmental stage has a tremendous influence on the appearance and functioning of the components of the head and neck.

Anatomy and Physiology Review

The structures of the head and neck include the skull, facial bones, vertebrae, hyoid bone, cartilage, muscles, thyroid gland, and major blood vessels found within the neck. In addition, many lymph nodes are located in the head and neck. Each of these structures is described in the following paragraphs (Marieb & Keller, 2018).

Head

The skull is a protective shell made up of the bones of the cranium (see Figure 13.1 ■) and face. The major bones of the cranium are the frontal, parietal, temporal, and occipital bones. These bones are connected to each other by means of **sutures**, or nonmovable joints. The solidification process of the sutures is completed by the second year of life. The primary function of the skull is to protect the brain. The bones of the skull are covered by the muscles and skin that are commonly called the scalp (Marieb & Keller, 2018). The bones provide landmarks for assessment. Fourteen bones form the anterior region of the skull, commonly called the face. They are the maxilla, the nasal, and the left and right frontal, zygomatic, ethmoid, lacrimal, sphenoid, and mandible bones. The intricate fusion of these bones provides structure for the face and cavities for the eyes, nose, and mouth. It also allows movement of the mandible at the temporomandibular joint (TMJ). The TMJ is located anterior to the tragus of the ear and allows a person to open and close the mouth, protract and retract the chin, and slide the lower jaw from side to side. These actions are used for chewing and speaking.

The skin, muscles, and bones of the face provide landmarks for assessment, as do the bones of the skull. The eyebrows are appendages of the skin and are located over the supraorbital margins of the skull. The lateral canthus of the eye forms a straight line with the pinna, and the nasolabial folds are equal (see Figure 13.2 ■).

Figure 13.3 ■ identifies the main muscles of the scalp, face, and neck. These muscles play a major role in expressing emotions through facial expressions. They also contribute to movement of the head and neck. Details regarding movement of the structures of the head and neck are discussed in Chapter 23. ∞ Cranial nerve innervation of muscles, senses, and balance are discussed in detail in Chapter 24. ∞

Neck

The neck is formed by the seven cervical vertebrae, along with the ligaments and muscles that support the cranium. The first cervical vertebra (C1), commonly called the **atlas**, carries the skull. The second cervical vertebra (C2), commonly called the **axis**, allows for movement of the head (see Figure 13.1). The greatest mobility is at the level of C4, C5, and C6. The seventh cervical vertebra (vertebra prominens) has the largest spinous process. This vertebral process is visible and easily palpated, making it a definite landmark during patient assessment.

The sternocleidomastoid and trapezius muscles are the primary muscles of the neck. The sternocleidomastoid muscles, innervated by cranial nerve XI (Accessory), originate at the manubrium of the sternum and the medial portion of the clavicles. The insertion of this muscle is at the mastoid process of the temporal bones.

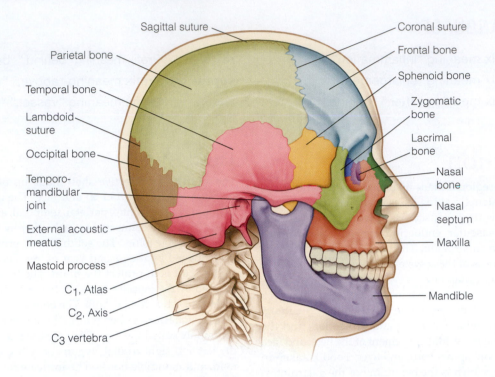

Figure 13.1 Bones of the head.

Each trapezius muscle, also innervated by cranial nerve XI (Accessory), originates on the occipital bone of the skull and spine of several vertebrae. The insertion of these muscles is on the scapulae and lateral third of the clavicles.

These two muscle groups form the anterior and posterior triangles of the neck. The mandible, the midline of the neck, and the anterior aspect of the sternocleidomastoid muscles border the **anterior triangle**. The trapezius muscle, the sternocleido-mastoid muscle, and the clavicle form the **posterior triangle** (see Figure 13.4 ■).

The **hyoid** bone is suspended in the neck (see Figure 13.5 ■) approximately 2 cm (1 in.) above the larynx. The hyoid is the only bone in the body that does not articulate directly with another bone. The base of the tongue rests on the curved body

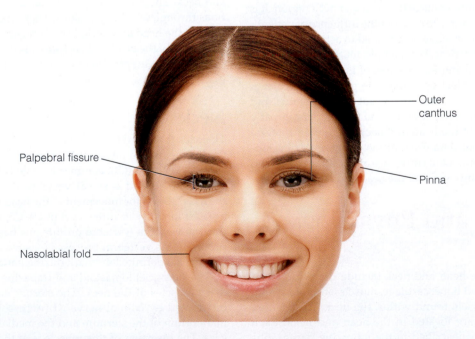

Figure 13.2 Facial landmarks.
Source: Syda Productions/Shutterstock.

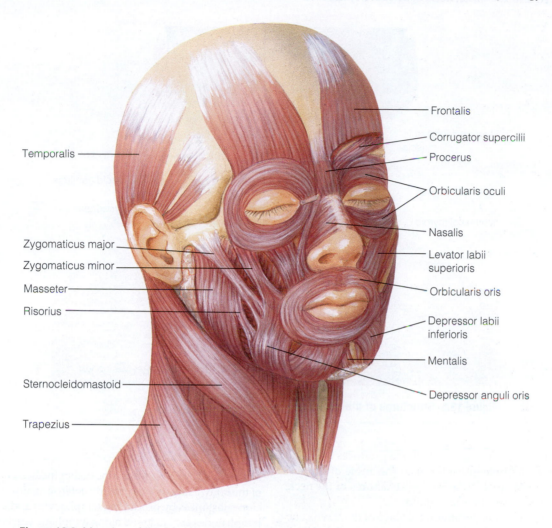

Figure 13.3 Muscles of the head and neck.

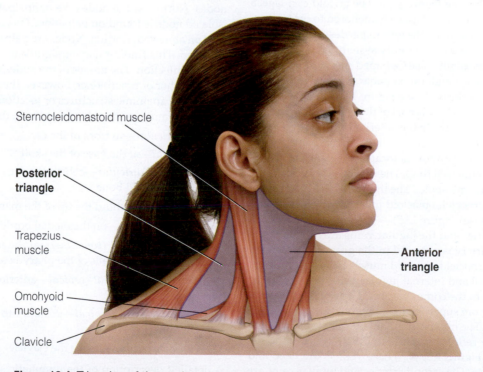

Figure 13.4 Triangles of the neck.

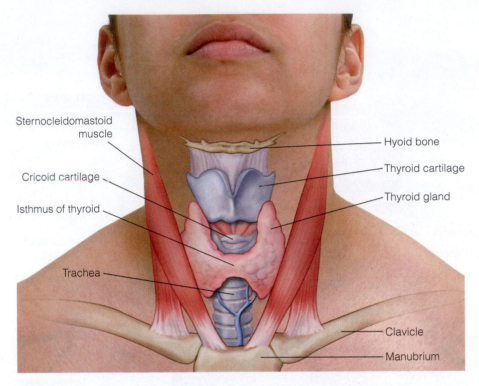

Sternocleidomastoid muscle

Cricoid cartilage

Isthmus of thyroid

Trachea

Hyoid bone

Thyroid cartilage

Thyroid gland

Clavicle

Manubrium

Figure 13.5 Structures of the neck.

of this bone. The curved shape of the bone produces a horn at each end that is palpable just inferior to the angle of the jaw. This serves as a landmark for assessing structures of the neck, especially the trachea and thyroid gland.

The thyroid cartilage is the largest cartilage of the larynx and is formed by the joining of two pieces of cartilage. This fusion forms a ridge called the Adam's apple. This ridge is significantly larger in males (see Figure 13.5). The cricoid cartilage, a C-shaped ring, is the first cartilage ring anchored to the trachea. The trachea, commonly called the windpipe, descends from the larynx to the bronchi of the respiratory system. The trachea has slight mobility and flexibility. The C-shaped rings help maintain the shape of the trachea and are palpable superior to the sternum at the midline of the neck (see Figure 13.5).

The **thyroid gland**, which is part of the endocrine system, is butterfly shaped. It is located in the anterior portion of the neck. The isthmus of the thyroid connects the right and left lobes of the thyroid gland. The isthmus is located beneath the cricoid cartilage (or the first tracheal ring). The isthmus is inferior to the thyroid cartilage (Adam's apple). The thyroid gland lies over the trachea, and the sternocleidomastoid muscles cover the lateral aspects of the lobes (see Figure 13.5).

The carotid arteries and the jugular veins are located in the neck. The carotid artery is palpated in the groove between the trachea and the sternocleidomastoid muscle below the angle of the jaw. The external and internal jugular veins are also in the neck, in proximity to the common carotid artery. The external jugular veins are more superficial and lateral to the sternocleidomastoid muscle. The internal jugular veins are larger and not visible; however, a reflection of the undulation is seen at the sternal notch (see Figure 13.6 ■). These vessels are deep and medial to the muscle. The carotid arteries and jugular veins are discussed in detail in Chapter 18. ∞

Lymphatics

Numerous lymph nodes are located in the head and neck region of the body. These nodes provide defense against invasion of foreign substances by producing lymphocytes and antibodies. The lymph nodes are clustered along lymphatic vessels that infiltrate tissue capillaries and pick up excess fluid called *lymph*. The nurse palpates various areas of the head and neck, looking for lymph nodes. Normally, the nodes are nonpalpable. Occasionally, an isolated node is found on palpation. This is usually not considered an abnormal finding. Nodes are palpable when infected or enlarged. This finding may be significant in recognizing signs of early infection. The names of the nodes may vary depending on the author or practitioner; however, they usually correspond to adjacent anatomic structures or locations (see Figure 13.7 ■). The nodes most commonly assessed are the following:

- *Preauricular*—in front of the ear
- *Occipital*—at the base of the skull
- *Posterior Auricular*—behind the ear, over the outer surface of the mastoid bone
- *Submental*—behind the tip of the mandible at the midline
- *Submandibular*—on the medial border of the mandible
- *Retropharyngeal (tonsillar)*—at the junction of the posterior and lateral walls of the pharynx at the angle of the jaw
- *Anterior/Superficial cervical*—anterior to the sternocleidomastoid muscle
- *Posterior/Deep cervical*—posterior to the sternocleidomastoid muscle
- *Supraclavicular*—above the clavicle

A detailed description of the lymphatic system is provided in Chapter 19. ∞

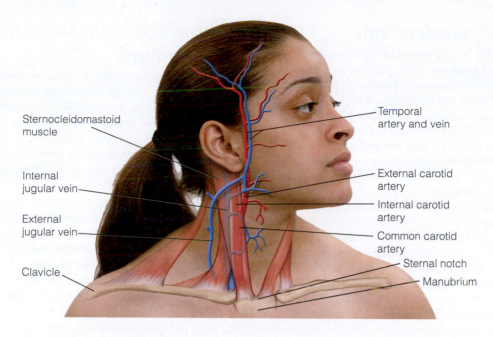

Figure 13.6 Vessels of the neck.

Sternocleidomastoid muscle

Internal jugular vein

External jugular vein

Clavicle

Temporal artery and vein

External carotid artery

Internal carotid artery

Common carotid artery

Sternal notch

Manubrium

Special Considerations

Throughout the assessment process, the nurse gathers subjective and objective data reflecting the patient's state of health. Using critical thinking and the nursing process, the nurse identifies many factors to be considered when collecting the data. Some of these factors include but are not limited to age, developmental level, race, ethnicity, work history, living conditions, social economics, and emotional well-being.

Lifespan Considerations

Growth and development are dynamic processes that describe change over time. It is important to understand data collection and interpretation of findings regarding growth and development in relation to normative values. Details about specific variations in the head and neck for different age groups is presented in Chapter 25, Chapter 26, and Chapter 27. ∞

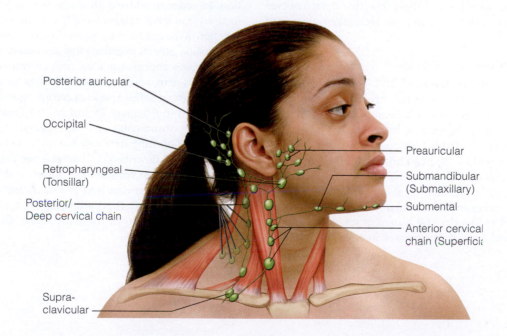

Posterior auricular

Occipital

Retropharyngeal (Tonsillar)

Posterior/ Deep cervical chain

Supra- clavicular

Preauricular

Submandibular (Submaxillary)

Submental

Anterior cervical chain (Superficial)

Figure 13.7 Lymph nodes of the head and neck.

Psychosocial Considerations

Stressors may affect the health status of a patient and result in symptoms such as headaches, neck pain, or mouth ulcers. Additional signs of stress or systemic conditions include pain in the TMJ because of unconscious clenching of the jaw during sleep or stressful situations, such as driving in heavy traffic or taking an exam. Chronic TMJ syndrome may eventually result in a wearing down of the teeth, and the patient may need to consult a dentist or orthodontist. Other indications of psychosocial disturbances include tics (involuntary muscle spasms), hair twisting or pulling, lip biting, and excessive blinking. The nurse will ask the patient about their perceived level of stress and the techniques used to relax or avoid the situations that cause stress.

The nurse should also be aware of psychosocial implications of face, head, and neck disorders that alter the appearance of the patient. The nurse must be knowledgeable about expected findings and variations that may be present. For example, hair loss may cause a patient to feel self-conscious about their appearance. The professional nurse understands that compassionate and thoughtful questioning can reveal information without causing more distress.

Cultural and Environmental Considerations

Cultural beliefs and practices about modesty may influence patient behaviors, and the nurse must be aware and respectful of the patient's needs. An example is that modesty is central to Islamic life and that segregation between men and women has direct implications for nurses caring for Muslim patients. The nurse must be diligent in asking permission before touching a patient and specifically before removing any head covering (Mujallad & Taylor, 2016).

Environmental impacts on the health status of components of the head and neck include patients' physical environment and access to food and other nutrients. Thyroid disease is common in areas where iodine is limited and may lead to deficiency disorders including **goiter** (enlarged thyroid) and hypothyroidism. Although the use of iodized salt has generally decreased iodine deficiencies in the United States, some individuals follow dietary practices that may result in clinical or subclinical deficiency of iodine (Sobiecki, Appleby, Bradbury, & Key, 2016).

Subjective Data—Health History

Assessment of the head and neck includes gathering subjective and objective data. Subjective data collection occurs during the patient interview, before the physical assessment. The nurse will use a variety of communication techniques to elicit general and specific information about the condition of the structures of the head and neck. Health records, the results of laboratory tests, and radiologic and imaging reports are important secondary sources to be reviewed and included in the data-gathering process. The questions in the focused interview form part of the subjective database. See Table 13.1 for information on potential secondary sources of patient data.

Focused Interview

The focused interview for the head and neck concerns data related to the head, the face, and the structures of the neck, including the thyroid, trachea, and lymph nodes. Subjective data are gathered during the focused interview when the nurse observes the patient and listens for cues related to the functions of structures within the head and neck. The nurse may use open-ended and closed questions to obtain information. Follow-up questions or requests for descriptions are required to clarify data or gather missing information. Follow-up questions are intended to identify the source of problems, explain the duration of problems, discuss ways to alleviate problems,

and provide clues about the patient's knowledge about his or her own health.

The information learned during the focused interview guides the physical assessment of the head and neck. The information is always considered in relation to normative values and expectations regarding function of the specific structure. Therefore, the nurse must consider age, gender, race, culture, environment, health practices, past and concurrent problems, and therapies when framing questions and using techniques to elicit information. In order to address all of the factors when conducting a focused interview, categories of questions related to status and function of the head and neck have been developed. These categories include general questions that are asked of all patients, such as questions addressing acute and chronic illness, infections, symptoms, pain, and behaviors, habits, or practices. Other questions that are specific to patients according to age and pregnancy are covered in Chapters 25 and 26. ∞ Finally, questions also address environmental or other special considerations. One approach to eliciting data about symptoms is the OLDCART & ICE method, as described in Chapter 5. See Figure 5.3. ∞

The nurse must consider the patient's ability to participate in the focused interview and physical assessment of the head and neck. If a patient is experiencing pain, stiffness, or anxiety that accompanies any of these problems, attention must focus on relief of symptoms.

Table 13.1 Potential Secondary Sources for Patient Data Related to the Head, Neck, and Related Lymphatics

LABORATORY TESTS	NORMAL VALUES
Thyroid	
TSH	0.3–5.0 mIU/L
T_3	80–190 ng/dL
T_4	5.0–12.5 mcg/dL
Calcitonin	Male: < 16 pg/mL
	Female: < 8 pg/mL
Lymph Nodes	
Complete Blood Count with Differential	Red blood cells (RBC)
	Male: 4.32–5.72 million/microliter (mcL)
	Female: 3.90–5.03 million/microliter (mcL)
	Hemoglobin (Hgb)
	Male: 13.5–17.5 g/dL
	Female: 12.0–15.5 g/dL
	Hematocrit (Hct)
	Male: 38%–50%
	Female: 34%–44.5%
	White blood cells
	Leukocytes 4,500–10,000/mcl
	Bands 0%–3%
	Basophils 0.5%–1%
	Eosinophils 1%–4%
	Lymphocytes 20%–40%
	B-Lymphocytes 4%–25%
	T-Lymphocytes 60%–95%
	Monocytes 2%–8%
	Neutrophils 40%–60%
	Platelets
	150–450 billion/L
	Erythrocyte Sedimentation Rate (ESR)
	Males: < 23 mm/hr
	Females: < 29 mm/hr
Diagnostic Tests	
Biopsy	
Chest X-ray	
Liver/Spleen Scan	
Lymph Nodes	
Biopsy	
Thyroid	
Thyroid Scan	
Ultrasonography	

Focused Interview Questions	Rationales and Evidence

The following section provides sample and follow-up questions in each of the previously mentioned categories. A rationale for each of the questions is provided. The list of questions is not inclusive but, rather, represents the types of questions required in a comprehensive focused interview related to the head and neck. The follow-up bulleted questions are asked in order to obtain additional information and clarification from the patient that will enhance the subjective database. The subjective data collected and the questions asked during the health history and the focused interview will provide data to help meet the goal of preventing head injuries and resulting disabilities.

General Questions

1. **Describe the condition of your scalp today.**
   - Is it different from 2 months ago? From 2 years ago?

   ▶ This question gives patients the opportunity to provide their own perceptions about the condition of the scalp.

2. **Do you have any problems that affect your scalp?**

   ▶ This question elicits information about localized or systemic problems or illnesses that impact the scalp. If the patient identifies any problems, follow-up is required to obtain descriptions and details about what, when, and how problems occur, as well as the duration of each problem.

3. **Has anyone in your family had a problem with his or her scalp or a problem that indirectly affected his or her scalp?**

   ▶ This question may elicit information about illnesses with a familial or genetic predisposition. Follow-up is required to obtain details about specific problems related to occurrence, treatment, and outcomes.

4. **Questions 1, 2, and 3 would be repeated for the skull, face, trachea, thyroid, and lymph nodes.**

(continued)

Focused Interview Questions	Rationales and Evidence

Questions Related to Illness, Infection, or Injury

1. **Have you ever been diagnosed with an illness affecting your head, face, or neck?**
   - When were you diagnosed with the problem?
   - What treatment was prescribed for the problem?
   - Do you use or have you used any strategies to minimize discomfort or otherwise cope with this problem? Was the strategy successful?
   - Has the problem ever recurred (acute)?
   - How are you managing the disease now (chronic)?

   ▶ The patient has an opportunity to provide information about specific illnesses. If a specific disease or illness is identified, follow-up about the date of diagnosis, treatment, and outcomes is required. Data about each illness identified by the patient are essential to an accurate health assessment. Illnesses are classified as acute or chronic, and follow-up regarding each classification will differ.

2. **Do you now have or have you ever had an infection affecting your head, face, or neck?**

   ▶ The patient has an opportunity to provide information about infectious processes. Follow-up would be carried out as in question 1.

3. **Have you ever had any problem with your thyroid gland? Have you had thyroid surgery? Are you currently taking thyroid medication? What symptoms do you associate with your thyroid problem?**

   ▶ Over- or undersecretion by the thyroid gland may cause rapid weight gain or loss, heat or cold intolerance, fatigue, mood swings, tremor, anxiety, tachycardia and palpitations, muscle weakness, changes in skin and hair, and other alterations in health (Dunn & Turner, 2016; Gaitonde, Rowley, & Sweeney, 2012).

4. **Describe any recent or past injury to your head.**
   - Did you lose consciousness?
   - How long were you unconscious?
   - How did it occur?
   - Have problems recurred (acute)?
   - How are you managing the problem now (chronic)?

   ▶ Head injury can result in acute or chronic neurologic problems.

Evidence-Based Practice

Concussion

- Sports injuries, specifically concussions, are a significant clinical and public health concern because of the potential long-term effects including cognitive impairment and mental health problems in some individuals (Manley et al., 2017). In addition to implementing evidence-based guidelines for recognition of concussion, researchers are looking for new ways to measure the severity of the injury and the time needed for recovery or return to play. There is a promising role for advanced brain imaging, a variety of biomarkers, and genetic testing in the assessment of concussion (McCrea et al., 2017).
- A novel method to objectively determine when an athlete can safely return to play after a concussion injury has been uncovered. Athletes who show an elevated plasma tau concentration within 6 hours of a concussive injury tend to have a prolonged return to play time (Gill, Merchant-Borna, Jeromin, Livingston, & Bazarian, 2017).
- In mild traumatic brain injury, researchers found several salivary markers that were up to 85% accurate in determining risk of prolonged post-concussion symptom risk in children (Johnson et al., 2018).

Questions Related to Symptoms, Pain, and Behaviors

When gathering information about symptoms, many questions are required to elicit details and descriptions. Questions are asked in relation to the significance of symptom, specific diseases or problems, and potential follow-up examination or referral. One rationale may be provided for a group of questions in this category.

Questions Related to Symptoms

The following questions refer to specific symptoms associated with the head and neck. For each symptom, questions and follow-up are required. The details to be elicited are the characteristics of the symptom; the onset, duration, and frequency of the symptom; the treatment or remedy for the symptom, including over-the-counter and home remedies; the determination if diagnosis has been sought; the effect of treatments; and family history associated with a symptom or illness.

1. **Have you had any dizziness, loss of consciousness, seizures, or blurred vision? When did each symptom occur? How long did the symptom last? What did you do to relieve the symptom? Does the treatment help?**

   ▶ These symptoms may indicate problems with carotid arteries, cerebral clots or bleeding, recent head injury, or neurologic disease (Osborn, Wraa, Watson, & Holleran, 2013).

Focused Interview Questions	Rationales and Evidence

Questions Related to Symptoms

2. **Have you noticed any swelling, lumps, bumps, or skin sores on your head that have not healed?**

3. **Have you noticed any lumps or swellings on your neck?**

▶ Swellings, masses, and lesions that do not heal may indicate cancer (Centers for Disease Control and Prevention [CDC], 2017).

▶ Lateral neck masses are usually because of enlargement of the cervical lymph nodes, indicative of infection or malignancy. Swelling in the medial aspect of the neck may be indicative of thyroid pathology (Berman, Snyder, & Frandsen, 2016).

Questions Related to Pain

1. **Do you have headaches? If so, please tell me about them.**
   - *Frequency:* How often?
   - *Onset:* How long have you been bothered with this type of headache? When does the headache begin?
   - *Duration:* How long does a typical headache last?
   - *Location:* Where is the pain? On one side of the head? Behind the eyes? In the sinus area?
   - *Character:* Is the pain throbbing, steady, dull, or sharp? On a scale of 0 to 10, with 10 being the strongest, how severe is the pain?
   - *Associated symptoms:* Do you experience any nausea, vomiting, sensitivity to light or noise, muscle pain, or other symptoms along with the headache?
   - *Precipitating factors:* Do you feel that the headaches usually are triggered by stress, alcohol intake, anxiety, menstrual cycle, allergies, or any other factors? Please describe.
   - *Treatment:* What seems to relieve the symptoms? Resting? Medication? Exercise?

2. **Do you experience any problems that precede the headache, such as visual problems?**

3. **Do your headaches occur in episodes? If so, describe the episodes.**
   - Do your headaches increase in severity with each episode?

4. **Have you recently had an infection or cold?**

5. **Has your neck been weak, sore, or stiff?**

▶ Questions 1, 2, and 3 encourage the patient to provide a detailed description of the headache, which is necessary to help determine the cause and possible treatments.

▶ Bright or rapidly changing lights, such as strobe lights, can trigger migraines. Migraines are often accompanied by visual symptoms such as blurry vision, photophobia, and eyelid ptosis (Kurlander, Punjabi, Liu, Sattar, & Guyuron, 2014).

▶ These conditions may be accompanied by headaches.

▶ Neck symptoms may indicate problems with the muscles of the neck or the cervical spinal cord or an infectious problem such as meningitis (Centers for Disease Control and Prevention [CDC], 2016).

Questions Related to Behaviors

1. **Do you now use or have you ever used alcohol, recreational drugs, tobacco products, or caffeine?**
   - How much of the product do you use?
   - When did you start using the product?
   - How long have you used the product?
   - Have you had problems associated with the product?
   - What have you done to deal with the problem?

▶ Use of alcohol, tobacco, and street drugs, as well as caffeine withdrawal, can affect neurologic and neurovascular function and increase headaches (Brust, 2014).

Questions Related to Age and Pregnancy

The focused interview must reflect the anatomic and physiologic differences in the head, neck, and related lymphatics that exist at different times during the age span as well as during pregnancy. Specific questions related to the head, neck, and related lymphatics for each of these groups are provided in Chapter 25, Chapter 26, and Chapter 27. ∞

Questions Related to the Environment

Environment refers to both the internal and external environments. Questions related to the internal environment include all of the previous questions and those associated with internal or physiologic responses. Questions regarding the external environment include those related to home, work, or social environments.

Internal Environment

1. **Are you now experiencing or have you ever had an experience of intermittent or prolonged anxiety or emotional upset?**

▶ Anxiety and situations of emotional upset impact the sympathetic nervous system, producing hormonal responses that affect vascular function. The resultant vasoconstriction can contribute to headache, hypertension, and risk for cardiovascular problems. Stress and tension may precipitate and increase neck pain or stiffness.

(continued)

Focused Interview Questions	Rationales and Evidence

Internal Environment, *continued*

2. Do you now use or have you ever used prescribed or over-the-counter (OTC) medications, home remedies, cultural treatments, or therapies for problems with your head and neck or for any other purpose?

▶ Medications can have side effects and interactions that exacerbate or enhance symptoms. Knowledge of medication usage provides information that assists in the analysis of patient situations and determination of the significance of findings in a comprehensive assessment (Shields, Fox, & Liebrecht, 2018).

External Environment

The following questions deal with substances and irritants found in the physical environment of the patient. These include the indoor and outdoor environments of the home and the workplace and those encountered during travel.

1. Have you ever had irradiation of the head or neck?

▶ Radiation exposure increases the risk for thyroid tumors (Veiga et al., 2016).

2. Are you exposed to chemicals or toxins in your home or work environment (e.g., radiation, acids, bases, detergents, pesticides, fertilizers, solvents, metals, etc.)?

▶ Environmental chemicals and toxins can be precipitating factors for headache and neurologic problems (Centers for Disease Control and Prevention [CDC], 2015).

Patient-Centered Interaction

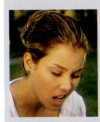

Ms. Dowd, a 20-year-old college sophomore, reports to the university health office with a "very bad headache." Following is part of the focused interview taken by the nurse.

Interview

Nurse: Ms. Dowd, you have already told me you have a headache, and I would like to know more about it. On a scale of zero to ten, with ten being the worst pain, please rate your headache.

Ms. Dowd: Right now my headache is an eight.

Nurse: During the interview, should you need to stop, close your eyes, and relax for a few minutes, let me know.

Ms. Dowd: Okay, but I should be all right.

Nurse: Tell me about your headaches.

Ms. Dowd: I have had this for two to three weeks, on and off. Now it feels like it is all the time, but it is not always eight. Sometimes it is five.

Nurse: Using one or two words, can you describe the pain?

Ms. Dowd: It is usually a dull, constant ache.

Nurse: Describe the location of this dull ache in your head.

Ms. Dowd: It always seems to start at the top of my neck. As it gets worse, it moves up to the top of my head.

Nurse: Are you talking about the right or left side?

Ms. Dowd: Right now it is both sides. That's why I'm here. I can't stand it anymore. Sometimes it's only one side. Sometimes it stays low (pointing to the occipital region) and doesn't come high.

Nurse: Have you always had headaches?

Ms. Dowd: I would have an occasional headache. Sometimes a day or two before my period and then it would go away. Nothing like this, though.

Nurse: What do you think is causing your headaches?

Ms. Dowd: I don't know. I have not been sleeping very well lately. I'm worried about this one course. I can't seem to "get it" and I'm afraid it will kill my GPA. If that happens I will lose my scholarship. I'm working so hard in this course that some of my other work is beginning to slide.

Analysis

The nurse begins the interview with confirmation of the reason for seeking help and then asks the patient to confirm the severity of the pain. The nurse acknowledges Ms. Dowd's pain before seeking more specific subjective data from the patient. Using an open-ended approach encourages Ms. Dowd to communicate more openly.

Objective Data—Physical Assessment

Assessment Techniques and Findings

Physical assessment of the head and neck requires the use of inspection, palpation, and auscultation. During each of the procedures, the nurse is gathering objective data related to the structures of the head and neck and the functions of the structures within them. Inspection includes looking at skin color, the scalp, the skull, and the face for symmetry of bones and structure. The trachea is palpated for position. The thyroid is palpated for movement, texture, and identification of size or abnormalities. The lymph nodes of the head and neck are palpated to evaluate enlargement, tenderness, and mobility. The temporal artery is auscultated. Knowledge of normal parameters and expected findings is essential to interpreting data as the nurse performs the assessment.

EQUIPMENT
- Examination gown
- Clean, nonsterile examination gloves
- Glass of water
- Stethoscope

In adults and children older than 12 to 18 months, the skull should be normocephalic—that is, rounded and symmetric. In all individuals, the frontal parietal and occipital prominences are present and symmetric. The scalp is clear and free of lesions; the hair is evenly distributed. The face is symmetric in shape; the eyes, ears, nose, and mouth are symmetrically placed. The facial movements are smooth and coordinated, and they demonstrate a variety of expressions. The temporal artery feels smooth and firm with no tenderness to palpation and without bruits on auscultation. The TMJ has nonpainful, full, and smooth range of motion. The head is held erect without tremors. The neck is symmetric without swelling and has full range of motion. Carotid artery pulsation is usually visible bilaterally when the patient is lying down. The trachea is midline, and the hyoid bone and tracheal cartilage move with swallowing. The thyroid is not enlarged and is without palpable nodules. The lymph nodes of the head and neck are nonpalpable in adults.

HELPFUL HINTS
- Explain what is expected of the patient for each step of the assessment. Obtain permission to touch the patient during the examination.
- Identify and remedy language or cultural barriers at the outset of the patient interaction.
- Tell the patient the purpose of each procedure and when and if discomfort will accompany any examination.
- Explain to the patient the need to remove any items that would interfere with the assessment, including jewelry, hats, scarves, veils, hairpieces, and wigs.
- Use Standard Precautions.

Techniques and Normal Findings	Abnormal Findings and Special Considerations

The Head

1. **Position the patient.**
   - Ask the patient to sit comfortably on the examination table (see Figure 13.8 ■).

Figure 13.8 Patient is positioned.

2. **Instruct the patient.**
   - Explain that you will be looking at the patient and touching the head, hair, and face. Explain that no discomfort should occur, but if the patient experiences pain or discomfort you will stop that part of the examination.

(continued)

Techniques and Normal Findings	Abnormal Findings and Special Considerations

3. Inspect the head and scalp.

- Note the size, shape, symmetry, and integrity of the head and scalp. Identify the prominences—frontal, parietal, and occipital—that determine the shape and symmetry of the head.
- Part the hair and look for scaliness of the scalp, lesions, infestations, or foreign bodies. (Refer to Chapter 12, Figure 12.14. ∞)
- Check hair distribution and hygiene.

4. Inspect the face.

- Note the facial expression and symmetry of structures. The eyes, ears, nose, and mouth should be symmetrically placed. Inspect the symmetry of the lips at rest and when speaking. The nasolabial folds should be equal. The palpebral fissures should be equal. The top of the pinnae of the ear should be at the level of the outer canthi of the eyes (refer to Figure 13.2).

5. Observe movements of the head, face, and eyes.

- All movements should be smooth and with purpose. Cranial nerves III (Oculomotor), IV (Trochlear), and VI (Abducens) control movement of the eye. Cranial nerve V (Trigeminal) stimulates movement for mastication. Cranial nerve VII (Facial) controls movement of the face. A detailed discussion of the cranial nerves is found in Chapter 24. ∞

▶ Jerky movements or tics may be the result of neurologic or psychologic disorders.

6. Palpate the head and scalp.

- Note the texture of the scalp and the contour and size of the head. Ask the patient to report any tenderness as you palpate. Normally there is no tenderness with palpation.

▶ Note any tenderness, swelling, edema, or masses, which require further evaluation. Ask permission before palpation because touching of the head is prohibited in some cultures.

7. Confirm skin and tissue integrity.

- The skin should be intact.

▶ Note any alteration in skin or tissue integrity related to ulcerations, rashes, discolorations, or swellings.

8. Palpate the temporal artery.

- Palpate between the eye and the top of the ear (see Figure 13.9 ■). The artery should feel smooth.

▶ Any thickening or tenderness could indicate inflammation of the artery.

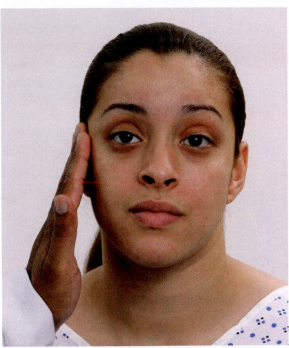

Figure 13.9 Palpating the temporal artery.

9. Auscultate the temporal artery.

- Use the bell of the stethoscope to auscultate for a bruit (a soft blowing sound). Bruits are not normally present.

▶ A bruit is indicative of stenosis (narrowing) of the vessel.

10. Test the range of motion of the TMJ.

- Place your fingers in front of each ear and ask the patient to open and close the mouth slowly. There should be no limitation of movement or tenderness. You should feel a slight indentation of the joint. For more detail on assessment of the TMJ, see Chapter 23. ∞
- Soft clicking noises on movement are sometimes heard and are considered normal.

▶ Any limitation of movement or tenderness on movement requires further evaluation. **Crepitation**, a crackling sound on movement, may indicate joint problems.

Techniques and Normal Findings	Abnormal Findings and Special Considerations

The Neck

1. Instruct the patient.
- Explain that you will be looking at and touching the front and sides of the patient's neck. Tell the patient that you will provide specific instructions for special tests. Advise the patient to inform you of any discomfort.

2. Inspect the neck for skin color, integrity, shape, and symmetry.
- Observe for any swelling of the lymph nodes below the angle of the jaw and along the sternocleidomastoid muscle.
- The head should be held erect with no tremors.

3. Test the range of motion of the neck.
- Ask the patient to slowly move the chin to the chest, turn the head right and left, then touch the left ear to left shoulder and the right ear to right shoulder (without raising the shoulders). Then ask the patient to extend the head back. There should be no pain and no limitation of movement. For further discussion, see Chapter 23 and Chapter 24. ∞

4. Observe the carotid arteries and jugular veins.
- The carotid artery runs just below the angle of the jaw, and its pulsations can frequently be seen. Assessment of the carotid arteries and jugular veins is discussed fully in Chapter 19. ∞

5. Palpate the trachea.
- Palpate the sternal notch. Move the finger pad of the palpating finger off the notch to the midline of the neck. Lightly palpate the area. You will feel the C rings (cricoid cartilage) of the trachea.
- Move the finger laterally, first to the right and then to the left. You have now identified the lateral borders of the trachea (see Figure 13.10 ■).

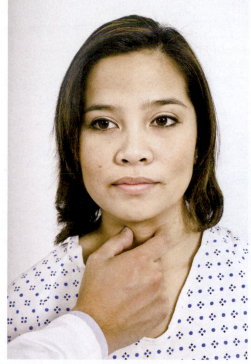

Figure 13.10 Palpating the trachea.

- The trachea should be midline, and the distance to the sternocleidomastoid muscles on each side should be equal. Place the thumb and index finger on each side of the trachea and slide them upward. As the trachea begins to widen, you have now identified the thyroid cartilage. Continue to slide your thumb and index finger high into the neck. Palpate the hyoid bone. The greater horns of the hyoid bone are most prominent. Confirm that the hyoid bone and tracheal cartilages move when the patient swallows.

▶ In the obese patient with a short neck, any assessments of structures in the neck can be difficult. Alternate methods may be required—for example, a Doppler stethoscope to assess pulses.

▶ Excessive rigidity of the neck may indicate arthritis. Inability to hold the neck erect may be because of muscle spasms. Swelling of the lymph nodes may indicate infection and requires further assessment.

▶ Any pain or limitation of movement could indicate arthritis, muscle spasm, or inflammation. Rapid movement and compression of the cerebral vertebrae may cause dizziness.

▶ Any distention or prominence may indicate a vascular disorder.

▶ Tracheal displacement is the result of masses in the neck or mediastinum, pneumothorax, or pulmonary fibrosis. Palpating the trachea may be difficult in the obese patient; ultrasound-guided identification of the structures is sometimes used (Kristensen et al., 2015).

(continued)

Techniques and Normal Findings	Abnormal Findings and Special Considerations

6. Inspect the thyroid gland.

- The thyroid is not observable normally until the patient swallows. Give the patient a cup of water.
- Distinguish the thyroid from other structures in the neck by asking the patient to drink a sip of water.
- The thyroid tissue is attached to the trachea, and, as the patient swallows, it moves superiorly. You may want to adjust the lighting in the room if possible so that shadows are not cast on the patient's neck. This may help you to visualize the thyroid.

7. Palpate the thyroid gland from behind the patient.

- Palpation of the thyroid gland is difficult and requires practice. Although not all nurses will be required to perform this assessment skill, the nurse should be familiar with the basic steps involved, as well as its purpose.
- Stand behind the patient.
- Ask the patient to sit up straight, lower the chin, and turn the head slightly to the right.
- This position causes the patient's neck muscles to relax.
- Using the fingers of your left hand, push the trachea to the right. Use light pressure during palpation to avoid obliterating findings.
- With the fingers of the right hand, palpate the area between the trachea and the sternocleidomastoid muscle. Slowly and gently retract the sternocleidomastoid muscle and then ask the patient to drink a sip of water. Palpate as the thyroid gland moves up during swallowing (see Figure 13.11 ■). Normally, you will not feel the thyroid gland, although in some patients with long, thin necks, you may be able to feel the isthmus. You may be able to feel the fullness of the thyroid as it moves up upon swallowing.
- Reverse the procedure for the left side.

▶ If the patient has any enlargement of the thyroid or masses near the thyroid, they appear as bulges when the patient swallows.

▶ An enlarged thyroid gland may be because of a metabolic disorder such as **hyperthyroidism** or **hypothyroidism**. Palpable masses of 5 mm or larger are alterations in health. Their location, size, and shape should be documented, and the patient should be evaluated further. In pregnancy, a slightly enlarged thyroid can be a normal finding. Most pathologic hyperthyroidism in pregnancy is caused by Graves disease, an autoimmune disorder that causes increased production of thyroid hormones.

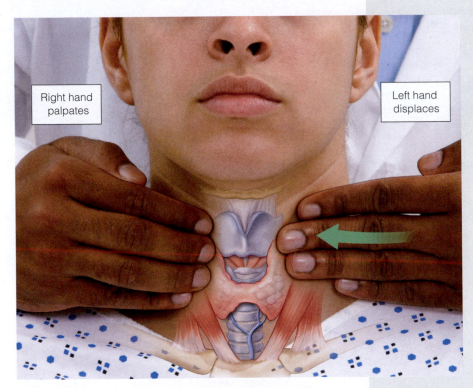

Right hand palpates

Left hand displaces

Figure 13.11 Palpating the thyroid using a posterior approach.

8. *Alternative Approach:* Palpate the thyroid gland from in front of the patient.

   - Stand in front of the patient. Ask the patient to lower the head and turn slightly to the right. Using the thumb of your right hand, push the trachea to the right (see Figure 13.12 ■).
   - Place your left thumb and fingers over the sternocleidomastoid muscle and feel for any enlargement of the right lobe as the patient swallows. Have water available to make swallowing easier. Reverse the procedure for the left side.

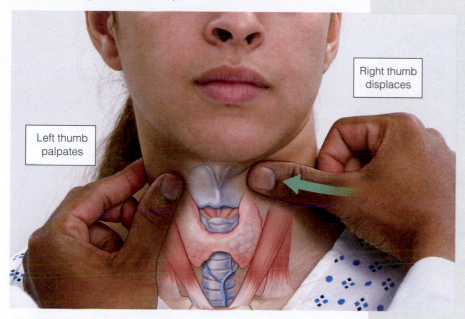

Right thumb displaces

Left thumb palpates

Figure 13.12 Alternative technique for palpating the thyroid.

9. **Auscultate the thyroid.**

   - If the thyroid is enlarged, the area over the thyroid is auscultated to detect any bruits. In an enlarged thyroid, blood flows through the arteries at an accelerated rate, producing a soft, rushing sound. This sound can best be detected with the bell of the stethoscope.

   ▶ The presence of a bruit is abnormal and is an indication of increased blood flow, caused by a partially blocked blood vessel.

10. **Palpate the lymph nodes of the head and neck.**

    - Palpate the lymph nodes by exerting gentle circular pressure with the finger pads of two or three fingers of both hands. It is important to avoid strong pressure, which can push the nodes into the muscle and underlying structures, making them difficult to find. It is also important to establish a routine for assessment; otherwise, it is possible to omit one or more of the groups of nodes.

    ▶ Enlargement of lymph nodes is called **lymphadenopathy** and can be because of infection, allergies, or a tumor.

(continued)

Techniques and Normal Findings	Abnormal Findings and Special Considerations

Techniques and Normal Findings

- The following is one suggested order of assessment (see Figure 13.13 ■).

  1. Preauricular
  2. Posterior auricular
  3. Occipital
  4. Retropharyngeal (tonsillar)
  5. Submandibular
  6. Submental (with one hand)
  7. Anterior/superficial cervical chain
  8. Posterior/deep cervical chain
  9. Supraclavicular

Abnormal Findings and Special Considerations

▶ Lymph nodes are normally nonpalpable in adults, infants, and adolescents. They may be palpable in children between the ages of 1 and 11 years (see Figure 13.13B ■).

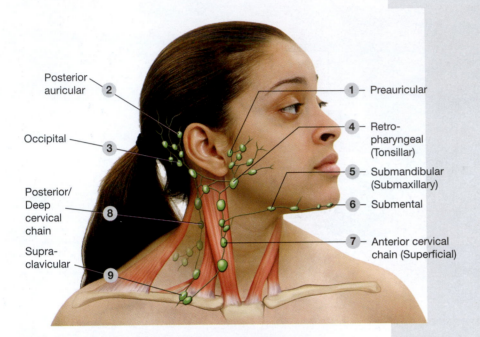

A.

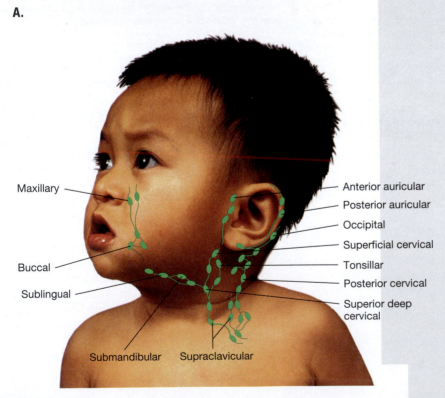

B.

Figure 13.13 A. Suggested sequence for palpating lymph nodes. B. Location of the head and neck lymph nodes in children.

Techniques and Normal Findings	Abnormal Findings and Special Considerations

- Ask the patient to relax the muscles of the neck to make the nodes easier to palpate. It is helpful to have the patient shrug the shoulders when palpating the supraclavicular nodes. If any lymph nodes are palpable, make a note of their location, size, shape, fixation or mobility, and tenderness (see Figure 13.14 ■).

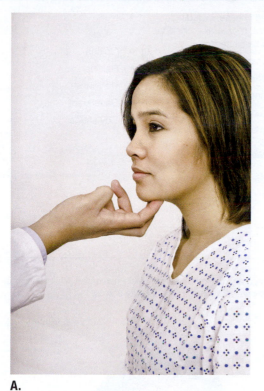

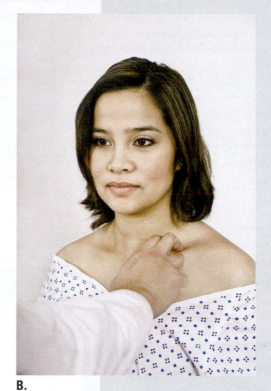

A.   **B.**

Figure 13.14 Palpating lymph nodes. A. Submental. B. Supraclavicular.

Documenting Your Findings

Documentation of assessment data—subjective and objective—must be accurate, professional, complete, and confidential. When documenting the information from the assessment of the head and neck, the nurse should use measurements where appropriate to ensure accuracy; use medical terminology rather than jargon; include all pertinent information; and avoid language that could identify the patient.

The use of measurements is relevant when documenting skin or scalp lesions, circumference of the head, and the size of any palpable lymph nodes. The nurse must use the metric measurements rather than comparison to some other object.

In addition, the documentation must be complete by including location, color, texture, size, tenderness, and any other descriptors as appropriate. Use the medical language that accurately communicates your findings to other healthcare professionals.

An example of effective documentation is *R anterior cervical lymph node, 1 cm, firm, mobile, non-tender.* An example of documentation that you should *not* use is *"Lymph node on R side of neck, size of small grape, moveable, squishy."* Please refer to the Key Terms at the beginning of the chapter to help you with language selection.

Abnormal Findings

Abnormal findings in the head and neck include headaches, abnormalities in the size and contour of the skull, malformations or abnormalities of the face and neck, and thyroid disorders. Table 13.2 provides an overview of skull and face abnormalities that are associated with common disorders. Headaches and thyroid disorders are discussed in the following sections.

Headaches

Headaches vary in terms of type and duration. Likewise, the cause of a headache, or its trigger, may vary among individuals. Especially with regard to migraine headaches, tyramine-rich foods and nitrates are believed to be potential headache triggers (see Box 13.1).

Box 13.1   Tyramine-Rich Foods

- Aged cheese, including Swiss, mozzarella, cheddar, and blue cheese
- Avocados
- Beer on tap
- Canned soup
- Cured meats
- Homemade yeast breads

- Nuts
- Olives
- Onions
- Raisins
- Red wine
- Sauerkraut
- Soy sauce

Sources: WebMD (2014, 2017).

Table 13.2 Abnormalities of the Head and Neck

Acromegaly	**Bell's Palsy**
Enlargement of the bones, facial features, hands, and feet because of the increased production of growth hormone by the pituitary gland.	A sudden, temporary disorder affecting cranial nerve VII (Facial) that produces unilateral facial paralysis. It may be caused by a virus.

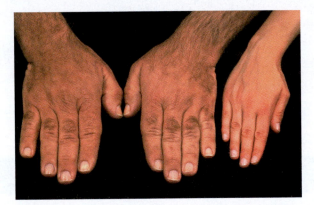

Figure 13.15 Acromegaly.
Source: Mediscan/Alamy Stock Photo.

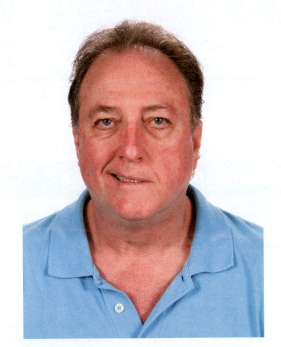

Figure 13.16 Bell's palsy.
Source: Steven Frame/123RF.

(continued)

Table 13.2 Abnormalities of the Head and Neck (continued)

Cerebrovascular Accident (CVA, stroke, brain attack)
As with Bell's palsy, neurologic deficits associated with CVA can include facial paralysis. However, unlike Bell's palsy, neurologic effects of a CVA extend to other body regions as well.

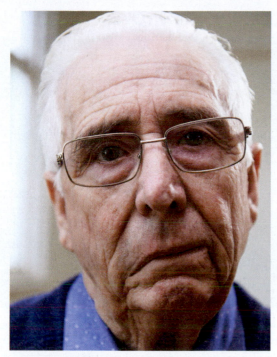

Figure 13.17 Cerebrovascular accident.
Source: Ian Allenden/123RF.

Craniosynostosis
Early closure of sagittal sutures causes the head to elongate; early closure of coronal sutures alters the head, face, and orbits.

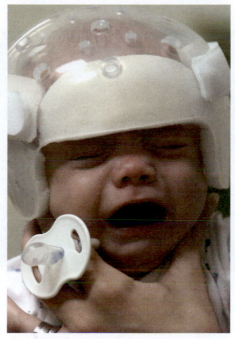

Figure 13.18 Craniosynostosis.
Source: ZUMA Press Inc/Alamy Stock Photo.

Cushing Syndrome
Increased cortisol production by the adrenal gland leads to a rounded "moon" face, ruddy cheeks, prominent jowls, pink or purple stretch marks, and excess facial hair.

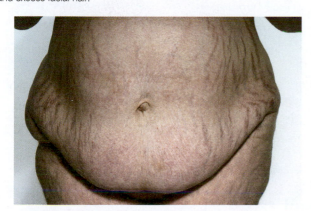

Figure 13.19 Cushing syndrome.
Source: Mediscan/Alamy Stock Photo.

Down Syndrome
A chromosomal defect causing varying degrees of intellectual disability and characteristic facial features such as slanted eyes; a flat nasal bridge; a flat nose; a protruding tongue; and a short, broad neck.

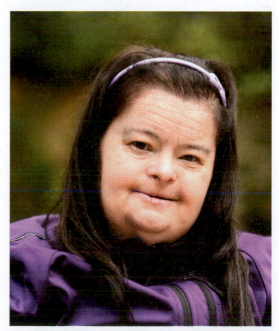

Figure 13.20 Down syndrome.
Source: Marcel Jancovic/Shutterstock.

(continued)

Table 13.2 Abnormalities of the Head and Neck (continued)

Fetal Alcohol Syndrome (FAS)

A disorder characterized by epicanthal folds, narrow palpebral fissures, a deformed upper lip below the septum of the nose, and some degree of intellectual disability; caused by fetal exposure to high levels of alcohol.

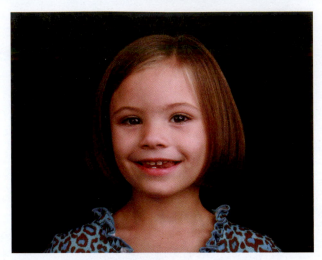

Figure 13.21 Fetal alcohol syndrome.

Source: Rick's Photography/Shutterstock.

Hydrocephalus

Enlargement of the head caused by inadequate drainage of cerebrospinal fluid, resulting in abnormal growth of the skull.

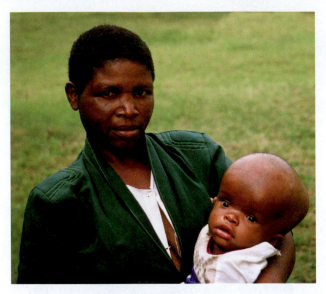

Figure 13.22 Hydrocephalus.

Source: Ulrich Doering/Alamy Stock Photo.

Parkinson Disease

A masklike expression occurs in Parkinson disease. The disease is the result of a decrease in the production of the neurotransmitter dopamine.

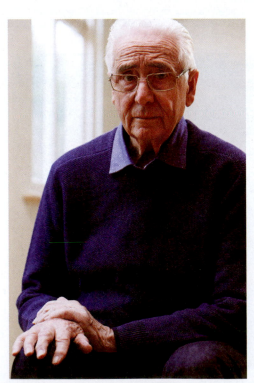

Figure 13.23 Parkinson disease.

Source: Ian Allenden/123RF.

Torticollis

A spasm of the muscles supplied by the spinal accessory nerve, causing lateral flexion contracture of the cervical spine musculature. Caused by cervical problems such as trauma, tumors, or scars.

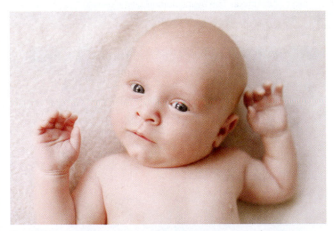

Figure 13.24 Torticollis.

Source: Bohemian soul/Shutterstock.

CLASSIC MIGRAINE

Migraine is an episodic primary headache disorder, affecting approximately 11% of adults worldwide. The most common type is migraine without aura with symptoms of headache, nausea, vomiting, photophobia, and phonophobia. Untreated or unsuccessfully treated migraines can last 4 to 72 hours and sometimes require the individual to stay in a dark, quiet room to rest. Approximately 25% of people with migraine experience an aura, or prodrome, of short-term and fully reversible neurological symptoms such as flashing lights, tingling or numbness, or changes in mood (Vetvik & MacGregor, 2017). The pain of the migraine itself may be mild or debilitating, requiring the patient to lie down in the darkness in silence. It is usually a pulsating pain that is localized to the side, front, or back of the head and may be accompanied by nausea, vertigo, tremors, and other symptoms. The acute phase of a classic migraine typically lasts from 4 to 6 hours.

CLUSTER HEADACHE

A cluster headache is so named because numerous episodes occur over a period of days or even months and then are followed by a period of remission during which no headaches occur. Cluster headaches have no aura. Their onset is sudden and may be associated with alcohol consumption, stress, or emotional distress. They often begin suddenly at night with an excruciating pain on one side of the face spreading upward behind one eye. The nose and affected eye water, and nasal congestion is common. A cluster headache may last for only a few minutes or up to a few hours.

TENSION HEADACHE

A tension headache, also known as a muscle contraction headache, occurs because of sustained contraction of the muscles in the head, neck, or upper back. The onset is gradual, not sudden, and the pain is usually steady, not throbbing. The pain may be unilateral or bilateral and typically ranges from the cervical region to the top of the head. Tension headaches may be associated with stress, overwork, position, dental problems, premenstrual syndrome, sinus inflammation, or other health problems.

Thyroid Abnormalities

Thyroid disorders may stem from various causes. The primary manifestations of a thyroid disorder depend on whether the thyroid is producing too much or too little thyroid hormones.

HYPERTHYROIDISM

Hyperthyroidism is excessive production of thyroid hormones.

Subjective findings:

- Irritability/nervousness
- Muscle weakness and fatigue
- Amenorrhea
- Insomnia
- Heat intolerance

Objective findings:

- Thyroid gland enlargement
- Exophthalmos (bulging eyes)
- Cardiac changes, including tachycardia (heart rate > 100 bpm) and cardiac dysrhythmias (abnormal heart rhythms)
- Integumentary changes, including skin thinning and fine, brittle hair
- Weight loss
- Increased diaphoresis (sweating)

HYPOTHYROIDISM

Hypothyroidism occurs when there is a decrease in production of thyroid hormones. The decrease in thyroid hormones results in lowered basal metabolism. The most common occurrence in hypothyroidism is loss of thyroid tissue as a result of iodine deficiency or an autoimmune response. It may be a result of decreased pituitary stimulation of the thyroid gland or lack of hypothalamic thyroid-releasing factor. Hypothyroidism occurs most frequently in females between ages 30 and 50.

Subjective findings:

- Weakness/feeling tired
- Depression
- Heavy menstrual periods
- Difficulty concentrating
- Cold intolerance

Objective findings:

- Constipation
- Integumentary changes, including dry skin and weak nails
- Weight gain
- Cool skin

THYROID-RELATED DISORDERS

Manifestations of thyroid disorders vary depending on whether the disorder involves hypothyroidism or hyperthyroidism. Goiter, which is an enlargement of the thyroid gland, may be caused by increased (hyper-) or decreased (hypo-) thyroid function. An overview of other selected thyroid disorders is provided in Table 13.3.

Table 13.3 Overview of Selected Thyroid Disorders

CONDITION	DESCRIPTION
Graves Disease	• Most common type of hyperthyroidism • No known cause; may be an autoimmune response or related to hereditary factors
Thyroid adenoma	• Benign thyroid nodules that occur most frequently in older adults • No known cause
Thyroid carcinoma	• Involves presence of malignant tumors in hormone-producing cells or supporting cells • Excess thyroid hormone production in the tumors • May occur following radiation of the thyroid, chronic goiter, or as a result of hereditary factors
Medication-induced hyperthyroidism	• Excessive iodine in some medications causing oversecretion of thyroid hormones
Congenital hypothyroidism	• Nonfunctioning thyroid at birth • Left untreated, results in retardation of physical and mental growth
Myxedema	• Severe form of hypothyroidism • Causes nonpitting edema throughout the body and thickening of facial features • Major organ systems possibly adversely affected by complications • Myxedema coma resulting in cardiovascular collapse, electrolyte disturbances, respiratory depression, and cerebral hypoxia
Thyroiditis	• Inflammation of the thyroid gland • Inflammation causing release of stored hormones, resulting in temporary hyperthyroidism that may last weeks or months • May manifest as hypothyroidism (American Thyroid Association, 2014)
Postpartum thyroiditis	• Temporary condition occurring in 5% to 9% of females postpartum • May manifest as temporary thyrotoxicosis (hyperthyroidism) followed by temporary hypothyroidism (American Thyroid Association, 2014)
Hashimoto thyroiditis	• Autoimmune disease that results in primary hypothyroidism • Occurs most frequently in females • Tends to be familial

Application Through Critical Thinking

CASE STUDY

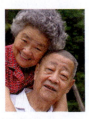

Source: Jack.Q/ Shutterstock.

A married couple has come to the clinic for renewal of prescriptions and annual flu shots. During the encounter, the husband mentions to the nurse that he is concerned about his 69-year-old wife. He tells the nurse that she has become very forgetful. She eats very little but has seemed to gain weight. She seems "down" all the time. When questioned, the wife states she "just hasn't been herself." She admits she doesn't have much of an appetite. She explains that she has not been as active as she used to be and as a result her bowels are not as regular. She thinks those are the reasons she feels "out of sorts." She chides her husband that his memory "isn't so hot either." He insists that she is forgetting simple things and that he has always forgotten to write down phone messages and birthdays and such.

The nurse is concerned about this patient and carries out a further interview, which reveals the following findings: The patient is generally cold, feels tired all of the time, and really doesn't have the energy to do much around the house. She finds the thought of going out exhausting. She tells the nurse that her tongue feels thick and she thinks her voice has changed.

The patient agrees to a physical examination. The findings include a weight gain of 10 lb from her last clinic visit, 6 months ago. Her thyroid is enlarged and palpable. Her skin is dry, she has edema of the lower extremities, and her speech is slow. Her abdomen is distended with bowel sounds in all quadrants.

The nurse recommends that this woman have laboratory testing for thyroid dysfunction and arranges for consultation with a physician. The nurse schedules a follow-up appointment and makes some recommendations for this patient that include increasing fluid intake and fiber to improve bowel function. The patient is advised to wear warm clothing and to rest frequently. The nurse explains the functions of the thyroid and that medication can improve all aspects of her current condition when taken regularly.

COMPLETE DOCUMENTATION

The following information is summarized from the case study.

Subjective Data "Just haven't been myself." Loss of appetite, decreased activity, irregular bowel function. Generally cold, tired, lack of energy, thick tongue, and change in voice. Husband states that wife is forgetful, eats very little, has gained weight, and seems "down."

Objective Data BP 120/76—P 64—T 98.4. Alert and oriented. Unable to repeat list of five words after 5 minutes. Weight gain 10 lb over 6 months. Thyroid enlarged and palpable. Skin cool, dry, edema lower extremities. Slow speech. Abdomen distended. Bowel sounds present all quadrants.

CRITICAL THINKING QUESTIONS

1. What may be responsible for the findings about this 69-year-old female?

2. What further data should the nurse collect?

3. What aspects of physical assessment and what tests are important in arriving at a diagnosis for this patient?

4. How could you determine if depression was causing the symptoms of "feeling down" and lack of energy?

5. How would you approach the situation if the patient and her husband are Muslim and she is required to keep her head covered?

REFERENCES

American Thyroid Association. (2014). *What is thyroiditis?* Retrieved from http://www.thyroid.org/what-is-thyroiditis

Berman, A., Snyder, S. J., & Frandsen, G. (2016). *Kozier & Erb's fundamentals of nursing: Concepts, process, and practice* (10th ed.). Hoboken, NJ: Pearson.

Brust, J. C. (2014). Neurological complications of illicit drug abuse. *CONTINUUM: Lifelong Learning in Neurology, 20*(3), 642–656. doi:10.1212/01.CON.0000450971.99322.cd

Centers for Disease Control and Prevention (CDC). (2015). *Workplace safety & health topics: Indoor environmental quality.* Retrieved from http://www.cdc.gov/niosh/topics/indoorenv/chemicalsodors.html

Centers for Disease Control and Prevention (CDC). (2016). *Meningitis: Viral meningitis.* Retrieved from http://www.cdc.gov/meningitis/viral.html

Centers for Disease Control and Prevention (CDC). (2017). *Skin cancer—what are the symptoms?* Retrieved from http://www.cdc.gov/cancer/skin/basic_info/symptoms.htm

Dunn, D., & Turner, C. (2016). Hypothyroidism in women. *Nursing for Women's Health, 20*(1), 93–98. doi:10.1016/j.nwh.2015.12.002

Gaitonde, D. Y., Rowley, K. D., & Sweeney, L. B. (2012). Hypothyroidism: An update. *South African Family Practice, 54*(5), 384–390. doi:10.1080/20786204.2012.10874256

Gill, J., Merchant-Borna, K., Jeromin, A., Livingston, W., & Bazarian, J. (2017). Acute plasma tau relates to prolonged return to play after concussion. *Neurology, 88*(6), 595–602. doi:10.1212/WNL.0000000000003587

Johnson, J. J., Loeffert, A. C., Stokes, J., Olympia, R. P., Bramley, H., & Hicks, S. D. (2018). Association of salivary microRNA changes with prolonged concussion symptoms. *JAMA Pediatrics, 172*(1), 65–73. doi:10.1001/jamapediatrics.2017.3884

Kristensen, M. S., Teoh, W. H., Rudolph, S. S., Tvede, M. F., Hesselfeldt, R. , Borglum, J., . . . Hansen, L. N. (2015). Structured approach to ultrasound-guided identification of the cricothyroid membrane: a randomized comparison with the palpation method in the morbidly obese. *British Journal of Anaesthesia, 114*(6), 1003–1004. doi:10.1093/bja/aev123

Kurlander, D. E., Punjabi, A., Liu, M. T., Sattar, A., & Guyuron, B. (2014). In-depth review of symptoms, triggers, and treatment of temporal migraine headaches (Site II). *Plastic and Reconstructive Surgery, 133*(4), 897–903. doi:10.1097/PRS.0000000000000045

Manley, G., Gardner, A. J., Schneider, K. J., Guskiewicz, K. M., Bailes, J., Cantu, R. C., . . . Iverson, G. L. (2017). A systematic review of potential long-term effects of sport-related concussion. *British Journal of Sports Medicine, 51*(12), 969–977. doi:10.1136/bjsports-2017-097791)

Marieb, E., & Keller, S. (2018). *Essentials of human anatomy and physiology* (12th ed.). New York, NY: Pearson

McCrea, M., Meier, T., Huber, D., Ptito, A., Bigler, E., Debert, C. T., . . . McAllister, T. (2017). Role of advanced neuroimaging, fluid biomarkers and genetic testing in the assessment of sport-related concussion: A systematic review. *British Journal of Sports Medicine, 51*(12), 919–929. doi:10.1136/bjsports-2016-097447

Mujallad, A., & Taylor, E. J. (2016). Modesty among Muslim women: Implications for nursing care. *MEDSURG Nursing, 25*(3), 169–172. Retrieved from http://www.ajj.com/services/pblshng/msnj/default.htm

Osborn, K. S., Wraa, C. E., Watson, A., & Holleran, R. S. (2013). *Medical-surgical nursing: Preparation for practice* (2nd ed.). Upper Saddle River, NJ: Pearson.

Shields, K. M., Fox, K. L., & Liebrecht, C. (2018). *Pearson nurse's drug guide.* Hoboken, NJ: Pearson.

Sobiecki, J. G., Appleby, P. N., Bradbury, K. E., & Key, T. J. (2016). High compliance with dietary recommendations in a cohort of meat eaters, fish eaters, vegetarians, and vegans: Results from the European Prospective Investigation into Cancer and Nutrition–Oxford Study. *Nutrition Research*, *36*(5), 464–477. doi:10.1016/j.nutres.2015.12.016

Veiga, L. H., Holmberg, E., Anderson, H., Pottern, L., Sadetzki, S., Adams, J. M., . . . Lubin, J. H. (2016). Thyroid cancer after childhood exposure to external radiation: An updated pooled analysis of 12 studies. *Radiation Research*, *185*(5), 473–484. doi:10.1667/RR14213.1

Vetvik, K. G., & MacGregor, E. A. (2017). Sex differences in the epidemiology, clinical features, and pathophysiology of migraine. *The Lancet Neurology*, *16*(1), 76–87. doi:10.1016/S1474-4422(16)30293-9

WebMD. (2014). *Frequently asked questions about food triggers, migraines, and headaches*. Retrieved from http://www.webmd.com/migraines-headaches/guide/triggers-specific-foods

WebMD. (2017). *Tyramine and migraines*. Retrieved from http://www.webmd.com/migraines-headaches/guide/tyramine-and-migraines

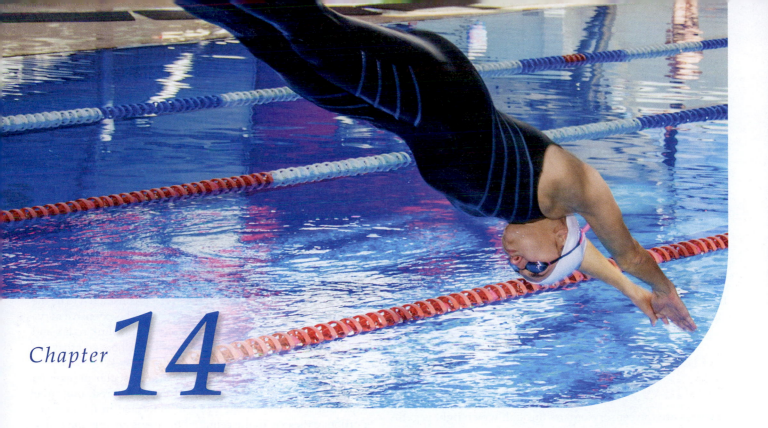

Chapter 14

Eyes

LEARNING OUTCOMES

Upon completion of this chapter, you will be able to:

1. Describe the anatomy and physiology of the eyes.

2. Identify the anatomic, physiologic, developmental, psychosocial, and cultural variations that guide assessment of the eyes.

3. Determine which questions about the eyes to use for the focused interview.

4. Outline the techniques for assessment of the eyes.

5. Generate the appropriate documentation to describe the assessment of the eyes.

6. Identify abnormal findings in the physical assessment of the eyes.

KEY TERMS

MEDICAL LANGUAGE

extra-	Prefix meaning "outside"	**ophthalm-**	Prefix meaning "eye"
-graphy	Suffix meaning "process of recording"	**-opia**	Suffix meaning "vision condition"
-itis	Suffix meaning "inflammation"	**photo-**	Prefix meaning "light"

Introduction

The eyes are an important part of the sensory perception of the human body. The special senses—smell, taste, touch, hearing, and vision—give humans the ability to process complex stimuli from the environment. The eyes are complex sensory organs containing nearly 70% of all of the sensory receptors in the body. Together with the neurologic system, our eyes help us process the world around us (Marieb & Keller, 2018).

Anatomy and Physiology Review

The eyes are the sensory organs through which light is gathered and sent to the brain for interpretation to produce vision. Located in the orbital cavities of the skull, only the anterior aspect of the eye is exposed. The various parts of the eye along with the accessory structures, enable vision, provide protection, and are responsible for movement of the eye. Each of these anatomic structures is described in the following sections.

Eye

The eye, commonly called the eyeball, is a fluid-filled sphere having a diameter of approximately 2.5 cm (1 in.). The eye receives light waves and transmits these waves to the brain for interpretation as visual images. Only a small portion of the eye is seen. Most of the eye is set into and protected by the bony orbit of the skull (see Figure 14.1 ■).

The eye is composed of three layers: the sclera, the choroids, and the retina. The **sclera**, the outermost layer, is an extremely dense, hard, fibrous membrane that helps to maintain the shape of the eye. It is the white fibrous part of the eye that is seen anteriorly. Its primary function is to support and protect the structures of the eye (see Figure 14.2 ■).

The **cornea** is the clear, transparent part of the sclera and forms the anterior one-sixth of the eye. It is considered to be the window of the eye, allowing light to enter. The extensive nerve endings in the cornea are responsible for the blink reflex and an increase in the secretion of tears for protection, and they are most sensitive to pain.

The **choroid**, the middle layer, is the vascular-pigmented layer of the eye. The **iris** is the circular, colored, muscular aspect of this layer of the eye and is located in the anterior portion of the eye. In the center of the iris is an opening called the **pupil**, which allows light to travel inside the eye. The iris responds to light by making the pupil larger or smaller, thereby controlling the amount of light that enters the eye. A dim light will cause the iris to respond, enlarging the pupil size (**mydriasis**). This increases the amount of light entering the eye, enhancing distance vision. A bright light causes the iris to respond by decreasing pupil size (**miosis**), thus decreasing the amount of light entering the eye and accommodating near vision. The third cranial nerve controls pupillary constriction and dilation. The parasympathetic branch of this nerve stimulates pupillary constriction; the sympathetic branch stimulates dilation of the pupil.

The third and innermost membrane, the **retina**, is the sensory portion of the eye. The retina, a direct extension of the optic nerve,

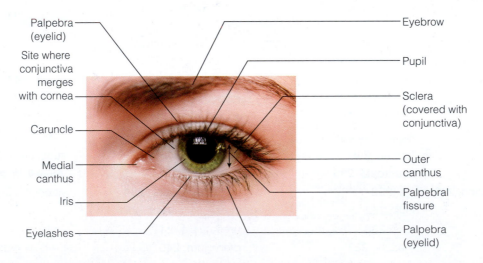

Figure 14.1 Structures of the external eye.
Source: Bo Valentino/Shutterstock.

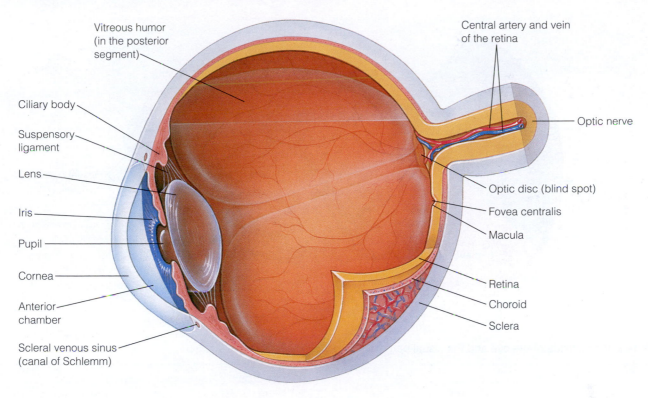

Ciliary body

Suspensory ligament

Lens

Iris

Pupil

Cornea

Anterior chamber

Scleral venous sinus (canal of Schlemm)

Vitreous humor (in the posterior segment)

Central artery and vein of the retina

Optic nerve

Optic disc (blind spot)

Fovea centralis

Macula

Retina

Choroid

Sclera

Figure 14.2 Interior of the eye.

helps to change light waves to neuroimpulses for interpretation as visual impulses by the brain. The retina contains many rods and cones; the rods function in dim light and are also considered to be peripheral vision receptors; the cones function in bright light, are central vision receptors, and provide color to sight.

The **optic disc**, on the nasal aspect of the retina, is round with clear margins. It is usually creamy yellow and is the point at which the optic nerve and retina meet. The color of the disc and the retinal background differ according to skin color. The color is lighter in persons with light skin color and darker in individuals with darker skin color. The center of this disc, the physiologic cup, is the point at which the vascular network enters the eye.

The **macula** is responsible for central vision. The macula, with its yellow, pitlike center called the *fovea centralis*, appears as a hyperpigmented spot on the temporal aspect of the retina.

Refraction of the Eye

Light rays travel in a straight line. For vision to occur, light rays must be reflected off an object and then transmitted through the cornea. The cornea refracts (bends) the light rays, directing them to pass through the pupil and into the eye. As light travels through the eye, each structure in its pathway has a different density. Several structures of the eye help with the deflection or refraction of the light rays. The structures responsible for refraction include the cornea, aqueous humor, crystalline lens, and vitreous humor.

Refraction allows the light rays to enter the eye and be aimed (reflected) to the correct part of the retina for most accurate vision. **Emmetropia** is the normal refractive condition of the

eye. **Myopia** (nearsightedness) is a condition in which the light rays focus in front of the retina. In **hyperopia** (farsightedness) the light rays focus behind the retina.

The **aqueous humor** is a clear, fluidlike substance found in the anterior segment of the eye that helps maintain ocular pressure. The aqueous humor is a refractory medium of the eye that is constantly being formed and is always flowing through the pupil and draining into the venous system. The **vitreous humor**, another refractory medium, is a clear gel located in the posterior segment of the eye. This gel helps maintain the intraocular pressure and the shape of the eye, and it transmits light rays through the eye.

The **lens**, situated directly behind the pupil, is a biconvex (convex on both surfaces), transparent, and flexible structure. It separates the anterior and posterior segments of the eye. The ability of the lens to accommodate or change its shape permits light to focus properly on the retina and enhances fine focusing of images.

Visual Pathways

An object external to the body is perceived by the eye, which creates an image. Via light waves, this image is transported to the brain for interpretation as vision. Light waves must bend to focus correctly on the retina. The refractory structures—the cornea, aqueous humor, anterior and posterior chambers, lens, and vitreous humor—help bend the light waves onto the retina. This retinal image, via the nerve fibers, is conducted to the optic nerve (cranial nerve II). At the optic chiasm, the optic fibers of the nerves cross over and join the temporal fibers from the opposite eye.

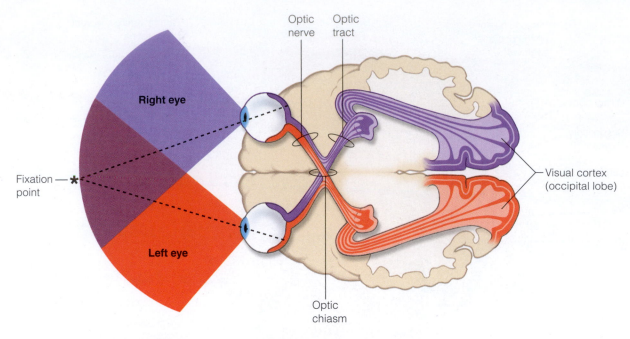

Figure 14.3 Visual fields of the eye and the visual pathway to the brain.

Optic tracts encircle the brain and the impulse is transmitted to the occipital lobe of the brain for interpretation (see Figure 14.3 ■).

Accessory Structures of the Eye

The eye has several external accessory structures. The eyebrows are the coarse short hairs that are located on the lower portion of the forehead at the orbital margins. The primary function of the eyebrow is to protect the eye (see Figure 14.1).

The eyelids, or **palpebrae**, are the movable folds of skin that cover and protect the eyes. The opening between the upper and lower eyelids is called the **palpebral fissure**. The eyelids meet medially and laterally to form the medial canthus and the outer canthus. The meibomian glands, embedded in the eyelids, are modified sebaceous glands that produce an oily substance to help lubricate the eyes and eyelids. The eyelashes are hairs that project from the eyelids and curl outward. The high supply of nerve fibers helps support the blink reflex, thereby protecting the eye.

The conjunctiva, a thin mucous membrane, lines the interior of the eyelids and continues over the anterior portion of the eye, meeting the cornea but not covering it. The conjunctiva protects the eye by preventing foreign objects from entering the eye. The conjunctiva also produces a lubricating fluid that prevents the eyes from drying.

The lacrimal apparatus consists of the lacrimal gland, punctum, canal, sac, and ducts. Lacrimal secretions, commonly called tears, are secreted and spread over the conjunctiva when blinking. The tears enter the lacrimal punctum and drain via the many ducts into the posterior nasal passage (see Figure 14.4 ■).

Each eye has six extrinsic or extraocular muscles. They help hold the eye in place within the bony orbit. These muscles are the lateral rectus, medial rectus, superior rectus, inferior rectus, inferior oblique, and superior oblique (see Figure 14.5 ■). With the coordination of these muscles, the individual experiences one single image. These muscles are innervated by cranial

nerves III, IV, and VI. Figure 14.6 ■ depicts the correlation of eye movement with eye muscles and cranial nerves.

Special Considerations

Throughout the assessment process, the nurse gathers subjective and objective data reflecting the patient's state of health. Using critical thinking and the nursing process, the nurse identifies many factors to be considered when collecting the data. Vision and eye health are influenced by a number of factors,

Evidence-Based Practice

Eye Health

For most of the population, eyesight is taken for granted and is part of one's everyday activity, occupational and educational pursuits, entertainment, and personal interactions. Among the many benefits of the ability to see, it allows us to interpret the environment and reduces risks from falls and injuries as well as from social isolation and depression. The National Academies of Sciences, Engineering, and Medicine propose to bring a greater awareness about eye health to the public through their report *Making Eye Health a Population Health Imperative: Vision for Tomorrow*. This framework will guide an overarching program in pursuit of improved eye and vision health and health equity in the United States (Higginbotham, Coleman, & Teutsch, 2017; Teutsch, McCoy, Woodbury, & Welp, 2016).

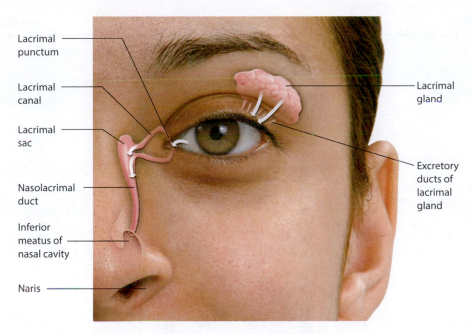

Figure 14.4 Lacrimal glands of the eye.

including age, developmental level, race, ethnicity, occupation, socioeconomics, and emotional well-being. The nurse must consider these factors when gathering subjective and objective data during a comprehensive health assessment.

Health Promotion Considerations

Vision is essential to overall health, yet the eyes often are overlooked during health assessment. Health promotion related to vision and eye health includes prevention of eye diseases, disorders, and injuries. For individuals who experience eye disorders

and vision impairment, nursing interventions may include early detection, prompt treatment, and rehabilitation.

Lifespan Considerations

Growth and development are dynamic processes that describe change over time. It is important to understand data collection and interpretation of findings regarding growth and development in relation to normative values. Details about specific variations in vision and eye health for different age groups are presented in Chapter 25, Chapter 26, and Chapter 27. ∞

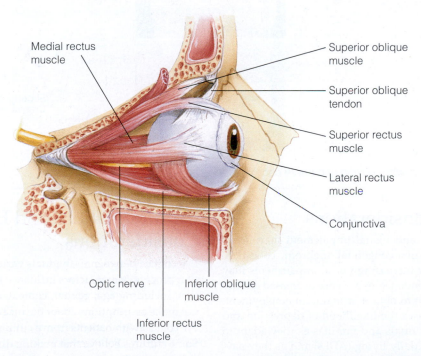

Figure 14.5 Extraocular muscles.

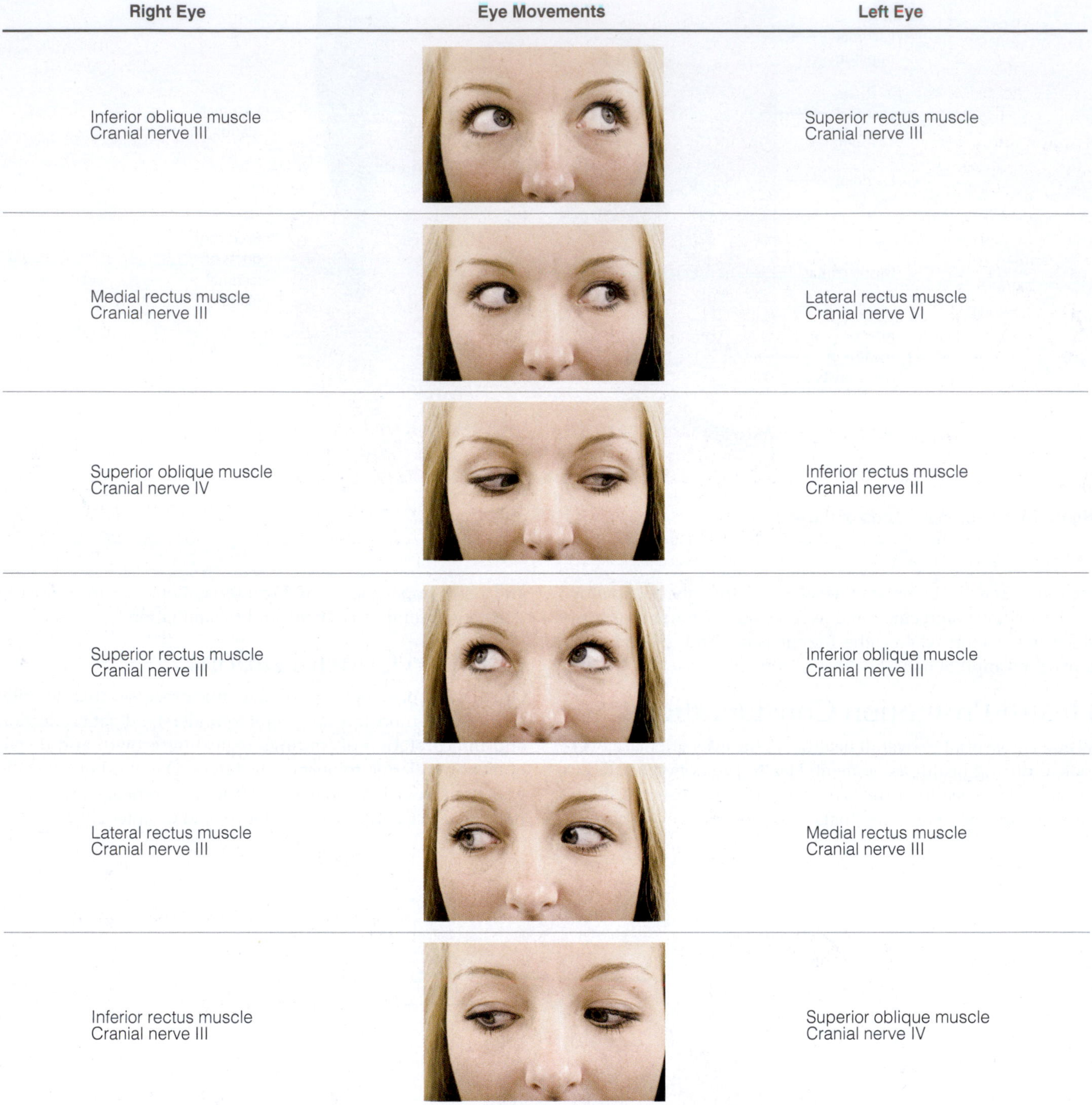

Right Eye	Eye Movements	Left Eye

Inferior oblique muscle
Cranial nerve III

Superior rectus muscle
Cranial nerve III

Medial rectus muscle
Cranial nerve III

Lateral rectus muscle
Cranial nerve VI

Superior oblique muscle
Cranial nerve IV

Inferior rectus muscle
Cranial nerve III

Superior rectus muscle
Cranial nerve III

Inferior oblique muscle
Cranial nerve III

Lateral rectus muscle
Cranial nerve III

Medial rectus muscle
Cranial nerve III

Inferior rectus muscle
Cranial nerve III

Superior oblique muscle
Cranial nerve IV

Figure 14.6 Eye movements with muscle and nerve coordination.

Psychosocial Considerations

Decreased visual acuity and visual impairment may occur suddenly or be the result of a congenital or chronic condition. Adults with new onset or increasing visual impairments may lose some personal independence, experience decreased quality of life, and find it difficult to obtain or maintain employment. Visual impairment increases the likelihood of depression and results in stress for individuals and families as they adapt to alterations in activities of daily living (ADLs) and as they navigate the healthcare and social service systems for diagnosis, treatment, and assistance (Choi, Lee, & Lee, 2018).

Cultural, Ethnic, and Environmental Considerations

Eye contact between individuals varies during the communication process. Many factors influence this aspect of communication, including age, gender, context, and culture. Nurses must not make assumptions about the meaning of direct or nondirect eye contact with patients from a culture different from their own. Some cultures believe that making direct eye contact is a sign of disrespect, whereas others perceive it as a sign of engagement. Further, for some individuals with posttraumatic stress disorder, direct eye contact may be perceived subconsciously as threatening behavior (Lanius et al., 2017). The nurse must be aware and considerate of the patient's condition and background.

The incidence and prevalence of eye-related disorders varies across individuals from different ethnic backgrounds. For example, among older adults, age-related macular degeneration occurs more frequently among Caucasians than in other groups (Fenwick et al., 2017). Among African Americans, cataracts are the leading cause of blindness, followed by glaucoma (Glaucoma Research Foundation [GRF], 2017). Glaucoma is approximately five times more common among African Americans than in individuals of other ethnic backgrounds (GRF, 2017).

Where the patient lives, diet, medication, and personal habits play an important role in eye health. Excessive sun exposure without the use of sunglasses may promote cataract formation (World Health Organization [WHO], n.d.). A deficiency of vitamin A in the diet may cause night blindness (Gilbert, 2013). Some medications have side effects that may cause excessive corneal dryness, vision changes, or increased intraocular pressure (Shields, Fox, & Liebrecht, 2018). When assessing a patient who wears contact lenses, it is important to determine what type of contact lens is worn (hard versus soft, extended wear versus daily) and evaluate the patient's cleansing routine (WebMD, 2017a). Eye makeup and applicators should be discarded after 3 months and, to reduce the risk of infection, makeup should not be shared.

Trauma or damage to the eye can occur in work, recreational, and social environments. Safety glasses or protective goggles are recommended when the eye is at risk. For example, protective eyewear is used in carpentry, welding, chemical laboratories, and in many healthcare fields to prevent debris or splashes from entering the eye.

Subjective Data—Health History

Health assessment of the eye includes the gathering of subjective and objective data. The subjective data are collected during the interview in which the professional nurse uses a variety of communication techniques to elicit general and specific information about the health of the eye. Health records combine subjective and objective data. The results of laboratory tests and radiologic studies are important secondary sources of objective data. Physical assessment of the eye, during which objective data are collected, includes the technique of inspection, the application of specific tests of vision and structures of the eye, and the use of the ophthalmoscope to assess the inner eye. See Table 14.1 for information on potential secondary sources of patient data.

Focused Interview

The focused interview for assessment of eye health and vision includes data related to the structures of the internal and external eye and visual acuity. The nurse will observe the patient and listen for cues that relate to the status and function of the eyes. The nurse may use open-ended and closed questions to obtain information. Follow-up questions or requests for descriptions are required to clarify data or to supply missing information. Follow-up questions are used to identify the source of problems, duration of difficulties, measures to alleviate problems, and cues about the patient's knowledge of his or her own health and health practices.

The focused interview guides the physical assessment of the eyes. The information obtained is considered in relation to norms and expectations about the function of the eye and structures of the eye. Therefore, the nurse must consider age, gender, race, culture, environment, health practices, past and current problems, and therapies when framing questions and using techniques to elicit information. The focused interview comprises six categories of questions: general questions that are asked of all patients; those addressing illness and infection; questions related to symptoms, pain, and behaviors; those related to habits or practices; questions that are specific to patients according to age and for the pregnant female; and questions to address environmental concerns. One method to elicit information about symptoms is the OLDCART & ICE method, described in Chapter 5. ∞

The nurse must consider the patient's ability to participate in the focused interview and physical assessment of the eyes. The ability to communicate is essential to the focused interview. If language barriers exist, a translator must be used. If the patient is experiencing discomfort or anxiety, efforts to address those problems have priority over other aspects of health assessment.

Table 14.1 Potential Secondary Sources for Patient Data Related to the Eye

DIAGNOSTIC TESTING
Automated perimetry examination
Electroretinography
Fluorescein angiography
Fluorescein eye stain
Refraction test
Retinal imaging
Tonometry (intraocular pressure [IOP] measurement)—Normal range: 12 to 22 mmHg
Ultrasonography of the eye and orbit

Focused Interview Questions	Rationales and Evidence

The following section provides sample questions and bulleted follow-up questions in each of the previously mentioned categories. A rationale for each of the questions is provided. The list of questions is not all-inclusive but, rather, represents the types of questions required in a comprehensive focused interview related to the eye.

General Questions

1. **Describe your vision today.**

▶ Open-ended discussion provides an opportunity for patients to describe their own perceptions about vision.

Focused Interview Questions	Rationales and Evidence

2. **What was the date of your last eye examination? What were the results of that examination? Have you had any vision changes or problems in the past few months? If so, please describe your vision problems.**
   - What medications were prescribed or measures taken to relieve the problem?
   - Have the medications or measures been effective in relieving the problem?
   - Has the problem affected your activities of daily living?

▶ These questions provide specific information about healthcare practices and identify any known visual problems.

▶ Follow-up questions would be required when a problem with vision or with the structures of the eye has been identified as a result of an eye examination.

3. **Do you wear glasses or contact lenses?**
   - How long have you used glasses or contact lenses?
   - Describe your vision with and without the use of glasses or contact lenses.

▶ These questions elicit information about vision correction and the effectiveness of the correction.

4. **Have you or any member of your family been diagnosed with hypertension, diabetes, or glaucoma?**

▶ This question may reveal information about diseases associated with genetic or familial predisposition. Each of the diseases mentioned can lead to vision problems. Hypertension can cause arteriosclerosis of the retina. Diabetes can cause bleeding in the capillaries of the retina (Folsom, Lutsey, Klein, Klein, & Tang, 2017).

Questions Related to Illness or Infection

1. **Have you ever been diagnosed with a disease of the eye?**
   - When were you diagnosed with the problem?
   - What treatment was prescribed for the problem?
   - Was the treatment helpful?
   - Describe things you have done or currently do to cope with this problem.
   - Has the problem ever recurred (acute)?
   - How are you managing the disease now (chronic)?

▶ The patient has an opportunity to provide information about a specific eye disease or problem. If a diagnosed illness is identified, follow-up is required about the date of diagnosis, treatment, and outcomes. Data about each illness identified by the patient are essential to an accurate health assessment. Illnesses can be classified as acute or chronic, and follow-up about each classification will differ.

2. *Alternative to question 1:* **List possible eye diseases, such as glaucoma, cataracts, corneal injury, Horner syndrome, and exophthalmos, and ask the patient to respond "yes" or "no" as each is stated.**

▶ This is a comprehensive and efficient way to elicit information about all eye-related diseases. Follow-up would be carried out for each identified diagnosis as in question 1.

3. **Do you now have or have you had an infection of the eye?**

▶ If an infection is identified, follow-up about the date of the infection, treatment, and outcomes is required. Data about each infection identified by the patient are essential to an accurate health assessment. Infections can be classified as acute or chronic, and follow-up about each classification will differ.

4. *Alternative to question 3:* **List possible eye infections, such as conjunctivitis, iritis, uveitis, blepharitis, dacryocystitis, stye (hordeolum), and episcleritis, and ask the patient to respond "yes" or "no" as each is stated.**

▶ This is a comprehensive and efficient way to elicit information about all eye infections. Follow-up would be carried out for each identified infection as in question 3.

5. **Have you had an injury to the eye?**

6. **Have you had eye surgery?**

▶ Questions 5 and 6 require follow-up regarding the type of injury or surgery, the causes and treatments, and the adaptations the individual has made to overcome visual or other deficits as a result of the injury or surgery.

Questions Related to Symptoms, Pain, and Behaviors

When gathering information about symptoms, many questions are required to elicit details and descriptions that assist in analysis of the data. Discrimination is made in relation to the significance of the symptom associated with a specific disease or problem, or in association with the need for referrals and follow-up. One rationale may be provided for a group of questions about symptoms.

The following questions refer to specific symptoms and behaviors associated with the eyes and vision. For each symptom, questions and follow-up are required. The details to be elicited are the characteristics of the symptom; the onset, duration, and frequency of the symptom; the treatment or remedy for the symptom, including over-the-counter and home remedies; the determination if diagnosis has been sought; the effect of treatments; and family history associated with a symptom or illness.

Questions 1 through 14 refer to blurred vision as a symptom. The rationales and follow-up questions provide examples of the number and types of questions required in a focused interview when symptoms exist. The remaining questions refer to other symptoms associated with problems with the eyes or vision. Follow-up is included only when required for clarification.

Questions Related to Symptoms

1. **Have you ever experienced blurred vision?**

2. **How long have you had blurred vision?**

▶ Determining the duration of symptoms is helpful in determining the significance of symptoms in relation to specific diseases and problems. Blurred vision can be an indication of a neurologic, cardiovascular, or endocrine problem; a need for corrective lenses; or cataracts (Berman, Snyder, & Frandsen, 2016; Osborn, Wraa, Watson, & Holleran, 2013).

Focused Interview Questions	Rationales and Evidence
3. Is your vision blurred all of the time?	▶ It is important to determine if a symptom is constant or intermittent.
4. Do you know what causes the blurred vision?	▶ This question permits patients to identify whether an actual diagnosis has been made in regard to the symptom or to express their beliefs or perceptions about the cause of the symptom.
5. Describe your blurred vision.	▶ Descriptions provide information about symptoms in the patient's own words. The descriptions often provide cues for further follow-up questions.
6. Have you sought treatment for the blurred vision?	▶ Questions 6 through 10 provide information about the need for diagnosis, referral, or continued evaluation of the symptom as well as information about the patient's knowledge of a current diagnosis and the response to intervention.
7. When was that treatment sought?	
8. What occurred when you sought treatment?	
9. Was something recommended or prescribed to help with the blurred vision?	
10. What was the effect of the treatment?	
11. Do you use any over-the-counter or home remedies for the blurred vision?	▶ Questions 11 through 14 provide information about drugs and/or remedies that may relieve symptoms or provide comfort. Conversely, some remedies may interfere with the effect of prescribed treatments or medications and may harm the patient.
12. What are the remedies that you use?	
13. How often do you use them?	
14. How much of them do you use?	
15. Have you ever experienced double vision?	▶ Double vision can be caused by muscle or nerve complications and some medications (Osborn et al., 2013).
16. Are you now or have you ever been sensitive to light?	▶ Sensitivity to light (photophobia) may indicate an eye disorder. However, other disorders and certain medications may also cause photophobia.
17. Do you experience burning or itching of the eyes?	▶ Burning and itching of the eyes are often associated with altered tear production and allergies (Scadding et al., 2017).
18. Do you ever see small black dots that seem to move when you are looking at something?	▶ Black dots or spots are known as floaters. Floaters are considered normal unless they obstruct vision (WebMD, 2017b).
19. Do you see halos around lights?	▶ Halos around lights are associated with cataracts, glaucoma, and digoxin drug toxicity (Mayo Clinic, 2015; Shields et al., 2018; WebMD, 2016).
20. Do you have trouble seeing at night?	▶ If the patient responds affirmatively to any of these questions, follow-up is required. Follow-up would include determination of onset, duration, and frequency of the symptom; identification of the treatment and effectiveness of the treatment; and determination of a diagnosis for the problem.
21. Do you have trouble driving at night?	

Questions Related to Pain

1. Have you had any eye pain?	▶ Eye pain can be superficial, affecting the outer eye only, or deep and throbbing, possibly associated with glaucoma. Any sudden onset of eye pain should be referred immediately to a physician.
2. Where is the pain?	▶ Questions 2 through 11 are standard questions associated with pain to determine the duration, location, frequency, and intensity of the pain.
3. How often do you experience the pain?	
4. How long does the pain last?	
5. How long have you had the pain?	
6. How would you rate the pain on a scale of 0 to 10?	
7. Is there a trigger for the pain?	
8. Can you describe the pain?	
9. Does the pain radiate to any other areas?	
10. What do you do to relieve the pain?	
11. Is this treatment effective?	

Focused Interview Questions	Rationales and Evidence

Questions Related to Behaviors

1. How do you clean and care for your eyes?

2. If you use eye makeup, how do you apply it and remove it? How often do you replace the makeup and applicators?

3. How do you clean and care for your contact lenses, if used?

4. Do you wear sunglasses when outside?

5. Do you use a tanning salon?

▶ Some eye care products, facial cleansers, and skin care products can be irritating to the eyes. Products used in applying makeup to the eyes and improper care of contact lenses can irritate the eye or cause infection if they are not cleaned or changed frequently (WebMD, 2017a).

▶ Ultraviolet (UV) radiation can cause temporary loss of vision, often referred to as "snow blindness," and **pterygium** (WHO, n.d.). Ultraviolet (UV) radiation (particularly UVA) can cause browning of the lens or loss of elasticity.

Overexposure to UVB radiation can cause cataracts (WHO, n.d.). Tanning indoors, through tanning salons and sunlamps, can result in eye injuries because of exposure to UV and visible light from sunlamp products.

Questions Related to Age and Pregnancy

The focused interview must reflect the anatomic and physiologic differences in the eyes that exist along the age span as well as during pregnancy. Specific questions related to the eyes for each of these groups are provided in Chapter 25, Chapter 26, and Chapter 27. ∞

Questions Related to the Environment

Environment refers to both the internal and external environments. Questions related to the internal environment include all of the previous questions and those associated with internal or physiologic responses. Questions regarding the external environment include those related to home, work, or social environments.

Internal Environment

1. What medications are you taking?

▶ Some medications have side effects that impact the eye (Shields et al., 2018).

2. Are you taking any medications specifically for the eyes?

3. Have you or any family member had diabetes, hypertension, or glaucoma?

▶ All of these diseases can be hereditary and can cause visual difficulties. Hypertension can cause arteriosclerosis of the retina. Diabetes can cause bleeding of the capillaries of the retina, eventually affecting vision (Folsom et al., 2017).

External Environment

The following questions deal with substances, irritants, and other factors found in the physical environment of the patient that could impact the eyes or vision. The physical environment includes the indoor and outdoor environments of the home and the workplace, those encountered for social engagements, and any encountered during travel.

1. Have you been exposed to inhalants such as dust, pollen, chemical fumes, or flying debris that caused eye irritation?

▶ Substances such as dust and pollen can cause eye irritation. Debris can cause a variety of eye injuries, including corneal abrasion. Exposure to chemical fumes can cause corneal burns and other eye injuries.

2. What were those irritants?

3. What was the effect on your eyes?

4. What have you done to remedy the eye problem?

5. What have you done to decrease the exposure to the irritant?

6. What kinds of activities do you perform at work?

7. Do you need or wear safety glasses at work?

8. How many hours in the workday are you using a computer?

9. What sports or hobbies do you participate in?

▶ Use of equipment at work or at home may require the use of safety glasses to prevent eye injury from debris. Prolonged work under bright lights or at a computer screen can cause eyestrain. Some athletic activities put the patient at risk for eye injury, and shields or masks are recommended to prevent or reduce the risk for injury.

10. Do you routinely wear sunglasses when outside in bright light?
   - Follow-up questions would include all of the questions previously mentioned that address symptoms and problems.

▶ Excess sun exposure may increase risk of short-term and long-term eye problems. UV rays can burn the cornea, causing temporary blindness; long-term exposure is linked to increased risk of cataracts (American Academy of Ophthalmology, 2016).

Patient-Centered Interaction

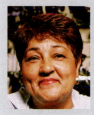

Sophia Rodriguez, a 62-year-old woman, is employed as a sewing machine operator at the local shirt factory. The operators are paid based on work production. Sophia has always received a monthly bonus for her production. Lately, her productivity has decreased, and her supervisor has been trying to help determine the reason. Sophia tells the supervisor she needs a better, stronger light on the sewing machine because it is very hard to see the stitches and thread. Sophia is directed to the local eye clinic. Following is an excerpt of the focused interview.

Source: George Doyle/Stockbyte/Getty Images.

Interview

Nurse: Mrs. Rodriguez, tell me your reason for coming to the eye clinic today.

Mrs. Rodriguez: I can't see the thread or the stitches like I used to. I don't sew as many sleeves anymore either. I make mistakes now, and that slows me down.

Nurse: Have you ever had your eyes examined?

Mrs. Rodriguez: Yes, several years ago. They told me everything was okay. No glasses.

Nurse: Describe your vision.

Mrs. Rodriguez: I don't know what you want me to say. I just can't see like I used to.

Nurse: Can you see to read the newspaper?

Mrs. Rodriguez: Yes.

Nurse: Do you need to hold the newspaper closer to your eyes or farther away when reading?

Mrs. Rodriguez: A little farther away. But I can't read it at night unless I'm next to the light in the room.

Nurse: Can you see the street signs when you are driving?

Mrs. Rodriguez: Yes, that is not a problem.

Nurse: Is your vision blurred?

Mrs. Rodriguez: Sometimes, especially if I'm tired.

Nurse: Do you ever see black spots floating in your eyes?

Mrs. Rodriguez: No.

Nurse: Are your eyes sensitive to light?

Mrs. Rodriguez: No.

Nurse: Do you see halos or rings around lights?

Mrs. Rodriguez: No.

Nurse: Do you have any pain or burning in your eyes?

Mrs. Rodriguez: No.

Analysis

The nurse knows **presbyopia** is a common change of the eye associated with aging. The nurse begins the interview using open-ended statements to gather data associated with presbyopia and other medical diagnoses. Using open-ended statements, the nurse obtains clear baseline data. When the patient indicates she is not clear how to respond, the nurse proceeds using closed-ended statements. This allows the patient to respond "yes" or "no." The nurse must be sure to present the many questions in a nonthreatening manner.

Objective Data—Physical Assessment

Assessment Techniques and Findings

Physical assessment of the eyes requires the use of inspection, palpation, and tests of the function of the eyes. The ophthalmoscope is used to assess the internal eye. During each of the assessments, the nurse is gathering data related to the patient's vision and the internal and external structures and functions of the eye. Inspection includes looking at the size, shape, and symmetry of the eye, eyelids, eyebrows, and eye movements. Knowledge of the norms and expectations related to the eyes and vision according to age and development is essential in determining the meaning of the data.

Presbyopia, the inability to accommodate for near vision, is common in patients over age 45. The size, shape, and position of the eyes should be symmetric. The sclerae are white, the cornea is clear, and the pupils are round and symmetric in size

EQUIPMENT
- Visual acuity charts (Snellen or E for distance vision, Rosenbaum for near vision). For patients who cannot read, including children, charts with pictures or numbers are used (MedlinePlus, 2018).
- Opaque card or eye cover
- Penlight
- Cotton-tipped applicator
- Ophthalmoscope

HELPFUL HINTS
- Provide specific instructions about what is expected of the patient. This includes telling the patient clearly which eye to cover when conducting an assessment of visual acuity.

and respond briskly to light. The eyebrows are located equally above the eyes; the eyelashes are full and everted. The eyes are moist, indicating tear production. The movements of the eye are smooth and symmetric. Upon ophthalmoscopic examination, the red reflex is visible in each eye, and the retinae are a uniform yellowish pink with a sharply defined disc and visible vessels.

Physical assessment of the eyes follows an organized pattern. It begins with assessment of visual acuity and is followed by assessments of visual fields, muscle function, and external eye structures. The assessment of the eye concludes with the ophthalmoscopic examination. Additional information about the eye, vision screening, and assessment can be obtained through the National Eye Institute at www.nei.nih.gov.

- The ability to read letters will determine the type of acuity chart to be used. Children and non–English-speaking patients can use the E chart or a chart with figures and images for visual acuity.
- An opaque card or eye cover is used for covering the eye in several assessments. The patient must be instructed not to close or apply pressure to the covered eye.
- Several types of lighting are required. Visual acuity requires bright lighting, in addition to which the room is darkened at times to assess pupillary responses and the internal eye.
- The room must provide 20 feet from the Snellen chart.
- The assessment may be conducted with the patient seated or standing. The nurse stands or sits at eye level with the patient.
- Use Standard Precautions.

Techniques and Normal Findings	Abnormal Findings and Special Considerations

Vision

Testing Distance Vision

1. **Position the patient.**
   - Position the patient exactly 20 ft (6.1 m) from the Snellen chart. The patient may be standing or seated. The chart should be at the patient's eye level.

▶ Most Americans believe that good vision is crucial to overall health with many individuals saying that losing visual acuity would greatly decrease their quality of life. Because of the importance of good vision to health and personal independence, the nurse must be skilled at assessment of both far and near vision (Higginbotham et al., 2017).

2. **Instruct the patient.**
   - Explain that you are testing distance vision. Explain that the patient will read the letters from the top of the chart down to the smallest line of letters that the patient can see, reading each line left to right. Explain that each line of the chart has a number that indicates what the patient's vision is in relation to that of a person with normal vision.

▶ Any findings other than 20/20 are considered abnormal. For example, 20/40 means that the line the patient can read at 20 feet (6 m) away can be read by a person with normal vision at 40 feet (12 m) away. Any abnormal result should prompt the nurse to recommend referral to a specialty provider (MedlinePlus, 2018).

3. **Ask the patient to cover one eye with the opaque card or eye cover (see Figure 14.7 ■). Tell the patient to read, left to right, from the top of the chart down to the smallest line of letters that the patient can see.**

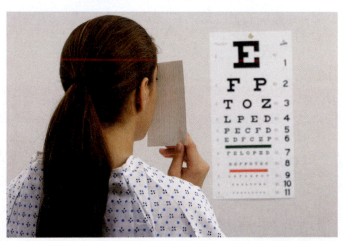

Figure 14.7 Testing distance vision.

4. **Ask the patient to cover the other eye and to read from the top of the chart down to the smallest line of letters that the patient can see.**

5. **Ask the patient to read from the top of the chart down to the smallest line of letters that the patient can see with both eyes uncovered.**

Techniques and Normal Findings	Abnormal Findings and Special Considerations

6. **If a patient uses corrective lenses for distance vision, test first with eyeglasses or contact lenses. Then test without glasses or contact lenses.**
   - The results are recorded as a fraction. The numerator indicates the distance from the chart (20 ft). The denominator indicates the distance at which a person with normal vision can read the last line.
   - Normal vision is 20/20; therefore, at 20 ft the patient can read the line numbered 20. If a patient's vision is 20/30, the patient reads at 20 ft what a person with normal vision reads at 30 ft. Observe while the patient is reading the chart.
   - If the patient is unable to read more than one half of the letters on a line, record the number of the line above.

▶ Frowning, leaning forward, and squinting indicate visual or reading difficulties.

The Snellen E Chart
The Snellen E chart has the letter *E* pointing in different directions (see Figure 14.8 ■). For patients who cannot read, including children, charts that feature numbers or pictures are used (MedlinePlus, 2018).

▶ Inability to see objects at a distance is myopia. The smaller the fraction, the worse the vision. Vision of 20/200 is considered legal blindness. Changes in vision may be related to dysfunction of cranial nerve II.

▶ The nurse should be aware that there are a variety of vision testing systems in addition to the Snellen and Snellen E charts. These may be used for children and individuals who cannot read or who read languages that use non-English alphabets. For example, there are vision charts with easily identifiable pictures, standardized symbols, or letters from non-English alphabets (Berman et al., 2016).

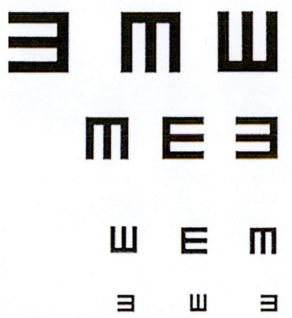

Figure 14.8 E chart for testing distance vision.

- The letter *E* becomes smaller as one proceeds from the top to the bottom of the chart. Numbers on each line correspond to the patient's vision in relation to what a person with normal vision would see when being tested for distance vision with the E chart.
- Repeat steps 1 to 6 as previously noted, but ask the patient to start at the top of the chart and to point in the direction the letter faces on each line until the patient can no longer see the Es.
- Observe while the patient is reading the chart.

Testing Near Vision

1. **Position the patient.**
   - The patient is sitting with a Jaeger or Rosenbaum chart held at a distance of 12 to 14 in. (30.5 to 35.5 cm) from the eyes.

2. **Instruct the patient.**
   - Explain that you are testing near vision, and the patient will read the letters from the top of the card down to the smallest line the patient can see. Tell the patient to hold the card at the same distance throughout the test. Explain that each line on the card has a number that indicates what the patient's vision is in relation to that of a person with normal vision (see Figure 14.9 ■).

▶ A Rosenbaum chart is used to test near vision in a similar way that the Snellen chart is used for far vision. The nurse must be sure the patient's literacy level is appropriate for the chart being used (Berman et al., 2016).

3. **Ask the patient to cover one eye with the opaque card or eye cover.**

▶ Inability to see objects at close range is called hyperopia. Presbyopia, the inability to accommodate for near vision, is common in persons over 45 years of age; however, this condition also may occur among individuals of other ages.

Techniques and Normal Findings	Abnormal Findings and Special Considerations

4. Repeat the test with the other eye and then with both eyes uncovered. The results are recorded as a fraction. A normal result is 14/14 in each eye.

5. If a patient uses corrective lenses for reading, test with the corrective lenses.

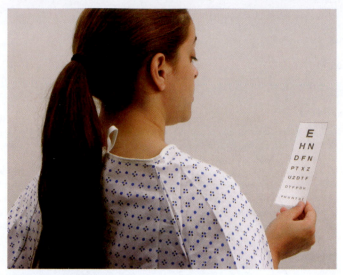

Figure 14.9 Testing near vision.

Testing Peripheral Vision

1. **Position the patient.**
   - For direct confrontation visual field testing, the patient and examiner sit facing one another. To test peripheral vision, the patient should be sitting 2 to 3 ft (0.6 to 0.9 m) from you and at eye level.

2. **Instruct the patient.**
   - Explain that you are testing peripheral vision. In this test, the patient's peripheral visual fields are compared with that of the examiner. The patient will alternately cover an eye and must look directly into your open eye. A pen or penlight will be moved into the patient's field of vision, sequentially from four directions. The patient is to indicate by saying "now" or "yes" when the object is first seen.

3. **Ask the patient to cover one eye with a card while you cover your opposite eye with a card.**

4. **Holding a penlight in one hand, extend your arm upward, and advance it in from the periphery to the midline point (see Figure 14.10 ■).**

▶ If the patient is not able to see the object at the same time that the examiner does, there may be some peripheral vision loss. The patient should be evaluated further.

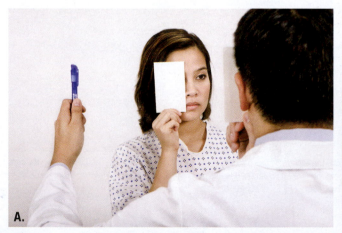
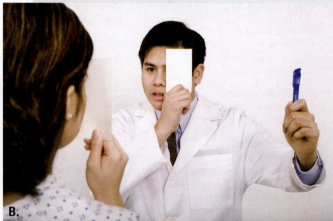

Figure 14.10 A. Testing visual fields by confrontation, nurse's view. B. Testing visual fields by confrontation, patient's view.

5. **Be sure to keep the penlight equidistant between the patient and yourself.**

6. **Ask the patient to report when the object is first seen. Repeat the procedure upward, toward the nose, and downward. Then repeat the entire procedure with the other eye covered. This test assumes the examiner has normal peripheral vision.**

Techniques and Normal Findings	Abnormal Findings and Special Considerations

Extraocular Movements (EOM)

Testing the Six Cardinal Fields of Gaze

1. **Position the patient.**
   - The patient is sitting in a comfortable position. You are at eye level with the patient.

2. **Instruct the patient.**
   - Explain that you will be testing eye movements and the muscles of the eye. Explain that the patient must keep the head still while following a pen or penlight that you will move in several directions in front of the patient's eyes.

3. **Stand about 2 ft (0.6 m) in front of the patient.**

4. **Letter "H" method.**
   - Starting at midline, move the penlight to the right, then straight up, then straight down past the midline.
   - Drop your hand. Again, position the penlight against the midline.
   - Now move the penlight to the left, then straight up, then straight down past the midline (see Figure 14.11 ▪).

▶ Be sure to move the penlight slowly and smoothly, keeping it in a consistent plane approximately 18 inches from the patient's face. Briefly stop the movement at each location to assess for nystagmus.

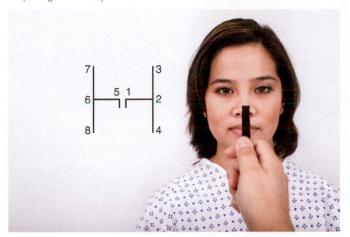

Figure 14.11 Testing cardinal fields of gaze.

5. **Wagon wheel method.**
   - Starting at the midline, move the pen or light to form a star or wagon wheel.
   - Use a random direction pattern to create the movement.
   - Always return the light or pen to the center before changing direction (see Figure 14.12 ▪).

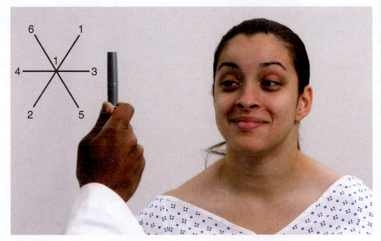

Figure 14.12 Alternative method of testing cardinal field of gaze.

Techniques and Normal Findings	Abnormal Findings and Special Considerations

6. Assess the patient's ability to follow your movements with the eyes (see Figure 14.11). Nystagmus, rapid fluttering of the eyeball, occurs at completion of rapid lateral eye movement.

▶ If **nystagmus** occurs during testing, there could be a weakness in the extraocular muscles or cranial nerve III.

Assessing Corneal Light Reflex

1. **Position the patient.**
   • You will sit at eye level with the patient.

2. **Instruct the patient.**
   • Explain that you are examining the cornea of the eyes. Instruct the patient to stare straight ahead while you hold a penlight 12 in. (30.5 cm) from both eyes.

3. **Shine the light into the eyes from a distance of 12 in. (see Figure 14.13 ■).**
   • The reflection of light should appear in the same spot on both pupils. This appears as a "twinkle" in the eye.

▶ If the reflection of light is not symmetric, there could be a weakness in the extraocular muscles.

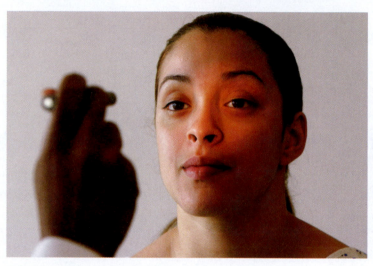

Figure 14.13 Testing the corneal light reflex.

▶ The corneal light reflex is also called the Hirschberg test. A positive Hirschberg sign indicates an abnormal finding.

Performing the Cover/Uncover Test

1. **Position the patient.**
   • You should be sitting at eye level with the patient.

2. **Instruct the patient.**
   • Explain that this test determines the balance mechanism (fusion reflex) that keeps the eyes parallel. Explain that the patient will look at a fixed point while covering each eye. You will observe the eyes.

3. **Cover one eye with a card and observe the uncovered eye, which should remain focused on the designated point (see Figure 14.14 ■).**

▶ If there is a weakness in one of the eye muscles, the fusion reflex is blocked when one eye is covered and the weakness of the eye can be observed.

Techniques and Normal Findings	**Abnormal Findings and Special Considerations**

▶ An abnormal finding is called strabismus, commonly referred to as cross-eye. There are a variety of causes, and any patient with this condition should be referred for specialty examination by an optometrist or ophthalmologist (Berman et al., 2016).

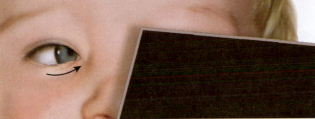

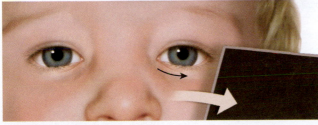

A. Right, or uncovered eye, is weaker.

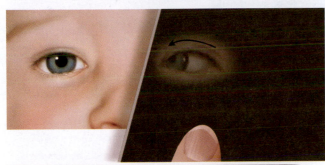

B. Left, or covered eye, is weaker.

Figure 14.14 Cover/Uncover test. A. Right, or uncovered eye, is weaker. B. Left, or covered eye, is weaker.

4. Quickly remove the card from the covered eye and observe the newly uncovered eye for movement. It should focus straight ahead.

5. Repeat the procedure with the other eye.

Inspection of the Eyes

Assessing the Eye

1. **Instruct the patient.**
   - Explain that you will be examining the patient's eye. You will be looking at the patient's eyes and touching them to see inside the lids. Explain that you will provide specific instructions before each test.

2. **Stand directly in front of the patient and focus on the external structures of the eye.**
   - The eyebrows should be symmetric in shape and the eyelashes similar in quantity and distribution. The eyebrows and eyelashes should be free of flakes and drainage.

▶ Absence of the lateral third of the eyebrow is associated with hypothyroidism. Absent eyelashes may indicate pulling or plucking associated with obsessive-compulsive behavior.

Techniques and Normal Findings | ## Abnormal Findings and Special Considerations

3. **Ask the patient to open the eyes.**
   - The distances between the palpebral fissures should be equal.
   - The upper eyelid covers a small arc of the iris.

4. **Ask the patient to close the eyes.**
   - The eyelids should symmetrically cover the eyeballs when closed.
   - The eyeball should be neither protruding nor sunken.

5. **Gently separate the eyelids and ask the patient to look up, down, and to each side.**
   - The conjunctiva should be moist and clear, with no redness or drainage, and with small blood vessels visible beneath the conjunctival surface.
   - The lens should be clear, and the sclera white.
   - The irises should be round and both of the same color, although irises of different colors can be a normal finding.

6. **Inspect the cornea by shining a penlight from the side across the cornea.**
   - The cornea should be clear with no irregularities.
   - The pupils should be round and equal in size (see Figure 14.15 ■).

▶ One eyelid drooping (**ptosis**) can be caused by a dysfunction of cranial nerve III (oculomotor). Eyes that protrude beyond the supraorbital ridge can indicate a thyroid disorder; however, this trait may be normal for the patient. Edema of the eyelids can be caused by allergies, heart disease, or kidney disease. Inability to move the eyelids can indicate dysfunction of the nervous system, including facial nerve paralysis.

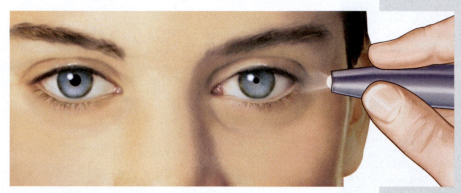

Figure 14.15 Inspecting the cornea.

7. **Observe the constriction in the illuminated pupil.**
   - Also observe the simultaneous reaction (**consensual constriction**) of the other pupil. The direct reaction should be faster and greater than the consensual reaction.

▶ If the illuminated pupil fails to constrict, there is a defect in the direct pupillary response. If the nonilluminated pupil fails to constrict, there is a defect in the consensual response, controlled by cranial nerve III (oculomotor).

Testing Accommodation

1. **Instruct the patient.**
   - Explain that you are testing muscles of the eye. Explain that the patient will shift the gaze from the far wall to an object held 4 to 5 in. (10 to 12 cm) from the patient's nose.

2. **Ask the patient to stare straight ahead at a distant point.**

3. **Hold a penlight about 4 to 5 in. (10 to 12 cm) from the patient's nose; then ask the patient to shift the gaze from the distant point to the penlight.**
   - The eyes should converge (turn inward), and the pupils should constrict as the eyes focus on the penlight. This pupillary change is **accommodation**, a change in size to adjust vision from far to near.
   - A normal response to pupillary testing is recorded as PERRLA (pupils equal, round, react to light, and accommodation).

▶ Lack of **convergence** (turning inward of the eye) and failure of the pupils to constrict indicates dysfunction of cranial nerves III, IV, and VI.

Palpation of the Eye

1. **Ask the patient to close both eyes.**

2. **Using the first two or three fingers, gently palpate the lacrimal sacs, the eyelids, and erythematous areas for warmth or tenderness.**

3. **Confirm that there is no swelling or tenderness and that the eyeballs feel firm.**

▶ Erythema may be a symptom of injury or infection, cardiovascular problems, or renal problems.

Appendix C: Advanced Skills *Appendix C provides step-by-step instructions on the ophthalmoscope exam of the fundus of the eye.*

Documenting Your Findings

Documentation of assessment data—subjective and objective—must be accurate, professional, complete, and confidential. When documenting the information from the focused assessment of each body system, the nurse should use measurements where appropriate to ensure accuracy, use medical terminology rather than jargon, include all pertinent information, and avoid language that could identify the patient. The subjective information in the documentation of the Review of Systems (ROS) should make it clear what questions were asked and should use language to indicate whether it is the patient's response or the nurse's findings. For patient responses the documentation will say "denies," "states," or "reports," and the nurse's findings will simply list the findings as fact or indicate "no" along with the condition—for example, patient "reports Lasik eye surgery at age 37 yrs" and the nurse found "distance vision 20/40 uncorrected OU." An example of normal results for the vision and eye health follows.

Sample Documentation: Vision and Eye Health Assessment

Focused History (Subjective Data)

Denies blurry vision or changes to vision. Denies personal or family history of glaucoma, macular degeneration, hypertension, or diabetes. Reports Lasik eye surgery at age 37 yrs. Denies floaters, flashes, halos, or blurred vision. Denies history of infections of the eye. Reports occasional "itchy" eyes for several weeks each spring when the trees bloom. Reports using "allergy eye drops" during this time period. Denies smoking or exposure to environmental toxins. Reports last eye exam was 6 months ago, when his vision was "20/20."

Physical Assessment (Objective Data)

Eyebrows and lashes are evenly distributed, free of flaking or drainage. Distance between palpebral fissures is symmetric and eyelids close completely. No ptosis. Eyeballs are not protruding or sunken. The conjunctivae and sclera are clear, smooth, no erythema. Irises are light blue and round. PERRLA, no corneal abnormalities. Visual acuity is 20/20 OD, 20/30 OS, 20/20 OU uncorrected.

Abnormal Findings

Abnormalities of the eye arise for a variety of reasons and can be associated with vision, eye movement, and the internal and external structures of the eye. The following sections address abnormal findings associated with the eyelids (see Table 14.2), the eye (see Table 14.3), and the **fundus** (see Table 14.4). In addition, an overview of conditions that may be associated with an impaired pupillary response is provided (see Table 14.5).

Table 14.2 Abnormalities of the Eyelids

Blepharitis **Blepharitis** is inflammation of the eyelids. Staphylococcal infection leads to red, scaly, and crusted lids. The eye burns, itches, and tears.	**Basal Cell Carcinoma** Usually seen on the lower lid and medial canthus. It has a papular appearance.

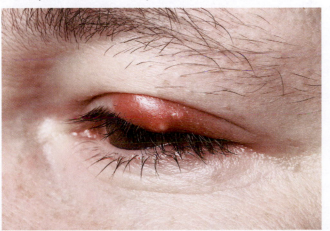

Blepharitis.
Source: Gromovataya/Shutterstock.

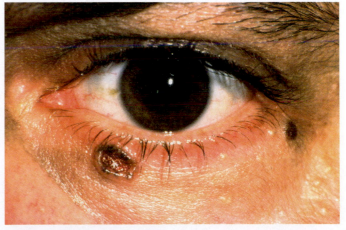

Basal cell carcinoma on lower eyelid.
Source: DR ZARA/BSIP SA/Alamy Stock Photo.

Table 14.2 Abnormalities of the Eyelids (continued)

Chalazion
A firm, nontender nodule on the eyelid, arising from infection of the meibomian gland. Not painful unless inflamed.

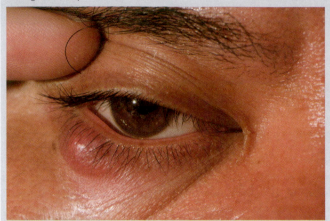

Chalazion.
Source: ARZTSAMUI/Shutterstock.

Hordeolum
The result of a staphylococcal infection of hair follicles on the margin of the lids. Affected eye is swollen, red, and painful. Also called a stye.

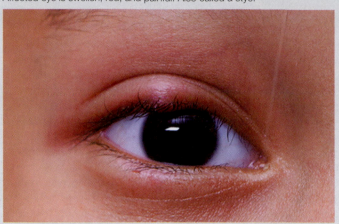

Hordeolum (stye).
Source: panachai cherdchucheep/123RF.

Entropion
Entropion is an inversion of the lid and lashes caused by muscle spasm of the eyelid. Friction from lashes can cause corneal irritation.

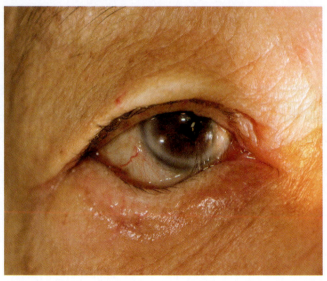

Entropion.
Source: Arztsamui/Shutterstock.

Ectropion
Ectropion is eversion of the lower eyelid caused by muscle weakness, exposing the palpebral conjunctiva.

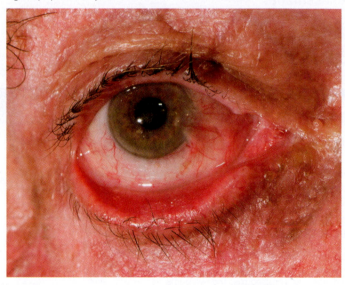

Ectropion.
Source: Arztsamui/Shutterstock.

Table 14.2 Abnormalities of the Eyelids (continued)

Ptosis

Drooping of the eyelid; occurs with cranial nerve damage or systemic neuro-muscular weakness.

Periorbital Edema

Periorbital edema refers to swollen, puffy lids; occurs with crying, infection, trauma, and systemic problems including kidney failure, heart failure, and allergy.

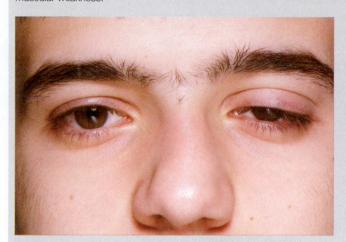

Ptosis.
Source: Mediscan/Alamy Stock Photo.

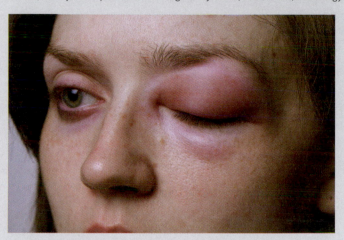

Periorbital edema.
Source: Oleg Iandubaev/123RF.

Exophthalmos

Abnormal protrusion of one or both eyeballs; usually occurs secondary to Graves disease; causes also may include infectious disease, certain forms of cancer, and other disorders (Medscape, 2016).

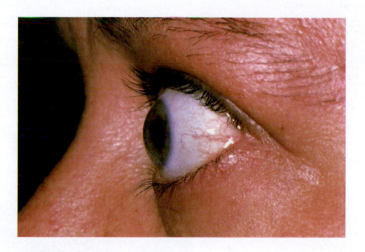

Exophthalmos.
Source: Dr P. Marazzi/Science Source.

Table 14.3 Abnormalities of the Eye

Conjunctivitis
Infection of the conjunctiva usually because of bacteria or virus but which may result from chemical exposure. It is commonly called pink eye.

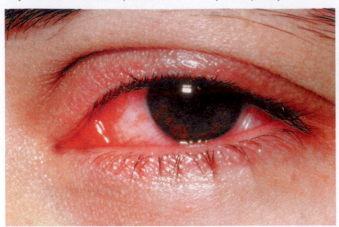

Conjunctivitis.
Source: Mediscan/Alamy Stock Photo.

Iritis
Iritis is a serious disorder characterized by redness around the iris and cornea, decreased vision, and deep, aching pain; pupil is often irregular.

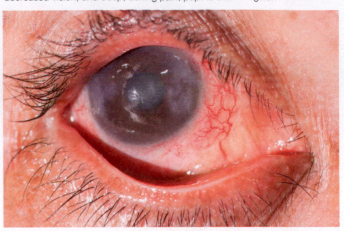

Iritis.
Source: PHUCHONG CHOKSAMAI/123RF.

Subconjunctival Hemorrhage
Results from ruptured blood vessel that leads to blood accumulation in the subconjunctival space. Causes include trauma, anticoagulant therapy, hypertension, and elevated venous pressure (Tarlan & Kiratli, 2013).

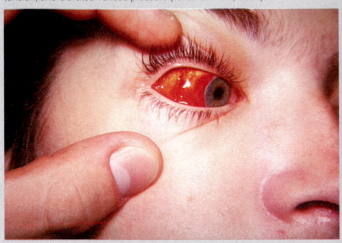

Subconjunctival hemorrhage.
Source: Dr. Thomas F. Sellers/Emory University/Centers for Disease Control and Prevention (CDC).

Pterygium
Noncancerous growth that develops from the conjunctiva and extends onto the sclera; may also extend to the cornea (MedlinePlus, 2016).

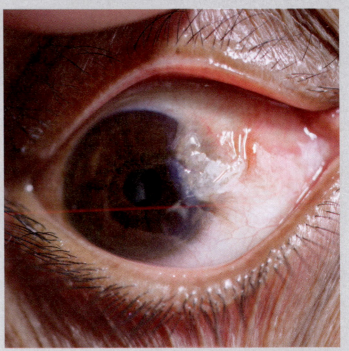

Pterygium.
Source: Arztsamui/Shutterstock.

Table 14.3 Abnormalities of the Eye (continued)

Hyphema

Collection of blood in the anterior chamber of the eye that is most often caused by blunt trauma to the eye. Additional causes include eye surgery, blood vessel abnormalities, and medical problems (cancer).

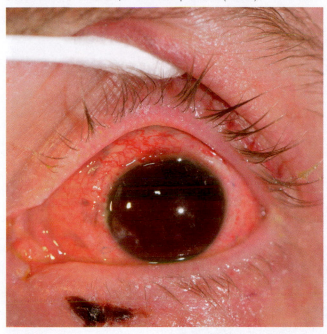

Hyphema.
Source: Arztsamui/Shutterstock.

Acute Glaucoma

The result of a sudden increase in intraocular pressure resulting from blocked flow of fluid from the anterior chamber. Pupil is oval shaped and dilated; cornea appears cloudy with circumcorneal redness. Pain onset is sudden and accompanied by halos around lights and a decrease in vision. Acute glaucoma requires immediate intervention.

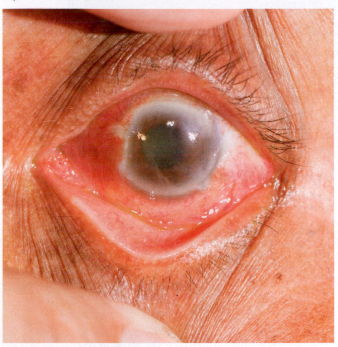

Acute glaucoma.
Source: Arztsamui/Shutterstock.

Cataract

An opacity in the lens; usually develops later in life.

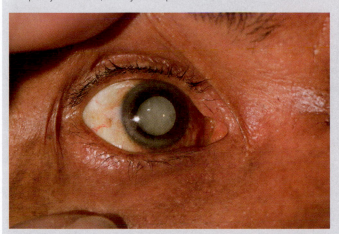

Cataract.
Source: Arztsamui/Shutterstock.

Pingueculae

Yellowish nodules that are thickened areas of the bulbar conjunctiva. Caused by prolonged exposure to sun, wind, and dust.

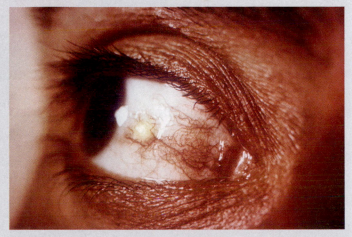

Pinguecula.
Source: Centers for Disease Control and Prevention (CDC).

Table 14.4 Abnormalities of the Fundus

Diabetic Retinopathy
Refers to the changes that occur in the retina and its vasculature, including microaneurysms, hemorrhages, macular edema, and retinal exudates.

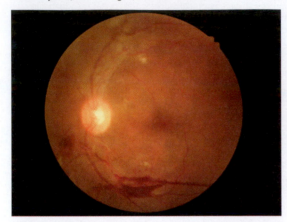

Diabetic retinopathy.
Source: Satit Umong/123RF.

Hypertensive Retinopathy
Refers to changes in the retina and its vasculature in response to high blood pressure. Includes flame hemorrhages, nicking of vessels, and "cotton wool" spots that arise from nerve fiber infarction.

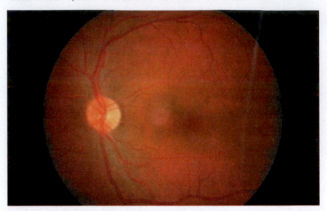

Hypertensive retinopathy.
Source: Santibhavank P/shutterstock.

Age-Related Macular Degeneration (ARMD)
A degenerative condition of the macula, the central retina, causing the gradual loss of central vision while peripheral vision remains intact. The eyes are affected at different rates. Risk factors for macular degeneration include hypertension and cigarette smoking. Protective factors include an increased consumption of fruits and vegetables (Kim, Kim, Vijayakumar, Kwon, & Chang, 2017).

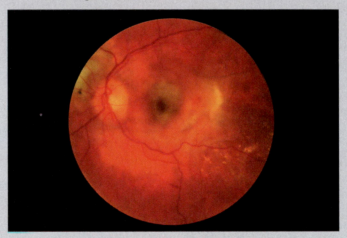

Macular degeneration.
Source: Terence Mendoza/Shutterstock.

Table 14.5 Conditions Associated with Impaired Pupillary Response

Adie's Pupil
Also known as tonic pupil, Adie's pupil is a sluggish pupillary response. Usually unilateral but can be bilateral. Occurs because of damage to parasympathetic nerves that innervate the eye.

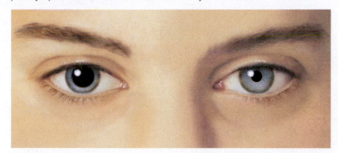

Adie's pupil.

Argyll Robertson Pupils
Small, irregular pupils that exist bilaterally and are nonreactive to light. Occur with central nervous system (CNS) disorders such as tumor, syphilis, and narcotic use.

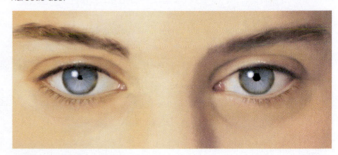

Argyll Robertson pupils.

Anisocoria
Unequal pupillary size, which may be a normal finding or may indicate CNS disease.

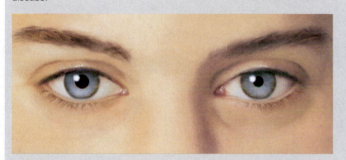

Anisocoria.

Cranial Nerve III Damage
Results in a unilaterally dilated pupil. There is no reaction to light. Ptosis may be seen.

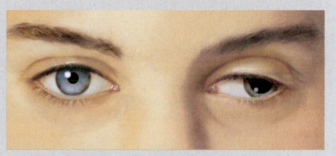

Cranial nerve III damage.

Horner Syndrome
A result of blockage of sympathetic nerve stimulation. Findings include a unilateral, small regular pupil that is nonreactive to light. Ptosis and anhidrosis of the same side accompany the pupillary signs.

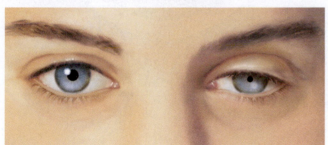

Horner syndrome.

Mydriasis
Refers to fixed and dilated pupils; may occur with sympathetic nerve stimulation, glaucoma, CNS damage, or deep anesthesia.

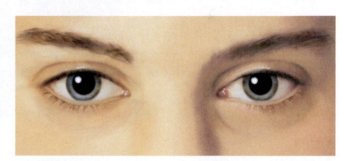

Mydriasis.

Monocular Blindness
Results in direct and consensual response to light directed in the normal eye and absence of response in either eye when light is directed in the blind eye.

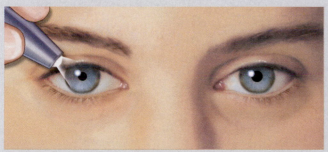

Monocular blindness.

Table 14.5 Conditions Associated with Impaired Pupillary Response (continued)

Miosis
Miosis refers to fixed and constricted pupils; may occur with the use of narcotics, with damage to the pons, or as a result of treatment for glaucoma.

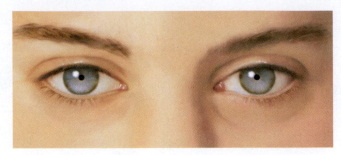

Miosis.

Disorders of Visual Acuity

Visual acuity is dependent on the ability of the eye to refract light rays and focus them on the retina. The shape of the eye is one determinant in the refractive and focusing processes of vision.

Emmetropia is the normal refractive condition of the eye in which light rays are brought into sharp focus on the retina (see Figure 14.16 ■).

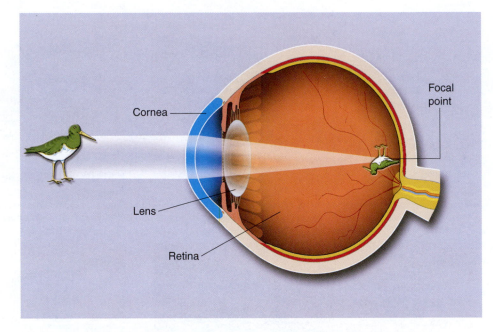

Figure 14.16 Emmetropia.

Myopia

Myopia (nearsightedness) is generally inherited and occurs when the eye is longer than normal. As a result, light rays focus in front of the retina (see Figure 14.17 ■).

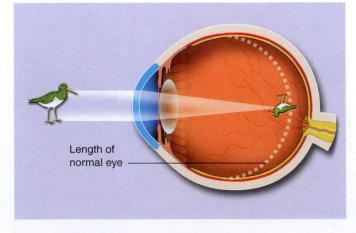

Figure 14.17 Myopia.

Hyperopia

Hyperopia (farsightedness) is also an inherited condition in which the eye is shorter than normal. In hyperopia the light rays focus behind the retina (see Figure 14.18 ■).

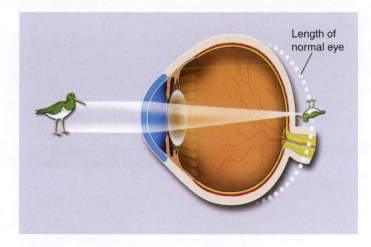

Figure 14.18 Hyperopia.

Astigmatism

Astigmatism is often a familial condition in which the refraction of light is spread over a wide area rather than on a distinct point on the retina. In the normal eye, the cornea is round in shape, whereas in astigmatism the cornea curves more in one direction than another. As a result, light is refracted and focused on two focal points on or near the retina. Vision in astigmatism may be blurred or doubled (see Figure 14.19 ■).

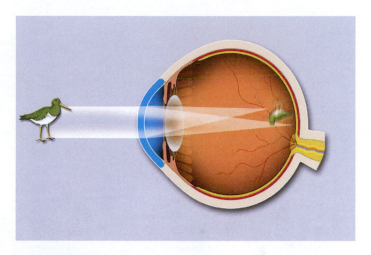

Figure 14.19 Astigmatism.

Presbyopia

Presbyopia is an age-related condition in which the lens of the eye loses the ability to accommodate. As a result, light is focused behind the retina, and focus on near objects becomes difficult.

Visual Fields

The **visual field** refers to the total area in which objects can be seen in the periphery while the eye remains focused on a central point. Testing visual fields enables the examiner to detect and map losses in peripheral vision. The mapping aids in determination of the problem. Changes in visual fields accompany damage to the retina, lesions in the optic nerve or chiasm, increased intraocular pressure, and retinal vascular damage. The normal visual pathways and loss of visual fields in relation to the previously mentioned conditions are depicted in Figure 14.20 ■ and Figure 14.21 ■, respectively.

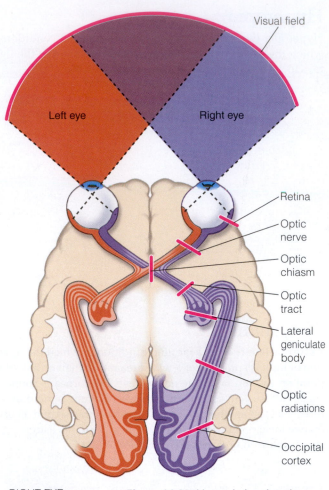

Figure 14.20 Normal visual pathways.

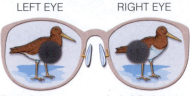

Retinal damage—results in blind spots in localized damaged areas.

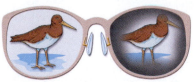

Increased intraocular pressure resulting in decreased peripheral vision.

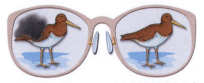

Retinal detachment—vision diminishes in affected area.

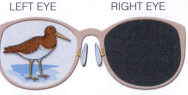

Optic nerve or globe lesion results in unilateral blindness.

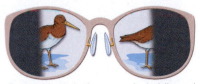

Optic chiasm lesion—results in bilateral heteronymous hemianopsia (loss of temporal visual fields).

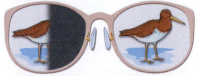

Lesion occurs in uncrossed fibers of optic chiasm resulting in left hemianopsia (nasal).

Right optic tract or optic radiation lesion resulting in loss of right nasal and left temporal fields. Homonymous hemianopsia.

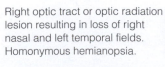

Figure 14.21 Patient's view with visual field loss.

Cardinal Fields of Gaze

Eye movement is controlled by six extraocular muscles and by cranial nerves III, IV, and VI. Muscle weakness or dysfunction of a cranial nerve can be identified by assessing the fields of gaze, assessing corneal light reflex, and performing the cover test.

Strabismus is a condition in which the axes of the eyes cannot be directed at the same object. Strabismus can be classified as convergent (esotropia), in which the eye deviates inward, and divergent (exotropia), in which the deviation is outward. In strabismus, light can be seen to reflect in different axes (see Figure 14.22A ■).

Esophoria (inward turning of the eye) and **exophoria** (outward turning of the eye) are detected in the cover test. Esotropic findings are depicted in Figure 14.22B. Unlike esotropia and exotropia, which are associated with strabismus, the eye misalignment that is associated with esophoria and exophoria is not always apparent. Instead, with esophoria and exophoria, the eye deviation is a tendency, and the eyes tend to function normally. However, if the misalignment is significant, it may cause eye strain and headache.

Nonparallel eye movements and failure of the eyes to follow in a certain direction are indicative of problems with extraocular muscles or cranial nerves. Figure 14.23 ■ provides details about the specific muscles and nerves associated with abnormal eye movement.

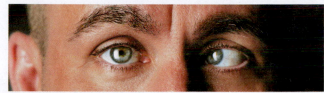

A. Esotropia
Source: Andrey Kiselev/123RF.

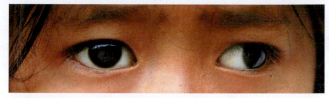

B. Exotropia
Source: photography by david price/Alamy Stock Photo.

Figure 14.22 Strabismus (esotropia and exotropia).

Disruption of Function		
Muscle	**Cranial Nerve**	**Results**
Superior rectus	Oculomotor	Inability to move eye upward or temporally
Superior oblique	Trochlear	Inability to move eye down or nasally
Lateral rectus	Abducens	Inability to move eye temporally
Inferior oblique	Oculomotor	Inability to move eye upward or temporally
Inferior rectus	Oculomotor	Inability to move eye downward or temporally
Medial rectus	Oculomotor	Inability to move eye nasally

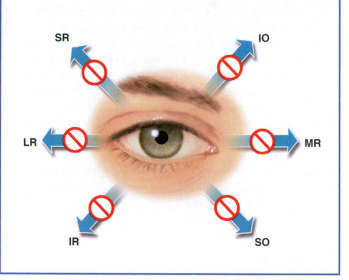

Figure 14.23 Extraocular muscle abnormalities.

Application Through Critical Thinking

CASE STUDY

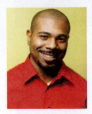

Source: logoboom/ Shutterstock.

John Jerome is a 45-year-old male who made an appointment for an annual employment physical assessment. Mr. Jerome completed a written questionnaire in preparation for his meeting with a healthcare professional. He checked "none" for all categories of family history of disease except diabetes. He indicated that he knew of no changes in his health since his last assessment.

The focused history reveals the following:

A male wearing eyeglasses entered the room; he appears his stated age of 45 yrs. He turned his head to the left and right and looked about the room before sitting across from the examiner. The patient had some redness in the sclera of both eyes. During the interview, the patient reveals that his last eye examination occurred 6 months ago, and he received a prescription for new glasses. He states that he is still having a problem with the new glasses and needs to have them checked. When asked to describe the problem, Mr. Jerome replies, "I just don't feel right with these glasses, and these are the second pair in a little over a year." He further states, "I just think I am overworking my eyes lately. I need to rest them more than ever, and I have had some headaches. I thought the glasses would help, but it hasn't gotten better." The patient denies any other problems. In response to inquiries about family history, he reports that his mother had diabetes but had no problems with her eyes. He doesn't know of any other eye problems in his family, except his mother had told him that an aunt of hers had been blind for some time. He reiterates that his only problem of late has been "this thing with my glasses, otherwise I feel fine."

The physical assessment reveals the following:

- Vital signs: BP 128/84—P 88—RR 22
- Height 6′3″, weight 188 lb
- Eyeballs firm to palpation
- Moderately dilated pupils

SAMPLE DOCUMENTATION

The following information is summarized from the case study.

SUBJECTIVE DATA: Visit for annual employment physical assessment. Negative family history except diabetes. No changes in health since last assessment. Last eye assessment 6 months ago—result prescription for new glasses. Stated he was having a problem with the new glasses. "I don't feel right with them." Stated, "I think I'm overworking my eyes lately. I thought the new glasses would help, but it hasn't gotten better." History of aunt with blindness.

OBJECTIVE DATA: Turns head to left and right and looked around room before sitting across from examiner. Scleral redness bilaterally. Eyeballs firm to palpation. Pupils moderate dilation. Cupping of optic discs. Height 6′3″, weight 188 lb. VS: BP 128/84—P 88—RR 22.

CRITICAL THINKING QUESTIONS

1. What conclusions would the nurse reach based on the data?
2. How was this conclusion formulated?
3. What information is missing?
4. What is the priority for this patient, and what options would apply?
5. As Mr. Jerome ages, for what age-related vision changes will he be at risk?

REFERENCES

American Academy of Ophthalmology. (2016). *Five tips from ophthalmologists that will protect your eyes from sun damage.* Retrieved from https://www.aao.org/newsroom/news-releases/detail/five-tips-to-protect-your-eyes-from-sun-damage

Berman, A., Snyder, S. J., & Frandsen, G. (2016). *Kozier and Erb's fundamentals of nursing: Concepts, process, and practice* (10th ed.). Hoboken, NJ: Pearson.

Choi, H. G., Lee, M. J., & Lee, S. (2018). Visual impairment and risk of depression: A longitudinal follow-up study using a national sample cohort. *Nature, Scientific Reports, 8*(2083). doi:10.1038/s41598-018-20374-5

Fenwick, E. K., Man, R. E., Cheung, C. M., Sabanayagam, C., Cheng, C., Neelam, K., . . . Lamoreux, E. L. (2017). Ethnic differ-ences in the association between age-related macular degener-ation and vision-specific functioning. *JAMA Ophthalmology, 135*(5), 469–476. doi:10.1001/jamaophthalmol.2017.0266

Folsom, A. R., Lutsey, P. L., Klein, R., Klein, B. E., & Tang, W. (2017). Retinal microvascular signs and incidence of abdom-inal aortic aneurysm: The Atherosclerosis Risk in Commu-nities Study. *Ophthalmic Epidemiology, 2017,* 1–4. doi:10.1080/09286586.2017.1418387

Gilbert, C. (2013). The eye signs of vitamin A deficiency. *Com-munity Eye Health Journal, 26*(84), 66–67. Retrieved from https://www.ncbi.nlm.nih.gov/pmc/journals/291

Glaucoma Research Foundation (GRF). (2017). *African Americans and glaucoma.* Retrieved from http://www.glaucoma.org/glaucoma/african-americans-and-glaucoma.php

Higginbotham, E. J., Coleman, A. L., & Teutsch, S. (2017). Eye health needs to be a population health priority. *American Journal of Ophthalmology, 173,* vii–viii. doi:10.1016/j.ajo.2016.10.003

Kim, E., Kim, H., Vijayakumar, A., Kwon, O., & Chang, N. (2017). Associations between fruit and vegetable, and antioxidant nutrient intake and age-related macular degeneration by smoking status in elderly Korean men. *Nutrition Journal, 77*(16), 1–9. doi:10.1186/s12937-017-0301-2

Lanius, R. A., Rabellino, D., Boyd, J. E., Harricharan, S., Frewen, P. A., & McKinnon, M. C. (2017). The innate alarm system in PTSD: Conscious and subconscious processing of threat. *Current Opinion in Psychology, 14,* 109–115. doi:10.1016/j.copsyc.2016.11.006

Marieb, E. N., & Keller, S. M. (2018). *Essentials of human anatomy and physiology* (12th ed.). New York, NY: Pearson Education.

Mayo Clinic. (2015). *Glaucoma: Symptoms.* Retrieved from http://www.mayoclinic.org/diseases-conditions/glaucoma/basics/symptoms/con-20024042

MedlinePlus. (2016). *Pterygium.* Retrieved from http://www.nlm.nih.gov/medlineplus/ency/article/001011.htm

MedlinePlus. (2018). *Visual acuity test.* Retrieved from http://www.nlm.nih.gov/medlineplus/ency/article/003396.htm

Medscape. (2016). *Exophthalmos clinical presentation.* Retrieved from http://emedicine.medscape.com/article/1218575-overview

Osborn, K. S., Wraa, C. E., Watson, A., & Holleran, R. S. (2013). *Medical-surgical nursing: Preparation for practice* (2nd ed.). Upper Saddle River, NJ: Pearson.

Scadding, G. K., Hariyawasam, H. H., Scadding, G., Mirakian, R., Buckley, R. J., Dixon, T., . . . Clark, A. T. (2017). BSACI guideline for the diagnosis and management of allergic and non-allergic rhinitis (1st ed., 2007; rev. ed., 2017). *Clinical & Experimental Allergy, 47*(7), 856–889. doi:10.1111/cea.12953

Shields, K. M., Fox, K. L., & Liebrecht, C. (2018). *Pearson nurse's drug guide.* Hoboken, NJ: Pearson.

Tarlan, B., & Kiratli, H. (2013). Subconjunctival hemorrhage: Risk factors and potential indicators. *Clinical Ophthalmology, 7,* 1163–1170. doi:10.2147/OPTH.S35062

Teutsch, S. M., McCoy, M. A., Woodbury, R. B., & Welp, A. (2016). *Making eye health a population health imperative: Vision for tomorrow.* Washington, DC: The National Academies Press. Retrieved from http://nap.edu/23471

WebMD. (2016). *Halos and glare: Why can't I see well at night?* Retrieved from https://www.webmd.com/eye-health/halos-and-glare-causes-prevention-treatment#1

WebMD. (2017a). *Caring for your contact lenses and your eyes.* Retrieved from http://www.webmd.com/eye-health/caring-contact-lens

WebMD. (2017b). *Eye floaters: Benign.* Retrieved from http://www.webmd.com/eye-health/benign-eye-floaters

World Health Organization (WHO). (n.d.). *Ultraviolet radiation and the INTERSUN programme: Health effects of UV radiation.* Retrieved from http://www.who.int/uv/health/en

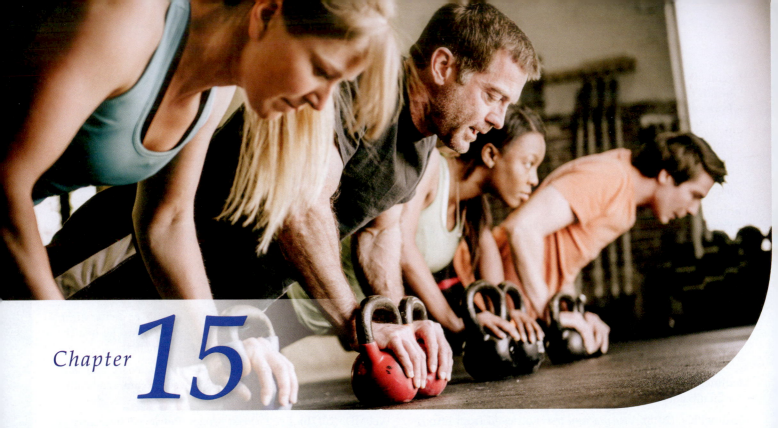

Chapter 15

Ears, Nose, Mouth, and Throat

LEARNING OUTCOMES

Upon completion of this chapter, you will be able to:

1. Describe the anatomy and physiology of the ears, nose, mouth, and throat.

2. Identify the anatomic, physiologic, developmental, psychosocial, and cultural variations that guide assessment of the ears, nose, mouth, and throat.

3. Determine which questions about the ears, nose, mouth, and throat to use for the focused interview.

4. Outline the techniques for assessment of the ears, nose, mouth, and throat.

5. Generate the appropriate documentation to describe the assessment of the ears, nose, mouth, and throat.

6. Identify abnormal findings in the physical assessment of the ears, nose, mouth, and throat.

KEY TERMS

air conduction, 277	eustachian tube, 263	ossicles, 263	tragus, 263
auricle, 263	fever blisters, 283	otitis externa, 271	tympanic membrane, 263
bone conduction, 277	helix, 263	otitis media, 287	uvula, 266
cerumen, 263	lobule, 263	palate, 266	
cochlea, 263	mastoiditis, 275	paranasal sinuses, 265	
cold sore, 283	nasal polyps, 281	pinna, 263	

MEDICAL LANGUAGE

gloss-	Prefix meaning "tongue"
-itis	Suffix meaning "inflammation"
naso-	Prefix meaning "nose"
oro-	Prefix meaning "mouth"

ot-	Prefix meaning "ear"
post-	Prefix meaning "after," "behind"
sub-	Prefix meaning "under," "below"

Introduction

This chapter describes the assessment of the ears, nose, mouth, and throat. Together with the head and eyes, these make up what is sometimes referred to as head, eyes, ears, nose, and throat, also known as HEENT. These structures include complex features that enable the senses of hearing, smell, and taste. In addition, the structures of the nose, mouth, and throat mark the beginning of both the respiratory and gastrointestinal systems. Assessment of each of these body systems is discussed in this chapter and will be further explored in Chapter 24 ∞

Anatomy and Physiology Review

The anatomic structures of the ears, nose, mouth, and throat include the internal and external ear, the nose and sinuses, the oral cavity, and the pharynx (throat). Each of the structures is described in the following sections.

Ear

The ear is the sensory organ that functions in hearing and equilibrium. It is divided into the external ear, middle ear, and inner ear. The external portion, or what most people think of as the ear, is called the **auricle** or **pinna**. It has a shell of cartilage covered with skin that funnels sound into the meatus (opening) of the external auditory canal. The major functions of the ears are collecting and transporting sound vibrations to the brain and maintaining the sense of equilibrium.

External Ear Figure 15.1 ■ depicts the surface anatomy of the external ear. The external large rim of the auricle is called the **helix**. The **tragus** is a stiff projection that protects the anterior meatus of the auditory canal. The **lobule** or earlobe of the ear is a small flap of flesh at the inferior end of the auricle. The external auditory canal is about 1 in. (2.54 cm) in length, is S-shaped, and leads to the middle ear. It is lined with glands that secrete a yellow-brown wax called **cerumen**. These secretions lubricate and protect the ear. The functions of chewing and talking help move the cerumen in the canal. The mastoid process, part of the temporal bone of the skull, is adjacent to the cavity of the middle ear. It contains many air cells and is assessed with the ear. This process has no role in hearing or balance. The mastoid process may become infected following ear infections in the adult.

Middle Ear The external ear and middle ear are separated by the **tympanic membrane** or eardrum (see Figure 15.2 ■). This thin, translucent membrane is pearly gray in color and lies obliquely in the canal. Sound waves entering the auditory

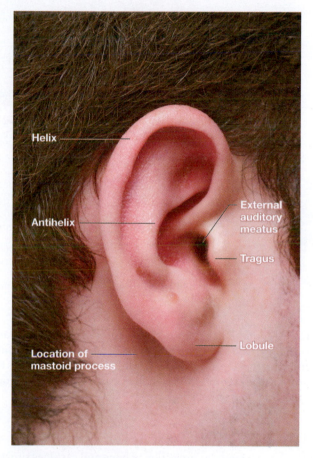

Figure 15.1 External ear.

canal strike the membrane, causing it to vibrate. The vibrations are transferred to the **ossicles**, or bones of the middle ear: the malleus, the incus, and the stapes. The ossicles, in turn, transfer the vibration to the oval window of the inner ear. Note that the malleus projects inferiorly and laterally and can be seen through the translucent tympanic membrane when viewed with the otoscope. The **eustachian tube** or auditory tube connects the middle ear with the nasopharynx. These tubes help to equalize air pressure on both sides of the tympanic membrane. The middle ear functions to conduct sound vibrations from the external ear to the inner ear. It also protects the inner ear by reducing loud sound vibrations.

Inner Ear The inner ear contains the bony labyrinth, which consists of a central cavity called the vestibule; three semicircular canals responsible for the sense of equilibrium; and the **cochlea**, a spiraling chamber that contains the receptors for hearing. Impulses from the equilibrium receptors of the inner ear are sent via the auditory nerve (cranial nerve VIII) to the

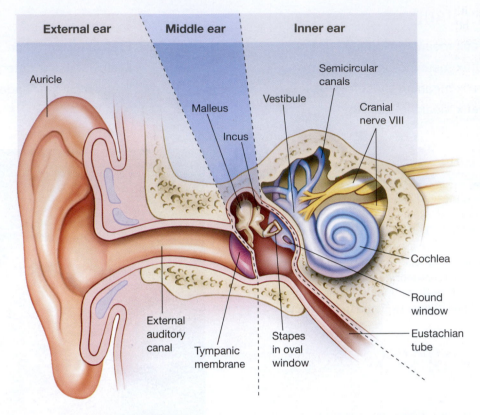

Figure 15.2 The three parts of the ear.

brain. Responses are then initiated to activate the eyes and muscles of the body to maintain balance. The cochlea transmits sound vibrations to the auditory nerve, which in turn carries the impulse to the auditory cortex in the temporal lobe of the brain for interpretation as hearing.

Nose and Sinuses

The nose is a triangular projection of bone and cartilage situated midline on the face (see Figure 15.3 ■). It is the only externally visible organ of the respiratory system. During inspiration, air enters the nasal cavity where it is filtered, warmed, and moistened before it moves toward the trachea and lungs.

The nose consists of external and internal structures. Externally, the bridge of the nose is on the superior aspect of the nose, medial to each orbit of the eyes. Inferior to the bridge and free of attachment to the face is the tip of the nose. The nares, two oval external openings at the base of the nose, are surrounded by the columella and ala structures of cartilage. Each nare widens into the internal vestibule and nasal cavity. The nasal septum is a continuation of the columella, dividing the nose into a right and left side.

The nasal mucosa with its rich blood supply helps filter inspired air and has a redder appearance than the oral mucosa. Three turbinates (superior, middle, and inferior) project from the medial wall into each side of the nasal cavity. These bony

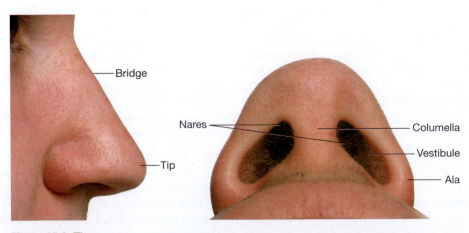

Figure 15.3 The nose.

projections, covered with nasal mucosa, add surface area for cleaning, moistening, and warming air entering the respiratory tract. Each side of the posterior nasal cavity opens into the naso-pharynx (see Figure 15.4 ■).

The olfactory cells, located in the roof of the nasal cavity, form filaments that connect to the olfactory nerve (cranial nerve I) and are responsible for the sense of smell.

The **paranasal sinuses** are mucus-lined, air-filled cavities that surround the nasal cavity and perform the air-processing functions of filtration, moistening, and warming. They are named for the bones of the skull in which they are contained:

sphenoid, frontal, ethmoid, and maxillary. The frontal and max-illary sinuses are accessible to examination and are discussed later in this chapter (see Figure 15.5 ■).

The major functions of the nose and sinuses are the following:

- Providing an airway for respiration
- Filtering, warming, and humidifying air flowing into the respiratory tract
- Providing resonance for the voice
- Housing the receptors for olfaction

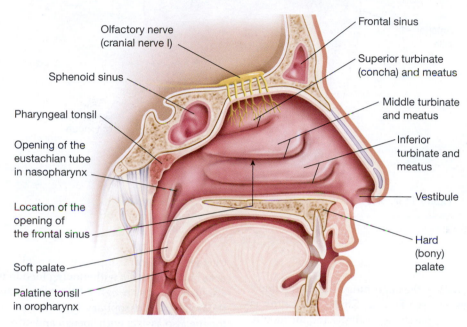

Figure 15.4 Internal structure of the nose—lateral view.

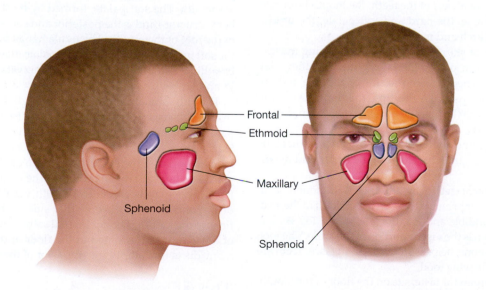

Figure 15.5 Nasal sinuses.

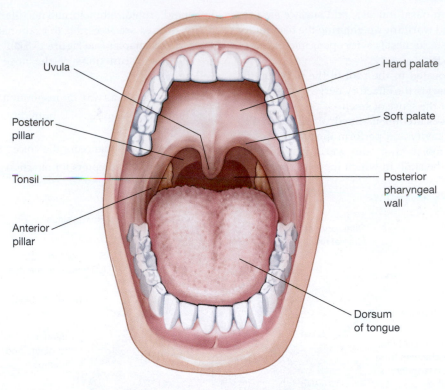

Uvula

Posterior pillar

Tonsil

Anterior pillar

Hard palate

Soft palate

Posterior pharyngeal wall

Dorsum of tongue

Figure 15.6 Oral cavity.

Mouth

The oval-shaped oral cavity is the beginning of the alimentary canal and digestive system (see Figure 15.6 ■). The cavity is divided by the teeth into two parts: the vestibule and the mouth. The vestibule, the anterior and smaller of the two regions, is composed of the lips, the buccal mucosa (the inner lining of the cheeks and lips), the outer surface of the gums and teeth, and the cheeks. At the posterior aspect of the teeth, the mouth is formed and includes the tongue, the hard and soft palate, the **uvula**, and the mandibular arch and maxillary arch.

The lips are folds of skin that cover the underlying muscle. They help keep food in place when chewing, and they play a role in speech. The cheeks form the side of the face and are continuous with the lips. Like the lips, the skin covers the underlying muscle. Both the lips and cheeks are lined internally with the buccal mucosa.

The gingivae or gums are bands of fibrous tissue that surround each tooth. The gums cover the mandibular and maxillary arches.

Thirty-two permanent teeth in the adult and 20 deciduous teeth (also called baby teeth or primary teeth) in the child sit in the alveoli sockets of the mandible and maxilla (see Figure 15.7 ■). The enamel-covered crown is the visible portion of the tooth. The root, embedded in the jawbone, helps hold the tooth in place. Teeth are used for biting and chewing food.

The tongue, the organ for taste, sits on the floor of the mouth. Its base sits on the hyoid bone (see Figure 13.5). The anterior portion of the tongue is attached to the floor of the mouth by the frenulum. The ventral surface (undersurface) of the tongue is smooth with visible vessels. The dorsal (top) surface of the tongue is rough and supports the papillae. Papillae contain the taste buds and assist with moving food in the mouth. Taste buds are distributed throughout the tongue and are innervated by the facial and glossopharyngeal nerves (see Figure 15.8 ■). The tongue also assists with speech and swallowing. These actions are stimulated by the hypoglossal nerve (cranial nerve XII).

Hard and soft palates form the roof of the mouth. The hard **palate**, formed by bones, is the anterior portion of the roof of the mouth. The soft palate, formed by muscle, does not have a bony structure and is the posterior and somewhat mobile aspect of the roof of the mouth. The uvula hangs from the free edge of the soft palate. The uvula and soft palate move with swallowing, breathing, and phonation and are innervated by cranial nerves IX and X.

Parotid, submandibular, and sublingual salivary glands are responsible for the production of saliva (see Figure 15.9 ■). The parotid glands are situated anterior to the ear within the cheek. Saliva enters the mouth via Stensen's duct located in the buccal mucosa opposite the second upper molar. The submandibular glands sit beneath the mandible at the angle of the jaw. Saliva from these glands enters the mouth via Wharton's duct. The orifice of these ducts is on either side of the frenulum on the floor of the mouth. The sublingual salivary glands, the smallest of the glands, are situated in the floor of the mouth and have many ducts that empty into the floor of the mouth.

Throat

The throat, known as the pharynx, connects the nose, mouth, larynx, and esophagus. The three sections of the throat are the nasopharynx (behind the nose), the oropharynx (behind

Upper deciduous teeth

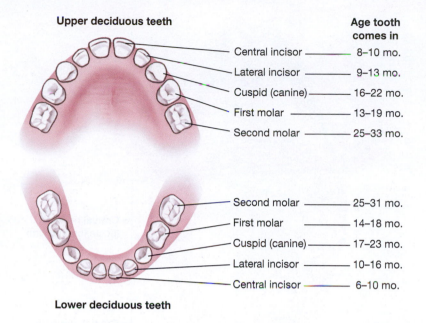

	Age tooth comes in
Central incisor	8–10 mo.
Lateral incisor	9–13 mo.
Cuspid (canine)	16–22 mo.
First molar	13–19 mo.
Second molar	25–33 mo.
Second molar	25–31 mo.
First molar	14–18 mo.
Cuspid (canine)	17–23 mo.
Lateral incisor	10–16 mo.
Central incisor	6–10 mo.

Lower deciduous teeth

Upper permanent teeth

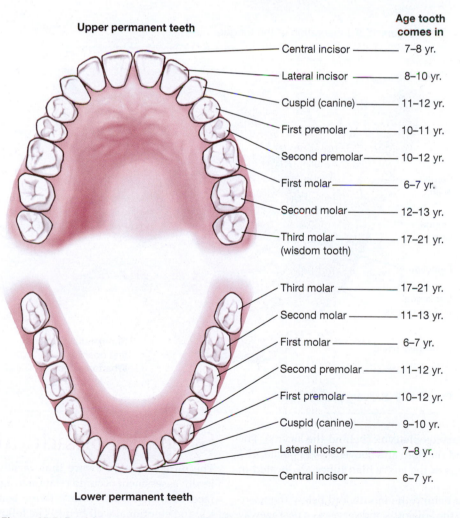

	Age tooth comes in
Central incisor	7–8 yr.
Lateral incisor	8–10 yr.
Cuspid (canine)	11–12 yr.
First premolar	10–11 yr.
Second premolar	10–12 yr.
First molar	6–7 yr.
Second molar	12–13 yr.
Third molar (wisdom tooth)	17–21 yr.
Third molar	17–21 yr.
Second molar	11–13 yr.
First molar	6–7 yr.
Second premolar	11–12 yr.
First premolar	10–12 yr.
Cuspid (canine)	9–10 yr.
Lateral incisor	7–8 yr.
Central incisor	6–7 yr.

Lower permanent teeth

Figure 15.7 Deciduous and permanent teeth.

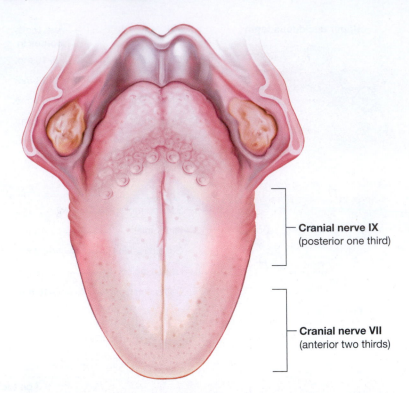

Figure 15.8 Innervation of the tongue.

Cranial nerve IX
(posterior one third)

Cranial nerve VII
(anterior two thirds)

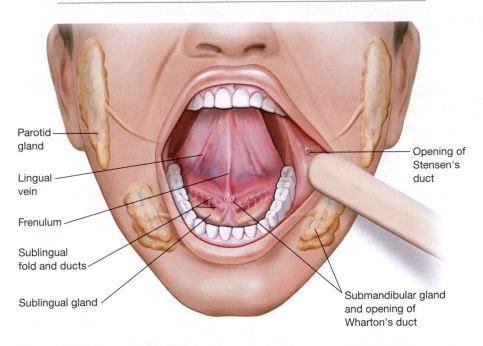

Figure 15.9 Salivary glands.

Parotid gland

Lingual vein

Frenulum

Sublingual fold and ducts

Sublingual gland

Opening of Stensen's duct

Submandibular gland and opening of Wharton's duct

the mouth), and the laryngopharynx (behind the larynx). The nasopharynx is behind the nose and above the soft palate. The adenoids and openings of the eustachian tubes are located in the nasopharynx.

The oropharynx is behind the mouth and below the nasopharynx. It extends to the epiglottis and serves as a passageway for air and food. The tonsils are located behind the pillars (palatopharyngeal folds) on either side.

Special Considerations

The nurse must be aware that variations in findings from health assessment occur in relation to age, developmental level, race, ethnicity, work history, living conditions, socioeconomics, and emotional well-being. The following sections describe some factors to consider when collecting subjective and objective data.

Lifespan Considerations

Growth and development are dynamic processes that describe change over time. It is important to understand data collection and interpretation of findings regarding growth and development in relation to normative values. Details about specific variations in ear, nose, mouth, and throat health for different age groups are presented in Chapter 25, Chapter 26, and Chapter 27. ∞

Psychosocial Considerations

A patient who is under a great deal of stress may be prone to mouth ulcers and lip biting. Tics (involuntary muscle spasms) and unconscious clenching of the jaw may indicate psychosocial disturbances. Relaxation techniques such as meditation and guided imagery may help relieve these stress-related behaviors.

Ethnic and Environmental Considerations

Cerumen or "earwax" is a waxy substance that is a combination of substances secreted by apocrine sweat glands and sebaceous glands in the external ear canal. The consistency ranges from white or grey to yellow, orange-brown, or dark brown; it may be flaky, crumbly, wet, sticky, or hard. The type of cerumen in an individual is linked to ethnicity. The dry type is more common in East Asian populations and rare in European and African populations. Native North American, Pacific Islander, and Central Asian populations may have a mix of dry and wet types (Mason, 2013; Shokry & Filho, 2017).

A patient's occupation or hobbies may increase the risk for hearing loss if the nature of the work or work environment exposes the patient to high noise levels. For example, construction workers, welders, groundskeepers, and musicians should be evaluated for hearing acuity and also should be advised to use earplugs. The nurse will ask detailed questions about the patient's exposure to noisy environments, including work, play, and home. Some studies are showing some negative connections between exposure to noise, such as from aircraft or traffic, and cardiovascular conditions and hypertension in adults, as well as with cognitive conditions in children (Dimakopoulou et al., 2017; Weyde et al., 2017).

Subjective Data—Health History

Health assessment of the ears, nose, mouth, and throat includes gathering subjective and objective data. Recall that subjective data collection occurs during the patient interview before the actual physical assessment. During the interview, the nurse uses a variety of communication techniques to elicit general and specific information about the state of health or illness of the patient's ears, nose, mouth, and throat. Health records, the results of laboratory tests, and x-rays are important secondary sources to be reviewed and included in the data-gathering process. The techniques of inspection, palpation, and percussion will be used in the physical assessment of the ears, nose, mouth, and throat. Before proceeding, it may be helpful to review the information about each of the data-gathering processes and practice the techniques of health assessment. Some special equipment and assessments are included—for example, the use of the otoscope. See Table 15.1 for information on potential secondary sources of patient data.

Table 15.1 Potential Secondary Sources for Patient Data Related to the Ears, Nose, Mouth, and Throat

LABORATORY TESTS FOR THE EAR, NOSE, MOUTH, AND THROAT
Diagnostic Tests
Ear
Audiometric Screening
Auditory Screening
Electronystagmography
X-ray
Nose and Sinuses
Computed Tomography (CT)
X-ray
Teeth
X-ray
Throat
Laryngoscopy

Focused Interview

The focused interview concerns data related to the structures and functions of the ears, nose, mouth, and throat. Subjective data related to these structures are gathered during the focused interview. The nurse must be prepared to observe the patient and listen for cues related to the functions of these structures. The nurse may use open-ended and closed questions to obtain information. Follow-up questions or requests for descriptions are required to clarify data or gather missing information. Follow-up questions identify the source of problems, duration of difficulties, and measures to alleviate problems. They also provide clues regarding the patient's knowledge about his or her own health.

The focused interview guides the physical assessment of the ears, nose, mouth, and throat. The information is always considered in relation to normative parameters and expectations about function. Therefore, the nurse must consider age, gender, race, culture, environment, health practices, past and concurrent problems, and therapies when framing questions and using techniques to elicit information. In order to address all of the factors when conducting a focused interview, categories of questions have been developed. These categories include general questions that are asked of all patients; those addressing illness, infection; questions related to symptoms, pain, behaviors; those related to habits or practices; and questions that address environmental concerns. One method to elicit information about symptoms is the OLDCART & ICE method, described in Chapter 5. ∞

The nurse must consider the patient's ability to participate in the focused interview and physical assessment of the ears, nose, mouth, and throat. If a patient is experiencing pain, discomfort, or anxiety, attention must focus on relief of symptoms.

Focused Interview Questions	Rationales and Evidence

The following section provides sample questions and bulleted follow-up questions in each of the previously identified categories. For assessment of the ears, a rationale for each of the questions is provided. The list of questions is not all inclusive but represents the types of questions required in a comprehensive focused interview related to the ears. Questions for the nose, mouth, and throat are included. These questions would follow the same format and be categorized as those for the ear. The bulleted follow-up questions are asked in order to obtain additional information and clarification from the patient that will enhance the subjective database.

EAR

General Questions

1. **Describe your hearing. Have you noticed any change in your hearing? If so, tell me about:**
   - *Onset:* Gradual or sudden?
   - *Character:* Just certain sounds or tones, or all hearing?
   - *Situations:* When using a telephone? Watching television? During conversations?

   ▶ The patient's failure to respond to questions, or asking the nurse to repeat questions, may indicate a hearing loss. Hearing acuity decreases gradually with age. Any sudden loss of hearing should be investigated.

2. **When was your last hearing test?**
   - What were the results?
   - Does your hearing seem better in one ear than the other?
   - Which ear?

   ▶ Individuals who live or work in noisy environments should have annual hearing tests (Carroll et al., 2017; Centers for Disease Control and Prevention [CDC], 2016). Hearing loss in one ear could indicate an obstruction with cerumen or a ruptured tympanic membrane (American Speech Language Hearing Association [ASHA], n.d.).

3. **Has any member of your family had ear problems or hearing loss?**

   ▶ Hearing loss can be hereditary (Shearer, Hildebrand, & Smith, 2017).

Questions Related to Illness or Infection

1. **Have you ever been diagnosed with a disease affecting the ears?**
   - When were you diagnosed with the problem?
   - What treatment was prescribed for the problem?
   - What kinds of things do you do to help with the problem?
   - Has the problem ever recurred (acute)?
   - How are you managing the disease now (chronic)?

   ▶ The patient has an opportunity to provide information about specific illnesses affecting the ears. If a diagnosed illness is identified, follow-up about the diagnosis, treatment, and outcomes is required. Data about each illness identified by the patient are essential to an accurate health assessment. Illnesses are classified as acute or chronic, and follow-up regarding each classification will differ.

2. *Alternative to question 1:* List possible illnesses of the ears, such as Ménière's disease, vertigo, and acoustic neuroma, and ask the patient to respond "yes" or "no" as each is stated.

   ▶ This is a comprehensive and easy way to elicit information about all diagnoses related to the ear. Follow-up would be carried out for each identified diagnosis as in question 1.

3. **Do you now have or have you had an ear infection?**
   - When were you diagnosed with the infection?
   - What treatment was prescribed for the problem?
   - Was the treatment helpful?
   - What kinds of things do you do to help with the problem?
   - Has the problem ever recurred (acute)?
   - How are you managing the infection now (chronic)?

   ▶ If an infection is identified, follow-up about the date of infection, treatment, and outcomes is required. Data about each infection identified by the patient are essential to an accurate health assessment. Infections can be classified as acute or chronic, and follow-up regarding each classification will differ.

4. *Alternative to question 3:* List possible ear infections, such as external otitis, otitis media, labyrinthitis, and mastoiditis, and ask the patient to respond "yes" or "no" as each is stated.

   ▶ This is a comprehensive and easy way to elicit information about all ear infections. Follow-up would be carried out for each identified infection as in question 3.

Questions Related to Symptoms, Pain, and Behaviors

When gathering information about symptoms, many questions are required to elicit details and descriptions that assist in the analysis of the data. Discrimination is made in relation to the significance of a symptom, in relation to specific diseases or problems, and in relation to potential follow-up examination or referral. One rationale may be provided for a group of questions in this category.

The following questions refer to specific symptoms and behaviors associated with the ear. For each symptom, questions and follow-up are required. The details to be elicited are the characteristics of the symptom; the onset, duration, and frequency of the symptom; the treatment or remedy for the symptom, including over-the-counter and home remedies; the determination if diagnosis has been sought; the effect of treatments; and family history associated with a symptom or illness.

Questions Related to Symptoms

1. **Have you had any ear drainage? If so, describe it.**

   ▶ Ear drainage may indicate an infection. Bloody or purulent drainage could indicate otitis media, or infection of the middle ear. Serous drainage could indicate allergic reaction. Clear drainage could be cerebrospinal fluid following trauma (Osborn, Wraa, Watson, & Holleran, 2013).

Focused Interview Questions	Rationales and Evidence
2. Have you had dizziness, nausea, vomiting, or ringing in your ears?	▶ These symptoms could indicate a problem with the inner ear, could be related to a neurologic problem, or could be drug related (ASHA, n.d.).
Questions Related to Pain	
1. Do you have any pain in your ears? • If so, describe it. If yes, have you recently had a cold or sore throat? • Have you had any problems lately with your sinuses or your teeth? • Have you had any ear trauma or ear surgery?	▶ Pain in one or both ears may be caused by acute otitis media, otitis externa, foreign bodies or trauma, temporomandibular joint syndrome, dental problems, pharyngitis, tonsillitis, and other diseases (Earwood, Rogers, & Rathjen, 2018).
Questions Related to Behaviors	
1. How do you clean your ears?	▶ Many people use cotton-tipped applicators to remove cerumen. This practice can cause trauma to the eardrum and cause cerumen to become impacted. Ear canals should never be cleaned. Cerumen moves to the outside naturally. Commercial cerumen removal products are available but should be used with the guidance of a healthcare provider (Mason, 2013).
2. Do you either own or use a hearing aid?	▶ Some patients have hearing aids but will not use them because of increased background noise, embarrassment, or inability to pay for the necessary batteries.

Questions Related to the Environment

Environment refers to both the internal and external environments. Questions related to the internal environment include all of the previous questions and those associated with internal or physiologic responses. Questions regarding the external environment include those related to home, work, or social environments.

Internal Environment

1. Are you taking any medications? • What are they? • How often do you take them?	▶ Certain medicines affect the ears. Aspirin can cause ringing in the ears (tinnitus). Some antibiotics can cause hearing loss and dizziness (Shields, Fox, & Liebrecht, 2018).

External Environment

The following questions deal with substances and irritants found in the physical environment of the patient. The physical environment includes the indoor and outdoor environments of the home and workplace, those encountered for social engagements, and any encountered during travel.

1. Are you frequently exposed to loud noise? • When? • How often? • Are protective devices available and do you use them?	▶ Long-term exposure to loud noise can result in hearing loss. Patients at risk are those with jobs in noisy factories; jobs at airports; jobs requiring the use of explosives, firearms, jackhammers, or other loud equipment; and jobs in nightclubs. Frequent exposure to loud music, either live or from stereos or headphones, can also contribute to hearing loss (CDC, 2016).
2. Do you experience ear infections or irritations after swimming or being exposed to dust or smoke? If so, describe them.	▶ Contaminated water left in the ear may cause **otitis externa**, or swimmer's ear. Irritation of the ear after exposure to certain substances may indicate an allergy to such substances (Osborn et al., 2013).

Questions Related to Age and Pregnancy

The focused interview must reflect the anatomic and physiologic differences in the ears, nose, mouth, and throat that exist along the age span as well as during pregnancy. Specific questions related to these systems for each of these groups are provided in Chapter 25, Chapter 26, and Chapter 27. ∞

NOSE AND SINUSES
General Questions

1. Are you having any problems with your nose or sinuses? If so, describe them. Are you able to breathe through your nose? • Can you breathe through both nostrils? • Is one side obstructed? • Describe any problems you have had breathing in the last few days and in the last few weeks.	▶ A history of frequent respiratory problems may indicate an underlying respiratory problem such as allergies or recurring infections.
2. Do you have nasal discharge? • If so, is it continuous or occasional? • Describe the discharge.	▶ A thin, watery discharge is the result of acute rhinitis from either a viral infection, such as the common cold, or an allergic reaction. Allergies that cause nasal discharge can also produce itchy eyes, postnasal drip, sore throats, ear infections, or headaches. Some allergies are seasonal; others are constant.

Focused Interview Questions	Rationales and Evidence
3. Do you have nosebleeds? • How often? • What is your usual blood pressure? • Do you use nasal sprays? • How do you treat your nosebleeds?	▶ Nosebleeds can occur as a result of high blood pressure, overuse of nasal sprays, and certain blood disorders (Mayo Clinic, 2018).
4. Have you ever had any nose injury or nose surgery? • If so, describe it. • How was the injury treated? • Do you have any residual problems from the injury or surgery?	
5. Describe your sense of smell. • Are there any circumstances, objects, places, or activities that affect your sense of smell? If so, describe them.	▶ Anosmia, the inability to smell, may be neurologic, hereditary, or because of a deficiency of zinc in the diet (CDC, 2018).
6. What prescribed or over-the-counter drugs do you take to relieve your nasal symptoms? • Do you use a nasal inhalant, oxygen, or a humidifier to help you breathe? • What other medications do you take regularly?	▶ Certain medications can produce unpleasant side effects in the nose, such as nasal stuffiness or nosebleeds. Many drugs administered by nasal inhalers may irritate the nasal mucosa and cause nosebleeds. Steroid inhalers can cause growth of *Candida* in the nose, mouth, or throat (Shields et al., 2018).
7. Do you use recreational drugs? • If so, what drugs? How often?	▶ Some inhaled drugs, such as cocaine, gradually break down the nasal lining by vasoconstriction. Regular nasal inhalation of cocaine may cause nasal perforation (Gold, Boyack, Caputo, & Pearlman, 2017).

MOUTH AND THROAT

General Questions

1. How would you describe the condition of your mouth and teeth? • Have you noticed any changes in the last few months?	
2. Do you have any problems swallowing?	▶ Dysphagia, or difficulty in swallowing, is frequently related to age-related changes in swallowing physiology; stroke; dementia and other neurological diseases; cancers of the head, neck, or esophagus; and other disorders. Achalasia is a motility disorder associated with loss of esophageal peristalsis and failure of the lower esophageal sphincter to relax upon swallowing; the cause of achalasia is unknown (O'Neill, Johnston, & Coleman, 2013).
3. Do you have any sores or lesions in your mouth or on your tongue? • If so, describe them. • Are they present constantly, or do they come and go periodically?	▶ Lesions of the mouth or tongue may be cold sores, mouth ulcers, or cysts. They may accompany gum infections, viral infections such as HIV or HPV, trauma, or inflammatory reactions. Lesions are frequently found in chronic tobacco users. Lesions may be benign or malignant, so any lesion of the mouth that does not heal should be evaluated for oral cancer (Hill, Devine & Renton, 2017).
4. Do your gums bleed frequently?	▶ Gum diseases such as gingivitis and periodontitis may cause gums to bleed easily. Gums may also bleed easily with ill-fitting braces or dentures (Osborn et al., 2013).
5. Have you noticed a change in your sense of taste recently?	▶ Loss of the sense of taste commonly accompanies colds. A foul taste in the mouth may signal a gum infection or inadequate care of teeth or dentures.
6. What dental problems, surgeries, or procedures have you had in the past? • Describe them.	
7. Do you wear dentures, partial plates, retainers, or any other removable or permanent dental appliance? • Does it fit well? Is it comfortable? • Why are you wearing the appliance? • Does it help resolve the problem? • Are any of your teeth capped? Which ones?	
8. How often do you brush your teeth or dentures? • Do you use floss regularly?	▶ Regular mouth care is important in maintaining healthy teeth and gums and preventing gum diseases such as gingivitis and periodontitis.
9. When was your last dental examination? • Are you unable to eat some foods because of problems with your teeth? • Do you have any pain in one or more teeth?	

Focused Interview Questions

10. Do you have frequent sore throats?

11. Have you noticed any hoarseness or loss of your voice?

12. Do you now or did you ever smoke a pipe, cigarettes, or cigars?
    - Chew tobacco or dip snuff?
    - How much? How often?

Rationales and Evidence

▶ A sore throat may be the result of irritation from sinus drainage, viral or bacterial infection, or the first sign of throat cancer (National Cancer Institute [NCI], 2017)

▶ Hoarseness is a common finding in disorders of the throat. Recurrent or persistent hoarseness may indicate cancer of the larynx (NCI, 2017). Hoarseness may also be because of anxiety, overuse of the voice, or a cold. Smoking and drinking alcohol can lead to inflammation of the vocal cords and result in hoarseness.

▶ Smoking, dipping snuff, or chewing tobacco may result in cancer of the lips, mouth, and throat (NCI, 2017).

Patient-Centered Interaction

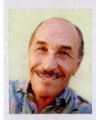

Source:
Diego Cervo/
Shutterstock.

Mr. Sanji, age 65, comes to the Medi-Center with a chief complaint of "having trouble hearing." The intake sheet that Mr. Sanji completed reveals a slow progressive loss of hearing with no pain in the ears or head. Following is an excerpt of the focused interview.

Interview

Nurse: Good morning, Mr. Sanji. Please have a seat and tell me about your deafness.

[The nurse and Mr. Sanji sit down across the desk from each other. During the interview, the nurse's head is down. The nurse maintains some eye contact by looking over the rim of the eyeglasses.]

Mr. Sanji: **I'm not deaf. I just can't hear like before.**

Nurse: How long have you noticed this progressive loss of hearing?

Mr. Sanji: **I'm not sure. A while. But I'm not deaf!**

Nurse: Have you had any purulent drainage from your ears?

Mr. Sanji: **Hmm!**

Nurse: Do you have a history of having otitis media or a tympanoplasty?

Mr. Sanji [Does not answer the question.]

Nurse: Would you like me to repeat the question?

Mr. Sanji: **Yeah, louder and in simple language!**

Analysis

In this situation the nurse has used several strategies that act as a hindrance to effective communication. The first problem is the nurse's body position and lack of eye contact. Keeping the head down muffles the sound for any person, especially one with a hearing deficit. The nurse should look up, speak directly to the patient, and maintain eye contact. Twice the patient says he is not deaf and the nurse does not seek clarification. Using language and terminology the individual does not understand is another obstacle. Mr. Sanji tells the nurse to speak louder and in simple terms.

Objective Data—Physical Assessment

Assessment Techniques and Findings

Physical assessment of the ears, nose, mouth, and throat requires the use of inspection, palpation, percussion, and transillumination of the sinuses. In addition, special examination techniques include the use of the otoscope, tuning fork, and nasal speculum. These techniques are used to gather objective data. Knowledge of normal or expected findings is essential in determining the meaning of data as the nurse proceeds.

Adults and children normally have binaural hearing, meaning that the brain is capable of simultaneously integrating information that is received from both ears. The ears are symmetric in size, shape, color, and configuration. The external

EQUIPMENT
- Examination gown
- Clean, nonsterile exam gloves
- Otoscope with specula of various sizes
- Tuning fork, 512 or 1024 Hz
- Nasal speculum
- Penlight
- Gauze pads
- Tongue blade

auditory canal is patent and free of drainage. The external ear and mastoid process are free of lesions, and the tragus is movable. Under otoscopic examination the external ear canal is open, nontender, and free of lesions, inflammation, or foreign substances. Cerumen, if present, is soft and in small amounts. The tympanic membrane is flat, gray, and translucent without lesions. The malleolar process and reflected light are visible on the tympanic membrane. The tympanic membrane flutters with the Valsalva maneuver. During hearing tests, air conduction is longer than bone conduction. Adults and healthy children other than infants are able to maintain balance.

The external nose is free of lesions, the nares are patent, and the mucosa of the nasal cavity is dark pink and smooth. The nasal septum is midline, straight, and intact. The sinuses are nontender and transilluminate.

The lips are smooth, symmetric, and lesion free. Typically, children begin losing their deciduous teeth by age 6 years. On average, most children lose their last deciduous tooth at approximately age 12 to 13 (Mayo Clinic, 2017). Healthy adults and children who are age 13 and older have 32 permanent teeth, including four wisdom teeth, all of which are white with smooth edges. The tongue is mobile, is pink, and has papillae on the dorsum. The oral mucosa is pink, moist, and smooth. Salivary ducts are visible and not inflamed. The membranes and structures of the throat are pink and moist. The uvula is midline and, like the soft palate, rises when the patient says "aah." This movement is related to the proper functioning of cranial nerves IX and X.

HELPFUL HINTS

- Provide specific instructions about what is expected of the patient. The nurse would state whether the head must be turned or the mouth opened.
- Consider the age of the patient. Response to directions varies across the lifespan.
- Pay attention to nonverbal cues throughout the assessment.
- Hearing difficulties may affect the data-gathering process. Clarify problems and possible remedies before beginning the assessment. The patient may use sign language, hearing aids, lip reading, or written communication.
- Explain the use of each piece of equipment throughout the assessment.
- Use Standard Precautions.

Physical assessment of the ears, nose, mouth, and throat follows an organized pattern. It begins with instruction of the patient and proceeds through inspection, palpation, and otoscopic examination of the ears, followed by hearing assessment and the Romberg test. The nose is inspected and the internal aspect visualized while using a speculum. The sinuses are palpated, percussed, and transilluminated. The assessment concludes with inspection of the external mouth, the internal structures of the mouth, and assessment of the throat.

Techniques and Normal Findings	Abnormal Findings and Special Considerations

Ear

1. Position the patient.
- The patient should be in a sitting position. Lighting must be adequate to detect skin color changes, discharge, and lesions.

▶ Ensure that the ear examination is conducted in a quiet place and that the patient is in a comfortable position.

2. Instruct the patient.
- Explain that you will be carrying out a variety of assessments of the ear. Tell the patient you will be touching the ear areas, that it should cause no discomfort, and that any pain or discomfort should be reported.

3. Note that you will have begun to evaluate the patient's hearing while taking the health history.
- Did the patient hear the questions you asked?
- Did the patient answer appropriately?
- Generally, the formal evaluation of hearing is performed after otoscopic examination so that physical barriers to hearing, such as large amounts of cerumen, can be identified.

4. Inspect the external ear for symmetry, proportion, color, and integrity.
- Confirm that the external auditory meatus is patent with no drainage. The color of the ear should match that of the surrounding area and the face, with no redness, nodules, swelling, or lesions.

▶ Any discharge, redness, or swelling may indicate an infection or allergy.

Techniques and Normal Findings	Abnormal Findings and Special Considerations

5. Palpate the auricle and push on the tragus (Figure 15.10 ■).
- Confirm that there are no hard nodules, lesions, or swelling. The tragus should be movable.
- This technique should not cause pain.

▶ Lesions accompanied by a history of long-term exposure to the sun may be cancerous.

▶ Pain could be the result of an infection of the external ear (otitis externa). Pain could also indicate temporomandibular joint dysfunction with pressure on the tragus. Hard nodules (tophi) are uric acid crystal deposits, which are a sign of gout.

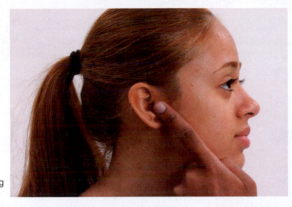

Figure 15.10 Palpating the tragus.

6. Palpate the mastoid process lying directly behind the ear (see Figure 15.11 ■).
- Confirm that there are no lesions, pain, or swelling.

▶ **Mastoiditis** refers to inflammation or infection of the mastoid bone. It is a complication of either a middle ear infection or a throat infection. Mastoiditis is very difficult to treat. It spreads easily to the brain because the mastoid area is separated from the brain by only a thin, bony plate.

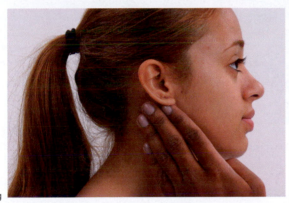

Figure 15.11 Palpating the mastoid process.

7. Inspect the auditory canal using the otoscope.
- For the best visualization, use the largest speculum that will fit into the auditory canal.
- Ask the patient to tilt the head away from you toward the opposite shoulder.
- Hold the otoscope between the palm and first two fingers of the dominant hand. The handle may be positioned upward or downward.
- Use your other hand to straighten the canal.
- In the adult patient, pull the pinna up, back, and out to straighten the canal (see Figure 15.12 ■).

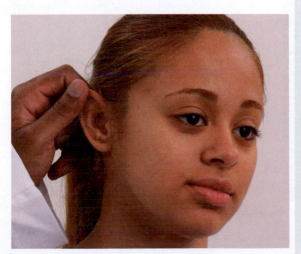

Figure 15.12 Pulling the pinna to straighten the canal.

Techniques and Normal Findings	Abnormal Findings and Special Considerations

- Be sure to maintain this position until the speculum is removed.
- Instruct the patient to tell you if any discomfort is experienced but not to move the head or suddenly pull away.

ALERT!   *The nurse must use care when inserting the speculum of the otoscope into the ear. The inner two-thirds of the ear are very sensitive, and pressing the speculum against either side of the auditory canal will cause pain.*

- With the light on, use the upward or downward position of the handle to insert the speculum into the ear (see Figure 15.13A and Figure 15.13B ■). Brace the otoscope with the dorsal surface of the fingers or hand. The external canal should be open and without tenderness, inflammation, lesions, growths, discharge, or foreign substances.
- Note the amount, color, and texture of the cerumen that is present.

▶ If the ear canal is occluded with cerumen, the cerumen must be removed. Most cerumen can be removed with a cerumen spoon. If the cerumen is dry, the external canal should be irrigated using a bulb syringe and a warmed solution of mineral oil and hydrogen peroxide, followed by warm water.

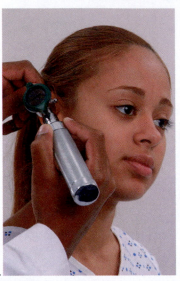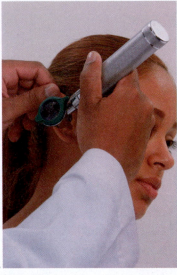

A.   B.

Figure 15.13 Two techniques for holding and inserting an otoscope.
A. Otoscopic examination with otoscope handle in downward position. B. Otoscopic examination with otoscope handle in upward position.

8. **Examine the tympanic membrane using the otoscope.**
   - The membrane should be flat, gray, and translucent with no scars (see Figure 15.14 ■). A cone-shaped reflection of the otoscope light should be visible at the 5 o'clock position in the right ear and the 7 o'clock position in the left ear. The short process of the malleus should be seen as a shadow behind the tympanic membrane. The membrane should be intact.
   - If you cannot visualize the tympanic membrane, remove the otoscope, reposition the auricle, and reinsert the otoscope. Do not reposition the auricle with the otoscope in place.

▶ White patches on the tympanic membrane indicate scars from prior infections. If the membrane is yellow or reddish, it could indicate an infection of the middle ear. A bulging membrane may indicate increased pressure in the middle ear, whereas a retracted membrane may indicate a vacuum in the middle ear because of a blocked eustachian tube. Failure to visualize the tympanic membrane may result from cerumen impaction. If needed, clean out the cerumen before attempting to visualize the tympanic membrane again.

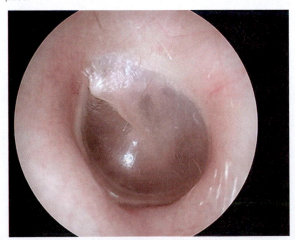

Figure 15.14 Normal tympanic membrane with cone of light and process of malleus.
Source: PROFESSOR TONY WRIGHT, INSTITUTE OF LARYNGOLOGY & OTOLOGY/ Science Source.

Techniques and Normal Findings	Abnormal Findings and Special Considerations

9. Perform the whisper test.
- This test evaluates hearing acuity of high frequency sounds.
- Ask the patient to occlude the left ear or the ear may be occluded by the nurse.
- Cover your mouth or stand where the patient cannot see your lips.
- Standing at a distance of 1 to 2 ft from the patient, (approximately 0.3 to 0.6 m), whisper a simple phrase such as, "The weather is hot today." Ask the patient to repeat the phrase. Then do the same procedure to test the right ear using a different phrase. The patient should be able to repeat the phrases correctly (Figure 15.15 ■).

▶ Inability to repeat the phrases may indicate a loss of the ability to hear high-frequency sounds.

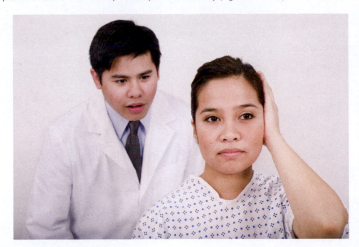

Figure 15.15 Performing the whisper test.

- Tuning forks are also used to evaluate auditory acuity. The tines of the fork, when activated, produce sound waves. The frequency, or cycles per second (cps), is the expression used to describe the action of the instrument. A fork with 512 cps vibrates 512 times per second and is the size of choice for auditory evaluations. The tines are set into motion by squeezing, stroking, or lightly tapping against your hand. The fork must be held at the handle to prevent interference with the vibration of the tines (see Figure 15.16 ■).

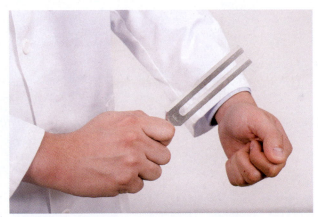

Figure 15.16 Activating the tuning fork.

- The following tests use a tuning fork primarily to evaluate conductive versus perceptive hearing loss. **Air conduction** (AC) is the transmission of sound through the tympanic membrane to the cochlea and auditory nerve. **Bone conduction** (BC) is the transmission of sound through the bones of the skull to the cochlea and auditory nerve.

Techniques and Normal Findings	Abnormal Findings and Special Considerations

10. Perform the Rinne test.

- The Rinne test compares air and bone conduction. This is an advanced assessment technique. Hold the tuning fork by the handle and gently strike the fork on the palm of your hand to set it vibrating.
- Place the base of the fork on the patient's mastoid process (see Figure 15.17A ■).
- Ask the patient to tell you when the sound is no longer heard.
- Note the number of seconds. Then immediately move the tines of the still-vibrating fork in front of the external auditory meatus (see Figure 15.17B ■). It should be 1 cm to 2 cm (about 1/2 in.) from the meatus.
- Ask the patient to tell you again when the sound is no longer heard. Again, note the number of seconds. Normally, the sound is heard twice as long by air conduction as by bone conduction after bone conduction stops. For example, a normal finding is AC 30 seconds, BC 15 seconds.

▶ If the patient hears the bone conducted sound as long as or longer than the air conducted sound, the patient may have some degree of conductive hearing loss.

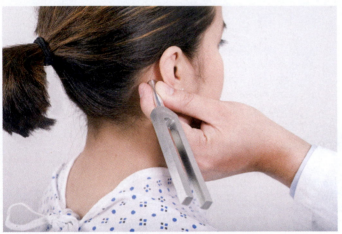

Figure 15.17A Rinne test. Bone conduction.

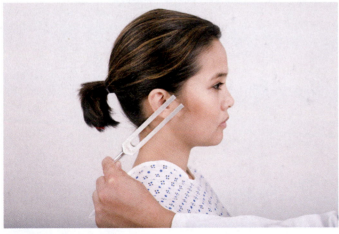

Figure 15.17B Rinne test. Air conduction.

Techniques and Normal Findings	Abnormal Findings and Special Considerations

11. Perform the Weber test.

- The Weber test uses bone conduction to evaluate hearing in a person who hears better in one ear than in the other. Hold the tuning fork by the handle and strike the fork on the palm of the hand. Place the base of the vibrating fork against the patient's skull. The midline of the anterior portion of the frontal bone is used (Figure 15.18 ■). The midline of the forehead is an alternative choice.

▶ If the patient hears the sound in one ear better than the other ear, the hearing loss may be because of either poor conduction or nerve damage. If the patient has poor conduction in one ear, the sound is heard better in the impaired ear because the sound is being conducted directly through the bone to the ear, and the extraneous sounds in the environment are not being picked up. Conductive loss in one ear may be because of impacted cerumen, infection, or a perforated eardrum. If the patient has a hearing loss because of nerve damage, the sound is referred to the better ear, in which the cochlea or auditory nerve is functioning better.

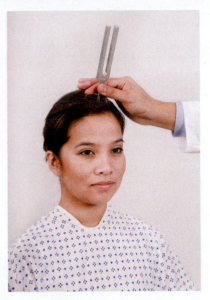

Figure 15.18 Weber test.

- Ask the patient if the sound is heard equally on both sides, or better in one ear than the other. The normal response is bilaterally equal sound, which is recorded as "no lateralization." If the sound is lateralized, ask the patient to tell you which ear hears the sound better.

▶ The abnormal findings are recorded as "sound lateralizes to (right or left) ear."

12. Perform the Romberg test.

- The Romberg test assesses equilibrium. Ask the patient to stand with feet together and arms at sides, first with eyes opened and then with eyes closed (Figure 15.19 ■).

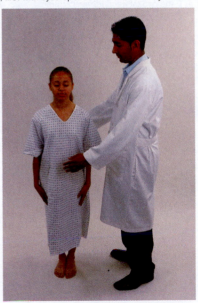

Figure 15.19 Romberg test.

- Wait about 20 seconds. The person should be able to maintain this position, although some mild swaying may occur. Mild swaying is documented as a negative Romberg. It is important to stand nearby and prepare to support the patient if there is a loss of balance. Hearing and balance are functions of cranial nerve VIII and are discussed in Chapter 24. ∞

▶ If the patient is unable to maintain balance or needs to have the feet farther apart, there may be a problem with functioning of the vestibular apparatus.

Techniques and Normal Findings	Abnormal Findings and Special Considerations

Nose and Sinuses

Note: The sense of smell and function of cranial nerve I are evaluated with the neurologic assessment presented in Chapter 24. ∞

1. **Instruct the patient.**
   - Explain that you will be looking at and touching the patient's nose. Tell the patient to inform you of discomfort.

2. **Inspect the nose for size, symmetry, shape, skin lesions, or signs of infection in frontal and lateral views.**
   - Confirm that the nose is straight, in proportion to the other facial structures, midline, without deformities; the nares are equal in size; the skin is intact; and no drainage or inflammation is present (see Figure 15.20 ■).

▶ If breathing is noisy or a discharge is present, the patient may have an obstruction or an infection.

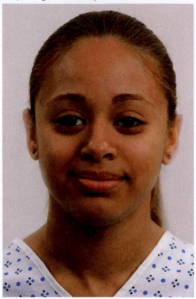

Figure 15.20 Inspection of the nose.

3. **Test for patency.**
   - Press your finger on the patient's nostril to occlude one naris and ask the patient to breathe through the opposite side with the mouth closed.
   - Repeat with the other nostril.
   - The patient should be able to breathe through each naris.

▶ If the patient cannot breathe through each naris, severe inflammation or an obstruction may be present.

▶ Ineffective breathing patterns or mouth breathing may be related to nasal swelling or trauma.

4. **Palpate the external nose for tenderness, swelling, and stability.**
   - Using two fingers, palpate the nose from the bridge to the tip and along the entire lateral surfaces, around the nares, and along the columella.
   - Note the smoothness and stability of the underlying soft tissue and cartilage.

5. **Inspect the nasal cavity using an otoscope.**
   - Apply a disposable cover to the tip of the otoscope. With your nondominant hand, stabilize the patient's head. With the otoscope in your dominant hand, gently insert the speculum horizontally into the naris (see Figure 15.21 ■). The speculum should be in the dominant hand for better control at the time of insertion to avoid hitting the sensitive septum.

Techniques and Normal Findings	**Abnormal Findings and Special Considerations**

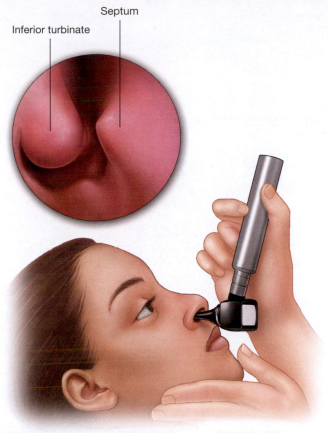

Septum

Inferior turbinate

Figure 15.21 Using the otoscope for nasal inspection.

- With the patient's head erect, inspect the vestibule and then the inferior turbinates (see Figure 15.22).
- With the patient's head tilted back, inspect the middle meatus and middle turbinates. Mucosa should be dark pink and smooth ithout swelling, discharge, bleeding, or foreign bodies. The septum should be midline, straight, and intact.
- When finished with inspection, gently remove the speculum. Again, do not hit the sensitive septum.
- Repeat on other side.

6. **Palpate the sinuses.**
   - Begin by pressing your thumbs over the frontal sinuses below the superior orbital ridge. Palpate the maxillary sinuses below the zygomatic arches of the cheekbones (see Figure 15.22A and Figure 15.22B ■).
   - Observe the patient for signs of discomfort. Ask the patient to inform you of pain.

▶ If the mucosa is swollen and red, the patient may have an upper respiratory infection. If the mucosa is pale and boggy or swollen, the patient may have chronic allergies. A *deviated septum* appears as an irregular lump in one nasal cavity. Slight deviations do not present problems for most patients. **Nasal polyps** are smooth, pale, benign growths found in many patients with chronic allergies.

▶ Tenderness upon palpation may indicate chronic allergies or sinusitis.

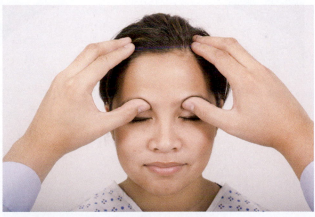

Figure 15.22A Palpating the frontal sinuses.

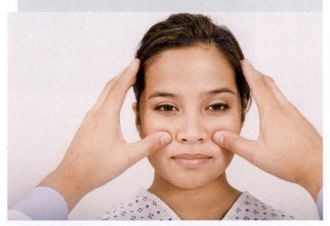

Figure 15.22B Palpating the maxillary sinuses.

Techniques and Normal Findings	Abnormal Findings and Special Considerations

7. Percuss the sinuses.
- To determine if there is pain in the sinuses, directly percuss over the maxillary and frontal sinuses by lightly tapping with one finger (see Figure 15.23A and Figure 15.23B ▪).

▸ Pain may indicate sinus fullness, allergies, or infection.

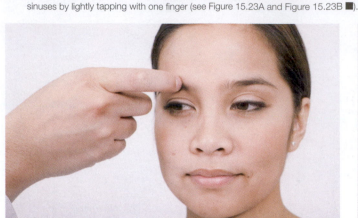

Figure 15.23A Percussion of frontal sinuses.

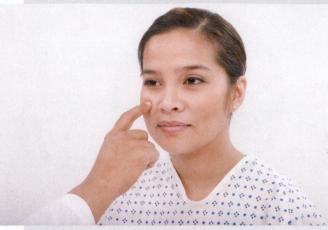

Figure 15.23B Percussion of maxillary sinuses.

8. Transilluminate the sinuses.
- If you suspect a sinus infection, the maxillary and frontal sinuses may be transilluminated.
- To transilluminate the frontal sinus, darken the room and hold a penlight under the superior orbit ridge against the frontal sinus area (see Figure 15.24A ▪).
- Cover the frontal sinus with your hand. There should be a red glow over the frontal sinus area (see Figure 15.24B ▪).

▸ If the sinus is filled with fluid, it will not transilluminate.

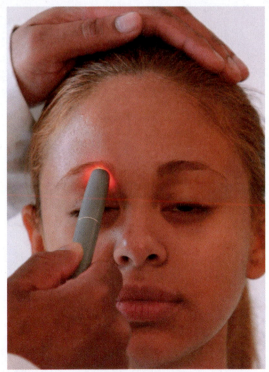

Figure 15.24A Transillumination of the frontal sinuses.

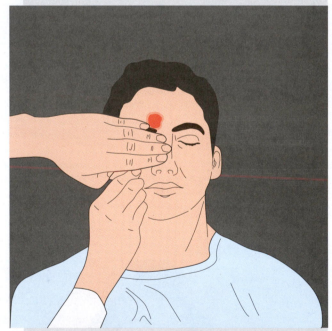

Figure 15.24B Observing transillumination of the frontal sinuses.

Techniques and Normal Findings	Abnormal Findings and Special Considerations

- To test the maxillary sinus, place a clean penlight in the patient's mouth and shine the light on one side of the hard palate, then the other. Gently cover the patient's mouth with one hand.
- There should be a red glow over the cheeks (see Figure 15.25A ■). Make sure the penlight is cleaned before using it again.
- An alternate technique is to place the penlight directly on the cheek and observe the glow of light on the hard palate (see Figure 15.25B ■).

▶ If there is no red glow under the eyes, the sinuses may be inflamed.

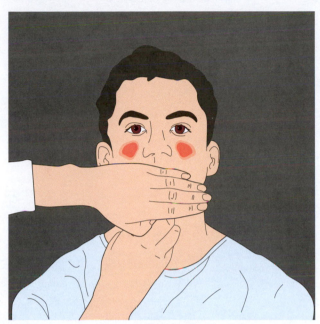

Figure 15.25A Transillumination of the maxillary sinuses.

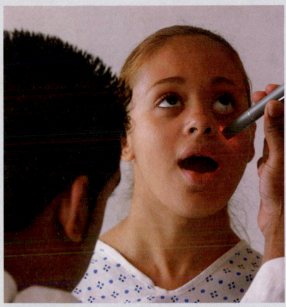

Figure 15.25B Transillumination of the maxillary sinuses using alternate technique.

Mouth and Throat

Note: Be sure to wear clean, nonsterile examination gloves for this part of the assessment.

1. **Inspect and palpate the lips.**
   - Confirm that the lips are symmetric, smooth, pink, moist, and without lesions. Makeup or lipstick should be removed.

   - Note the presence, shape, and color of the vermilion border, which is the darker line that forms a boundary between the lips and the skin.

2. **Inspect the teeth.**
   - Observe the patient's dental hygiene. Ask the patient to clench the teeth and smile while you observe occlusion (see Figure 15.26 ■).
   - Note dentures and caps at this time.
   - The teeth should be white, with smooth edges, and free of debris. Adults should have 32 permanent teeth, if wisdom teeth are intact.

▶ Lesions or blisters on the lips may be caused by the herpes simplex virus. These lesions are also known as **fever blisters** or **cold sores**. However, because cancer of the lip is the most common oral cancer, lesions must be evaluated for cancer. Pallor or cyanosis of the lips may indicate hypoxia.

▶ A thin vermilion border may be a sign of fetal alcohol syndrome. The vermilion border may also be absent after reconstructive surgery for cleft lip or hemangioma resection.

▶ Loose, painful, broken, or misaligned teeth; malocclusion; and inflamed gums need further evaluation.

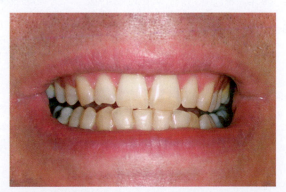

Figure 15.26 Inspecting the teeth.

Techniques and Normal Findings	Abnormal Findings and Special Considerations

3. Inspect and palpate the buccal mucosa, gums, and tongue.
- Look into the patient's mouth under a strong light.
- Confirm that the tongue is pink and moist with papillae on the dorsal surface.

- Ask the patient to touch the roof of the mouth with the tip of the tongue. The ventral surface should be smooth and pink. Palpate the area under the tongue.
- Check for lesions or nodules. Using a gauze pad, grasp the patient's tongue and inspect for any lumps or nodules (see Figure 15.27 ■). The tissue should be smooth.

▶ Abnormal findings of the gums include bleeding, pale color, retraction of gum tissue from teeth, edema, and lesions (Berman et al., 2016).

▶ A smooth, coated, or hairy tongue is usually related to dehydration or disease. A small tongue may indicate undernutrition. Tremor of the tongue may indicate a dysfunction of the hypoglossal nerve (cranial nerve XII).

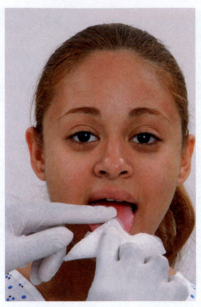

Figure 15.27 Palpating the tongue.

- Use a tongue blade to hold the tongue aside while you inspect the mucous lining of the mouth and the gums.
- Confirm that these areas are pink, moist, smooth, and free of lesions.
- Confirm the integrity of both the soft and the hard palate.

- Inspect the frenula of the tongue, upper lip, and lower lip. The frenulum is the small flap of tissue connecting the protruding portion of the lip or tongue to the rest of the mouth.
- The sense of taste (cranial nerves VII and IX) and movement of the tongue (cranial nerve XII) are discussed in detail in Chapter 24. ∞

▶ Persistent lesions on the tongue must be evaluated further. Cancerous lesions occur most commonly on the sides or at the base of the tongue. The gums are diseased if there is bleeding, retraction, or overgrowth onto the teeth.
▶ The frenula are delicate flaps of skin and are easily damaged by a direct blow to the mouth during abuse or other trauma.

4. Inspect the salivary glands.
- The salivary glands open into the mouth. Wharton's salivary ducts (submandibular) open close to the lingual frenulum. Stensen's salivary ducts (parotid) open opposite the second upper molars. Both ducts are visible, whereas the ducts of the sublingual glands are not visible.
- Confirm that Wharton's and Stenson's salivary ducts are visible, with no pain, tenderness, swelling, or redness.
- Touch the area close to the ducts with a sterile applicator, and confirm the flow of saliva.

▶ Pain or the lack of saliva can indicate infection or an obstruction.

Techniques and Normal Findings	**Abnormal Findings and Special Considerations**

5. Inspect the throat.

- Use a tongue blade and penlight to inspect the throat (see Figure 15.28 ■).

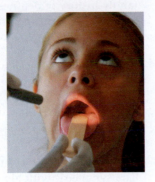

Figure 15.28 Inspecting the throat.

- Ask the patient to open the mouth wide, tilt the head back, and say *aah*. The uvula should rise in the midline.
- Use the tongue blade to depress the middle of the arched tongue enough so that you can clearly visualize the throat but not so much that the patient gags. Ask the patient to say *aah* again.
- Confirm the rising of the soft palate, which is a test for cranial nerve X.
- Confirm that the tonsils, uvula, and posterior pharynx are pink and are without inflammation, swelling, or lesions. Observe the tonsils behind the anterior tonsillar pillar. The color should be pink with slight vascularity present. Tonsils may be partially or totally absent.
- Visualization of tonsils may be described based on size (Figure 15.29 ■) as follows:

  0: Absent

  1+ (normal): Tonsils are hidden behind the tonsillar pillars

  2+: Tonsils extend to the edges of the tonsillar pillars

  3+: Tonsils extend beyond the edges of the tonsillar pillars but not to the midline

  4+: Tonsils extend to the midline and may touch.

- As you inspect the throat, note any mouth odors.
- Discard the tongue blade.

▶ Viral pharyngitis may accompany a cold. Tonsils may be bright red and swollen and may have white spots on them.

▶ Patients with sinus infections may have visible exudate at the posterior pharynx.

▶ Patients with diabetic acidosis may have sweet, fruity-smelling breath. The breath of patients with kidney disease smells of ammonia.

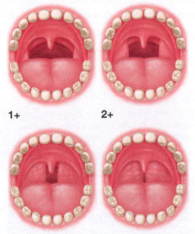

Figure 15.29 Tonsil size grading. 1+   2+   3+   4+

Documenting Your Findings

Documentation of assessment data—subjective and objective—must be accurate, professional, complete, and confidential. When documenting the information from the focused assessment of each body system, the nurse should use measurements where appropriate to ensure accuracy, use medical terminology rather than jargon, include all pertinent information, and avoid language that could identify the patient. The information in the documentation should make it clear what questions were asked and use language to indicate whether it is the patient's response or the nurse's findings. For patient responses, the documentation will say "denies," "states," or "reports," whereas the nurse's findings will simply list the findings as fact or say "no" along with the condition. For example: patient "runny nose, watery eyes, and changes in sense of smell" and the nurse found "32 teeth, white, smooth, no caries." An example of normal results for the ears, nose, mouth, and throat follows.

Sample Documentation: Ears, Nose, Mouth, and Throat Health Assessment

Focused History (Subjective Data)

This is information from Review of Systems (ROS) and other pertinent history information that is or could be related to the patient's ears and hearing, nose, mouth, and throat.

Denies changes in hearing ability. Denies personal or family history of deafness, ear infections, or vertigo. Denies dizziness or ringing in the ears. Denies history of exposure to loud noises except for one summer working at a warehouse in 2005. Reports "broken nose" at age 19 from skateboarding accident. Denies use of ear drops, nasal spray. Denies history of nosebleeds, sinus infection, use of OTC cold medicines. Denies changes in voice, sore throat, or postnasal drip. Reports last dental exam and teeth cleaning was 6 months ago.

Physical Assessment (Objective Data)

Ears symmetric with top of pinna even with outer canthus of eyes bilaterally. No pain on palpation of tragus, mastoid process, or pinna; no lesions. External ear canal open, no erythema or cerumen. TMs grey with cone of light at R: 5 o'clock and L: 7 o'clock positions. Hearing grossly normal. Romberg negative. Nose symmetrical, smooth skin, no lesions or discharge. Nares patent, mucosa pink, moist. No pain on palpation of sinuses. Lips smooth, pink, moist, no lesions. 32 teeth present, white, smooth, no caries. Mucous membranes moist, pink, no lesions. Tonsils 2+ no erythema or exudate.

Abnormal Findings

Abnormal findings in the ears, nose, mouth, and throat include lesions, deformities, infectious processes, and dental problems. See Table 15.2 and Table 15.3 for an overview of disorders related to the ear. Table 15.4 provides examples of disorders of the nose and sinuses. An overview of disorders of the mouth and throat is presented in Table 15.5.

Table 15.2 Overview of Disorders of the External Ear

Keloid
Scar tissue that forms following tissue injury. Keloid tissue may be pink, red, or flesh colored.

Otitis Externa
Infection of the outer ear that causes redness and swelling of the auricle and ear canal and scanty drainage; may be accompanied by itching, fever, and enlarged lymph nodes. Also called swimmer's ear.

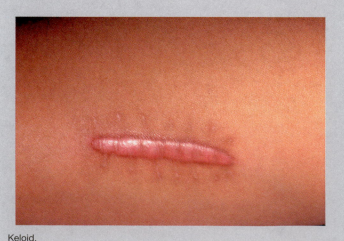

Keloid.
Source: Mediscan/Alamy Stock Photo.

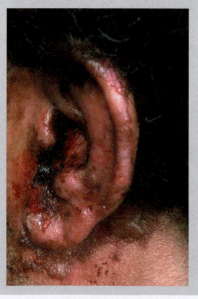

Otitis externa (swimmer's ear).
Source: Mediscan/Alamy Stock Photo.

(continued)

Table 15.2 Overview of Disorders of the External Ear (continued)

Tophi
Small white nodules on the helix or antihelix of the ear that contain uric acid crystals and are a sign of gout, which is a type of arthritis that is caused by a buildup of uric acid in the joints. Tophi may also occur in the olecranon process (elbow), knee joint, palm, and Achilles tendon.

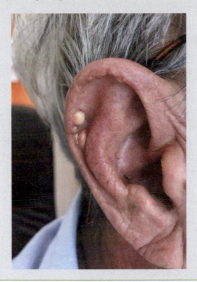

Tophi.
Source: TisforThan/Shutterstock.

Table 15.3 Overview of Disorders of the Middle and Internal Ear

Otitis Media
Infection of the middle ear producing a red, bulging eardrum; fever; and hearing loss. Otoscopic examination reveals absent light reflex.

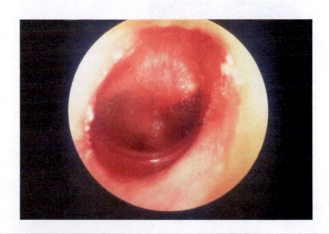

Otitis media.
Source: Mediscan/Alamy Stock Photo.

Perforation of the Tympanic Membrane
A rupturing of the eardrum because of trauma or infection. During otoscopic inspection, the perforation may be seen as a dark spot on the eardrum.

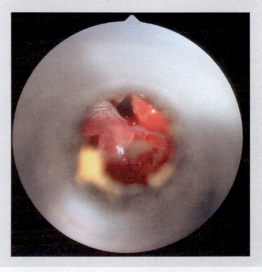

Perforation of the tympanic membrane.
Source: Mediscan/Alamy Stock Photo.

Table 15.3 Overview of Disorders of the Middle and Internal Ear (continued)

Scarred Tympanic Membrane

A condition in which the eardrum has white patches of scar tissue because of repeated ear infections. Chronic irritation of the tympanic membrane without infection also can cause scarring. In most cases, this condition does not cause hearing loss.

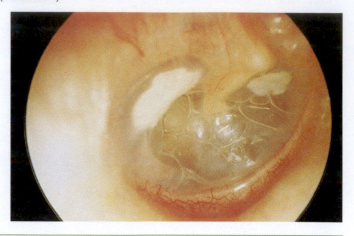

Scarred tympanic membrane.
Source: Prof. Tony Wright/Inst. of Laryngology & Otology/Science Source.

Table 15.4 Overview of Disorders of the Nose and Sinuses

Deviated Septum

A displacement of the lower nasal septum. When viewed with a nasal speculum, one nasal cavity appears to have an outgrowth or shelf.

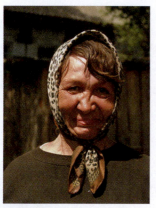

Deviated septum.
Source: Zaichiki/Alamy Stock Photo.

Epistaxis

A nosebleed may follow trauma, such as a blow to the nose, or it may accompany another alteration in health, such as rhinitis, hypertension, or a blood coagulation disorder.

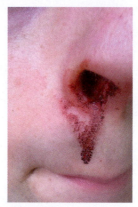

Epistaxis (nosebleed).
Source: Chris Harvey/123RF.

Nasal Polyp

Pale, round, firm, nonpainful overgrowth of nasal mucosa usually caused by chronic allergic rhinitis.

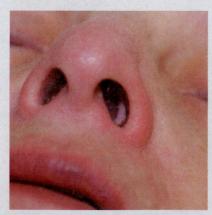

Nasal polyp.
Source: Anthony Ricci/Shutterstock.

Perforated Septum

A hole in the septum caused by chronic infection, trauma, or sniffing cocaine. It can be detected by shining a penlight through the naris on the other side.

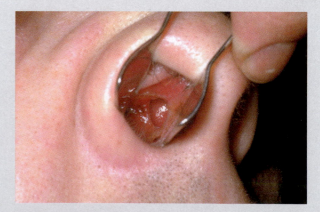

Perforated nasal septum.
Source: Mediscan/Alamy Stock Photo.

Table 15.4 Overview of Disorders of the Nose and Sinuses (continued)

Rhinitis

Nasal inflammation usually because of a viral infection or allergy, accompanied by watery and often copious discharge, sneezing, and congestion. *Acute rhinitis* is caused by a virus, whereas *allergic rhinitis* results from contact with allergens such as pollen and dust.

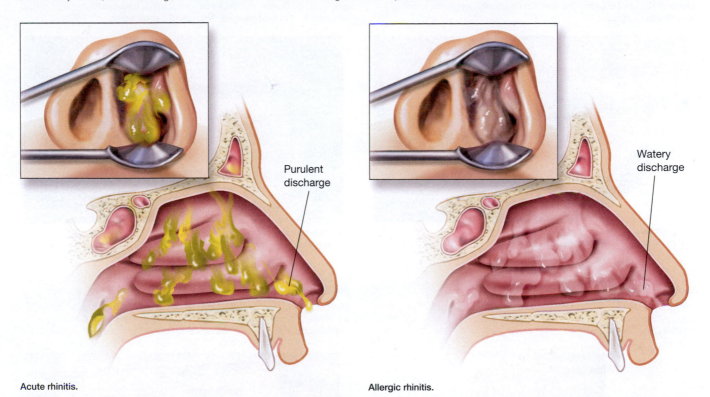

Purulent discharge

Watery discharge

Acute rhinitis.

Allergic rhinitis.

Sinusitis

Inflammation of the sinuses usually following an upper respiratory infection. The inflammation causes facial pain and discharge. Fever, chills, frontal headache, or a dull, pulsating pain in the cheeks or teeth may accompany sinusitis.

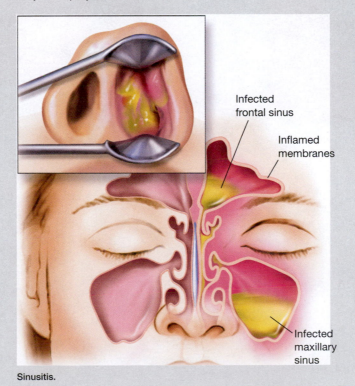

Infected frontal sinus

Inflamed membranes

Infected maxillary sinus

Sinusitis.

Table 15.5 Overview of Disorders of the Mouth and Throat

Ankyloglossia

Fixation of the tip of the tongue to the floor of the mouth because of a shortened lingual frenulum. The condition is usually congenital and may be corrected surgically.

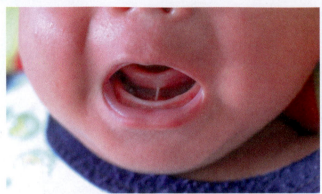

Ankyloglossia.
Source: Akkalak Aiempradit/Shutterstock.

Aphthous Ulcers

Small, round, white, painful lesions occurring singularly or in clusters on the oral mucosa. Commonly result from oral trauma; also associated with stress, exhaustion, and food allergies. Also called canker sores.

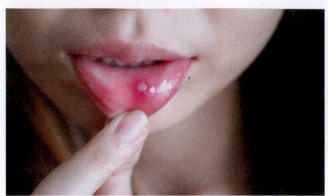

Aphthous ulcers.
Source: Pipat Chotchoung/123RF.

Black Hairy Tongue

A temporary condition caused by the inhibition of normal bacteria and the overgrowth of fungus on the papillae of the tongue. It is usually associated with the use of antibiotics.

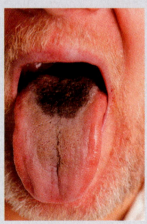

Black hairy tongue.
Source: Voyagerix/Shutterstock.

Oral Carcinoma

Most commonly found on the lower lip or the base of the tongue. Cancer is suspected if a sore or lesion does not heal within a few weeks. Heavy smoking, chewing tobacco, and chronic heavy alcohol use increase the risk.

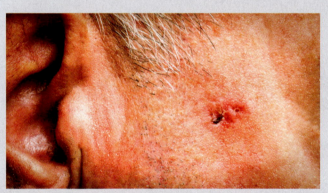

Basil cell carcinoma.
Source: flik47/123RF.

(continued)

Table 15.5 Overview of Disorders of the Mouth and Throat (continued)

Cleft Lip

A separation or splitting of the two sides of the upper lip; appears as a gap or narrow opening in the skin of the upper lip. May occur alone or along with cleft palate.

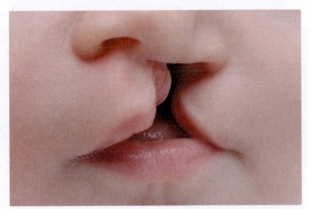

Cleft lip.
Source: malost/Shutterstock.

Cleft Palate

An opening or separation in the roof of the mouth; may involve the hard palate, the soft palate, or both of these structures. May or may not occur along with cleft lip.

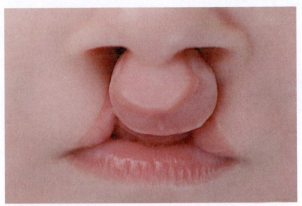

Cleft palate.
Source: malost/Shutterstock.

Gingival Hyperplasia

An enlargement of the gums; frequently seen in pregnancy, leukemia, or after prolonged use of phenytoin (Dilantin).

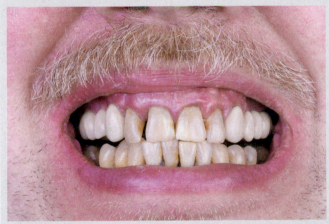

Gingival hyperplasia.
Source: vilax/Shutterstock.

Gingivitis

Gum inflammation that may be caused by poor dental hygiene or vitamin C deficiency. Untreated, it may progress to periodontal disease and tooth loss.*(continued)*

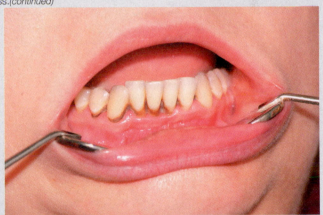

Gingivitis.
Source: drtrig/123RF.

Table 15.5 Overview of Disorders of the Mouth and Throat (continued)

Herpes Simplex

A virus that is often accompanied by clear vesicles (cold sores, fever blisters) usually at the junction of the skin and the lip that erupt, crust over, and heal within 2 weeks. Usually recur, especially after heavy exposure to bright sunlight.

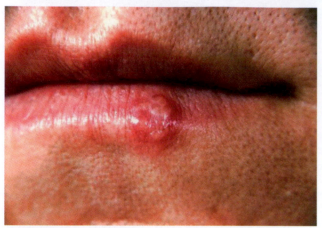

Herpes simplex.
Source: Dr. Herrmann/Centers for Disease Control and Prevention (CDC).

Leukoplakia

A whitish thickening of the mucous membrane in the mouth or tongue that cannot be scraped off. Most often associated with heavy smoking or drinking, it can be a precancerous condition.

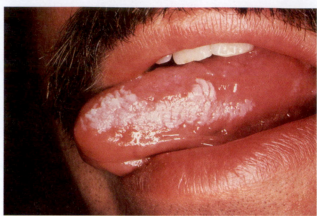

Leukoplakia.
Source: J.S. Greenspan, B.D.S., University of California, San Francisco; Sol Silverman, Jr., D.D.S Centers for Disease Control and Prevention (CDC).

GLOSSITIS

The surface of the tongue is smooth and red with a shiny appearance; occurs as a result of vitamin B and iron deficiency.

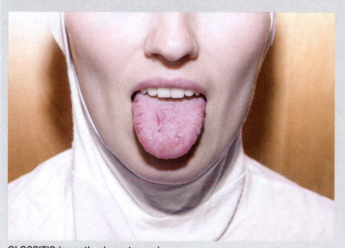

GLOSSITIS (smooth, glossy tongue).
Source: Gabdrakipova Dilyara/Shutterstock.

Tonsillitis

Inflammation of the tonsils. The throat is red and the tonsils are swollen and covered by white or yellow patches (exudate); may include high fever and enlarged cervical chain lymph nodes.

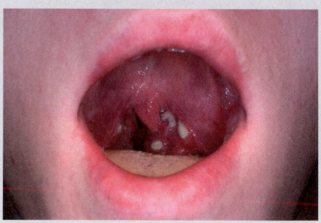

Tonsillitis.
Source: Scott Camazine/Alamy Stock Photo.

Application Through Critical Thinking

CASE STUDY

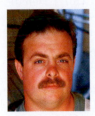

Source: Ryan McVay/Getty Images.

Harold Chandler is a 35-year-old executive in a computer firm who comes to the employees' wellness center complaining of a marked loss of hearing in his left ear. He says that he woke up yesterday with a "feeling of fullness" in his left ear but no pain. He further relates that his 3-year-old daughter has a "bad cold and an earache," and he wonders if he has "the same thing." He denies any other symptoms of infection, has had no discharge from either ear, and is not taking any medicine at this time. He has not had an audiometric assessment since his last physical 3 years ago. He further volunteers that he has just returned from a business trip to Europe and wonders whether the pressurized atmosphere of the airplane "created a problem with his hearing." He also tells you he spent summers working construction jobs when he was in college.

Nurse Michael Navarro's assessment of Mr. Chandler reveals normal vital signs. His left ear's external canal is of a uniform pink color with no redness, swelling, lesions, or discharge. The Weber test reveals lateralization to the left ear. The otoscopic assessment reveals a left ear impacted with brown-gray cerumen, and the tympanic membrane cannot be visualized. Assessment of the right ear shows the external canal is of a uniform pink color with no redness, swelling, lesions, or discharge. During the otoscopic assessment, the tympanic membrane is easily visualized. It is translucent and pearl-gray with the cone of light at the 5 o'clock position. No perforations are noted.

To visualize the tympanic membrane of the left ear, Mr. Navarro prepares a solution of mineral oil and hydrogen peroxide and instills the solution into the left ear canal to soften the cerumen. Then he irrigates the canal with warm water using a bulb syringe. After Mr. Navarro completes the irrigation, Mr. Chandler is surprised to discover that his hearing has returned in his left ear. Now Mr. Navarro completes the otoscopic assessment. He is able to visualize the tympanic membrane, which is translucent and pearl-gray with the cone of light at the 7 o'clock position. No perforations are noted.

To be sure that Mr. Chandler's hearing has been restored, Mr. Navarro performs a screening evaluation of his auditory function. He is able to hear a low whisper at 2 feet. His Rinne test is positive, and his Weber test indicates equal lateralization.

SAMPLE DOCUMENTATION

The following is sample documentation for Harold Chandler.

SUBJECTIVE DATA 35-year-old c/o hearing loss (Left) ear. Woke up yesterday with fullness, no pain (Left) ear. His 3-year-old daughter has "bad cold and earache," wonders if he has the same. Denies signs of infection, no discharge, and no medication. Audiometric assessment 3 years ago. Recent air travel, wonders if pressurized atmosphere created hearing problem.

OBJECTIVE DATA Ears, equal in size, shape. Tragus mobile, nontender bilaterally. Left ear canal pink, no redness, edema, lesions, discharge. Weber—lateralization to left. Otoscopic assessment: Left ear impacted—brown-gray cerumen, no visualization tympanic membrane. Right ear—canal pink, clear, no edema, tympanic membrane gray with no lesions.

CRITICAL THINKING QUESTIONS

1. Describe the application of critical thinking to the situation.
2. How was information clustered to guide decision making?
3. What recommendations should the nurse provide for this patient?
4. What special considerations should the nurse take into account in this situation?
5. Why is it important to understand whether the hearing loss was acute or gradual?

REFERENCES

American Speech-Language-Hearing Association (ASHA). (n.d.) Causes of hearing loss in adults. Retrieved from http://www.asha.org/public/hearing/Causes-of-Hearing-Loss-in-Adults

Carroll, Y. I., Eichwald, J., Scinicariello, F., Hoffma, H. J., Deitchman, S., Radke, M. S., . . . Breysse, P. (2017). Vital signs: Noise-induced hearing loss among adults—United States 2011–2012. *Morbidity and Mortality Weekly Report, 66*(5), 139–144. doi:10.15585/mmwr.mm6605e3

Centers for Disease Control and Prevention (CDC). (2016). *Workplace safety & health topics: Noise and hearing loss prevention.* Retrieved from http://www.cdc.gov/niosh/topics/noise/faq.html

Centers for Disease Control and Prevention (CDC). (2018). *Loss of smell (anosmia)—causes.* Retrieved from http://www.mayoclinic.org/symptoms/loss-of-smell/basics/causes/sym-20050804

Dimakopoulou, K., Koutentakis, K., Papageorgiou, I., Kasdagli, M., Haralabidis, A. S., Sourtzi, P., . . . Katsouyanni, K. (2017). Is aircraft noise exposure associated with cardiovascular disease and hypertension? Results from a cohort study in Athens, Greece. *Occupational & Environmental Medicine, 74*(11), 830–837. doi:10.1136/oemed-2016-104180

Earwood, J. S., Rogers, T. S., & Rathjen, N. A. (2018). Ear pain: Diagnosing common and uncommon causes. *American Family Physician*, 97(1), 20–27. Retrieved from https://www.aafp.org/afp/2018/0101/p20.html

Gold, M., Boyack, I., Caputo, N., & Pearlman, A. (2017). Imaging prevalence of nasal septal perforation in an urban population. *Clinical Imaging*, 43, 80–82. doi:10.1016/j.clinimag.2017.02.002

Hill, C. M., Devine, M., & Renton, T. (2017). Oral surgery II: Part 4. Common oral lesions. *British Dental Journal*, 223(10), 769–779. doi:10.1038/sj.bdj.2017.985

Mason, P. (2013). Nothing smaller than your elbows, please [Web log post]. Retrieved from http://blog.asha.org/2013/01/08/nothing-smaller-than-your-elbow-please

Mayo Clinic. (2017). *At what age do children start losing their baby teeth?* Retrieved from http://www.mayoclinic.org/healthy-living/childrens-health/expert-answers/baby-teeth/faq-20058532

Mayo Clinic. (2018). *Nosebleeds: Causes*. Retrieved from http://www.mayoclinic.org/symptoms/nosebleeds/basics/causes/sym-20050914

National Cancer Institute (NCI). (2017). *Head and neck cancer.* Retrieved from http://www.cancer.gov/cancertopics/factsheet/Sites-Types/head-and-neck

O'Neill, O. M., Johnston, B. T., & Coleman, H. G. (2013). Achalasia: A review of clinical diagnosis, epidemiology, treatment and outcomes. *World Journal of Gastroenterology*, 19(35), 5808–5812. doi:10.3748/wjg.v19.i35.5806

Osborn, K. S., Wraa, C. E., Watson, A., & Holleran, R. S. (2013). *Medical-surgical nursing: Preparation for practice* (2nd ed.). Upper Saddle River, NJ: Pearson.

Shearer, A. E., Hildebrand, M. S., & Smith, R. J. (2017). Hereditary hearing loss and deafness overview. *GeneReviews* [Internet]. Retrieved from http://www.genereviews.org

Shields, K. M., Fox, K. L., & Liebrecht, C. (2018). *Pearson nurse's drug guide*. Hoboken, NJ: Pearson.

Shokry, E., & Filho, N. R. (2017). Insights into cerumen and application in diagnostics: Past, present and future prospective. *Biochemia Medica*, 27(3), 030503. doi:10.11613/BM.2017.030503

Weyde, K. V., Krog, N. H., Oftedal, B., Magnus, P., Overland, S., Stansfeld, S., . . . Aasvang, G. M. (2017). Road traffic noise and children's inattention. *Environmental Health*, 16(127). doi:10.1186/s12940-017-0337-y

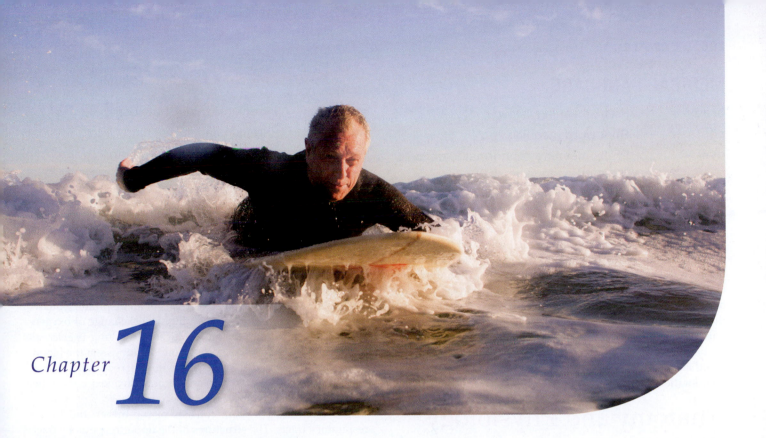

Chapter 16

Lungs and Thorax

LEARNING OUTCOMES

Upon completion of this chapter, you will be able to:

1. Describe the anatomy and physiology of the lungs and thorax.

2. Identify anatomic, physiologic, developmental, psychosocial, and cultural variations that guide assessment of the lungs and thorax.

3. Determine which questions about the lungs and thorax to use for the focused interview.

4. Outline the techniques for assessment of the lungs and thorax.

5. Generate the appropriate documentation to describe the assessment of the lungs and thorax.

6. Identify abnormal findings in the physical assessment of the lungs and thorax.

KEY TERMS

adventitious sounds, 319
angle of Louis, 300
atelectasis, 325
bronchial sounds, 317
bronchophony, 320
bronchovesicular sounds, 317

crackles, 319
dyspnea, 298
egophony, 320
eupnea, 298
fremitus, 316
friction rub, 319

landmarks, 299
manubrium, 299
mediastinum, 296
orthopnea, 307
rales, 319
respiratory cycle, 296

rhonchi, 319
stridor, 319
tracheal sounds, 317
vesicular sounds, 317
wheezes, 319
whispered pectoriloquy, 320

MEDICAL LANGUAGE

brady-	Prefix meaning "slow"
costa	Root word meaning "rib"
dys-	Prefix meaning "abnormal," "difficult," "painful"
inter-	Prefix meaning "between"
intra-	Prefix meaning "within," "into"
-pnea	Suffix meaning "breathing"
pneum-	Prefix meaning "lung," "air," "gas"

Introduction

The fundamental responsibility of the lungs and thorax—the primary organs of the respiratory system—is the exchange of gases in the body. Exchange of oxygen and carbon dioxide is essential to the homeostatic and hemodynamic processes of the body. Assessment of respiratory function is an integral aspect of the total patient assessment performed by the professional nurse with the goal of detecting any actual or potential respiratory problems. Changes in a patient's respiratory status are recognized as a sensitive indicator of concern and possible physical deterioration.

Anatomy and Physiology Review

The thorax or thoracic cavity, commonly called the chest, is a closed cavity of the body, containing structures needed for respiration. The thorax is surrounded by ribs and muscles and extends from the base of the neck to the diaphragm. It has three sections: the mediastinum and the right and left pleural cavities. The **mediastinum** contains the heart, trachea, esophagus, and major blood vessels of the body. Each pleural cavity contains a lung (see Figure 16.1 ■).

The major structures of the respiratory system are situated in the thoracic cavity. The main function of the respiratory system is to supply the body with oxygen and expel carbon dioxide. Air moves in and out of the lungs with each respiratory cycle. A complete **respiratory cycle** consists of an inspiratory phase and an expiratory phase of breathing. The exchange of oxygen and carbon dioxide at the alveoli level of the lung is *external respiration*. Gases are transported from the lungs via the blood to the cells of the body. As the gases move across the systemic capillaries, exchange of oxygen and carbon dioxide occurs at the cellular level and *internal respiration* occurs.

The respiratory system consists of the upper and lower respiratory tracts. The structures of the upper respiratory tract include the nose, the mouth, the sinuses, the pharynx, the larynx, and the proximal portion of the trachea. The lower respiratory tract includes the distal portion of the trachea, as well as the bronchi and lungs. Pleural membranes, the muscles of respiration, and the mediastinum complete the lower respiratory tract.

The anatomy, physiology, and assessment of the structures of the upper respiratory tract are discussed in Chapter 13. ∞ Before proceeding, it may be helpful to review that information.

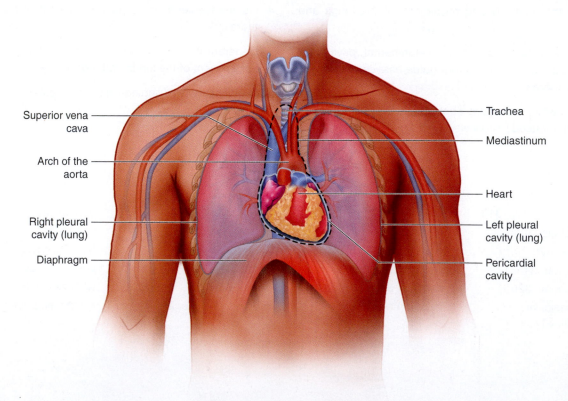

Figure 16.1 Anatomy of the respiratory system.

Lower Respiratory Tract

The lower respiratory tract includes the trachea, bronchi, and lungs. Additional structures of the pleural membranes, the mediastinum, and the muscles of respiration are also discussed at this time during the assessment. Consideration must be given to all structures during the assessment process.

Trachea The trachea, located in the mediastinum, descends from the larynx in the neck to the main bronchi at the distal point. In adults, the trachea is approximately 10 cm to 12 cm (4 in.) long and 2.5 cm (1 in.) in diameter. The trachea is a flexible and mobile structure, bifurcating anteriorly at about the sternal angle and posteriorly at about vertebrae T3 to T5. The trachea contains 16 to 20 rings of hyaline cartilage. These C-shaped rings help maintain the shape of the trachea and prevent its collapse during inspiration and expiration. Just above the point of bifurcation, the last tracheal cartilage, known as the carina, is expanded. The carina separates the openings of the two main bronchi. The trachea, like other structures of the respiratory tract, is lined with a mucus-producing membrane that traps dust, bacteria, and other foreign bodies. This membrane at the level of the carina is most sensitive to foreign substances. The cilia—hairlike projections of the membrane—and coughing help sweep debris toward the mouth for removal.

Bronchi Anteriorly, the trachea bifurcates at about the level of the sternal angle, forming the right and left main bronchi (see Figure 16.2 ■). The main bronchus enters each lung at the hilus (medial depression) and maintains an oblique position in the mediastinum. The right main bronchus is shorter, wider, and more vertical than the left main bronchus; therefore, aspirated objects are more likely to enter the right lung. The bronchi continue to divide within each lobe of the lung. The terminal bronchioles are less than 0.5 mm (0.019 in.) in diameter. The bronchi and the many branches continue to warm and moisten air as it moves along the respiratory tract to the alveoli in the lungs.

Lungs The lungs are cone-shaped, elastic, spongy, air-filled structures that are situated in the pleural cavities of the thorax on either side of the mediastinum (see Figure 16.3 ■). The apex of each lung is slightly superior to the inner third of the clavicle, and the base of each lung is at the level of the diaphragm. The left lung has two lobes (upper and lower) and tends to be longer and narrower than the right lung. The left lung accommodates the heart at the medial surface. The oblique fissure separates the two lobes of this lung. The right lung has three lobes (upper, middle, and lower) and is slightly larger, wider, and shorter than the left lung. The horizontal and oblique fissures separate the lobes of the right lung. Within each lung, the numerous terminal bronchioles branch into the alveolar ducts, which lead into alveolar sacs and alveoli. The single-layered cells of the alveoli permit simple diffusion and gas exchanges to occur (see Figure 16.4 ■).

Pleural Membranes The pleura is a thin, double-layered, serous membrane that lines each pleural cavity. The parietal membrane lines the superior aspect of the diaphragm and the thoracic wall. The visceral membrane covers the outer surface of the lung. A pleural fluid produced by these membranes acts as a lubricant, allowing the lung to glide during the respiratory cycle of inspiration and expiration. The surface tension created by the fluid and the negative pressure between the membranes helps keep the lungs expanded. As the negative pressure changes, one is able to move air into and out of the lungs.

Mediastinum The mediastinum is the middle section of the thoracic cavity and is surrounded by the right and left pleural cavities. The mediastinum contains the heart, the trachea, the esophagus, the proximal portion of the right and left main bronchi, and the great vessels of the body. (See Figure 16.1)

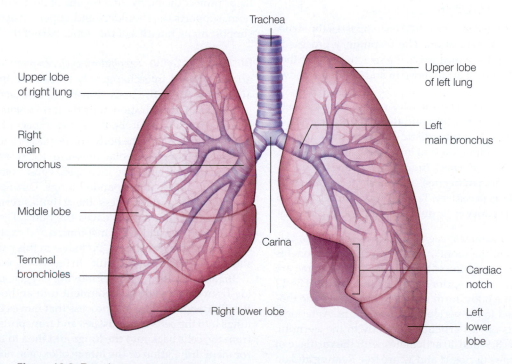

Figure 16.2 Respiratory passages.

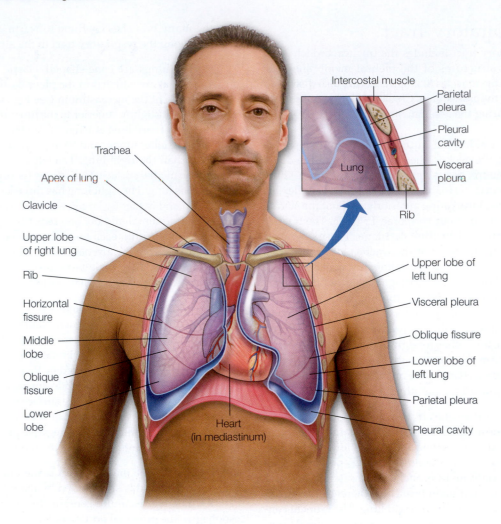

Figure 16.3 Anterior view of thorax and lungs.

Respiratory Process

Respiratory process is a general term that encompasses the structures and activities of respiration. The respiratory process is dependent on the muscles of the thorax, the structures of the thoracic cage, and the ability of air to move in and out of the body.

Muscles of Respiration   The muscles of the thoracic cage (internal and external intercostals) and the diaphragm assist in the breathing process. The synergistic action of these muscle groups aids in the respiratory cycle of inspiration and expiration. The accessory muscles of the neck (trapezius, scalenes, and sternocleidomastoid), abdomen (rectus), and chest (pectorals) assist the respiratory cycle as necessary. The accessory muscles play a major role in the respiratory cycle during distress and pathology.

Thoracic Cage   The thoracic cage consists of the bones, cartilage, and muscles of the thorax. The sternum (breastbone) is located in the anterior midline of the thorax. The vertebrae are located at the dorsal or posterior aspect of the thorax. The 12 pairs of ribs circle the body, form the lateral aspects of the thorax, and are attached to the vertebrae and sternum. Anteriorly, the first seven pairs of ribs articulate directly to the sternum. The cartilage of ribs 8, 9, and 10 articulates with the cartilage of rib 7, whereas the pairs of ribs 11 and 12 are free floating and do not articulate anteriorly. The costal cartilage and external intercostal muscles help to complete the thoracic cage. This bony cage helps protect the many vital organs of the pleura and mediastinum, supports the shoulders and upper extremities, and helps support many muscles of the upper part of the body.

Respiratory Cycle   *Respiratory cycle, respirations,* and *breathing* are terms used interchangeably to indicate the movement of air in and out of the body. Breathing consists of two phases: inspiration and expiration, thus the term *respiratory cycle*. Inspiration is considered to be the active aspect of the respiratory cycle. For air to enter the body, the respiratory muscles contract, the chest expands, alveolar pressure decreases, and the negative intrapleural pressure increases. These combined activities allow air to enter the expanded lungs. During expiration, the passive phase of the process, the activities reverse themselves: the lungs recoil, and air leaves the body. The regular, even-depth, rhythmic pattern of inspiration and expiration describes **eupnea** (normal breathing). A change in this pattern, producing shortness of breath or difficulty in breathing, is called **dyspnea**.

Breathing is the action of moving oxygen and carbon dioxide from the outside environment into and out of the lungs. Respiration is a metabolic process that moves oxygen from the lungs into the cells of the tissues and transports carbon dioxide from the cells back into the lungs and then to the outside environment. Inhalation or the intake of oxygen needed for metabolism and exhalation or the release of carbon dioxide, which is the waste product of metabolism, occur with each respiratory

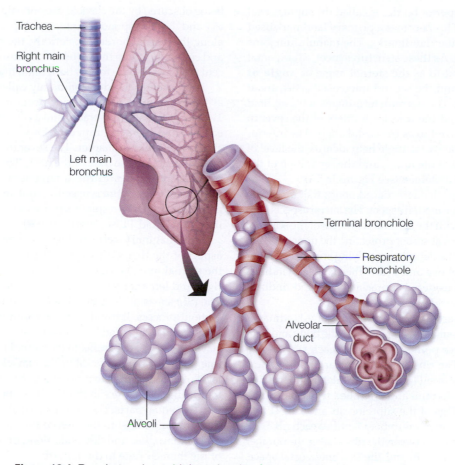

Figure 16.4 Respiratory bronchioles, alveolar ducts, and alveoli.

cycle. This delicate balance of gas exchange is influenced by the nervous system, the cardiovascular system, and the musculoskeletal system. The central nervous system, influenced by the concentration of gases in the blood, regulates the rate and depth of each respiratory cycle. The cardiovascular system is responsible for transporting the gases throughout the body. The musculoskeletal system provides the bones to protect the structures of the respiratory system, and muscular activity allows for the rhythmic movement of the thoracic cavity. This coordinated movement, together with pressure changes in the thoracic cavity, leads to the exchange of the oxygen and carbon dioxide.

The respiratory system has a major role in helping the body to maintain acid–base balance. The concentration of carbon dioxide in the blood directly influences the blood concentration of carbonic acid and hydrogen ions. The respiratory system responds to the needs of the body to either retain or excrete carbon dioxide. This action will help maintain the delicate balance of carbonic acid and bicarbonate ions at the 1:20 ratio, keeping the plasma pH between 7.35 and 7.45, which is the normal range.

The respiratory system is also influential in the production of vocal sounds. The sounds commonly referred to as speech are produced as air moves out of the lungs and passes over the vocal cords. The pitch and volume of one's speech are influenced by the length and tension of the vocal cords, the movement of the glottis, and the force of the air across the vocal cords. The quality of the voice is further influenced by other structures including the pharynx, tongue, palate, mouth, and lips.

Landmarks

Identification and location of **landmarks** help the professional nurse develop a mental picture of the structures being assessed. Thoracic reference points and specific anatomic structures are used as landmarks (see Figure 16.5 ■). They help provide an exact location for the assessment findings and an accurate orientation for documentation of findings. Landmark identification for the thorax includes bony structures, horizontal and vertical lines, and the division of the thorax.

The thorax may be divided into two or three sections for assessment. Two sections include the anterior thorax and posterior thorax, and three sections include the anterior, lateral, and posterior aspects. This text uses the former option: The lateral areas are incorporated into the anterior and posterior sections. The bony structures include the sternum, clavicles, ribs, and vertebrae. At the horizontal plane, the landmarks are the clavicles, the ribs, and the corresponding intercostal spaces. Anteriorly, the vertical lines start at the sternum and are strategically drawn parallel to this structure. Posteriorly, the vertical lines start at the vertebral column, and additional lines are drawn parallel to this reference point.

The first bony landmark to be considered is the sternum, commonly called the breastbone. It is a flat, elongated bone located in the midline of the anterior thoracic cage and consists of three parts: the manubrium, the body, and the xiphoid process. The clavicles and some of the pairs of ribs articulate with the sternum. The **manubrium** is the superior portion of the sternum.

The depression at the superior border is called the suprasternal notch or jugular notch. This becomes a primary landmark used to identify and locate other landmarks. The manubrium joins the body of the sternum. As these structures meet, a horizontal ridge is formed, referred to as the sternal angle or **angle of Louis**. The second rib and the second intercostal space are at this level of the sternum. The sternum terminates at the xiphoid process. This process and the inferior borders of the seventh ribs form a triangle referred to as the costal angle. The inferior border of the ribs and the costal angle help identify the level of the diaphragm, the base of the lungs, and the separation of the thoracic cavity from the abdomen (see Figure 16.5A).

The clavicles are long, slender, curved bones that articulate with the manubrium at the medial aspect. The lateral aspects help form the shoulder joint with the acromion process of the scapula. The clavicles act as a shock absorber protecting the upper portion of the thoracic cage and the delicate underlying structures. Lung tissue will be assessed above and below the clavicles. Findings above the clavicle are considered supraclavicular, and findings below the clavicle are considered infraclavicular.

The 12 pairs of ribs are another group of bony landmarks used in respiratory assessment. The ribs circle the body and help form horizontal reference points. Posteriorly, each rib attaches to a thoracic vertebra. The ribs curve downward and forward as they become anterior (see Figure 16.5B). Bilaterally, the first seven ribs attach to the sternum and are called true ribs. Ribs 8, 9, and 10 attach to cartilage of the superior rib, and ribs 11 and 12 are free floating anteriorly. A number identifies each rib. Each intercostal space—the space between the ribs—takes the number of the superior rib. The first rib and the first intercostal space,

being obscured by the clavicle, are not palpable. Anteriorly, ribs 2 to 7 and the corresponding intercostal spaces are easily palpated along the sternal border. Posteriorly, the ribs are best palpated and counted close to the vertebral column. Each rib and its adjacent intercostal space form a horizontal line used as a landmark.

The vertebral column, commonly called the spine, is located at the midline of the posterior portion of the thoracic cage. Twelve vertebrae are thoracic, and a pair of ribs articulates with each. The vertebral column contributes to the vertical lines discussed later in this chapter. The seventh cervical vertebra (C7) is most visible at the base of the neck. The much larger spinous process contributes to the uniqueness of the vertebra. This prominent C7 vertebra is used to count and locate other spinous processes. When two spinous processes are equally prominent, they are C7 and T1 (see Figure 16.6 ■).

Five imaginary vertical lines are identified on the anterior aspect of the thoracic cage (see Figure 16.7 ■). These lines are the sternal line, the right and left midclavicular lines, and the right and left anterior axillary lines. The sternal or midsternal line (SL) starts at the sternal notch and descends through the xiphoid process. It divides the sternum in half and ultimately identifies the right and left thoracic cage. The right and left midclavicular lines are parallel to the sternal line. The midclavicular line begins at the midpoint of the clavicle and descends to the level of the 12th rib. The nipples of the breast are slightly lateral to this line. This line subdivides the right and left thoracic cage into two equal parts. The anterior axillary line (AAL) is another line drawn parallel to the sternal line. It begins at the anterior fold of the axillae and descends along the anterior lateral aspect of the thoracic cage to the 12th rib.

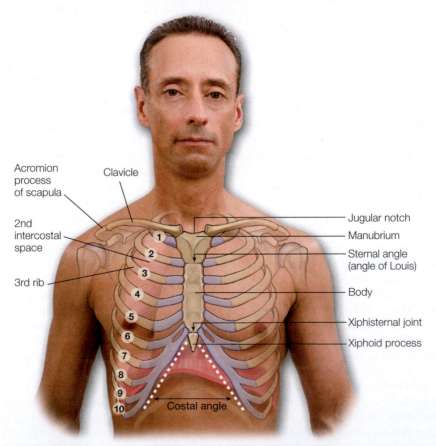

Figure 16.5A Landmarks of the anterior thorax, anterior view.

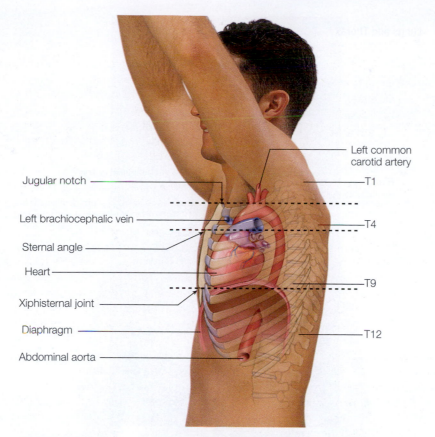

Figure 16.5B Landmarks of the anterior thorax, left lateral view, showing relationship of anterior landmarks to the vertebral column.

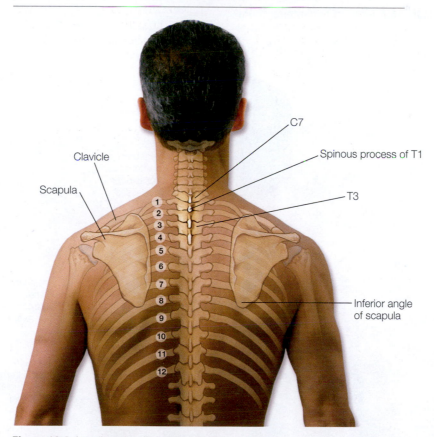

Figure 16.6 Landmarks: Posterior thorax.

Five imaginary lines are located on the posterior aspect of the thoracic cage (see Figure 16.8 ■). The vertebral line, the right and left scapular lines, and the right and left posterior axillary lines are used as landmarks on the posterior aspect of the thoracic cage. The vertebral or midspinous line commences at C7 and descends through the spinous process of each thoracic vertebra. It divides the vertebral column in half, forming the posterior right and left thoracic cage.

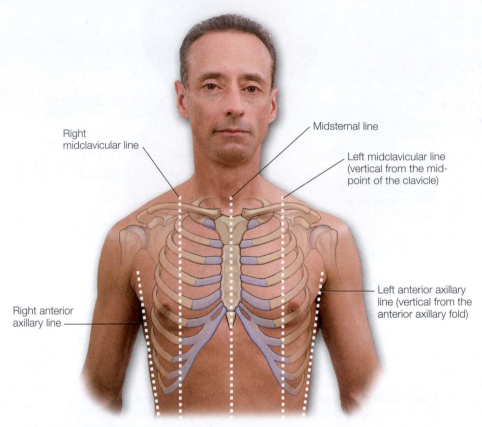

Right
midclavicular line

Midsternal line

Left midclavicular line
(vertical from the mid-
point of the clavicle)

Right anterior
axillary line

Left anterior axillary
line (vertical from the
anterior axillary fold)

Figure 16.7 Lines of the anterior thorax.

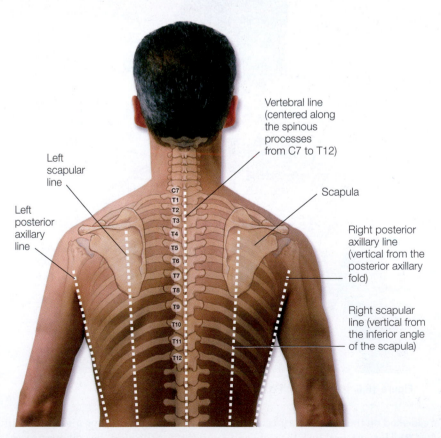

Left
scapular
line

Left
posterior
axillary
line

Vertebral line
(centered along
the spinous
processes
from C7 to T12)

Scapula

Right posterior
axillary line
(vertical from the
posterior axillary
fold)

Right scapular
line (vertical from
the inferior angle
of the scapula)

C7
T1
T2
T3
T4
T5
T6
T7
T8
T9
T10
T11
T12

Figure 16.8 Lines of the posterior thorax.

The scapular line, parallel to the vertebral line, is drawn from the inferior angle of the scapula to the level of the 12th rib. This line subdivides the right and left thoracic cage into two equal parts. The posterior axillary line (PAL) is parallel to the vertebral line. It starts at the posterior axillary fold and descends along the lateral aspect of the thoracic cage to the 12th rib.

The lateral aspect of the thoracic cage is the third section to be considered. Three imaginary lines are identified in this section (see Figure 16.9 ■). They are the anterior axillary, posterior axillary, and midaxillary lines. Two of these lines, the anterior and posterior lines, have been described. The midaxillary line is parallel to the anterior and posterior axillary lines. This line descends from the middle of the axillae to the level of the 12th rib. It forms the frontal plane, dividing the thorax into the anterior and posterior portions.

The described landmarks serve as a reference point for internal structures of the respiratory system. Recall that the trachea bifurcates, forming the right and left main bronchi. Anteriorly, this occurs at the level of the angle of Louis or sternal angle. Posteriorly, this bifurcation occurs between the third and fifth thoracic vertebrae.

The apices of the lung extend 2 cm to 4 cm (0.78–1.57 in.) above the inner third of the clavicle anteriorly. Posteriorly, the apices of the lungs are located superior to the scapula between the vertebral line and midscapular line. The base of the lung has three reference points. The lung is cone shaped, and the base of the lung is located at the sixth intercostal space at the midclavicular line. At the midaxillary line, the base of the lung is at the eighth intercostal space. At the scapular line on the posterior thorax, the base of the lung is at the 10th intercostal space.

Using external landmarks and drawing imaginary lines can also identify the five lobes of the lungs. Remember that the right lung has three lobes and the left lung has two lobes. The right and left oblique fissure divides the lung into upper and lower lobes: Starting at C7, identify T3. Draw an imaginary line from T3 at the vertebral line to the fifth intercostal space at the midaxillary line. This line follows the border of the scapula when the arms are extended over the head. It reflects the oblique fissure on the posterior wall of the thorax (see Figure 16.10 ■). On the left side continue this line to the sixth intercostal at the left midclavicular line. The two lobes of the left lung have been identified at the posterior, lateral, and anterior aspects of the left thorax.

Anteriorly, on the right side, draw two lines from the fifth intercostal space at the midaxillary line. One line descends to the sixth intercostal space at the right midclavicular line. The second line transverses the right thorax to the sternal border inferior to the fourth rib. These lines identify the oblique fissure and the horizontal fissure, forming the three lobes of the right lung (see Figure 16.11 ■, Figure 16.12A ■, and Figure 16.12B ■).

The clavicle, the scapula, and the lateral base of the neck form a triangle at the superior aspect of the thorax. This triangle, also known as Kronig's area, is used for palpation of muscles and lymph nodes and for percussion and auscultation of the apex and the lungs.

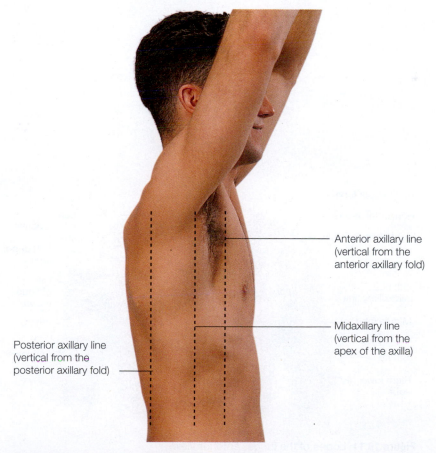

Posterior axillary line (vertical from the posterior axillary fold)

Anterior axillary line (vertical from the anterior axillary fold)

Midaxillary line (vertical from the apex of the axilla)

Figure 16.9 Lines of the lateral thorax.

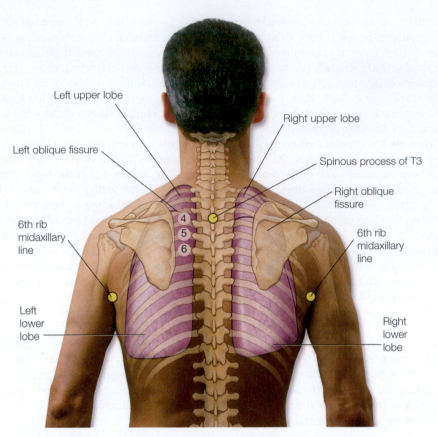

Figure 16.10 Lobes of the lungs: Posterior view.

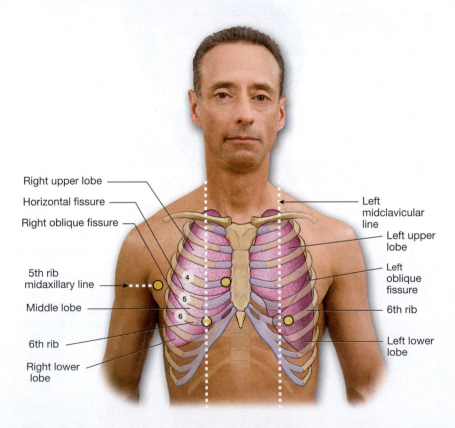

Figure 16.11 Lobes of the lungs: Anterior view.

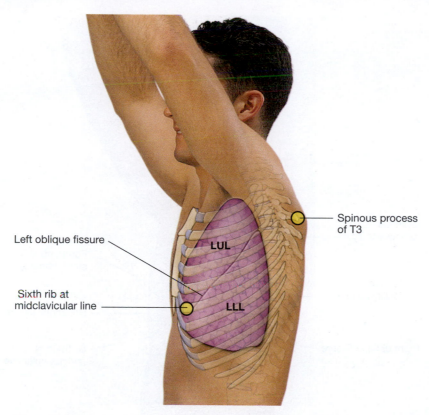

Left oblique fissure

Sixth rib at
midclavicular line

Spinous process
of T3

LUL

LLL

Figure 16.12A Lateral view of lobes of the left lung.

Special Considerations

Throughout the assessment process, the nurse gathers subjective and objective data reflecting the patient's state of health. Using critical thinking and the nursing process, the nurse identifies many factors to be considered when collecting the data. Some of these factors include but are not limited to age, developmental level, race, ethnicity, work history, living conditions, socioeconomic status, and emotional wellness.

Health Promotion Considerations

Oxygen is essential to life. Respiratory disorders and diseases include pathophysiological conditions that impair the respiratory system's ability to obtain oxygen (O_2) and expel, or get rid of, carbon dioxide (CO_2). Examples of common respiratory disorders include asthma and chronic obstructive pulmonary disease (COPD), which comprises two respiratory disorders: chronic bronchitis and emphysema.

Patients with allergies or asthma should be encouraged to explore the possibility of allergens in their work or home environment. For example, pets, dust, and molds are common allergens found in the home. Secondhand smoke in the home or work environment can also lead to respiratory distress. Research has established a link between exposure to secondhand smoke and the development of lung cancer (Hagstad et al., 2014; Manning et al., 2017). Communities that have comprehensive laws regulating smoke-free public environments have shown a greater reduction in hospitalizations for serious lung disease, like COPD, than communities with less stringent laws (Hahn et al., 2014).

Workers in some industries may be exposed to substances that are hazardous to their respiratory health, such as caustic fumes, fungi, asbestos, coal tar, nickel, silver, textile fibers, chromate, and vinyl chlorides. All of these substances are known carcinogens. Exposure to large amounts of dust in a granary or mine may lead to the development of silicosis. Coal miners are susceptible to pneumoconiosis, a form of black lung disease. People working in an office building may need to be concerned with air conditioners and forced hot-air heat. The ducts of the cooling and heating systems can carry airborne organisms, increasing the risk for respiratory infections.

Lifespan Considerations

Growth and development are dynamic processes that describe change over time. The collection of data and the interpretation of findings in relation to normative values are important. Developmental factors are considered during assessment of the respiratory system. For example, newborns have a high respiratory rate. In the pediatric patient, respirations are abdominal in nature. In pregnant patients, as the uterus enlarges, increasing pressure in the abdominal cavity limits diaphragmatic excursion and can result in more rapid and shallow respirations. See Chapter 25, Chapter 26, and Chapter 27 for more lifespan considerations. ∞

Psychosocial Considerations

Stress, anxiety, pain, and fatigue may exacerbate respiratory problems. Patients experiencing acute or chronic respiratory problems will have a physiologic alteration with gas exchange. These changes can limit or restrict the individual's ability to independently perform the activities of daily living and to participate in activities, exercise, and sports. This limitation contributes to social isolation, changes role activities, lowers self-esteem, and increases the dependency factor with support systems.

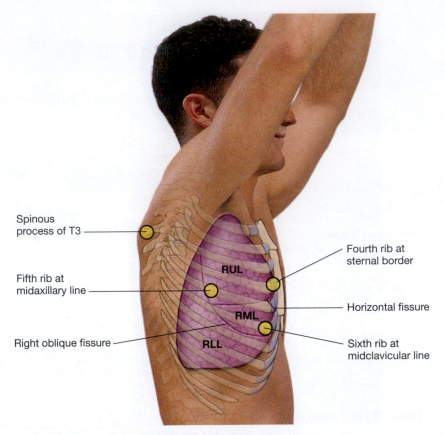

Spinous
process of T3

Fifth rib at
midaxillary line

Right oblique fissure

RUL

RML

RLL

Fourth rib at
sternal border

Horizontal fissure

Sixth rib at
midclavicular line

Figure 16.12B Lateral view of lobes of the right lung.

Certain drugs, such as bronchodilators, are used in the treatment of respiratory conditions and may cause the hands to tremble visibly. The nurse should not confuse this sign with nervousness. Even mild respiratory distress is frightening for the patient and family. Proceeding in a calm and reassuring manner helps reduce the patient's fear. Parents of young children who have experienced severe asthmatic attacks in the past may be extremely anxious any time the child develops a cold, seasonal allergy, or any other respiratory problem. A calm and careful assessment of the current health status helps to decrease the anxiety level of all involved individuals.

Ethnic, Cultural, and Environmental Considerations

Ethnicity, culture, and environment are significant factors in respiratory health. For example, with regard to heritage, the prevalence of asthma is highest among individuals who are Hispanic of Puerto Rican descent, American Indians, Alaska Natives, non-Hispanic Blacks, Filipinos, and non-Hispanic Whites. The lowest prevalence of asthma is found among Asian Americans and Asian Pacific Islanders (Tran, Siu, Iribarren, Udaltsova, & Klatsky, 2011). Chronic obstructive pulmonary disease (COPD), although primarily caused by either direct or indirect exposure to cigarette smoke, has been found to occur at higher rates in non-Hispanic Whites than in Blacks and at lower rates in Hispanics (Diaz et al., 2014; Tran et al., 2011).

For patients of any cultural background, a thorough assessment of the respiratory system is best accomplished when the patient is disrobed and the surfaces of the anterior and posterior chest can be visualized, touched, and auscultated. However, some cultural or religious practices, including the wearing or prohibition of removal of symbolic icons, jewelry, undergarments, or clothing, may interfere with physical examination. In addition, the requirement of a same-sex examiner or the presence of a companion during the assessment is an issue that must be addressed. Careful questioning of the patient during the interview, with the assistance of a translator when necessary, will allow for clarification, negotiation, and decision making about the assessment process.

The geographic location of an individual's environment will also influence respiratory health. Factors to be considered are temperature, moisture, altitude, and pollution. A cold environment encourages vasoconstriction and, ultimately, a decreased need for oxygen. An environment with increased moisture or humidity has heavy air. Individuals will tire easily, increasing the need for oxygen. As the altitude increases, the partial pressure of oxygen decreases. The individual must adapt by increasing the rate and depth of the respiratory cycle. Air pollution with smog, industrial wastes, or exhaust fumes contributes to respiratory problems in all people.

Factors within the home and social environment will influence respiratory health. Forced hot air heat is very drying to the membranes of the body. Individuals are encouraged to add moisture or use a humidifier to keep the air moist and support respiratory health. In the hot, humid, hazy days of summer, an air conditioner or dehumidifier may be necessary to help decrease the moisture in the air. Secondhand smoke, certain foods, dust, pets, and stress may also contribute to respiratory changes.

Subjective Data—Health History

Respiratory health assessment includes the gathering of subjective data during the patient interview before the actual physical assessment. During the interview the nurse uses a variety of communication techniques to elicit general and specific information about the patient's state of respiratory health or illness.

Focused Interview

The focused interview for the respiratory system concerns data related to the structures and functions of that system. Subjective data related to respiratory status are gathered during the focused interview. The nurse must be prepared to observe the patient and listen for cues related to the function of the respiratory system. The nurse may use open-ended and closed questions to obtain information. Often a number of follow-up questions or requests for descriptions are required to clarify data or gather missing information. The subjective data collected and the questions asked during the health history and focused interview will provide information intended to identify the source of problems, the duration of difficulties, and measures taken to alleviate problems. Follow-up questions also provide clues about the patient's knowledge of his or her own health.

The focused interview guides the physical assessment of the respiratory system. The information is always considered in relation to norms and expectations about respiratory function. Therefore, the nurse must consider age, gender, race, culture, environment, health practices, past and concurrent problems, and therapies when framing questions and using techniques to elicit information. In order to address all of the factors when conducting a focused interview, categories of questions related to respiratory status and function have been developed. These categories include general questions that are asked of all patients: those questions addressing illness or infection; those related to symptoms, pain, or behaviors; those related to habits or practices; those that are specific to patients according to age; those for pregnant females; and those that address environmental concerns. One method to elicit information about symptoms is OLDCART & ICE, as described in Chapter 5. ∞

The nurse must consider the patient's ability to participate in the focused interview and physical assessment of the respiratory system. If a patient is experiencing dyspnea, cyanosis, difficulty with speech, and the anxiety that accompanies any of these problems, attention must focus on relief of symptoms and restoration of oxygenation.

Focused Interview Questions	Rationales and Evidence

The following sections provide sample questions and bulleted follow-up questions in each of the previously mentioned categories. A rationale for each of the questions is provided. The list of questions is not all-inclusive but, rather, represents the types of questions required in a comprehensive focused interview related to the respiratory system.

General Questions

1. **Describe your breathing today. Is it different from 2 months ago? From 2 years ago?**

   ▶ These questions give patients the opportunity to provide their own perceptions about breathing.

2. **Do you breathe through your mouth or through your nose?**
   - Have you always breathed through your mouth?
   - Do you have a problem with your nose?
   - How long have you had the problem?
   - Have you received any treatment for the problem?
   - Did the treatment help?

   ▶ Nose breathing allows inhaled air to be warmed, moistened, and filtered before entering the lung and is considered the norm. Patients who identify themselves as mouth breathers require follow-up. Mouth breathing is associated with problems in the nose, habit, or air hunger (Goodman, Lynm, & Livingston, 2013).

3. **Are you able to carry out all of your regular activities without a change in your breathing?**
   - Describe the change in your breathing.
   - Do you know what causes the change?
   - What do you do when this occurs?
   - How long has this been happening?
   - Have you discussed this with a healthcare professional?

   ▶ This provides an opportunity to elicit information about typical breathing patterns and changes related to normal activities of daily living. A "yes" would be considered the norm. Any other response requires follow-up questions to determine the type of change and factors that contribute to or predispose the patient to changes in breathing.

4. **Describe your breathing when you are engaged in exercise or vigorous activity.**
   - Describe the breathing problem that occurs when you are exercising or very active.
   - How long has this been happening?
   - What do you do when it happens?
   - Do your actions relieve the problem?

   ▶ A normal expectation is that the patient will describe his or her breathing as becoming more rapid or deeper with activity but quickly returning to normal upon completion of the exercise or activity. Follow-up is required when the patient describes dyspnea during, or slow recovery from, exercise or activity (Berman & Snyder, 2015).

5. **When you sleep do you lie down flat, prop yourself up with pillows, or sit up?**
   - Tell me why you prefer to sit up.
   - How many pillows do you use?
   - Does the position or number of pillows help with your breathing?
   - How long have you slept like this?
   - Have you discussed this with a healthcare professional?
   - What treatment was recommended?
   - Did the treatment help?

   ▶ The norm is for a patient to sleep fully reclined with a pillow. The number of pillows for propping oneself up should be determined. Patients who must prop themselves up or sit up while sleeping may have **orthopnea**—that is, dyspnea when lying down (Dumitru & Baker, 2014). It is important to determine if the propping up or sitting up is simply a preference or because of breathing problems or some other cause.

Focused Interview Questions	Rationales and Evidence

6. **Do you have any physical problems that affect your breathing?**
   - Describe the way your breathing is affected.
   - How long has this been occurring?
   - Have you sought treatment for the problem?
   - What was the treatment?
   - Did the treatment help?

   ▶ This is a general question to elicit information about respiratory or other problems that impact breathing. For example, pain from an injury to the upper body may impact breathing but not be directly related to respiratory structures. If the patient identifies any problems that affect breathing, follow-up is required. The nurse should ask for clear descriptions and details about what, when, and how problems occur and impact breathing as well as the duration of the problems.

7. **Is there anyone in your family who has or has had a respiratory disease or problem?**
   - What is/was the disease or problem?
   - Who in the family has/had the disease?
   - When was it diagnosed?
   - How has it been treated?
   - How effective is/was the treatment?

   ▶ This information may reveal information about respiratory diseases associated with familial or genetic predisposition. Follow-up is required to obtain details about specific problems and their occurrence, treatment, and outcomes.

Questions Related to Illness or Infection

1. **Have you ever been diagnosed with a respiratory disease?**
   - When were you diagnosed with the problem?
   - What treatment was prescribed for the problem?
   - Was the treatment helpful?
   - What kinds of things do you do to help with the problem?
   - Has the problem ever recurred (acute)?
   - How are you managing the disease now (chronic)?

   ▶ The patient has an opportunity to provide information about specific respiratory illnesses. If a diagnosed illness is identified, follow-up about the date of diagnosis, treatment, and outcomes is required. Data about each illness identified by the patient are essential to an accurate health assessment. Illnesses can be classified as acute or chronic, and follow-up regarding each classification will differ.

2. *Alternative to question 1: List possible respiratory illnesses, such as asthma, chronic obstructive pulmonary disease (COPD), and emphysema, and ask the patient to respond yes or no as each is stated.*

   ▶ This is a comprehensive and easy way to elicit information about all respiratory diagnoses. Follow-up would be carried out for each identified diagnosis as in question 1.

3. **Do you now have or have you had a respiratory infection?**
   - When were you diagnosed with the infection?
   - What treatment was prescribed for the problem?
   - Was the treatment helpful?
   - What kinds of things do you do to help with the problem?
   - Has the problem ever recurred (acute)?
   - How are you managing the infection now (chronic)?

   ▶ If an infection is identified, follow-up about the date of infection, treatment, and outcomes is required. Data about each infection identified by the patient are essential to an accurate health assessment. Infections can be classified as acute or chronic, and follow-up regarding each classification will differ.

4. *Alternative to question 3: List possible respiratory infections, such as bronchitis, pneumonia, and pleurisy, and ask the patient to respond yes or no as each is stated.*

   ▶ This is a comprehensive and easy way to elicit information about all respiratory infections. Follow-up would be carried out for each identified infection as in question 3.

Questions Related to Symptoms, Pain, and Behaviors

When gathering information about symptoms, many questions are required to elicit details and descriptions that assist in the analysis of the data. Discrimination is made in relation to the significance of a symptom, specific diseases or problems, and potential follow-up examination or referral. One rationale may be provided for a group of questions in this category.

The following questions refer to specific symptoms and behaviors associated with the respiratory system. For each symptom, questions and follow-up are required. The details to be elicited are the characteristics of the symptom; the onset, duration, and frequency of the symptom; the treatment or remedy for the symptom, including over-the-counter (OTC) and home remedies; the determination if diagnosis has been sought; the effect of treatments; and family history associated with a symptom or illness.

Questions 1 through 23 refer to coughing as a symptom associated with respiratory diseases or problems and are comprehensive enough to provide an example of the number and types of questions required in a focused interview when a symptom exists. The remaining questions refer to other symptoms associated with respiratory problems. The number and types of questions are limited to identification of the symptom. Follow-up is included only when required for clarification.

Questions Related to Symptoms

1. **Do you have a cough?**

   ▶ Question 1 identifies the existence of a symptom, and questions 2 through 7 add knowledge about the symptom.

2. **How long have you had the cough?**

   ▶ Determining the duration of symptoms is helpful in determining the significance of symptoms in relation to specific diseases and problems.

3. **How often are you coughing?**

4. **Do you know what causes the cough?**

5. **Is there a difference in the cough at different times of the day?**

6. **Describe your cough.**

Focused Interview Questions	Rationales and Evidence
7. Is it dry, hacking, hoarse, moist, or barking?	▶ The type of cough may indicate a symptom associated with a specific disease or problem. For example, wet or moist coughs are most often associated with lung infection (Foltz-Gray, 2017).
8. Are you coughing up mucus or phlegm?	
9. What does the mucus look like?	▶ The color and odor of any mucus or phlegm (sputum) is associated with specific diseases or problems. For example, pink or reddish-colored mucus is associated with tuberculosis (TB), and green or yellow mucus often signals lung infection (Marcin, 2017).
10. Does the mucus have any odor?	
11. Has the amount of mucus changed?	▶ A change in the amount or character of sputum is often a sign of a respiratory disease (Marcin, 2017).
12. Has the consistency or thickness of the mucus changed?	
13. Do you have pain when you cough? • Describe the type, severity, and location of the pain. • What do you do for the cough or the pain? • Is the remedy effective?	▶ Painful coughing may occur because of muscle pain or may be indicative of an underlying lung disease (Berman & Snyder, 2015). Follow-up elicits details that assist in data analysis.
14. Have you sought treatment for the cough?	▶ Questions 14 through 18 provide information about the need for diagnosis, referral, or continued evaluation of the symptom; information about the patient's knowledge of a current diagnosis or underlying problem, and information about the patient's response to intervention.
15. When was that treatment sought?	
16. What occurred when you sought that treatment?	
17. Was something prescribed or recommended to help with the cough?	
18. What was the effect of the remedy?	
19. Do you use OTC or home remedies for the cough?	▶ Questions 19 through 22 provide information about drugs and substances that may relieve symptoms or provide comfort. Some substances may mask symptoms, interfere with the effect of prescribed medications, or harm the patient (Shields et al., 2018).
20. What are those OTC medications or remedies that you use?	
21. How often do you use them?	
22. How much of them do you use?	
23. Do you now have or have you ever had any wheezing?	
24. Have you had a change in your weight recently? • How much weight have you gained or lost? • Over what period of time did this change occur? • Was the change purposeful? • Can you associate the change with any event or problem?	▶ Weight loss or gain may be associated with lung or cardiac diseases (Berman & Snyder, 2015).
25. Describe your diet. Do you use any nutritional supplements?	▶ Questions about nutritional intake are important to determine the contribution to production of red blood cells (erythropoiesis) and hemoglobin, which are essential to oxygenation (Berman & Snyder, 2015).
26. Do you ever become light-headed or dizzy? • When did or does that occur? • How often? • Do you associate this with any event or activity? • What do you do when this happens?	▶ Light-headedness or dizziness may be associated with hypoxia (Berman & Snyder, 2015).

Questions Related to Pain

1. Do you have pain anywhere in your chest?	▶ Chest pain may be related to cardiac or respiratory problems.
2. Where is the pain?	▶ Questions 2 through 6 are standard questions associated with pain to determine the location, frequency, duration, and intensity of the pain.
3. How often do you experience the pain?	
4. How long does the pain last?	
5. How long have you had the pain?	
6. How would you rate the pain on a scale of 0 to 10, with 10 being the worst?	

Focused Interview Questions	Rationales and Evidence

7. **Does the pain affect your breathing?**
  • Are you short of breath?
  • Are you able to take a deep breath?
  • What do you do when this happens?
 	
8. **Does the pain occur when you are taking a breath or when you are exhaling, or both?**
 	
9. **Is there a trigger for the pain, such as a cough or movement?**
 	
10. **Can you describe the pain?**
 	
11. **Does the pain radiate to other areas?**
 	
12. **What do you do to relieve the pain?**
 	
13. **Is this treatment effective?**
	▶ Follow-up questions relate to the ways in which breathing is affected.
	▶ Questions 7 through 11 are intended to discriminate the characteristics of pain associated with underlying acute or chronic respiratory disease from muscular pain that can occur with cough or maintaining a posture to ease breathing.
	
	▶ Questions 12 and 13 are intended to determine if the patient has selected a treatment based on past experience, knowledge of respiratory illness, or use of complementary care and its effectiveness.

Questions Related to Behaviors

1. **Do you now smoke or have you ever smoked tobacco products?**
 	
2. **What type of tobacco product do/did you smoke?**
 	
3. **How much of the product do/did you smoke?**
 	
4. **When did you start smoking?**
 	
5. **When did you stop smoking?**
 	
6. **Have you tried to stop smoking?**
 	
7. **What did you do to stop smoking?**
 	
8. **Do you have any symptoms related to smoking?**
 	
9. **Do you smoke or inhale marijuana, other herbal products, or chemical preparations such as glue or spray paint? Have you done so in the past?**
  • What is the substance you inhale?
  • How much do you use?
  • How often do you inhale the substance?
  • For those patients who state they have inhaled substances in the past, ask: When did you stop using the substance?
 	
10. **Have you received immunization for respiratory illnesses such as flu or pneumonia?**
  • What immunizations have you had?
  • When was each given? Were there any adverse effects?
	▶ Tobacco products include cigarettes, cigars, and pipe tobacco.
	
	▶ Smoking tobacco products is associated with respiratory diseases including emphysema and lung cancer. If the patient exhibits or affirms that respiratory symptoms exist, questions for any symptom as previously described would be asked.
	
	▶ Inhalation of marijuana, herbal substances, and/or chemicals may result in respiratory problems associated with incidental or continuous irritation of the linings of the respiratory organs (Centers for Disease Control and Prevention [CDC], 2013).
	
	▶ Immunization reduces the risk of infection from flu or pneumonia.

Questions Related to Age

The focused interview must reflect the anatomic and physiologic differences in lung and thorax health that exist along the age span as well as during pregnancy. Specific questions related to lung and thorax health for each of these groups are provided in Chapter 25, Chapter 26, and Chapter 27. ∞

Patient-Centered Interaction

Source: GUIZIOU Franck/hemis .fr/Alamy Stock Photo.

Mr. Loi is a 78-year-old with a history of COPD who recently moved from another state to live with his daughter, Anita. His daughter scheduled an appointment for Mr. Loi with her healthcare group. When Anita called to arrange the appointment, she explained that her father was widowed 3 years ago and had been doing well in his own home, but he seemed lonely and was not participating in activities in his neighborhood and community as he had been. He also did not say much when she phoned. Anita stated that he has COPD. Although it did not seem to affect his activity in the past, she was concerned about him. She visited him and suggested he move in with her family and was relieved that he agreed. Since the move, he has been quiet and resting in his room most of the time. His respirations are regular and nonlabored. He has had a cough once in a while, but she thought she had better get him set up with a doctor just in case something happened.

Mr. Loi completed several forms before his health interview. These forms included biographic information, personal and family health history, and information about his current diagnosis and medications.

Interview

Because Mr. Loi's only diagnosed health problem is COPD, the nurse begins the interview with questions related to his respiratory system. The nurse greets Mr. Loi, offers him a seat, and explains the interview process. Mr. Loi takes a seat, smiles, and nods.

Nurse: Tell me about your breathing.

Mr. Loi: I'm doing fine. I take all my medications.

Nurse: Has your breathing changed in the last two months?

Mr. Loi: Oh, I moved here to be with my daughter a month ago.
The nurse realizes that Mr. Loi has not answered the question. It is not clear if Mr. Loi did not hear the question, misunderstood the question, or is seeking an opportunity to discuss his move. The nurse uses an open-ended statement to allow him to discuss the move.

Nurse: Tell me a little about your move.
Mr. Loi leans forward and focuses on the nurse's lips while listening to the question.

Mr. Loi: Well, my daughter wanted me here. She worries that I don't get out and see people. You know I have COPD, but it's been okay as long as I take my pills.

Mr. Loi's posture and focus while the nurse spoke suggests that Mr. Loi is having difficulty hearing. Further, Mr. Loi's daughter was concerned about her father's diminished social contact and decreasing phone communication, which are additional signs of hearing deficit.

In order to complete the health assessment, the nurse will use techniques appropriate for those patients with hearing impairment.

The nurse faces Mr. Loi, uses a low-pitched voice at normal loudness, and speaks in short sentences to conduct the interview. The nurse pauses after each statement so Mr. Loi can interpret the statement.

Nurse: What do you think of the move?

Mr. Loi: So far, so good. She's been great and so has her family. It's all pretty different, but I think I'll be okay. I don't want her to worry, so I agreed to come and get checked out here. You know . . . my COPD and all.

Nurse: Tell me about the COPD.

Mr. Loi: Well, it started about 5 years ago. I was getting winded with just a little work around the house. Then I got bronchitis and it just took off from there.

Objective Data—Physical Assessment

In the physical assessment of the respiratory system, the techniques of inspection, palpation, and auscultation will be used. Percussion is a more advanced skill, which is discussed in Chapter 7 and in Appendix C. ∞ Before proceeding, it may be helpful to review the information about each of the data-gathering processes and practice the techniques of health assessment. Health records, the results of laboratory tests, and x-rays are important secondary sources to be reviewed and included in the data-gathering process. See Table 16.1 for information on potential secondary sources of patient data.

the patient's breathing and level of oxygenation. The nurse inspects skin color, structures of the thoracic cavity, chest configuration, and respiratory rate rhythm and effort. Knowledge of norms or expected findings is essential in determining the meaning of the data as one proceeds.

HELPFUL HINTS

- Provide an environment that is comfortable and private.
- Explain each step of the procedure.
- Provide specific instructions about what is expected of the patient—for example, whether deep or regular breathing will be required.
- Tell patient the purpose of each procedure and when and if discomfort will accompany any examination.
- Pay attention to nonverbal cues that may indicate discomfort and ask the patient to indicate if he or she experiences any difficulties or discomforts.
- An organized and professional approach goes a long way toward putting the patient at ease.
- Use Standard Precautions.

EQUIPMENT

- Examination gown and drape
- Examination gloves
- Examination light
- Stethoscope
- Tissues
- Face mask for nurse, if indicated

Assessment Techniques and Findings

Physical assessment of the respiratory system requires the use of inspection, palpation, percussion, and auscultation. During each of the procedures, the nurse is gathering data related to

Adults normally breathe at a rate of 12 to 20 breaths per minute. The respiratory cycle includes full inspiration (I) and expiration (E). The ratio of the length of inspiration to expiration is

Table 16.1 Potential Secondary Sources for Patient Data Related to the Respiratory System

LABORATORY TESTS	NORMAL VALUES
Arterial Blood Gases (ABGs)	pH 7.35–7.45 pH units PO_2 80–100 mmHg PCO_2 35–45 mmHg HCO_3 22–26 mEq/L
Complete Blood Count (CBC) Red Blood Cells (RBCs)	Male 4.32–5.72 million/mcL Female 3.90–5.03 million/mcL
Hemoglobin (Hgb)	Male 13.5–17.5 g/dL Female 12.0–15.5 g/dL
Hematocrit (Hct)	Male 38.8%–50.0% Female 34.9%–44.5%

White Blood Cells (WBCs)
    Leukocytes
    Bands
    Basophils
    Eosinophils
    Lymphocytes
    B-Lymphocytes
    T-Lymphocytes
    Monocytes
    Neutrophils
Platelets
Erythrocyte Sedimentation Rate (ESR)
	4,500–10,000/mcL
	0%–3%
	0.5%–1%
	1%–4%
	20%–40%
	4%–25%
	60%–95%
	2%–8%
	40%–60%
	150–450 billion/L
	Males less than 23 mm/hr
	Females less than 29 mm/hr (MedlinePlus, 2017)

DIAGNOSTIC TESTS	
O_2 Saturation Normal Value ≥ 95% Chest x-ray Fiberoptic Bronchoscopy Pulmonary Function Testing Sputum Evaluation Tuberculin Skin Testing Ventilation Perfusion (VQ) Scan (Pagana & Pagana, 2017)	

about 1:2 (I:E). Breathing should be even, regular, and coordinated. Chest movement should be uniform; the structures of the thorax should be aligned, and the thorax should be symmetric. The sternum is midline and flat. The costal angle is less than 90° in an adult. The vertebrae are midline and follow the pattern of cervical, thoracic, and lumbar curves. The anterior to posterior diameter of the chest should be half of the lateral diameter. Pink skin or pink undertones indicate normal oxygenation. Assessment for pink-colored tongue or oral mucous membranes may be required in dark-skinned individuals. The color of the skin of the thorax should be consistent with that of the rest of the body.

Physical assessment of the respiratory system follows an organized pattern. It begins with a patient survey followed by inspection of the anterior thorax and complete assessment of the posterior thorax. The assessment ends with palpation and auscultation of the anterior thorax. The nurse includes the anterior, posterior, and lateral aspects of the thorax when conducting each of the assessments.

Techniques and Normal Findings	Abnormal Findings and Special Considerations

Survey

A quick survey of the patient enables the nurse to identify any immediate problems as well as the patient's ability to participate in the assessment.

▶ Patients experiencing anxiety may demonstrate pallor and shallow breathing. Acknowledgment of the problem and discussion of the procedures often provide some relief. If a patient is in obvious respiratory distress, the problem must be addressed. The patient may require referral to a medical care provider or emergency care facility.

ALERT! *Individuals experiencing pain and dyspnea, who are restless, anxious, and unable to follow directions, may need immediate medical assistance.*

Inspect the overall appearance, posture, and position of the patient. Note the skin color and respiratory effort. Observe for signs of anxiety or distress.

▶ Circumoral cyanosis, evidenced by bluish mucous membranes in the mouth, is often an early warning sign of respiratory distress or hypoxia. Therefore, patients with circumoral cyanosis should be immediately evaluated for the source of respiratory distress and treated appropriately.

Techniques and Normal Findings	Abnormal Findings and Special Considerations

Inspection of the Anterior and Lateral Thorax

ALERT! *Be sensitive to the patient's privacy, and limit exposure of body parts.*

1. Position the patient.
- The patient should be in a sitting position with clothing removed except for an examination gown and drape (see Figure 16.13 ■).

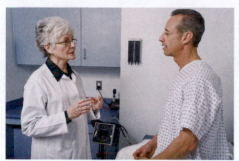

Figure 16.13 Patient positioned and gowned for assessment.

- Stand in front of the patient for anterior inspection and to the side of the patient for lateral inspection. Lighting must be adequate to detect color differences, lesions, and chest movement.

2. Instruct the patient.
- Explain that you are going to be looking at the patient's chest structures. Tell the patient to breathe normally.

3. Observe skin color.
- Skin color varies among individuals, but pink undertones indicate normal oxygenation. Skin color of the thorax should be consistent with that of the rest of the body.

▶ Pigments and levels of oxygenation influence skin color. Pallor, cyanosis, erythema, or grayness requires further evaluation.

4. Inspect the structures of the thorax.
- The clavicles should be at the same height. The sternum should be midline. The costal angle should be less than 90°.

▶ Misalignment of clavicles may be caused by deviations in the vertebral column such as scoliosis. An increase in the costal angle in an adult may indicate COPD. The thorax of children is rounder than that of adults.

5. Inspect for symmetry.
- The structures of the chest and chest movement should be symmetric.

▶ Asymmetry may indicate postural problems or underlying respiratory dysfunction.

6. Inspect chest configuration.
- The adult transverse (T) diameter is approximately twice that of the anteroposterior (AP) diameter (AP:T = 1:2). See Box 16.1.

▶ A change in the ratio requires further evaluation. Remember: Older adults have a decreased ratio. See Box 16.2.

Box 16.1 Normal Chest Configurations

Adult

- The adult chest is elliptical in shape with a lateral diameter that is larger than the anteroposterior diameter in a 2:1 ratio.

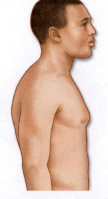

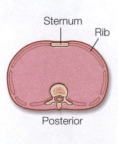

Sternum

Rib

Posterior

Box 16.2 Abnormal Chest Configurations

Barrel Chest

The anteroposterior diameter is equal to the lateral diameter, and the ribs are horizontal. A barrel chest occurs normally with aging and accompanies COPD.

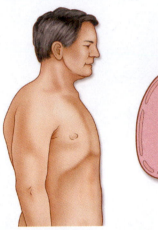
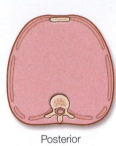

Posterior

Funnel Chest (Pectus Excavatum)

This is a congenital deformity characterized by depression of the sternum and adjacent costal cartilage. All or part of the sternum may be involved, but predominant depression is at the lower portion where the body meets the xiphoid process.

   If the condition is severe, chest compression may interfere with respiration. Murmurs may be present with cardiac compression.

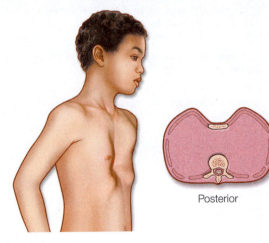

Posterior

Scoliosis

Scoliosis is a condition in which there is lateral curvature and rotation of the thoracic and lumbar spine. It occurs more frequently in females. Scoliosis may result in elevation of the shoulder and pelvis.

   Deviation greater than 45° may cause distortion of the lung, which results in decreased lung volume or difficulty in interpretation of findings from physical assessment.

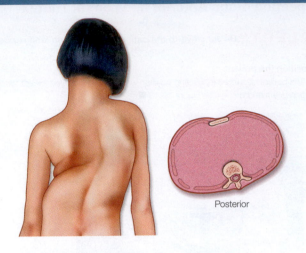

Posterior

Pigeon Chest (Pectus Carinatum)

This congenital deformity is characterized by forward displacement of the sternum with depression of the adjacent costal cartilage. This condition generally requires no treatment.

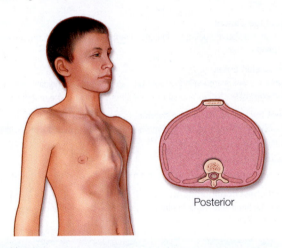

Posterior

Kyphosis

Kyphosis is exaggerated posterior curvature of the thoracic spine. It is associated with aging. Severe kyphosis may decrease lung expansion and increase cardiac problems.

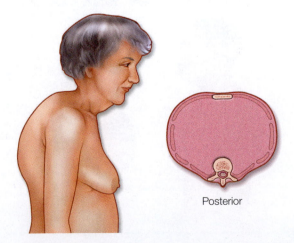

Posterior

Techniques and Normal Findings	**Abnormal Findings and Special Considerations**

7. Count the respiratory rate.

- Count the number of respiratory cycles per minute. Normal adult respiratory rate is 12 to 20.
- Observe chest movement.
- Observe the muscles of the chest and neck, including the intercostal muscles and sternocleidomastoids.
- Do not tell the patient that you are counting respirations; it may alter the normal breathing pattern.
- Respirations should be even and smooth. Chest movement should be symmetric.
- Males tend to breathe abdominally.
- Females breathe more thoracically.

Inspection of the Posterior Thorax

1. Instruct the patient.

- Explain to the patient that you will be performing several assessments and that you will provide instructions as you move from one step to the next. Tell the patient to try to relax and breathe normally to begin the examination.

2. Observe skin color.

- Skin color of the posterior thorax should be consistent with that of the rest of the body.

3. Inspect the structures of the posterior thorax.

- The height of the scapulae should be even; the vertebrae should be midline.

4. Inspect for symmetry.

- The structures of the chest and chest movement should be symmetric.

5. Observe respirations.

- Respirations should be smooth and even.

▶ Lateral deviation of the spine and elevation of one scapula are indicative of scoliosis.

▶ Asymmetry may indicate postural problems or underlying respiratory problems.

▶ Respirations in the obese patient may be shallow and rapid.

Palpation of the Posterior Thorax

1. Instruct the patient.

- Explain that you will be touching the patient's back to determine if there are any areas of tenderness. Tell the patient to breathe normally during this part of the examination and to tell you if pain or discomfort is felt at any area.

2. Lightly palpate the posterior thorax.

- Use the finger pads to lightly palpate symmetric areas on the posterior thorax. Include the entire thorax by starting at the areas above each scapula and move from side to side to below the 12th rib and laterally to the midaxillary line on each side (see Figure 16.14 ■).

▶ Pain may occur with inflammation of fibrous tissue or underlying structures such as the pleura. Crepitus is a crunching feeling under the skin caused by air leaking into subcutaneous tissue.

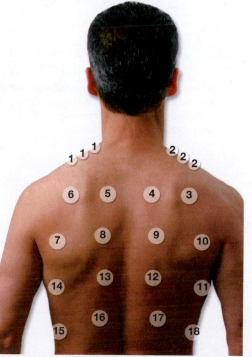

Figure 16.14 Pattern for palpating the posterior thorax.

Techniques and Normal Findings	Abnormal Findings and Special Considerations

- Assess muscle mass.
- Assess for growths, nodules, and masses.
- Assess for tenderness.
- Muscle mass should be firm and underlying tissue smooth. The chest should be free of lesions or masses. The area should be nontender to palpation.

3. **Palpate and count ribs and intercostal spaces.**
   - Instruct the patient to flex the neck, round the shoulders, and lean forward. Tell the patient you will be applying light pressure to the spine and rib areas. Instruct the patient to breathe normally and to tell you of pain or discomfort.
   - When the neck is flexed, the spinous process of C_7 is most prominent. When two spinous processes are equally prominent, they are C_7 and T_1. Use the finger pads to palpate each spinous process. The spinous processes should form a straight line. Further assessment is discussed in Chapter 23. ∞ Move to the left and right to identify ribs and intercostal spaces from C_7 through T_{12}.

▶ Lateral deviation of the thoracic spinous processes indicates scoliosis.

4. **Palpate for respiratory expansion.**
   - Explain that you will be assessing the movement of the chest during breathing by placing your hands on the lower chest and asking the patient to take a deep breath.
   - Place the palmar surface of your hands, with thumbs close to the vertebrae, on the chest at the level of T_{10}. Pinch up some skin between your thumbs. Ask the patient to take a deep breath (see Figure 16.15 ■).

▶ Unilateral decrease or delay in expansion may indicate underlying fibrotic or obstructive lung disease or may result from splinting associated with pleural pain or pneumothorax.

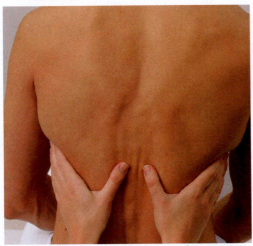

Figure 16.15 Palpation for respiratory expansion.

   - The movement and pressure of the chest against your hands should feel smooth and even. Your thumbs should move away from the spine, and the skin should move smoothly as the chest moves with inspiration. Your hands should lift symmetrically outward when the patient takes a deep breath.

5. **Palpate for tactile fremitus.**
   - **Fremitus** is the palpable vibration on the chest wall when the patient speaks. Fremitus is strongest over the trachea, diminishes over the bronchi, and becomes almost nonexistent over the alveoli of the lungs.
   - Explain that you will be feeling for vibrations on the chest while the patient speaks. Tell the patient you will be placing your hands on various areas of the chest while he or she repeats "ninety-nine" or "one, two, three" in a clear, loud voice.
   - Use the ulnar surface of the hand or the palmar surface of the hand at the base of the fingers at the metacarpophalangeal joints when palpating (see Figure 16.16 ■). Palpate and compare symmetric areas of the lungs by moving from side to side, from apices to bases. Using one hand to palpate for fremitus is believed to increase accuracy of findings. Two-handed methods may, however, increase speed and facilitate identification of asymmetry.

▶ Decreased or absent fremitus may result from a soft voice, from a very thick chest wall, from obesity, or from underlying diseases, including COPD and pleural effusion. Increased fremitus occurs with fluid in the lungs, fibrosis, tumor, or infection.

Techniques and Normal Findings	Abnormal Findings and Special Considerations

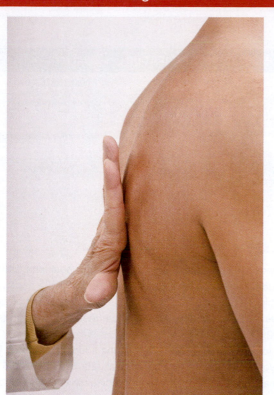

Figure 16.16 Palpation for tactile fremitus using metacarpo-phalangeal joint area.

Auscultation of the Posterior Thorax

Auscultation of the respiratory system refers to listening to the sounds of breathing through the stethoscope. The sounds are produced by air moving through the airways. Sounds change as the airway size changes or with the presence of fluid or mucus.

- Use the diaphragm of the stethoscope and listen through the full respiratory cycle. When auscultating, classify each sound according to intensity, location, pitch, duration, and characteristic.

▶ Auscultation through clothing or coarse chest hair may produce deceptive sounds. Thick, coarse chest hair may be matted with a damp cloth or lotion to prevent interference with auscultation.

▶ In the obese patient, the skin folds must be moved and the stethoscope placed firmly on the chest wall for auscultation. Asking overweight and obese patients to put the arm over the head and lean toward the opposite side is often helpful in accessing the chest wall during auscultation.

ALERT! *It is important to monitor the patient's breathing to prevent hyperventilation.*

Four normal breath sounds are heard during respiratory auscultation. **Tracheal sounds** are harsh, high-pitched sounds heard over the trachea when the patient inhales and exhales. **Bronchial sounds** are loud, high-pitched sounds heard next to the trachea and are longer on exhalation. **Bronchovesicular sounds** are medium in loudness and pitch. They are heard between the scapulae, posteriorly and next to the sternum, and anteriorly upon inhalation and exhalation. **Vesicular sounds** are soft and low pitched and heard over the remainder of the lungs. Vesicular sounds are longer on inhalation than exhalation (see Table 16.2).

Table 16.2 Normal Breath Sounds

SOUND	LOCATION	RATIO INSPIRATION TO EXPIRATION	QUALITY
Tracheal	Over trachea	I < E	Harsh, high pitched
Bronchial	Next to trachea, superior to each clavicle and in the first intercostal space	E > I	Loud, high pitched
Bronchovesicular	Over major bronchi in the second and third intercostal spaces between scapulae	I = E	Medium loudness, medium pitch
Vesicular	Remainder of lungs	I > E	Soft, low pitched

Evidence-Based Practice

Auscultating Lung Sounds

- A small study looked at the effect of body position on lung sounds in healthy males, examined in four positions: sitting, supine, prone, and lateral decubitus. A slight increase in the loudness of the lung sounds was found over the dependent lung in the lateral decubitus position, with no differences found in the other positions. Because patients are not always able to be in an upright position during lung auscultation, knowing position changes have little effect on lung sounds is important (Fiz, Gnitecki, Kraman, Wodicka, & Pasterkamp, 2008).
- Studies have shown a lack of agreement by healthcare professionals regarding auscultated lung sounds, unrelated to experience (Berry, Marti, & Ntoumenopoulos, 2016; Eseonu-Ewoh & Sterling, 2016; Leuppi et al., 2005). Leuppi et al. (2005) concluded that the absence of abnormal lung sounds is a predictor for not having lung disease and wheezing is a predictor for having lung disease. The research recommends using all the findings from the lung exam and a thorough health history to ensure the accuracy of the patient's diagnosis (Berry et al., 2016; Eseonu-Ewoh & Sterling, 2016; Leuppi et al., 2005).
- It is important to assess the lungs and thorax by removing the patient's clothing and completing the examination directly on skin as the clothing interferes with inspection, palpation, and percussion (Kraman, 2008; Sherman, 2009). Kraman (2008) studied the sensitivity of the stethoscope when used over clothing and found the clothing needed to be removed in order to complete an accurate exam; however, if clothing cannot be removed, it is possible to auscultate over it. Medium to heavy pressure is needed over a single or double layer of fabric to ensure accurate sound transmission (Kraman, 2008).

1. **Instruct the patient.**
   - Explain that you will be listening to the patient's breathing with the stethoscope.
   - The patient will be in either a supine or a seated position. Ask the patient to breathe deeply through the mouth each time the stethoscope is placed on a new spot. Tell the patient to let you know if he or she is becoming tired, short of breath, or dizzy and, if so, that you will stop and allow time to rest.

2. **Visualize the landmarks.**
   - Observe the posterior thorax and visualize the horizontal and vertical lines, the level of the diaphragm, and the fissures of the lungs.

3. **Auscultate for bronchovesicular sounds.**
   - The right and left primary bronchi are located at the level of T_3 and T_5. Auscultate at the right and left of the vertebrae at those levels. The breath sounds will be bronchovesicular.

▶ The obese patient may be unable to take deep breaths because of the weight of the chest wall and the fatty deposits in the intercostal muscles and the diaphragm.

▶ Auscultation of diminished breath sounds in both lungs may indicate emphysema, bronchospasm, or shallow breathing. Atelectasis, which is reflective of collapse or impaired expansion of one or more areas of the lung, also may produce diminished breath sounds (National Heart, Lung, & Blood Institute [NHLBI], 2013). In some cases, atelectasis will be accompanied by a faint "popping" sound at end-inspiration, if the atelectatic alveoli re-expand. Breath sounds heard in just one lung may indicate pleural effusion, pneumothorax, tumor, or mucous plugs in the airways in the other lung. Hearing bronchial or bronchovesicular sounds in areas where one would normally hear vesicular sounds may be reflective of fluid or exudate in the alveoli and small bronchioles. Fluid and exudate decrease the movement of air through small airways and result in loss of vesicular sounds.

Techniques and Normal Findings	Abnormal Findings and Special Considerations

4. Auscultate for vesicular sounds.

- Auscultate the apex of the left lung, then the apex of the right lung. Move the stethoscope from side to side while comparing sounds. Start at the apices and move to the bases of the lungs and laterally to the midaxillary line. The breath sounds over most of the posterior surface are vesicular. See Figure 16.17 ■.

▶ Added or **adventitious sounds** are superimposed on normal breath sounds and are often indicative of underlying airway problems or diseases of the cardiovascular or respiratory systems (see Table 16.3). Adventitious sounds are classified as discontinuous or continuous.

Discontinuous sounds are **crackles**, which are intermittent, nonmusical, and brief. These sounds are commonly referred to as **rales**. Fine rales are soft, high pitched, and very brief. Coarse rales/crackles are louder, lower in pitch, and longer.

Continuous sounds are musical and longer than rales but do not necessarily persist through the entire respiratory cycle. The two types are wheezes/sibilant wheezes and rhonchi (sonorous wheezes). **Wheezes** (sibilant) are high pitched with a shrill quality. **Rhonchi** are low pitched with a snoring quality.

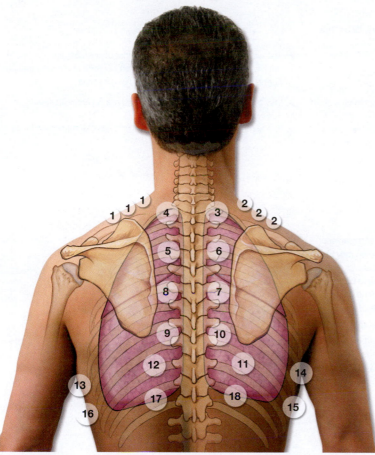

Figure 16.17 Pattern for auscultation: Posterior thorax.

Table 16.3 Adventitious Breath Sounds

SOUND	OCCURRENCE	QUALITY	CAUSES
Rales/Crackles			
Fine	End inspiration, do not clear with cough	High pitched, short, crackling	Collapsed or fluid-filled alveoli open
Coarse	End inspiration, do not clear with cough	Loud, moist, low pitched, bubbling	Collapsed or fluid-filled alveoli open
Rhonchi			
Wheezes (sibilant)	Expiration/inspiration when severe	High pitched, continuous	Blocked airflow as in asthma, infection, foreign body obstruction
Rhonchi (sonorous)	Expiration/inspiration Change/disappear with cough	Low pitched, continuous, snoring, rattling	Fluid-blocked airways
Stridor	Inspiration	Loud, high-pitched crowing heard without stethoscope	Obstructed upper airway
Friction rub	Inhalation/exhalation	Low-pitched grating, rubbing	Pleural inflammation

Techniques and Normal Findings	Abnormal Findings and Special Considerations

Assessment of Voice Sounds

The spoken voice can be heard over the chest wall. The sound is produced by vibrations as the patient speaks.

1. **Instruct the patient.**
   - The patient will remain in the same position as for auscultation. Explain that you will be listening to the chest while the patient says certain words, letters, or numbers.

2. **Auscultation of voice sounds.**
   - Use the same pattern for evaluating voice sounds as for auscultation of the lungs. This sequence will be followed for three different findings.
   - **Bronchophony.** Ask the patient to say "ninety-nine" each time you place the stethoscope on the chest. In normal lung tissue the sound will be muffled.

   - **Egophony.** Ask the patient to say "E" each time you place the stethoscope on the chest. In normal lung tissue you should hear "eeeeee" through the stethoscope.
   - **Whispered pectoriloquy.** Ask the patient to whisper "one, two, three" each time you place the stethoscope on the chest. In normal lung tissue the sound will be faint, almost indistinguishable.
   - Voice sounds are heard as muffled sounds in the normal lung.

▶ The words sound loud and more distinct over areas of lung consolidation. Lung consolidation occurs when portions of the lung that are normally filled with air instead contain fluid or tissue.

▶ The "E" sounds like "aaaaay" over areas of lung consolidation.

▶ The numbers sound loud and clear over areas of lung consolidation.

Palpation of the Anterior and Lateral Thorax

1. **Position the patient.**
   - The patient is usually in a supine position for palpation and auscultation of the anterior thorax. If the patient is experiencing discomfort or dyspnea, a sitting position may be used, or the patient may be in a Fowler position. The breasts of female patients normally flatten when in a supine position. Large and pendulous breasts may have to be moved to perform a complete assessment. Explain this to the patient and inform her that she may move and lift her own breasts if that will make her more comfortable.

2. **Instruct the patient.**
   - Explain to the patient that you will be performing several assessments and that you will continue to provide explanations as you move from one assessment to the next. Tell the patient to breathe normally throughout this initial examination and to tell you if pain or discomfort is felt at any area.

3. **Palpate the sternum, ribs, and intercostal spaces.**
   - Locate the suprasternal notch; palpate downward to the sternal angle (angle of Louis) where the manubrium meets the body of the sternum. Palpate laterally to the left and right to locate the second rib and second intercostal space. Continue palpating the sternum to the xiphoid process and to the left and right of the sternum to count the ribs.
   - The sternum should feel flat except for the ridge of the sternal angle and should taper to the xiphoid. The ribs should feel smooth and the spacing of ribs and intercostal spaces should be symmetric.

4. **Lightly palpate the anterior and lateral thorax.**
   - Use the finger pads to lightly palpate symmetric areas of the anterior thorax. Include the entire thorax by starting at the areas above each clavicle and move from side to side to below the costal angle and laterally to the midaxillary line (see Figure 16.18 ■).

▶ The obese patient may be unable to lie flat during assessment of the anterior thorax.

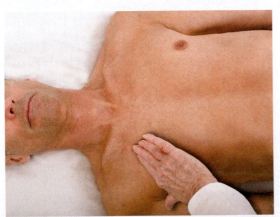

Figure 16.18 Palpation of the anterior thorax.

Techniques and Normal Findings	Abnormal Findings and Special Considerations

- Assess muscle mass.
- Assess for growths, nodules, and masses.
- Assess for tenderness.
- Muscle mass should be firm and the underlying tissue should be smooth. The thorax should be free of lesions or masses. The area should be nontender to palpation.

5. Palpate for respiratory expansion.
- Explain that you will be assessing movement of the chest during breathing by placing your hands on the lower chest and asking the patient to take a breath.
- Place the palmar surface of your hands along each costal margin with thumbs close to the midsternal line. Pinch up some skin between your thumbs. Ask the patient to take a deep breath (see Figure 16.19 ■).

▶ Pain may occur with inflammation of fibrous tissue or underlying structures. Crepitus may be felt if there is air in the subcutaneous tissue.

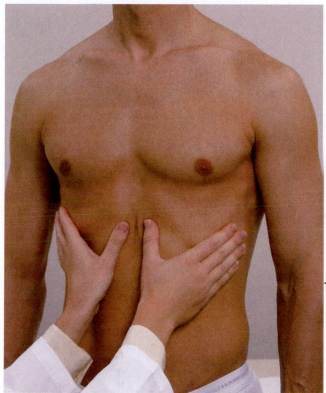

Figure 16.19 Palpation for respiratory expansion: Anterior view.

- The movement of the chest beneath your hands should feel smooth and even. Your thumbs should move apart and the skin move smoothly as the chest expands with inspiration.

6. Palpate for tactile fremitus.
- Explain that you will be feeling for vibrations on the chest wall while the patient speaks. Explain that you will be placing your hands on various areas of the chest while the patient repeats "ninety-nine" or "one, two, three" in a clear, loud voice.
- Use the ulnar surface of the hand or the palmar surface of the hand at the base of the metacarpophalangeal joints when palpating for fremitus. Palpate and compare symmetric areas of the lungs by moving from side to side from apices to bases (see Figure 16.20 ■). Displace female breasts as required.

▶ Unilateral decrease or delay in expansion may indicate fibrotic or obstructive lung disease or may result from splinting associated with pleural pain.

Techniques and Normal Findings	Abnormal Findings and Special Considerations

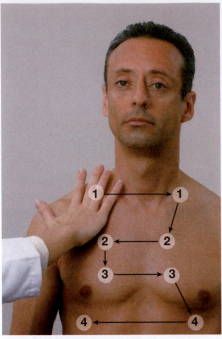

Figure 16.20 Palpation for tactile fremitus: Anterior thorax.

- Fremitus normally diminishes as you move from large to small airways and is decreased or absent over the precordium.

▶ Absent or decreased fremitus in other areas may result from underlying diseases, including emphysema, pleural effusion, or fibrosis.

Auscultation of the Anterior and Lateral Thorax

Auscultation is used to identify and discriminate between and among normal and adventitious breath sounds. Listen to the full respiratory cycle with each placement of the stethoscope (see Figure 16.21 ■).

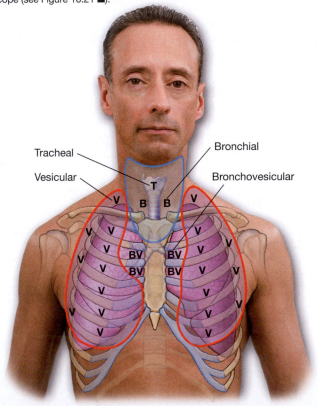

Figure 16.21 Auscultatory sounds: Anterior thorax.

Techniques and Normal Findings	Abnormal Findings and Special Considerations
1. Instruct the patient. • Explain that you will be listening to the patient's breathing with the stethoscope. Ask the patient to breathe deeply through the mouth each time the stethoscope is placed on the chest and to let you know if he or she is becoming short of breath or tired. **2. Auscultate the trachea.** • Place the stethoscope over the trachea above the suprasternal notch. You will hear tracheal breath sounds. Move the stethoscope to the left, then the right side of the trachea, just above each sternoclavicular joint. You will hear bronchial breath sounds. **3. Auscultate the apices.** • Place the stethoscope in the triangular areas just superior to each clavicle. You will hear bronchial sounds. **4. Auscultate the bronchi.** • The bronchi are auscultated at the first intercostal space at the manubrium and left and right sternal borders. You will hear bronchial sounds. Auscultation of the major bronchi in the second and third intercostal spaces and the interscapular area will result in you hearing bronchovesicular sounds. **5. Auscultate the anterior and lateral lungs.** • Visualize the landmarks. • Observe the anterior thorax and visualize the horizontal and vertical lines, the level of the diaphragm, and the fissures of the lungs. • Auscultate the lungs by beginning at the apices of the lungs (see Figure 16.21). Move the stethoscope from side to side as you compare sounds. Move down to the sixth intercostal space and laterally to the midaxillary line. You will hear vesicular sounds. When auscultating the lateral lungs, ask the patient to sit up straight with the patient's arms raised over his or her head. **6. Interpret the findings.** • Refer to the descriptions and interpretations of normal and adventitious breath sounds described in auscultation of the posterior thorax. Also, see Box 16.3.	▶ Lateral auscultation of the fourth to sixth intercostal spaces is required to hear breath sounds from the right middle lobe, which is a frequent site of aspiration pneumonia. ▶ Because of the small size of the chest, breath sounds may be difficult to distinguish in newborns, especially preterm infants, as sounds may transmit to distant parts of the chest. ▶ Breath sounds may be diminished in the obese patient because of poor inspiratory effort resulting from the weight of the chest and fatty deposits in the respiratory musculature.

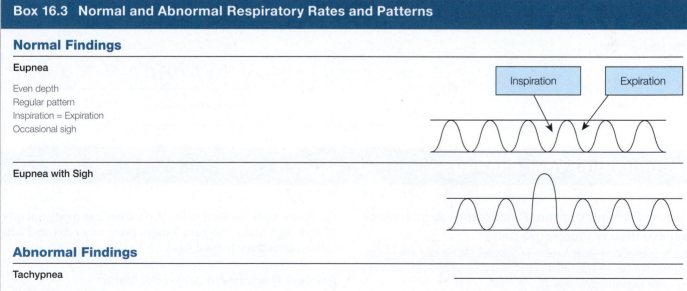

Box 16.3 Normal and Abnormal Respiratory Rates and Patterns

Normal Findings

Eupnea

Even depth
Regular pattern
Inspiration = Expiration
Occasional sigh

Inspiration   Expiration

Eupnea with Sigh

Abnormal Findings

Tachypnea

Rapid, shallow respirations
Rate > 24
Precipitating factors: fever, fear, exercise, respiratory insufficiency, pleuritic pain, alkalosis, pneumonia

Box 16.3   Normal and Abnormal Respiratory Rates and Patterns (continued)

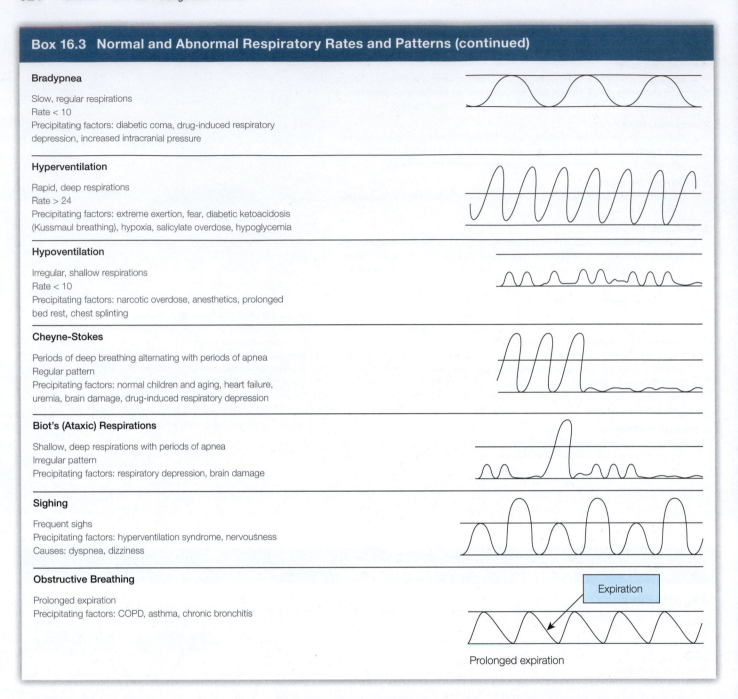

Bradypnea

Slow, regular respirations
Rate < 10
Precipitating factors: diabetic coma, drug-induced respiratory
depression, increased intracranial pressure

Hyperventilation

Rapid, deep respirations
Rate > 24
Precipitating factors: extreme exertion, fear, diabetic ketoacidosis
(Kussmaul breathing), hypoxia, salicylate overdose, hypoglycemia

Hypoventilation

Irregular, shallow respirations
Rate < 10
Precipitating factors: narcotic overdose, anesthetics, prolonged
bed rest, chest splinting

Cheyne-Stokes

Periods of deep breathing alternating with periods of apnea
Regular pattern
Precipitating factors: normal children and aging, heart failure,
uremia, brain damage, drug-induced respiratory depression

Biot's (Ataxic) Respirations

Shallow, deep respirations with periods of apnea
Irregular pattern
Precipitating factors: respiratory depression, brain damage

Sighing

Frequent sighs
Precipitating factors: hyperventilation syndrome, nervousness
Causes: dyspnea, dizziness

Obstructive Breathing

Prolonged expiration
Precipitating factors: COPD, asthma, chronic bronchitis

Expiration

Prolonged expiration

Documenting Your Findings

Sample Documentation: Respiratory Assessment
Focused History (Subjective Data)

*This is information from Review of Systems (ROS) and other perti-
nent history information that is or could be related to the patient's
lungs and respiratory system.*

Denies cough or sputum, shortness of breath, dyspnea, and
chest pain with breathing. Denies history of respiratory infections other than occasional colds. Reports environmental
allergy to ragweed, which causes nasal congestion. Denies
other environmental exposures to toxins. Denies history of TB
or asthma. TB test done 2 years ago was negative. Immunizations are up to date. Denies having the pneumococcal vaccine.

Pt. reports smoking for 5 years, ½ pack per day (ppd), but quit
15 years ago. States she runs 3 miles every other day and lifts
light weights three times a week.

Physical Assessment (Objective Data)

Skin and nails free of cyanosis. No respiratory distress or use
of accessory muscles noted. Respiratory rate 16 breaths per
minute and regular. Trachea midline. AP: Transverse diameter
1:2. Ribs and thorax free of pain or lumps or lesions. Thoracic
expansion equal bilaterally. Tactile fremitus symmetrical.
Lungs sounds clear in all lung fields. Voice sounds muffled
throughout.

Abnormal Findings

Respiratory Disorders

ASTHMA

A chronic hyperreactive condition resulting in bronchospasm, mucosal edema, and increased mucus secretion. This condition usually occurs in response to inhaled irritants or allergens (see Figure 16.22 ■).

Subjective findings:
- Dyspnea (shortness of breath)
- Anxiety
- Chest pain

Objective findings:
- Wheezing
- Diminished breath sounds
- Absent breath sounds (with severe asthma)
- Increased respiratory rate
- Increased use of accessory muscles
- Decreased oxygen saturation

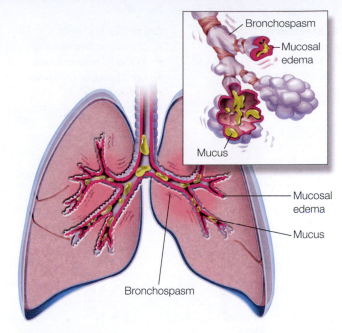

Figure 16.22 Asthma.

ATELECTASIS

A collapse or impaired inflation of one or more areas of the lung (NHLBI, 2013). During **atelectasis**, the alveoli or an entire lung may collapse from airway obstruction, such as a mucous plug, lack of surfactant, or a compressed chest wall (see Figure 16.23 ■).

Subjective findings:
- Absence of symptoms, if only a small portion of the lung is affected
- Dyspnea, if significant portions of the lung are affected

Objective findings:
- Decreased or absent breath sounds over the affected area
- Increased respiratory rate
- Decreased oxygen saturation
- Cyanosis (if severe)

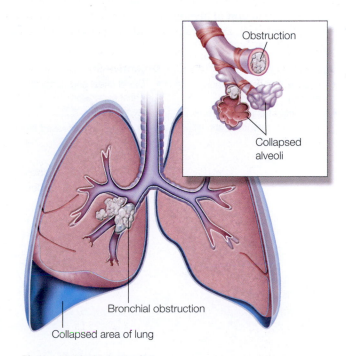

Figure 16.23 Atelectasis.

CHRONIC BRONCHITIS

Chronic inflammation of the tracheobronchial tree leads to increased mucus production and blocked airways. A productive cough is present (see Figure 16.24 ■).

Subjective findings:

* Dyspnea
* Fatigue (related to increased work of breathing)

Objective findings:

* Chronic productive cough
* Increased respiratory rate
* Use of accessory muscles
* Wheezes
* Rhonchi

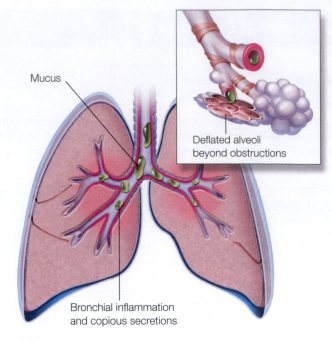

Mucus

Deflated alveoli beyond obstructions

Bronchial inflammation and copious secretions

Figure 16.24 Chronic bronchitis.

EMPHYSEMA

A condition in which chronic inflammation of the lungs leads to destruction of alveoli and decreased elasticity of the lungs. As a result, air is trapped and lungs hyperinflate (see Figure 16.25 ■).

Subjective findings:

* Dypsnea, especially upon exertion
* Air hunger (related to hypoxemia, CO_2 retention, and air trapping)

Objective findings:

* Barrel chest and decreased chest expansion
* Cyanosis
* Hypercarbia (increased blood concentration of CO_2)
* Clubbing of fingers
* Use of accessory muscles
* Diminished breath sounds

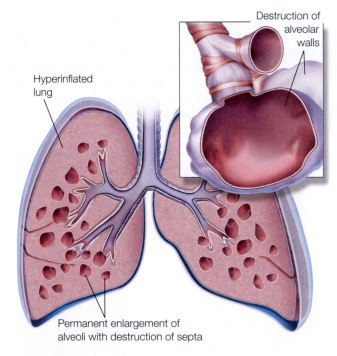

Destruction of alveolar walls

Hyperinflated lung

Permanent enlargement of alveoli with destruction of septa

Figure 16.25 Emphysema.

LOBAR PNEUMONIA

An infection that causes fluid, bacteria, and cellular debris to fill the alveoli (see Figure 16.26 ■).

Subjective findings:
- Dyspnea
- Fatigue
- Chills

Objective findings:
- Increased respiratory rate
- Fever
- Productive cough
- Decreased oxygen saturation
- Bronchial breath sounds and crackles

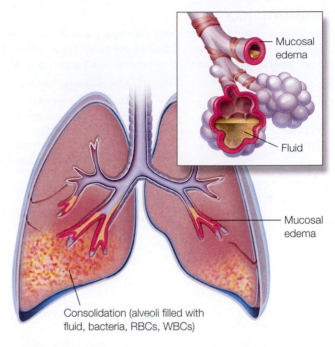

Mucosal edema

Fluid

Mucosal edema

Consolidation (alveoli filled with fluid, bacteria, RBCs, WBCs)

Figure 16.26 Lobar pneumonia.

PLEURAL EFFUSION

A fluid accumulation in the pleural space (see Figure 16.27 ■). Pleural effusion may be asymptomatic, or it could present with common signs and symptoms (Saguil, Wyrick, & Hallgren, 2014).

Subjective findings:
- Dyspnea
- Occasional sharp, nonradiating chest pain

Objective findings:
- Cough
- Diminished or absent breath sounds
- Decreased or absent tactile fremitus
- No voice transmission

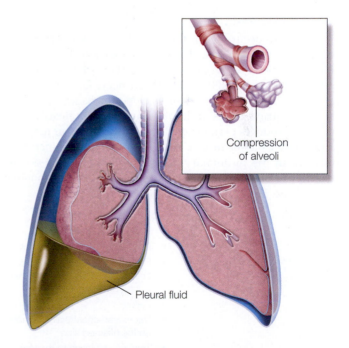

Compression of alveoli

Pleural fluid

Figure 16.27 Pleural effusion.

PNEUMOTHORAX

A condition in which air moves into the pleural space and causes partial or complete collapse of the lung. Pneumothorax can be spontaneous, traumatic, or tension (see Figure 16.28 ■).

Subjective findings:

- Dyspnea
- Sharp chest pain with inspiration
- Anxiety

Objective findings:

- Increased respiratory rate
- Decreased oxygen saturation
- Diminished or absent breath sounds over the affected area
- Decreased chest wall expansion on the affected side
- Tracheal deviation to the unaffected side

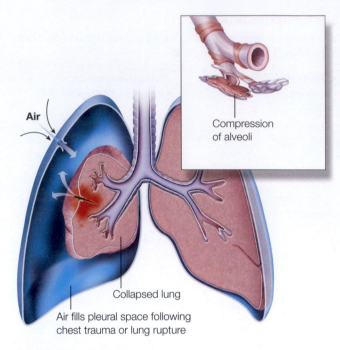

Air

Compression of alveoli

Collapsed lung

Air fills pleural space following chest trauma or lung rupture

Figure 16.28 Pneumothorax.

LEFT HEART FAILURE

Heart failure occurs when the heart is unable to effectively pump oxygen-rich blood. Heart failure may affect one or both sides of the heart. Most often, both the left and right sides of the heart are affected (NHLBI, 2014). Left heart failure typically produces respiratory symptoms as blood that is not ejected by the left ventricle backs up into the lungs. Right heart failure typically produces peripheral edema, as well as other manifestations (see Chapter 18 ∞). With left heart failure, increased pressure in the pulmonary veins causes interstitial edema around the alveoli and may cause edema of the bronchial mucosa (see- Figure 16.29 ■).

Subjective findings:

- Dyspnea, especially upon exertion
- Orthopnea
- Anxiety

Objective findings:

- Increased respiratory rate
- Decreased oxygen saturation
- Pulmonary congestion with auscultation of wheezes or crackles in lung bases
- Pallor
- Decreased chest wall expansion on the affected side
- Tracheal deviation to the unaffected side

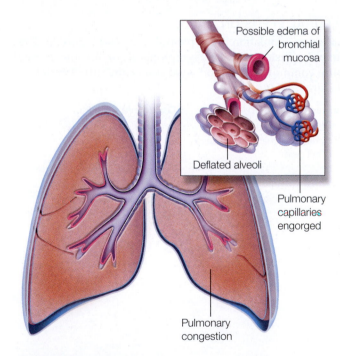

Possible edema of bronchial mucosa

Deflated alveoli

Pulmonary capillaries engorged

Pulmonary congestion

Figure 16.29 Left heart failure.

Application Through Critical Thinking

CASE STUDY

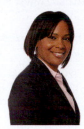

Source: Carlos E. Santa Maria/ Shutterstock.

Tamara Robinson, a 44-year-old female, has been seen regularly in the clinic for chronic asthma. Mrs. Robinson has required two visits to the emergency department (ED) for severe wheezing in the month since her last clinic visit.

The physical assessment reveals that the patient is in mild distress with soft expiratory wheezes on the right. Her vital signs are BP 126/82—P 84—RR 20. Her skin is warm, dry, and pink in color. Mrs. Robinson can speak clearly but appears to have slight dyspnea.

While completing the health history, the nurse learns that the patient has been following her prescribed treatments but has not been able to be completely symptom free for the last month and has had some mild shortness of breath and wheezing. The symptoms worsened, requiring the two ED visits.

The nurse learns that each ED visit occurred in the early evening. The patient experienced severe shortness of breath and wheezing that was unrelieved by rest or use of her inhalers. ED treatment consisted of injection of epinephrine, administration of oxygen, intravenous (IV) fluids, Benadryl, and steroids. Each ED visit lasted approximately 6 hours. The patient's breathing was restored to near normal at discharge, and she was given a prescription for a course of prednisone.

When asked if she could identify any precipitating factors, Mrs. Robinson replies, "I know they happened on days that I cleaned the basement." The nurse asks if she had any changes in her routines, activities, or environments. She says, "No, not that I can think of." The patient then adds, "I need to get this under control. I can't afford to miss any more work."

The nurse asks more details about the condition of the basement and the timing of her symptoms after she cleaned and the patient says, "The basement flooded from a burst water pipe a month or so ago. This caused the carpet to be completely saturated. My husband removed as much water as he could and then put fans all over the basement, hoping we could get the carpet to dry. Things looked dry after a few days, but about a week later we noticed a moldy smell. I can see mold on some of the walls too." The nurse asks if the work in the basement coincided with her recent attacks. The patient says, "Gee, I don't know, I never thought about it."

SAMPLE DOCUMENTATION

The following is a sample documentation from the assessment of Tamara Robinson.

SUBJECTIVE DATA Visit to clinic for a checkup, 44-year-old female asthmatic. Required two ED visits for severe wheezing in month since last clinic visit. Following prescribed treatments but continuing to have shortness of breath and wheezing. ED visits occurred on days when patient had been cleaning in her basement where a flood from a burst pipe caused the carpets to be saturated. Mold was said to be seen and smelled. Severe wheezing started approximately an hour after cleaning the basement and increased in severity requiring epinephrine, IV, Benadryl, and steroids. Patient discharged with course of oral steroids after each visit. Resumed normal treatment and activity after episodes.

OBJECTIVE DATA Breathing pattern regular with slight dyspnea. No audible wheezing noted on inspection. Thorax AP 1:2. Trachea midline. Expansion equal bilaterally. Tactile fremitus symmetrical. Breath sounds with expiratory wheezes in the upper lobes bilaterally, anteriorly and posteriorly. VS: BP 126/82—P 84—RR 20.

CRITICAL THINKING QUESTIONS

1. Describe the nurse's thoughts and actions as the nurse applies the steps of the critical thinking process in this situation.

2. In interpreting the data, how would they be clustered?

3. What are the options that could be developed for this patient?

4. What special considerations should the nurse pay attention to in this situation?

REFERENCES

Berman, A., & Snyder, S. J. (2015). *Kozier and Erb's fundamentals of nursing: Concepts, process and practice* (10th ed.). Upper Saddle River, NJ: Prentice Hall.

Berry, M. P., Marti, J-D., & Ntoumenopoulos, G. (2016). Inter-rater agreement of auscultation, palpable fremitus, and ventilator waveform sawtooth patterns between clinicians. *Respiratory Care, 61*(10), 1374–1383. doi:10.4187/respcare.04214

Centers for Disease Control and Prevention (CDC). (2013). *Smoking & tobacco use: Hookahs.* Retrieved from http://www.cdc.gov/tobacco/data_statistics/fact_sheets/tobacco_industry/hookahs

Diaz, A. A., Come, C. E., Mannino, D. M., Pinto-Plata, V., Divo, M. J., Bigelow, C., . . . Washko, G. R. (2014). Obstructive lung disease in Mexican Americans and Non-Hispanic Whites: An analysis of diagnosis and survival in the National Health and Nutritional Examination survey follow-up study. *Chest, 145*(2), 282–289.

Dumitru, I., & Baker, M. M. (2014). *Heart failure: Clinical presentation*. Retrieved from http://emedicine.medscape.com/article/163062-clinical

Eseonu-Ewoh, N., & Sterling, K. (2016). Can clinicians reliably auscultate crackles on lung exam and differentiate between fine and course crackles? *Evidence-Based Practice, 19*(6), E2–E3.

Fiz, J. A., Gnitecki, J., Kraman, S. S., Wodicka, G. R., & Pasterkamp, H. (2008). Effect of body position on lung sounds in healthy young men. *Chest, 133*(3), 729–736.

Foltz-Gray, D. (2017). Types of coughs and what they mean. How to decode 10 types of coughs. Retrieved from http://www.lifescript.com/health/centers/allergies/articles/decoding_your_cough.aspx

Goodman, D. M., Lynm, C., & Livingston, E. L. (2013). Adult sinusitis. *Journal of the American Medical Association, 309*(8), 837–837.

Hagstad, S., Bjerg, A., Ekerlijung, L., Backman, H., Lindberg, A., Ronmark, E., & Lundback, B. (2014). Passive smoking exposure is associated with increased risk of COPD in never smokers. *Chest, 145*(6), 1298–1304. doi:10.1378/chest.13-1349

Hahn, E. J., Rayens, M. K., Adkins, S., Simpson, N., Frazier, S., & Mannino, D. M. (2014). Fewer hospitalizations for chronic obstructive pulmonary disease in communities with smoke-free public policies. *American Journal of Public Health, 104*(6), 1059–1065.

Kraman, S. S. (2008). Transmission of lung sounds over light clothing. *Respiration, 75*, 85–88. doi:10.1159/000098404

Leuppi, J. D., Dieterle, T., Koch, G., Martina, B., Tamm, M., Perruchoud, A. P., . . . Leimenstoll, B. M. (2005). Diagnostic value of lung auscultation in an emergency room setting. *Swiss Medicine Weekly, 135*, 520–524.

Manning, M., Wojda, M., Hamel, L., Salkowski, A., Schwartz, A. G., & Harper, F. W. K. (2017). Understanding the role of family dynamics, perceived norms, and lung cancer worry in predicting second-hand smoke avoidance among high-risk lung cancer families. *Journal of Health Psychology, 22*(12), 1493–1509. doi:10.1177/1359105316630132

Marcin, A. (2017). *Yellow, brown, green, and more: What does the color of my phlegm mean?* Retrieved from https://www.healthline.com/health/green-phlegm#modal-close

MedlinePlus. *Blood differential.* (2017). Retrieved from http://www.nlm.nih.gov/medlineplus/ency/article/003657.htm

National Heart, Lung, & Blood Institute (NHLBI). (2013). *What is atelectasis?* Retrieved from http://www.nhlbi.nih.gov/health/health-topics/topics/atl

National Heart, Lung, and Blood Institute (NHLBI). (2014). *What is heart failure?* Retrieved from http://www.nhlbi.nih.gov/health/health-topics/topics/hf

Pagana, K. D., & Pagana, T. J. (2017). *Mosby's manual of diagnostic and laboratory tests* (6th ed.). St. Louis, MO: Elsevier.

Saguil, A., Wyrick, K., & Hallgren, J. (2014). Diagnostic approach to pleural effusion. *American Family Physician, 90*(2), 99–104.

Sherman, F. T. (2009). Auscultation with fabric upon lungs (AWFUL) Editorial. *Geriatrics, 64*(6) 7–8.

Shields, K. M., Fox, K. L., & Liebrecht, C. (2018). *Pearson nurse's drug guide.* Hoboken, NJ: Pearson.

Tran, H. N., Siu, S., Iribarren, C., Udaltsova, N., & Klatsky, A. (2011). Ethnicity and risk of hospitalization for asthma and chronic obstructive pulmonary disease. *Annals of Epidemiology, 21*(8), 615–622. doi:10.1016/j.annepidem.2010.10.015

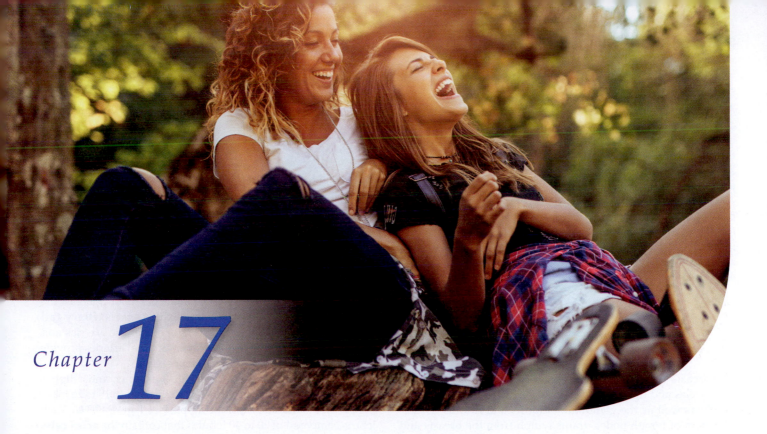

Chapter 17

Breasts and Axillae

LEARNING OUTCOMES

Upon completion of this chapter, you will be able to:

1. Describe the anatomy and physiology of the breasts and axillae.

2. Identify the anatomic, physiologic, developmental, psychosocial, and cultural variations that guide assessment of the breast and axillae.

3. Determine which questions about the breasts and axillae to use for the focused interview.

4. Outline the techniques for assessment of the breasts and axillae.

5. Generate the appropriate documentation to describe the assessment of the breasts and axillae.

6. Identify abnormal findings in the physical assessment of the breasts and axillae.

KEY TERMS

acini cells, 332	breast self-awareness, 335	mammary ridge, 333	peau d'orange, 342
areola, 332	galactorrhea, 347	mastalgia, 337	suspensory ligaments, 333
axillary tail, 332	gynecomastia, 348	Montgomery's glands, 332	

MEDICAL LANGUAGE

-algia	Suffix meaning "pain"
-ectomy	Suffix meaning "removal," "excision," "resection"
mamm-	Prefix meaning "breast"

mast-	Prefix meaning "breast"
-oma	Suffix meaning "tumor," "mass," "fluid collection"
-rrhea	Suffix meaning "flow," "discharge"

Introduction

Assessment of the breasts, axillae, and relevant lymph node chains is essential to assisting the nurse in determining breast health. Throughout the lifespan, many changes occur within the breasts of the female patient. The nurse must have thorough knowledge of the anatomy, physiology, and health history and physical assessment techniques for the breasts and axillae. Although focus on breasts and axillae typically is on the female patient, nurses also should be aware of the need for asking questions and examination related to male breasts. Understanding and acceptance of different individuals' feelings, beliefs, and practices regarding the breasts and breast care are also essential.

Anatomy and Physiology Review

The breasts are located on the anterior chest and supported by muscles and ligaments. The breast includes the areola and nipple as well as the glandular, adipose, and fibrous tissues. A system of lymph nodes drains lymph from the breasts and axillae. These tissues and structures are described in the following sections.

Breasts

The breasts are paired mammary glands located on the anterior chest wall (Marieb & Keller, 2018). Breast tissue extends from the second or third rib to the sixth or seventh rib and from the sternal margin to the midaxillary line, depending on body shape and size (see Figure 17.1 ■). The breasts lie anterior to the pectoralis major and serratus anterior muscles. The nipple is centrally located within a circular pigmented field of wrinkled skin called the **areola**. The surface of the areola is speckled with tiny sebaceous glands known as **Montgomery's glands** or Montgomery's tubercles (see Figure 17.2 ■). Hair follicles are normally seen around the periphery of the areola. Commonly, breast tissue extends superolaterally into the axilla as the **axillary tail** (tail of Spence). The internal and lateral thoracic arteries and cutaneous branches of the posterior intercostal arteries provide an abundant supply of blood to the breasts.

Breasts are composed of glandular, fibrous, and adipose (fat) tissues. The glandular tissue is arranged into 15 to 20 lobes per breast that radiate from the nipple (see Figure 17.3 ■). Each lobe is composed of 20 to 40 lobules that contain the **acini cells**

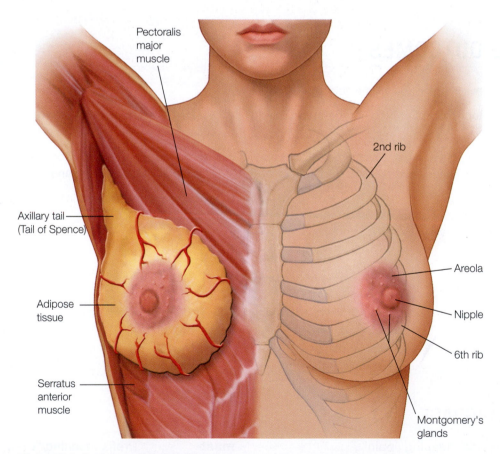

Figure 17.1 Anatomy of the breast.

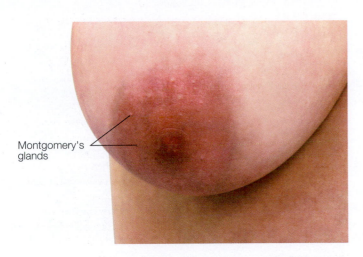

Montgomery's glands

Figure 17.2 Montgomery's glands.

(or alveoli) that produce milk. These cells empty into the lactiferous ducts, which carry milk from each lobe to the nipple. The fibrous tissue provides support for the glandular tissue. **Suspensory ligaments** (Cooper's ligaments) extend from the connective tissue layer, through the breast, and attach to the fascia underlying the breast. Subcutaneous and retromammary adipose tissue make up the remainder of the breast. The proportions of these three components vary with the patient's age, weight, genetics, general health, menstrual cycle, pregnancy, and lactation. Supernumerary nipples or breast tissue may be present along the **mammary ridge**, or "milk line," which extends from each axilla to the groin (see Figure 17.4 ■). Usually this tissue atrophies during fetal development, but occasionally a nipple persists and is visible. It needs to be differentiated from a mole (see Figure 17.5 ■). The major functions of the breasts include producing, storing, and supplying milk for the process of lactation. In the male, the breast is composed of a small nipple and flat areola superior to a thin disk of undeveloped breast

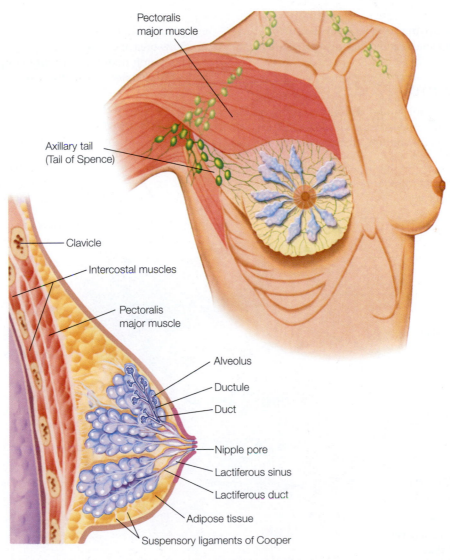

Pectoralis major muscle

Axillary tail (Tail of Spence)

Clavicle

Intercostal muscles

Pectoralis major muscle

Alveolus

Ductule

Duct

Nipple pore

Lactiferous sinus

Lactiferous duct

Adipose tissue

Suspensory ligaments of Cooper

Figure 17.3 Anterior and lateral views of breast anatomy.

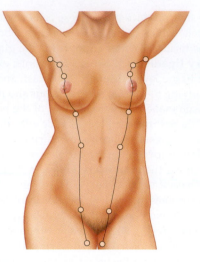

Figure 17.4 Mammary ridge.

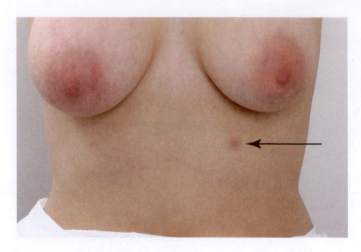

Figure 17.5 Supernumerary nipple.

tissue that may not be distinguishable from the surrounding tissues. Breasts, in both females and males, also provide a mechanism for sexual arousal.

Axillae and Lymph Nodes

A complex system of lymph nodes drains lymph from the breasts and axillae and returns it to the blood. Superficial lymph nodes drain the skin, and deep lymph nodes drain the

mammary lobules. Figure 17.6 ■ depicts the groups of nodes that drain the breasts and axillae.

The lymph nodes are usually nonpalpable. The following nodes are palpated during the assessment:

1. Internal mammary nodes
2. Supraclavicular nodes
3. Subclavicular (infraclavicular) nodes

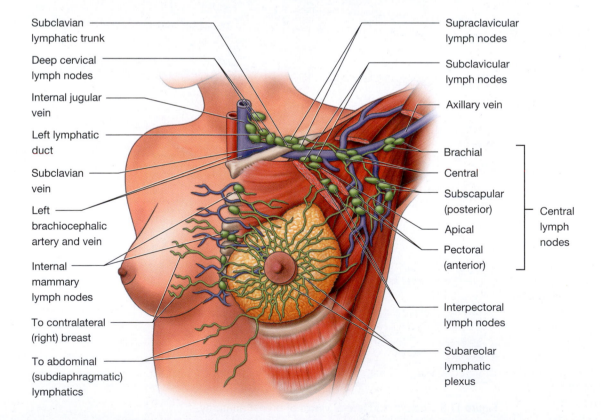

Subclavian lymphatic trunk
Deep cervical lymph nodes
Internal jugular vein
Left lymphatic duct
Subclavian vein
Left brachiocephalic artery and vein
Internal mammary lymph nodes
To contralateral (right) breast
To abdominal (subdiaphragmatic) lymphatics

Supraclavicular lymph nodes
Subclavicular lymph nodes
Axillary vein
Brachial
Central
Subscapular (posterior)
Apical
Pectoral (anterior)
Central lymph nodes
Interpectoral lymph nodes
Subareolar lymphatic plexus

Figure 17.6 Lymphatic drainage of the breast.

4. Interpectoral nodes
5. Central axillary nodes
6. Brachial (lateral axillary) nodes
7. Subscapular (posterior axillary) nodes
8. Pectoral (anterior axillary) nodes

The internal mammary nodes drain toward the abdomen and the opposite breast. Most of the lymph from the rest of the breast drains toward the axilla and subclavicular region. Thus, a cancerous lesion can spread via the lymphatic system to the subclavicular nodes, into deep channels within the chest or abdomen, and even to the opposite breast. The male breast has the same potential and needs to be examined as well. The major functions of the lymphatic system include returning water and proteins from the interstitial spaces to the blood, thus helping to maintain blood osmotic pressure and body fluid balance. It also helps filter out microorganisms and other body debris.

Muscles of the Chest Wall

The major muscles of the chest wall, which support the breast and contribute to its shape, are the pectoralis major and serratus anterior muscles (see Figure 17.1). The overall contour of the breasts is determined by the suspensory ligaments, which provide support. The major function of the muscles of the chest wall is to support breast and lymphatic tissue.

Special Considerations

Age, developmental level, race, ethnicity, work history, living conditions, socioeconomic status, and emotional well-being are among the factors that influence breast health. These factors must be considered when collecting subjective and objective data during the comprehensive health assessment. The nurse applies critical thinking to assess the patient's state of health and to identify the factors that may influence breast health.

Health Promotion Considerations

Health promotion in relation to breast health is commonly focused on screening and prevention of breast cancer. In the United States, breast cancer is the most common type of cancer in women and is second only to lung cancer as a cause of cancer deaths in women (Centers for Disease Control and Prevention [CDC], 2017b). Approximately 12%, or 1 in 8 women, will be diagnosed with breast cancer in their lifetimes. Rates of death from breast cancer are approximately 1 in 37 women (American Cancer Society [ACS], 2017b).

Recommendations for breast cancer screening have been updated in recent years, and to date there is no clear consensus among certain healthcare groups, such as the ACS, American College of Obstetricians and Gynecologists (ACOG, 2017a), American Academy of Family Physicians (AAFP, 2016), and U.S. Preventive Services Task Force (USPSTF, 2009, 2016) regarding breast cancer screening. However, all groups promote avoidance or elimination of modifiable breast cancer risk factors (e.g., diet, physical activity, alcohol intake, overweight, and obesity) and early detection through screening measures such as mammography. The ACS (2018) cites evidence-based changes to their breast cancer screening guidelines from a yearly mammogram starting at age 40 to yearly starting at age 45 for women at average risk for breast cancer. Other groups such as ACOG,

AAFP, and USPSTF recommend a patient-centered approach and shared decision making among care providers and their patients to determine the most appropriate time to begin screening based on an individual's history and risk factors (ACOG, 2017a; AAFP, 2016). The ACS (2018) does state that although the recommendation is to start screening with mammography at 45 years old, "women should have the choice to start screening with yearly mammograms as early as age 40 if they want to" (para. 2). For women ages 55 and over, ACS (2018) recommends mammography screening every 2 years but leaves the option up to the individual to continue yearly screening.

Breast examination, whether performed by a care provider (i.e., clinical breast exam [CBE]) or through breast self-examination (BSE), is another screening measure that has recently undergone changes to recommendations. The ACS (2017a) has removed this guideline from its breast cancer screening recommendations for average-risk asymptomatic women, citing that there is a lack of evidence in the research to show they provide clear benefit. The ACS does recommend that **breast self-awareness** (i.e., becoming familiar with the appearance and feel of one's own breasts) is important and that changes from an individual's norm should be reported promptly to a care provider. ACOG (2017a) recommends continuation of CBE, citing "different interpretation of data and the weight assigned to the harms versus the benefits" (para. 2). Their recommendation is CBE every 1 to 3 years for women ages 29 to 39 and yearly for women ages 40 and over (ACOG, 2017b). ACOG (2017a) agrees with the importance of breast self-awareness and no longer refers to BSE as a recommended practice.

Lifespan Considerations

A patient's age and developmental stage have tremendous influence on the appearance and functioning of the breasts. Growth and development are dynamic processes that cause changes over time. Data collection and interpretation of these findings in relation to expected values are important. Details about differences in the assessment of the breasts and axillae are located in Chapter 25, Chapter 26, and Chapter 27.

Psychosocial Considerations

A woman's overall sense of self-esteem may be reflected in the way she feels about her breasts. In fact, some women may view their breasts as a badge of femininity. Media portrayal of idealized images of "perfect" breasts, especially by advertisers, may increase this feeling. Thus, patients whose breasts are smaller or larger than average, patients with asymmetric breasts, and patients who have had a mastectomy or other breast surgery or trauma are at an increased risk for body image disturbance, self-esteem disturbance, and dysfunctional grieving.

Lack of access to care is a common reason among women who do not receive recommended breast cancer screening. Factors contributing to the lack of screening include no regular healthcare, no health insurance, lower socioeconomic status, and lack of education (CDC, 2017c). Other factors that may contribute to lack of screening may include anxiety and fear of cancer or surgery, a body image change, a change in significant relationships, denial, feelings of powerlessness, or a lack of knowledge about breast disorders. During the assessment of the breasts and axillae, the nurse needs to encourage the patient to share her fears and concerns.

Several of the risk factors for breast cancer related to personal lifestyle behaviors are modifiable. For example, a link between alcohol intake and breast cancer has been established (ACS, 2017d). The more drinks a woman has per day, the higher her risk of developing breast cancer. Therefore, the ACS recommends women limit alcohol intake to no more than one drink per day. Research also indicates that a high-fat diet and lack of physical activity may increase a woman's risk of developing breast cancer. Obesity has been linked with higher risks of breast cancer (ACS, 2017a). However, severely obese women are less likely to comply with recommendations about breast health screening than are nonobese women (Friedman, Hemler, Rossetti, Clemow, & Ferrante, 2012). It is suggested that embarrassment in the examination room, concern about negative reactions from healthcare providers, fear of being lectured about obesity, and the small size of examination gowns, tables, and equipment are among the reasons that prevent obese women from seeking breast screening.

Although breast cancer is normally seen as a woman's disease, men can also develop breast cancer. Men should be taught the importance of reporting lumps in their breasts and seeking follow-up and treatment as needed. Men may delay reporting lumps because of social stigmas or embarrassment. Therefore, the nurse needs to encourage male patients to report any abnormalities they discover and discuss fears or other emotions that accompany the possible diagnosis of breast cancer.

Race, Ethnicity, and Environmental Considerations

The nurse must be aware of variations in breast development related to race, ethnicity, and environment. For example, women of African ancestry may develop secondary sexual characteristics earlier than women of European ancestry (Susman et al., 2010). The time of appearance, texture, and distribution of axillary and pubic hair also vary according to race and ethnicity.

Diagnosis and mortality rates related to breast cancer vary across different groups. In the United States, breast cancer is more often diagnosed in White women, followed by women of Black, Hispanic, Asian/Pacific Islander, and American Indian/Alaska Native heritage (CDC, 2016). However, in women younger than age 45, breast cancer is more common among African Americans (CDC, 2017a). Likewise, African American women are more likely to die of breast cancer (ACS, 2017e).

Geographic disparities in breast health, particularly related to breast cancer, are another issue of concern about which nurses should be aware (ACS, 2017a). In north-central and western parts of the United States and some Mid-Atlantic states, breast cancer deaths are more prevalent in White women. Death rates for Black women are highest in some parts of the south-central United States, some Mid-Atlantic states, and California. Lack of access to screening and treatment are common reasons for disparities in these areas. Access issues are frequently affected by socioeconomic factors, legislative policies, and the need to travel far distances to obtain medical services. Other environmental factors commonly known to increase breast cancer risk include exposure to radiation, diethylstilbestrol (DES; a drug thought to reduce miscarriages that was commonly given to pregnant women from the 1940s into the 1960s), and other environmental pollutants (e.g., in utero exposure to dichlorodiphenyltrichloroethane [DDT] linked to breast cancer later in life) (ACS, 2017a).

Subjective Data—Health History

Breast health assessment includes the gathering of subjective and objective data. Subjective data collection occurs during the patient health history interview, before the actual physical assessment. During the interview the nurse uses a variety of communication techniques to elicit general and specific information about the patient's state of breast health or illness. Before proceeding, it may be helpful to review the information about each of the data-gathering processes of taking a health history for breasts and axillae.

Focused Interview

The focused interview for the breasts and axillae concerns data related to the structures and functions of the breasts and lymphatic system. Subjective data related to breast health are gathered during the focused interview. The nurse must be prepared to observe the patient and listen for cues related to the breasts and axillae. The nurse may use open- and closed-ended questions to obtain information. Often a number of follow-up questions or requests for descriptions are required to clarify data or gather missing information. Follow-up questions are aimed at identifying the source of problems, duration of difficulties, measures to alleviate problems, and clues about the patient's knowledge of his or her own health. The subjective data collected and the questions asked during the health history and focused interview provide information to help meet the goals of improving breast health and preventing and controlling breast disease.

The focused interview guides physical assessment of the breasts and axillae. The information is always considered in relation to norms and expectations about breast and lymphatic function. Therefore, the nurse must consider age, gender, race, culture, environment, health practices, and past and concurrent problems and therapies when framing questions and using techniques to elicit information. In order to address all the factors involved when conducting a focused interview, categories of questions related to the breasts and axillae have been developed. These categories include general questions that are asked of all patients, those addressing illness and infection, questions related to symptoms and behaviors, those related to habits or practices, questions that are specific to patients according to age, those for the pregnant woman, and questions that address environmental concerns. One approach to elicit information about symptoms is the OLDCART & ICE method, which is described in Chapter 5. See Figure 5.3. ∞

The nurse must consider the patient's ability to participate in the focused interview and physical assessment of the breasts and axillae. Patients who are experiencing breast discomfort or pain may require immediate assessment by the primary health-care provider. Breast pain, or **mastalgia**, is most often associated with the menstrual cycle (WebMD, 2018a). In some cases, however, referred pain from cardiac, pulmonary, and gastrointestinal causes must be ruled out. See Table 17.1 for an overview of the two primary categories of mastalgia.

Table 17.1 Overview of Mastalgia

TYPE OF MASTALGIA	DESCRIPTION
Cyclic	• Most common form of mastalgia • Typically associated with the menstrual cycle; onset of pain occurs in the days before menstruation and gradually increases, then subsides once menstruation begins • Most commonly affects younger women • Usually occurs in both breasts (bilateral) • Typically disappears after menopause
Noncyclic	• Not associated with the menstrual cycle • Has no apparent precipitating factor, although can be related to large breasts that are not supported sufficiently • Most commonly affects women ages 30 to 50 • Often occurs in one breast (unilateral) • Pain is often described as sharp or burning sensation that occurs in one region of the breast • Often results from changes to breast structure, including fibroadenoma, cysts, and trauma, or from pain in the chest cavity and neck that radiates to the breast • May require diagnostic studies, such as mammogram or biopsy

Sources: Adapted from Mayo Clinic (2017a); Salzman, Fleegle, & Tully (2012); WebMD (2018a); and Johns Hopkins Medicine (n.d.a).

Focused Interview Questions	Rationales and Evidence

The following section provides sample questions and bulleted follow-up questions in each of the categories previously mentioned. A rationale for each of the questions is provided. The list of questions is not all-inclusive but represents the types of questions required in a comprehensive focused interview related to the breasts and axillae.

General Questions

1. **Describe your breasts today. How do they differ, if at all, from 3 months ago? From 3 years ago?**

   ▶ This question gives the patient the opportunity to share her perception of her breasts and any changes she has experienced that may be related to breast health.

2. **Are you still menstruating?**
   • If so, have you noticed any changes in your breasts that seem to be related to your normal menstrual cycle, such as tenderness, swelling, pain, or enlarged nodes? If so, please describe.

   ▶ These changes may occur with changing hormone levels, or they may be related to the use of oral, transdermal, and injectable contraceptives (Johns Hopkins Medicine, n.d.b). "Lumpy breasts" occurring monthly before the onset of menses and resolving at the end of menstruation may be because of a benign condition called fibrocystic breasts (WebMD, 2018b).

3. **What was the date of your last menstrual period?**

   ▶ This information, if applicable, helps correlate the current status of the breasts to the cycle.

Questions Related to Illness or Infection

1. **Have you ever had any breast disease, such as cancer, fibrocystic breast disease, benign breast disease, or fibroadenoma?**

   ▶ A history of breast cancer poses the risk of a second primary breast cancer (Susan G. Koman Breast Cancer Foundation, 2018b). Both fibroadenoma and the general lumpiness of fibrocystic breast disease must be differentiated from cancer. Increased risk for breast cancer is associated with some benign breast lesions (Susan G. Koman Breast Cancer Foundation, 2018a).

2. **Have you ever had breast surgery?**
   • If so, what type and when?
   • How do you feel about it?
   • How has it affected you?
   • Has it affected your sex life? If so, how?

   ▶ Previous breast surgery has implications for physical and psychologic well-being. Breast surgery includes lumpectomy, mastectomy, breast reconstruction, breast reduction, and breast augmentation.

3. **Has your mother or sister had breast cancer?**

   ▶ Having a first-degree relative (mother, sister, or daughter) who has experienced breast cancer approximately doubles a woman's risk for developing the disorder (ACS, 2017b).

Focused Interview Questions	Rationales and Evidence
4. Has one of your grandmothers or an aunt had breast cancer?	▶ Although the risk is higher for women whose first-degree relative has experienced breast cancer, a history of this disorder in a second-degree relative (e.g., grandmother or aunt) also increases the risk (American Society of Clinical Oncology [ASCO], 2017).
5. Has anyone in your family been found to have a genetic mutation linked to breast cancer?	▶ BRCA1 and BRCA2, which are genetic proteins that help repair damaged DNA, are especially important in terms of cancer development. Approximately 72% of women who inherit BRCA1 mutations and 69% who inherit BRCA2 mutations will develop breast cancer by the age of 80 (National Cancer Institute [NCI], 2018). Further information about genetic mutation and heredity in breast cancer is available through the National Cancer Institute at www.cancer.gov/cancertopics/factsheet/risk/BRCA.
6. Have you had radiation therapy to the chest area for cancer other than breast cancer?	▶ Radiation to the chest increases the risk for breast cancer (ACS, 2017a).

Questions Related to Symptoms or Behaviors

When gathering information about symptoms, many questions are required to elicit details and descriptions that assist in analysis of the data. The questions are intended to determine the significance of a symptom in relation to specific diseases and problems and to identify the need for follow-up examination or referral.

The following questions refer to specific symptoms and behaviors associated with the breasts and axillae. For each symptom, questions and follow-up are required. The details to be elicited are the characteristics of the symptom; the onset, duration, and frequency of the symptom; the treatment or remedy for the symptom, including home remedies; the determination if a diagnosis has been sought; the effects of treatments; and family history associated with a symptom or illness.

Questions Related to Symptoms

1. **Have you noticed any changes in breast characteristics, such as size, symmetry, shape, thickening, lumps, swelling, temperature, color of skin or vessels, or sensations such as tingling or tenderness?**
   - If so, how long have you had them? Please describe them.

2. **Have you noticed any changes in nipple and areola characteristics, such as size, shape, open sores, lumps, pain, tenderness, discharge, skin changes, or retractions?**
   - If so, how long have you had them? Please describe them.

3. **Have you ever experienced any trauma or injury to your breasts?**
   - If so, please describe.

▶ Breast self-awareness (becoming familiar with the appearance and feel of one's own breasts) is important, and changes should be reported promptly to a care provider (ACS, 2017a; ACOG, 2017b).

▶ Pain and tenderness can be caused by fibrocystic breast changes, pregnancy, lactation, cancer, or other disorders. A lump may indicate a benign cyst, a fibroadenoma, fatty necrosis, or a malignant tumor (Mayo Clinic, 2018b). Skin irritation may occur because of pendulous breasts or friction from a bra. In older patients, decreased estrogen levels may cause the breasts to sag (MedlinePlus: National Library of Medicine, 2018a).

▶ Nipple discharge resulting from medication is usually clear. A bloody drainage is always a concern and must be further evaluated, especially in the presence of a lump (Mayo Clinic, 2018c). Eczematous changes of the skin of the nipples and areola may indicate Paget disease, a rare form of breast cancer (Mayo Clinic, 2017e). Dimpling of skin or retraction of the nipple also suggests cancer (MedlinePlus: National Library of Medicine, 2018b).

▶ Contact sports, automobile accidents, and physical abuse can cause bruising of the breast and tissue changes (Healthline, 2017).

Questions Related to Behaviors

1. **Do you exercise?**
   - If so, describe your routine.
   - What kind of bra do you wear when you exercise?

2. **Have you ever had a mammogram?**
   - If so, when was your most recent one?

3. **Do you see your healthcare provider regularly for a physical examination?**

▶ Physical activity, in the form of exercise, decreases the risk for breast cancer (ACS, 2017a). Firm support is recommended during exercise to prevent loss of tissue elasticity (Yu & Zhou, 2016).

▶ Mammography can detect a cancer before it is detectable by palpation. Screening guidelines are discussed earlier in this chapter under "Health Promotion Considerations."

▶ Patients from lower socioeconomic brackets may have reduced access to healthcare (ACS, 2017a).

▶ Patients who see their provider regularly may have better outcomes for many diseases because of early detection (ACS, 2017a).

Focused Interview Questions	Rationales and Evidence

Questions Related to Age and Pregnancy

The focused interview must reflect the anatomic and physiologic differences in the breasts and axillae that exist along the age span as well as during pregnancy. Specific questions related to breasts and axillae for each of these groups are located provided in Chapter 25, Chapter 26, and Chapter 27.

Questions Related to the Environment

Environment refers to both the internal and external environments. Questions regarding the internal environment include all of the previous questions and those associated with internal or physiologic responses. Questions regarding the external environment include those related to home, work, or social environments.

Internal Environment

1. What medications are you presently taking?

2. How do you feel about your breasts?

3. Do you have breast implants?

4. How old were you when you started to menstruate?

5. Do you have children?
   - How old were you when they were born?
6. Did you breastfeed your children? Are you currently breastfeeding?

7. Have you gone through menopause?
   - If so, at what age?
   - Did you experience any residual problems?

8. Have you been treated with hormone therapy during or since menopause?

9. Describe your weight from childhood up until now.
   - Describe your dietary intake.

- ► Hormone replacement therapy is associated with an increased risk of cancer. Women taking these drugs must be monitored very carefully (ACS, 2017a).
- ► Answers to this question may reveal a body image disturbance, self-esteem disturbance, dysfunctional grieving (in a woman who has had a mastectomy or lumpectomy), or ineffective breastfeeding (in a lactating woman).
- ► Breast implants do not increase the risk for breast cancer but may create difficulties in visualizing breast tissue on standard mammograms (ACS, 2017c).
- ► Patients with a history of menarche before age 12 are at greater risk for breast cancer (ASCO, 2017).
- ► Women who have never had children or who had their first child after age 30 are at greater risk for breast cancer (ACS, 2017a).
- ► Breastfeeding, especially for 1.5 to 2 years, decreases the risk for breast cancer (ACS, 2017a).
- ► Women who undergo menopause after age 55 are at greater risk for breast cancer. Postmenopausal weight gain may increase the risk of breast cancer (ACS, 2017a). After menopause, decreased estrogen levels may result in decreased firmness of breast tissue (MedlinePlus: National Library of Medicine, 2018a). The patient should be reassured that this is normal.
- ► Combined hormone replacement therapy places patients at increased risk for breast cancer. (ACS, 2017a)
- ► Obesity is considered a predisposing factor in breast cancer (ACS, 2017a).

External Environment

1. Have you been exposed to any environmental carcinogens, such as benzene or asbestos, or to excessive radiation, such as frequent, repeated x-rays?
2. Have you or your mother taken diethylstilbestrol (DES)?

3. Do you work at night?

- ► Such exposures may increase the risk of breast cancer (ACS, 2017a).
- ► A history of DES use is linked with increased risk for breast cancer (ACS, 2017a).
- ► An increased risk for breast cancer has been linked with night-shift work. This may be related to disruption in melatonin, a hormone affected by light (ACS, 2017a).

Patient-Centered Interaction

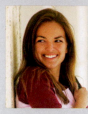

Miranda Cowan, a 22-year-old college student, makes an appointment with her gynecologist for a routine examination. Ms. Cowan indicates that she is concerned because breast cancer seems to run in her family. Following is part of the focused interview taken by the nurse working in the office.

Source: Stockbyte/ Getty Images.

Interview

Nurse: Hello, Ms. Cowan, I see you are here for your routine examination.

Ms. Cowan: Yes, that is correct.

Nurse: Before the physical examination, I need to get some information from you, and I will be asking you questions. You indicated a concern regarding breast cancer in your family. Would you like to begin with your concern?

Ms. Cowan: No. I just don't know where to begin. You ask your questions first. I'm sure we will talk about my concerns.

Nurse: How would you describe your breasts?

Ms. Cowan: They are small and firm. My left breast is a little bigger than my right breast.

Nurse: Have your breasts changed in the past several months?

Ms. Cowan: No, I think they are the same. Maybe a little fuller before my period, but that's it.

Nurse: Describe your nipples and the skin around them.

Ms. Cowan: They are small, equal in size, and stick out a little. The skin around my nipples is round and pink, almost the same color as my nipple.

Nurse: Have you noticed any changes to your breasts, nipples, or areolae, the skin around your nipples?

Ms. Cowan: No, no changes.

Nurse: Tell me about your family and breast cancer.

Ms. Cowan: My grandmother (maternal) and my aunt (paternal) both have been diagnosed, and that worries me.

Nurse: What about your mother, your older sister, and your maternal aunt?

Ms. Cowan: No, they're fine. No problems.

Nurse: Your grandmother— do you know how old she was when diagnosed?

Ms. Cowan: No, I don't. I guess she was in her late sixties. She was diagnosed three or four years ago, and now she's seventy-three years old. She had surgery and seems to be doing all right.

Analysis

The nurse sets the tone and sequence of events for Ms. Cowan's visit. Ms. Cowan declines the offer from the nurse to begin with her concerns of familial cancer. The nurse knows it will be beneficial to reduce any anxiety the patient may have regarding her concern. Taking the lead from Ms. Cowan, the nurse proceeds with the focused interview using open-ended statements and introduces the family questions later in the interview.

Objective Data—Physical Assessment

Assessment Techniques and Findings

Physical examination of the breasts and axillae requires the use of inspection and palpation. This portion of the exam may be incorporated into the total body assessment along with the heart and lung assessments when the patient is sitting and again when supine. Although the majority of the material in this chapter assumes that the patient is female, it is important to incorporate assessment of the male patient's breasts during the physical assessment, usually when assessing the thorax. During each of the procedures, the nurse is gathering data related to the breasts and axillae. Inspection includes looking at skin color, structures of the breast, and the appearance of the axillae. Knowledge of norms or expected findings is essential in determining the meaning of the data. Before proceeding, it may be helpful to practice the techniques of physical assessment of the breasts and axillae. In addition, health records, the results of

EQUIPMENT
- Examination gown and drape
- Clean nonsterile examination gloves
- Small pillow or rolled towel
- Metric ruler

laboratory tests, mammography, and magnetic resonance imaging (MRI) are important secondary sources of objective data to be reviewed and included in the data-gathering process. See Table 17.2 for information on potential secondary sources of patient data.

Adult breasts are generally symmetric, although one breast is typically slightly larger than the other. The areolae should be round or oval and nearly equal in size. The nipples are the

Table 17.2 Potential Secondary Sources for Patient Data Related to the Breast and Axillae

LABORATORY TESTS

Genetic Screen for BRCA1 and BRCA2

DIAGNOSTIC TESTS

Breast Ultrasound
Excisional Biopsy
Fine-Needle Aspiration Biopsy
Mammography
MRI
Stereotactic Biopsy

same color as the areolae. The nipples are in the center of the breast, point outward and upward, and are free of discharge, ulcerations, and crust. The breasts should move away from the chest wall with ease and symmetrically. The texture of the skin is smooth, and the breast tissue is slightly granular. The axillae are clean and hair is present or removed. The skin is moist. Lymph nodes are nonpalpable.

Physical assessment of the breasts and axillae follows an organized pattern. It begins with a patient survey followed by inspection of the breasts while the patient assumes a variety of positions. Palpation includes the entire surface of each breast, including the axillary tail, as well as the lymph nodes of the axillae.

HELPFUL HINTS

- To relieve patient anxiety, provide an environment that is warm, comfortable, and private.
- Ask the patient if she prefers a nurse who is the same gender; some cultures only allow female healthcare workers to assess females, and some women may be uncomfortable having a male complete a breast examination.
- Provide specific instructions to the patient; state whether the patient must sit, stand, or lie down during a procedure.
- Exposure of the breasts is uncomfortable for many women. Use draping techniques to maintain the patient's dignity.
- Explore cultural and language barriers at the onset of the interaction.
- Nonsterile examination gloves may be required to prevent infection when patients have lesions or drainage in and around the breasts.
- Use Standard Precautions.

Techniques and Normal Findings	Abnormal Findings and Special Considerations

Inspection of the Breast

1. **Instruct the patient.**
   - Explain to the patient that you will be assessing her breasts in a variety of ways. First, you will have the patient sit and then assume several positions that move the breasts away from the chest wall so that differences in size, shape, symmetry, contour, and color can be detected. Inform the patient that she will then lie down and you will assess each breast by palpating the breast tissue and nipple. Also be sure to assess her axillae. Explain the purpose of each assessment in terms the patient will understand. Tell the patient that none of the assessments should be painful; however, she must inform you of any tenderness or discomfort as the examination proceeds.

2. **Position the patient.**
   - The patient should sit comfortably and erect, with the gown at the waist so both breasts are exposed (see Figure 17.7 ■).

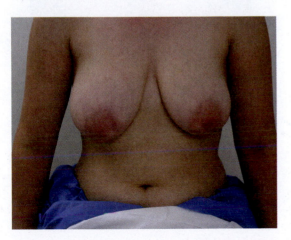

Figure 17.7 The patient is seated at the beginning of the breast examination.

3. **Inspect and compare size and symmetry of the breasts.**
   - One breast may normally be slightly larger than the other.

▶ Obvious masses, flattening of the breast in one area, dimpling, or a recent increase in the size of one breast may indicate abnormal growth or inflammation.

| Techniques and Normal Findings | Abnormal Findings and Special Considerations |

4. Inspect for skin color.
- Color should be consistent with the rest of the body. Observe for thickening, tautness, redness, rash, or ulceration.

▶ Inflamed skin is red and warm. Edema from blocked lymphatic drainage in advanced cancer causes an "orange peel" appearance called **peau d'orange** (see Figure 17.8 ■).

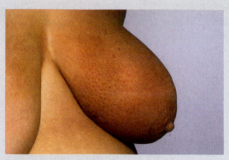

Figure 17.8 Peau d'orange sign.
Source: Mediscan/Alamy Stock Photo.

5. Inspect for venous patterns.
- Venous patterns are the same bilaterally. Venous patterns may be more predominant in pregnancy or obesity.

▶ Pronounced unilateral venous patterns may indicate increased blood flow to a malignancy.

6. Inspect for moles or other markings.
- Moles that are unchanged, nontender, and long-standing are of no concern. Striae that are present in pregnancy or recent weight loss or gain may appear purple in color. Striae become silvery white over time.

▶ Moles that have changed or appear suddenly require further evaluation. A mole along the milk line may be a supernumerary nipple (see Figure 17.5).

7. Inspect the areolae.
- The areolae are normally round or oval and almost equal in size. Areolae are pink in light-skinned people and brown in dark-skinned people. The areolae darken in pregnancy.

▶ Peau d'orange associated with cancer may be seen first on the areolae. Redness and fissures may develop with breastfeeding.

8. Inspect the nipples.
- Nipples are normally the same color as the areolae and are equal in size and shape. Nipples are generally everted but may be flat or inverted. Nipples should point in the same direction outward and slightly upward. Nipples should be free of cracks, crust, erosions, ulcerations, pigment changes, or discharge.

▶ Recent retraction or inversion of a nipple or change in the direction of the nipple is suggestive of malignancy. Discharge requires cytologic examination. A red, scaly, eczema-like area over the nipple could indicate Paget disease, a rare type of breast cancer. The area may exude fluid, scale, or crust (see Figure 17.9 ■).

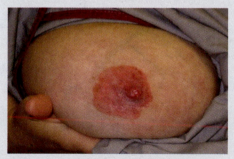

Figure 17.9 Paget disease of the nipple.
Source: PJF Military Collection/Alamy Stock Photo.

9. Observe the breasts for shape, surface characteristics, and bilateral pull of suspensory ligaments.
- Ask the patient to assume the following positions while you continue to inspect the breasts.

Techniques and Normal Findings	Abnormal Findings and Special Considerations

10. **Inspect with the patient's arms over the head (see Figure 17.10 ■).**

▶ Dimpling of the skin over a mass is usually a visible sign of breast cancer. Dimpling is accentuated in this position. Variations in contour and symmetry may also indicate breast cancer (Mayo Clinic, 2018a).

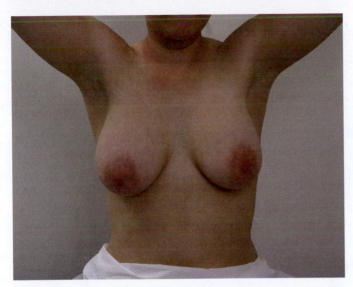

Figure 17.10 Inspection of the breasts with the patient's arms above her head.

11. **Inspect with the patient's hands pressed against her waist (see Figure 17.11 ■).**

▶ Tightening of the pectoral muscles may help to accentuate dimpling.

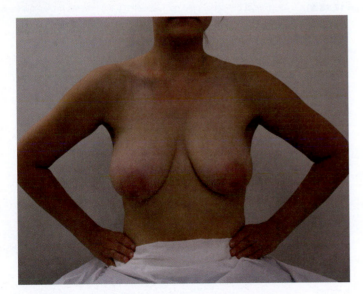

Figure 17.11 Inspection of the breasts with the patient's hands pressed against her waist.

Techniques and Normal Findings	Abnormal Findings and Special Considerations

12. **Inspect with the patient's hands pressed together at the level of the waist (see Figure 17.12 ■).**

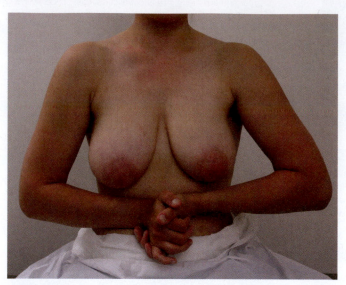

Figure 17.12 Inspection of the breasts with the patient's hands pressed together at the level of her waist.

13. **Inspect with the patient leaning forward from the waist (see Figure 17.13 ■).**
   - The breasts normally fall freely and evenly from the chest.

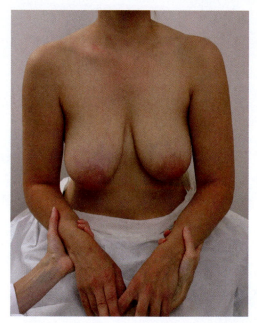

Figure 17.13 Assisting the patient to lean forward for inspection.

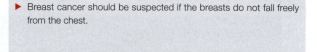

▶ Breast cancer should be suspected if the breasts do not fall freely from the chest.

| **Techniques and Normal Findings** | **Abnormal Findings and Special Considerations** |

Palpation of the Breast

1. **Position the patient.**
   * Ask the patient to lie down. Cover the breast that is not being examined. Place a small pillow or rolled towel under the shoulder of the side to be palpated and position the patient's arm over her head. This maneuver flattens the breast tissue over the chest wall.

2. **Instruct the patient.**
   * Explain that you will be touching the entire breast and nipple. Tell the patient to inform you of any discomfort or tenderness.

3. **Palpate skin texture.**
   * Skin texture should be smooth with uninterrupted contour.

4. **Palpate the breast.**
   * Use the finger pads of the first three fingers in dime-size circular motions to press the breast tissue against the chest wall (see Figure 17.14 ■). Be sure to palpate the entire breast.

▶ Thickening of the skin suggests an underlying carcinoma (Mayo Clinic, 2018a).

▶ The incidence of breast cancers is highest in the upper outer quadrant, including the axillary tail of Spence. Masses in the tail must be distinguished from enlarged lymph nodes.

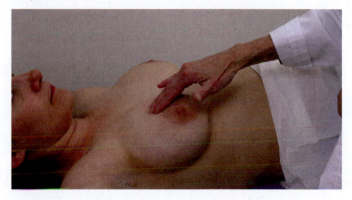

Figure 17.14 Palpating the breast.

The vertical strip pattern is the recommended method for breast palpation. (See Figure 17.15A ■).
* The following landmarks are used to be sure the entire breast is assessed: down the midaxillary line, across the inframammary ridge at the fifth or sixth rib, up at the lateral edge of the sternum, across the clavicle, and back to the midaxillary.
* As each area is examined, three levels of pressure should be applied in sequence. These are light for subcutaneous tissue, medium at the midlevel tissues, and deep to the chest wall. Pressure is adapted according to the size, shape, and consistency of the breast tissue. In addition, pressure will vary in relation to breast size and the presence of breast implants. Implants are placed behind breast tissue; therefore, the steps for breast examination are the same as for palpation of breasts in women without implants.

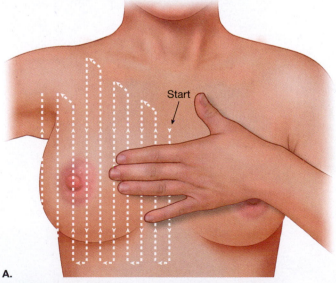

A.

Figure 17.15A A. The vertical strip method for palpation of the breast.

Techniques and Normal Findings	Abnormal Findings and Special Considerations

Additional patterns include the concentric circles or back-and-forth techniques (see Figure 17.15B ■).

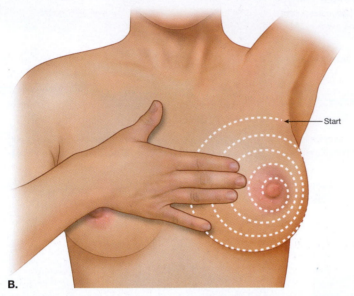

B.

Figure 17.15B B. The concentric circle pattern for palpation of the breast.

- In women with pendulous breasts, palpate with one hand under the breast to support it and the other hand pushing against breast tissue in a downward motion (see Figure 17.16 ■).

▶ Breasts that are heavy and pendulous can cause stretching of ligaments and tissues, leading to ongoing breast, shoulder, back, and neck pain (Harvard Medical School, 2018). Some women may find relief from this pain through breast reduction surgery.

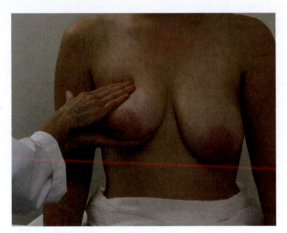

Figure 17.16 Palpating a pendulous breast.

- In obese women with large breasts, palpation with two hands should be performed with the patient in the sitting and supine positions.

Techniques and Normal Findings	Abnormal Findings and Special Considerations

5. Palpate the nipple and areolae.
- The area beneath and at the nipple should be palpated, not squeezed, to observe for drainage (see Figure 17.17 ■). Squeezing may result in discharge and discomfort. Confirm that the nipple is free of discharge, that it is nontender, and that the areola is free of masses.

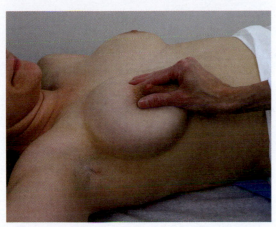

Figure 17.17 Palpating the nipple.

- Repeat steps 1 through 5 on the other breast.

Examination of the Axillae

1. Instruct the patient.
- Explain that you will be examining the axillae by looking and palpating. Tell the patient that she will sit for this examination and you will support the arm while palpating with the other hand. Explain that relaxation will make the examination more comfortable. Tell the patient to inform you of any discomfort.

2. Position the patient.
- Ask the patient or assist the patient to assume a sitting position. Flex the arm at the elbow and support it on your arm. Note the presence of axillary hair. Confirm that the axilla is free of redness, rashes, lumps, or lesions. With the palmar surface of your fingers, reach deep into the axilla (see Figure 17.18 ■). Gently palpate the anterior border of the axilla (anterior or subpectoral nodes), the central aspect along the rib cage (central nodes), the posterior border (subscapular/posterior nodes), and along the inner aspect of the upper arm (lateral nodes).

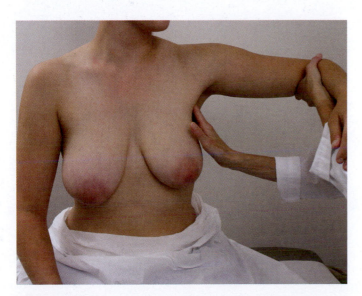

Figure 17.18 Palpating the axilla. Note that the nurse is supporting the woman's arm with her own nondominant arm.

▶ Lactation not associated with childbearing is called **galactorrhea**. It can be present in women, men, and even infants. It occurs most commonly with endocrine disorders or medications, including some sedatives, antidepressants, antipsychotics, and antihypertensives (Mayo Clinic, 2017d).

▶ Unilateral discharge from the nipple is suggestive of benign breast disease, an intraductal papilloma, or cancer. Spontaneous discharge from the nipple warrants further evaluation.

▶ Infections of the breast, arm, and hand cause enlargement and tenderness of the axillary lymph nodes. Hard, fixed nodes are suggestive of cancer or lymphoma. Patients who have had a wide local excision (removal of tumor and narrow margin of normal tissue) or mastectomy (removal of tumor and extensive areas of surrounding tissue) need to be examined carefully. The remaining tissue on the chest wall should be palpated as it would be for nonsurgical patients.

Techniques and Normal Findings	Abnormal Findings and Special Considerations

Inspection of the Male Breast

1. **Instruct the patient.**
   - Explain all aspects of the procedure and the purpose for each part of the examination.

2. **Position the patient.**
   - The patient is in the sitting position with the gown at the waist.

3. **Inspect the male breasts.**
   - Observe that breasts are flat and free of lumps or lesions.

Palpation of the Male Breast and Axillae

1. **Position the patient.**
   - Place the patient in a supine position.

2. **Instruct the patient.**
   - Explain that you will be using the pads of your fingers to gently palpate the breast area. Instruct the patient to report any discomfort.

3. **Palpate the male breasts.**
   - Using the finger pads of the first three fingers, gently palpate the breast tissue, using concentric circles until you reach the nipple (see Figure 17.19 ■). The male breast feels like a thin disk of tissue under a flat nipple and areola.

▶ **Gynecomastia** (breast enlargement in males) is a temporary condition seen in infants, at puberty, and in older males (Mayo Clinic, 2017b). In older males, it may accompany hormonal treatment for prostate cancer. Breast cancer in the male is usually identified as a hard nodule fixed to the nipple and underlying tissue. Nipple discharge may be present. Pseudogynecomastia, an increase in subcutaneous fat, may occur in obese males. On palpation, breast tissue is more firm than fat. A mammogram may be required to distinguish enlarged or changed breast tissue from increased subcutaneous fat.

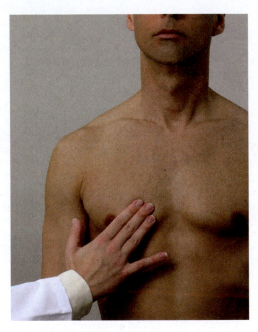

Figure 17.19 Palpation of the male breast.

4. **Palpate the nipple.**
   - Compress the nipple between your thumb and forefinger.
   - The nipple should be free of discharge.

5. **Repeat on the other breast.**

6. **Palpate the axillae.**
   - Palpate axillary nodes in men as you would for women.

Documenting Your Findings

Documentation of assessment data—subjective and objective—must be accurate, professional, complete, and confidential. When documenting the information from the focused assessment of each body system, the nurse should use measurements where appropriate to ensure accuracy, use medical terminology rather than jargon, include all pertinent information, and avoid language that could identify the patient. The information in the documentation should make it clear what questions were asked, and the language used should indicate whether it is the patient's response or the nurse's findings.

For the purpose of documenting assessment findings, the breast is divided into four quadrants defined by a vertical line and a horizontal line that intersect at the nipple (see Figure 17.20 ■). The location of clinical findings may be described according to clock positions, for example, at the 2 o'clock position, 5cm (1.95 in.) from the nipple. The following is an example of normal results for the breasts.

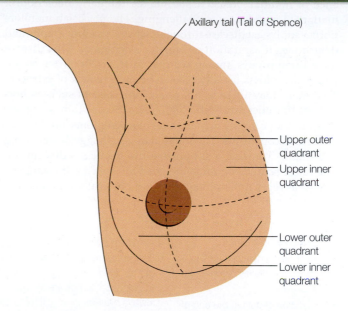

Figure 17.20 Breast quadrants.

Sample Documentation: Breasts and Axillae Assessment

Focused History (Subjective Data)

This is information from the Review of Systems (ROS) and other pertinent history information that is or could be related to the patient's breast and axillae.

Denies lumps, pain, or other notable changes to the breast. Denies nipple discharge. Reports cyclical breast tenderness around the time of ovulation and the start of a period. Currently denies tenderness. Denies personal or family history of breast disease.

Physical Assessment (Objective Data)

Breasts are smooth, symmetric, and with even skin tone. No masses, tenderness, lesions, or nipple discharge. No lymphadenopathy in axillary region.

Abnormal Findings

Some of the problems identified during the physical assessment are entirely within the realm of nursing and are addressed with appropriate nursing interventions. Some problems, however, require collaborative management.

Abnormalities of the Female Breast

Benign breast disease, fibroadenoma, intraductal papilloma, mammary duct ectasia, and breast cancer are the most common breast conditions that will challenge the nurse and the rest of the healthcare team. These common abnormalities are discussed in the following sections.

BENIGN BREAST DISEASE (FIBROCYSTIC BREAST DISEASE)

One of the most common benign breast problems, this disorder is caused by *fibrosis*, a thickening of the normal breast tissue; it is not usually clinically significant, and there is no direct link between fibrocystic tissue changes and the incidence of cancer (see Figure 17.21 ■). In some cases, it may result in ductal hyperplasia and dysplasia, which may eventually develop into

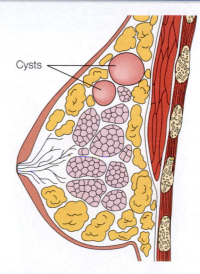

Figure 17.21 Fibrocystic breast disease.

noninvasive intraductal, lobular, or intraepithelial carcinoma. This can be a potential focus for invasive carcinoma. The presence of nodular breast tissue makes the early detection of malignant nodules more challenging. The physician monitors fibrocystic breast disease through periodic mammography and determines if aspiration or biopsy is necessary. This disease most often occurs among women in their 20s. After menopause, symptoms usually resolve because of lack of estrogen. Treatment may include pharmacologic agents such as hormones, diuretics, and mild analgesics. Some studies suggest that limiting caffeine may help relieve symptoms, but the evidence is inconclusive. The nurse may also suggest decreasing salt intake. Wearing a supportive bra decreases discomfort. The nurse should reinforce the need for breast self-awareness as well as regular mammography and physical examination.

Subjective findings:
- Breast pain or tenderness that begins immediately before onset of menses.
- Resolution of pain at the end of menses.

Objective findings:
- Soft breast lumps that are well demarcated and freely movable to palpation; lumps are almost always bilateral.
- Nipple discharge (clear, straw colored, milky, or green).
- Cysts also may be present (usually located in the upper outer quadrant).

FIBROADENOMA

A benign tumor of the glandular tissue of the breast, fibroadenoma is most common in adolescent girls and women ages 15 to 35 (Mayo Clinic, 2017c) (see Figure 17.22 ■). Its development in adolescents appears to be linked to breast hypertrophy, which may occur during the growth spurt of puberty. The usual treatment is careful observation over time. Biopsy or excision of the lump is indicated if the findings are inconclusive. No relationship has been established between fibroadenomas and malignant neoplasms.

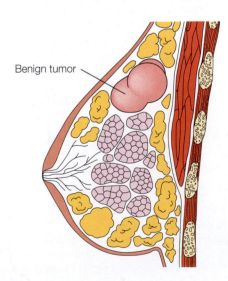

Benign tumor

Figure 17.22 Fibroadenoma.

Subjective findings:
- None; aside from the breast mass, the individual usually is asymptomatic.
- Often discovered through BSE or during clinical breast examination.

Objective findings:
- Presence of well-defined, round, firm tumors, about 1 to 5 cm (0.39 to 1.95 in.) in diameter, that can be moved freely within the breast tissue.
- Usually involves a single tumor near the nipple or in the upper outer quadrant of the breast.

INTRADUCTAL PAPILLOMA

Intraductal papillomas are tiny growths of epithelial cells that project into the lumen of the lactiferous ducts (see Figure 17.23 ■). They are the primary cause of nipple discharge in women who are not pregnant or lactating and are more commonly found in menopausal women but may occur at any age. Treatment usually involves surgical removal (excision) and biopsy of the affected ducts.

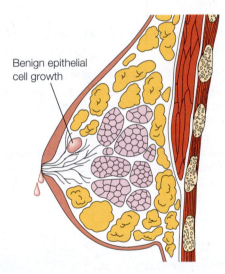

Benign epithelial cell growth

Figure 17.23 Intraductal papilloma.

Subjective findings:
- Breast enlargement.
- Breast pain.

Objective findings:
- One or more lumps in the breast.
- Nipple discharge. Because the growths are fragile, even minimal trauma causes leakage of blood or serum into the involved duct and subsequent discharge (MedlinePlus, 2018c).

MAMMARY DUCT ECTASIA

Mammary duct ectasia is an inflammation of the lactiferous ducts behind the nipple. As cellular debris and fluid collect in the involved ducts, they become enlarged and can form a palpable, painful mass (see Figure 17.24 ■). Because there may be some nipple retraction, a careful assessment is required to distinguish the condition from breast cancer. Although the disorder is painful, it is not associated with cancer and usually resolves spontaneously.

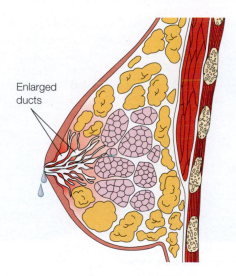

Figure 17.24 Mammary duct ectasia.

determines which protocol is used for treatment. Treatment may consist of surgery, radiation therapy, chemotherapy, or a combination of these modalities.

Subjective findings:
- Perceived change in breast size.
- Perceived change in breast shape. Irregular shape of one breast as compared with the other, such as a flattening of one quadrant.
- Breast pain or tenderness.
- Nipple pain or tenderness.

Objective findings:
- Breast lump or thickening of local area of breast tissue.
- Dimpling of the skin over the tumor caused by a retraction or pulling inward of breast tissue. This results primarily from tissue fibrosis. Retraction is also caused by fat necrosis and mammary duct ectasia.
- Deviation of the breast or nipple from its normal alignment. Deviation is also caused by retraction. The nipple typically deviates toward the underlying cancer.
- Nipple retraction. The nipple flattens or even turns inward. Retraction is also caused by tissue fibrosis.
- Edema, which may result in a peau d'orange appearance, especially near the nipple. Edema is caused by blockage of the lymphatic ducts that normally drain the breast.
- Discharge, which may be bloody or clear.

Subjective findings:
- Thick, sticky nipple discharge.
- Nipple retraction (Mayo Clinic, 2015b).

Objective findings:
- Often asymptomatic.
- Breast tenderness or inflammation of the clogged duct (periductal mastitis) may be present (Mayo Clinic, 2015b).

CARCINOMA (CANCER)

Among women in the United States, carcinoma of the breast, or breast cancer, is the most commonly diagnosed form of cancer CDC, 2017b). Although breast cancer can occur in both men and women, it is much more common in women. The screening examination and studies for breast cancer are physical examination and mammography. A positive diagnosis of cancer is made by histologic examination following an open or closed (needle) biopsy. The tumor is then staged to determine its characteristics, nodal involvement, and the presence or absence of distant metastasis (see Figure 17.25 ■). The outcome of this staging

Abnormalities of the Male Breast

Male breast tissue is similar to that of the female. Therefore, changes in relation to hormone secretion and disease occur. The following sections describe abnormalities in the male breast.

GYNECOMASTIA

This enlargement of the male breast tissue can occur at birth in response to maternal hormones. In addition, at the onset of puberty more than 30% of males have enlargement of one or both breasts in response to hormonal changes, which can be a cause of embarrassment or shame. Gynecomastia may also occur in males over age 50 because of pituitary or testicular tumors and in males taking estrogenic medication for prostate cancer. It may occur in cirrhosis of the liver and with adrenal and thyroid diseases (see Figure 17.26 ■).

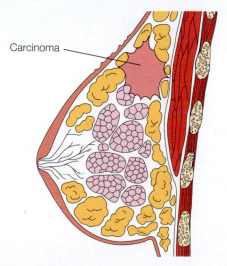

Figure 17.25 Breast cancer.

Subjective findings:
- Perceived swelling or increase in size of breast tissue.
- Pain or tenderness in breast tissue (Mayo Clinic, 2017b).

Objective findings:
- Swelling of breast tissue.
- If gynecomastia occurs secondary to another condition, such as hyperthyroidism, manifestations also will include those related to the primary condition (Mayo Clinic, 2017b).

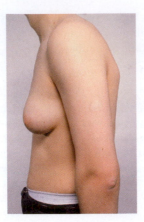

Figure 17.26 Gynecomastia.
Source: Mediscan/Alamy Stock Photo.

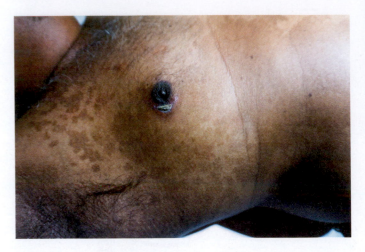

Figure 17.27 Carcinoma of the breast.
Source: Alan Nissa/Shutterstock.

CARCINOMA (CANCER)

Male breast cancer is rare. Less than 1% of all breast cancer occurs in men. Predisposing factors include radiation exposure, cirrhosis, and estrogen medications. Increased rates have been seen in males with a familial history of breast cancer in primary female relatives (see Figure 17.27 ■). Men who are diagnosed with early-stage breast cancer typically have a high likelihood of being cured. However, many men delay seeking treatment for unusual signs or symptoms, such as a breast lump. As a result, for many men, breast cancer is not diagnosed until the disease is more advanced (Mayo Clinic, 2015a).

Subjective findings:

- Perceived change in breast size.
- Perceived change in breast shape.
- Pain or tenderness (Mayo Clinic, 2015a).

Objective findings:

- Breast lump or thickening of local area of breast tissue.
- Bloody or clear nipple discharge.
- Swelling of breast tissue.
- Dimpling of the breast skin.
- Nipple inversion.
- Scaling, peeling, or flaking of the nipple or breast skin.
- Redness or pitting of the breast skin, like the skin of an orange (Mayo Clinic, 2015a).

Application Through Critical Thinking

CASE STUDY

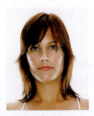

Source: Digital Vision/Photodisc/ Getty Images.

Carol Jenkins is a 29-year-old female who has come to the clinic today because of complaints of increasing breast tenderness. Carol is an avid runner and has been training for a marathon but is experiencing significant tenderness in her breasts during running. When you start to question Carol, she tells you she has had breast tenderness associated with her periods for most of her adult life. Upon further questioning, you discover the tenderness has increased over the past several months and is not just associated with running. Her breasts seem swollen and heavy, and what used to hurt in the outer portion of the breast has changed to discomfort all over. The physical assessment revealed round, tender, mobile masses with smooth borders in all quadrants. The nipples are everted, round, and free of lesions. The breasts are symmetric in shape and contour.

Complete Documentation   The following is sample documentation for Carol Jenkins.

SUBJECTIVE DATA   Breast tenderness "with periods" for most of her adult life. Tenderness increasing over past several months. Breasts seem "swollen and heavy." Discomfort in outer breast now "discomfort all over."

OBJECTIVE DATA Round, mobile masses with smooth borders in all quadrants bilaterally. Nipples everted, round, free of lesions. Breasts symmetric in shape and contour.

CRITICAL THINKING QUESTIONS

1. What is most likely the cause of the patient's symptoms?

2. Identify several differential diagnoses.

3. What information is required to validate the diagnoses?

4. What recommendations should the nurse make for this patient?

5. What do you think Carol's greatest concern was when she came to the clinic?

REFERENCES

American Academy of Family Physicians (AAFP). (2016). *USPSTF, AAFP issue final breast cancer screening recommendations.* Retrieved from https://www.aafp.org/news/health-of-the-public/20160115uspstffinalbrstcascreen.html

American Cancer Society (ACS). (2017a). *Breast cancer facts and figures: 2017–2018.* Retrieved from https://www.cancer.org/content/dam/cancer-org/research/cancer-facts-and-statistics/breast-cancer-facts-and-figures/breast-cancer-facts-and-figures-2017-2018.pdf

American Cancer Society (ACS). (2017b). *Breast cancer risk factors you cannot change.* Retrieved from https://www.cancer.org/cancer/breast-cancer/risk-and-prevention/breast-cancer-risk-factors-you-cannot-change.html

American Cancer Society (ACS). (2017c). *Disproven or controversial breast cancer risk factors.* Retrieved from https://www.cancer.org/cancer/breast-cancer/risk-and-prevention/disproven-or-controversial-breast-cancer-risk-factors.html

American Cancer Society (ACS). (2017d). *Lifestyle-related breast cancer risk factors.* Retrieved from https://www.cancer.org/cancer/breast-cancer/risk-and-prevention/lifestyle-related-breast-cancer-risk-factors.html

American Cancer Society (ACS). (2017e). *Study: Lack of insurance linked to higher breast cancer death rates in black women.* Retrieved from https://www.cancer.org/latest-news/study-lack-of-insurance-linked-to-higher-breast-cancer-death-rates-in-black-women.html

American Cancer Society (ACS). (2018). *Breast cancer screening guideline.* Retrieved from https://www.cancer.org/latest-news/special-coverage/american-cancer-society-breast-cancer-screening-guidelines.html

American College of Obstetricians and Gynecologists (ACOG). (2017a). *ACOG revises breast cancer screening guidance: Ob-Gyns promote shared decision making.* Retrieved from https://www.acog.org/About-ACOG/News-Room/News-Releases/2017/ACOG-Revises-Breast-Cancer-Screening-Guidance--ObGyns-Promote-Shared-Decision-Making

American College of Obstetricians and Gynecologists (ACOG). (2017b). *Clinical breast examination.* Retrieved from https://www.acog.org/About-ACOG/ACOG-Departments/Annual-Womens-Health-Care/Well-Woman-Recommendations/Clinical-Breast-Examination

American Society of Clinical Oncology (ASCO). (2017). *Breast cancer: Risk factors and prevention.* Retrieved from https://www.cancer.net/cancer-types/breast-cancer/risk-factors-and-prevention

Centers for Disease Control and Prevention (CDC). (2016). *Breast cancer rates by race and ethnicity.* Retrieved from https://www.cdc.gov/cancer/breast/statistics/race.htm

Centers for Disease Control and Prevention (CDC). (2017a). *Breast cancer in young African American women.* Retrieved from https://www.cdc.gov/cancer/dcpc/data/women.htm

Centers for Disease Control and Prevention (CDC). (2017b). *Cancer among women.* Retrieved from https://www.cdc.gov/cancer/dcpc/data/women.htm

Centers for Disease Control and Prevention (CDC). (2017c). Cancer screening test use — United States, 2015. *Morbidity and Mortality Weekly Report, 66*(8), 201–206. Retrieved from https://www.cdc.gov/mmwr/volumes/66/wr/mm6608a1.htm

Friedman, A. M., Hemler, J. R., Rossetti, E., Clemow, L. P., & Ferrante, J. M. (2012). Obese women's barriers to mammography and Pap smear: The possible role of personality. *Obesity (Silver Spring), 20*(8), 1611–1617. doi:10.1038/oby.2012.50

Harvard Medical School. (2018). *Breast pain: Not just a premenopausal complaint.* Retrieved from https://www.health.harvard.edu/pain/breast-pain-not-just-a-premenopausal-complaint

Healthline. (2017). *Traumatic breast injuries: Should you see a doctor?* Retrieved from https://www.healthline.com/health/breast-injury-trauma

Johns Hopkins Medicine. (n.d.a). *Breast pain: Mastalgia.* Retrieved from http://www.hopkinsmedicine.org/healthlibrary/conditions/breast_health/mastalgia_breast_pain_85,P00154

Johns Hopkins Medicine. (n.d.b). *Normal breast development and changes.* Retrieved from https://www.hopkinsmedicine.org/healthlibrary/conditions/breast_health/normal_breast_development_and_changes_85,P00151

Marieb, E. N., & Keller, S. M. (2018). *Essentials of human anatomy and physiology* (12th ed.). New York, NY: Pearson

Mayo Clinic. (2015a). *Male breast cancer.* Retrieved from http://www.mayoclinic.org/diseases-conditions/male-breast-cancer/basics/definition/con-20025972

Mayo Clinic. (2015b). *Mammary duct ectasia*. Retrieved from http://www.mayoclinic.org/diseases-conditions/mammary-duct-ectasia/basics/definition/con-20025073

Mayo Clinic. (2017a). *Breast pain*. Retrieved from https://www.mayoclinic.org/diseases-conditions/breast-pain/symptoms-causes/syc-20350423

Mayo Clinic. (2017b). *Enlarged breasts in men: Gynecomastia*. Retrieved from https://www.mayoclinic.org/diseases-conditions/gynecomastia/symptoms-causes/syc-20351793

Mayo Clinic. (2017c). *Fibroadenoma*. Retrieved from https://www.mayoclinic.org/diseases-conditions/fibroadenoma/symptoms-causes/syc-20352752

Mayo Clinic. (2017d). *Galactorrhea*. Retrieved from https://www.mayoclinic.org/diseases-conditions/galactorrhea/symptoms-causes/syc-20350431

Mayo Clinic. (2017e). *Paget's disease of the breast*. Retrieved from https://www.mayoclinic.org/diseases-conditions/pagets-disease-of-the-breast/symptoms-causes/syc-20351079

Mayo Clinic. (2018a). *Breast cancer*. Retrieved from https://www.mayoclinic.org/diseases-conditions/breast-cancer/symptoms-causes/syc-20352470

Mayo Clinic. (2018b). *Breast lumps*. Retrieved from https://www.mayoclinic.org/symptoms/breast-lumps/basics/causes/sym-20050619

Mayo Clinic. (2018c). *Nipple discharge*. Retrieved from https://www.mayoclinic.org/symptoms/nipple-discharge/basics/causes/sym-20050946

MedlinePlus: National Library of Medicine. (2018a). *Aging changes in the breast*. Retrieved from https://medlineplus.gov/ency/article/003999.htm

MedlinePlus: National Library of Medicine. (2018b). *Breast skin and nipple changes*. Retrieved from http://www.nlm.nih.gov/medlineplus/ency/patientinstructions/000622.htm

MedlinePlus: National Library of Medicine. (2018c). *Intraductal papilloma*. Retrieved from http://www.nlm.nih.gov/medlineplus/ency/article/001238.htm

National Cancer Institute (NCI). (2018). *BRCA mutations: Cancer risk and genetic testing*. Retrieved from https://www.cancer.gov/about-cancer/causes-prevention/genetics/brca-fact-sheet

Salzman, B., Fleegle, S., & Tully, A. S. (2012). Common breast problems. *American Family Physician, 86*(4), 343–349.

Susan G. Koman Breast Cancer Foundation. (2018a). *Facts and statistics*. Retrieved from https://ww5.komen.org/BreastCancer/FactsandStatistics.html

Susan G. Koman Breast Cancer Foundation. (2018b). *Personal history of breast cancer or other cancers*. Retrieved from https://ww5.komen.org/BreastCancer/PersonalHistoryofBreastCancer.html

Susman, E. J., Houts, R. M., Steinberg, L., Belsky, J., Cauffman, E., DeHart, G., . . . Halpern-Felsher, B. L. (2010). Longitudinal development of secondary sexual characteristics in girls and boys between ages 9½ and 15½ years. *Archives of Pediatrics & Adolescent Medicine, 164*(2), 166–173.

U.S. Preventive Services Task Force (USPSTF). (2009). Archived: *Breast cancer: Screening*. Retrieved from http://www.uspreventiveservicestaskforce.org/uspstf14/breastcancer/breastcancerfaq.htm

U.S. Preventive Services Task Force (USPSTF). (2016). *Breast cancer: Screening*. Retrieved from https://www.uspreventiveservicestaskforce.org/Page/Document/RecommendationStatementFinal/breast-cancer-screening1

WebMD. (2018a). *Breast pain (mastalgia)—Topic overview: What do I need to know about breast pain?* Retrieved from https://www.webmd.com/women/tc/breast-pain-mastalgia-topic-overview#1

WebMD. (2018b). *Fibrocystic breasts: Topic overview*. Retrieved from https://www.webmd.com/women/tc/fibrocystic-breasts-topic-overview#1

Yu, W., & Zhou, J. (2016). Sports bras and breast kinetics. In W. Yu (Ed.), *Advances in women's intimate apparel technology* (pp. 135–146). Sawston, UK: Woodhead Publishing.

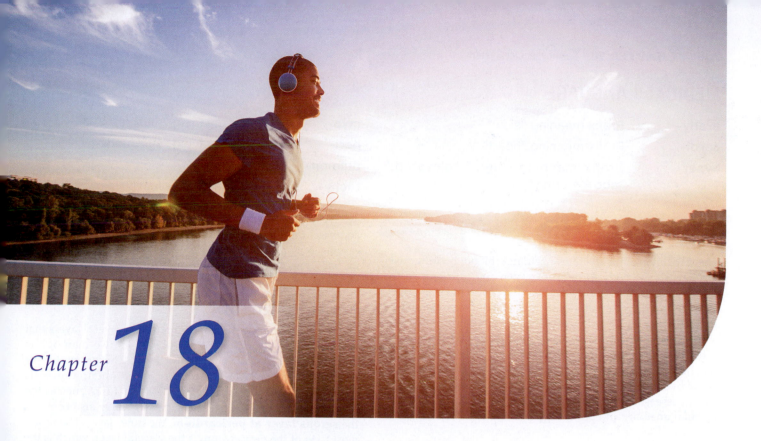

Chapter 18

Cardiovascular System

LEARNING OUTCOMES

Upon completion of this chapter, you will be able to:

1. Describe the anatomy and physiology of the cardiovascular system.

2. Identify the anatomic, physiologic, developmental, psychosocial, and cultural variations that guide assessment of the cardiovascular system.

3. Determine which questions about the cardiovascular system to use for the focused interview.

4. Outline the techniques for assessment of the cardiovascular system.

5. Generate the appropriate documentation to describe the assessment of the cardiovascular system.

6. Identify abnormal findings in the physical assessment of the cardiovascular system.

KEY TERMS

MEDICAL LANGUAGE

brady-	Prefix meaning "slow"	**myo-**	Prefix meaning "muscle"
cardi-	Prefix meaning "heart"	**peri-**	Prefix meaning "surrounding"
hyper-	Prefix meaning "high," "elevated," "above normal"	**pulmon-**	Prefix meaning "lung"
		tachy-	Prefix meaning "fast"

Introduction

The cardiovascular system circulates blood continuously throughout the body to deliver oxygen and nutrients to the body's organs and tissues and to dispose of their excreted wastes. The delicate balance of this system is vulnerable to stress, trauma, and a variety of pathologic mechanisms that may impair its ability to function. Inadequate tissue perfusion results in both a diminished supply of nutrients necessary for metabolic functions and a buildup of metabolic wastes. The assessment of cardiac function is an essential component of the complete patient assessment, so having a solid understanding of cardiovascular anatomy and physiology is essential.

Anatomy and Physiology Review

The cardiovascular system is composed of the heart and the vascular system. The heart includes the cardiac muscle, atria, ventricles, valves, coronary arteries, cardiac veins, electrical conducting structures, and cardiac nerves. The vascular system is composed of the blood vessels of the body: the arteries, arterioles, veins, venules, and capillaries. In this chapter, only the coronary blood vessels are considered in detail. Chapter 19

addresses the peripheral vessels. ∞ The major functions of the cardiovascular system are transporting nutrients and oxygen to the body, removing wastes and carbon dioxide, and maintaining adequate perfusion of organs and tissues.

Pericardium

The **pericardium** is a thin sac composed of several layers that surrounds the heart (see Figure 18.1 ■). Its two main layers are the parietal layer and visceral layer. The parietal layer contains the outer layer, the fibrous pericardium; it protects the heart and anchors it to the adjacent structures, such as the diaphragm and great vessels. The parietal layer also contains the **serous layer of pericardium**, the inner layer. The innermost layer of the pericardium is the visceral layer, which is the same as the epicardium. The **visceral layer of pericardium** lines the surface of the heart. Fluid between the fibrous and the serous layers of pericardium lubricates the layers and allows for a gliding motion between them with each heartbeat.

Heart

The **heart** is an intricately designed pump composed of a meticulous network of synchronized structures. It lies behind the sternum and typically extends from the second rib to the fifth intercostal space(ICS) (see Figure 18.2A–C ■). The heart sits obliquely within the thoracic cavity between the lungs and

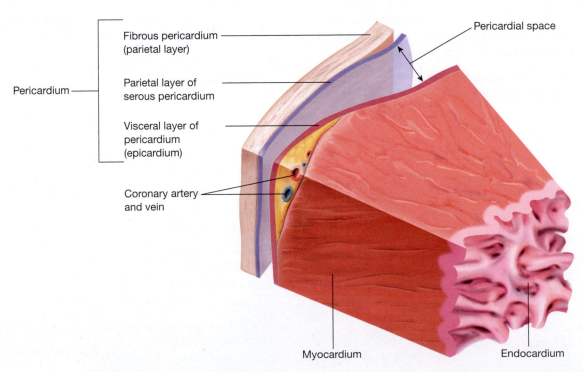

Fibrous pericardium
(parietal layer)

Pericardial space

Pericardium

Parietal layer of
serous pericardium

Visceral layer of
pericardium
(epicardium)

Coronary artery
and vein

Myocardium

Endocardium

Figure 18.1 Layers of the heart.

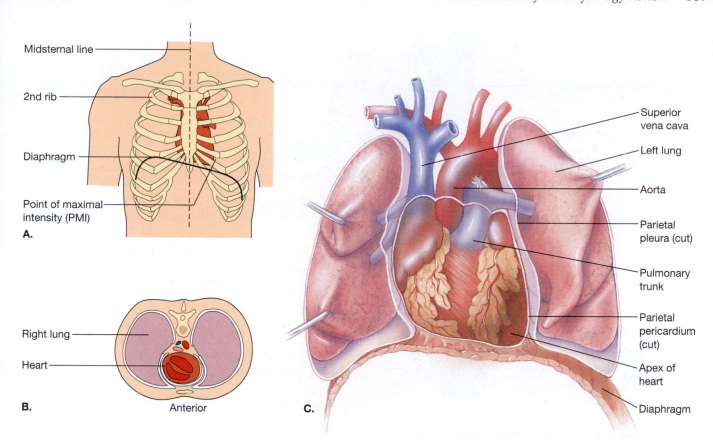

Figure 18.2 Location of the heart in the mediastinum of the thorax. A. Relationship of the heart to the sternum, ribs, and diaphragm. B. Cross-sectional view showing relative position of the heart in the thorax. C. Relationship of the heart and great vessels to the lungs.

above the diaphragm in an area called the **mediastinal space,** or mediastinum. Ventrally, the right side of the heart is more forward than the left. The heartbeat is most easily palpated over the apex; thus, this point is referred to as the **apical impulse** or point of maximum impulse (PMI).

The heart is approximately 12.8 cm (5 in.) long, 9 cm (3.5 in.) across, and 6.4 cm (2.5 in.) thick. It is slightly larger than the patient's clenched fist. The heart of the female typically is smaller and weighs less than the heart of the male.

Heart Wall   The heart wall is composed of three layers: epicardium, myocardium, and endocardium (see Figure 18.1). The outer layer, called the **epicardium**, is anatomically identical to the visceral pericardium. The **myocardium** is the thick, muscular layer. It is made up of bundles of cardiac muscle fibers reinforced by a branching network of connective tissue fibers called the fibrous skeleton of the heart. The innermost layer is the **endocardium**, a smooth layer that provides an inner lining for the chambers of the heart. The endocardium is continuous with the linings of the blood vessels that enter and leave the cardiac chambers.

Cardiac muscle is quite different from skeletal muscle. The muscle cells are shorter, interconnected, branched structures. Mitochondria, the cell's energy-producing organelles, comprise about 25% of cardiac muscle fibers versus only about 2% of skeletal muscle fibers. This higher ratio is related to the much higher energy requirements of cardiac muscle. Unlike

the independently functioning fibers of skeletal muscle, the fibers of cardiac muscle are interconnected by special junctions that provide for the conduction of impulses across the entire myocardium. This property allows the heart to contract as a single unit.

Heart Chambers   The heart is composed of four chambers: two smaller, superior chambers called atria, and two larger, inferior chambers called ventricles (see Figure 18.3 ■). One atrium is located on the right side of the heart and one on the left side. These serve as receiving chambers for blood returning to the heart from the major blood vessels of the body. The atria then pump the blood into the right and left ventricles, which lie directly below them. The ventricles also are located on each side of the heart. They eject blood into the vessels leaving the heart. A longitudinal partition separates the heart chambers. The *interatrial septum* separates the two atria, and the *interventricular septum* divides the ventricles.

RIGHT ATRIUM   The **right atrium** (RA) is a thin-walled chamber located above and slightly to the right of the right ventricle. It forms the right border of the heart. Deoxygenated venous blood from the systemic circulation enters the right atrium via the inferior and superior venae cavae (two main structures of the venous system) and the coronary sinus. The blood is then ejected from the right atrium through the tricuspid valve into the right ventricle.

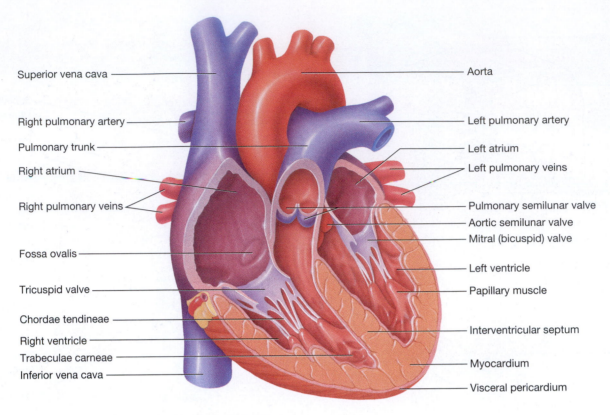

Superior vena cava

Right pulmonary artery

Pulmonary trunk

Right atrium

Right pulmonary veins

Fossa ovalis

Tricuspid valve

Chordae tendineae

Right ventricle

Trabeculae carneae

Inferior vena cava

Aorta

Left pulmonary artery

Left atrium

Left pulmonary veins

Pulmonary semilunar valve

Aortic semilunar valve

Mitral (bicuspid) valve

Left ventricle

Papillary muscle

Interventricular septum

Myocardium

Visceral pericardium

Figure 18.3 Structural components of the heart.

RIGHT VENTRICLE The **right ventricle** (RV) is formed triangularly and comprises much of the anterior or sternocostal surface of the heart. After receiving deoxygenated blood from the right atrium, the right ventricle ejects it through the pulmonary semilunar valve to the trunk of the pulmonary arteries so that the blood may be oxygenated within the lungs. Its wall is much thinner than that of the left ventricle, reflecting the relatively low vascular pressure in the vessels of the lungs.

LEFT ATRIUM The **left atrium** (LA) forms the posterior aspect of the heart. Its muscular structure is slightly thicker than that of the right atrium. It receives oxygenated blood from the pulmonary vasculature via the pulmonary veins. From here, the blood is pumped through the mitral, or bicuspid, valve into the left ventricle.

LEFT VENTRICLE The **left ventricle** (LV) is located behind the right ventricle and forms the left border of the heart. The left ventricle, which is egg shaped, is the most muscular chamber of the heart. The thick wall of ventricular muscle permits the pumping of blood through the aortic semilunar valve into the aorta against high systemic vascular resistance. This causes the left ventricle to develop more mass than the right ventricle. The left ventricle of a female has about 10% less mass compared with that of a male.

Valves

The valves of the heart are structures through which blood is ejected either from one chamber to another or from a chamber into a blood vessel. The flow of blood in a healthy individual with competent valves is mostly unidirectional. When valves are diseased or *incompetent* (**incompetent valve**), forward blood flow is restricted, resulting in **regurgitation** (backflow) of blood into the chambers of the heart. Valves can also demonstrate **stenosis** if the valve does not open completely and creates a narrowed opening. Both *regurgitation* and *stenosis* are assessed as murmurs. Valves are classified by their location as either atrioventricular or semilunar.

Atrioventricular Valves The **atrioventricular (AV) valves**—the tricuspid and mitral (bicuspic) valves—separate the atria from the ventricles. The tricuspid valve lies between the right atrium and the right ventricle, whereas the thicker mitral (bicuspid) valve lies between the left atrium and left ventricle.

The AV valves open as a direct result of atrial contraction and the concomitant buildup of pressure within the atria. This pressure forces the valvular leaflets to open. When the ventricles contract, the increased ventricular pressure forces the valvular leaflets shut, thus preventing the blood from flowing back into the atria.

Semilunar Valves The **semilunar valves**—the pulmonary and aortic semilunar valves—separate the ventricles from the vascular system. The pulmonary semilunar valve (pulmonic valve) separates the right ventricle from the trunk of the pulmonary arteries, whereas the aortic semilunar valve (aortic valve) separates the left ventricle from the aorta.

The semilunar valves open in response to rising pressure within the contracting ventricles. When the pressure is great enough, the cusps open, allowing blood to be ejected into either the pulmonary trunk or the aorta. Upon relaxation of the ventricles, the valves close, allowing for ventricular filling and preventing backflow into the chambers.

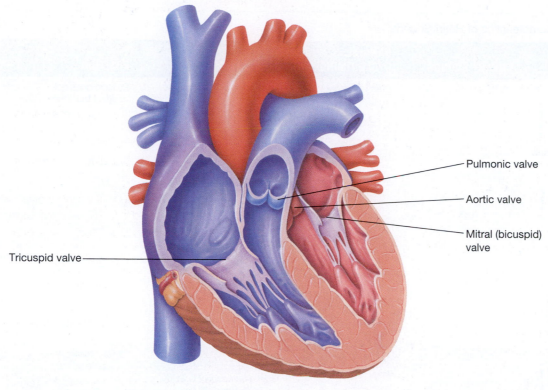

Figure 18.4 Valves of the heart.

Heart Sounds

Closure of the valves of the heart gives rise to heart sounds (see Figure 18.4 ■). Expected heart sounds include **S1** and **S2**. These are heard as the *lub-dub* of the heart when auscultated over the precordium, the area of the chest that lies over the heart. The first heart sound, S1 (*lub*), is heard when the AV valves close. Closure of these valves occurs when the ventricles have been filled. The second heart sound, S2 (*dub*), occurs when the aortic and pulmonic valves close. These semilunar valves close when the ventricles have emptied their blood into the aorta and pulmonary arteries.

The heart sounds are associated with the contraction and relaxation phases of the heart. **Systole** refers to the phase of ventricular contraction. In the systolic phase, the ventricles have been filled and then contract to expel blood into the aorta and pulmonary arteries. Systole begins with the closure of the AV valves (S1) and ends with the closure of the aortic and pulmonic valves (S2).

Diastole refers to the phase of ventricular relaxation. In the diastolic phase the ventricles relax and are filled as the atria contract. Diastole begins with the closure of the aortic and pulmonic valves (S2) and ends with the closure of the AV valves (S1) (see Figure 18.5 ■).

Splitting of S2 occurs toward the end of inspiration in some individuals. This results from a slight difference in the time in which the semilunar valves close. The increase in intrathoracic pressure during inspiration is a normal splitting of S2. The aortic valve closes just slightly faster than the pulmonic valve. As a result, a split sound is heard (instead of *dub*, one hears *t-dub*). The valves close at the same time during expiration, and the sound of S2 is *dub*.

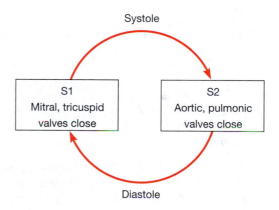

Figure 18.5 Heart sounds in systole and diastole.

Two other heart sounds that may be present in some healthy individuals are S3 and S4. S3 may be heard in children, in young adults, or in pregnant females in their third trimester. It is heard after S2 and is termed a *ventricular gallop*. When the AV valves open, blood flow into the ventricles may cause vibrations. These vibrations create the S3 sound during diastole. The S4 sound may also be heard in children, well-conditioned athletes, and even healthy elderly individuals without cardiac disease. It is caused by atrial contraction and ejection of blood into the ventricles in late diastole. S4 is heard before S1 and is termed an *atrial gallop*.

Heart sounds are interpreted according to the characteristics of pitch, duration, intensity, phase, and location on the precordium. Table 18.1 provides information about the characteristics of heart sounds.

Table 18.1 Characteristics of Heart Sounds

		HEART SOUNDS	CARDIAC CYCLE TIMING	AUSCULTATION SITE	POSITION	PITCH
S1 — LUB	S2 — dub	S1	Start of systole	Best at apex with diaphragm	Position does not affect the sound	High
S1 — lub	S2 — DUB	S2	End of systole	Both at 2nd ICS; pulmonary component best at LSB; aortic component best at RSB with diaphragm	Sitting or supine	High
S1 T	S2	Split S1	Beginning of systole	If normal, at 2nd ICS, LSB; abnormal if heard at apex	Better heard in the supine position	High
S1	S2	Fixed Split S2	End of systole	Both at 2nd ICS; pulmonary component best at LSB; aortic component best at RSB with diaphragm	Better heard in the supine position	High
S1	S2 P2A2	Expiration Paradoxical Split S2	End of systole	Both at 2nd ICS; pulmonary component best at LSB; aortic component best at RSB with diaphragm	Better heard in the supine position	High
S1 / S1	S2 / S2	Expiration Wide Split S2 Inspiration	End of systole	Both at 2nd ICS; pulmonary component best at LSB; aortic component best at RSB with diaphragm	Better heard in the supine position	High
S1	S2 S3	S3	Early diastole right after S2	Apex with the bell	Auscultated better in left lateral position or supine	Low
S4 S1	S2	S4	Late diastole right before S1	Apex with the bell	Auscultated in almost a left lateral position or supine	Low

ICS = Intercostal space. LSB = Left sternal border. RSB = Right sternal border.

Additional Heart Sounds

Although S3 and S4 sounds are sometimes heard in healthy individuals, they are more commonly associated with pathologic conditions such as myocardial infarction (MI) or heart failure. S3 occurs when the ventricle reaches its elastic limit, rapidly causing the blood flow from the atrium to slow. This may occur in the presence of systolic or diastolic ventricular dysfunction; ischemic heart disease; tricuspid, mitral, or aortic regurgitation; volume overload; and hypertension. Patients with heart failure who have S3 sounds often have a poor prognosis. S4 sounds are associated with active atrial contractions that cause late ventricular filling, such as occurs with ventricular hypertrophy, acute MI, angina, ventricular aneurysm, and hyperkinetic states (Mangla & Gupta, 2014).

The valves of the heart open quietly and without sound unless the tissue has been damaged. Clicks and snaps may be heard in patients with valvular disease. An opening snap may be heard in mitral stenosis. Ejection clicks occur in damaged pulmonic and aortic valves, and nonejection clicks are heard in prolapse of the mitral valve.

Friction rubs result from inflammation of the pericardial sac. The surfaces of the parietal and visceral layers of the pericardium cannot slide smoothly and thus produce the rubbing or grating sound. Table 18.2 includes information regarding interpretation of additional heart sounds.

Heart murmurs are harsh, blowing sounds caused by disruption of blood flow into the heart, between the chambers of the heart, or from the heart into the pulmonary or aortic systems. Methods to distinguish murmurs and classification of heart murmurs are provided in Table 18.3 and Table 18.4, respectively.

Coronary Arteries

The word *coronary* comes from the Latin word meaning "crown," which accurately describes this extensive network of arteries supplying the heart (see Figure 18.6A–B ■). The coronary arteries are visible initially on the external surface of the heart but descend deep into the myocardial tissue layers. Their function is to transport blood bringing nutrients and oxygen to the myocardial muscle. The coronary arteries fill during diastole.

The main coronary arteries are the left main coronary artery, the right coronary artery, the left anterior descending coronary artery, and the circumflex coronary artery. These arteries and those that branch from them may vary in size and configuration among individuals. The coronary arteries are located above the aortic valve. The right and left main coronary arteries originate from the aorta and then diverge to provide blood to different surfaces. Atherosclerotic plaque in these arteries as well as in their branches contributes significantly to the development of ischemic and injury processes and the potential for death.

Table 18.2 Additional Heart Sounds

CLICKS	HEART SOUNDS	CARDIAC CYCLE TIMING	AUSCULTATION SITE	POSITION	PITCH
	Aortic Click	Early systole	2nd ICS, RSB for aortic click and apex with diaphragm	Sitting or supine position may increase sound	High
	Pulmonic	Early systole	2nd ICS, LSB for pulmonic click with diaphragm	Sitting	High
	Opening Snap	Early diastole	3rd to 4th ICS, LSB with diaphragm	Sitting or supine position may increase the sound	High
	Friction Rub	Can occur at any time	Best heard with the diaphragm, location variable	May be heard in any position, but best when the patient sits forward	High, harsh in sound, grating

ICS = Intercostal space. LSB = Left sternal border.

Table 18.3 Distinguishing Heart Murmurs

ASK YOURSELF	INFORMATION
1. How loud is the murmur?	Murmurs are graded on a rather subjective scale of 1 to 6: • Grade 1: Barely audible with stethoscope, often considered physiologic, not pathologic. Requires concentration and a quiet environment. • Grade 2: Very soft but distinctly audible. • Grade 3: Moderately loud; there is no thrill or thrusting motion associated with the murmur. (**Thrills** are soft vibratory sensations best assessed with either the fingertips or the palm flattened on the chest.) • Grade 4: Distinctly loud, in addition to a palpable thrill. • Grade 5: Very loud, can actually hear with part of the diaphragm of the stethoscope off the chest; palpable thrust and thrill present. • Grade 6: Loudest, can hear with the diaphragm off the chest; visible thrill and thrust.
2. Where does it occur in the cardiac cycle: systole, diastole, or both?	Location in cardiac cycle: • Systole: early systole, midsystole, late systole • Diastole: early diastole, mid-diastole, late diastole • Both
3a. Is the sound continuous throughout systole, diastole, or only heard for part of the cycle?	Duration of murmur: • Continuous through systole only • Continuous through diastole only • Continuous through systole and diastole *Systolic murmurs* may be of two types: • Midsystolic: Murmur is heard after S1 and stops before S2. • Pansystolic/holosystolic: Murmur begins with S1 and stops at S2. *Diastolic murmurs* may be one of three types: • Early diastolic: Murmur auscultated immediately after S2 and then stops. There is a gap where this murmur stops and S1 is heard. • Mid-diastolic: Murmur begins a short time after S2 and stops well before S1 is auscultated. • Late diastolic: This murmur starts well after S2 and stops immediately before S1 is heard.
3b. What does the configuration of the sound look like? *Potential configurations:* S1 ▨▨▨▨ S2 **Pansystolic/holosystolic** S1 ▨▨▨ S2 ▨▨▨ S1 **Continuous** S2 ▨▨ S1 **Crescendo (Systolic represented)**	S2 ◁▨ S1 **Decrescendo (Diastolic represented)** S1 ◁▨▷ S2 **Crescendo Decrescendo (Systole represented)** S1 ▨▨ S2 **Rumble**
4. What is the quality of the sound of the murmur?	• Blowing • Harsh • Musical • Raspy • Rumbling

ASK YOURSELF	INFORMATION
5. What is the pitch or frequency of the sound?	• Low • Medium • High
6. In which landmark(s) do you best hear the murmur?	Use the five landmarks for auscultation: • Pulmonic areas 1 and 2 • Aortic area • Tricuspid area • Mitral area • Apex
7. Does it radiate?	• To the throat? • To the axilla?
8. Is there any change in pattern with respirations?	• Increases/decreases with inspiration • Increases/decreases with expiration
9. Is it associated with variations in heart sounds?	• Associated with split S1? • Associated with split S2? • Associated with S3? • Associated with S4? • Associated with a click or ejection sound?
10. Does intensity of murmur change with position?	• Increases/decreases with squatting? • Increases/decreases with patient in the left lateral position? (Do not have the patient perform the Valsalva maneuver or any abrupt positional changes because some patients do not tolerate position changes well.)

Table 18.4 Classifications of Heart Murmurs

MURMUR	CARDIAC CYCLE TIMING	AUSCULTATION SITE	CONFIGURATION OF SOUND	CONTINUITY
Aortic stenosis	Midsystolic	RSB, 2nd ICS	S1 — S2	Crescendo-decrescendo, continuous
Pulmonary stenosis	Midsystolic	LSB, 2nd to 3rd ICS	S1 — S2	Crescendo-decrescendo, continuous
Mitral regurgitation	Systole	Apex	S1 — S2	Holosystolic, continuous
Tricuspid regurgitation	Systole	4th ICS, LSB	S2 — S1	Holosystolic, continuous

RSB = Right sternal border. ICS = Intercostal space. LSB = Left sternal border. MCL = Midclavicular line.

(continued)

Table 18.4 Classifications of Heart Murmurs *(continued)*

MURMUR	CARDIAC CYCLE TIMING	AUSCULTATION SITE	CONFIGURATION OF SOUND	CONTINUITY
Mitral stenosis	Diastole	Apical	S1 ... S2	Rumble that increases in sound toward the end, continuous
Tricuspid stenosis	Diastole	Lower LSB	S2 ... S1	Rumble that increases in sound toward the end, continuous
Ventricular septal defect (left-to-right shunt)	Systole	3rd, 4th, 5th ICS, LSB	S1 ... S2	Holosystolic, continuous
Aortic regurgitation	Diastole (early)	3rd ICS, LSB	S2 ... S1	Decrescendo, continuous
Pulmonic regurgitation	Diastole (early)	3rd ICS, LSB	S2 ... S1	Decrescendo, continuous

MURMUR	QUALITY	PITCH	RADIATION	CHANGES WITH RESPIRATIONS
Aortic stenosis	Usually harsh, coarse	Medium	Most commonly into neck into carotid area and down LSB, possibly apex	Expiration may intensify the murmur
Pulmonary stenosis	Usually harsh	Medium	Toward the left upper neck and shoulder areas	Inspiration may intensify the murmur
Mitral regurgitation	Blowing and can be harsh in sound quality	High	Usually to left axilla, LSB, and base	Expiration may intensify the murmur
Tricuspid regurgitation	Blowing	High	May radiate to LSB and MCL but not to axilla	Inspiration may intensify the murmur
Mitral stenosis	Rumbling	Low and best heard with bell	Rare	Expiration may intensify the murmur
Tricuspid stenosis	Rumbling	Low	Rare	Inspiration may intensify the murmur
Ventricular septal defect (left-to-right shunt)	Harsh	High	May radiate across precordium but not to axilla	Expiration may intensify the murmur
Aortic regurgitation	Blowing	High, best auscultated with diaphragm unless patient is sitting up and leaning forward	May radiate to 2nd ICS, RSB and may proceed to apex	Expiration may intensify the murmur if the patient leans forward and sits up
Pulmonic regurgitation	Blowing	High, best auscultated with diaphragm	May radiate to 2nd ICS, RSB and may proceed to apex	Inspiration may intensify the murmur

RSB = Right sternal border. ICS = Intercostal space. LSB = Left sternal border. MCL = Midclavicular line.

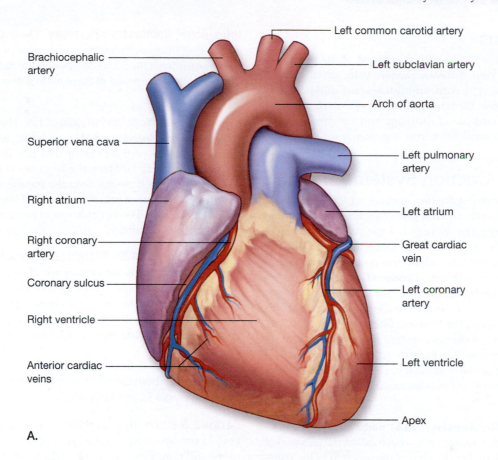

Left common carotid artery

Brachiocephalic artery

Left subclavian artery

Arch of aorta

Superior vena cava

Left pulmonary artery

Right atrium

Left atrium

Right coronary artery

Great cardiac vein

Coronary sulcus

Left coronary artery

Right ventricle

Anterior cardiac veins

Left ventricle

Apex

A.

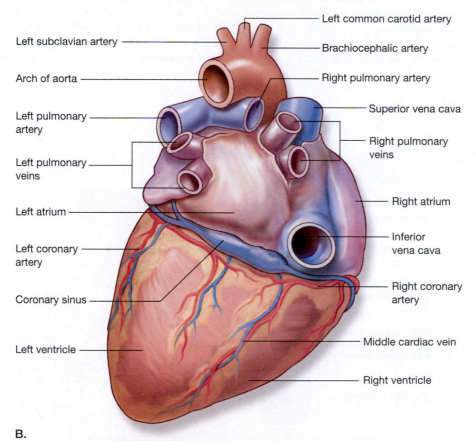

Left common carotid artery

Left subclavian artery

Brachiocephalic artery

Arch of aorta

Right pulmonary artery

Left pulmonary artery

Superior vena cava

Left pulmonary veins

Right pulmonary veins

Left atrium

Right atrium

Left coronary artery

Inferior vena cava

Coronary sinus

Right coronary artery

Left ventricle

Middle cardiac vein

Right ventricle

B.

Figure 18.6 Vessels of the heart. A. Anterior. B. Posterior.

Cardiac Veins

The venous system of the heart is composed of the great cardiac vein, oblique vein, anterior cardiac vein, small cardiac vein, middle cardiac vein, cordis minimae veins, and posterior cardiac vein. The great cardiac vein serves as the tributary for the majority of venous blood drainage and empties into the coronary sinus. The small venae cordis minimae drain into the cardiac chambers.

Cardiac Conduction System

The heart has its own conduction system, which can initiate an electrical charge and transmit that charge via cardiac muscle fibers throughout the myocardial tissue. This electrical charge stimulates the heart to contract, causing the propulsion of blood throughout the heart chambers and vascular system. The main structures of the **cardiac conduction system** are the sinoatrial node (SA node), the intra-atrial conducting pathways, the atrioventricular (AV) node, the bundle of His, the right and left bundle branches, and the Purkinje fibers (see Figure 18.7 ■). Because the cardiac conduction system relies on muscle contraction, it is very susceptible to dysregulation during electrolyte imbalances, particularly imbalances in calcium, potassium, and sodium. Therefore, electrolytes are an integral part of normal cardiac function.

Sinoatrial Node The **sinoatrial (SA) node** initiates the electrical impulse. For this reason, it has been called the pacemaker of the heart. The SA node is located at the junction of the superior vena cava and right atrium. The autonomic nervous system feeds into the SA node and can influence it to either speed up or slow down the discharge of electrical current. In the healthy individual, the SA node discharges an average of 60 to 100 times a minute.

Intra-Atrial Conduction Pathway These loosely organized conducting fibers assist in the propagation of the electrical current emitted from the SA node through the right and left atrium. The network is composed of three main pathways: anterior, middle, and posterior.

Atrioventricular Node and Bundle of His The **atrioventricular (AV) node** and **bundle of His** are intricately connected and function to receive the current that has finished spreading throughout the atria. Here the impulse is slowed for about 0.1 second before it passes onto the bundle branches. The AV node is also capable of initiating electrical impulses in the event of SA node failure. The intrinsic rate of firing is slower and averages about 60 per minute.

Right and Left Bundle Branches and Purkinje Fibers The right and left **bundle branches** are like expressways of conducting fibers that spread the electrical current through the ventricular myocardial tissue. Arising from the right and left bundle branches are the **Purkinje fibers**. These fibers fan out and penetrate into the myocardial tissue to spread the current into the tissues.

The bundle branches are also capable of initiating electrical charges in case both the SA node and AV node fail. Their intrinsic rate averages 40 to 60 per minute.

Cardiac Nerves Just as there is an extensive network of vessels transporting oxygen and nutrients to the myocardial tissue and removing waste products, an equally important network of autonomic nerves is present. Both sympathetic nervous fibers and parasympathetic nervous fibers interact with the myocardial tissue. The sympathetic fibers stimulate the heart, increasing the heart rate, force of contraction, and dilation of the coronary arteries. Conversely, the parasympathetic

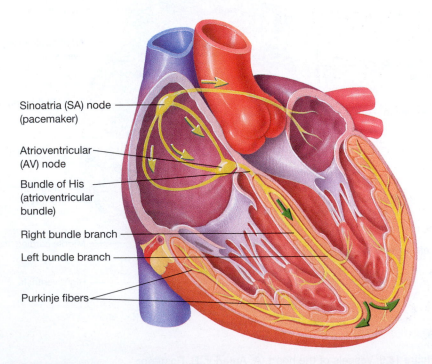

Sinoatria (SA) node (pacemaker)

Atrioventricular (AV) node

Bundle of His (atrioventricular bundle)

Right bundle branch

Left bundle branch

Purkinje fibers

Figure 18.7 Conduction system of the heart.

fibers, such as the vagus nerve, exercise the opposite effect. The central nervous system influences the activation and interaction of these nerves through the information supplied by the cardiac plexus.

Pulmonary Circulation

The vessels of the pulmonary circulation include arteries, veins, and an expansive network of pulmonary capillaries. This vascular system carries deoxygenated blood to the lungs, where carbon dioxide is exchanged for oxygen. Deoxygenated blood from the veins of the body enters this network by passing into the right atrium. It is then ejected through the tricuspid valve into the right ventricle and passes through the pulmonic valve into the pulmonary artery and pulmonary circulation. The pulmonary artery is the only artery to carry unoxygenated blood. After going through the pulmonary capillary network, oxygenated blood returns to the left atrium via the pulmonary veins (see Figure 18.8 ■). Pulmonary veins are the only veins to carry oxygenated blood.

Systemic Circulation

The vessels of the systemic circulation also include arteries, veins, and capillaries. This vascular system supplies freshly oxygenated blood to the body's periphery and returns deoxygenated blood to the pulmonary circuit. The arteries of the systemic circulation are composed of elastic tissue and smooth muscle, which allows their walls to stretch during systole. During systole, the elasticity of the walls propels the blood forward into the systemic circulation. The left ventricle propels freshly oxygenated blood into the aorta. As the blood moves toward the body periphery, the major arteries of the body subdivide into arterioles, which carry the nutrients and oxygen to the smallest blood vessels of the body, the capillaries. Oxygen and nutrients are exchanged in the capillaries for carbon dioxide and metabolites, which are then carried into the venules, then veins, and finally the superior and inferior venae cavae, which carry the deoxygenated blood into the right atrium of the heart (see Figure 18.8).

Landmarks for Cardiovascular Assessment

Landmarks for assessing the cardiovascular system include the sternum, clavicles, ribs, and intercostal spaces. By correlating assessment findings with the overlying body landmarks, the nurse may gain vital information concerning underlying pathologic mechanisms. Many landmarks identified during the respiratory assessment also are used when performing a cardiac assessment. These include but are not limited to the sternum and the second through fifth intercostal spaces. It may be helpful to review the landmarks in Chapter 16 before proceeding. ∞

The **sternum** is the flat, narrow center bone of the upper anterior chest (see Figure 18.9 ■). There are three portions of the adult sternum. The upper sternum is called the manubrium, the middle part is the body, and the inferior piece is the xiphoid process. The average sternal length in an adult is 18 cm (7 in.). During cardiovascular assessment, the sternum is used as a vertical landmark, and the angle of Louis is used to locate the second intercostal space.

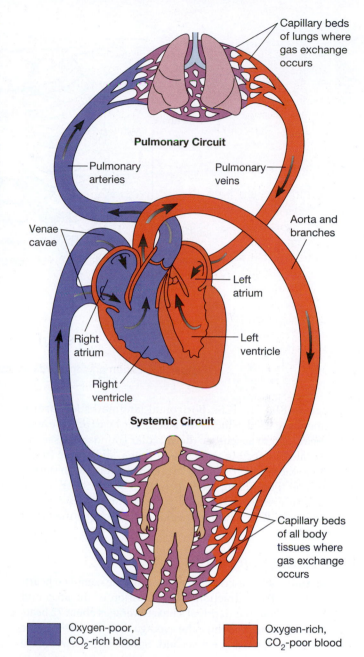

Figure 18.8 Pulmonary and systemic circulation. The left side of the heart pumps oxygenated blood (indicated in red) into the arteries of the systemic circulation, which provides oxygen and nutrients to the cells. Deoxygenated blood (indicated in blue) returns via the venous system into the right side of the heart, where it is transported to the pulmonary arterial system to be reoxygenated.

The clavicles are bones that attach at the top of the manubrium of the sternum above the first rib (see Figure 18.9). The left midclavicular line (LMCL) is used as a landmark for cardiovascular assessment.

The ribs are flat, arched bones that form the thoracic cage. There are 12 pairs of ribs. Between each rib is an intercostal space (ICS). The first ICS lies between the first and the second rib, and each remaining ICS is numbered successively

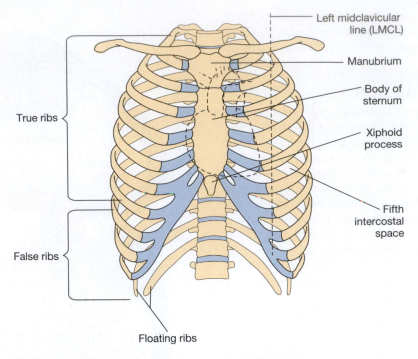

Figure 18.9 Landmarks for cardiovascular assessment.

(see Figure 18.9). The ICSs, horizontal landmarks for cardiac assessment, are used to locate the base of the heart and the apex of the heart and to auscultate the valvular sounds. The second ICS is located by feeling the angle of Louis, sliding the finger laterally to the second rib at the left (LSB) or right (RSB) sternal borders, and then sliding the finger down below the rib to the ICS. Each succeeding ICS is located by sliding the finger over the rib into the ICS. Additional landmarks are identified later in this chapter.

Cardiac Cycle

The **cardiac cycle** describes the events of one complete heartbeat—that is, the contraction and relaxation of the atria and ventricles. A healthy individual's heart averages about 72 beats per minute (beats/min); thus, the average time for each cardiac cycle to be completed is 0.8 second. Synchrony between the

mechanical and electrical events of the cycle is imperative. Any interruption in this balance affects the ability of the heart to provide oxygen and nutrients to the body. Significant disruptions in synchrony can be fatal.

Electrical and Mechanical Events The cardiac cycle can be divided into three periods (see Figure 18.10 ■): the period of ventricular filling, ventricular systole, and isovolumetric relaxation.

PERIOD OF VENTRICULAR FILLING This is the start of the cardiac cycle. Blood enters passively into the ventricles from the atria. About 70% of the blood that eventually ends up in the ventricles enters at this time. As this blood is entering the ventricles, the atria are stimulated to contract by the electrical current emanating from the SA node. Another 30% volume of blood exits the atria into the ventricles. This extra 30% volume is termed the *atrial kick.*

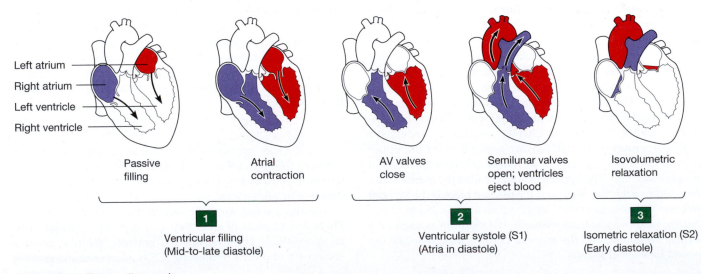

Figure 18.10 The cardiac cycle.

VENTRICULAR SYSTOLE The electrical current stimulates the ventricles, and they respond by contracting. The force of contraction increases the pressure within both ventricles. The mitral and tricuspid valves respond to this increased pressure by snapping shut (S1). The ventricular pressure continues to increase until it causes the aortic and pulmonic valves to open. Blood rushes out of the ventricles into the systemic and pulmonary circulation.

ISOVOLUMETRIC RELAXATION Once the majority of blood is ejected, the pressure in the aorta and pulmonary artery becomes higher than in the ventricles, causing the aortic and pulmonic valves to shut (S2). During ventricular systole, the atria have been filling with blood returning from the systemic and pulmonary circulation. When the pressure in the atria becomes higher than in the ventricles, the mitral and tricuspid valves open, and the cycle begins again.

Electrical Representation of the Cardiac Cycle Electrical representations of the cardiac cycle are documented by deflections on recording paper. A straight horizontal line means the absence of electrical activity. Deflections representing the flow of electrical current toward or away from an electrode record the timing of the electrical events in the cardiac cycle. The terms describing the electrical deflections are *P wave*, *PR interval*, *QRS complex*, and *T wave*. They are recorded as an **electrocardiogram (ECG)** (see Figure 18.11 ■). When the cardiac cell is in a resting state, it is more positively charged on the outside of the cell and more negatively charged on the inside of the cell. This spread of electrical current, called *depolarization*, causes the inside of the cardiac cell to become more positively charged. Depolarization occurs when the electrical current normally initiated in the SA

node spreads across the atria. Contraction of the atria follows after stimulation by the electrical current. After contraction, the cardiac cells experience *repolarization*, during which the inside of the cell returns to its more negatively charged state. The same process occurs in the ventricles.

P WAVE The P wave represents part of atrial depolarization. The pacemaker of the heart, the SA node, emits an electrical charge that initially spreads throughout the right and left atria. As a result of the electrical stimulation, the myocardial cells contract. The initial P wave deflection is caused by the initiation of the electrical current and atrial response to the current. It lasts an average 0.08 second.

PR INTERVAL The PR interval represents the time needed for the electrical current to travel across both atria and arrive at the AV node. The normal PR interval averages 0.12 to 0.20 second.

QRS COMPLEX The QRS complex represents ventricular depolarization. Atrial repolarization is hidden in the QRS complex. The ventricular myocardial cells also respond to the spread of electrical current by becoming more positively charged. This change in polarity is ventricular depolarization. The QRS complex should range from 0.08 to 0.11 second.

T WAVE The T wave represents ventricular repolarization. Once the ventricular myocardial cells have been stimulated by the electrical current and contract, they return to their original electrical potential state. This change in polarity is repolarization. The atria also repolarize, but that is not recorded because it occurs at the same time as ventricular repolarization; therefore, the QRS complex covers it.

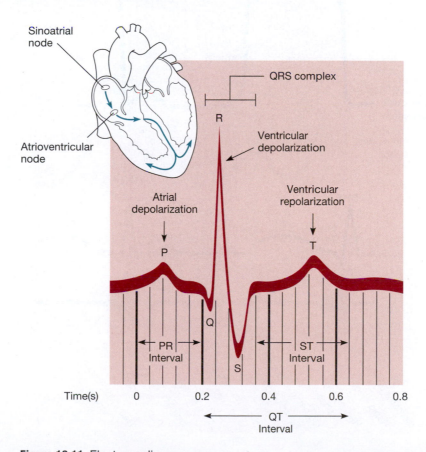

Figure 18.11 Electrocardiogram wave.

QT INTERVAL The QT interval represents the period from the beginning of ventricular depolarization to the moment of repolarization. Thus, it represents ventricular contraction. Electrical events in the heart occur slightly ahead of the mechanical events. Figure 18.12 ■ illustrates the events of the cardiac cycle in relation to heart sounds, pressure waves, and the ECG.

Measurements of Cardiac Function

When the heart is functioning at optimal level, the synchrony of the events of the cardiac cycle produces an outflow of blood with oxygen and nutrients to every cell in the body. The terms that describe the effectiveness of the action of the cardiac cycle are *stroke volume*, *cardiac output*, and *cardiac index*.

Stroke volume describes the amount of blood that is ejected with every heartbeat. Normal stroke volume is 55 to 100 mL/beat. The formula for calculating stroke volume is:

Stroke Volume = Cardiac Output/Heart Rate

Cardiac output describes the amount of blood ejected from the left ventricle over 1 minute. Normal adult cardiac output is 4 to 8 L/min. The following is the formula for calculating cardiac output:

Cardiac Output = Stroke Volume × Heart Rate

The cardiac index is a valuable diagnostic measurement of the effectiveness of the pumping action of the heart. The cardiac index takes into consideration the individual's weight, which is a significant factor in judging the effectiveness of the pumping action. For example, suppose a cardiac output of 4 L/min is obtained for two patients: an elderly female who weighs 60 kg (132.3 lb) and a middle-aged male who weighs 130 kg (286.6 lb). The elderly female's cardiac index is significantly higher than that of the male, whose pumping effectiveness is significantly compromised. The formula for calculating cardiac index is:

Cardiac Index = Cardiac Output/Body Surface Area

The body surface area (BSA) measurement is obtained and determined from published tables.

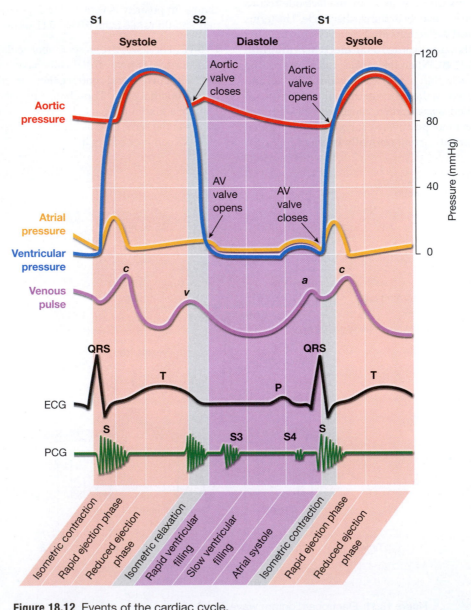

Figure 18.12 Events of the cardiac cycle.

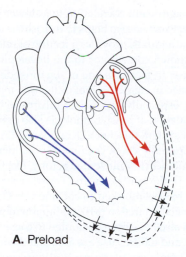

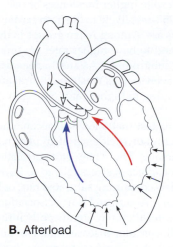

A. Preload

B. Afterload

Figure 18.13 A. Preload is related to the amount of blood and stretching of the ventricular myocardial fibers. B. Afterload is the pressure that the ventricles must overcome in order to open the aortic and pulmonic valvular cusps.

There are two strong influences on pumping action: preload and afterload. Preload is influenced by the volume of the blood in the ventricles and relates to the length of ventricular fiber stretch at the end of diastole. The Frank-Starling law states that an increasingly greater contractile ability is provided with greater stretching of the ventricular muscle fibers. Thus, the greater the stretch, the greater the contractile force, and the greater the volume of blood ejected with each contraction. Afterload is the amount of stress or tension present in the ventricular wall during systole. It is interrelated to the pressure in the aorta because the pressure in the ventricular wall must be greater than that in the aorta and pulmonary trunk for the semilunar valves to open (Marieb, 2015). (See Figure 18.13A–B ■).

Special Considerations

Many factors influence the patient's health status. Among these are age, developmental level, race, ethnicity, work history, living conditions, socioeconomics, and emotional well-being. Each of the factors must be addressed while gathering subjective and objective data during a comprehensive health assessment.

Health Promotion Considerations

Goals related to cardiovascular health are focused on prevention, early diagnosis, and reduction of risk factors. By asking appropriate questions during the focused interview, the nurse uncovers clues to the patient's health status and any cardiovascular problems. Assessment of the patient's psychosocial and physical health, self-care habits, culture, ethnicity, and environment are important aspects of health promotion. Enhancing public awareness and screening of risk factors is important to help reduce mortalities from heart disease and stroke. The health of the cardiovascular system may be promoted throughout the lifespan by means of self-care habits such as eating a low-fat diet, exercising, and not smoking. The nurse plays a key role in teaching the healthy patient the facts about preventing cardiovascular disease. For the patient with cardiovascular disease, the nurse provides teaching to promote optimum health according to the patient's individual needs.

Lifespan Considerations

Growth and development are dynamic processes that describe change over time. The collection of data and the interpretation of findings in relation to normative values are important. Developmental factors are considered during assessment of the cardiac system. For example, newborns have a higher heart rate than adults. In pregnant patients, as the uterus enlarges, the heart is displaced to the left and upward, and the apex is pushed laterally and to the left. See Chapter 25, Chapter 26, and Chapter 27 for more lifespan considerations. ∞

Psychosocial Considerations

Stress causes an individual to experience longer periods of sympathetic stimulation, which increases the workload on the heart. Systemic vascular resistance may be elevated for longer periods, especially in situations of excessive stress. Counseling, relaxation, yoga, meditation, and biofeedback techniques are usually helpful to reduce stress level (Hagstrom et al., 2018).

Cultural and Environmental Considerations

In the United States adults, regardless of race or ethnicity, are more likely to die from heart disease than any other cause. It is important to recognize that racial and ethnic differences are present and that much of the overall risk comes from environmental influences on health. Some differences in risk of cardiovascular disease do exist among certain groups of people, and the risks appear to come from higher incidences of high blood pressure, diabetes, and obesity when compared with Caucasians (Harvard Heart Letter, 2015).

Nearly half of all African American adults have some type of cardiovascular disease, compared with about one-third of Caucasians. African Americans are genetically predisposed to high blood pressure; there appears to be a genetic predisposition to being sensitive to salt, leading to more sodium retention, which in turn leads to an elevation in blood pressure. Hispanics and Latinos have a higher risk of cardiovascular disease than Caucasians do because of higher rates of the risk factors of obesity and diabetes; despite higher incidences of risk factors, they are approximately 25% less likely to die from cardiovascular disease than Caucasians are. Among Asian groups in the United States, South Asians tend to have higher rates of coronary artery disease than other subgroups of Asians. Increases in all subgroups of Asians have been seen as Western cultural and diet practices are adopted, leading to higher rates of obesity (Harvard Heart Letter, 2015).

Some data suggest that a low socioeconomic bracket is correlated with a higher incidence of hypertension, especially among adult females. There may be a correlation between this situation and the effect of stress related to lower incomes, limited exercise, diets containing saturated fats, or lack of access to quality healthcare (American Heart Association [AHA], 2017).

Diet is one factor that may significantly influence the development of cardiovascular disease. Intake of fat, especially saturated fat, contributes significantly to cardiovascular disease. *Couch potato* is a popular term that describes a lifestyle of inactivity. Studies on individuals who perform continuous aerobic exercise for at least 30 to 45 minutes at least three times a week have shown a significant correlation to a slower progression of atherosclerosis. Exercise also helps to diffuse the effects of stress and, in most individuals, provides a feeling of relaxation. Smoking is a well-known contributor to the development of cardiovascular disease. In fact, it is one of the most devastating. The chemicals inhaled in cigarette smoke alter and injure the linings of the arteries, especially in areas of bifurcation (division into branches). Inhalation of passive smoke is also detrimental to the cardiovascular system (Fischer & Kraemer, 2015).

Cocaine, especially crack cocaine, causes increased oxygen demands on the heart. Ventricular ectopy, electrical impulses that originate in the ventricles and cause early contraction of the ventricles, has been linked to cocaine use. Coronary artery spasm, myocardial infarction (MI), malignant hypertension, and ruptured aorta also have been attributed to cocaine (AHA, 2017).

Alcoholism and tobacco use are associated with the development of many cardiovascular complications, such as cardiomyopathy and coronary artery disease. Alcohol consumption may also cause ventricular ectopy, which contributes to decreased cardiac output and may be life threatening (AHA, 2017).

Subjective Data—Health History

Cardiovascular assessment includes the gathering of subjective and objective data. Subjective data collection occurs during the patient interview, before the actual physical assessment. During the interview, the nurse uses a variety of communication techniques to elicit general and specific information about the patient's state of cardiovascular health or illness. Health records, the results of laboratory tests, cardiograms, and other tests are important secondary sources to be reviewed and included in the data-gathering process. See Table 18.5 for information on potential secondary sources of patient data.

Focused Interview

The focused interview for the cardiovascular system concerns data related to the structures and functions of that system. Subjective data related to cardiac status are gathered during the focused interview. The nurse must be prepared to observe the patient and listen for cues related to the function of the cardiovascular system. The nurse may use open-ended and closed questions to obtain information. Often a number of follow-up questions or requests for descriptions are required to clarify data or gather missing information.

The focused interview guides the physical assessment of the cardiovascular system. The information is always considered in relation to normal parameters and expectations about cardiovascular function. Therefore, the nurse must consider age, gender, race, culture, environment, health practices, past and concurrent problems, and therapies when framing questions and using techniques to elicit information. Categories of questions related to cardiovascular status and function have been developed to address all of the factors when conducting a focused interview. These categories include general questions that are asked of all patients; those addressing illness and infection; questions related to symptoms, pain, and behaviors; those related to habits or practices; questions that are specific to patients according to age; those for the pregnant female;

Table 18.5 Potential Secondary Sources for Patient Data Related to the Cardiovascular System

LABORATORY TESTS	NORMAL VALUE
Cholesterol	< 200 mg/dL
Triglycerides	< 150 mg/dL
HDL (high-density lipoprotein)	> 60 mg/dL
LDL (low-density lipoprotein)	< 50 mg/dL
CPK (creatinine phosphokinase)	Males: 52–336 Units/L Females: 38–176 Units/L
CPK-MB	0–3 mcg/mL
Myoglobin	≤ 90 mcg/mL
Troponin I	< 0.04 nanogram/mL
LDH	122–222 Units/L
SGOT	Males: 8–48 Units/L Females: 8–43 Units/L
DIAGNOSTIC TESTS	
Cardiac Catheterization	
Echocardiography	
Electrocardiography	
Electrophysiologic Testing	
Exercise Stress Test	
Holter Monitor	

and questions that address internal and external environmental concerns. One approach to questioning about symptoms is the OLDCART & ICE method, which is described in Chapter 5. ∞ See Figure 5.3.

As these questions are asked and subjective data are obtained during the focused interview, the data will be used to help determine if the patient's lifestyle will help to improve their cardiovascular health and decrease their risk for developing cardiovascular disease. The nurse must consider the patient's ability to participate in the focused interview and physical assessment of the cardiovascular system. If a patient is experiencing pain, dyspnea, cyanosis, difficulty with speech, and the anxiety that accompanies any of these problems, attention must focus on relief of symptoms and improvement of oxygenation.

Focused Interview Questions	Rationales and Evidence

The following section provides sample questions and bulleted follow-up questions in each of the previously mentioned categories. A rationale for each of the questions is provided. The list of questions is not all-inclusive but represents the types of questions required in a comprehensive focused interview related to the cardiovascular system.

General Questions

1. **Describe how you are feeling. Has your sense of well-being changed in the last 2 months? Is your sense of well-being different than it was 2 years ago?**
   * Describe the change.
   * How long have you experienced the change?
   * Do you know what caused the change?
   * Have you seen a healthcare provider?
   * Was a diagnosis made?
   * Was treatment prescribed?
   * What have you done to deal with the change?

   ▶ This question gives patients the opportunity to provide their own perceptions about their health. Statements about fatigue, weakness, dizziness, or shortness of breath, especially after activity, may indicate problems with cardiovascular health.

2. **Are you able to perform all of the activities needed to meet your personal and work-related responsibilities?**
   * Describe the changes in your abilities.
   * Do you know what is causing the difficulty?
   * How long have you had this problem?
   * What have you done about the problem?
   * Have you discussed this with a healthcare professional?

   ▶ Inability to carry out or perform personal or work-related activities can be indicative of problems in the cardiovascular system.

3. **Is there anyone in your family who has had a cardiovascular problem or disease?**
   * What is the disease or problem?
   * Who in the family now has or has ever had the problem?
   * When was it diagnosed?
   * How has the problem been treated?
   * What was the outcome?

   ▶ This may reveal information about cardiovascular diseases associated with familial predisposition. Follow-up is required to obtain details about specific problems, occurrence, treatment, and outcomes.

4. **What is your weight? Have you experienced a change in your weight?**
   * How much weight have you gained or lost?
   * Over what period of time did the change occur?
   * Do you know what caused the change?
   * Have you done anything to address the change in your weight?
   * Have you discussed the change with a healthcare provider?

   ▶ Obesity and a high percentage of body fat are risk factors for cardiovascular disease. Weight gain or loss may accompany physical problems, including systemic diseases such as diabetes, which increases risk for cardiovascular disease. Psychosocial problems, including stress, can affect weight gain or loss and also contribute to cardiovascular problems (AHA, 2017).

Questions Related to Illness

1. **Have you ever been diagnosed with a cardiovascular disease?**
   * When were you diagnosed with the problem?
   * What treatment was prescribed for the problem?
   * Was the treatment helpful?
   * Describe things you have done or currently do to cope with the problem?
   * Has the problem ever recurred (acute)?
   * How are you managing the problem now (chronic)?

   ▶ The patient has an opportunity to provide information about specific cardiovascular illnesses. If a diagnosed illness is identified, follow-up about the date of diagnosis, treatment, and outcomes is required. Data about each illness identified by the patient are essential to an accurate health assessment.
   ▶ Illnesses can be classified as acute or chronic, and follow-up regarding each classification will differ.

2. ***Alternative to question 1:*** List possible cardiovascular problems, such as MI, congestive heart failure, arteriosclerosis, coronary artery disease, angina, arrhythmia, and valvular disease, and ask the patient to respond "yes" or "no" as each is stated.

   ▶ This is a comprehensive and easy way to elicit information about all diagnoses. Follow-up would be carried out for each identified diagnosis as in question 1.

3. **Do you now have or have you ever had an infection or viral illness affecting the cardiovascular system?**
   * When were you diagnosed with the infection?
   * What treatment was prescribed?
   * Has the treatment helped?
   * What kind of things do you do to help with the problem?
   * Has the infection recurred (acute)?
   * How are you managing the problem now (chronic)?

   ▶ If an infection is identified, follow-up about the date of infection, treatment, and outcome is required.

4. *Alternative to question 3:* List possible infections, such as rheumatic fever, viral illness, endocarditis, and pericarditis, and ask the patient to respond "yes" or "no" as each is stated.

5. **Have you ever had a diagnostic test, such as an electrocardiogram, stress test, echocardiogram, or a surgical procedure for a cardiovascular problem?**

6. *Alternative to question 5:* List possible surgical procedures, such as coronary artery bypass graft, angioplasty, pacemaker insertion, insertion of a defibrillator, and valve replacement, and ask the patient to respond "yes" or "no" as each is stated.

7. **Do you have hypertension, diabetes, or thyroid disorders?**

8. **Do you know your cholesterol and triglyceride levels?**

▶ This is a comprehensive and easy way to elicit information about all infections related to the cardiovascular system. Follow-up would be required as in question 3.

▶ The patient has the opportunity to provide information about diagnostic testing or surgical procedures related to cardiovascular problems. If a surgical procedure is identified, follow-up about the date of surgery, outcome, and effectiveness is required.

▶ This is a comprehensive and easy way to elicit information about surgeries. Follow-up would be required as in question 5.

▶ Medical conditions such as diabetes, hypertension, or thyroid dysfunction can contribute to cardiovascular problems (Berman & Snyder, 2016).

▶ Elevated cholesterol and triglyceride levels are associated with cardiovascular disease (AHA, 2017).

Questions Related to Symptoms or Behaviors

When gathering information about symptoms, many questions are required to elicit details and descriptions that assist in the analysis of the data. Discrimination is implemented in relation to the significance of a symptom, in relation to specific diseases or problems, and in relation to potential follow-up examination or referral. One rationale may be provided for a group of questions in this category.

The following questions refer to specific symptoms and behaviors associated with the cardiovascular system. For each symptom, questions and follow-up are required. The details to be elicited are the characteristics of the symptom; the onset, duration, and frequency of the symptom; the treatment or remedy for the symptom, including over-the-counter and home remedies; the determination if diagnosis has been sought; the effect of treatments; and family history associated with a symptom or illness.

Questions Related to Symptoms

1. **Have you experienced any symptoms that may suggest the presence of cardiovascular disease: activity intolerance, loss of appetite, bloody sputum (mucus), changes in sexual activities or performance, confusion or difficulty with thinking or concentrating, chest discomfort, coughing, dizziness, dyspnea (difficulty breathing), fatigue, fever, hoarseness, frequent urination at night, leg pains after activity, sleeping pattern alteration, syncope (fainting), palpitations, or swelling?**

2. **Does a change in position increase, decrease, or do nothing to change the symptoms?**
   • Can you identify precipitating factors for the symptoms?

3. **Describe the quality of the symptom.**
   • Does it feel sharp, dull, or like pressure, piercing, or ripping?

4. **Does the feeling radiate to other parts of the body?**

5. **Where do you feel the symptom on the body?**

▶ For any of these symptoms, the nurse should gather objective information on the specific characteristics and ask patients to describe their own subjective experience. If the nurse prompts the patient, valuable clues may be missed.

▶ The nurse should look for activity, emotion, stress, or drugs as a precipitating factor. However, heart symptoms may have no precipitating factors.

▶ The description of the quality offers clues to the potential origin of the disease, especially when chest discomfort is present.

▶ Radiation of pain may occur with chest discomfort.

▶ If the symptom or one of the symptoms is chest discomfort, the patient should be asked to show the nurse the location on the body. Often, the patient identifies chest discomfort of cardiac origin by placing a clenched fist over the precordium. When the patient points one or more fingers to a limited area on the chest wall, it is generally more indicative of pain with a pulmonary or muscular origin. Females may experience less severe cardiac pain over the precordium, back pain, or fatigue. Angina pectoris—oppressive chest pain caused by decreased oxygenation of the myocardium—is typical in patients with coronary artery disease. Females with angina often experience "atypical" symptoms, including burning or tenderness to touch in the back, shoulder, or jaw, and may have no chest discomfort (Mayo Clinic, 2013). In MI, the loss of myocardium because of coronary artery occlusion produces the following typical symptoms in males: prolonged, dull chest pain radiating to the shoulder or jaw accompanied by diaphoresis; shortness of breath; and nausea. Females may experience nausea and vomiting, indigestion, shortness of breath or extreme fatigue, with no chest pain (Mayo Clinic, 2013).

6. **What relieves the symptoms?**

7. **Rate the severity of the symptoms on a scale of 0 to 10, with 1 being hardly noticeable and 10 being the worst discomfort you have ever experienced.**
   - What is the timing of the symptoms?
   - Is the timing predictable?
   - What is the duration of the symptoms?
   - Is it constant during that time or does it wax and wane?
   - Are the symptoms isolated or do they occur in combinations?
   - Have you seen your healthcare provider about these symptoms?
   - What is being done for these symptoms?

▶ This technique leaves out the nurse's opinion on the degree of discomfort.

Questions Related to Behaviors

1. **Describe your diet.**
   - What types of food do you eat? How often? How much?

▶ Diet is one of the key interventions that a patient can control when working to minimize the effects of aging, slow the progression of disease, or maintain optimum health while experiencing cardiac disease (AHA, 2015). Supplementing the diet with vitamins under proper supervision may be beneficial. Unfortunately, without proper supervision, the patient who is poorly informed may ingest an unbalanced proportion of supplements and compromise a healthy state. The nurse must be alert if the patient has been dieting to reduce weight. Many diets deplete valuable electrolytes and subject the patient to potential complications. Muscle wasting may occur if the diet is deficient in protein. Lack of protein may compromise cardiac function (Osborn, Wraa, Watson, & Holleran, 2013).

2. **Do you keep track of the amount of fat, protein, and carbohydrates you eat?**

3. **Do you know the difference between saturated and unsaturated fat?**
   - How much daily fiber do you consume?

4. **Do you add salt or other flavor enhancers to your food? If so, how much and how often?**
   - Do you taste the food before adding these flavor enhancers?

▶ Awareness of nutrient intake will help determine if patients need to alter their diet to include healthier foods. Knowledge of proper nutrition, the difference between types of fats, and the harmful effects of too much salt will determine how much patient education is needed in the area of nutrition. The nurse may need to refer the patient to a nutrition specialist or dietitian.

5. **Do you eat differently when you travel, when at social functions, when under stress, or when on vacation?**

6. **Have you tried to lose weight? If so, describe the type of diet, the duration of the diet, and any diet supplements you take.**
   - Do you diet under the care of a healthcare provider?
   - Do you supplement your diet with vitamins, protein supplements, or antioxidants?
   - Do you use weight-loss supplements or medications?
   - What type of nonalcoholic liquids do you drink? How much, and how often?
   - Do you exercise to lose weight?

7. **Do you smoke or are you frequently exposed to secondhand smoke?**
   - If you smoke, what type of product (cigarette, cigar, pipe) do you use?
   - How long have you smoked?
   - How many packs per day and what brand?
   - If you are exposed to secondhand smoke, where and for how long each day?
   - Did you ever smoke? When did you quit?

▶ Smoking has been linked to hypertension and is strongly suspected of contributing to injury in the walls of arteries, thus accelerating the development of atherosclerotic plaques. It is believed that the chemical contained in the cigarette smoke injures the inner wall of arterial vessels, thus contributing to the subsequent development of a coronary artery plaque (AHA, 2017).

8. **Do you take any drugs such as cocaine?**
   - If so, describe the type, amount, frequency, and duration of use.
   - Do you drink alcohol? If so, describe the type, amount, frequency, and duration of use.

▶ Substance abuse, especially of cocaine, is associated with coronary artery spasm and potential development of ischemia or injury of myocardial tissue (Katikaneni, Akkus, Tandon, & Modi, 2013).

9. **Do you exercise? What type of exercise do you perform?**
   - How many times a week?
   - What is the duration of exercise?
   - The intensity?
   - What is your total exercising time?
   - Is the exercise continuous or interspersed with breaks?
   - What amount of aerobic exercise versus nonaerobic do you do?
   - Do you exercise with a partner or alone? Is the exercise pattern regular or sporadic?
   - What is your understanding about the benefits of exercise and the type of exercise selected?
   - What was your reason for choosing the specific exercise routines and patterns?
   - Is your exercise tolerance increasing, staying the same, or decreasing?
   - If it is decreasing, how has the tolerance decreased?
   - What were you able to do before versus what you are able to do now?
   - How rapidly has this change occurred?
   - What symptoms contribute to the decreased tolerance?
   - Do you know the causes of the decreased tolerance?

▶ The benefits of exercise are well documented, yet the type, duration, and frequency of the exercise regimen produce variable results. It is important for the patient to have a basic understanding of the benefits of aerobic versus nonaerobic exercise. One is not better than the other, and, ultimately, a blending of routines is invaluable whether the patient is a well-conditioned athlete or an individual trying to stay healthy. Studies suggest that both aerobic exercise and resistance or weight training may increase high-density lipoprotein (HDL) levels in adults (AHA, 2017).

Questions Related to Age and Pregnancy

The focused interview must reflect the anatomic and physiologic differences in the cardiovascular system that exist along the lifespan as well as during pregnancy. Specific questions related to the cardiovascular system for each of these groups are provided in Chapter 25, Chapter 26, and Chapter 27. ∞

Questions Related to the Environment

Environment refers to both the internal and external environments. Questions related to the internal environment include all of the previous questions and those associated with internal or physiologic responses. Questions regarding the external environment include those related to home, work, or social environments.

Internal Environment

1. **What medications do you take?**
   - Are they prescribed or self-ordered?
   - What are the dose and brand of each medication?
   - How often do you take them?

   ▶ It is important to assess the patient's knowledge, compliance, and ability to administer medication accurately, whether ordered by a physician or not. Medication actions may vary depending on the mix of medications; diet; and vitamins, herbs, or dietary supplements.

2. **Why do you take these drugs?**

3. **Do you take these medications as prescribed?**
   - If you miss a dose, do you double up the next time?

4. **Who ordered these medications?**
   - If more than one person, does each know what the others have ordered?

5. **Do you know how the medications you are taking react with each other?**

6. **Do you know the side effects of the medications?**

7. **Are you experiencing any side effects that you think might be related to medications?**

   The nurse should ask female patients the following questions.

1. **Do you take oral contraceptives?**

   ▶ The risk of developing cardiovascular disease significantly increases in the female patient over age 35 who smokes and takes oral contraceptives containing high doses of synthetic estrogen and progesterone (AHA, 2017).

2. **Are you still menstruating?**
   - If not, at what age did menopause start?
   - Did you have a hysterectomy?
   - Were your ovaries removed?

   ▶ The earlier menopause starts, the greater the risk for development of heart disease. Coronary artery disease may be increased eightfold in the patient who has had her ovaries removed before menopause (Kim et al., 2015).

External Environment

The following questions deal with substances and irritants found in the physical environment of the patient. That includes the indoor and outdoor environments of the home and the workplace, those encountered for social engagements, and any encountered during travel.

1. **What is your present occupation?**
   - What is your work environment like?

   ▶ Jobs with long hours, stress, deadlines, and tension are thought to contribute to the development of cardiovascular disease (Hagstrom et al., 2018).

2. **What were your previous occupations?**

3. **Have you been exposed to passive smoking in your environment?**

   ▶ Inhalation of secondhand cigarette smoke in a closed environment is currently thought to contribute to the development of coronary artery plaque (Fischer & Kraemer, 2015).

4. **Have you been exposed to chemicals or other hazardous substances?**

   ▶ Such exposure may correlate to stress, alterations in eating habits and exercise habits, recreational drug use, and alterations in sleep patterns.

Patient-Centered Interaction

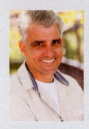

Source: HONGQI ZHANG/123RF.

Mr. Ameen Abo-Hamzy reports to the office of his internist for his yearly physical examination. He is 53 years old and has worked for the same company for 22 years. At this time, he is part of the management team and is concerned regarding company layoffs and general downsizing. He tells the nurse, "I feel fine. I think I'm in good health. I have an occasional gas bubble or pressure right here [pointing to the xiphoid process on his chest], and then I can sometimes feel my heart beat real fast." The following is an excerpt from the focused interview with Mr. Abo-Hamzy:

Interview

Nurse: Good morning, Mr. Abo-Hamzy. I see from the record you were last here a year ago for your physical.

Mr. Abo-Hamzy: Yes, that is right.

Nurse: Let's talk about your state of health.

Mr. Abo-Hamzy: I consider myself a really healthy person. I haven't missed a day of work all year. I never got a cold when everybody at work seemed to catch one this past winter. It is just the pressure that I get right here.

Again, Mr. Abo-Hamzy points to the xiphoid process on his chest.

Nurse: Tell me more about this pressure.

Mr. Abo-Hamzy: It is just here, and not all the time.

Nurse: Does the pressure get worse before or after you eat?

Mr. Abo-Hamzy: I have not noticed any change when I eat.

Nurse: When do you notice the change?

Mr. Abo-Hamzy: I'm usually at work. I can always count on the pressure starting either during or after our management meetings.

Nurse: Do you find work stressful these days?

Mr. Abo-Hamzy: I guess you could call it that. Somebody is always getting a pink slip. You know, being let go. I don't know what I will do if it happens to me. I have a family, a mortgage, and I carry the health insurance for all of us. My wife tells me I worry too much.

Nurse: And you? Do you think you worry too much?

Analysis

Throughout the interview the nurse used open-ended and close-ended questions to collect detailed subjective data from Mr. Abo-Hamzy. The patient mentioned subxiphoid pressure several times. The nurse picked up on this cue, sought clarification, ruled out gastrointestinal involvement, and ascertained the source of the pressure as being stress related before discussing another concern. The nurse used open-ended statements, allowing Mr. Abo-Hamzy to discuss pertinent information about his chest discomfort. The nurse stayed with one topic before directing the response to another area of concern.

Objective Data—Physical Assessment

Assessment Techniques and Findings

Physical assessment of the cardiovascular system requires the use of inspection, palpation, and auscultation. During each of the procedures, the nurse is gathering objective data related to the function of the heart as determined by the heart rate and the quality and characteristics of the heart sounds. In addition, the nurse observes for signs of appropriate cardiac function in relation to oxygen perfusion by assessing skin color and temperature, abnormal pulsations, and the characteristics of the patient's respiratory effort. Knowledge of normal parameters and expected findings is essential in determining the meaning of the data during a physical health assessment.

Skin is uniform in color on the face, trunk, and extremities. The eyes are symmetric. The periorbital area is flat, and the eyes do not bulge. The sclera of the eye should be white, the cornea clear, and the conjunctiva pink. The lips should be smooth and noncyanotic. The head should be steady and the skull proportional to the face. The earlobes should be smooth and without creases. The jugular veins are not visible when the chest is

EQUIPMENT

- Examination gown
- Metric rulers
- Examination drape
- Stethoscope with bell and diaphragm

HELPFUL HINTS

- Provide specific instructions throughout the assessment. Explain what is expected of the patient and that he or she will be able to breathe regularly throughout the assessment.
- Assessment of the heart will require several position changes. The nurse should assist the patient, if necessary; allow time for movement if the patient is uncomfortable; and explain the purpose of the position changes.
- The nurse's hands and the stethoscope should be warmed before beginning the assessment.
- The room should be quiet so that subtle sounds may be heard.

upright. Carotid pulsations are visible bilaterally. The fingers should be round and even with flat pink nails. The respiratory pattern is even, regular, and unlabored. ICSs and clavicles are visible, chest veins are evenly distributed and flat, and no bulges or masses are visible. Pulsations over the pericardium are absent; however, aortic pulsations in the epigastric area are visible in thin patients. The lower extremities are of uniform color and temperature with even hair distribution. The skeleton should be free of deformity and the neck and extremities in proportion to the torso. Palpation over the pericardium reveals slight vibration at the apical area only. Carotid pulses are palpable and equal in intensity. S2 is louder than S1 at the aortic and pulmonic auscultatory areas. S1 and S2 are heard equally at Erb's point (third left ICS). S1 is louder than S2 at the tricuspid and apical areas. Murmurs are absent. The carotid pulse is synchronous with the apical pulse.

- Provide adequate draping to prevent unnecessary exposure of the female breasts.
- Use Standard Precautions.

Physical assessment of the cardiovascular system follows an organized pattern. It begins with inspection of the patient's head and neck, including the eyes, ears, lips, face, skull, and neck vessels. The upper extremities, chest, abdomen, and lower extremities are also inspected. Palpation includes the precordium and carotid pulses. Auscultation includes the heart in five areas with the diaphragm and the bell of the stethoscope. The carotid arteries and the apical pulse are auscultated.

Techniques and Normal Findings	Abnormal Findings and Special Considerations

Inspection

1. **Instruct the patient.**
   - Explain that you will be looking at the head, neck, and extremities to provide clues to cardiac function.
   - Explain that you will ask the patient to sit up and lie down as part of the examination and that you will provide specific instructions and assistance as required throughout the examination. Explain that you will be touching the neck and chest as well as tapping on the chest and listening with the stethoscope. Tell the patient that none of the procedures should cause discomfort, but assure the patient that you will stop any time if discomfort occurs or the examination is causing fatigue.
2. **Position the patient.**
   - Begin the examination with the patient seated upright with the chest exposed (see Figure 18.14 ■).

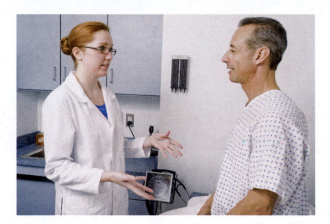

Figure 18.14 Begin the exam by having the patient sit upright.

3. **Inspect the patient's face, lips, ears, and scalp.**
   - These structures can provide valuable clues to the patient's cardiovascular health. Begin with the facial skin. The skin color should be uniform.

   ▶ Flushed skin may indicate rheumatic heart disease or presence of a fever. Grayish undertones are often seen in patients with coronary artery disease or those in shock. A ruddy color may indicate *polycythemia*, a condition in which there is a significantly increased number of red blood cells, or *Cushing syndrome*, a hormonal disorder caused by prolonged exposure of the tissues of the body to cortisol, a product of the adrenal glands.

   - Examine the eyes and the tissue surrounding the eyes (periorbital area). The eyes should be uniform and not have a protruding appearance.

   ▶ Protruding eyes are seen in *hyperthyroidism*. In hyperthyroidism, excessive hormone secretion results in high cardiac output, a tendency toward tachycardia (rapid heart rate), and potential for congestive heart failure.

   - The periorbital area should be relatively flat. No puffiness should be present.

   ▶ Periorbital puffiness may result from fluid retention (edema).

Techniques and Normal Findings	Abnormal Findings and Special Considerations

- The sclera should be whitish in color. The cornea should be without an *arcus*, which is a ringlike structure.

▶ A blue color in the sclera is often associated with *Marfan syndrome*, a degenerative disease of the connective tissue, which over time may cause the ascending aorta to either dilate or dissect, leading to abrupt death. An arcus in a young person may indicate hypercholesterolemia; however, in people of African descent or in adults over age 60, it may be normal.

- The conjunctiva should be clear, and underlying tissue should be pinkish in color. The eyelid should be smooth. For information on how to examine the conjunctiva, see Chapter 14. ∞

▶ **Xanthelasma** are yellowish cholesterol deposits seen on the eyelids and are indicative of premature atherosclerosis.

- Inspect the lips. They should be uniform in color without any underlying tinge of blueness. The buccal mucosa, gums, and tongue are also inspected for cyanosis.

▶ Blue-tinged lips may indicate cyanosis, which is often a late sign of inadequate tissue perfusion.

- Assess the general appearance of the face. It should be symmetric with uniform contours.

▶ Patients with *Down syndrome* may exhibit a large protruding tongue, low-set ears, and an underdeveloped mandible. Children with Down syndrome often have congenital heart disease. Wide-set eyes may be seen in a child with *Noonan syndrome*, which is accompanied by pulmonic stenosis (narrowing).

- Examine the head. Look first for the ability of the patient to hold the head steady. Rhythmic head bobbing should not be present.

▶ Head bobbing up and down in synchrony with the heartbeat is characteristic of severe aortic regurgitation. This bobbing is created by the pulsatile waves of regurgitated blood, which reverberate upward toward the head.

- Assess the structure of the skull and the proportion of the skull to the face.

▶ A protruding skull is seen in *Paget disease*, a rare bone disease characterized by localized loss of calcium from the bone and replacement with a porous bone formation, which leads to distorted, thickened contours. Paget disease is also characterized by a high cardiac output, which may lead to heart failure.

4. **Inspect the jugular veins.**

- Examination of the jugular veins can provide essential information about the patient's central venous pressure and the heart's pumping efficiency.

- With the patient sitting upright, adjust the gooseneck lamp to cast shadows on the patient's neck. Tangential lighting is effective in visualizing the jugular vessels.

- Be sure that the patient's head is turned slightly away from the side you are examining. Look for the external and internal jugular veins.

- Note that the jugular veins are not normally visible when the patient sits upright. The external jugular vein is located over the sternocleidomastoid muscle. The internal jugular vein, which is the best indicator of central venous pressure, is located behind this muscle, medial to the external jugular and lateral to the carotid artery.

- If you are able to visualize the jugular veins, measure their distance superior to the clavicle. (Be sure not to confuse the carotid pulse with pulsations of the jugular veins. The carotid pulse is lateral to the trachea.) If jugular vein pulsations are visible, palpate the patient's radial pulse and determine whether the jugular vein pulsations coincide with the palpated radial pulse.

▶ Obvious pulsations that are present during both inspiration and expiration and coincide with the arterial pulse are commonly seen with severe congestive heart failure.

- Next, have the patient lie at a 45-degree angle if the patient can tolerate this position without pain and is able to breathe comfortably.

- Place the first of the metric rulers vertically at the angle of Louis. Place the second metric ruler horizontally at a 90-degree angle to the first ruler. One end of this ruler should be at the angle of Louis and the other end in the jugular area on the lateral aspect of the neck (see Figure 18.15 ■).

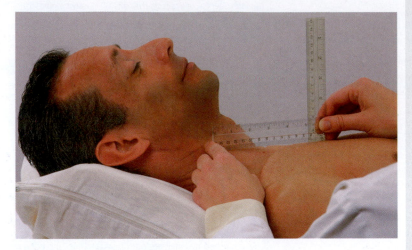

Figure 18.15 Assessment of central venous pressure.

- Inspect the neck for distention of the jugular veins. Raise the lateral portion of the horizontal ruler until it is at the top of the height of the distention and assess the height in centimeters of the elevation from the vertical ruler.

▶ Distention of the neck veins indicates elevation of central venous pressure commonly seen with congestive heart failure, fluid overload, or pressure on the superior vena cava.

- The jugular veins normally distend only 3 cm (1.18 in.) above the sternal angle when the patient is lying at a 45-degree angle (see Figure 18.15). You need to measure the distention only on one side.

5. Inspect the carotid arteries.
- The carotid arteries are located lateral to the patient's trachea in a groove that is medial to the sternocleidomastoid muscle.

- With the patient still lying at a 45-degree angle, using tangential lighting, inspect the carotid arteries for pulsations. Pulsations should be visible bilaterally. Carotid pulsations may be difficult to assess in the obese patient because of the thick neck and because breathing difficulties require an upright position.

▶ Bounding pulses are not normal findings and may indicate fever. The absence of a pulsation may indicate an obstruction either internal or external to the artery.

- When you finish, help the patient back to an upright sitting position.

6. Inspect the patient's hands and fingers.
- Help the patient to resume a sitting position. Confirm that the fingertips are rounded and even. The fingernails should be relatively pink, with white crescents at the base of each nail.

▶ Fingertips and nails that are clubbed bilaterally are characteristic of congenital heart disease. Clubbing may be associated with many respiratory and cardiac disorders. Thin red lines or splinter hemorrhages in the nail beds are associated with **infective endocarditis** (see Figure 18.16 ■), a condition caused by bacterial infiltration of the lining of the heart's chambers.

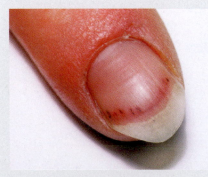

Figure 18.16 Splinter hemorrhage.
Source: Mediscan/Alamy Stock Photo.

Techniques and Normal Findings	Abnormal Findings and Special Considerations

7. **Inspect the patient's chest.**
   - Observe the respiratory pattern, which should be even, regular, and unlabored, with no retractions.

   - Observe the veins on the chest, which should be evenly distributed and relatively flat.

   - Inspect the entire chest for bulges and masses. The ICSs and clavicles should be even.

   - Inspect the entire chest for pulsations. Observe the patient first in an upright position and then at a 30-degree angle, which is a low- to mid-Fowler position. In particular, observe for pulsations over the five key landmarks (see Figure 18.17 ■).

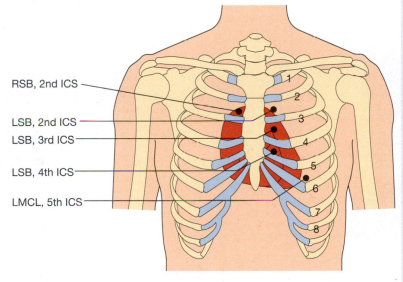

RSB, 2nd ICS

LSB, 2nd ICS
LSB, 3rd ICS

LSB, 4th ICS

LMCL, 5th ICS

Figure 18.17 Landmarks in precordial assessments.

   - Start by observing the RSB, second ICS. Next, observe the LSB, second ICS. The angle of Louis can be used to mark the second ICS.

   - Then observe the LSB, third to fifth ICS.
   - Move on to the apex: fifth ICS, MCL.
   - Finish with the epigastric area below the xiphoid process.

   - Confirm that the apical impulse/*point of maximum impulse* (PMI) is located at the fifth ICS in the left MCL.

   - Inspect the entire chest for heaves or lifts while the patient is sitting upright and again with the patient at a 30-degree angle.

   - *Heaves* or *lifts* are forceful risings of the landmark area.

   - In particular, make sure you observe over the five key landmarks previously listed.

8. **Inspect the patient's legs.**
   - Help the patient to a sitting position.

   - Inspect the legs for skin color. The skin color should be even and uniform.

   - Inspect the legs for hair distribution. The distribution should be even without bare patches devoid of hair.

▶ Fingernails and tips may be stained yellow when the patient is a smoker. Smoking is one of the main contributors to the development of atherosclerosis.

▶ Respiratory distress may be precipitated by various disorders. Pulmonary edema is often a severe complication of cardiovascular disease.

▶ Dilated, distended veins on the chest indicate an obstructive process, as seen with obstruction of the superior vena cava.

▶ Bulges are abnormal and may indicate obstructions or aneurysms. Masses may indicate obstructions or presence of tumors.

▶ If the entire precordium (anterior chest) pulsates and shakes with every heartbeat, extreme valvular regurgitation or shunting (redirection of blood flow that does not follow the normal physiologic pathway) may be present.

▶ Pulsations present in the LSB, second ICS indicate pulmonary artery dilation or excessive blood flow.

▶ Pulsations present in the LSB, third to fifth ICS may indicate right ventricular overload.

▶ If left ventricular hypertrophy is present, the PMI is displaced laterally in the fifth ICS from the LMCL.

▶ A heave or lift found in the LSB, third to fifth ICS, may indicate right ventricular hypertrophy or respiratory disease, such as pulmonary hypertension.

▶ Patches of lighter color may indicate compromised circulation. Mottling indicates severe hemodynamic compromise.

▶ Patchy hair distribution is often a sign of circulatory compromise that has occurred over time. The patient should be asked if the hair distribution on the legs has changed over time.

Techniques and Normal Findings	Abnormal Findings and Special Considerations

9. **Inspect the patient's skeletal structure.**
   - Ask the patient to stand.

   - Observe the skeletal structure, which should be free of deformities.

   - Observe the neck and extremities, which should be in proportion to the torso.

▶ *Scoliosis* is associated with prolapsed mitral valve.

▶ A patient who is tall and thin with an elongated neck and extremities should be evaluated further for the presence of Marfan syndrome.

Palpation

Palpate the chest in the six designated areas (see Figure 18.18 ■). Note that palpation may be performed with the patient sitting upright, reclining at a 45-degree or 30-degree angle, or lying flat. Start by palpating with the patient sitting upright and then in the lowest position that the patient can comfortably tolerate.

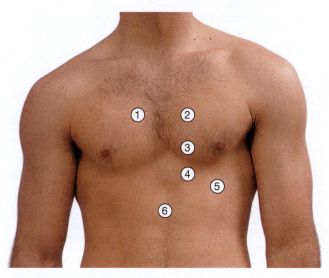

Figure 18.18 Landmarks for palpation of the chest.

1. **Palpate the chest.**
   - Place your right hand over the RSB, second ICS. Palpate with the base of your fingers.

   - You should not feel any pulsation, heave, or vibratory sensation against your palm in this location.

   - Place your hand on the LSB, second ICS.

   - You should not feel any pulsation, heave, or vibratory sensation against your palm in this location in anyone other than some very thin patients who are nervous about the examination.

   - Move your hand to the LSB, third then fourth ICS. No pulsations, heaves, or vibratory sensations should be felt.

   - Place your right hand over the apex: LMCL, fifth ICS.

   - When palpating over the LMCL, fifth ICS, you should feel a soft vibration, a tapping sensation, with each heartbeat. The vibration felt in this location should be isolated to an area no more than 1 cm (0.39 in.) in diameter.

   - Palpate the epigastric area, below the xiphoid process.

▶ Pulsations or heaves in the RSB, second ICS, indicate the presence of ascending aortic enlargement or aneurysm, aortic stenosis, or systemic hypertension.

▶ Pulsations or heaves in the LSB, second ICS, are associated with pulmonary hypertension, pulmonary stenosis, right ventricular enlargement, atrial septal defect, enlarged left atrium, and large posterior left ventricular aneurysm.

▶ Pulsations or heaves over the LSB, third or fourth ICS, may indicate right ventricular enlargement or pressure overload on this ventricle, pulmonary stenosis, or pulmonary hypertension.

▶ The presence of a heave, which is a forceful thrust over the fifth ICS, LMCL, indicates the potential presence of increased right ventricular stroke volume or pressure and mild-to-moderate aortic regurgitation. If vibration is felt in a downward and lateral position from where the normal PMI should be palpated, or if it can be palpated in an area greater than 1 cm (0.39 in.) in diameter, these conditions may be present: left ventricular hypertrophy, severe left ventricular volume overload, or severe aortic regurgitation.

▶ The presence of heaves or thrills in the subxiphoid area suggests the presence of elevated right ventricular volume or pressure overload.

Techniques and Normal Findings	**Abnormal Findings and Special Considerations**

- Repeat the palpation technique, with the patient at either a 30-degree angle or lying flat.

> **ALERT!** *Some patients are unable to lie flat. The patient should be placed in the lowest angle that is comfortably tolerated. It is necessary to be alert to any physical distress experienced by the patient during examination and to stop activity immediately if distress is experienced.*

- Palpation with the patient lying flat normally reveals either no pulsation or very faint taps in a localized area. No thrills, heaves, or lifts should be palpated in any of the five locations.

2. **Palpate the patient's carotid pulses.**
- The carotid artery is located in the groove between the trachea and sternocleidomastoid muscle beneath the angle of the jaw.

- It is important to palpate carotid pulses to assess their presence, strength, and equality. The patient may remain supine, or you may help the patient to sit upright.

- Ask the patient to look straight ahead and keep the neck straight (see Figure 18.19 ■).

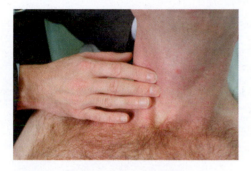

Figure 18.19 Palpating the carotid artery.
Source: Mediscan/Alamy Stock Photo.

- Palpate each carotid pulse separately. Normal findings bilaterally should demonstrate equality in intensity and regular pattern. The pulses should be strong but not bounding. If the pulse is difficult to palpate, ask the patient to turn the head slightly to the examining side.

▶ Diminished or absent carotid pulses may be found in patients with carotid disease or dissecting ascending aneurysm. Absence of both pulses indicates *asystole* (absent heart rate). If the patient is in critical care and has an arterial line, a printout of the arterial waveform should be obtained.

> **ALERT!** *The carotid pulses must never be palpated simultaneously because this may obstruct blood flow to the brain, resulting in severe bradycardia (slow heart rate) or asystole (absent heart rate).*

Auscultation

The position of the patient affects objective data collected from auscultatory examination. A full examination includes auscultation with the patient sitting upright, leaning forward when upright, supine, and in the left lateral position. Have the patient breathe normally initially. If you recognize the presence of abnormal sounds, have the patient slow down the respirations so that you may listen to the effects of inspirations and expiratory efforts on the heart sounds. You may want to have some patients perform a forced expiration. When preparing to auscultate a child's chest, you may want to let the child listen to the parent's heart sounds with the stethoscope to reduce or prevent fear of this unfamiliar object. Use a stethoscope with a smaller bell and diaphragm when you examine a child. In obese patients, heart sounds are best heard at the apical area with the patient in the left lateral position and at the aortic and pulmonic areas.

1. **Auscultate the patient's chest with the diaphragm of the stethoscope.**
   - Start the auscultation with the patient sitting upright.
   - Inch the stethoscope slowly across the chest and listen over each of the five key landmarks (see Figure 18.20 ■).
   - Listen over the RSB, second ICS.
   - In this location, the S2 sound should be louder than the S1 sound because this site is over the aortic valve.
   - Listen over the LSB, second ICS.
   - Also in this location, the S2 sound should be louder than the S1 sound because this site is over the pulmonic valve.
   - Listen over the LSB, third ICS, also called Erb's point.
   - You should hear both the S1 and S2 heart tones, relatively equal in intensity.
   - Listen at the LSB at the fourth ICS.
   - In this location the S1 sound should be louder than the S2 sound because the closure of the tricuspid valve is best auscultated here.
   - Listen over the apex: fifth ICS, LMCL.
   - In this location the S1 sound should also be louder than the S2 sound because the closure of the mitral valve is best auscultated here.

2. **Auscultate the patient's chest with the bell of the stethoscope.**
   - Place the bell of the stethoscope lightly on each of the five key landmark positions shown with step 1.
   - Listen for softer sounds over the five key landmarks. Then listen for murmurs.

3. **Auscultate the carotid arteries.**
   - Listen with the diaphragm and bell of the stethoscope. Have the patient hold the breath briefly. You may hear heart tones. This finding is normal.
   - You should not hear any turbulent sounds, such as murmurs.

4. **Compare the apical pulse with a carotid pulse.**
   - Auscultate the apical pulse.
   - Simultaneously palpate a carotid pulse.
   - Compare the findings. The two pulses should be synchronous. The carotid artery is used because it is closest to the heart and most accessible (see Figure 18.21 ■).

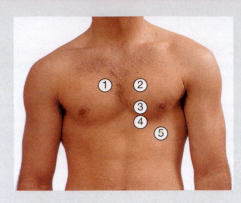

Figure 18.20 Auscultating the chest over five key landmarks.

▶ Low-pitched sounds are best auscultated with light application of the bell. Sounds such as S3, S4, murmurs (originating from stenotic valves), and gallops are best heard with the bell.

▶ A **bruit**, a loud blowing sound, is an abnormal finding. It is most often associated with a narrowing or stricture of the carotid artery and usually associated with atherosclerotic plaque.

▶ An apical pulse greater than the carotid rate indicates a pulse deficit. The rate, rhythm, and regularity must be evaluated.

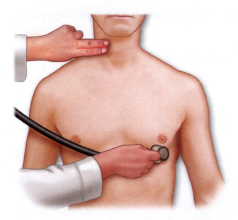

Figure 18.21 Comparing the carotid and apical pulses.

Techniques and Normal Findings	Abnormal Findings and Special Considerations

5. Repeat the auscultation of the patient's chest.

- This time have the patient lean forward, then lie supine, and finally lie in the left lateral position. Remember that not all patients will be able to tolerate all positions. In such cases, do not perform the technique (see Figure 18.22A–C ■).

- Listen with both the diaphragm and the bell in all five positions with the patient lying supine.

- With the bell lightly placed over the mitral area, have the patient roll onto the left side. Listen before, during, and after the patient moves for an S3, S4, or gallop.

▶ The S3 and S4 sounds will be easiest to hear during and just after the patient rolls to the left side.

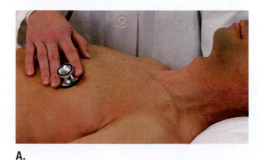
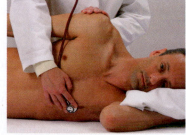
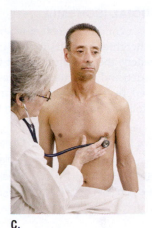

A.   B.   C.

Figure 18.22 Positions for auscultation of the heart. A. Supine, B. Lateral, C. Sitting.

Evidence-Based Practice:

Gender Bias in Cardiac Exam

Auscultation of the tricuspid and mitral areas and palpation of the point of maximal impulse (PMI) in a mature or maturing female patient require the examiner to have contact with the breasts. This may result in the examiner either not performing those aspects of the exam correctly or not at all. A study by Chakkalakal et al. (2012) looked at 110 resident physicians performing a cardiac examination on a standardized patient (SP). The results showed the residents were significantly less likely to correctly perform auscultation of the tricuspid and mitral valve regions and palpate the PMI on a female standardized patient. Male residents were significantly more likely than female residents to correctly perform the skills on a female SP. Because the auscultation of S3 and S4 is done at the mitral area, detection of these findings can be important in the case of cardiovascular disease. Having an awareness that this bias may exist could encourage complete and accurate assessments.

Documenting Your Findings

Documentation of assessment data—subjective and objective—must be accurate, professional, complete, and confidential. When documenting the information from the assessment of the cardiac system, the nurse should clearly describe abnormal or unexpected findings. For example, if a murmur is detected, be sure to include the location(s) where it is heard, the type, timing, quality, and grade. Use medical terminology rather than jargon, include all pertinent information, and avoid language that could identify the patient. An example of effective documentation is "Grade 2, holosystolic, blowing murmur heard best at the apex and radiates to the axilla." Please refer to the Key Terms at the beginning of the chapter to help you with language selection.

Focused History (SUBJECTIVE DATA)

No c/o SOB, chest pain or pressure, or fatigue. No history of angina or myocardial infarction. Diagnosed with hypertension 10 years ago. Taking hydrochlorothiazide daily. States current BP is around 130/70. Runs 3 miles every other day, which takes approximately 30 minutes. Nonsmoker. Enjoys fried foods but limits them to once a week. States unaware of lipid levels. Drinks 2 glasses of beer every weekend. Family history of hypertension and myocardial infarction.

Physical Assessment (OBJECTIVE DATA)

Skin color on chest consistent throughout, no cyanosis. No heaves, lifts, or thrills noted. S1, S2 clear and crisp. No splits, murmurs, S3 or S4. No JVD noted at 45 degrees. No carotid bruits.

Abnormal Findings

Abnormal findings in the cardiovascular system include murmurs (see Table 18.4), diseases of the myocardium and pumping capacity, valvular heart disease, septal defects, congenital heart disease, and electrical rhythm disturbances.

Diseases of the Myocardium and Pumping Capacity of the Heart

MYOCARDIAL ISCHEMIA

Ischemia is a common problem where the oxygen needs of the body are heightened, thus increasing the work of the heart. Unfortunately, the oxygen needs of the heart are not met as it works harder, and an ischemic process ensues. Ischemia is usually caused by the presence of an atherosclerotic plaque. A blood clot may be associated with the plaque.

Subjective findings:
- Pain in the chest, neck, jaw, or other region
- Shortness of breath
- Nausea
- Anxiety

Objective findings:
- Diaphoresis
- Pallor
- Vomiting
- Changes or abnormalities on electrocardiogram (EKG) may or may not be present

MYOCARDIAL INFARCTION (MI)

During infarction, there is complete disruption of oxygen and nutrient flow to the myocardial tissue in the area below a total occlusion. Infarction leads to the death of the myocardial tissue unless flow of blood is reestablished. MI is caused by ischemia to the cardiac muscle. As such, manifestations associated with myocardial infarction mirror those seen with myocardial ischemia.

Subjective findings:
- Pain in the chest, neck, jaw, or other region
- Shortness of breath
- Nausea
- Anxiety

Objective findings:
- Diaphoresis
- Pallor
- Vomiting
- Changes or abnormalities on EKG may or may not be present.

Right-sided heart failure causes backup of the blood into the systemic circulation.

Subjective findings:
- Fatigue
- Weakness
- Mental confusion
- Loss of appetite

Objective findings
- Jugular venous distention (JVD)
- Hypertension
- Liver congestion
- Peripheral edema

HEART FAILURE

This condition is the inability of the heart to produce a sufficient pumping effort. Most commonly, both left-sided and right-sided heart failure are present.

Left-sided heart failure causes blood to back up into the pulmonary system and results in pulmonary edema.

Subjective findings:
- Dyspnea
- Shortness of breath

Objective findings
- Frothy sputum
- Adventitious breath sounds, including rhonchi or rales (crackles)
- Decreased oxygen saturation

VENTRICULAR HYPERTROPHY

Ventricular hypertrophy occurs in response to pumping against high pressures. Right ventricular hypertrophy occurs with pulmonary hypertension, congenital heart disease, pulmonary disease, pulmonary stenosis, and right ventricular infarction.

Left ventricular hypertrophy occurs in the presence of systemic hypertension, congenital heart disease, aortic stenosis, or MI to the left ventricle.

Subjective findings:
- Chest pain
- Dizziness, especially after activity
- Shortness of breath

Objective findings
- Cardiac dysrhythmias
- Tachycardia

Valvular Heart Disease

Disease of the valves denotes either narrowing (stenosis) of the valve leaflets or incompetence (regurgitation) of these same leaflets. Valvular disease may be caused by rheumatic fever, congenital defects, MI, and normal aging. Common forms of valvular heart disease are described in Table 18.6.

Septal Defects

An atrial septal defect is an opening between the right and left atria, whereas a ventricular septal defect is an opening between the right and left ventricles. Both of these septal defects may result from congenital heart disease and MI. The two primary septal defects are described in Table 18.7.

Table 18.6 Overview of Valvular Heart Disease

Mitral Stenosis

A narrowing of the left mitral valve.
Etiology: Rheumatic fever or cardiac infection
Findings: Murmur heard at the apical area with the patient in left lateral position

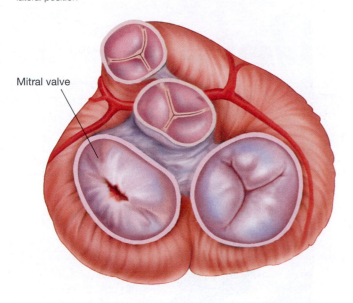

Mitral stenosis.

Aortic Stenosis

A narrowing of the aortic valve.
Etiology: Congenital bicuspid valves, rheumatic heart disease, atherosclerosis.
Findings: Murmur at aortic area, RSB, second ICS.9

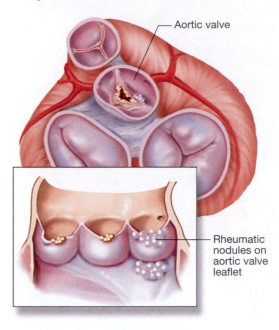

Aortic stenosis.

Mitral Regurgitation

The backflow of blood from the left ventricle into the left atrium.
Etiology: Rheumatic fever, MI, rupture of chordae tendineae.
Findings: Murmur at apex. Sound is transmitted to (L) axillae.

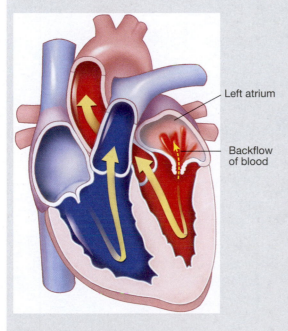

Mitral regurgitation.

Pulmonic Stenosis

The narrowing of the opening between the pulmonary artery and the right ventricle.
Etiology: Congenital.
Findings: Murmur at pulmonic area radiates to neck. Thrill in (L) second and third ICS.

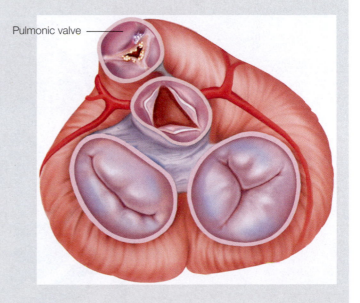

Pulmonic stenosis.

(continued)

Tricuspid Stenosis

The narrowing or stricture of the tricuspid valve of the heart.
Etiology: Rheumatic heart disease, congenital defect, right atrial myxoma (tumor).
Findings: Murmur heard with the bell of the stethoscope over the tricuspid area.

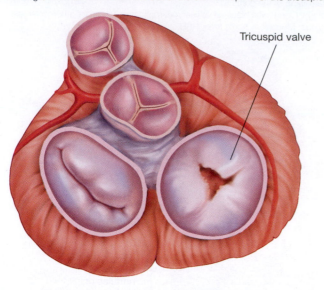

Tricuspid valve

Tricuspid stenosis.

Mitral Valve Prolapse

The mitral valve leaflets so they prolapse into the left atrium.
Etiology: May occur with pectus excavatum, often unknown.
Findings: Murmur, nonejection clicks heard (L) lower sternal border in upright position.

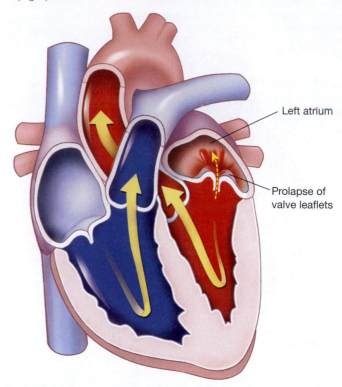

Left atrium

Prolapse of valve leaflets

Mitral valve prolapse.

Aortic Regurgitation

The backflow of blood from the aorta into the left ventricle.
Etiology: Rheumatic heart disease, endocarditis, Marfan syndrome, syphilis.
Findings: Murmur with patient leaning forward; click in second ICS.

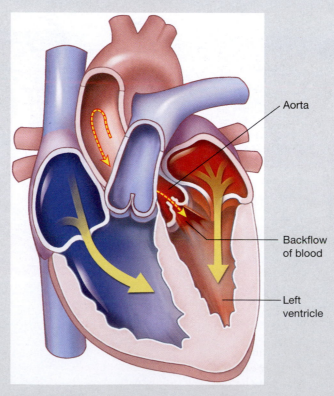

Aorta

Backflow of blood

Left ventricle

Aortic regurgitation.

Table 18.7 Overview of Septal Defects

Ventricular Septal Defect

Regurgitation occurs through the defect, resulting in a holosystolic murmur that is loud, coarse, high-pitched, and heard at the LSB, third to fifth ICS.

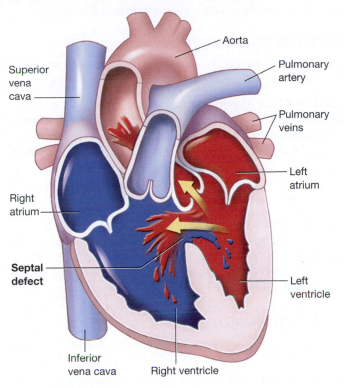

Ventricular septal defect.

Atrial Septal Defect

Regurgitation occurs through the defect, resulting in a harsh, loud, high-pitched murmur heard at the LSB, second ICS.

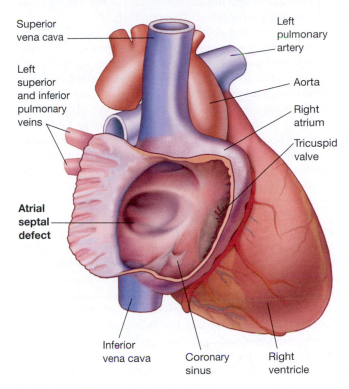

Atrial septal defect.

Application Through Critical Thinking

CASE STUDY

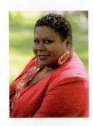

Source: Jeff Cleveland/ Shutterstock.

Jayla Tibbs, a 56-year-old African American female, presents to the emergency room with reports of shortness of breath, tingling in her left arm, and nausea. Mrs. Tibbs's medical history includes hypertension and type 1 diabetes mellitus, which she controls with diet and insulin injections.

Mrs. Tibbs states her signs and symptoms began this morning while she was taking a walk. Mrs. Tibbs reports that she fatigued quickly and had difficulty catching her breath. Subsequently, she felt a little nauseated and experienced a faint burning sensation in her left shoulder. Mrs. Tibbs states that when she returned to her home, her husband told her she "did not look right." Mrs. Tibbs further states she felt that there was no cause for concern and told her husband, "It will go away if I rest." Despite Mrs. Tibbs's attempts to reassure her husband that she did not need medical care, her husband insisted that she go to the hospital.

First, the nurse must determine if Mrs. Tibbs is in acute distress by gathering objective and subjective data. The nurse will assess for indications of respiratory distress, chest pain, pallor or cyanosis, abnormal vital signs, and anxiety. Priorities of care include promoting adequate oxygenation and perfusion.

The nurse knows that hypertension and diabetes are risk factors for cardiovascular disease and that the symptoms of nausea, breathlessness, and unusual sensations in the shoulder may be indicators of a myocardial infarction (MI).

Using an organized approach, the nurse begins the assessment. Mrs. Tibbs denies chest pain or chest pressure but continues to report a burning sensation in her left shoulder and nausea. She states the burning sensation is constant and very uncomfortable, rating it an 8 on a 1 to 10 pain scale. This pain has been consistent since her arrival in the ED. Mrs. Tibbs is complaining of shortness of breath that seems to be getting worse. She is also experiencing mild nausea without any emesis.

The physical assessment reveals that Mrs. Tibbs is diaphoretic, is dyspneic, appears anxious, and her skin is gray-tinged, especially around the eyes. Her vital signs are B/P 144/72—P 102—RR 28. Her oxygen saturation (SaO_2) is 92% on room air. No heaves or lifts observable. No heaves or thrills present with palpation. Heart sounds are rapid with a regular rhythm. No extra heart sounds or murmurs auscultated. Her jugular veins were slightly distended when she was sitting at a 45-degree angle. Mrs. Tibbs is in acute distress. Rapid data interpretation and prompt implementation of collaborative nursing interventions are required. Her complaints include a burning sensation in her left shoulder, nausea, and shortness of breath. Her skin color suggests altered tissue perfusion. Her blood pressure is within normal limits, but her heart rate and respiratory rate are increased.

Collectively, the assessment data may be indicative of an acute cardiovascular problem. Collaborative goals of care include promoting oxygenation and perfusion, as well as preventing further systemic compromise.

The nurse administers O_2 via nasal cannula to Mrs. Tibbs and applies a cardiac monitor. Mrs. Tibbs's electrocardiogram (EKG) shows no obvious abnormalities; however, the nurse is aware that impaired cardiac perfusion does not always produce immediate EKG changes. Nitroglycerin sublingual (SL) as ordered by the ER physician is administered.

Two minutes after receiving nitroglycerin SL, Mrs. Tibbs's B/P is 120/64, and her heart rate (HR) is 84. Her respiratory rate is 22. She continues to receive supplemental O_2 via nasal cannula at a rate of 4 L/min. Her oxygen saturation has increased to 97%. Mrs. Tibbs states, "I'm not short of breath anymore, and that burning in my shoulder is gone now."

Mrs. Tibbs occasionally rubs her left arm but denies tingling or pain. She continues to report mild nausea. She states, "This is all probably from something I ate or an insulin reaction. I'd like to go home."

The physician orders a 12-lead EKG and laboratory diagnostics, including cardiac enzyme tests. Mrs. Tibbs is scheduled for admission to the hospital's coronary care unit (CCU).

SAMPLE DOCUMENTATION

The following is sample documentation for Jayla Tibbs on admission to the ED.

SUBJECTIVE DATA History of hypertension and type 1 diabetes, controlled with diet and insulin. Fatigued quickly during morning walk, worsening shortness of breath, slight nausea without emesis, constant burning sensation in left shoulder, rated pain 8 on 1-to-10 scale. She felt it was nothing to worry about and stated, "It will go away if I rest." Husband stated Mrs. Tibbs "did not look right" upon returning from her morning walk.

OBJECTIVE DATA 56-year-old African American female. Diaphoresis, dyspnea, gray-tinged skin, especially around eyes. VS: B/P left 144/72—P 102—RR 28—SaO_2 92% on room air. No heaves, lifts, or thrills. S1 and S2 rapid, regular. No extra sounds or murmurs. JVD 3 cm at 45 degrees.

CRITICAL THINKING QUESTIONS

1. What additional information will be required to formulate a plan of care for Mrs. Tibbs in the CCU?

2. How should the nurse interpret the patient's desire "to go home" and statement that "This is all probably from something I ate or an insulin reaction"?

3. How does the absence of chest pain support or refute the possibility that Mrs. Tibbs is experiencing a myocardial infarction (MI)?

4. Explain the following conclusions about the patient's physical condition:
   a. Impaired oxygenation
   b. Alteration in peripheral perfusion
   c. Fatigue
   d. Nausea

5. What special considerations should the nurse consider when evaluating Mrs. Tibbs's situation?

REFERENCES

American Heart Association (AHA). (2015). *The American Heart Association's diet and lifestyle recommendations.* Retrieved from http://www.heart.org/HEARTORG/HealthyLiving/HealthyEating/Nutrition/The-American-Heart-Associations-Diet-and-Lifestyle-Recommendations_UCM_305855_Article.jsp#.WqVxImrwbX4

American Heart Association (AHA). (2017). AHA statistical update: Heart disease and stroke statistics—2017 update. *Circulation, 135,* E146-E603. doi:10.1161/CIR.0000000000000485

Berman, A., & Snyder, S. J. (2016). *Kozier and Erb's fundamentals of nursing: Concepts, process, and practice* (10th ed.). Upper Saddle River, NJ: Prentice Hall.

Chakkalakal, R. J., Higgins, S. M., Bernstein, L. B., Lundberg, K. L., Wu, V., Green, J., Long, Q., & Doyle, J. P. (2012). Does patient gender impact resident physicians' approach to the cardiac exam? *Journal of General Internal Medicine, 28*(4), 561–566. doi:10.1007/s11606-012-2256-5

Fischer, F., & Kraemer, A. (2015). Meta-analysis of the association between second-hand smoke exposure and ischaemic heart diseases, COPD and stroke. *BMC Public Health, 15,* 1–18. doi:10.1186/s12889-015-2489-4

Hagstrom, E., Norlund, F., Stebbins, A., Armstrong, P. W., Chiswell, K., Granger, C. B., . . . Held, C. (2018). Psychosocial stress and major cardiovascular events in patients with stable coronary heart disease. *The Association for the Publication of the Journal of Internal Medicine, 283,* 83–92. doi:10.1111/joim.12692

Harvard Heart Letter. (2015). *Race and ethnicity: Clues to your heart disease risk?* Retrieved from https://www.health.harvard.edu/heart-health/race-and-ethnicity-clues-to-your-heart-disease-risk

Katikaneni, P. K., Akkus, N. I., Tandon, N., & Modi, K. (2013). Cocaine-induced postpartum coronary artery dissection: A case report and 80-year review of literature. *Journal of Invasive Cardiology, 25*(8), E163–E166.

Kim, C., Cushman, M., Khodneva, Y., Lisabeth, L., Judd, S., Kleindorfer, D., . . . Safford, M. (2015). Risk of incident coronary heart disease events in men compared to women by menopause type and race. *Journal of the American Heart Association, 4* (E001881), 1–10. doi:10.1161/JAHA.115.001881

Mangla, A., & Gupta, S. (2014). *Heart sounds.* Retrieved from http://emedicine.medscape.com/article/1894036-overview#a1

Marieb, E. (2015). *Essentials of human anatomy and physiology* (10th ed.). Redwood City, CA: Benjamin/Cummings/Pearson Education.

Mayo Clinic. (2013). *Angina: Symptoms.* Retrieved from http://www.mayoclinic.org/diseases-conditions/angina/basics/symptoms/con-20031194

Osborn, K. S., Wraa, C. E., Watson, A., & Holleran, R. S. (2013). *Medical-surgical nursing: Preparation for practice* (2nd ed.). Upper Saddle River, NJ: Pearson.

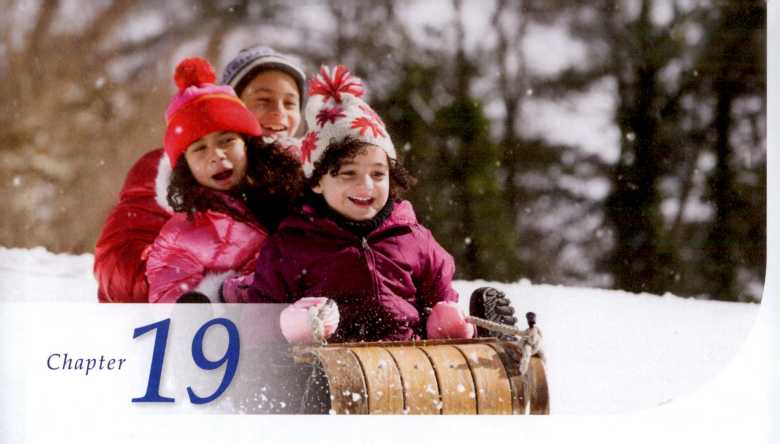

Chapter 19

Peripheral Vascular System

LEARNING OUTCOMES

Upon completion of this chapter, you will be able to:

1. Describe the anatomy and physiology of the peripheral vascular system.

2. Identify the anatomic, physiologic, developmental, psychosocial, and cultural variations that guide assessment of the peripheral vascular system.

3. Determine which questions about the peripheral vascular system to use for the focused interview.

4. Outline the techniques for assessment of the peripheral vascular system.

5. Plan the patient education related to the assessment on the peripheral vascular system.

6. Generate the appropriate documentation to describe the assessment of the peripheral vascular system.

7. Identify abnormal findings in the physical assessment of the peripheral vascular system.

KEY TERMS

arterial aneurysm, 414
arterial insufficiency, 413
arteries, 393
bruit, 403
capillaries, 394

claudication, 413
clubbing, 403
edema, 403
epitrochlear node, 395
lymph, 395

lymphatic vessels, 394
lymph nodes, 395
peripheral vascular system, 393
pulse, 393

Raynaud disease, 415
varicosities, 405
veins, 394
venous insufficiency, 398

MEDICAL LANGUAGE

hyper-	Prefix meaning "high," "elevated," "above normal"	**sclerosis**	Root word meaning "hardening"
		thromb-	Prefix meaning "clot"
hypo-	Prefix meaning "below," "deficient"	**vaso-**	Prefix meaning "vessel," "duct"
-itis	Suffix meaning "inflammation"		

Introduction

The **peripheral vascular system** is made up of the blood vessels of the body. Together with the heart and the lymphatic vessels, they make up the body's circulatory system, which transports blood and lymph throughout the body. This chapter discusses assessment of the 60,000-mile network of veins and arteries that make up the peripheral vascular system and assessment of the peripheral lymphatic system.

The vascular system plays a key role in the development of heart disease, one of the leading causes of death. People with high blood pressure have an increased risk of developing heart disease and stroke. Hypertension, "the silent killer," produces many physiologic changes before any symptoms are experienced. This characteristic has tended to undermine efforts at treatment. Therefore, the healthcare professional's role includes educating patients and consumers about the prevention of peripheral vascular disorders. Factors that influence a patient's vascular health include psychosocial wellness, self-care practices, and considerations related to the patient's family, culture, and environment.

Anatomy and Physiology Review

The peripheral vascular system is composed of arteries, veins, and lymphatics. Each of these is described in the following sections.

Arteries

The **arteries** of the peripheral vascular system receive oxygen-rich blood from the heart and carry it to the organs and tissues of the body. The pumping heart (ventricular systole) creates a high-pressure wave or **pulse** that causes the arteries to expand and contract. This pulse propels the blood through the vessels and is palpable in arteries near the skin or over a bony surface. The thickness and elasticity of arterial walls help them to withstand these constant waves of pressure and to propel the blood to the body periphery. The thickness or viscosity of blood, the heart rate or cardiac output, and the ability of the vessels to expand and contract influence the arterial pulse. It is described as a smooth wave with a forceful ascending portion that domes and becomes less forceful as it descends. Review Chapter 18 for more detailed information. ∞

In the arm, the pulsations of the *brachial artery* can be palpated in the antecubital region. The divisions of the brachial artery, the *radial* and *ulnar arteries,* can be palpated for pulsations over the anterior wrist. The major arteries of the arm are shown in Figure 19.1 ■.

In the leg, the pulsations of the femoral artery can be palpated inferior to the inguinal ligament, about halfway between the anterior superior iliac spine and the symphysis pubis. The *femoral artery* continues down the thigh and becomes the *popliteal artery* as it passes behind the knee. Pulsations of the popliteal artery are palpable over the popliteal region. Below the knee, the popliteal artery divides into the anterior and posterior tibial arteries. The *anterior tibial artery* travels to the dorsum of the foot, and its pulsation can be felt just lateral to the prominent extensor tendon of the big toe close to the ankle. This pulse is known as the dorsalis pedis. Pulsations of the *posterior tibial artery* can be felt where it passes behind the medial malleolus of the ankle. The major arteries of the leg are illustrated in Figure 19.2 ■.

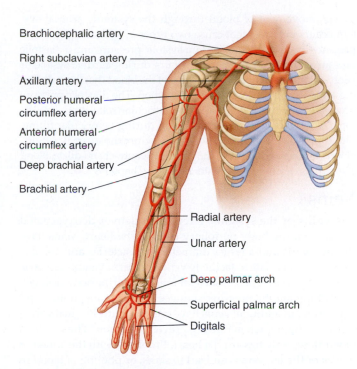

Figure 19.1 Main arteries of the arm.

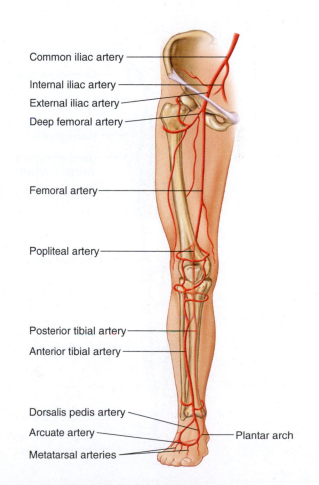

Figure 19.2 Main arteries of the leg.

The movement of blood through the systemic arterial system occurs in waves that cause two types of pressure. The blood pressure has two distinct parts, a systolic pressure and a diastolic pressure. The systolic pressure occurs during cardiac systole or ventricular contraction. It is the force of the blood that is exerted on the arterial wall during this cardiac action. The diastolic pressure occurs during cardiac diastole or ventricular relaxation. It is the force of the blood on the arterial wall during ventricular filling. Blood pressure is influenced by age, sympathoadrenal activity, blood volume, and ability of the vessels to contract and dilate. Blood pressure is discussed in greater detail in Chapter 8. ∞

Veins

The **veins** of the systemic circulation deliver deoxygenated blood from the body periphery back to the heart. Veins have thinner walls and a larger diameter than arteries and are able to stretch and dilate to facilitate venous return. Venous return is assisted by contraction of skeletal muscles during activities such as walking and by pressure changes related to inspiration and expiration. In addition, veins have one-way intraluminal valves that close tightly when filled to prevent backflow. Thus, venous blood flows only toward the heart. Problems with the lumen or valves of the leg veins can lead to *stasis*, or pooling of blood in the veins of the lower extremities.

The femoral and the popliteal veins are deep veins of the legs and carry about 90% of the venous return from the legs. The great and small saphenous veins are superficial veins that are not as well supported as the deep veins by surrounding tissues and, therefore, are more susceptible to venous stasis. The major veins of the leg are depicted in Figure 19.3 ∎.

Capillaries

The **capillaries** are the smallest vessels of the circulatory system and where exchanges of gases and nutrients between the arterial and venous systems occur. Blood pressure in the arterial end of the capillary bed forces fluid out across the capillary membrane and into the body tissues.

Lymphatic System

The lymphatic system consists of a vast network of vessels, fluid, tissues, and organs throughout the body. These vessels help transport escaped fluid back to the vascular system. The lymphoid organs have a major role regarding body defenses and the immune system. These structures help fight infection and provide the individual immunocompetence. The spleen, tonsils, and thymus gland are examples of lymphoid organs.

The **lymphatic vessels** form their own circulatory system in which their collected fluid flows to the heart. The vessels extend

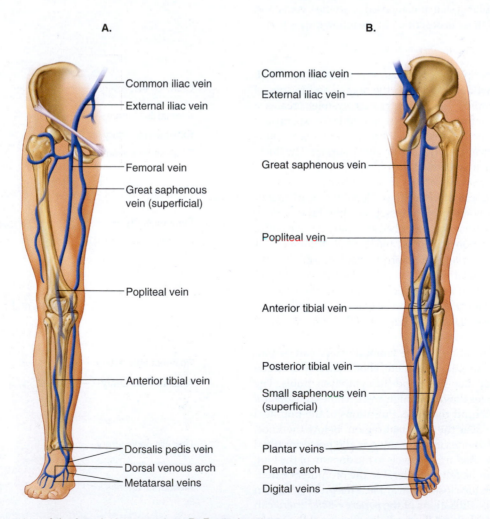

A.
- Common iliac vein
- External iliac vein
- Femoral vein
- Great saphenous vein (superficial)
- Popliteal vein
- Anterior tibial vein
- Dorsalis pedis vein
- Dorsal venous arch
- Metatarsal veins

B.
- Common iliac vein
- External iliac vein
- Great saphenous vein
- Popliteal vein
- Anterior tibial vein
- Posterior tibial vein
- Small saphenous vein (superficial)
- Plantar veins
- Plantar arch
- Digital veins

Figure 19.3 The main veins of the leg. A. Anterior view. B. Posterior view.

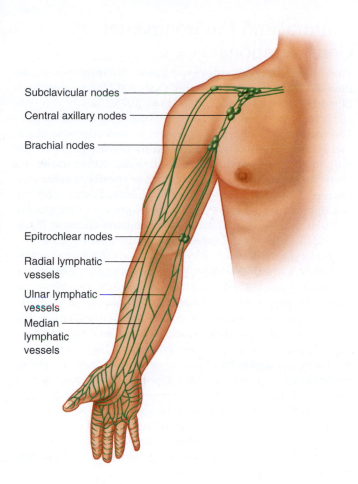

Figure 19.4 Main lymph nodes of the arm.

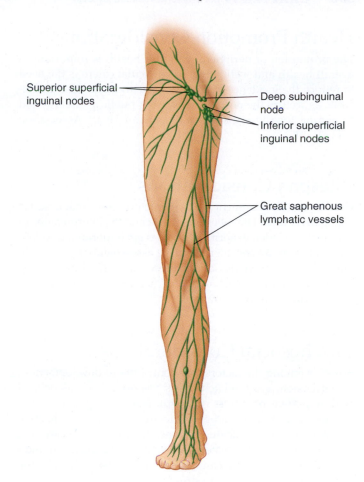

Figure 19.5 Main lymph nodes of the leg.

from the capillaries of their system to the two main lymphatic trunks. The *right lymphatic duct* collects lymph from the right upper extremity, which is the right side of the thorax and head. The *thoracic duct* collects lymph from the remaining part of the body. The thoracic duct responds to the protein and fluid pressure at the capillary end of the vessels that help keep the lymph properly circulated. During circulation, as blood continues through the capillary bed toward the smallest veins, the *venules,* more fluid leaves the capillaries than can be absorbed by the veins. The lymphatic system retrieves this excess fluid, called **lymph**, from the tissue spaces and carries it to the lymph nodes throughout the body. **Lymph nodes** are clumps of tissue located along the lymphatic vessels and are either deep or superficial in the body. The lymph nodes usually are covered and protected by connective tissue and are, therefore, not palpable. Some of the more superficial nodes are located in the neck, the axillary region, and the inguinal region. Deeper clusters are located in the abdomen and thoracic cavity. The lymph nodes filter lymph fluid, removing any pathogens before the fluid is returned to the bloodstream.

The **epitrochlear node** located on the medial surface of the arm above the elbow drains the ulnar surface of the forearm and the third, fourth, and fifth digits. The nodes in the axilla of the arm drain the rest of the arm. The major lymph nodes of the arm are shown in Figure 19.4 ∎.

The legs have two sets of superficial inguinal nodes, a vertical group and a horizontal group. The vertical group is located close to the saphenous vein and drains that area of the leg. The horizontal group of nodes is found below the inguinal ligament. These nodes drain the skin of the abdominal wall, the external genitals, the anal canal, and the gluteal area. The major lymph nodes of the leg are illustrated in Figure 19.5 ∎.

The functions of the peripheral vascular system are the following:

- Delivering oxygen and nutrients to tissues of the body
- Transporting carbon dioxide and other waste products from the tissues for excretion
- Removing pathogens from the body fluid by filtering lymph

Special Considerations

The nurse must use critical thinking and the nursing process to identify factors to consider when conducting a comprehensive health assessment. Factors that impact the patient's health status include but are not limited to age, developmental level, race, ethnicity, work history, living conditions, socioeconomics, and emotional well-being.

Health Promotion Considerations

The promotion of peripheral vascular health is important to overall health and well-being. In particular, there is the need to reduce the incidence of hypertension and hypercholesterolemia, as well as the need for increasing public awareness and screening for these disorders (American Heart Association [AHA], 2017).

Lifespan Considerations

Growth and development are dynamic processes that describe change over time. The collection of data and the interpretation of findings in relation to normative values are important. Developmental factors are considered during assessment of the peripheral vascular system. Blood pressure values differ based on age and health status. See Chapter 25, Chapter 26, and Chapter 27 for more lifespan considerations. ∞

Psychosocial Considerations

Stress is among the factors that contribute to development of hypertension. Work-related stress has often been associated with hypertension. Stress can result from the rigors of everyday life in a complex and ever-changing world. Globalization and resulting economic fluctuations, the spread of disease, and terrorist threats have created a stressful environment. An individual's ability to cope can determine the risk of developing hypertension in response to stress.

Cultural and Environmental Considerations

There is a greater incidence of hypertension in African Americans than in Caucasians or Hispanics (National Heart, Lung, and Blood Institute [NHLBI], 2014; AHA, 2017). Obesity is a risk factor for hypertension and is increasing in the United States. The incidence of obesity is greatest in non-Hispanic Black and Hispanic individuals, followed by non-Hispanic White individuals. In comparison, non-Hispanic Asian individuals demonstrate the lowest incidence of obesity (Centers for Disease Control and Prevention [CDC], 2014). Diabetes, which is a significant risk factor for the development of peripheral vascular disease, is most common among non-Hispanic Black individuals (American Diabetes Association [ADA], 2014).

Smoking is a risk factor for hypertension and peripheral vascular disease. In the United States, smoking is most prevalent among American Indian/Alaska Natives, followed by non-Hispanic Whites, Hispanics, African Americans, and Asians (AHA, 2017).

Risk factors for varicose veins include Irish and German descent, family history of varicosities, a sedentary lifestyle, obesity, and multiple pregnancies. Patients whose jobs require them to stand for most of the day, such as hairdressers and cashiers, are at greater risk for developing varicose veins. Desk jobs that require sitting for prolonged periods also contribute to venous stasis and varicose veins.

Skin color variations across ethnic groups may affect assessment of circulation. The nurse must use skin temperature, capillary refill, the color of the palms of the hands and soles of the feet, the color of the oral mucosa, and pulse characteristics when pink undertones are not easily detected.

Subjective Data—Health History

Health assessment of the peripheral vascular system includes gathering subjective and objective data. During the interview, the nurse uses a variety of communication techniques to elicit general and specific information about the patient's state of health or illness. Health records and the results of laboratory tests are important secondary sources to be reviewed and included in the data-gathering process. See Table 19.1 for information on potential secondary sources of patient data.

Focused Interview

The focused interview for the peripheral vascular system concerns data related to the structures and functions of that system. Subjective data are gathered during the focused interview. The nurse must be prepared to observe the patient and listen for cues related to the functions of the systems. The nurse may use open- and closed-ended questions to obtain information. Often a number of follow-up questions or requests for descriptions are required to clarify data or gather missing information.

The focused interview guides the physical assessment of the peripheral vascular system. The information is always

Table 19.1 Potential Secondary Sources for Patient Data Related to the Peripheral Vascular System

LABORATORY TESTS	NORMAL VALUES
PT (prothrombin time)	10–12 seconds
Platelets	150,000–300,000/mm³
Thrombin Time	15–23 seconds
ACT (Activated Clotting Time)	90–130 seconds
aPTT (Activated Partial Thromboplastin Time)	28–38 seconds
INR (International Normalized Ratio)	0.8–1.2 (if not taking warfarin)
	2.5–3.5 (if taking warfarin)
DIAGNOSTIC TESTS	
Arterial Blood Flow Studies	
Doppler Ultrasonography	
Venous Ultrasonography	
Ankle Brachial Index (ABI)	

considered in relation to normal parameters and expectations. Therefore, the nurse must consider age, gender, race, culture, environment, health practices, past and concurrent problems, and therapies when framing questions and using techniques to elicit information. In order to address all of the factors when conducting a focused interview, categories of questions related to the peripheral vascular system status and function have been developed. These categories include general questions that are asked of all patients; those addressing illness and infection; questions related to symptoms, pain, and behaviors;

those related to habits or practices; questions that are specific to patients according to age; those for the pregnant female; and questions that address environmental concerns. One approach to eliciting information about symptoms is the OLDCART & ICE method as described in Chapter 5. See Figure 5.3. ∞ The data will be used to help improve peripheral vascular health.

The nurse must consider the patient's ability to participate in the focused interview and physical assessment. If a patient is experiencing pain or anxiety, attention must focus on relief of symptoms.

Focused Interview Questions	Rationales and Evidence

The following section provides sample questions and bulleted follow-up questions in each of the previously mentioned categories. A rationale for each of the questions is provided. The list of questions is not all-inclusive but represents the types of questions required in a comprehensive focused interview related to the peripheral vascular and lymphatic systems.

General Questions

1. **Describe your circulation.**
   - Have you felt cold or hot?
   - Have you had numbness anywhere?
   - Has your skin been pale or blue?
   - Has your circulation changed in the last 2 months or 2 years?

▶ This gives patients the opportunity to provide subjective data about circulatory status.

2. **Have you or any member of your family ever had heart problems, respiratory disease, diabetes, varicose veins, or blood clots?**

▶ These problems can damage the peripheral circulation, and they tend to be hereditary (AHA, 2017).

Questions Related to Illness

1. **Have you ever been diagnosed with a disease of your circulatory or lymphatic system?**
   - When were you diagnosed with the problem?
   - What treatment was prescribed for the problem?
   - Was the treatment helpful?
   - Describe things you have done or currently do to cope with this problem.
   - Has the problem ever recurred (acute)?
   - How are you managing the disease now (chronic)?

▶ The patient has an opportunity to provide information about specific illnesses. If a diagnosed illness is identified, follow-up about the date of diagnosis, treatment, and outcomes is required. Data about each illness identified by the patient are essential to an accurate health assessment. Illnesses can be classified as acute or chronic, and follow-up regarding each classification will differ.

2. *Alternative to question 1:* List possible illnesses—such as hypertension, arteriosclerosis, Raynaud disease, varicose veins, thrombophlebitis, and aneurysms—and to ask the patient to respond "yes" or "no" as each is stated.

▶ This is a comprehensive and easy way to elicit information about all diagnoses. Follow-up would be carried out for each identified diagnosis as in question 1.

Questions Related to Symptoms, Pain, and Behaviors

When gathering information about symptoms, many questions are required to elicit details and descriptions that assist in the analysis of the data. Discrimination is made in relation to the significance of a symptom, in relation to specific diseases or problems, and in relation to potential follow-up examination or referral. One rationale may be provided for a group of questions in this category.

The following questions refer to specific symptoms and behaviors associated with the peripheral vascular and lymphatic systems. For each symptom, questions and follow-up are required. The details to be elicited are the characteristics of the symptom; the onset, duration, and frequency of the symptom; the treatment or remedy for the symptom, including over-the-counter and home remedies; the determination if diagnosis has been sought; the effect of treatments; and family history associated with a symptom or illness.

Questions Related to Symptoms

1. **Have you noticed any skin changes on your arms, hands, fingers, legs, feet, or toes?**
   - If so, describe the changes.
   - Have you noticed any swelling or shiny skin, particularly on your legs?

▶ Shiny skin and swelling are sometimes caused by fluid leaking into tissue spaces because of incompetent valves in the veins (University of Rochester Medical Center [URMC], 2014).

▶ Peripheral arterial insufficiency can result in hair loss or skin changes (Johns Hopkins University, n.d.).

Focused Interview Questions	Rationales and Evidence
2. If the patient reports swelling: Is the swelling in one leg or both legs? • When did this swelling start? • Is the swelling worse in the morning or at the end of the day, or is the swelling constant? • What relieves the swelling?	▶ Answers to these questions may help the nurse collect data that will be useful in determining the reason for the swelling.
3. Have you noticed any changes in temperature in your arms or legs, such as extreme coolness or heat?	▶ Extreme coolness may indicate arterial insufficiency (URMC, 2014).
4. Have you noticed any skin changes such as sores or ulcers on your legs? • If so, is there any pain associated with the sores?	▶ Leg ulcers can be an indication of chronic arterial or venous problems (Cleveland Clinic, 2017).
5. Have you noticed any changes in the feeling in your legs, such as numbness or tingling?	▶ Decreased circulation in the lower extremities can cause a loss of sensation, particularly in persons with diabetes (URMC, 2014).
6. Have you noticed a change in the growth of hair on your legs?	▶ Hair loss or slowed hair growth on the legs may be a manifestation of peripheral vascular disease (URMC, 2014).
7. Do you have any swollen glands? If so, where are they in your body? • How long have they been swollen? • Is there any pain or redness associated with these swollen glands? • Have you had any other symptoms, such as fever, fatigue, or bleeding?	▶ Enlarged lymph glands usually are associated with an infectious process in the body. Older adults have fewer and smaller lymph glands as a result of a decrease in lymphatic tissue (Mayo Clinic, 2018).
8. For male patients: Have you experienced any difficulty in achieving an erection?	▶ Impotence may occur as a result of a diminished arterial flow to the pelvic arteries (URMC, 2014). This condition is a common finding in peripheral vascular disease and is not always reported because of patient embarrassment.

Questions Related to Pain

1. Do you ever have pains in your legs or leg cramps? Is the sensation in one or both legs? • If so, please describe the pain or cramp, the location, and the time it most often occurs.	▶ Pain associated with arterial insufficiency is usually described as gnawing, sharp, or stabbing and increases with exercise (Ustundag, Gul, & Findik, 2016). Pain is relieved with the cessation of movement and when legs are dangling. The pain is most commonly in the calf of the leg, but it also may be in the lower leg or top of the foot. **Venous insufficiency** is described as aching or a feeling of fullness. It intensifies with prolonged standing or sitting in one position. Swelling and varicosities in the legs may also be present. The condition is relieved by elevating the legs or by walking.

Questions Related to Behaviors

1. Do you smoke? Do you use smokeless tobacco? • If so, how long have you smoked? • How many cigarettes, cigars, or pipes of tobacco do you smoke per day? How much smokeless tobacco do you use?	▶ Nicotine is a vasoconstrictor and aggravates peripheral vascular disease.
2. Do you exercise regularly? • If so, describe your exercise routine. • How often do you exercise? • For how long?	▶ Exercise not only helps to prevent vascular disease but also improves the survival rate of people who have already suffered a heart attack and reduces the likelihood of their suffering a second attack. Even modest levels of physical activity are beneficial, according to the American Heart Association (AHA, 2017).

Questions Related to Age and Pregnancy

The focused interview must reflect the anatomic and physiologic differences in the peripheral vascular system that exist along the age span as well as during pregnancy. Specific questions related to the peripheral vascular system for each of these groups are provided in Chapter 25, Chapter 26, and Chapter 27. ∞

Questions Related to the Environment

Environment refers to both the internal and external environments. Questions related to the internal environment include all of the previous questions and those associated with internal or physiologic responses. Questions regarding the external environment include those related to home, work, or social environments.

Focused Interview Questions	**Rationales and Evidence**

Internal Environment

1. **Are you now experiencing or have you ever had an experience of intermittent or prolonged anxiety or emotional upset?**
   - Describe the situation.
   - Can you determine precipitating factors?
   - Have you sought care or treatment for the problem?
   - What do you do when the problem arises?

   ▶ Anxiety and situations of emotion impact the sympathetic nervous system, producing hormonal responses that affect vascular function.

2. **What medications are you taking, either over the counter or prescription?**

   ▶ Contraceptive medications have been associated with blood clots in the peripheral vascular system (AHA, 2017). Aspirin is an anticoagulant.

External Environment

The following questions deal with the physical environment of the patient. That includes the indoor and outdoor environments of the home and the workplace, those encountered for social engagements, and any encountered during travel.

1. **Describe your daily activities.**

   ▶ Sedentary activities and prolonged periods of sitting and standing at work or in the home can promote peripheral vascular problems, varicosities, or problems associated with venous stasis.

Patient-Centered Interaction

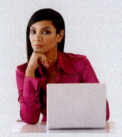

Source: George Doyle/ Stockbyte/Getty Images.

Ms. Mercedes Carlos, age 35, is an accountant at a local firm. She is married and has two children, ages 6 and 4. The family recently returned from a 10-day vacation in Florida where they visited many of the theme parks. The flight home was delayed 2 hours, and they were seated on the plane for more than 4 hours. Ms. C. reports to the employee health office complaining of right leg pain and edema of the right ankle and foot that seem to be worse when standing or sitting at the desk. Following is an excerpt of the nurse–patient interaction.

Interview

Nurse: Good morning, Ms. Carlos. What brings you here?

Ms. Carlos: I've been having some trouble with my leg. I just got back from vacation at a theme park in Florida. Our trip was great. Some of the lines at the parks were long. We did a lot of standing, walking, and sitting.

Nurse: How long was your trip?

Ms. Carlos: We were away for ten days. We got home Saturday night, and here I am Tuesday morning seeing you.

Nurse: Tell me about the swelling in your right leg.

Ms. Carlos: The swelling started in my lower right leg about the fifth day of our trip. After our flight home, I noticed my foot was really swollen. My right leg was almost double the size of the left leg. It is a little better now, but when I rub or push on the skin above my ankle, I leave fingerprints. It takes a few seconds for them to go away. I have never seen that before.

Nurse: Can you describe the type and severity of the pain you are feeling?

Ms. Carlos: The pain has been pretty bad. It is achy and constant, except when I put my leg up. Whenever I can put my leg up, the pain mostly goes away. As soon as I get up and start moving, the pain comes back again. It doesn't seem to be going away.

Nurse: Have you noticed any redness or heat around the swollen area?

Ms. Carlos: No, I have not.

Nurse: Have you ever had a problem like this before?

Ms. Carlos: During my last pregnancy I had a problem like this. The doctor told me I could be developing varicose veins. After the birth, I never had a problem until now. I'm too young to have varicose veins.

Analysis

Throughout the interview, the nurse uses open- and closed-ended questions to obtain information. The opening question by the nurse was to determine the patient's problem or chief complaint. Additional statements by the nurse give direction to the patient to provide specific subjective data.

Objective Data—Physical Assessment

In physical assessment of the peripheral vascular system, the techniques of inspection, palpation, and auscultation will be used. Before proceeding, it may be helpful to review the information about each of these data-gathering processes and practice the techniques of physical assessment.

EQUIPMENT

- Examination gown
- Sphygmomanometer
- Stethoscope
- Doppler stethoscope

HELPFUL HINTS

- The patient should don an examination gown, but undergarments may remain in place.
- The patient should remove watches and jewelry that may interfere with assessment.
- Socks and stockings must be removed.
- The patient will sit, stand, and lie in a supine position during various aspects of the assessment. The nurse should provide assistance and support when required and ensure that the patient's respiratory effort will not be affected by moving about or when lying flat.
- Use Standard Precautions.

Assessment Techniques and Findings

Physical assessment of the peripheral vascular and lymphatic systems requires the use of inspection, palpation, auscultation, and assessment of blood pressure. During each aspect of the assessment, the nurse is gathering objective data about circulation. Inspection includes looking at skin color, appearance of superficial vasculature, and shape and size of the extremities and nails. Palpation of pulses and auscultation of blood pressure and arteries provide information about vascular status. Knowledge of normal parameters and expected findings is essential in determining the meaning of the data as the physical assessment is performed.

An adult younger than age 60 or an adult older than age 60 with diabetes should have a normal systolic blood pressure of less than 140 and normal diastolic blood pressure below 90. (Normal pediatric blood pressure ranges are listed in Table 8.3.) The carotid pulses are palpable, symmetric, and synchronous with S1 of the heart. Auscultation of carotid arteries yields a soft sound, occasionally with transmission of heart sounds, but absence of bruits. The upper extremities are of equal size and warm with pink undertones and no edema. Capillary refill occurs in less than 2 seconds. The fingernails are pink and without clubbing. The brachial and radial arteries are equal in rate and symmetric in amplitude. The epitrochlear nodes are not palpable. The lower extremities are warm and equal in size, and the color is consistent with the rest of the body; hair is evenly distributed; and the extremities have no edema, lesions, or varicosities. The inguinal nodes are nonpalpable. The femoral, popliteal, posterior tibial, and dorsalis pedis pulses are equal and symmetric in rate and amplitude. The toes have hair, and the toenails are pink and not thickened or opaque.

Physical assessment of the peripheral vascular and lymphatic systems proceeds in an organized pattern. Blood pressure is assessed in the upper extremities. A cephalocaudal pattern for assessment of the vascular and lymphatic system begins with the carotid arteries and follows through inspection of the upper and lower extremities and palpation of pulses and lymph nodes within them.

Techniques and Normal Findings	Abnormal Findings and Special Considerations

Blood Pressure

1. **Instruct the patient.**
   - Explain that you will be assessing blood pressure in the arms. Tell the patient you will inflate the cuff twice for each location. The first time you will only touch a pulse area, and the second time you will use the stethoscope. Tell the patient to breathe normally and relax the extremity. The only discomfort should occur when the cuff is fully inflated and will be relieved as the cuff deflates. Tell the patient to report any other problems.
   - Ask the patient to remain still and not to speak during the auscultation because you will not hear well when the stethoscope is in place for the blood pressure reading.
   - Explain that you will take the blood pressure while the patient is sitting and then when lying down. The readings will be compared.

▶ Be sure to select the correct cuff size, especially for children or for obese patients. Inappropriate cuff size can alter the blood pressure reading.

Techniques and Normal Findings	Abnormal Findings and Special Considerations

2. **Position the patient.**
   - Place the patient in a sitting position on the examination table (see Figure 19.6 ■).

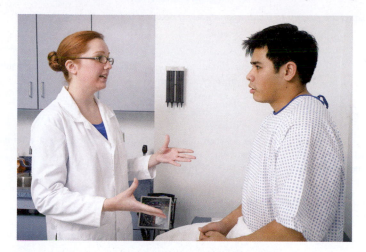

Figure 19.6 The patient is positioned for the examination.

- Take the blood pressure in both arms. Assess the palpable systolic pressure (see Figure 19.7A ■).
- Auscultate the blood pressure (see Figure 19.7B ■).

▶ Assessing the palpable systolic pressure helps to avoid an inaccuracy because of auscultatory gap when auscultating blood pressure.

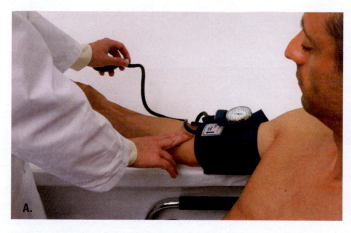 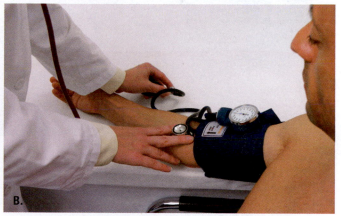

Figure 19.7 Blood pressure measurements. A. Palpable blood pressure. B. Auscultation of blood pressure.

- The blood pressure normally does not vary more than 5 mmHg to 10 mmHg in each arm.

▶ A difference of 10 mmHg or more between the arms may indicate an obstruction of arterial flow to one arm (The Consensus Committee of the American Autonomic Society and the American Academy of Neurology, 1996).

- Table 19.2 includes current guidelines regarding interpretation of blood pressure readings for individuals age 18 and older.

▶ A systolic reading below 90 or a diastolic reading under 60 may be an early indication of shock, which requires immediate medical attention.

Table 19.2 Classification of Blood Pressure for Adults 18 Years and Older

CLASSIFICATION	SYSTOLIC	DIASTOLIC
Adult	Less than 140	60–90
Older adult	Less than 150	60–90

Source: Charbek (2015); James et al. (2014).

Techniques and Normal Findings	Abnormal Findings and Special Considerations

3. Assist the patient to a supine position.

> **ALERT!** *When caring for older adults, it is important to assist the patient to a sitting or standing position before retaking the blood pressure and to be cautious that the patient does not fall.*

4. Take the blood pressure in both arms.
- Pressures are lower when taken in the supine position.
- Standards for blood pressure are set for patients in the sitting position.

▶ It is important to document the patient's position for each assessment of blood pressure.

Carotid Arteries

1. Inspect the neck for carotid pulsations.
- With the patient in a supine or sitting position, inspect the neck from the hyoid bone to the clavicles. Bilateral pulsations will be seen between the trachea and sternocleidomastoid muscle.

▶ The absence of pulsation may indicate internal or external obstruction.

2. Palpate the carotid pulses.
- Place the pads of your first two or three fingers on the patient's neck between the trachea and the sternocleidomastoid muscle below the angle of the jaw (see Figure 19.8 ■).

▶ Assessment of the carotid pulses may be difficult in obese patients with short, thick necks.

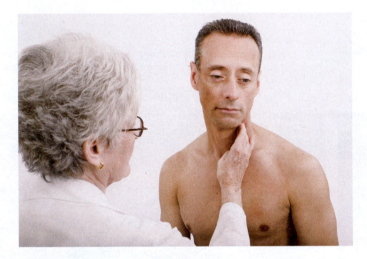

Figure 19.8 Palpating the carotid artery.

- Ask the patient to turn the head slightly toward your hand to relax the sternocleidomastoid muscle.
- Palpate firmly but not so hard that you occlude the artery.
- Palpate one side of the neck at a time. If you are having difficulty finding the pulse, try varying the pressure of your fingers, feeling carefully below the angle.

- Note the rate, rhythm, amplitude, and symmetry of the carotid pulses. Compare this rate to the apical pulse.

▶ If both carotid arteries are palpated at the same time, the result can be a drop in blood pressure or a reduction in the pulse rate from the stimulation of baroreceptors (Berman & Snyder, 2016).

▶ A rate over 90 beats/min is considered abnormal unless the patient is anxious or has recently been exercising or smoking. A rate below 60 is also considered abnormal. (Some athletes have a resting pulse as low as 50 beats/min.)

▶ An irregular rhythm or a pulse with extra beats or missed beats is considered abnormal. An exaggerated pulse or a weak, thready pulse is abnormal. A discrepancy between the two carotid pulses is abnormal.

3. Auscultate the carotid pulses.
- Using the diaphragm and bell of the stethoscope, auscultate each carotid artery inferior to the angle of the jaw and medial to the sternocleidomastoid muscle. Ask the patient to hold his or her breath for several seconds to decrease tracheal sounds. You may need to have the patient turn the head slightly to the side not being examined.
- Repeat the procedure using the bell of the stethoscope.

> **ALERT!** *It is important not to put pressure on the bell of the stethoscope because this may occlude the sounds in the blood vessel.*

Techniques and Normal Findings	Abnormal Findings and Special Considerations

- While auscultating, you should hear a very quiet sound. Normal heart sounds could be transmitted to the neck, but there should be no swishing sounds.

▶ A swishing sound indicates the presence of a **bruit**, an obstruction causing turbulence, such as a narrowing of the vessel because of the buildup of cholesterol.

▶ An increased cardiac output such as that seen in hyperthyroidism or anemia also will produce a bruit.

Arms

1. **Assess the hands.**
   - Take the patient's hands in your hands. Note the color of the skin and nail beds, the temperature and texture of the skin, and the presence of any lesions or swelling. Look at the fingers and nails from the side and observe the angle of the nail base. The angle should be about 160 degrees.

▶ Flattening of the angle of the nail and enlargement of the tips of the fingers (**clubbing**) is a sign of oxygen deprivation in the extremities. In patients with chronic hypoxia (oxygen deprivation), there may be a rounding of the tip of the finger described as "turkey drumsticks." The nail may feel spongy instead of firm, and there may be a blue discoloration of the nail.

2. **Observe for capillary refill in both hands.**
   - Holding one of the patient's hands in your hand, apply pressure to one of the patient's fingernails for 5 seconds.
   - The area under pressure should turn pale. Release the pressure and note how rapidly the normal color returns.
   - In a healthy patient, the color should return in less than 2 seconds.
   - Repeat the procedure for the other hand.

▶ A delayed capillary refill could indicate decreased cardiac output or constriction of the peripheral vessels. However, cigarette smoking, anemia, or cold temperatures can also cause delayed capillary refill.

3. **Place both arms together and compare their size.**
   - They should be nearly equal in size.

▶ **Edema** (increased accumulation of fluid) in the arms could indicate an obstruction of the lymphatic system.

4. **Palpate the radial pulse.**
   - The radial pulses are found on the ventral and medial side of each wrist. Ask the patient to extend one hand, palm up.
   - Palpate with two fingers over the radial bone (see Figure 19.9 ■).

▶ You may need to add more pressure to palpate if the patient is obese and has thick wrists.

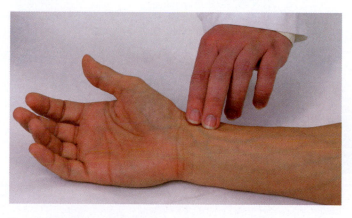

Figure 19.9 Palpating the radial pulse.

- Repeat the procedure for the other arm. Note the rate, rhythm, amplitude, and symmetry of the pulses.

▶ It is not necessary to palpate the ulnar pulses, located medial to the ulna on the flexor surface of the wrist. They are deeper than the radial pulses and are difficult to palpate.

Techniques and Normal Findings	Abnormal Findings and Special Considerations

- Characteristics of the peripheral pulse are included in Box 19.1.

Box 19.1 Assessing Peripheral Pulses

Assess peripheral pulses by palpating with gentle pressure over the artery. Use the pads of your first three fingers.

Note the following characteristics:

- Rate—the number of beats per minute
- Rhythm—the regularity of the beats
- Symmetry—pulses on both sides of body should be similar
- Amplitude—the strength of the beat, assessed on a scale of 0 to 4:

    0 = Absent or nonpalpable

    d = Doppler

    1 = Weak

    2 = Normal

    3 = Increased

    4 = Bounding

---

5. **Palpate both brachial pulses.**
    - The brachial pulses are found just medial to the biceps tendon.
    - Ask the patient to extend the arm.
    - Palpate over the brachial artery just superior to the antecubital region (see Figure 19.10 ■).
    - Repeat the procedure for the other arm.
    - Note the rate, rhythm, amplitude, and symmetry of the pulses.
    - Grade the amplitude on the 4-point scale as before.

▶ If a pulse is not palpable, a Doppler stethoscope should be used to palpate. When positioned over a patent artery, this device emits pulsing sound waves as the blood moves through the artery. If the Doppler is needed, document a lower case "d" to note the amplitude. Document a 0 if no pulsing sound is heard with the Doppler.

▶ Peripheral pulses may be difficult to assess in obese patients. It may require application of firmer pressure to the area in order to feel the pulse.

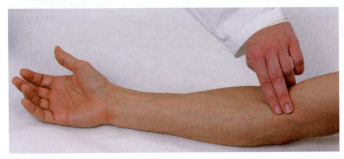

Figure 19.10 Palpating the brachial pulse.

6. **Palpate the epitrochlear lymph nodes in each arm.**
    - The epitrochlear node drains the forearm and the third, fourth, and fifth fingers.
    - Hold the patient's right hand in your right hand. With your left hand, reach behind the elbow to the groove between the biceps and triceps muscles (see Figure 19.11 ■).

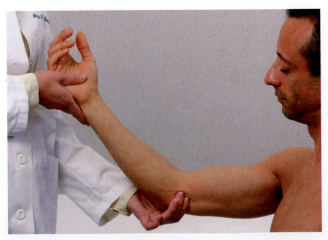

Figure 19.11 Palpating the epitrochlear lymph nodes.

Techniques and Normal Findings	Abnormal Findings and Special Considerations
• Note the size and consistency of the node. Normally, it is not palpable or is barely palpable. • Repeat the procedure for the left arm. **7. Palpate the axillary lymph nodes.** • With the palmar surface of your fingers, reach deep into the axilla. Gently palpate the anterior border of the axilla (anterior or subpectoral nodes), the central aspect along the rib cage (central nodes), the posterior border (subscapular/posterior nodes), and along the inner aspect of the upper arm (lateral nodes). Palpation of the axillary nodes is often part of the breast examination. Refer to Chapter 17, Table 17.18, for a depiction of palpating the axillary lymph nodes. **∞**	▶ An enlarged node may indicate an infection in the hand or forearm (Mayo Clinic, 2018).

Appendix C: Advanced Skills *Appendix C provides step-by-step instructions on performing Allen's Test.* **∞**

Legs

1. Inspect both legs. • Observe skin color, hair distribution, and any skin lesions. • Skin color should match the skin tone of the rest of the body. Hair is normally present on the legs. • If the hair has been removed, there is still usually hair on the dorsal surface of the great toes. Hair growth should be symmetric.	▶ If peripheral vessels are constricted, the skin will be paler than the rest of the body. If the vessels are dilated, the skin will have a reddish tone.
	▶ A rusty discoloration over the anterior tibial surface with the skin intact is associated with venous disease. The characteristic color stems from blood leaking out of a vessel with decreased capacity for it to be reabsorbed. Unintentional absence of hair on the legs may be a manifestation of peripheral vascular disease (URMC, 2014).
• The skin should be intact with no lesions.	▶ If skin lesions or ulcerations are present, the size and location should be noted. Ulcers occurring as a result of arterial deficit tend to occur on pressure points, such as tips of toes and lateral malleoli. Venous ulcers occur at medial malleoli because of fragile tissue with poor drainage.
	▶ If any blackened tissue is discovered, the patient must be referred to a physician immediately. The presence of blackened tissue can indicate tissue death (necrosis).
2. Compare the size of the legs. • The legs should be symmetric in size. If they are unequal in size, measure the circumference of each leg at the widest point. It is important to measure each leg at the same point.	▶ A discrepancy in the size of the legs could indicate an accumulation of fluid (edema) resulting from increased pressure in the capillaries or an obstruction of a lymph vessel. Unequal size of the legs could also indicate a blood clot in the deep vessels of the leg.
3. Palpate the legs for temperature. • Palpate from the feet up the legs, using the dorsal surface of your hands. • Note any discrepancies. • The skin should be the same temperature on both legs.	▶ If the peripheral vessels are constricted, the skin will feel cool. If the peripheral vessels are dilated, the skin will feel warm. A difference in the temperature of the feet may be a sign of arterial insufficiency.
4. Assess the legs for the presence of superficial veins. • With the patient in a sitting position and legs dangling from the examination table, inspect the legs. • Now ask the patient to elevate the legs. • The veins may appear as nodular bulges when the legs are in the dependent position, but any bulges should disappear when the legs are elevated.	▶ **Varicosities** (distended veins) frequently occur in the anterolateral aspect of the thigh and lower leg or on the posterolateral aspect of the calf. These bulging veins do not disappear when legs are elevated. Varicose veins are dilated but have a diminished blood flow and an increased intravenous pressure. An incompetent valve, a weakness in the vein wall, or an obstruction in a proximal vein causes varicosities (Marieb, 2017).
• Palpate the veins for tenderness or inflammation.	▶ Tenderness or inflammation could be a sign of phlebitis, especially if redness and swelling are present.
5. Perform the manual compression test. • If varicose veins are present, you can determine the length of the varicose vein and the competency of its valves with the manual compression test. • Ask the patient to stand. • With the fingers of one hand, palpate the lower part of the varicose vein.	

Techniques and Normal Findings	Abnormal Findings and Special Considerations

- Keeping that hand on the vein, compress the vein firmly at least 15 cm to 20 cm higher with the fingers of your other hand (see Figure 19.12 ■).

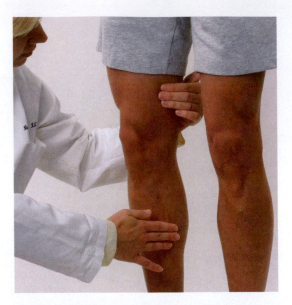

Figure 19.12 Performing the manual compression test.

- You will not feel any pulsation beneath your lower fingers if the valves of the varicose vein are still competent.

▶ If the valves are incompetent, an impulse in the vein will be felt between your two hands.

6. Palpate the inguinal lymph nodes.
- Move the patient's gown aside over the inguinal region. Palpate over the top of the medial thigh (see Figure 19.13 ■).

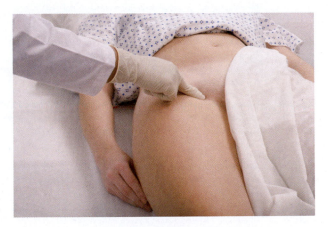

Figure 19.13 Palpating the inguinal lymph nodes.

- If the nodes can be palpated, they should be movable and not tender.
- Repeat the procedure for the other leg.

▶ Generally, lymph nodes that are larger than 1 cm (0.39 in.) or tender are considered to be abnormal and may be an indication of an infection in the legs or a sexually transmitted infection (Cleveland Clinic, 2013).

7. Palpate both femoral pulses.
- The femoral pulses are inferior and medial to the inguinal ligament.
- Ask the patient to flex the knee and externally rotate the hip. Palpate over the femoral artery (see Figure 19.14 ■).

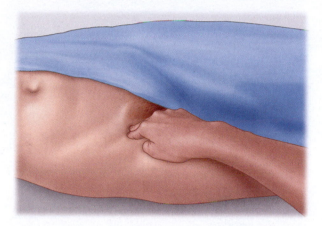

Figure 19.14 Palpating the femoral artery.

- The femoral artery is deep, and you may need to place one hand on top of the other to locate the pulse. Repeat the procedure for the other leg.
- Note the rate, rhythm, amplitude, and symmetry of the pulses.
- Grade the amplitude on the 4-point scale.

8. Palpate both popliteal pulses.
- The pulsations of the popliteal artery can be palpated deep in the popliteal fossa lateral to the midline.
- Ask the patient to flex the knee and relax the leg.
- Palpate the popliteal pulse.
- If you cannot locate the pulse, ask the patient to roll onto the abdomen and flex the knee (see Figure 19.15 ■).
- Palpate deeply for the pulse.
- Repeat the procedure for the other leg.
- Note the rate, rhythm, amplitude, and symmetry of the pulses.
- Grade the amplitude on the 4-point scale.
- Grade the amplitude on the 4-point scale.

▶ If it is not possible to palpate the femoral pulse, an artery may be occluded.

▶ If the popliteal pulse cannot be palpated, an artery may be occluded.

▶ A Doppler ultrasound may be required to assess popliteal pulses.

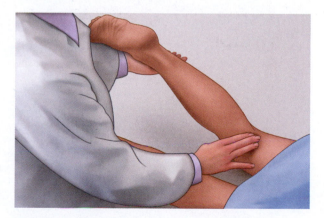

Figure 19.15 Palpating the popliteal pulse.

Techniques and Normal Findings	Abnormal Findings and Special Considerations

9. Palpate both dorsalis pedis pulses.
- The dorsalis pedis pulses may be felt on the medial side of the dorsum of the foot.
- Palpate the pulse lateral to the extensor tendon of the great toe (see Figure 19.16 ■).
- Use light pressure.
- Repeat the procedure for the other foot.
- Note the rate, rhythm, amplitude, and symmetry of the pulses.
- Grade the amplitude on the 4-point scale.

▶ The absence of a dorsalis pedis pulse may not be indicative of occlusion because another artery may be supplying blood to this area of the foot. Edema in the foot will make palpation difficult. A Doppler ultrasound device may be used to assess the pulse in an obese or edematous area.

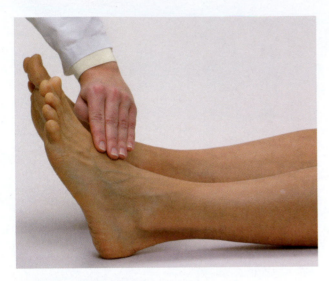

Figure 19.16 Palpating the dorsalis pedis pulse.

10. Palpate both posterior tibial pulses.
- The posterior tibial pulses may be palpated behind and slightly inferior to the medial malleolus of the ankle, in the groove between the malleolus and the Achilles tendon.
- Palpate the pulse by curving your fingers around the medial malleolus (see Figure 19.17 ■).
- Repeat the procedure for the other foot. Note the rate, rhythm, amplitude, and symmetry of the pulses.
- Grade the amplitude on the 4-point scale.

▶ If it is not possible to palpate the posterior tibial pulse, an artery may be occluded. If the patient has edematous ankles, this pulse may be difficult to palpate.

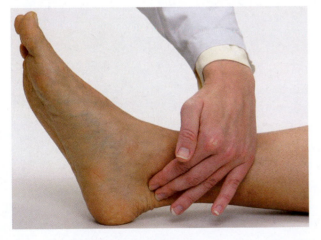

Figure 19.17 Palpating the posterior tibial pulse.

Techniques and Normal Findings	Abnormal Findings and Special Considerations

11. Assess for arterial supply to the lower legs and feet.
- If you suspect an arterial deficiency, test for arterial supply to the lower extremities. Ask the patient to remain supine.
- Elevate the patient's legs 12 inches above the heart (see Figure 19.18 ■).

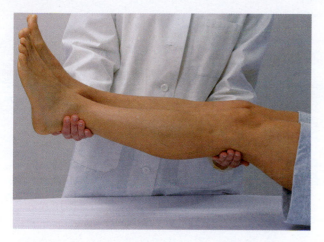

Figure 19.18 Testing the arterial supply to the lower extremities.

- Ask the patient to move the feet up and down at the ankles for 60 seconds to drain the venous blood.
- The skin will be blanched in color because only arterial blood is present.
- Now ask the patient to sit up and dangle the feet.
- Compare the color of both feet.
- The original color should return in about 10 seconds.
- The superficial veins in the feet should fill in about 15 seconds.

- The feet of a dark-skinned person may be difficult to evaluate, but the soles of the feet should reflect a change in color.

▶ Marked pallor of the elevated extremities may indicate arterial insufficiency.

▶ A marked bluish-red color of the dependent feet occurs with severe arterial insufficiency. This color is because of a lack of oxygenated blood to the area, which leads to a loss of vasomotor tone and venous stasis.

▶ Delayed filling of the superficial veins of the feet also could indicate arterial insufficiency. Motor loss may occur with arterial insufficiency.

▶ Sensory loss may occur with arterial insufficiency.

▶ Pitting edema can be related to a failure of the right side of the heart or an obstruction of the lymphatic system. Edema in only one leg may indicate an occlusion of a large vein in the leg. Diminished arterial flow thickens toenails, which often become yellow and loosely attached to the nail bed. Patients with diabetes often acquire fungal and bacterial infections of the nail because of increased glucose collecting in the skin under the nail. Careful examination of the feet is essential in the patient with diabetes because of the potential decrease in sensitivity to pain or injury and altered capacity for healing.

12. Test the lower legs for muscle strength.
- With the patient in a sitting position, instruct the patient to extend each knee while you apply opposing force. Instruct the patient to flex the knees again. The patient should be able to perform the movement against resistance. The strength of the muscles in both legs is equal. Testing of muscle strength is discussed in greater detail in Chapter 23. ∞

Techniques and Normal Findings	Abnormal Findings and Special Considerations

13. Test the lower legs for sensation.

- To assess light touch, use a cotton wisp lightly applied to symmetric areas on each lower extremity. The rounded end and the sharp end of a safety pin are used to assess pain sensation. The ends are applied to symmetric areas of the lower legs in a random pattern of sharp and dull to assess sensation. The patient should have eyes closed during the assessment. Ask the patient to state "Now" when the cotton wisp is felt, and "Sharp" or "Dull" when the ends of the safety pin are applied.

- The patient should sense touch and pain. Testing for the perception of sensation is discussed in greater detail in Chapter 24. ∞

14. Check for edema of the legs.

- For at least 5 seconds, press the skin over the tibia, behind the medial malleolus, and over the dorsum of each foot (see Figure 19.19 ■).

▶ Edema can be localized or generalized. It refers to a collection of fluid in the body tissues. It is classified as pitting or nonpitting. Edema can result from cardiac, vascular, or lymphatic problems; fluid and electrolyte disturbances; nutritional disturbances; renal failure; and in response to toxins and chemicals (Marieb, 2017).

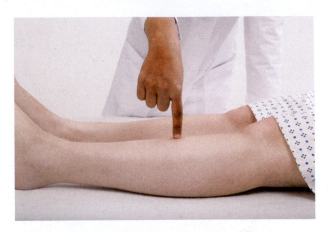

Figure 19.19 Palpating for edema over the tibia.

- Look for a depression in the skin (called pitting edema) caused by the pressure of your fingers (see Figure 19.20 ■).

▶ Pitting edema usually occurs in the extremities.

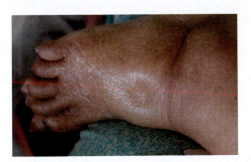

Figure 19.20 Pitting edema of the lower extremities.
Source: Akkalak Aiempradit/Shutterstock.

Techniques and Normal Findings	Abnormal Findings and Special Considerations

- If edema is present, you should grade it on a scale of 1+ (mild) to 4+ (severe) as shown in Figure 19.21 ■.

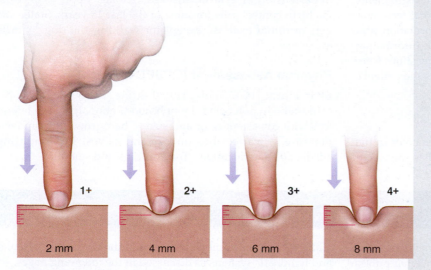

1+	2+	3+	4+
2 mm	4 mm	6 mm	8 mm

Figure 19.21 Grading pitting edema.

15. Inspect the toenails for color and thickness.
- Nails should be pink and not thickened. Clubbing should not be present.

Evidence-Based Practice:

Deep Vein Thrombosis

A deep vein thrombosis (DVT) is a frequently occurring condition that can have serious consequences, the most serious of which is a pulmonary embolus (PE). Assessment of a DVT can be difficult because the patient does not generally experience obvious symptoms. Decades ago the Homans sign was identified as a means of determining the presence or absence of a DVT. The procedure for eliciting a Homans sign has the examiner flex the patient's leg while simultaneously dorsiflexing the ankle, which if positive will cause calf pain. The pain occurs when the posterior tibial vein is inflamed, possibly from a DVT. Unfortunately, this pain can be caused by other factors, including short heel cords from wearing high-heel shoes, calf muscle spasms, and cellulitis (Mathewson, 1983; Urbano, 2001).

Over the years, belief that Homans sign was a reliable indicator of a DVT diminished as numerous sources showed problems with its accuracy. In patients with a confirmed DVT, positive Homans signs were found in as low as 8% and as high as 56% (Cranley, Canos, & Sull, 1976; Heick & Farris, 2017; Molloy, English, O'Dwyer, & O'Connell, 1982; Urbano, 2001). In addition, positive Homans signs were found in up to 50% of those who did not have a DVT (Cranley et al., 1976; Heick & Farris, 2017; Koepplinger & Jaeblon, 2010; Molloy et al., 1982; Urbano, 2001). The lack of reliability has led to a decline in the use of this test as a means to screen for DVT.

Heick and Farris (2017) surveyed physical therapy clinical instructors to determine the methods they used to assess for DVT. Over 80% of the instructors were taught to use the Homans sign, and 68% continued to use it in their own practice. Heick and Farris (2017) determined significant use of outdated screening methods suggesting a need to ensure evidence-based practice used to identify DVT.

Documenting Your Findings

Documentation of assessment data—subjective and objective—must be accurate, professional, complete, and confidential. When documenting the information from the focused assessment of each body system, the nurse should use measurements where appropriate to ensure accuracy, use medical terminology rather than jargon, include all pertinent information, and avoid language that could identify the patient. The information in the documentation should make it clear what questions were asked and use language to indicate whether it is the patient's response or the nurse's findings.

Focused History (SUBJECTIVE DATA)

Denies any change in temperature, sensation, or color in the legs. No ulcers or pain with activity. States she has some aching in her calves and swelling in her ankles after being on her feet at work. States she developed some varicose veins during her second pregnancy. No history or family history of hypertension or arterial disease. Smokes 1 ppd × 10 years. On birth control pills for most of the last 15 years. States she gets minimal exercise except for walking the dog $1/2$ mile every day.

Physical Assessment (OBJECTIVE DATA)

BP in R arm 114/82 lying, 110/80 sitting, 108/80 standing. No orthostatic hypotension. Lymph nodes nonpalpable. Bilateral legs with consistent color and size, + hair growth, warm temperature, + varicosities on bilateral calves, 1+ nonpitting edema on bilateral ankles. Toenails pink and smooth.

Abnormal Findings

Findings from physical assessment of the peripheral vascular and lymphatic systems include normal and abnormal pulses (Table 19.3) and common alterations of the peripheral vascular and lymphatic systems as discussed in the following pages.

Table 19.3 Normal and Abnormal Pulses

NAME OF PULSE	CHARACTERISTICS	ARTERIAL WAVEFORM PATTERN	CONTRIBUTING CONDITIONS
Normal	• Regular, even in intensity		• Normal
Absent	• No palpable pulse, no waveform		• Arterial line disconnected • Cardiac arrest
Weak/Thready	• Intensity of pulse is +1 • May wax and wane • May be difficult to find		• Shock • Severe peripheral vascular disease
Bounding	• Intensity of pulse is +4 • Very easy to observe in arterial locations near surface of skin • Very easy to palpate and difficult to obliterate with pressure from fingertips		• Hyperdynamic states such as seen with hyperthyroidism, exercise, anxiety, vasodilation seen in high cardiac output syndromes • May be because of normal aging secondary to arterial wall stiffening • Aortic regurgitation • Anemia
Biferiens	• Has two systolic peaks with a dip in between • Easier to detect in the carotid location • In the case of hypertrophic obstructive cardiomyopathy, only one systolic peak palpated but waveform demonstrates double systolic peak		• Aortic regurgitation • Combination of aortic regurgitation and stenosis • Hypertrophic obstructive cardiomyopathy
Pulsus Alternans	• Alternating strong and weak pulses • Equal interval between each pulse		• Aortic regurgitation • Terminal left ventricular heart failure • Systemic hypertension
Pulsus Bigeminus	• Alternating strong and weak pulses, but the weak pulse comes in *early* after the strong pulse		• Regular bigeminal dysrhythmias such as premature ventricular contractions (PVCs) and premature atrial contractions (PACs)

(continued)

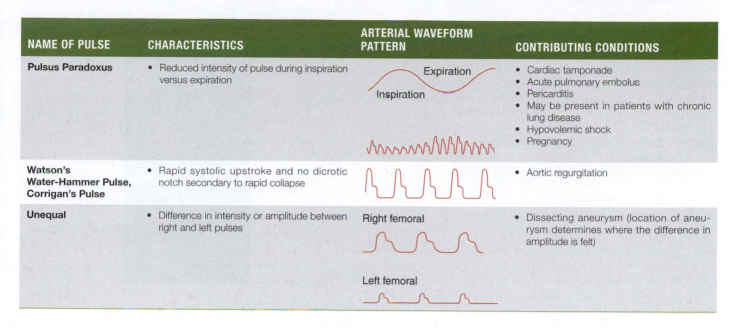

NAME OF PULSE	CHARACTERISTICS	ARTERIAL WAVEFORM PATTERN	CONTRIBUTING CONDITIONS
Pulsus Paradoxus	• Reduced intensity of pulse during inspiration versus expiration	Expiration / Inspiration	• Cardiac tamponade • Acute pulmonary embolus • Pericarditis • May be present in patients with chronic lung disease • Hypovolemic shock • Pregnancy
Watson's Water-Hammer Pulse, Corrigan's Pulse	• Rapid systolic upstroke and no dicrotic notch secondary to rapid collapse		• Aortic regurgitation
Unequal	• Difference in intensity or amplitude between right and left pulses	Right femoral Left femoral	• Dissecting aneurysm (location of aneurysm determines where the difference in amplitude is felt)

Arterial Insufficiency

Arterial insufficiency is inadequate circulation in the arterial system, usually because of the buildup of fatty plaque or calcification of the arterial wall. Narrowing or obstruction of the arteries in the legs, aorta, or both regions causes a reduction in oxygenated blood flow to the lower extremities. When arterial insufficiency causes pain in the thigh, calf, or buttocks, this condition is referred to as **claudication**, which may be a symptom of peripheral arterial disease (PAD). In most cases, pain related to claudication is caused by ischemia in the cells of the tissues in the lower extremities, is triggered by walking, and resolves with rest. Oxygen requirements to the muscles is greater during activity (Johns Hopkins University, n.d.). Ulcers resulting from arterial insufficiency are usually seen on the toes or areas of trauma of the feet or lateral malleolus (see Figure 19.22 ■). The ulcer is pale in color with well-defined edges and no bleeding. The wounds are often difficult to heal because of the lack of oxygenated blood reaching the affected area.

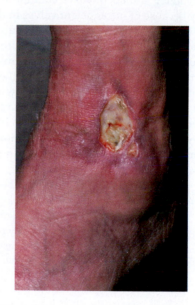

Figure 19.22 Ulcer because of arterial insufficiency.
Source: SPL/Science Source.

Subjective findings:
• Pain, aching, burning, or discomfort in the feet, calves, or thighs
• Numbness in legs or feet when at rest
• Appearance of symptoms only when walking uphill, walking at a brisk pace, or walking for extended periods (MedlinePlus, 2014)

Objective findings:
• Diminished pulses
• Cool, shiny skin
• Absence of hair on toes
• Pallor of lower extremities on elevation
• Red color (rubor) of lower extremities when dependent

Arterial Aneurysm

Arterial aneurysm is a bulging or dilation caused by a weakness in the wall of an artery (see Figure 19.23 ■). It can occur in the aorta and the abdominal, renal, or femoral arteries. Aneurysms can sometimes be detected by a characteristic bruit over the artery; however, if they are located deep in the abdomen, they can be difficult to discover. Both the subjective and objective findings vary greatly depending on the location of the aneurysm; some aneurysms are not discovered before rupturing.

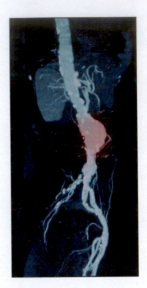

Figure 19.23 Arterial aneurysm.
Source: Suttha Burawonk/Shuttertstock.

Venous Insufficiency

Venous insufficiency is inadequate circulation in the venous system usually because of incompetent valves in deep veins or a blood clot in the veins. The valves in the veins are designed to keep the blood moving back to the heart and to prevent the blood from remaining in the veins or accumulating in the lower extremities. As the valves are damaged, the blood flows backward and pools in the legs, especially with standing. Ulcers related to venous insufficiency are often found on the medial malleolus and are characterized by bleeding and uneven edges (see Figure 19.24 ■). There is minimal pain associated with the ulcer, and the skin surrounding the ulcer is coarse.

Subjective findings:
- Feeling of fullness or discomfort in the legs
- Exacerbation of leg discomfort caused by prolonged standing or sitting
- Discomfort relieved by several hours of rest

Objective findings:
- Normal skin temperature
- Edema usually present
- Thickening and brown discoloration of skin around the ankles

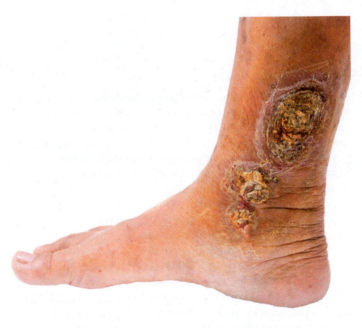

Figure 19.24 Ulcer related to venous insufficiency.
Source: myibean/123RF.

Orthostatic Hypotension

Orthostatic hypotension is a temporary drop in blood pressure that occurs after standing up rapidly from a sitting or lying position. This results from abrupt peripheral vasodilation without a compensatory increase in cardiac output. Causes of orthostatic hypotension include dehydration; decrease in blood volume; neurologic, cardiovascular, or endocrine disorders; and some medications.

Subjective findings:

- Dizziness or lightheadedness
- Blurred vision
- Weakness
- Nausea
- Headache or chest, neck, or shoulder pain

Objective findings:

- A decrease in systolic blood pressure of 20 mmHg or more or a decrease in diastolic blood pressure of 10 mmHg or more within three minutes of standing compared with the blood pressure taken from the sitting or supine position (The Consensus Committee of the American Autonomic Society and the American Academy of Neurology, 1996)
- Palpitations
- Syncope

Varicose Veins

Varicose veins (varicosities) are veins that have become dilated and have a diminished rate of blood flow and increased intravenous pressure (see Figure 19.25 ■). The condition may be the result of incompetent valves that permit the reflux of blood or an obstruction of a proximal vein.

Subjective findings:

- Aching, burning, heaviness, tiredness, or pain in legs
- Exacerbation of symptoms because of extended periods of sitting or standing
- Burning or itching over affected veins

Objective findings:

- Distended, twisted veins near the skin's surface
- Edema in feet or ankles
- Skin changes, including discoloration, dryness, or scaling
- Skin ulceration
- Bleeding after minor trauma

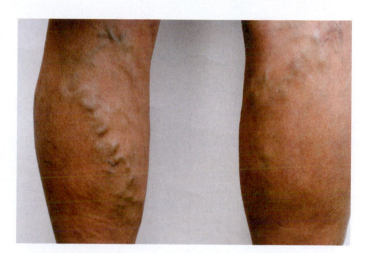

Figure 19.25 Varicose veins.
Source: Mark Boulton/Alamy Stock Photo.

Raynaud Disease

Raynaud disease is a condition in which the arterioles in the fingers develop spasms, causing intermittent skin pallor or cyanosis and then rubor (red color). This condition is seen most commonly in young, otherwise healthy females, frequently secondary to connective tissue disease, drug intoxication, pulmonary hypertension, or trauma (see Figure 19.26 ■).

Subjective findings:

- Bilateral spasms lasting from minutes to hours
- Numbness or pain during the pallor or cyanotic state
- Burning or throbbing pain during the rubor (Mayo Clinic, 2017b)

Objective findings:

- Skin pallor or cyanosis that may progress to rubor
- Swelling of affected digits or areas (Mayo Clinic, 2017b)

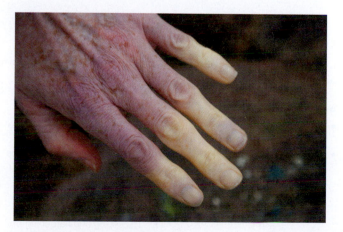

Figure 19.26 Raynaud disease.
Source: Richard Newton/Alamy Stock Photo.

Deep Vein Thrombosis

Deep vein thrombosis (DVT) is the occlusion of a deep vein, such as in the femoral or pelvic circulation, by a blood clot (see Figure 19.27 ■). This condition requires immediate referral because of the danger of the clot becoming a venous thrombo-embolism (VTE) and migrating to the lung, resulting in a pulmonary embolism (PE).

Subjective findings:

- Absence of symptoms, or the patient may describe intense, sharp pain along the iliac vessels, in the popliteal space, or in the calf muscles

Objective findings:

- Unilateral edema
- Low-grade fever
- Tachycardia (rapid heartbeat)
- Venous distention

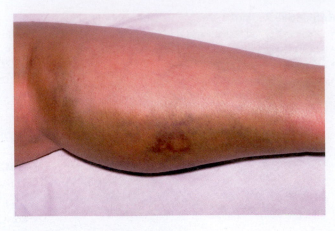

Figure 19.27 Deep vein thrombosis.
Source: Mediscan/Alamy Stock Photo.

Arteriovenous Fistula

An arteriovenous (AV) fistula is an abnormal connection between an artery and vein. This is commonly caused by piercing injuries, such as stab or gunshot wounds that occur in a location where a vein and artery lie close together. However, it can also be congenital, genetic, or the result of a procedure such as cardiac catheterization. An AV fistula may be surgically formed if needed for kidney dialysis.

Subjective findings:

- Fatigue
- Difficulty breathing
- Dizziness
- Lightheadedness

Objective findings:

- Machinery murmur (a sound like the clicking or humming of machinery) when auscultated
- Bulging veins near the surface of the skin
- Decreased blood pressure, increased heart rate, and heart failure
- Cyanosis
- Clubbing of fingers (Mayo Clinic, 2015)

Lymphedema

Lymphedema is unilateral swelling associated with an obstruction in lymph nodes (see Figure 19.28 ■).

Subjective findings:

- Sensation of heaviness or tightness in the associated limb
- Discomfort or aching in the associated limb (Mayo Clinic, 2017a)

Objective findings:

- Limited range of motion in the associated limb
- Swelling of all or part of the associated arm or leg, including fingers or toes
- Chronic, recurrent infections in the associated limb
- Thickening and hardening of the skin of the associated limb (Mayo Clinic, 2017a)

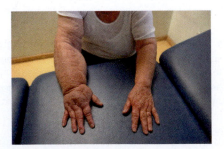

Figure 19.28 Lymphedema.
Source: Sergio Azenha/Alamy Stock Photo.

Application Through Critical Thinking

CASE STUDY

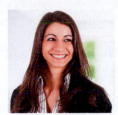

Source: Minerva Studio/ Shutterstock.

Jenny Battaglia, a 26-year-old female, is seen in the emergency department (ED) for pain in her lower legs. The patient states that she has had pain in her calves for about 48 hours, starting when she got home from vacation. She does not recall any injury. She says it started like cramping but has not improved with rest or taking Tylenol. She thinks there is a little swelling and some tenderness.

The nurse knows that an organized approach to data collection is essential. Further, every effort must be made to get a comprehensive picture of the situation and to avoid missing pieces of information that will guide decision making for the patient.

The approach to care of the patient will be determined by the patient's condition. When a patient is in acute distress—for example, with dyspnea, with a bleeding injury, in shock, or in severe pain—data gathering focuses on the immediate problem and its resolution.

Ms. Battaglia is uncomfortable but does not appear to be in acute distress and denies severe discomfort. She states, "I'm a little nervous. I've never really been sick and have only been in the emergency department once before for a couple of stitches when I was ten." The nurse tells Ms. Battaglia that they will begin an examination to determine the cause of her problem.

The assessment reveals the following: A thin female. The patient is suntanned, and without pink undertone to her skin. B/P 116/64 (R) arm, sitting—radial pulse 3+ bilaterally rate 88, RR 16—temperature 99.2°F. Upper extremities symmetric in size, no edema; radial and brachial pulses equal, regular; lower extremities, edema, rubor (redness) bilateral posterior lower legs, warm and tender to touch. Radial and pedal pulses present, equal, 3+.

The nurse considers the data and determines that Ms. Battaglia is not in acute distress. However, pallor, edema in lower extremities suggests a vascular problem. The nurse decides to continue the health assessment by further interview for missing subjective information.

The interview reveals that Ms. Battaglia has no personal or family history of vascular problems, cardiovascular disease, or diabetes. She is not married and lives with her boyfriend. She takes aspirin or Tylenol occasionally for headaches or menstrual cramps. She has no allergies. She is para 0 gravida 0, LMP 2 weeks before ED visit, regular menses, has taken birth control pills for 3 years.

The nurse asks Ms. Battaglia several questions about the leg pain. The patient states it is 5 to 7 on a scale of 1 to 10 and continuous. Nothing she has done has relieved the pain. It started 48 hours ago "at the end of my vacation" and wakes her at night.

The nurse asks if travel was involved in the vacation. Ms. Battaglia says, "Yes, we flew to Aruba for six days. That's how I got a tan. We had a great time, and I was feeling rested, ready to go back to work, and looked forward to seeing family and friends." Further questions reveal that the flight was 6 hours and Ms. Battaglia "slept almost all the way back—I never really moved."

The data suggest to the nurse that Ms. Battaglia has deep vein thrombosis. Ms. Battaglia is admitted to a medical unit. She will be on bed rest and receive anticoagulation therapy.

COMPLETE DOCUMENTATION

The following is a sample narrative complete documentation for Jenny Battaglia.

SUBJECTIVE DATA: Pain in lower legs for about 48 hr. Started when she got home from vacation. No recall of injury. Started as cramping, no improvement with rest or Tylenol. She thinks there is some swelling and tenderness. "A little nervous." No personal or family history of vascular problems, cardiac disease, or diabetes. Single, lives with boyfriend. Tylenol or aspirin occasionally for headache or menstrual cramps. No allergies. Gravida 0, Para 0, LMP 2 weeks before ED visit, regular menses. Oral contraceptives for 3 years. Air travel—flight of 6 hr—Jenny slept almost all the time.

OBJECTIVE DATA: Suntanned, without pink undertone. Vital signs: B/P 116/64 right, sitting. Radial pulse 3+ bilaterally rate 88, RR 16. Temperature 99.2°F. Pain: 5 to 7 on a scale of 1 to 10, continuous, wakes at night. Upper extremities symmetric in size, no edema, warm, brachial and radial pulses = regular. Cap refill < 2 sec L & R. Extremities—below knees, posterior bilateral rubor, edema 1+, warm, tender to touch. Pulses present, 3+. No lesions, no visible superficial vessels. Feet warm, no edema. Toenails—polish—unable to assess.

CRITICAL THINKING QUESTIONS

1. Identify the data that suggest the presence of DVT.

2. How would the data be clustered?

3. Describe the areas for patient education derived from this case study.

4. What would you recommend the patient do to prevent a future occurrence?

5. What additional factors would put the patient at even greater risk for DVT?

REFERENCES

American Diabetes Association. (2014). *Statistics about diabetes.* Retrieved from http://www.diabetes.org/diabetes-basics/statistics/

American Heart Association (AHA). (2017). AHA statistical update: Heart disease and stroke statistics—2017 update. *Circulation,*135,E146-E603.doi:10.1161/CIR.0000000000000485

Berman, A., & Snyder, S. (2016). *Kozier and Erb's fundamentals of nursing: Concepts, process, and practice* (9th ed.). Upper Saddle River, NJ: Prentice Hall.

Centers for Disease Control and Prevention (CDC). (2014). *Overweight and obesity: Adult obesity facts.* Retrieved from http://www.cdc.gov/obesity/data/adult.html

Charbek, E. (2015). *Normal vital signs.* Retrieved from https://emedicine.medscape.com/article/2172054-overview

Cleveland Clinic. (2013). *Diseases & conditions: Swollen lymph nodes.* Retrieved from http://my.clevelandclinic.org/disorders/lymph-nodes/hic-swollen-lymph-nodes.aspx

Cleveland Clinic. (2017). *Leg and foot ulcers.*https://my.clevelandclinic.org/health/diseases/17169-leg-and-foot-ulcers

The Consensus Committee of the American Autonomic Society and the American Academy of Neurology. (1996). Consensus statement on the definition of orthostatic hypotension, pure autonomic failure, and multiple system atrophy. *Neurology,*46 (5), 1470.

Cranley, J., Canos, A. J., & Sull, W. J. (1976). The diagnosis of deep venous thrombosis: Fallibility of clinical symptoms and signs. *Archives of Surgery,*111, 34–36.

Heick, J. D., & Farris, J. W. (2017). Survey of methods used to determine if a patient has a deep vein thrombosis: An exploratory research report. *Physiotherapy Theory and Practice,*33 (9), 733–742. doi:10.1080/09593985.2017.1345023

James, P. A., Oparil, S., Carter, B. L., Cushman, W. C., Dennison-Himmelfarb, C., Handler, J., . . . Ortiz, E. (2014). 2014 Evidence-Based Guideline for the Management of High Blood Pressure in Adults Report From the Panel Members Appointed to the Eighth Joint National Committee (JNC 8) [Abstract].JAMA,311(5),507–520. doi:10.1001/jama.2013.284427

Johns Hopkins University. (n.d.). *Claudication: What is claudication?* Retrieved from http://www.hopkinsmedicine.org/healthlibrary/conditions/cardiovascular_diseases/claudication_85,P08251

Koepplinger, M. E., & Jaeblon, T. D. (2010). Venous thromboembolism diagnosis and prophylaxis in the trauma population. *Current Orthopaedic Practice,* 21(3), 301–305.

Marieb, E. (2017). *Essentials of human anatomy and physiology* (9th ed.). San Francisco, CA: Benjamin/Cummings/Pearson Education.

Mathewson, M. (1983). A Homan's sign is an effective method of diagnosing thrombophlebitis in bedridden patients. *Critical Care Nurse,* July/August, 64–65.

Mayo Clinic. (2015). *Arteriovenous fistula.* Retrieved from https://www.mayoclinic.org/diseases-conditions/arteriovenous-fistula/symptoms-causes/syc-20369567

Mayo Clinic. (2017a). *Lymphedema: Symptoms.* Retrieved from https://www.mayoclinic.org/diseases-conditions/lymphedema/symptoms-causes/syc-20374682

Mayo Clinic. (2017b). *Raynaud's disease: Symptoms.* Retrieved from https://www.mayoclinic.org/diseases-conditions/raynauds-disease/symptoms-causes/syc-20363571

Mayo Clinic. (2018). *Swollen lymph nodes.* Retrieved from https://www.mayoclinic.org/diseases-conditions/swollen-lymph-nodes/symptoms-causes/syc-20353902

MedlinePlus. (2014). Peripheral artery disease – Legs. Retrieved from http://www.nlm.nih.gov/medlineplus/ency/article/000170.htm

Molloy, W., English, J., O'Dwyer, R., & O'Connell, J. (1982). Clinical findings in the diagnosis of proximal deep vein thrombosis. *Irish Medical Journal,*75, 119–120.

University of Rochester Medical Center (URMC). (2014). *Peripheral vascular disease: What is peripheral vascular disease (PVD)?* Retrieved from http://www.urmc.rochester.edu/Encyclopedia/Content.aspx?ContentTypeID=85&ContentID=P00

Urbano, F. (2001, March). Homans' sign in the diagnosis of deep venous thrombosis. *Hospital Physician,* 22–24.

Ustundag, H., Gul, A., & Findik, U. Y. (2016). Quality of life and pain in patients with peripheral arterial disease. *International Journal of Caring Sciences,*9 (3), 838–845.

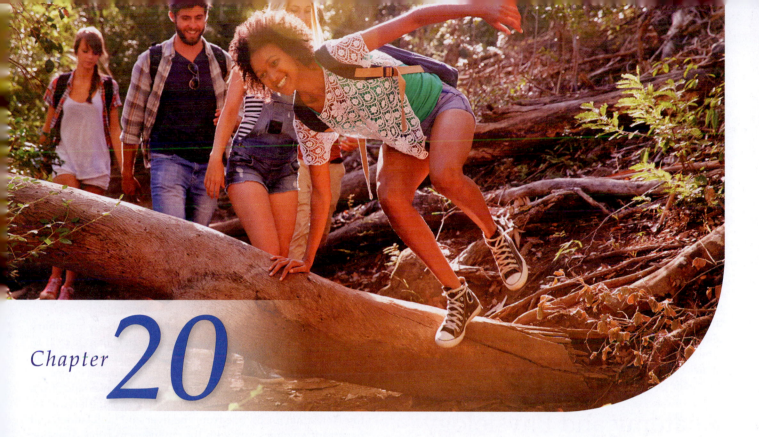

Chapter 20

Abdomen

LEARNING OUTCOMES

Upon completion of this chapter, you will be able to:

1. Describe the anatomy and physiology of the abdomen.

2. Identify the anatomic, physiologic, developmental, psychosocial, and cultural variations that guide assessment of the abdomen.

3. Determine which questions about the abdomen to use for the focused interview.

4. Outline the techniques for assessment of the abdomen.

5. Generate the appropriate documentation to describe the assessment of the abdomen.

6. Identify abnormal findings in the physical assessment of the abdomen.

KEY TERMS

abdomen, 420
accessory digestive organs, 420
alimentary canal, 420
ascites, 441

Blumberg's sign, 438
borborygmi, 435
dysphagia, 442
esophagitis, 443
friction rub, 435

hepatitis, 443
hernia, 442
mapping, 423
peritoneum, 421
peritonitis, 443

referred pain, 439
striae, 434
ulcerative colitis, 443
umbilical hernia, 442

MEDICAL LANGUAGE

bi-	Prefix meaning "two"
dys-	Prefix meaning "abnormal," "difficult," "painful"
gastro-	Prefix meaning "stomach"
hyper-	Prefix meaning "high," "elevated," "above normal"
hypo-	Prefix meaning "below," "deficient"
peri-	Prefix meaning "around"
post-	Prefix meaning "after," "behind"

Introduction

The **abdomen** is not a system unto itself. It is the largest cavity of the body and contains many organs and structures that belong to various systems of the body. For example, the liver, gallbladder, and stomach belong to the digestive system. The kidneys, ureters, and bladder belong to the urinary system. These structures and many other structures are assessed when performing an abdominal assessment. The primary focus of this chapter is the assessment of the structures of the digestive system. The secondary focus is the abdominal structures of other systems.

The primary responsibility of the digestive system is to take in, break down, and absorb nutrients to be used by all cells of the body. The ability to perform these functions is influenced by the health of many other body systems. The parasympathetic fibers of the nervous system increase digestion, whereas the sympathetic fibers inhibit the process. The respiratory system provides oxygen needed for the metabolic processes and removes the carbon dioxide created by metabolism. The hormones of the endocrine system help regulate digestion and the metabolic processes.

Anatomy and Physiology Review

The abdomen is composed of the alimentary canal, the intestines, the accessory digestive organs, the urinary system, the spleen, and the reproductive organs. Each of these structures or systems is discussed in the following sections.

Abdomen

The abdomen is situated in the anterior region of the body. It is inferior to the diaphragm of the respiratory system and superior to the pelvic floor. The abdominal muscles, the intercostal margins, and the pelvis form the anterior borders of the abdomen. The vertebral column and the lumbar muscles form the posterior borders of the abdomen.

This anatomy and physiology review of the abdomen also has a two-point focus: The primary focus is the gastrointestinal system, and the secondary focus is the abdominal structures of other systems. The gastrointestinal system consists of the alimentary canal and the accessory organs of the digestive system. The **alimentary canal**, a continuous, hollow, muscular tube, begins at the mouth and terminates at the anus. The accessory organs include the teeth, salivary glands, liver, gallbladder, and pancreas (see Figure 20.1 ■).

The anatomy, physiology, and assessment of the mouth, teeth, tongue, salivary glands, and pharynx are discussed in Chapter 15 of this text. ∞ Before proceeding with the assessment of the abdomen, it may be helpful to review the information in that chapter.

Alimentary Canal

The alimentary canal is the continuous hollow tube extending from the mouth to the anus. The boundaries include the mouth, pharynx, esophagus, stomach, small and large intestines, rectum, and anus.

Esophagus The esophagus, a collapsible tube, connects the pharynx to the stomach. Approximately 25 cm (10 in.) in length, it passes through the mediastinum and diaphragm to meet the stomach at the cardiac sphincter. The primary function of the esophagus is to propel food and fluid from the mouth to the stomach.

Stomach The stomach extends from the esophagus at the cardiac sphincter to the duodenum at the pyloric sphincter. Located in the left side of the upper abdomen, the stomach is directly inferior to the diaphragm. The diameter and volume of the stomach are directly related to the food it contains. Food mixes with digestive juices in the stomach and becomes chyme before entering the small intestine. The primary function of the stomach is the chemical and mechanical breakdown of food.

Small Intestine The small intestine is the body's primary digestive and absorptive organ. Approximately 6 m (18 to 21 ft) in length, it has three subdivisions. The first segment, the duodenum, meets the stomach at the pyloric sphincter and extends to the middle region, called the jejunum. The ileum extends from the jejunum to the ileocecal valve at the cecum of the large intestine. Intestinal juices, bile from the liver and gallbladder, and pancreatic enzymes mix with the chyme to promote digestion and facilitate the absorption of nutrients. The primary functions of the small intestine are the continuing chemical breakdown of food and the absorption of digested foods.

Large Intestine The last portion of the alimentary canal is the large intestine, which extends from the ileocecal valve to the anus. The large intestine is approximately 1.5 m (5 to 5.5 ft) in length. It consists of the cecum, ascending colon, transverse colon, descending colon, sigmoid colon, rectum, and anus. The vermiform appendix is attached to the large intestine at the cecum. The appendix contains masses of lymphoid tissue that make only a minor contribution to immunity; however, when inflamed, the appendix causes significant health problems. The large intestine is wider and shorter than the small intestine. It is on the periphery of the abdominal cavity, surrounding the small intestine and other structures. The main functions of the large intestine are absorbing water from indigestible food residue and eliminating the residue in the form of feces.

Accessory Digestive Organs

The **accessory digestive organs**—the liver, gallbladder, and pancreas—contribute to the digestive process of foods. These structures connect to the alimentary canal by ducts.

Liver The largest gland of the body, the liver is located in the right upper portion of the abdominal cavity, directly inferior to the diaphragm to just below the costal margin and extends into the left side of the abdomen. The lower portion of the rib cage, which makes only the lower border of the liver palpable, protects the liver. The only digestive function of the liver is the production and secretion of bile for fat emulsification. It has a major role in the metabolism of proteins, fats, and carbohydrates. The liver has the ability to store some vitamins, produce substances for coagulation of blood, produce antibodies, and detoxify harmful substances.

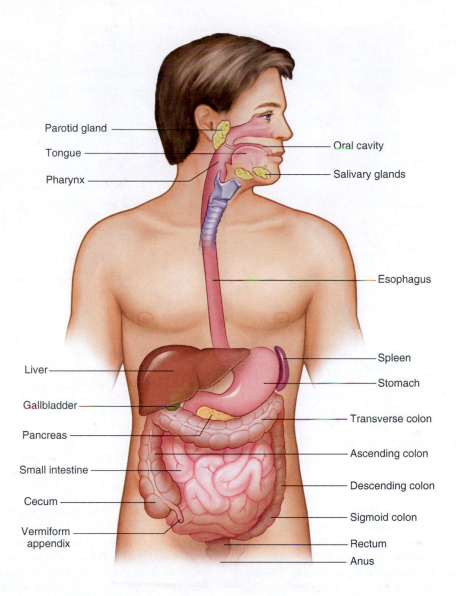

Parotid gland

Tongue

Pharynx

Oral cavity

Salivary glands

Esophagus

Liver

Gallbladder

Pancreas

Small intestine

Cecum

Vermiform appendix

Spleen

Stomach

Transverse colon

Ascending colon

Descending colon

Sigmoid colon

Rectum

Anus

Figure 20.1 Organs of the alimentary canal and related accessory organs.

Gallbladder Chiefly a storage organ for bile, the gallbladder, a thin-walled sac, is nestled in a shallow depression on the ventral surface of the liver. The main functions of the gallbladder are storing of bile and assisting in the digestion of fats. The gallbladder releases stored bile into the duodenum when stimulated and thus promotes the emulsification of fats.

Pancreas An accessory digestive organ, the pancreas is a triangular-shaped gland located in the left upper portion of the abdomen. The head of the pancreas is nestled in the C curve of the duodenum, and the body and tail of the pancreas lie deep to the left of the stomach and extend toward the spleen at the lateral aspect of the abdomen. The pancreas is an endocrine and exocrine gland. As an endocrine gland, it secretes insulin, an important factor in carbohydrate metabolism. As an exocrine gland, it releases pancreatic juice, which contains a broad spectrum of enzymes that mixes with bile in the duodenum. The main function of the pancreas is assisting with the digestion of proteins, fats, and carbohydrates.

Other Related Structures

Some structures located in the abdomen have no connection to the digestive process. They are part of other systems and are considered with the general assessment of the abdomen.

Peritoneum The **peritoneum** is a thin, double layer of serous membrane in the abdominal cavity. The visceral peritoneum covers the external surface of most digestive organs. The parietal peritoneum lines the walls of the abdominal cavity. The serous fluid secreted by the membranes helps lubricate the surface of the organs, allowing motion of structures without friction.

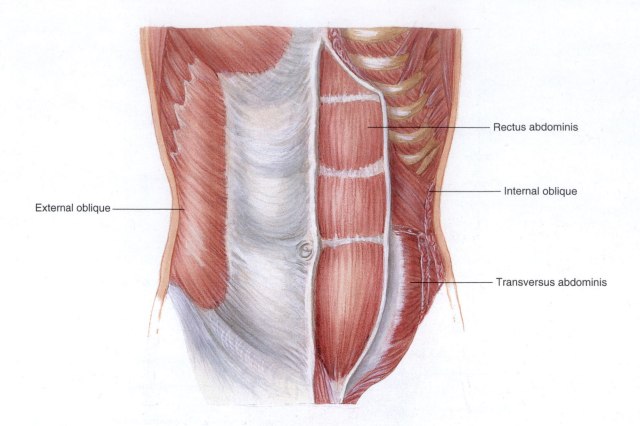

Figure 20.2 Muscles of the abdominal wall.

Muscles of the Abdominal Wall Having no bony reinforcements, the anterior and lateral abdominal walls depend on the musculature for support and protection. The four pairs of abdominal muscles, when well toned, support and protect the abdominal viscera most effectively (see Figure 20.2 ■). The muscle groups include the rectus abdominis, external oblique, internal oblique, and transverse abdominis. Secondary functions of these muscle groups include lateral flexion, rotation, and anterior flexion of the trunk. Simultaneous contraction of the muscle groups increases intra-abdominal pressure by compressing the abdominal wall. Weakness in the muscular structure will produce herniation of structures.

Aorta As the descending aorta passes through the diaphragm and enters the abdominal cavity, it becomes the abdominal aorta. This penetration occurs at the T12 level of the vertebral column slightly to the left of the midline of the body. The abdominal aorta continues to the L4 level of the vertebral column, where it bifurcates to form the right and left common iliac arteries. The many branches of the abdominal aorta serve all the parietal and visceral structures (see Figure 20.3 ■).

Kidneys, Ureters, and Bladder The kidneys are located in the posterior abdomen on either side of the spine, protected by the lower ribs. Besides filtering nitrogenous wastes from blood and producing urine, the kidneys produce a biologically active form of vitamin D. The kidneys also secrete erythropoietin and renin. The slender tubelike structures that carry the urine from the kidneys to the bladder are the ureters. The urinary bladder, a smooth, collapsible muscular sac, is located in the pelvis of the abdominal cavity. The primary function of the bladder is to store urine until it can be released. As the bladder fills with urine, it may rise above the symphysis pubis into the abdominal cavity. Assessment of the kidneys, ureters, and bladder is discussed in Chapter 21 and Chapter 22. ∞

Spleen The spleen, the largest of the lymphoid organs, is located in the left upper portion of the abdomen directly inferior to the diaphragm. Surrounded by a fibrous capsule, the spleen provides a site for lymphocyte proliferation and immune surveillance and response. It filters and cleanses blood, destroying worn-out red blood cells and returning their breakdown products to the liver.

Reproductive Organs In the female, the uterus, fallopian tubes, and ovaries are in the pelvic portion of the abdominal cavity. In the male, the prostate gland surrounds the urethra just below the bladder. The assessment of these structures is discussed in Chapter 21 and Chapter 22. ∞

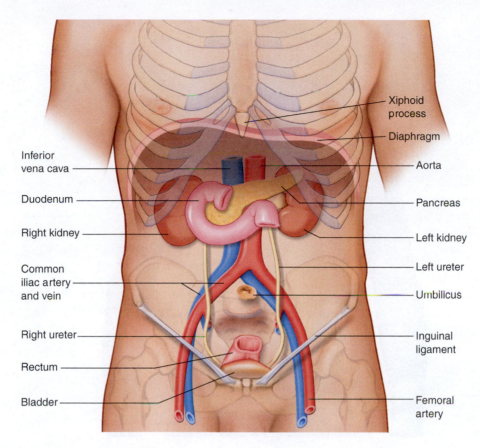

Figure 20.3 Abdominal vasculature and deep structures.

Landmarks

Reference points and anatomic structures must be identified when assessing the abdomen. Defined landmarks help to identify specific underlying structures and provide a source for description and recording of findings. Landmarks for the abdomen include the xiphoid process, umbilicus, costal margin, iliac crests, and pubic bone.

Mapping is the process of dividing the abdomen into quadrants or regions for the purpose of examination. To obtain the four quadrants, the nurse extends the midsternal line from the xiphoid process through the umbilicus to the pubic bone and then draws a horizontal line perpendicular to the first line through the umbilicus. These two perpendicular lines form four equal quadrants of the abdomen, as illustrated in Figure 20.4 ■. The quadrants are simply named right upper quadrant (RUQ), right lower quadrant (RLQ), left upper quadrant (LUQ), and left lower quadrant (LLQ).

The second mapping method divides the abdomen into nine regions. To obtain these abdominal regions, one extends the right and left midclavicular lines to the groin and then draws a horizontal line across the lowest edge of the costal margin. The final step is to draw another horizontal line at the level of the iliac crests. The abdomen has now been divided into nine

regions as shown in Figure 20.5 ■. The names of the regions are right hypochondriac, epigastric, left hypochondriac, right lumbar, umbilical, left lumbar, right inguinal, hypogastric or pubic, and left inguinal.

Of the two methods described, the quadrant method is more commonly used. When using the quadrant method, it is important to pay attention to structures that are in the midline of the abdomen and do not belong to any specific quadrant. These structures include the abdominal aorta, urinary bladder, and uterus.

The nurse should select one mapping method and use it consistently. Once a method has been selected, the nurse visualizes the underlying structures before proceeding (see Figure 20.6 ■). The gallbladder sits in the upper right quadrant of the abdomen inferior to the liver and lateral to the right midclavicular line (RMCL). The kidneys are posterior to the abdominal contents and situated in the retroperitoneal space, protected by the 11th and 12th pairs of ribs. The costovertebral angle is formed as the ribs articulate with the vertebra. The liver displaces the right kidney, thus making the lower pole palpable. The spleen, part of the lymphatic system, is at the level of the 10th rib lateral to the left midaxillary line (LMAL). The lower pole of the spleen moves into the abdomen toward the midline when enlarged.

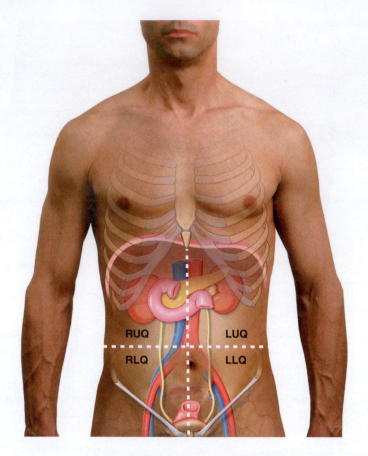

Figure 20.4 Mapping of the abdomen into four quadrants.

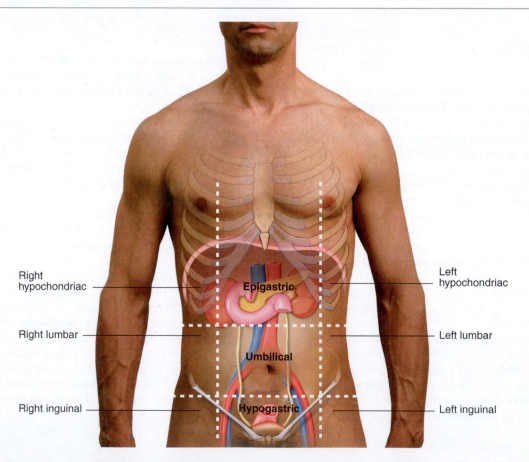

Figure 20.5 Mapping of the abdomen into nine regions.

FOUR ABDOMINAL QUADRANTS

A
Right Upper Quadrant
Liver and gallbladder
Pyloric sphincter
Duodenum
Head of pancreas
Right adrenal gland
Portion of right kidney
Hepatic flexure of colon
Portions of ascending and transverse colon

B
Left Upper Quadrant
Left lobe of liver
Spleen
Stomach
Body of pancreas
Left adrenal gland
Portion of left kidney
Splenic flexure of colon
Portions of transverse and descending colon

C
Right Lower Quadrant
Lower pole of right kidney
Cecum and appendix
Portion of ascending colon
Ovary and uterine tube
Right spermatic cord
Right ureter

D
Left Lower Quadrant
Lower pole of left kidney
Sigmoid colon
Portion of descending colon
Ovary and uterine tube
Left spermatic cord
Left ureter

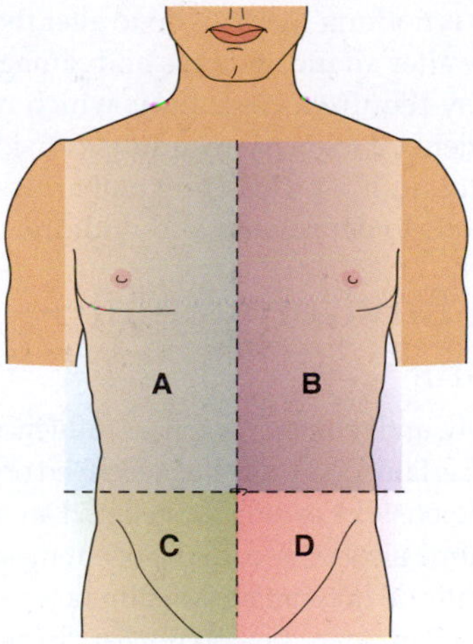

Midline
Aorta
Bladder
Uterus

◯ = Umbilicus

NINE ABDOMINAL REGIONS

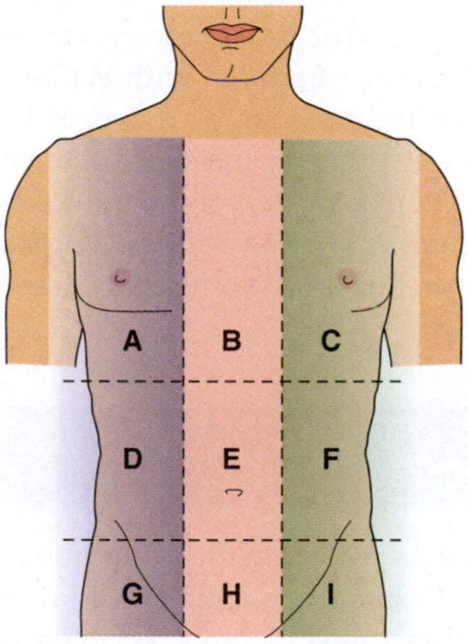

A
Right Hypochondriac
Right lobe of liver
Gallbladder
Portion of duodenum
Hepatic flexure of colon
Portion of right kidney
Right adrenal gland

B
Epigastric
Pyloric sphincter
Duodenum
Pancreas
Portion of liver
Aorta

C
Left Hypochondriac
Stomach
Spleen
Tail of pancreas
Splenic flexure of colon
Upper pole of left kidney
Left adrenal gland

D
Right Lumbar
Ascending colon
Lower half of right kidney
Portion of duodenum and jejunum

E
Umbilical
Lower part of duodenum
Jejunum and ileum

F
Left Lumbar
Descending colon
Lower half of left kidney
Portions of jejunum and ileum

G
Right Inguinal
Cecum
Appendix
Lower end of ileum
Right ureter
Right spermatic cord
Right ovary and uterine tube

H
Hypogastric (Pubic)
Ileum
Bladder
Uterus (in pregnancy)

I
Left Inguinal
Sigmoid colon
Left ureter
Left spermatic cord
Left ovary and uterine tube

Figure 20.6 Upper torso: Organs of the four abdominal quadrants. Lower torso: Organs of the nine abdominal regions.

Special Considerations

Subjective and objective data inform the nurse about the patient's health status. A variety of factors may influence health, including age, developmental level, race, ethnicity, work history, living conditions, socioeconomics, and emotional well-being. These factors are discussed in the following sections.

Health Promotion Considerations

A healthy digestive system promotes efficient nutrient absorption, which is essential for healthy growth and development. Digestive health also allows for adequate elimination of wastes and toxins from the body. Objectives related to digestive health include reducing the incidence of colorectal cancer, which in 2014 was the fourth-leading cause of cancer-related deaths in the United States (Centers for Disease Control and Prevention [CDC], 2017a). In addition, national objectives include increasing food safety measures and reducing the incidence of foodborne illnesses, such as *Listeria*, *Salmonella*, and *E. coli* (CDC, 2017b).

Lifespan Considerations

Growth and development are dynamic processes that describe change over time. The collection of data and the interpretation of findings in relation to normative values are important. Developmental factors are considered during assessment of the abdomen. For example, the size of the abdomen at all ages is an indication of the nutritional state of the child. During pregnancy the abdomen undergoes many changes as the growing uterus compresses many abdominal structures.

Expected variations in the abdomen for different age groups are discussed in Chapter 25, Chapter 26, and Chapter 27. ∞

Psychosocial Considerations

High stress levels may cause or aggravate abdominal problems. Gastritis, gastric or duodenal ulcers, and ulcerative colitis are examples of stress-related problems.

Self-perception may have a subtle influence on the patient's weight. Patients who perceive themselves as naturally thin may show greater dedication to restricting their caloric intake and exercising to maintain that self-image. Conversely, patients who perceive themselves as naturally fat may overeat and avoid exercise, feeling that there is nothing they can do to alter their weight.

Surgical scars may alter an individual's body image. Gastrointestinal surgery may require a colostomy, which might be a temporary or permanent change. Many adults consider "wearing a bag" a significant limitation, causing embarrassment and anxiety. This often leads to depression and withdrawal.

Cultural and Environmental Considerations

Culture, customs, family, and religious practices influence the foods patients choose to eat. Certain foods may be prescribed or avoided in certain cultures or religions. For example, Seventh Day Adventists generally do not consume alcohol or caffeine or eat meat; the Diné (Navajo Indians) typically do not eat fish; Muslims are expected not to eat pork, and during Ramadan they do not eat, drink, or smoke between sunrise and sunset; Hindus may abstain from eating meat and fish; and Buddhists are often vegetarians. However, a healthy diet usually can be achieved even with significant food restrictions. Patients accustomed to a diet of meat and potatoes may not fully appreciate the value of fresh fruits and vegetables.

The financial security of the patient also has an impact on eating habits. In some areas, certain foods may not be available year-round or may be much more costly than in other areas. For example, fresh fruits and vegetables typically increase in price in many regions in winter months. Unfortunately, highly processed foods, which are usually less expensive than whole fresh foods, are often lower in fiber than their fresh counterparts.

Cultural factors also may affect the incidence of gastrointestinal disorders. For example, African Americans experience a higher rate of colorectal cancer compared with White, Asian/Pacific Islander, American Indian/Alaska Native, or Hispanic individuals (CDC, 2017c). Likewise, the incidence of infection by *Helicobacter pylori*, which is a major cause of peptic ulcer disease, is highest among individuals of African American heritage and Mexican Americans (Mapel, Roberts, Overhiser, & Mason, 2013).

Subjective Data—Health History

Health assessment of the abdomen includes the gathering of subjective and objective data. Subjective data collection occurs during the patient interview before the actual physical assessment. During the interview, the nurse uses a variety of communication techniques to elicit general and specific information about the patient's state of abdominal health or illness. Health records, the results of laboratory tests, and radiologic studies are important secondary sources to be reviewed and included in the data-gathering process.

See Table 20.1 for information on potential secondary sources of patient data.

Focused Interview

The focused interview for assessment of the abdomen concerns data related to the structures and functions of organs within the abdomen. Subjective data related to the status and function of the structures within the abdomen are gathered during the focused interview. The nurse must be prepared to observe the patient and listen for cues related to the function of the organs and systems within the abdomen. The nurse may use open-ended and closed questions to obtain information. Often a number of follow-up questions or requests for descriptions are required to clarify data or gather missing information.

The focused interview guides the physical assessment of the abdomen. The information is always considered in relation to norms and expectations about the function of organs and systems within the abdomen. Therefore, the nurse must consider age, gender, race, culture, environment, health practices, past and concurrent problems, and therapies when framing questions and using techniques to elicit information. In order to

Table 20.1 Potential Secondary Sources for Patient Data Related to the Digestive System

LABORATORY TESTS	NORMAL VALUES
Stomach	
Helicobacter Pylori	Negative for antibody, antigen
Liver	
ALT (alanine aminotransferase)	Males: 7–55 Units/L
	Females: 7–45 Units/L
AST (aspartate aminotransferase)	Males: 8–48 Units/L
	Females: 8–43 Units/L
ALP (alkaline phosphatase)	44–147 Units/L
LDH (lactic dehydrogenase)	122–222 Units/L
Hepatic antigens	Negative
Serum vitamin B12	180–914 nanograms/L
Serum total bilirubin	≤ 1.2 mg/dL
Serum ammonia	15–45 mcg/dL
Serum albumin	3.5–5 g/dL
Pancreas	26–102 Units/L
Amylase	10–73 Units/L
Lipase	70–140 mg/dL
Glucose	8.9–10.1 mg/dL
Calcium	
Diagnostic Tests	
Abdominal X-ray	
Barium Swallow	
Colonoscopy	
Computed Tomography (CT)	
Endoscopic Retrograde Cholangiography (ECP)	
Esophagoscopy	
Fecal Occult Blood Testing	
Gallbladder Ultrasonography	
Gastric Analysis	
Gastroscopy	
Liver Biopsy	
Magnetic Resonance Imaging (MRI)	
Percutaneous Transhepatic Cholangiography (PTCA)	

address all of the factors when conducting a focused interview, categories of questions related to status and function of organs and systems within the abdomen have been developed. These categories include general questions that are asked of all patients, those addressing illness and infection, questions related to symptoms and behaviors, those related to habits or practices, questions that are specific to patients according to age, those for the pregnant female, and questions that address environmental concerns. One method to elicit information about symptoms is

OLDCART & ICE as described in Chapter 5. ∞ See Figure 5.3.

The nurse must consider the patient's ability to participate in the focused interview and physical assessment of the abdomen. If a patient is experiencing pain, cramping, problems with elimination (including frequency or urgency), difficulty swallowing, nausea and vomiting, or the anxiety that accompanies any of these problems, attention must focus on identification of immediate problems and relief of symptoms.

Focused Interview Questions	Rationales and Evidence

The following section provides sample questions and bulleted follow-up questions in each of the previously mentioned categories. A rationale for each of the questions is provided. The list of questions is not all-inclusive but represents the types of questions required in a comprehensive focused interview related to the abdomen.

General Questions

1. **Describe your appetite. Has it changed in the last 24 hours? In the last month? In the last year?**
   - What do you believe has caused the change in your appetite?
   - Have you done anything to address the change?
   - Have you spoken to a healthcare professional about the change?
   - Has anything else occurred with the change in appetite?

▶ These questions elicit basic information about the patient's eating habits. In addition, appetite change can be indicative of underlying physical and emotional problems. If a change has occurred, it is important to elicit the patient's perception of the change and to identify factors that may have contributed to the change.

Focused Interview Questions	Rationales and Evidence

2. What is your weight? Has your weight changed?
- Over what period of time did the weight change occur?
- What do you believe has contributed to your weight change?
- Have any problems or symptoms accompanied the weight change?
- Have you discussed this with a healthcare professional?

▶ Weight loss or gain can accompany physical and emotional problems. Dietary consumption is one of the leading factors in weight control. The nurse should determine if weight gain is associated with a decrease in activity, changes in metabolic rates, hormonal factors, or fluid retention. Emotional problems may cause an individual to over- or underconsume foods. Weight loss may be an appropriate or desired outcome for some individuals. The nurse must determine if the weight loss was purposeful. Weight loss can accompany problems associated with diabetes, hyperthyroidism, and some cancers (Berman & Snyder, 2016).

- Questions about dietary intake can be included in the follow-up about weight or may be included in questions about behaviors. These questions would include the following: Tell me what you have had to eat and drink in the last 24 hours, including snacks. How much of each item did you consume? Is this a typical eating pattern for you?

▶ In addition to obtaining data about weight, the nurse is building on the nutritional data already collected. The nurse is establishing the patient's dietary patterns, paying special attention to overconsumption and underconsumption.

3. Describe your bowel habits. Describe the color and consistency of your stool.
- Have you experienced any changes in your elimination pattern or in your stool?
- What kind of change has occurred in your elimination pattern or stool?
- When did the change begin?
- Can you identify anything you believe may have caused the change?
- What have you done about the problem?
- Have you discussed the changes with a healthcare professional?
- Questions about the use of medications such as laxatives or antidiarrheals may be included as follow-up questions here. However, this information may have been obtained in the health history or can be included in questions about behaviors.

▶ These questions provide initial information about bowel functioning. The nurse determines if the patient has an established pattern for bowel elimination. If the patient indicates that there has been a change in the pattern of elimination or in the characteristics of the stool, follow-up questions are indicated. Tarry stool indicates bleeding in the upper part of the gastrointestinal tract. A clay color may indicate lack of bile in the stool (Sira, Salem, & Sira, 2013).

4. Do you have feelings of bloating or increased gas?
- What do you think causes this? Have any changes been made in your diet or medications?
- What do you do to decrease these feelings?
- What do you do to relieve the symptoms?
- Do you use antacids?
- Do you increase water intake?
- Do you exercise?

▶ Some foods (e.g., broccoli, cauliflower, figs) and intolerance to lactose will cause this feeling. Some medications are constipating (Wilson, Shannon, & Shields, 2018). Severe bloating and gas can be indicative of abdominal pathology.

5. Do you have any physical problems that affect your appetite, affect your bowel functioning, or contribute to abdominal problems?
- Describe the way your abdominal function is affected.
- How long has this been occurring?
- Have you sought relief for the problem?
- What have you done to relieve the problem?
- Did the remedy help?
- Have you sought advice from a healthcare professional?

▶ This question is used to elicit information about abdominal or other problems that may impact the structures and functions within the abdomen. For example, pain from any source may diminish appetite, and intake of medications for nonabdominal problems may affect digestion and abdominal comfort. If the patient identifies any problems that affect abdominal functions, follow-up is required for clear descriptions and details about what, when, and how problems occur; how abdominal function is impacted; and the duration of the problem.

6. Is there anyone in your family who has had an abdominal disease or problem?
- What is the disease or problem?
- Who in the family now has or has had the disease?
- When was it diagnosed?
- Describe the treatment.
- How effective was the treatment?

▶ This may reveal information about abdominal diseases associated with familial or genetic predisposition.

▶ Follow-up is required to obtain details about specific problems as well as their occurrence, treatment, and outcomes.

Questions Related to Illness or Infection

1. Have you ever been diagnosed with an abdominal disease?
- When were you diagnosed with the problem?
- What treatment was prescribed for the problem?
- Was the treatment helpful?
- What kinds of things do you do to help with the problem?
- Has the problem ever recurred (acute)?
- How are you managing the disease now (chronic)?

▶ The patient has an opportunity to provide information about specific abdominal diseases. If a diagnosed illness is identified, follow-up about the date of diagnosis, treatment, and outcomes is required. Data about each illness identified by the patient are essential to an accurate health assessment. Illness can be classified as acute or chronic, and follow-up regarding each classification will differ.

2. *Alternative to question 1:* List possible abdominal illnesses, such as cholecystitis, cholelithiasis, ulcers, diverticulosis, and cirrhosis, and ask the patient to respond "yes" or "no" as each is stated.
- Follow-up would be carried out for each identified diagnosis as in question 1.

▶ This is a comprehensive and easy way to elicit information about all abdominal diagnoses.

Focused Interview Questions	Rationales and Evidence
3. Do you now have or have you ever had an infection within the abdomen? • When were you diagnosed with the infection? • What treatment was prescribed for the problem? • Was the treatment helpful? • What kinds of things do you do to help with the problem? • Has the problem ever recurred (acute)? • How are you managing the infection now (chronic)?	▶ If an infection is identified, follow-up about the date of the infection, treatment, and outcomes is required. Data about each infection identified by the patient are essential to an accurate health assessment. Infections can be classified as acute or chronic, and follow-up regarding each classification will differ.
4. *Alternative to question 3:* List possible abdominal disorders, such as hepatitis, cholecystitis, and diverticulitis, and ask the patient to respond "yes" or "no" as each is stated.	▶ This is a comprehensive and easy way to elicit information about all abdominal disorders. Follow-up would be carried out for each identified diagnosis as in question 3.

Questions Related to Symptoms, Pain, and Behaviors

When gathering information about symptoms, many questions are required to elicit details and descriptions that assist in the analysis of the data. Discrimination is made in relation to the significance of a symptom, in relation to specific diseases or problems, and in relation to potential follow-up examination or referral. One rationale may be provided for a group of questions in this category.

The following questions refer to specific symptoms and behaviors associated with the organs and structures within the abdomen. For each symptom, questions and follow-up are required. The details to be elicited are the characteristics of the symptom; the onset, duration, and frequency of the symptom; the treatment or remedy for the symptom, including over-the-counter (OTC) and home remedies; the determination if a diagnosis has been sought; the effect of treatments; and family history associated with a symptom or illness.

Questions Related to Symptoms

Questions 1 through 20 refer to nausea as a symptom associated with abdominal problems and are comprehensive enough to provide an example of the number and types of questions required in a focused interview when a symptom exists. The remaining questions refer to other symptoms associated with abdominal problems. The number and types of questions are limited to identification of the symptom. Follow-up is included only when required for clarification.

1. Do you have nausea?	▶ Question 1 identifies the existence of a symptom, and questions 2 through 5 add knowledge about the symptom.
2. How long have you had the nausea?	▶ Determining the duration of symptoms is helpful in determining the significance of symptoms in relation to specific diseases and problems.
3. How often are you nauseated?	
4. Do you know what is causing the nausea?	
5. Is there a difference in the nausea at different times of the day?	
6. Describe your nausea.	
7. Is the nausea accompanied by burning, indigestion, or bloating?	▶ The description of the nausea may indicate a symptom associated with a specific disease or problem.
8. Do you vomit when you experience the nausea?	
9. What does the vomitus look like?	
10. Does the vomitus have any odor?	▶ The color and odor of vomitus may be associated with specific diseases or problems. For example, brown vomitus with a fecal odor can indicate an intestinal obstruction.
11. What was the cause, in your opinion?	
12. How frequently do you have this experience?	
13. What do you do to relieve the symptoms?	
14. When you vomit, describe what comes up and the amount.	▶ Vomiting can be related to a variety of pathologic conditions, such as food poisoning, ulcers, varices of the esophagus, hepatitis, and beginning of an intestinal obstruction. Medications, both those prescribed and OTC, may contribute to or cause vomiting (Wilson, et al., 2018).
15. Do you have pain with the nausea? • Describe the type, severity, and location of the pain. • What do you do for the pain? • Is the remedy effective?	▶ Pain associated with nausea and vomiting may be indicative of an underlying abdominal disease. Follow-up elicits details that assist in the data analysis.
16. Have you sought treatment for the nausea?	▶ These questions provide information about the need for diagnosis, referral, or continued evaluation of the symptom. They also provide information about the patient's knowledge of a current diagnosis or problem, as well as his or her response to intervention.
17. When was the treatment sought?	
18. What occurred when you sought that treatment?	
19. Was something prescribed or recommended for the nausea?	
20. What was the effect of the remedy?	

Focused Interview Questions	Rationales and Evidence
21. Do you use OTC or home remedies for the nausea?	▶ Questions 21 through 24 provide information about drugs and substances that may relieve symptoms or provide comfort. Some substances may mask symptoms, interfere with the effect of prescribed medications, or harm the patient.
22. What are the OTC or home remedies that you use?	
23. How often do you use them?	
24. How much of them do you use?	
25. Do you have any difficulty chewing or swallowing your food?	
26. Do you wear dentures?	▶ Ill-fitting dentures, failure to wear them, and missing or diseased teeth make chewing and swallowing difficult (Berman & Snyder, 2016). Disorders of the throat and esophagus can also make swallowing difficult.
27. Do you have any crowns?	
28. Do your gums bleed easily?	▶ Chronic dry mouth, periodontal disease, anticoagulant use, and decreased platelets can cause an older adult's gums to bleed easily. If a dose of anticoagulant is too high, such as with coumadin, bleeding of the mucous membranes may occur (Wilson et al., 2018). Bacterial growth from plaque can cause periodontal disease, which may not be easily diagnosed because of being painless until its late stages (American Dental Association, 2018).
29. Do you have indigestion? • Questions would address onset, frequency, and duration as well as knowledge about causative factors including food intolerance and discomfort associated with medications or treatments for other problems. For example, when did the indigestion start?	
30. Do you suffer from diarrhea or constipation?	
31. What do you think is the cause?	
32. What have you done to correct the situation?	
33. Have these measures helped the situation?	
34. Do you experience any rectal itching or bleeding?	▶ Dark, tarry stool indicates bleeding, usually in the upper or middle part of the intestinal tract. Bright red (frank) blood usually indicates lower tract bleeding (Berman & Snyder, 2016).

Questions Related to Pain

1. Are you having any abdominal pain at this time?	▶ Questions 2 through 12 are standard questions associated with pain to determine the location, frequency, duration, and intensity of the pain.
2. Where is the pain?	
3. How often do you experience the pain?	▶ Pain could indicate cardiac disease, ulcers, cholecystitis, renal calculi, diverticulitis, urinary cystitis, small bowel obstruction, or ectopic pregnancy (Marieb & Hoehn, 2019).
4. How long does the pain last?	
5. How long have you had the pain?	
6. How would you rate the pain on a scale of 0 to 10, with 10 being the worst pain?	
7. Does the pain radiate?	
8. Where does the pain radiate?	
9. Is there a trigger for the pain?	
10. Does the pain affect your breathing or any other functions?	
11. What do you think is causing the pain?	
12. What do you do to relieve the pain?	

Questions Related to Behaviors

1. What have you had to eat and drink in the last 24 hours?	
2. What snacks do you have in a 24-hour period?	
3. What size portions do you eat?	
4. Is the 24-hour pattern you described typical of the way you eat?	▶ This provides input about diet and nutrition, which may contribute to obesity or problems with weight loss. This also provides information about meeting nutritional requirements.
5. How much coffee, tea, cola, alcoholic beverages, or chocolate do you consume in a 24-hour period?	▶ Caffeine and alcohol irritate the gastrointestinal system and can contribute to ulcers and irritable bowel syndrome (Johns Hopkins Medicine, n.d.).

Focused Interview Questions	Rationales and Evidence

Questions Related to Age and Pregnancy

The focused interview must reflect the anatomic and physiologic differences in the abdomen that exist along the age span as well as during pregnancy. Specific questions related to the abdomen for each of these groups are provided in Chapter 25, Chapter 26, and Chapter 27. ∞

Questions Related to the Environment

Environment refers to both the internal and external environments. Questions related to the internal environment include all of the previous questions and those associated with internal or physiologic responses. Questions regarding the external environment include those related to home, work, or social environments.

Questions Related to the Internal Environment

1. How would you describe your stress level?

2. Do you think you are coping well?

3. Could your coping skills be better?

▶ Prolonged stress is linked to gastrointestinal disease (Melinder et al., 2017).

Questions Related to the External Environment

1. Do you work with any chemical irritants?

▶ Exposure to benzene, lead, or nickel may lead to gastric irritation (Cherian, Mulky, & Menon, 2014). Excessive exposure to chemical hepatotoxins such as carbon tetrachloride may lead to postnecrotic cirrhosis (Mayo Clinic, 2016).

2. Have you recently done any traveling?

3. Where did you travel?

▶ Water purification and food storage methods vary in different regions and different countries. Exposure to food- or waterborne microorganisms can lead to gastroenteritis, hepatitis, diarrhea, or parasite infestation.

▶ Follow-up questions would include all of the questions mentioned above that address symptoms and problems.

Patient-Centered Interaction

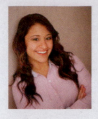

Source: aastock/Shutterstock.

Ms. Emily Zabriski is a 20-year-old college student living on campus. She has purchased the seven-day meal plan and has lunch and dinner in the student dining room. Breakfast is usually one cup of coffee and one glass of orange juice "to go." This is determined by the time of her first class and how late she gets up.

Not having slept last night, Ms. Zabriski reports to the health center on campus early in the morning with complaints of nausea, vomiting, diarrhea, abdominal pain, and cramping in the right and left lower quadrants. She has experienced these symptoms for approximately 18 hours. The following is an excerpt of the focused interview.

Interview

Nurse: Good morning, Ms. Zabriski. I see by your report you have had nausea, vomiting, diarrhea, lower abdominal pain, and cramping for about eighteen hours.

Ms. Zabriski: Yes, that is correct.

Nurse: First, I want you to rate and describe your pain. On a scale of zero to ten, with zero being no pain and ten being the most severe pain ever, choose a number that matches your pain.

Ms. Zabriski: Oh, it is a two to three right now. When I vomit or have diarrhea it goes up, maybe to eight, then comes down. I have a lot of cramps.

Nurse : With your pain at a two to three level, do you think you could answer a few questions?

Ms. Zabriski: Oh, that won't be a problem. It is only a problem when I'm going to vomit or have diarrhea. Right now I'm okay.

Nurse: These symptoms could occur for any number of reasons. What do you think is causing your problem?

Ms. Zabriski: I don't understand what you mean.

Nurse:: These symptoms could be caused by stress, food allergies, an intestinal disease such as Crohn disease, or pregnancy, just to mention a few.

Ms. Zabriski: It could be something I ate, or maybe it is a stomach virus. Five dorm mates on my floor have the same thing.

Nurse:: Let's talk about you. Because you indicated maybe it was something you ate, tell me about your eating before getting sick.

Ms. Zabriski: I had lunch in the student dining room. I had a glass of iced tea, cottage cheese with fruit salad, and a small bag of chips.

Nurse: What have you had to eat since lunch yesterday?

Ms. Zabriski: Well, I started to vomit and have cramps about an hour and a half after I ate. Now even crackers won't stay down.

Nurse: When was the last time you drank something?

Ms. Zabriski: I tried some diet cola after I vomited the first time, and that came up.

Nurse: What have you taken to try to stop the nausea, vomiting, and diarrhea?

Ms. Zabriski: Nothing, I thought it would stop and go away, but it hasn't. That's why I'm here.

Analysis

The nurse used several communication strategies to obtain information from Ms. Zabriski. First, the nurse determined Ms. Zabriski's level of pain and discomfort and ability to participate in the interview. When asked what could be causing the symptoms, Ms. Zabriski responded with uncertainty. The nurse provided clarity with some diagnoses that could contribute to the symptoms. Following the response by Ms. Zabriski, the nurse brought the focus to Ms. Zabriski and not the dorm mates. The interview continued with the nurse obtaining specific subjective data using open-ended questions.

Objective Data—Physical Assessment

Assessment Techniques and Findings

Physical assessment of the abdomen requires the use of inspection, auscultation, percussion, palpation. Percussion of the abdomen and palpation of the liver and spleen are considered advanced skills and are described in Appendix C. The order of the techniques for assessing the abdomen changes to inspection, auscultation, percussion, and palpation. Percussion and palpation could influence peristaltic activity thereby changing the findings upon auscultation. Delaying percussion and palpation prevents disturbance of the normal bowel sounds. The lateral aspects of the abdomen are included when conducting each of the assessments.

During each of the procedures, the nurse is gathering data related to problems with underlying abdominal organs and structures. Inspection includes looking at skin color, structures of the abdomen, abdominal contour, pulsations, and abdominal movements. Knowledge of normative values or expected find-ings is essential in determining the meaning of the data as the physical assessment is performed.

The skin of the abdomen should be consistent with the skin of the rest of the body. The umbilicus should be midline in an abdomen that may be round, flat, convex, or protuberant. The abdomen should be symmetric and free of bulges. Pulsations and wavelike movements below the xiphoid process are nor-mal in thin adults.

HELPFUL HINTS

- Provide an environment that is warm and comfortable.
- Place a small pillow under the patient's knees to help relax the abdominal muscles.
- Encourage the patient to void before the examination.
- Provide instructions about what is expected of the patient (e.g., taking several deep breaths to relax abdominal muscles).
- Pay attention to nonverbal cues that may indicate discomfort. Facial gestures, legs flexed at the knees, and abdominal guarding with the hands are all indices of discomfort.
- When a patient is experiencing abdominal pain, examine that area last.
- Stand on the right side of the patient, unless otherwise indi-cated, because the liver and right kidney are within the right side of the abdomen.
- Maintain the dignity of the patient through appropriate draping techniques.
- Use Standard Precautions.

EQUIPMENT

- Examination gown and drape
- Clean, nonsterile examination gloves
- Stethoscope
- Tissues
- Tape measure

Techniques and Normal Findings	Abnormal Findings and Special Considerations

Survey

A quick survey of the patient enables the nurse to identify any immediate problems as well as the patient's ability to participate in the assessment.

Inspect the overall appearance, posture, and position of the patient. Observe for signs of pain or discomfort and signs of anxiety or distress.

▶ Patients experiencing anxiety may demonstrate pallor and shal-low breathing. They may be diaphoretic and use their hands to guard their abdomen.

▶ Acknowledgment of the problem and a discussion of the pro-cedures often provide some relief. If the patient is experiencing severe pain or discomfort, the problem must be addressed, and a complete abdominal assessment may need to be delayed.

Inspection of the Abdomen

1. **Position the patient.**
   - The patient should be in a supine position with a small pillow placed beneath the head and knees. Drape the examination gown over the chest, exposing the abdomen. Place the drape at the symphysis pubis, covering the patient's pubic area and legs (see Figure 20.7 ■).
   - Stand at the right side of the patient. Lighting must be adequate to detect color differences, lesions, and movements of the abdomen.

▶ These measures relax the abdominal musculature and prevent unnecessary exposure of the patient.

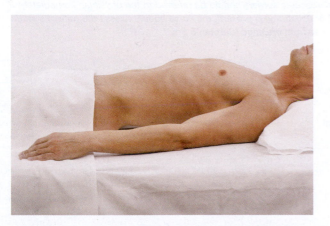

Figure 20.7 Patient positioned and draped.

Techniques and Normal Findings	Abnormal Findings and Special Considerations

2. **Instruct the patient.**
   - Explain that you will be looking at the patient's abdomen. Tell the patient to breathe normally.

3. **Map the abdomen.**
   - Visualize the imaginary horizontal and vertical lines delineating the abdominal quadrants and regions as identified in Figure 20.5 and Figure 20.6.
   - Visualize the underlying structures as identified in Figure 20.6.

4. **Determine the contour of the abdomen.**
   - Observe the profile of the abdomen between the costal margins and the symphysis pubis.
   - The abdominal profile should be viewed at eye level. You may need to sit or kneel to observe the abdominal profile.
   - Normal findings include flat, rounded, or scaphoid contours (see Figure 20.8 ■).

▶ If the patient is guarding the abdomen, demonstrated by posture or breathing, ask the patient to take several deep breaths. This assists in relaxation of abdominal musculature.

▶ A protuberant abdomen is normal in toddlers and in pregnancy. It may indicate obesity or ascites in a nonpregnant patient.

Flat. A straight horizontal line is observed from the costal margin to the symphysis pubis. This contour is common in a thin person.

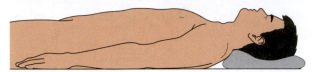

Rounded. Sometimes called a convex abdomen. The horizontal line now curves outward, indicating an increase in abdominal fat or a decrease in muscle tone. This contour is considered a normal variation in the toddler and the pregnant female.

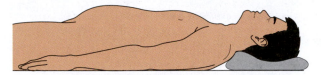

Figure 20.8 Contour of the abdomen.

Protuberant. Similar to the rounded abdomen, only greater. This contour is anticipated in pregnancy. It is also seen in the adult with obesity, ascites, and other conditions.

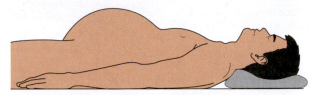

Scaphoid. Sometimes called a concave abdomen. The horizontal line now curves inward toward the vertebral column, giving the abdomen a sunken appearance. In the adult, this contour is seen in the very thin person.

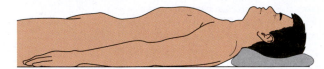

5. **Observe the position of the umbilicus.**
   - The umbilicus is normally in the center of the abdomen. It may be inverted or protruding. The umbilicus should be clean and free of inflammation or drainage.

▶ A protruding or displaced umbilicus is a normal variation in pregnant females. In the nonpregnant adult, it could indicate an abdominal mass or distended urinary bladder. Inflammation or drainage may indicate an infection or complication from recent laparoscopic surgery. A displaced or protruding umbilicus may be a sign of a hernia in a child.

ALERT! *A patient with drainage from the umbilicus following laparoscopic surgery should be referred to the physician immediately. If a bowel diversion ostomy (e.g., gastrostomy, colonostomy, jejunostomy, or ileostomy) is present, the nurse should assess the patient's stoma for color and presence of drainage. Usually, the stoma is red, moist, and free from drainage (Berman & Snyder, 2016).*

6. **Observe skin color.**
   - The abdominal skin should be consistent in color and luster with the skin of the rest of the body. The skin is smooth, moist, and free of lesions.

7. **Observe the location and characteristics of lesions, scars, and abdominal markings.**
   - Lesions such as macules, moles, and freckles are considered normal findings.

▶ Taut, glistening skin could indicate ascites.

▶ **Striae**, commonly called stretch marks, are silvery, shiny, irregular markings on the skin. These are seen in obesity, pregnancy, and ascites (refer to Figure 25.8A. ∞).

▶ Scars indicate previous surgery or trauma and the possibility of underlying adhesions. The location of all lesions must be documented as baseline data and for determination of change in future assessment.

8. **Observe the abdomen for symmetry, bulging, or masses.**
   - First, observe the abdomen while standing at the patient's side. Second, observe the abdomen while standing at the foot of the examination table. Compare the right and left sides. The sides should appear symmetric in shape, size, and contour.

▶ Asymmetry may indicate masses, adhesions, or strictures of underlying structures.

Techniques and Normal Findings	Abnormal Findings and Special Considerations

- Third, return to the patient's side and use a tangential light across the abdomen. No shadows should appear.
- Observe the abdomen from eye level, by sitting or kneeling, and shine the light across the abdomen. The abdomen should appear symmetric without bulges or masses.
- You may repeat all of the assessments above while asking the patient to take a deep breath and raise the head off the pillow.

9. **Observe the abdominal wall for movement.**
- Movements can include pulsations or peristaltic waves. In thin patients it is normal to observe a pulsation of the abdominal aorta below the xiphoid process. The observation of peristaltic waves in thin patients is normal.

▶ Shadows may indicate bulges or masses.

▶ Bulges could indicate tumors, cysts, or hernias.

▶ Deep breathing and head raising accentuate masses.

▶ Marked pulsations could indicate aortic aneurysm or increased pulse pressure. Increased peristaltic activity could indicate gastroenteritis or an obstructive process.

Auscultation of the Abdomen

Auscultation of the abdomen refers to listening to bowel sounds, vascular sounds, and friction rubs through the stethoscope.

ALERT! *It is important to auscultate before percussing and palpating, because the latter techniques could alter peristaltic action.*

The pattern for auscultation of bowel sounds is to begin in the RLQ and then proceed through each of the remaining quadrants. The diaphragm of the stethoscope is used to auscultate bowel sounds. The pattern for auscultation of vascular sounds is to begin at the midline below the xiphoid process for the aorta and to proceed from side to side over renal, iliac, and femoral arteries. The bell of the stethoscope is used to auscultate vascular sounds.

The pattern for auscultation for friction rubs is to begin in the RLQ and proceed through each of the remaining quadrants and to listen over the liver and spleen.

The normal bowel sounds heard upon auscultation of the abdomen are irregular, high-pitched, gurgling sounds.

Normal bowel sounds occur from 5 to 30 times per minute. **Borborygmi** typically refers to more frequent sounds heard in patients who have not eaten in a few hours.

Auscultation of the normal abdomen will not produce vascular sounds or friction rubs.

▶ Hyperactive bowel sounds are loud, high-pitched, and rushing. They may occur more frequently with gastroenteritis or diarrhea.

▶ Hypoactive sounds that are slow and sluggish are common following abdominal surgery or bowel obstruction. Absent bowel sounds may be indicative of paralytic ileus.

▶ Vascular sounds include bruits and venous hum. A bruit is pulsatile and blowing. A venous hum is soft, continuous, and low pitched. **Friction rub** refers to a rough, grating sound caused by the rubbing together of organs or an organ rubbing on the peritoneum.

1. **Instruct the patient.**
- Explain that you will be listening to the patient's abdomen with the stethoscope. The patient will be in the supine position. Tell the patient to breathe normally. Explain that you will be moving the stethoscope around the patient's abdomen and stopping to listen when the stethoscope is placed on the skin. Inform the patient that this will cause no discomfort.

2. **Auscultate for bowel sounds.**
- Use the diaphragm of the stethoscope. Start in the RLQ and move through the other quadrants. Note the character and frequency of the sounds. Count the sounds for at least 60 seconds (see Figure 20.9 ■).

- Normal bowel sounds are irregular, gurgling, and high pitched. They occur from 5 to 30 times per minute. Borborygmi is a normal finding.

▶ Hyperactive sounds are common in gastroenteritis and diarrhea.

▶ Hypoactive sounds are common following abdominal surgery and occur in end-stage intestinal obstruction.

▶ Absence of bowel sounds may indicate paralytic ileus or intestinal obstruction. Patients with paralytic ileus or intestinal obstruction require immediate attention.

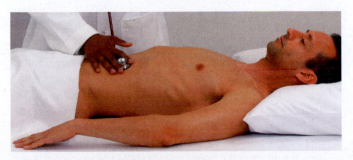

Figure 20.9 Auscultating the abdomen for bowel sounds.

Techniques and Normal Findings	Abnormal Findings and Special Considerations

ALERT! *It may be difficult for the novice nurse to hear bowel sounds in some patients. Bowel sounds may be difficult to hear in obese patients with large amounts of adipose tissue in the abdomen. All four quadrants are auscultated for a total of at least 5 minutes before documenting absent bowel sounds.*

3. **Auscultate for vascular sounds.**
   - Use the bell of the stethoscope. Listen at the midline below the xiphoid process for aortic sounds. Move the stethoscope from side to side as you listen over the renal, iliac, and femoral arteries (see Figure 20.10 ■).

▶ Bruits heard during systole and diastole may indicate arterial occlusion.

▶ A venous hum usually indicates increased portal tension.

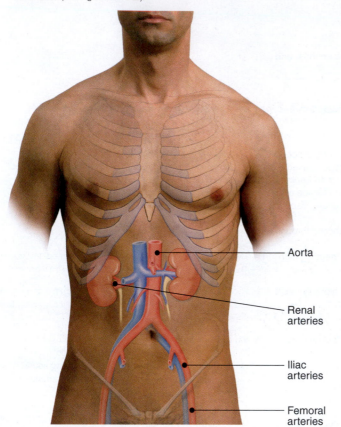

Aorta

Renal arteries

Iliac arteries

Femoral arteries

Figure 20.10 Auscultatory areas for vascular sounds.

4. **Auscultate for friction rubs.**
   - Auscultate the abdomen, listening for a coarse, grating sound. Listen carefully over the liver and spleen. Friction rubs are not normally heard.

Evidence-Based Practice:

Bowel Sounds

After abdominal surgery, it is common for most patients to experience a phenomenon called postoperative ileus (POI), in which there is a loss of gastrointestinal motility resulting in the absence of bowel sounds. Since the 1900s, healthcare providers, including nurses, have been instructed to listen for a full 5 minutes in each quadrant for the return of bowel sounds as an indication of the end of POI. Past research has failed to show any correlation between the return of bowel sounds, passing of flatus, and a bowel movement, thus leading to doubt that bowel sounds were a reliable indicator that the POI has resolved (Huge et al., 2000; Waldhausen & Schirmer, 1990; Waldausen, Shaffrey, Skenderis, Jones, & Schirmer, 1990). Massey (2012) found no significant correlation between the first passing of flatus and the return of bowel sounds in a study of 66 patients recovering from abdominal surgery. These findings suggest that in patients recovering from abdominal surgery, the return of the bowel sounds should be used cautiously as an indicator that the POI has resolved (Massie, 2012).

Palpation of the Abdomen

Palpation of the abdomen is conducted to determine organ size and placement, muscle tightness or guarding, masses, tenderness, and the presence of fluid. This is performed after auscultation to avoid changing the natural sounds and movements of the abdomen. Identify painful areas and palpate these areas last.

You will use both light and deep palpation.

▶ Muscle tightness or guarding may indicate abdominal pain. Guarding is involuntary contraction of abdominal muscles associated with peritonitis.

▶ Abdominal pain from an organ is often experienced as referred pain—that is, felt on the surface of the abdomen or back.

> **ALERT!** *Palpation of the abdomen is contraindicated in the following conditions: suspected appendicitis or dissecting abdominal aortic aneurysm, polycystic kidneys, and transplanted organs.*

Techniques and Normal Findings	Abnormal Findings and Special Considerations

1. **Instruct the patient.**
   - Explain that you will be touching the patient's abdomen with your hands. Explain that you are going to use light touch and then slight pressure to explore the abdomen. Instruct the patient to inform you of any discomfort. Observe the patient's facial expression for signs of pain. Also watch for the tendency to guard the abdomen with the hands or to flex the knees.
   - Instruct the patient to take several deep breaths to relax the muscles of the abdomen.

2. **Lightly palpate the abdomen.**
   - Place the palmar surface of your hand on the abdomen and extend your fingers. Lightly press into the abdomen with your fingers (see Figure 20.11 ■).
   - Move your hand over the four quadrants by lifting your hand and then placing it in another area. Do not drag or slide your hand over the surface of the skin.
   - The abdomen should be soft, smooth, nontender, and pain free.

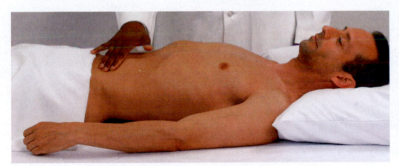

Figure 20.11 Light palpation of abdomen.

3. **Deeply palpate the abdomen.**
   - Proceed as for light palpation, described in the previous step. Exert pressure with your hand to depress the abdomen about 5 cm (2 in.).
   - Palpate all four quadrants in an organized sequence.
   - In an obese patient or a patient with an enlarged abdomen, use a bimanual technique. Place the fingers of your nondominant hand over your dominant hand (see Figure 20.12 ■).
   - Identify the size of the underlying organs and any masses for tenderness. The pancreas is nonpalpable because of its size and location.

▶ Masses, tumors, or obstructions may be palpated.

▶ In the pregnant female the uterus is palpable. The height of the fundus varies according to the week of gestation.

▶ A mass in the LLQ may be stool in the colon.

▶ A vaguely palpable sensation of fullness in the epigastric region may be pancreatic in origin.

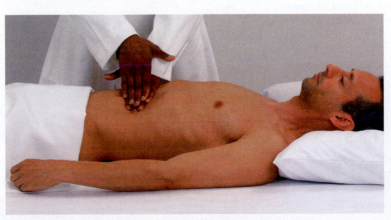

Figure 20.12 Deep palpation of abdomen using a bimanual technique.

Techniques and Normal Findings	Abnormal Findings and Special Considerations

Additional Procedures

1. **Palpate for rebound tenderness.**
   - With the patient in a supine position, hold your hand at a 90-degree angle to the abdominal wall in an area of no pain or discomfort. Press deeply into the abdomen, using a slow steady movement.
   - Rapidly remove your fingers from the patient's abdomen (see Figure 20.13 ■).
   - Ask if the patient feels any pain. Normally, the patient feels the pressure but no pain.

▶ The experience of sharp stabbing pain as the compressed area returns to a noncompressed state is known as **Blumberg's sign**. This finding occurs in peritoneal irritation and requires immediate medical attention.

▶ Pain referred to McBurney's point (2.5 to 5.1 cm [1 to 2 in.] above the anterosuperior iliac spine, on a line between the ileum and the umbilicus) on palpation of the left lower abdomen is Rovsing's sign (pain in the RLQ upon palpation of the LLQ), suggestive of peritoneal irritation in appendicitis.

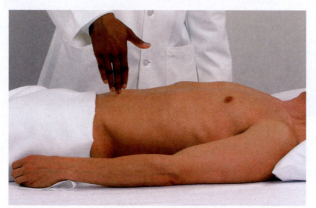

A.

B.

Figure 20.13 Palpating for rebound tenderness. A. Applying pressure. B. Rapid release of pressure.

ALERT! *To avoid causing unnecessary pain or discomfort, abdominal palpation for rebound tenderness should not be performed when assessing patients whose current subjective reports include abdominal pain or tenderness.*

2. **Test for psoas sign.**
   - Perform this test when lower abdominal pain is present and you suspect appendicitis.
   - With the patient in a supine position, place your left hand just above the level of the patient's right knee. Ask the patient to raise the leg to meet your hand. Flexion of the hip causes contraction of the psoas muscle (see Figure 20.14 ■).
   - Normally there is no abdominal pain associated with this maneuver.

▶ Pain during this maneuver is indicative of irritation of the psoas muscle associated with peritoneal inflammation or appendicitis.

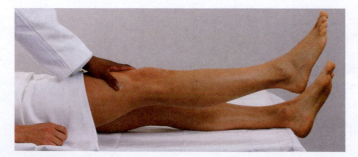

Figure 20.14 Psoas sign.

Techniques and Normal Findings	Abnormal Findings and Special Considerations
3. **Test for Murphy's sign.** • While palpating the liver, ask the patient to take a deep breath. The diaphragm descends, pushing the liver and gallbladder toward your hand. • In a healthy patient, liver palpation is painless.*(continued)*	▶ Sharp abdominal pain and the need to halt the examination is a positive Murphy's sign. This occurs in patients with cholecystitis.

Appendix C: Advanced Skills! *Appendix C provides step-by-step instructions on percussion of the abdomen, liver, and spleen.*

Documenting Your Findings

Documentation of assessment data—subjective and objective—must be accurate, professional, complete, and confidential. When documenting the information from the focused assessment of each body system, the nurse should use measurements whenever appropriate to ensure accuracy, use medical terminology rather than jargon, include all pertinent information, and avoid language that could identify the patient. The information in the documentation should make it clear what questions were asked and should use language to indicate whether it is the patient's response or the nurse's findings.

Sample Documentation: Abdomen
Focused History (Subjective Data)

Patient reports mild, cramping abdominal pain in the lower left quadrant. Rates pain as a 2 on 1–10 scale. Denies nausea, vomiting, heartburn, or diarrhea. Reports constipation over the last 2 weeks with last bowel movement 4 days ago. Has not taken any medication to help with constipation. History of irritable bowel disease for 10 years. Has tried numerous diets and medications to help without success. Appetite and weight are unchanged.

Physical Assessment (Objective Data)

Abdomen has a flat contour, skin color consistent, midline umbilicus, no scars, lesions, or striae. Hypoactive bowel sounds in all four quadrants. No bruits at the aorta, renal, iliac, or femoral arteries. Slight tenderness noted in the LLQ. Negative rebound, psoas, Murphy's sign.

Abnormal Findings

Abnormal findings in the abdomen occur in association with general health and in illness. For example, protrusion of the abdomen is seen in obese individuals and in pregnancy. Abdominal hernias are often seen in otherwise healthy adults and children. Untreated hernias, however, can lead to obstructive intestinal complications that give rise to acute symptoms and serious health problems. Further, alterations of the gastrointestinal tract include nutritional problems, eating disorders, cancers, ulcers, and inflammatory and infectious processes.

For accurate diagnosis in many abdominal and gastrointestinal problems, the health history and physical assessment are accompanied by observations of products of elimination and require diagnostic testing. Diagnostic testing includes laboratory studies of blood, urine, and feces as well as radiographic and magnetic resonance imaging (MRI). In appendicitis, for example, physical findings include facial expressions demonstrating pain, abdominal guarding, tenderness to palpation at McBurney's point, RLQ rebound tenderness, and a positive Rovsing's sign. Diagnosis is confirmed by an elevation in the white blood cell count and findings from an abdominal X-ray, ultrasound, or computerized tomography (CT) scan. Abnormal findings from abdominal assessment are presented in the following section.

Abnormal Abdominal Sounds

When conducting an abdominal assessment, the nurse auscultates for bowel sounds and for vascular sounds. Table 20.2 includes information for interpretation of abnormal abdominal sounds.

Abdominal Pain

Pain is associated with acute and chronic conditions that affect the digestive organs and abdominal structures. Table 20.3 provides information about several disorders that cause abdominal pain. Disruption of function of the abdominal structures may result in referred pain. **Referred pain** is pain or discomfort that is perceived in an area of the body other than the region or point from which the pain originates. For example, pain related to pancreatitis may be perceived in the individual's back. See Figure 9.5 ■ for an illustration of common sites of referred pain and their origins.

Abdominal Distention

Abdominal distention occurs for a variety of reasons including obesity, gaseous distention, and ascites. Each of these conditions is described in Table 20.4.

Table 20.2 Abnormal Abdominal Sounds

SOUND	LOCATION	CAUSATIVE FACTORS
Bowel Sounds		
Hyperactive sounds	Any quadrant	Gastroenteritis, diarrhea
Hyperactive sounds followed by absence of sound	Any quadrant	Paralytic ileus
High-pitched sounds with cramping	Any quadrant	Intestinal obstruction
Vascular Sounds		
Systolic bruit (blowing)	Midline below xiphoid	Aortic arterial obstruction
	Left and right lower costal borders at midclavicular line	Stenosis of renal arteries
	Left and right abdomen at midclavicular line between umbilicus and anterior iliac spine	Stenosis of iliac arteries
Venous hum (continuous tone)	Epigastrium and around umbilicus	Portal hypertension
Rubbing		
Friction rub (harsh, grating)	Left and right upper quadrants, over liver and spleen	Tumor or inflammation of organ

Table 20.3 Pain in Common Abdominal Disorders

DISORDER	DEFINITION	PAIN CHARACTERISTICS	PRECIPITATING FACTORS
Appendicitis	Acute inflammation of vermiform appendix	Epigastric and periumbilical Localizes to RLQ Sudden onset	Obstruction (fecal stone, adhesions)
Cholecystitis	Acute or chronic inflammation of wall of gallbladder	RUQ, radiates to right scapula Sudden onset	Fatty meals, obstruction of duct in cholelithiasis
Diverticulitis	Inflammation of diverticula (outpouches of mucosa through intestinal wall)	Cramping LLQ Radiates to back	Ingestion of fiber-rich diet, stress
Duodenal Ulcer	Breaks in mucosa of duodenum	Aching, gnawing, epigastric	Stress, use of nonsteroidal anti-inflammatory drugs (NSAIDs)
Ectopic Pregnancy	Implantation of blastocyte outside of the uterus, generally in the fallopian tube	Fullness in the rectal area Abdominal cramping, unilateral pain	Tubal damage, pelvic infection, hormonal disorders, lifting, bowel movements
Gastritis	Inflammation of mucosal lining of the stomach (acute and chronic)	Epigastric pain	*Acute:* NSAIDs, alcohol abuse, stress, infection *Chronic:* H. pylori Autoimmune responses
Gastroesophageal Reflux Disorder (GERD)	Backflow of gastric acid to the esophagus	Heartburn, chest pain	Food intake, lying down after meals
Intestinal Obstruction	Blockage of normal movement of bowel contents	*Small intestine:* aching *Large intestine:* spasmodic pain *Neurogenic:* diffuse abdominal discomfort *Mechanical:* colicky pain associated with distention	*Mechanical:* physical block from impaction, hernia, volvulus *Neurogenic:* manipulation of bowel during surgery, peritoneal irritation
Irritable Bowel Syndrome (Spastic Colon)	Problems with gastrointestinal (GI) motility	LLQ accompanied by diarrhea and/or constipation Pain increases after eating and decreases after bowel movement	Stress, untolerated foods, caffeine, lactose intolerance, alcohol, familial linkage
Pancreatitis	Inflammation of the pancreas	Upper abdominal, knifelike, deep epigastric or umbilical area pain	Ductal obstruction, alcohol abuse, use of acetaminophen, infection

Table 20.4 Selected Causes of Abdominal Distention

Obesity

Distention or protuberance of the abdomen. Abdomen's increased size is caused by a thickened abdominal wall and fat deposited in the mesentery and omentum. Percussion produces normal tympanic sounds.

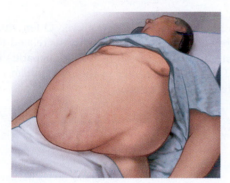

Obesity.

Gaseous Distention

A result of increased production of gas in the intestines, which occurs with the ingestion of some foods. In paralytic ileus and intestinal obstruction, it is also associated with altered peristalsis in which gas cannot move through the intestines. Can be localized or generalized. Percussion produces tympany over a large area.

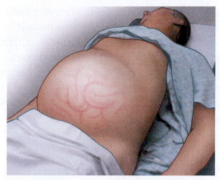

Distended abdomen.

Abdominal Tumor

Tumor produces abdominal distention. The abdomen is firm to palpation and dull to percussion. This type of distention is common in ovarian and uterine tumors.

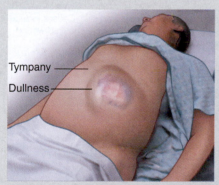

Abdominal tumor.

Ascites

The accumulation of fluid in the abdomen in which the abdomen becomes protuberant like bulging flasks. Fluid descends with gravity, resulting in dullness to percussion in the lower abdomen. May also be assessed by placing the patient in a lateral position and observing fluid shift to the dependent side. Occurs in cirrhosis, congestive heart failure (CHF), nephrosis, peritonitis, and neoplastic diseases.

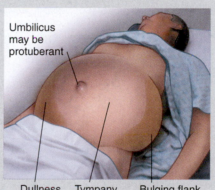

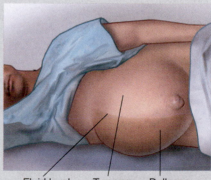

Ascites.

Abdominal Hernias

A **hernia**, commonly called a rupture, is a protrusion of an organ or structure through an abnormal opening or weakened area in a body wall. The abdominal wall is the most common site of hernias. This weakening could be congenital or acquired. If the protruding or displaced abdominal contents return to their normal position when the patient relaxes, the hernia is said to be reducible or reduced. When the displaced or protruding structures do not return to their normal position, the hernia is said to be incarcerated or nonreducible. An incarcerated hernia can become strangulated. In strangulated hernias, the blood supply to the displaced abdominal contents is compromised. The strangulated visceral contents can become gangrenous. Overstretched rectus muscles with weakened fascia cause an umbilical hernia. An overview of common types of hernias is presented in Table 20.5.

Alterations of the Gastrointestinal Tract

Alterations of the gastrointestinal tract include cancers and inflammatory diseases. These alterations are described in the following sections.

CANCERS

Cancer of the esophagus is a malignant growth of the esophagus, most common in males over 50 years of age. The lower third of the esophagus is most commonly involved. Patients commonly complain of weight loss, **dysphagia** (difficulty swallowing), and odynophagia (pain on swallowing). Alcohol abuse, smoking, and poor oral hygiene appear to be predisposing factors.

Hepatic Cancers

Hepatic cancer is a malignant growth of the liver. Often, this type of cancer is preceded by the onset of cirrhosis related to alcohol abuse, autoimmune diseases of the liver, or hepatitis B and C infections. The use of the liver in the metabolism of drugs leads to limited treatment options.

Subjective findings:
- Upper right quadrant abdominal pain
- Bruising or bleeding easily
- Nausea
- Fatigue

Objective findings:
- Ascites or fluid accumulation in the abdomen
- Jaundicing (yellowing) of the skin, eye sclera, and/or mucous membranes
- Vomiting
- Pale or white stools

Table 20.5 Overview of Common Types of Hernias

Umbilical Hernia
Occurs when the abdominal rectus muscle separates or weakens, allowing abdominal structures, usually the intestines, to push through and come closer to the skin. More common in children than in adults.

Ventral (Incisional) Hernias
Occurs at the site of an incision when the incision weakens the muscle, and the abdominal structures move closer to the skin. Causes include obesity, repeated surgeries, postoperative infection, impaired wound healing, and poor nutrition.

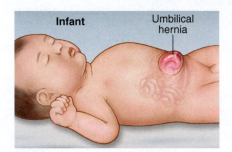

Umbilical hernia.

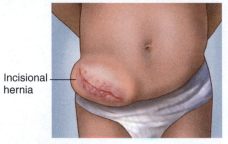

Ventral hernia.

Hiatal Hernia
Weakening in the diaphragm allows a portion of the stomach and esophagus to move into the thoracic cavity. Classified as sliding or rolling; more common in adults than children.

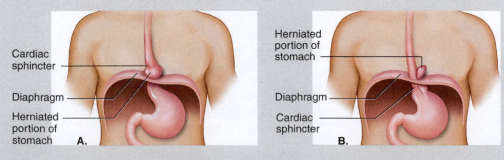

Abdominal hernias. A. Sliding hiatal hernia. B. Rolling hiatal hernia.

Pancreatic Cancer

Pancreatic cancer is a malignant growth of the pancreas. Because this type of cancer metastasizes very rapidly, pancreatic cancer offers a poor prognosis. The pancreas helps contribute to digestion, produces insulin, and produces hormones. Though smoking is a major risk factor in pancreatic cancer, additional risk factors are age, race, and genetic disposition.

Subjective findings:

- Upper middle to left quadrant abdominal pain that radiates to the back
- Nausea
- Pruritis (itching) (American Cancer Society [ACS], 2014a)

Objective findings:

- Extreme weight loss
- Jaundicing of the skin, eyes, or mucous membranes
- Dark-colored urine
- Diarrhea
- Greasy, pale-colored stools (ACS, 2014a)

Stomach Cancer

Cancer of the stomach is a malignant growth of the stomach. The disease is often in the advanced stages before a diagnosis is made. Dietary habits seem to be an influencing factor.

Subjective findings:

- Indigestion
- Loss of appetite
- Sense of abdominal bloating after eating
- Nausea
- Abdominal pain

Objective findings:

- Weight loss
- Vomiting
- Abdominal distention
- Gastrointestinal bleeding
- Cancerous lesions, most frequently located in the distal third of the stomach

Colorectal Cancer

Colorectal cancer is a malignant lesion involving any part of the large intestine, sigmoid colon, or rectum. Predisposing factors include poor dietary habits and chronic constipation. Signs and symptoms vary according to the location of the growth. Risk factors include age over 50, family history, preexisting disorder of the GI tract, diabetes, history of tobacco use, history of moderate alcohol use, obesity, diet high in red and/or processed meats, and lack of physical activity (ACS, 2014b).

Subjective findings:

- Variation in bowel habits or elimination patterns
- Abdominal cramping or pain
- Increased production of intestinal gas
- Fatigue

Objective findings:

- Rectal bleeding (occult or overt)
- Unexplained weight loss
- Intestinal obstruction, which requires surgical intervention and may necessitate permanent colostomy

Inflammatory Processes

Inflammatory processes may affect any organ in the digestive tract. Common gastrointestinal inflammatory processes include ulcerative colitis, esophagitis, peritonitis, hepatitis, and Crohn disease.

Ulcerative Colitis

Ulcerative colitis is a recurrent inflammatory process causing ulcer formation in the lower portions of the large intestine and rectum. This condition is common in adolescents and young adults. The distribution of the inflammatory process is diffuse. The ulcerative areas abscess and later become necrotic. Manifestations vary depending on the location of the inflammation.

Subjective findings:

- Rectal pain
- Urgency to move bowels with or without ability to pass stool
- Abdominal pain and cramping

Objective findings:

- Weight loss
- Diarrhea (which may be bloody)
- Fever

Esophagitis

Esophagitis is an inflammatory process of the esophagus. It is caused by a variety of irritants. The more common causes include smoking, alcohol abuse, reflux of gastric contents, and ingestion of extremely hot or cold foods and liquids.

Subjective findings:

- Dysphagia (difficulty swallowing)
- Chest pain
- Nausea

Objective findings:

- Vomiting
- Weight loss
- Esophageal obstruction (Mayo Clinic, 2011a)

Peritonitis

Peritonitis is a local or generalized inflammatory process of the peritoneal membrane of the abdomen. The precipitant can be an infectious process (pelvic inflammatory disease), perforation of an organ (ruptured duodenal ulcer), internal bleeding (ruptured ectopic pregnancy), or trauma (stab wound to abdomen).

Subjective findings:

- Abdominal pain or tenderness
- Abdominal bloating
- Nausea
- Decreased urine output

Objective findings:

- Abdominal distention
- Vomiting
- Decreased appetite
- Fever (Mayo Clinic, 2011b)

Hepatitis

Hepatitis is an inflammatory process of the liver. Manifestations of hepatitis vary, depending on the form of hepatitis that is contracted. Its causes include viruses, bacteria, chemicals, and drugs. Types of hepatitis include the following:

- **Hepatitis A virus** (HAV), infectious hepatitis, is transmitted via enteric routes (feces or oral routes).
- **Hepatitis B virus** (HBV) is transmitted parenterally, sexually, or perinatally.
- **Hepatitis C virus** (HCV) is transmitted via blood and blood products, parenterally, and through unknown factors.
- **Hepatitis D virus** (HDV) is the same as HBV and requires HBV to replicate.
- **Hepatitis E virus** (HEV) is a non-A, non-B type and is transmitted enterically. HEV is most common in those who travel to India, Africa, Asia, and Central America.

Crohn Disease

Crohn disease is a chronic inflammatory process of the intestine. It is sometimes called regional ileitis, which is a misnomer because it can involve any part of the lower intestinal tract. Crohn disease is characterized by "skipped" sections of involvement. It is most common in young adults and usually has an insidious onset. The inflammation involves all layers of the intestinal mucosa. Transverse fissures develop in the bowel, producing a characteristic cobblestone appearance.

Subjective findings:

- Abdominal pain or cramping
- Fatigue
- Decreased appetite

Objective findings:

- Diarrhea (which may be bloody)
- Weight loss
- Fever (Mayo Clinic, 2011c)

Application Through Critical Thinking

CASE STUDY

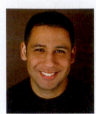

Source: Phase4Studios / Shutterstock

Luiz Hernandez, a 28-year-old Hispanic male, is seeking care in the neighborhood clinic for abdominal pain and weight loss. He has been seen here previously for employment physicals, which revealed no acute or chronic health problems.

During the interview, the nurse learns that the patient has had abdominal pain, on and off, for a couple of months and that the pain is getting worse. The pain is in the middle of his stomach and is like an ache. Mr. Hernandez says he also has had no interest in food, feels gassy, and has lost about 10 lb.

When asked about factors that precipitate or affect the pain, the patient reveals that the pain occurs most frequently late in the morning and afternoon and that he wakes up at night with the pain. When asked if he has tried any remedy for the pain, Mr. Hernandez states that he uses an antacid once in a while, which helps, and that he takes mint because that is what his mother gave to his family members when they had stomach troubles.

In response to questions about weight loss, Mr. Hernandez says that he thinks he has been losing weight because he just hasn't been feeling hungry and many of the foods he is used to eating do not appeal to him. He also states that he is starting to get nervous about the pain, and when he is nervous he never feels like eating. The nurse asks if he is nervous about this clinic visit. The patient replies that he was really nervous when he arrived but is feeling a little better now that he is talking about what is going on. He further states, "I am still scared about what might be causing this."

The nurse continues the interview with questions about the patient's past and family history. No acute or chronic problems are revealed. The nurse asks the patient about his use of medications and habits. Mr. Hernandez states that he uses Tylenol occasionally for a headache. He does not smoke and uses alcohol socially, mostly on weekends.

The physical assessment reveals vital signs of BP 132/84, P 88, RR 22. The skin is cool, dry, and pale. The abdomen is soft and not distended, bowel sounds are present in all quadrants, and there is no tenderness on palpation.

The plan for this patient is to begin antacids three times a day, after meals and at bedtime; schedule an endoscopy; obtain cultures for *H. pylori*; and arrange for a follow-up visit in 1 week.

SAMPLE DOCUMENTATION

The following is sample documentation for Luis Hernandez.

SUBJECTIVE DATA Aching midabdominal pain for several months, getting worse. Feels "gassy." No interest in food. Weight loss 10 lb. Pain occurs late in a.m. and p.m., wakes at night. Antacid used infrequently with relief. Uses mint for symptoms. Nervous about pain and what it might mean.

OBJECTIVE DATA Skin pale, cool, dry. Abdomen soft, nontender. BS + 4 Qs. VS: BP 132/84 Left, BP 130/83 Right—P 88—RR 22.

CRITICAL THINKING QUESTIONS

1. What data suggest the need for *H. pylori* cultures?
2. How would data be clustered to formulate nursing diagnoses?
3. What would be included in an educational plan for this patient?
4. Which psychosocial considerations would be important to evaluate?
5. What cultural considerations should be addressed?

REFERENCES

American Cancer Society (ACS). (2014a). *Signs and symptoms of pancreatic cancer.* Retrieved from http://www.cancer.org/cancer/pancreaticcancer/detailedguide/pancreatic-cancer-signs-and-symptoms

American Cancer Society (ACS). (2014b). *What are the risk factors for colorectal cancer?* Retrieved from http://www.cancer.org/cancer/colonandrectumcancer/detailedguide/colorectal-cancer-risk-factors

American Dental Association. (2018). *Adults over 60: Concerns.* Retrieved from http://www.mouthhealthy.org/en/adults-over-60/concerns

Berman, A., & Snyder, S. J. (2016). *Kozier and Erb's fundamentals of nursing: Concepts, process, and practice* (10th ed.). Upper Saddle River, NJ: Prentice Hall.

Centers for Disease Control and Prevention (CDC). (2017a). *Colorectal cancer rates by race and gender.* Retrieved from https://gis.cdc.gov/grasp/USCS/DataViz.html

Centers for Disease Control and Prevention (CDC). (2017b). *Food safety.* Retrieved from https://www.cdc.gov/foodsafety/index.html

Centers for Disease Control and Prevention (CDC). (2017c). *Colorectal cancer rates by gender and ethnicity*. Retrieved from https://gis.cdc.gov/grasp/USCS/DataViz.html

Cherian, K. M., Mulky, M. J., & Menon, K. K. G. (2014). Toxicological considerations in the use of consumer products. *Defence Science Journal, 37*(2), 143–159.

Huge, A., Kreis, M. E., Zittel, T. T., Becker, H. D., Starlinger, M. J., & Jehle, E. C. (2000). Postoperative colonic motility and tone in patients after colorectal surgery. *Diseases of the Colon and Rectum, 43*(7), 932–939.

Johns Hopkins Medicine. (n.d.). *Stomach and duodenal ulcers: Peptic ulcers*. Retrieved from http://www.hopkinsmedicine.org/healthlibrary/conditions/digestive_disorders/stomach_and_duodenal_ulcers_peptic_ulcers_85,P00394

Mapel, D., Roberts, M., Overhiser, A., & Mason, A. (2013). The epidemiology, diagnosis, and cost of dyspepsia and *Helicobacter pylori* gastritis: A case-control analysis in the southwestern United States. *Helicobacter, 18*(1), 54–65.

Marieb, E. N., & Hoehn, K. (2019). *Human anatomy and physiology* (11th ed.). Redwood City, CA: Benjamin/Cummings.

Massey, R. L. (2012). Return of bowel sounds indicating an end of postoperative ileus: Is it time to cease this long-standing nursing tradition? *Medsurg Nursing, 21*(3), 146–150.

Mayo Clinic. (2011a). *Esophagitis: Symptoms*. Retrieved from http://www.mayoclinic.org/diseases-conditions/esophagitis/basics/symptoms/con-20034313

Mayo Clinic. (2011b). *Peritonitis: Symptoms*. Retrieved from http://www.mayoclinic.org/diseases-conditions/peritonitis/basics/symptoms/con-20032165

Mayo Clinic. (2011c). *Crohn's disease: Symptoms*. Retrieved from http://www.mayoclinic.org/diseases-conditions/crohns-disease/basics/symptoms/con-20032061

Mayo Clinic. (2016). *Toxic hepatitis*. Retrieved from https://www.mayoclinic.org/diseases-conditions/toxic-hepatitis/symptoms-causes/syc-20352202

Melinder, C., Hiyoshi, A., Kasiga, T., Halfvarson, J., Fall, K., & Montgomery, S. (2017). Resilience to stress and risk of gastrointestinal infections. European Journal of Public Health, 28(2), 364–369.

Sira, M. M., Salem, T. A. H., & Sira, A. M. (2013). Biliary atresia: A challenging diagnosis. *Global Journal of Gastroenterology & Hepatology, 1*(1), 34–45.

Waldhausen, J. H., & Schirmer, B. D. (1990). The effect of ambulation on recovery from postoperative ileus. *Annals of Surgery, 212*(6), 671–677.

Waldhausen, J. H., Shaffrey, M. E., Skenderis, B. S., Jones, R. S., & Schirmer, B. D. (1990). Gastrointestinal myoelectric and clinical patterns of recovery after laparotomy. *Annals of Surgery, 211*(6), 777–784.

Wilson, B. A., Shannon, M. T., & Shields, K. M. (2018). *Pearson nurse's drug guide*. Upper Saddle River, NJ: Pearson.

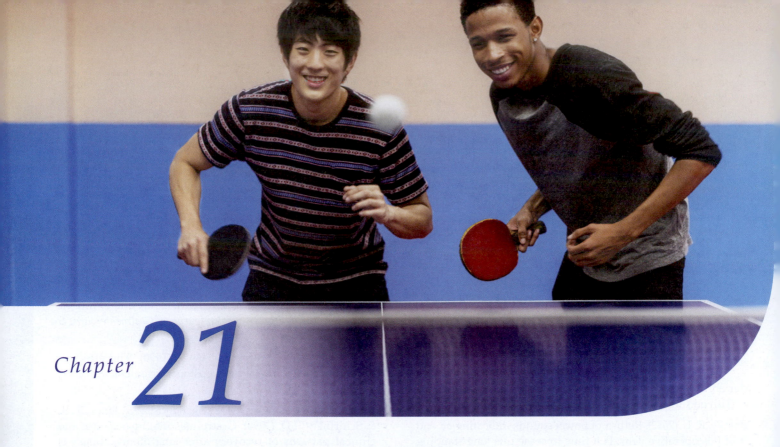

Chapter 21

Male Genitourinary System

LEARNING OUTCOMES

Upon completion of this chapter, you will be able to:

1. Describe the anatomy and physiology of the male genitourinary system.

2. Identify anatomic, physiologic, developmental, psychosocial, and cultural variations that guide assessment of the male genitourinary system.

3. Determine questions about the male genitourinary system to use for the focused interview.

4. Outline the techniques for assessment of the male genitourinary system.

5. Generate the appropriate documentation to describe the assessment of the male genitourinary system.

6. Identify abnormal findings in the physical assessment of the male genitourinary system.

KEY TERMS

MEDICAL LANGUAGE

bi-   Prefix meaning "two"

-cele   Suffix meaning "hernia"

erythr- Prefix meaning "red"

hem-   Prefix meaning "blood"

nephr-   Prefix meaning "kidney"

orch-   Prefix meaning "testis"

-uria   Suffix meaning "urine," "condition of urine"

Introduction

The male **genitourinary system** includes the urinary system and the reproductive organs: respectively, these are the kidneys, ureters, bladder, and urethra; the penis, scrotum, testes, spermatic cord, duct system, accessory glands, and inguinal and perianal areas. The functions of the genitourinary system include the function of the kidneys to prevent the accumulation of nitrogenous wastes, promote fluid and electrolyte balance, assist in maintenance of blood pressure, and contribute to *erythropoiesis* (development of mature red blood cells); in addition, the reproductive organs are integral for human reproduction and sexual gratification.

Male Genitourinary System Anatomy and Physiology Review

Urinary Anatomy and Physiology

The **urinary system** in both males and females is composed of the kidneys, renal vasculature (blood vessels), ureters, bladder, and urethra. The organs of the genitourinary system are distributed among the retroperitoneal space, abdomen, and genitals. The **glomeruli** (tufts of capillaries) of the kidneys filter more than 1 liter (L) of fluid each minute. As a result, wastes, toxins, and foreign matter are removed from the blood.

Kidneys The **kidneys** are bean-shaped organs located in the retroperitoneal space on either side of the vertebral column. Extending from the level of the 12th thoracic vertebra to the 3rd lumbar vertebra, the upper portion of the kidneys is protected by the lower rib cage (Marieb & Keller, 2018). The right kidney is displaced downward by the liver and sits slightly lower than the left kidney. A layer of fat cushions each kidney, and the kidney itself is surrounded by tissue called the renal capsule (see Figure 21.1 ■). The renal fascia connects the kidney and fatty layer to the posterior wall of the abdomen. Each adult kidney weighs approximately 150 g (5 oz) and is 11 to 13 cm (4 to 5 in.) long, 5 to 7 cm (2 to 3 in.) wide, and 2.5 to 3 cm (1 in.) thick. The lateral surface of the kidney is convex. The medial surface is concave and contains the hilus, a vertical cleft that opens into a space within the kidney referred to as the renal sinus. The ureters, renal blood vessels, nerves, and lymphatic vessels pass through the hilus into the renal sinus. The superior part of the kidney is referred to as the upper pole, whereas the inferior surface is called the lower pole.

The inner portion of the kidney is called the *renal medulla*. The renal **medulla** is composed of structures called pyramids

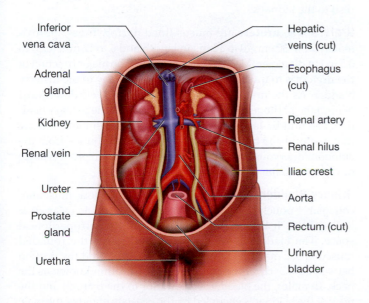

A.

Labels: Inferior vena cava, Adrenal gland, Kidney, Renal vein, Ureter, Prostate gland, Urethra, Hepatic veins (cut), Esophagus (cut), Renal artery, Renal hilus, Iliac crest, Aorta, Rectum (cut), Urinary bladder

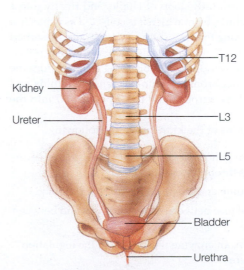

B.

Labels: Kidney, Ureter, T12, L3, L5, Bladder, Urethra

Figure 21.1 The urinary system. A. Anterior view of the urinary organs of a male. B. Relationship of the kidneys to the vertebrae.

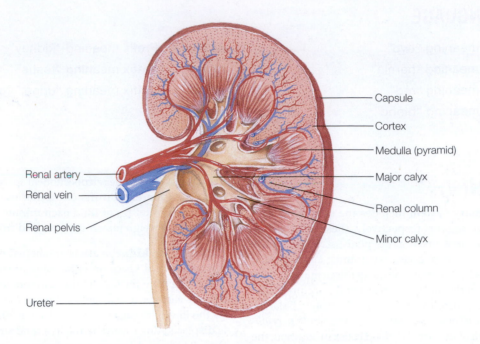

Capsule

Cortex

Medulla (pyramid)

Major calyx

Renal column

Minor calyx

Renal artery

Renal vein

Renal pelvis

Ureter

Figure 21.2 Internal anatomy of the kidney.

and calyces. The pyramids are wedgelike structures made up of bundles of urine-collecting tubules. At their apex, the pyramids have papillae that connect to the cuplike calyces. The calyces collect urine and transport it into the renal pelvis, which is the funnel-shaped superior end of the ureter (see Figure 21.2 ■).

The outer portion of each kidney is called the renal **cortex**. It is composed of over 1 million nephrons, which form urine. The first part of each nephron is the renal corpuscle, which consists of a tuft of capillaries called a glomerulus. These glomeruli begin the filtration of the blood. Larger blood components, such as red blood cells and larger proteins, are separated from most of the fluid, which passes into the glomerular capsule (or Bowman's capsule). The filtrate then moves into a proximal convoluted tubule, then into the loop of Henle, and finally into a distal convoluted tubule, from which it is collected as urine by a collecting tubule. Along the way, some of the filtrate is resorbed along with electrolytes and chemicals such as glucose, potassium, phosphate, and sodium. Each collecting tubule guides the urine from several nephrons out into the renal pyramids and calyces and from there through the renal pelvis and into the ureters.

The major functions of the kidneys are the following:

- Eliminating nitrogenous waste products, toxins, excess ions, and drugs through urine
- Regulating volume and chemical makeup of the blood
- Maintaining balance between water and salts and between acids and bases
- Producing renin, an enzyme that assists in the regulation of blood pressure
- Producing erythropoietin, a hormone that stimulates production of red blood cells in the bone marrow
- Assisting in the metabolism of vitamin D

Renal Arteries   The kidneys require a tremendous amount of oxygen and nutrients and receive about 25% of the cardiac output. Although not part of the urinary system, an extensive network of arteries intertwines within the renal network. These arteries include renal arteries, arcuate arteries, interlobular arteries, afferent arteries, and efferent arterioles. The vasa recta are looping capillaries that connect with the juxtamedullary nephrons and continue into the medulla alongside the loop of Henle. The vasa recta help to concentrate urine. The major function of the renal arteries is to provide a rich supply of blood (approximately 1,200 mL per minute when an individual is at rest) to the kidneys.

Ureters   The **ureters** are mucus-lined narrow tubes approximately 25 to 30 cm (10 to 12 in.) in length and 6 to 12 mm (0.25 to 0.5 in.) in diameter (Marieb & Keller, 2018). The major function of the ureters is to transport urine from the kidney to the urinary bladder. As the ureter leaves the kidney, it travels downward behind the peritoneum to the posterior wall of the urinary bladder. The middle layer of the ureters contains smooth muscle that is stimulated by transmission of electric impulses from the autonomic nervous system. Their peristaltic action propels urine downward to the urinary bladder.

Urinary Bladder   The urinary bladder is a hollow, muscular, collapsible pouch that acts as a reservoir for urine (Marieb & Keller, 2018). It lies on the pelvic floor in the retroperitoneal space. The bladder is composed of two parts: the rounded muscular sac made up of the detrusor muscle, and the portion between the body of the bladder and the urethra known as the neck. In males, the bladder lies anterior to the rectum, and the neck of the bladder is encircled by the prostate gland of the male reproductive system. The detrusor muscle allows the bladder to expand as it fills with urine and to contract to release urine to the outside of the body during micturition (voiding). When empty, the bladder collapses upon itself, forming a thick-walled, pyramidal organ that lies low in the pelvis behind the symphysis pubis. As urine accumulates, the fundus, the superior wall of the bladder, ascends in the abdominal cavity and assumes a rounded shape that is palpable. When moderately filled (500 mL), the bladder is approximately 12.5 cm (5 in.) long. When larger amounts of urine are present, the bladder becomes distended and rises above the symphysis pubis.

The major functions of the urinary bladder are the following:

- Storing urine temporarily
- Contracting to release urine during micturition

Urethra The **urethra** is a mucus-lined tube that transports urine from the urinary bladder to the exterior (Marieb & Keller, 2018). The male urethra is approximately 20 cm (8 in.) long and runs the length of the penis. It terminates in the external urethral orifice in the glans penis. The urethra serves as a conduit for the transportation of both urine and semen to the outside of the body. It is composed of three sections: the prostatic urethra, the membranous urethra, and the cavernous (penile) urethra (see Figure 21.3 ■).

Landmarks During assessment of the urinary system, the nurse uses three landmarks to locate and palpate the kidneys and urinary bladder. These landmarks are the costovertebral angle, the rectus abdominis muscle, and the symphysis pubis. The **costovertebral angle (CVA)** is the area on the lower back formed by the vertebral column and the downward curve

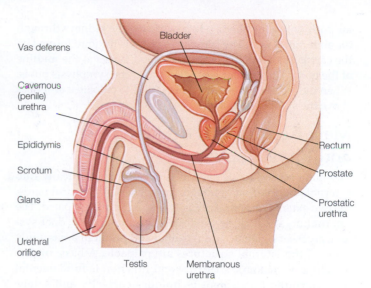

Figure 21.3 Anatomy of the male reproductive organs.

of the last posterior rib, as depicted in Figure 21.4A ■. It is an important anatomic landmark because the lower poles of the kidney and ureter lie below this surface. The rectus abdominis muscles are a longitudinal pair of muscles that extend from the pubis to the rib cage on either side of the midline, as illustrated in Figure 21.4B ■. These muscles are used as guidelines

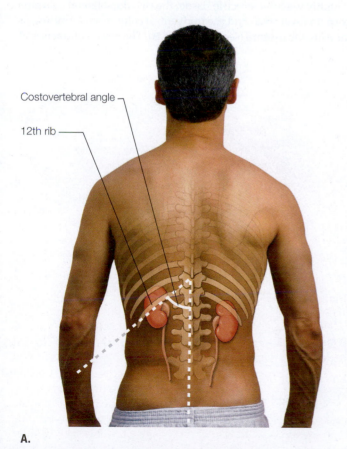

A.

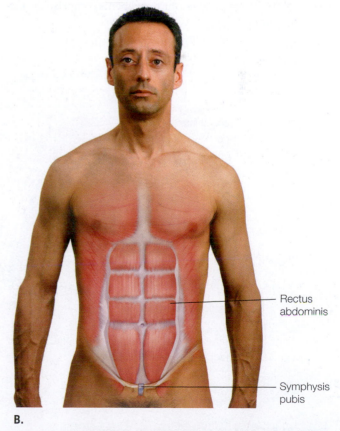

B.

Figure 21.4 Landmarks for urinary asessment. A. The costovertebral angle. B. The rectus abdominis muscle and the symphysis pubis.

for positioning the hands when palpating the kidneys through the abdominal wall. The symphysis pubis is the joint formed by the cartilaginous union of the two pubic bones at the midline of the body. The bladder is cradled under the symphysis pubis. When the bladder is full, the nurse is able to palpate it as it rises above the symphysis pubis.

Male Reproductive Anatomy and Physiology

The male reproductive system is divided anatomically into external and internal genital organs. The scrotum and penis, the two external organs, are easily inspected and palpated. The internal organs include the testes, spermatic cord, duct system, accessory glands, and inguinal and perianal areas. Only some of the internal structures are palpable. A basic understanding of anatomic structure and function is fundamental to performing assessment techniques correctly and safely. Figure 21.3 illustrates the gross anatomy of the male reproductive system.

Some of the male reproductive organs serve dual roles as part of both the reproductive system and the urinary system. The functions of the male reproductive system include the following:

- Manufacturing and protecting sperm for fertilization
- Transporting sperm to the female vagina
- Regulating hormonal production of and secretion of male sex hormones
- Providing sexual stimulation and pleasure

External Genitalia   The scrotum and penis comprise the external male genitalia.

SCROTUM   The **scrotum** is a loosely hanging, pliable, pear-shaped pouch of darkly pigmented skin that is located behind the penis. Pubic hair scantily covers the scrotum. It is visibly asymmetric, with the left side extending lower than the right because the left spermatic cord is longer. It contains the testes, which produce sperm. Spermatogenesis (sperm production) requires an environment in which the temperature is slightly lower than core body temperature; thus, the scrotum hangs outside of the abdominopelvic cavity and maintains a surface temperature of about 34°C (93.2°F), which is approximately 3°C cooler than core body temperature (Agarwal, Aitken, & Alvarez, 2012). A vertical septum within the scrotum divides it into two sections, each containing a testis, epididymis, vas deferens, and spermatic cord, as well as other functional structures (see Figure 21.5 ■). The major functions of the scrotum are protecting the testes, epididymides, and part of the spermatic cords, as well as protecting sperm production and viability through the maintenance of an appropriate surface temperature.

Below the scrotal surface lie two muscles, the cremaster muscle and the dartos muscle, which play a protective role in sperm production and viability. In cold temperatures, the dartos muscle wrinkles the scrotal skin, whereas the cremaster muscle contracts, causing the testes to elevate toward the body. Warmer temperatures cause the reverse reaction. The testes also become more wrinkled and contract toward the body during sexual arousal.

PENIS   The **penis** is centrally located between the left and right groin areas and lies directly in front of the scrotum. Internally, the penile shaft consists of the penile urethra and three columns of highly vascular, erectile tissue: the two dorsolateral columns (corpora cavernosa) and the midventral column surrounding or encasing the urethra (see Figure 21.6 ■). The penis contracts and

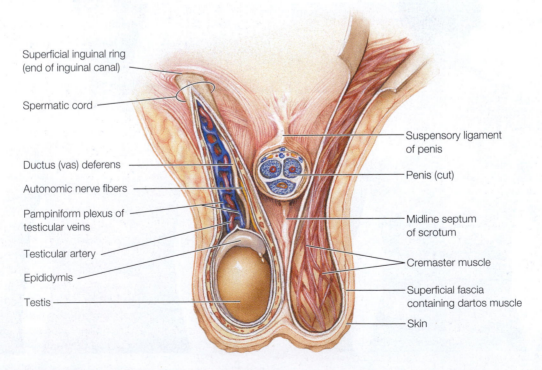

Figure 21.5 Contents of the scrotum, anterior view.

elongates during sexual arousal when its vasculature dilates as it fills with blood. This process allows the penis to become firm and erect so that it can deposit sperm into the female vagina. The distal end of the urethra (the external meatus) appears as a small opening centrally located on the glans of the penis, the cone-shaped distal end of the organ. In uncircumcised males, the glans is covered by a layer of skin called the foreskin. The major functions of the penis are serving as an exit for urine and as a passageway for sperm to exit and be deposited into the vagina during sexual intercourse.

Internal Genital Organs

The testes and spermatic cord comprise the internal male genital organs.

TESTES The **testes** are two firm, rubbery, olive-shaped structures that measure 4 to 5 cm (1.57 to 1.96 in.) long and 2 to 2.5 cm (0.78 to 0.98 in.) wide. They manufacture sperm and are, thus, the primary male sex organs. Each testis has two coats, the outer tunica vaginalis and the inner tunica albuginea, that separate it from the scrotal wall. Within each testis are the seminiferous tubules that produce sperm and Leydig's cells that produce testosterone. Testosterone plays a significant role in sperm production and the development of male sexual characteristics. The testes receive their blood supply from the testicular arteries. The testicular veins remove deoxygenated blood from the testes and also form a network called the pampiniform plexus (see Figure 21.5). This plays a crucial supportive role in regulating the temperature in the testes by cooling arterial blood before it passes into the testes. The major functions of the testes are producing spermatozoa and secreting testosterone.

SPERMATIC CORD The **spermatic cord** is composed of fibrous connective tissue. Its purpose is to form a protective sheath around the nerves, blood vessels, lymphatic structures, and muscle fibers associated with the scrotum (see Figure 21.5).

Duct System

The duct system plays a crucial role in the transportation of sperm. The three structures comprising the duct system are the epididymis, the ductus deferens, and the urethra (see Figure 21.5 and Figure 21.6).

EPIDIDYMIS Positioned on top of and just posterior to each testicle is a comma- or crescent-shaped **epididymis**, which is palpable upon physical examination. It is actually a long, coiled tube, about 18 to 20 ft (5.5 to 6 meters) in length, which forms the beginning of the duct system. Once immature sperm have been produced in the testes, they are transported into the epididymis, where they mature and become mobile. During orgasm, forceful contraction of muscles in this structure propels the sperm into the ductus deferens. The major functions of the epididymis are storing sperm as they mature and transporting sperm to the ductus deferens.

DUCTUS DEFERENS Also known as the vas deferens, this tubular structure stretches from the end of the epididymis to the ejaculatory duct. Extending about 46.15 cm (18 in.) long, the tube runs through the inguinal canal, on the backside of the bladder, and to the ejaculatory duct as it enters into the prostate gland. Mature sperm remain in the ductus deferens until ready for transport. The major functions of the ductus deferens are serving as an excretory duct in the transport of sperm and serving as a reservoir for mature sperm.

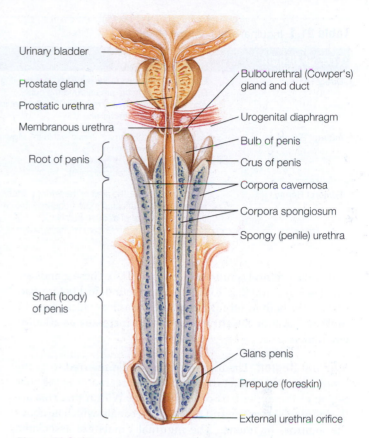

Urinary bladder

Prostate gland

Prostatic urethra

Membranous urethra

Root of penis

Shaft (body) of penis

Bulbourethral (Cowper's) gland and duct

Urogenital diaphragm

Bulb of penis

Crus of penis

Corpora cavernosa

Corpora spongiosum

Spongy (penile) urethra

Glans penis

Prepuce (foreskin)

External urethral orifice

Figure 21.6 Structure of the penis.

Accessory Glands

The accessory glands play a crucial role in the formation of semen. These glands include the seminal vesicles, the prostate gland, and the bulbourethral gland.

SEMINAL VESICLES The **seminal vesicles** are a pair of saclike glands, 7.5 cm (2.95 in.) long, located between the bladder and rectum. These vesicles are the source of 60% of the volume of semen produced. Semen, a thick yellow fluid, is composed of a high concentration of fructose, amino acids, prostaglandins, ascorbic acid, and fibrinogen. It is secreted into the ejaculatory duct, where it mixes with sperm, which has been propelled from the ductus deferens. Semen nourishes and dilutes the sperm, enhancing their motility. Seminal fluid is propelled from the ejaculatory duct into the prostatic urethra.

PROSTATE GLAND The **prostate gland** surrounds the urethra near the lower part of the bladder. A sphere-shaped organ, approximately 2 cm (0.784 in.) in diameter, it is partially palpable through the front wall of the rectum because it lies just anterior to the rectum (see Figure 21.3). The prostate is composed of glandular structures that continuously secrete a milky, alkaline solution. During sexual intercourse, glandular activity increases, and the alkaline secretions flow into the urethra. Because sperm motility is reduced in an acidic environment, these secretions aid sperm transport. Additionally, the prostate gland produces about one-third of the volume of the semen.

BULBOURETHRAL GLANDS Also referred to as Cowper's glands, the **bulbourethral glands** are located below the prostate and

Table 21.1 Inguinal and Femoral Hernias

TYPE OF HERNIA	CHARACTERISTICS	SIGNS AND SYMPTOMS
Direct Hernia	Extrusion of abdominal intestine into inguinal ring. Bulging occurs in the area around the pubis. Abdominal intestine may remain within the inguinal canal or extrude past the external ring.	Most often is painless. Appears as a swelling. During palpation, have the patient cough. You will feel pressure against the side of your finger.
Indirect Hernia	Abdominal intestine may remain within the inguinal canal or extrude past the external ring. Most common type of hernia. Located within the femoral canal.	Appears as a swelling. During palpation, have the patient cough. You will feel pressure against your fingertip. Palpate soft mass.
Femoral Hernia	Bulge occurs over the area of the femoral artery. The right femoral artery is affected more frequently than the left. Lowest incidence of all three hernias.	May not be painful; however, once strangulation occurs, pain is severe.

within the urethral sphincter (see Figure 21.6). These glands are small (4.5 to 5 mm [0.17 to 0.19 in.]) and round. Just before ejaculation, the bulbourethral glands secrete a clear mucus into the urethra that lubricates the urethra and increases its alkaline environment.

Inguinal Region   The inguinal areas, often referred to as the groin, are located laterally to the pubic region over the iliac region or the upper part of the hip bone. Within this area are the inguinal ligaments and the inguinal canals, which lie above the inguinal ligaments. The inguinal canals are associated with the abdominal muscles and actually represent a potential weak link in the abdominopelvic wall. When a separation of the abdominal muscles exists, the weak points of these canals afford an area for the protrusion of the intestine into the groin region. This is called an **inguinal hernia**. It is important to note that femoral hernias, which are more common in females, are another type of hernia occurring in the groin area. Inguinal and femoral hernias can be confused, leading to the need for a good understanding of these types of hernias and thorough examination. Table 21.1 describes types, characteristics, and signs and symptoms of inguinal and femoral hernias.

Anus and Perianal Area   The **anus** is the terminal end of the gastrointestinal system. The anal canal is between 2 and 4 cm (0.78 to 1.57 in.) long, opens onto the perineum at the midpoint of the gluteal folds, and has internal and external muscles. The external muscles are skeletal muscles, which form the part of the anal sphincter that voluntarily controls evacuation of stool. Above the anus is the rectum with the prostate gland in close proximity to the anterior surface of the rectum. The mucosa of the anus is moist, darkly pigmented, and hairless. Lying between the scrotum and the anus is the **perineum**, which has a smooth surface and should be free of lesions.

Special Considerations

The nurse uses effective communication, critical thinking, the nursing process, and appropriate assessment techniques throughout a comprehensive assessment process to determine the patient's health status. Health status is influenced by a number of factors, including age, developmental level, race, ethnicity, work history, living conditions, socioeconomics, and emotional well-being. These factors are described in the following sections.

Health Promotion Considerations

Healthcare professionals' efforts related to genitourinary health have a focus on reduction of chronic kidney disease. Chronic kidney disease (CKD) and end-stage renal disease (ESRD) impact a significant number of adults. More than 25% of Medicare dollars are spent on treatment of these diseases (Office of Disease Prevention and Health Promotion, n.d.). Individuals with any form of diabetes are at increased risk for kidney injury. Nurses can help improve patient outcomes by careful assessment of urinary function through a thorough focused interview and physical exam.

Lifespan Considerations

Growth and development are dynamic processes that describe change over time. It is important to understand data collection and interpretation of findings regarding growth and development in relation to normative values. Details about specific variations in male genitourinary system health for different age groups are presented in Chapter 26 and Chapter 27. ∞

Psychosocial Considerations

Urinary incontinence is less common in men than in women but has a significant impact on the quality of life and an individual's self-esteem. Stress urinary incontinence is a well-known complication following radical prostatectomy occurring in as many as 65% of patients. Many promising and successful treatments are available. The nurse should be sure to carefully assess for incontinence or other genitourinary symptoms in all men, especially in men who have had surgery for any genitourinary conditions (Wingate et al., 2018).

Cultural and Environmental Considerations

When considering the influence of culture on a patient's healthcare practices, the nurse must be open-minded and sensitive to the specific values and beliefs of the patient without passing judgment. Not all individuals adhere to the norms, values, and practices of their culture. Consideration for the patient's privacy and modesty is essential when obtaining subjective and objective data regarding urinary elimination. Though not every patient is embarrassed by these components of assessment, many individuals experience considerable uneasiness. It is essential to afford the patient as much privacy and dignity as possible. Some individuals will not disrobe or allow a physical examination by anyone of the opposite sex. Other patients will not allow a sample of their body fluids to be taken and examined by strangers.

Patients with hypertension or diabetes mellitus are especially vulnerable to kidney damage if they do not follow a strict medication and diet regimen. Hispanics and African Americans experience higher rates of hypertension and diabetes mellitus (Office of Minority Health, 2014); however, these conditions are not limited to these populations. The nurse can help all patients maintain optimal health by providing information on diet, prevention of hypertension, and the importance of compliance with medication regimens.

Religious and cultural beliefs may influence multiple aspects of reproductive health and sexuality, including the patient's preference for a same-gender examiner. Before assessment, the nurse should determine the patient's preference in this regard. Although general awareness of cultural influences is essential to patient care, the nurse should be careful to avoid making assumptions, including that all patients of a given cultural background share every belief or follow all practices of their religious or cultural group. Some cultures and religions have specific beliefs or encourage specific behaviors related to circumcision and sexual practices. For example, male circumcision is a common practice in some religions, such as Judaism and Islam (Spector, 2017).

Subjective Data—Health History

Health assessment of the male genitourinary system includes gathering subjective and objective data. Subjective data collection occurs during the patient interview, before the actual physical assessment. A variety of communication techniques are used to elicit general and specific information about the health of the male genitourinary system. Health records, the results of laboratory tests, and X-rays are important secondary sources to be reviewed and included in the data-gathering process (see Table 21.2).

Table 21.2 Potential Secondary Sources for Patient Data Related to the Male Genitourinary System

LABORATORY TESTS FOR THE MALE REPRODUCTIVE SYSTEM	NORMAL VALUES
Prostate Specific Antigen (PSA)	0–4 ng/dL
Testosterone	300–1,000 ng/dL
Serum Studies for Tumor Markers	
Serum Studies for STDs	
Urethral Discharge Smears	
Diagnostic Tests	
Residual Post-Void Urine Ultrasonography	0 mL
Transrectal Ultrasound and Biopsy of the Prostate	
Uroflometry	Normal 14 mL/second
LABORATORY TESTS FOR THE MALE URINARY SYSTEM	
Blood Chemistry	
Albumin	3.5–5 g/dL
Ammonia	15–45 mcg/dL
Blood urea nitrogen (BUN)	6–23 mg/dL
Creatinine	Male 0.7–1.3 mg/dL
Urinalysis	
Color	Yellow-straw
Specific Gravity	1.005–1.030
pH	5–8
Glucose	Negative
Sodium	10–40 mEq/L
Potassium	< 8 mEq/L
Chloride	25–40 mEq/L
Protein	negative–trace
Osmolality	500–800 mOsm/L

(continued)

Table 21.2 Potential Secondary Sources for Patient Data Related to the Male Genitourinary System (continued)

LABORATORY TESTS FOR THE MALE URINARY SYSTEM	NORMAL VALUES
Urine Culture, Colony Count, Sensitivity	Varies
Diagnostic Tests	
Angiography	
Computed Tomography (CT)	
Cystoscopy	
Cystourethography	
Intravenous urography	
Magnetic resonance imaging (MRI)	
Radionuclide scanning	
Tissue and cell sampling—kidney biopsy	
Ultrasonography	
Urine cytology	

Focused Interview

The focused interview for the male genitourinary system concerns data related to the structures and functions of the urinary and reproductive systems. Subjective data are gathered during the focused interview. The nurse should be prepared to observe the patient and listen for cues related to the function of this body system. Open-ended and closed questions are used to obtain information. Often a number of follow-up questions or requests for descriptions are required to clarify data or gather missing information. Follow-up questions are aimed at identifying the source of problems, duration of difficulties, measures to alleviate problems, and clues about the patient's knowledge of his own health.

Information about the urinary system, genital areas, reproduction, and sexual activity is generally considered very private. The nurse must be sensitive to the patient's need for privacy and carefully explain that all information is confidential. A conversational approach with the use of open-ended statements is often helpful in a situation that can promote anxiety and embarrassment. The patient's terminology about body parts and functions should guide the nurse's questions.

Because of the dual functions of some of the male reproductive structures, data gathered during the focused interview will relate to the status of the urinary system as well as the reproductive system. Some commonly reported problems are those related to altered patterns of voiding, the presence of masses or lesions, unusual discharge, pain and tenderness, changes in sexual

functioning, suspected contact with a sexual partner who may have an STD, and infertility. Examination of the anus and rectum is included in examination of the male genitourinary system. Related problems include hemorrhoids, fissures, and infectious processes.

The focused interview guides the physical assessment of the male reproductive system. The information is always considered in relation to normal parameters and expectations about the function of the system. Therefore, the nurse must consider age, gender, race, culture, environment, health practices, past and current problems, and therapies when framing questions and using techniques to elicit information. In order to address all of the factors when conducting a focused interview, categories of questions related to urinary and reproductive systems status and function have been developed. These categories include general questions that are asked of all patients, those addressing illness and infection, questions related to symptoms and behaviors, those related to habits or practices, those that are specific to patients according to age, and questions that address environmental concerns. One approach to elicit data about symptoms is the OLDCART & ICE method, described in Chapter 5. ∞ (See Figure 5.3.)

The nurse must consider the patient's ability to participate in the focused interview and physical assessment of the male reproductive system. If a patient is experiencing pain, urgency, incontinence, or the anxiety that accompanies any of these problems, attention must focus on relief of these symptoms.

Focused Interview Questions	Rationales and Evidence

The following section provides sample questions and bulleted follow-up questions in each of the categories previously mentioned. A rationale for each of the questions is provided. The list of questions is not all-inclusive but does represent the types of questions required in a comprehensive focused interview related to the male genitourinary system.

MALE URINARY SYSTEM

General Questions

1. **What are your normal patterns when you urinate?**
   - How often do you urinate each day?
   - How much urine do you pass each time you urinate? (Note: The nurse may use terms familiar to the patient, such as *pass water*, when asking about urination.)

▶ Many factors influence the number of times and amount that a patient voids. Among these are size of the bladder, amount of fluid intake, type of fluid or solid intake, medications, amount of perspiration, and the patient's temperature. The adult may void five or six times per day in amounts averaging 100 mL to 400 mL. For adults, daily urine output typically averages 1,500 mL (Berman, Snyder, & Frandsen, 2016). However, adults may urinate as much as 2 L of fluid. At minimum, the adult patient should produce urine at a rate of 30 mL/kg/hour. The child may void more frequently in smaller amounts. The key point is to determine the patient's normal patterns and to identify excess or insufficient urine output.

Focused Interview Questions	Rationales and Evidence

2. Have you noticed any change from your normal urination patterns?
- Have you noticed any changes in your pattern recently?
- Have you had any of these changes: urinating more often, urinating less often, urinating more fluid, or urinating less fluid?

▶ Changes in urinary elimination patterns signal fluid retention, which may indicate heart failure, kidney failure, or improper nutritional intake. Other considerations include obstructions, infections, and endocrine alterations (Devarajan, 2017).

3. When you urinate, do you feel you are able to empty your bladder completely?
- If not, describe your feeling.

▶ The feeling of being unable to empty the bladder may indicate that the patient is retaining urine or developing increased residual urine, which may contribute to the development of infection (National Institute of Diabetes and Digestive and Kidney Diseases [NIDDKD], 2014).

4. Are you always able to control when you are going to urinate?
- If not, do you have to hurry to the bathroom as soon as you feel the urge to urinate?
- When you feel the urge to urinate, are you able to get to the toilet?
- Have you ever had an "accident" and wet yourself?
- Have you ever urinated by accident when you have coughed, sneezed, or lifted a heavy object?

▶ Urgency and stress incontinence may be caused by an infection, an inflammatory process, or the loss of muscle control over urination (MacDonald, Colaco, & Terlecki, 2017).

5. Do you ever have to get up at night to urinate?
- If so, can you describe why?
- Is there any predictable pattern?
- How many times per night?
- Describe your fluid intake for a day.

▶ **Nocturia**, nighttime urination, may indicate the presence of aging changes in the older adult, cardiovascular changes, diuretic therapy, or habit. Nocturia can be influenced by the amount and timing of fluid intake.

6. Do you have difficulty starting the flow of the stream?
- Does the stream flow continuously, or does it start and stop?
- Do you need to strain or push during urination to empty your bladder completely?

▶ Difficulties of this sort may signify the presence of prostate disease in the male.

7. If you have urinary problems, have they caused you embarrassment or anxiety?
- Have your urinary problems affected your social, personal, or sexual relationships?

▶ These are important considerations because they may affect patients' abilities to function in other parts of their lives.

8. Has anyone in your family had a kidney disease or urinary problem?
- If so, when did they have it?
- How was it treated?
- Do they still have it?

▶ A family history of kidney disease may signify a genetic predisposition to the development of renal disorders in some individuals. (National Kidney Foundation, 2017).

9. Have you had a recent urinalysis or blood work evaluating your kidneys?
- If so, do you know the results?

▶ It is valuable for patients to know the results of laboratory work and to provide the healthcare professional with their impression of the results.

Questions Related to Illness or Infection

1. Have you ever been diagnosed with a disease of the kidney or bladder?
- When were you diagnosed with the problem?
- What treatment was prescribed for the problem?
- Was the treatment helpful?
- What kinds of things do you do to help with the problem?
- Has the problem ever recurred (acute)?
- How are you managing the disease now (chronic)?

▶ The patient has an opportunity to provide information about specific urinary illnesses. If a diagnosed illness is identified, follow-up about the date of diagnosis, treatment, and outcomes is required. Data about each illness identified by the patient are essential to an accurate health assessment. Illnesses can be classified as acute or chronic, and follow-up regarding each classification will differ.

2. *Alternative to question 1:* List possible illnesses of the urinary system, such as renal calculi, nephrosis, and renal failure, and ask the patient to respond "yes" or "no" as each is stated.

▶ This is a comprehensive and easy way to elicit information about all diagnoses. Follow-up would be carried out for each identified diagnosis as in question 1.

3. Do you now have or have you had an infection in the urinary system?
- When were you diagnosed with the infection?
- What treatment was prescribed for the problem?
- Was the treatment helpful?
- What kinds of things do you do to help with the problem?
- Has the problem ever recurred (acute)?
- How are you managing the infection now (chronic)?

▶ If an infection is identified, follow-up about the date of infection, treatment, and outcomes is required. Data about each infection identified by the patient are essential to an accurate health assessment. Infections can be classified as acute or chronic, and follow-up regarding each classification will differ.

4. *Alternative to question 3:* List possible urinary system infections, such as cystitis, pyelonephritis, and prostatitis, and ask the patient to respond "yes" or "no" as each is stated.

▶ This is a comprehensive and easy way to elicit information about all urinary system infections. Follow-up would be carried out for each identified infection as in question 2.

5. Have you ever had surgery on the urinary system?
- If so, describe the procedure. How long ago did you have it done? Is the problem corrected?
- If not, describe it.
- Has anyone in your family ever had surgery on the urinary system?
- If so, please describe.

▶ Previous surgeries help provide insight as to the patient's history of urological problems. Some urinary problems, such as overflow incontinence, are more common among patients who have had urological surgery.

Focused Interview Questions	Rationales and Evidence

6. Do you have any of these problems: high blood pressure, diabetes, frequent bladder infections, kidney stones?
- If so, how has the problem been treated?
- Describe any associated symptoms.
- Do you still have problems with this condition?
- Do you have any idea what causes this problem?

▶ High blood pressure may contribute to the development of renal disease (Centers for Disease Control and Prevention [CDC], 2018). Diabetes may significantly contribute to the development of renal disease (CDC, 2018). Infections may be caused by inadequate fluid intake, inadequate hygiene, and structural anomalies (Berman et al., 2016). Kidney stones may be an isolated event or a recurring condition. Parathyroid disorders and any condition that causes an increase in calcium may contribute to the formation of kidney stones.

7. Do you have any of these neurologic diseases: multiple sclerosis, Parkinson disease, spinal cord injury, or stroke?
- If so, which one?
- When was it diagnosed? How are you being treated?

▶ These conditions contribute to the retention and stasis of urine, thus placing the patient at risk for chronic urinary infections (Dellis, Mitsogiannis, & Mitsikostas, 2017).

8. Do you have any type of cardiovascular disease?
- If so, what was the diagnosis?
- When was it diagnosed?
- How are you being treated?

▶ Hypertension in particular may significantly contribute to the development of renal failure (CDC, 2018).

9. Have you had influenza, a skin infection, a respiratory tract infection, or other infection recently?
- If so, what was it?
- What medication did the physician prescribe?
- Did you take all of the medication?
- Is this a recurrent problem?

▶ If the infection was untreated, the patient may be at risk for developing a renal infection (Rodriguez-Iturbe, & Haas, 2016).

Questions Related to Symptoms, Pain, and Behaviors

When gathering information about symptoms, many questions are required to elicit details and descriptions that assist in the analysis of the data. Discrimination is made in relation to the significance of a symptom, in relation to specific diseases or problems, and in relation to potential follow-up examination or referral. One rationale may be provided for a group of questions in this category.

The following questions refer to specific symptoms and behaviors associated with the urinary system. For each symptom, questions and follow-up are required. The details to be elicited are the characteristics of the symptom; the onset, duration, and frequency of the symptom; the determination if diagnosis has been sought; the treatment or remedy used to treat the symptom, including over-the-counter (OTC) and home remedies; the effect of treatments; and family history associated with a symptom or illness.

Questions Related to Symptoms

1. Have you noticed any changes in the quality of the urine?
- If so, describe the change.
- Has your urine been cloudy?
- Does it have an odor?
- Has the color changed?
- If there has been a color change, what is it?
- Does the color change happen each time you urinate?
- Is there a pattern?
- Can you predict the color change?

▶ Color changes offer clues to the presence of infection, kidney stones, or neoplasm. The quantity of urine may indicate the presence of renal failure or may reflect hydration status (Berman et al., 2016).

2. If the urine is bloody (hematuria), the nurse should ask these questions:
- Have you fallen recently?
- Do you experience burning when the blood is present? Have you seen clots in the urine?
- Have you noticed any stones or other material in the urine?
- Have you noticed any granular material on the toilet paper after you wipe?

▶ The patient may offer valuable information about the source and characteristics of bleeding, because this symptom is present in a wide variety of conditions, including bladder cancer. Hematuria is a serious finding and warrants additional follow-up (Berman et al., 2016).

3. Is your urine foamy and amber in color?

▶ This finding may indicate the presence of kidney dysfunction or other illnesses (Sise, Lo, Goldstein, Allegretti, & Masia, 2017).

4. Have you had any weight gain recently?
- If so, describe it.
- Are you retaining fluid?
- Are your rings, clothing, or shoes becoming tighter?
- Has this change been gradual, or did it come on suddenly?

▶ This may alert the nurse to the presence of hypertension, associated heart failure, or endocrine problems. These ultimately affect the renal circulation and function of the kidneys.

5. Have you noticed any discharge from the urethra?
- If so, describe the color, odor, amount, and frequency.
- When did it start?
- Is this a recurrent problem? If so, what was the diagnosis?
- How was it treated?
- Did you follow the treatment as prescribed by the physician?

▶ Discharge signals the potential presence of an infective process.

Focused Interview Questions	Rationales and Evidence

6. Have you noticed any redness or other discoloration in the urethral area or penis? If so, describe the characteristics.

▶ Redness may indicate the presence of inflammation, irritation, or infection.

7. Has your skin changed recently?
   - Describe the change.
   - Has the color changed?
   - Is it itchy all the time?

▶ Patients with chronic renal failure have itchy skin (pruritus), and lichenification (a thickening of the skin) may develop (Asokan, Narasimhan, & Rajagopalan, 2017).

8. Have you recently had nausea, vomiting, diarrhea, or chills?
   - If so, which one? Describe it.
   - How was it treated?
   - Has it recurred?

▶ These conditions may indicate the presence of infection or recurring infection.

9. Have you had any shortness of breath or difficulty breathing lately? If so, describe it.

▶ This may alert the nurse to the presence of hypertension and associated heart failure. These ultimately affect the renal circulation and function of the kidneys.

10. Do you have difficulty concentrating, reading, or remembering things?

▶ Difficulty remembering may be associated with **azotemia**, which is a buildup of wastes in the bloodstream because of renal dysfunction (O'Lone et al., 2016).

Questions Related to Pain

When assessing pain, the nurse needs to gather information about the characteristics of the pain, which include quality, severity, location, duration, predictability, onset, relief, and radiation.

1. Do you ever have pain, burning, or other discomfort before, during, or after urination?
   - If so, describe the discomfort, location, and timing.
   - Do you have symptoms all of the time or some of the time?
   - Is the discomfort predictable? For instance, is it related to time of the day or to certain foods or beverages?
   - Do you feel it after sexual intercourse?

▶ Painful urination may indicate the presence of an infective process (Berman et al., 2016).

2. Do you have any pain or discomfort in your back, sides, or abdomen?
   - If so, show me where the pain or discomfort is located.
   - Describe the pain.
   - What aggravates or alleviates the symptoms?

▶ Back or abdominal pain often accompanies renal disease (Berman et al., 2016).

3. Have you noticed any pain or discomfort when your urine is bloody?
   - If so, describe the type, location, and timing of the discomfort.

▶ Hematuria without pain is often associated with benign tumors such as hemangioma (Ozkanli, Girgin, Kosemetin, & Zemheri, 2014).

Questions Related to Behaviors

1. Describe your diet.
   - Describe what you have eaten and drunk over the last week.
   - How is your appetite?
   - On a typical day, how much do you eat and drink?
   - Do you drink alcoholic beverages?
   - How many glasses of water do you drink each day?
   - Are there any foods or beverages that bother you?
   - Do any foods or beverages cause you discomfort either before or upon urination?
   - Do any foods or beverages cause you to feel bloated or gassy?
   - Do any foods or beverages affect the color, clarity, or smell of your urine?
   - How much salt do you use?
   - Do you retain fluid after consuming certain foods or beverages?

▶ Questions such as these may provide information regarding the patient's hydration status, potential allergic reaction to foods, and retention of fluid.

2. Do you smoke or are you exposed to passive smoke?
   - If so, what type of smoking (cigarette, cigar, pipe)?
   - For how long?
   - How many packs per day?

▶ Smoking has been linked to hypertension, which over time may contribute to the development of renal failure. Smoking also significantly increases an individual's risk for developing bladder cancer (American Cancer Society [ACS], 2018).

3. Do you use any recreational drugs?
   - If so, describe the type, amount, and frequency.
   - How long have you been using these drugs?

▶ Abuse of certain drugs over time may lead to kidney failure (National Institute on Drug Abuse, 2017), potential for inadequate nutrition and hydration, and susceptibility to infection.

4. How often do you have intercourse?
   - Do you urinate after intercourse?
   - Are you aware of any sexual partners who may have sexually transmitted diseases?

▶ Some patients may have a tendency to develop UTIs if they do not urinate after intercourse (Mayo Clinic, 2017d).

Focused Interview Questions	Rationales and Evidence

Questions Related to Age

The focused interview must reflect the anatomic and physiologic differences in the male genitourinary system that exist along the lifespan. Specific questions related to the urinary system can be found in Chapter 26 and Chapter 27. ∞

Questions Related to the Environment

Environment refers to both the internal and external environments. Questions related to the internal environment include all of the previous questions and those associated with internal or physiologic responses. Questions regarding the external environment include those related to home, work, or social environments.

Internal Environment

1. **What medications do you currently take?**
   - What medications have you been taking during the last several months?
   - Describe the type, the dose, and the reason why you are taking the medication.
   - How often do you take it?
   - Do you take it every day, as needed, or only when you remember?

▶ It is important to know the patient's compliance with the medication regimen. If the patient has not completed a regimen of antibiotic therapy to clear a UTI, kidney infection, or sexually transmitted disease, the infection may persist.

2. **Do you take any vitamins, protein powders, or dietary supplements?**
   - If so, which ones?
   - How much do you take?
   - How many days a week do you take it?
   - How many times a day do you take it?
   - Why do you take it?

▶ Excessive ingestion of certain nutritional supplements or herbal agents may contribute to the development of renal disorders (Shaw, Graeme, Pierre, Elizabeth, & Kelvin, 2012).

External Environment

The following questions deal with substances and irritants found in the physical environment of the patient. The physical environment includes the indoor and outdoor environments of the home and workplace, those encountered for social engagements, and any encountered during travel.

1. **Do you live in an environment or work in an industry that exposes you to toxic chemicals?**

▶ These may contribute to the development of cancer of the urinary system (ACS, 2018).

2. **Have you traveled recently to a foreign country or any unfamiliar place?**

▶ The patient may have been exposed to bacterial, viral, or fungal agents that affect renal function.

MALE REPRODUCTIVE SYSTEM

General Questions

1. **Do you have any concerns about your sexual health?**
   - Have you had concerns in the past? If so, please tell me about those concerns.

▶ These questions may prompt the male patient to discuss any concerns about reproductive health.

2. **Are you sexually active? If so, how would you describe your sexual relationship(s)?**

▶ The male patient may feel pressured to be in a sexual relationship. These pressures may be external (expectations of family, friends, or work associates) or internal (fear of being viewed by others as less than desirable or not of an accepted sexual orientation, fear of being alone, or fear of not being loved and accepted).

3. **Are there any obstacles to your ability to achieve sexual satisfaction?**

▶ Causes of inability to achieve sexual satisfaction include fear of acquiring an STD; fear of being unable to satisfy the partner; fear of pregnancy; confusion regarding sexual preference; unwillingness to participate in sexual activities enjoyed by the partner; job stress; financial considerations; crowded living conditions; loss of partner; attraction to or sexual involvement with individuals about whom the partner does not know; criticism of sexual performance by the partner; or history of sexual trauma.

4. **Have you noticed a change in your sex drive recently?**

▶ This may be indicative of some physical or psychologic problems that need follow-up (Holloway & Wylie, 2015). If the patient answers "yes," the nurse should ask the following question.

5. **Can you associate the change with anything in particular?**

▶ Often patients can relate a decrease in sex drive with stress, illness, drug therapy, or some other factor (Holloway & Wylie, 2015).

6. **For patients who are sexually active:**
   - What type of contraception do you use?
   - In what kind of sexual activities do you engage?

▶ Questions about types of sexual activities provide information related to risk for STDs.

7. **Do your family and friends support your relationship with your sexual partner?**

▶ The patient's family and friends can influence the patient's sexual relationship in a variety of ways. The patient may feel tension if the partner is not accepted.

Focused Interview Questions	Rationales and Evidence
8. Are you able to talk to your partner about your sexual needs? • Does your partner accept your needs and help you fulfill them? • Are you able to do the same for your partner?	▶ Communication with a sexual partner helps in establishing a fulfilling relationship (Frederick, Lever, Gillespie, & Garcia, 2017).
9. Some patients come to a healthcare provider to discuss sexual abuse. • Have you ever been forced to have sexual intercourse or other sexual contact against your will? • Have you ever been molested or raped?	▶ The opening statement lets the patient know that sexual abuse is a topic that can be addressed in this encounter. The questions allow the patient to describe abusive encounters in some detail.
10. If the patient answers "yes," the nurse should ask the following questions: • When did the abuse occur? • Who abused you? • What was the experience? • How often did this happen? • What was done about the situation and for you?	
11. For patients who are sexually active: • Are you in a relationship with one partner? • If not, how many sexual partners have you or your partner had over the last year?	▶ Sexual activity with many different partners increases the risk of acquiring STDs (Mayo Clinic, 2017c).
12. Do you have children? • If so, how many? • *If the patient answers "no":* Have you tried to have children? • *If the patient answers "yes":* How long have you been trying to have a child?	▶ The couple is not considered potentially infertile unless they have been unable to conceive for a year (World Health Organization, 2018).
13. If the patient indicates that his partner has shown inability to conceive after 1 year: How often do you and your partner have intercourse?	▶ For couples attempting to have a child, it is important to engage in intercourse routinely, two to three times a week (Mayo Clinic, 2016). Although nurses do not treat infertility, they may be involved in teaching the patient about certain measures that may be helpful, such as temperature tracking in the female partner, to determine the optimal time for intercourse. Concerns about infertility can produce great anxiety for many couples.
14. Have you ever had mumps?	▶ Mumps occurring after puberty has been linked to sterility in males (Johns Hopkins Medicine, n.d.).
15. Have you ever sought professional help for fertility problems? If so, describe this experience.	▶ This provides the opportunity to identify diagnostic testing and procedures for infertility. In addition, the patient can describe psychosocial or emotional issues surrounding the fertility problem.
16. Has an inability for your partner to conceive placed a strain on your relationship? • How has this problem affected your relationship? • How are you feeling about this?	▶ The patient has the opportunity to express emotional or psychosocial concerns surrounding a partner's infertility.
17. Are you able to be sexually aroused? • Has this ability changed over time or recently?	▶ A variety of factors may influence an individual's ability to become sexually aroused. These include use of prescribed or illicit drugs; disorders of the nervous system; diabetes; stress; and fear (e.g., of intimacy, inability to satisfy a partner, or acquiring an STD) (Byun et al., 2013).
18. Are you able to achieve and maintain an erection? • Have any aspects in your ability to achieve an erection changed? • Are you satisfied with the length of time it takes to achieve and maintain an erection?	▶ The ability to achieve an erection depends on both physiologic factors and state of mind (Byun et al., 2013).
19. When you have an erection, is the shaft of the penis straight or crooked?	▶ **Peyronie disease** causes the shaft of the penis to be crooked during an erection (Mayo Clinic, 2017a).
20. Are you able to achieve orgasm? • Are you satisfied with your ability to control the timing of your orgasms?	▶ Premature ejaculation is defined by some researchers as orgasm immediately after, or even before, penetration. It may also be defined as ejaculation before the male's sexual partner reaches orgasm in more than half of the male's sexual experiences. It is often a devastating disorder that may severely compromise sexual relationships. The patient can learn techniques to delay ejaculation (Mayo Clinic, 2017b).

Questions Related to Illness or Infection

1. Have you ever been diagnosed with an illness or disease of the reproductive organs? • When were you diagnosed with the problem? • What treatment was prescribed for the problem? • Was the treatment helpful? • What kinds of things do you do to help with the problem? • Has the problem ever recurred (acute)? • How are you managing the problem now (chronic)?	▶ The patient has an opportunity to provide information about specific illnesses. If a diagnosed illness is identified, follow-up about the date of diagnosis, treatment, and outcomes is required. Data about each illness identified by the patient are essential to an accurate health assessment. Illnesses can be classified as acute or chronic, and follow-up regarding each classification will differ.

Focused Interview Questions	Rationales and Evidence

2. *Alternative to question 1:* List possible disorders of the male reproductive system—such as benign prostatic disease, erectile dysfunction, and cancer of the penis, prostate, or testicles—and ask the patient to respond "yes" or "no" as each is stated.

▶ This is a comprehensive and easy way to elicit information about illnesses of the reproductive system. Follow-up would be required for each diagnosis as in question 1.

3. Have you ever had a sexually transmitted disease (such as herpes, gonorrhea, syphilis, or chlamydia)?
   - *If the patient answers "yes":* Was it treated?
   - Did you inform your partner?
   - Did you have sexual relations with your partner while you were infected?
   - *If the patient answers "yes":* Did you use condoms?
   - What treatment did you receive?

▶ Serious, sometimes fatal, complications can develop if treatment is delayed. For example, untreated syphilis can eventually involve the cardiovascular and central nervous systems, and genital herpes is contagious and may infect partners with every sexual encounter (Centers for Disease Control and Prevention [CDC], 2017b).

▶ The nurse should educate the patient regarding the risks and methods of STD transmission, as well as strategies for prevention of STD transmission.

4. Are you aware of having had any exposure to HIV?
   - *If the patient answers "yes":* Describe the situation and how you feel you were exposed.
   - Have you ever been tested for HIV?
   - What were the results?

▶ This question helps to determine at-risk practices and knowledge of the transmission of HIV.

5. Do you have sexual intercourse without condoms?
   - *If the patient answers "yes":* On one occasion or routinely?

▶ Consistent, correct use of latex condoms by males is a highly effective means by which to prevent the transmission of HIV, as well as to prevent the spread of numerous other STDs (Centers for Disease Control and Prevention [CDC], 2017a).

6. Have you had surgery on any of your reproductive organs?
   - If so, what was the surgery? When?
   - What was the outcome?

▶ Some surgeries, such as penile implants, require periodic follow-up for problems, including possible infection. Surgeries such as prostatectomy (removal of the prostate) or surgeries that alter body image, such as colostomy, may have bearing on sexual function as well as attitude about oneself in relation to sexuality.

Questions Related to Symptoms

1. Have you felt any lumps or masses on your penis, scrotum, or surrounding areas? If so, describe the mass.
   - Exactly where is it?
   - Describe the size.
   - Is it soft or hard?
   - Is it movable?
   - When did you first notice the mass?
   - Is it painful?
   - Has there been any pattern to the swelling: an increase, decrease, or unchanged pattern?
   - What treatments have you tried?

▶ This information helps the nurse to understand the nature of the mass or lump.

2. Have you noticed any swelling of your scrotum, penis, or surrounding areas?
   - If so, when did it start?
   - Is it painful?
   - Has there been any pattern to the swelling: an increase, decrease, or unchanged pattern?
   - What treatments have you tried?

▶ This information could help identify problems of rapid onset, which sometimes have the potential to be more detrimental. Swelling in the inguinal area may signal the presence of a hernia. Sources of swelling in the scrotal area include an acute or chronic inflammatory process, a hydrocele, scrotal edema, or scrotal hernia (Mayo Clinic, 2018).

3. Have you noticed any unusual discharge from your penis?
   - If so, of what color?
   - Is there any odor to the discharge?
   - Is it a small, moderate, or large amount?
   - When did you first notice the discharge?
   - Is there any burning or pain with the discharge?

▶ Discharge characteristics may indicate whether an infectious process is occurring (Berman et al., 2016).

4. Have you noticed any change in color of your penis or scrotum?
   - If so, describe the change and the location.

▶ Inflammatory processes may cause redness in the affected area (Berman et al., 2016).

5. Have you had any unusual itching in your genital area?
   - If so, where? Have you noticed any rash, scaling, or lumps?

▶ Causes may include environmental allergens, soaps, lotions, and the presence of pubic lice (crabs).

6. Have you had any problems with your rectal area, such as pain, itching, bruising, burning, or bleeding?
   - When did the problem begin?
   - Do you know the cause of the problem?
   - Have you sought healthcare for the problem?
   - Was a diagnosis made?
   - What treatment was prescribed?
   - What do you do to help with the problem?
   - Has the treatment helped?

▶ Pain, itching, bleeding, or burning may indicate the presence of infection, irritation, or injury to the anus or rectum. Bleeding, pain, and irritation may result from passing hard stools, from hemorrhoids, from injuries, or from trauma including anal sex. Fungal infection may result in chronic pruritus or irritation of the perianal area (Klein, 2014).

Focused Interview Questions	**Rationales and Evidence**
	▶ When symptoms involving the anorectal area are associated with hemorrhoids or hard stool, follow-up would include information about diet and bowel habits (Berman et al., 2016).
	▶ Irritation or injury to the perianal area can occur as a result of sexual practices or sexual abuse (Shamaskin-Garroway, Giordano, & Blakley, 2017). Sensitive questioning about these topics is required when sexual activity is described or when abuse is suspected or disclosed.
Questions Related to Pain 1. **Have you noticed any pain, tenderness, or soreness in the areas of your penis or scrotum?** • If so, describe the pain. • Is it dull? Sharp? Radiating? Intermittent? Continuous? • Does anything make the pain better or worse?	▶ Testicular torsion may cause excruciating acute pain in the testicular area. Often, the affected testicle will be higher in the scrotal sac than the unaffected testicle (Tang, Yeung, Chu, & Man, 2017). A dull, aching pain is a common symptom of **epididymitis**, which is swelling of the epididymis. This condition is most often caused by infection (Cek, Sturdza, & Pilatz, 2017).
2. **Are you having any pain in the area now?**	▶ This question helps the nurse determine if the problem is current, experienced in the past only, or chronic.
Questions Related to Behaviors 1. **Do you check your genitals on a routine basis?** • Do you know how to perform testicular self-exam? • How often do you perform this exam? • What technique do you use?	▶ Self-examination of the genitals should be performed at least monthly for early detection of changes that need follow-up. Teaching may be indicated if the patient is not performing self-examination. (See Evidence-Based Practice: Screening for Testicular Cancer and Evidence-Based Practice: Prostate Cancer Screening.)
2. **How often do you get physical examinations?**	▶ Screening for problems such as prostate or testicular cancer usually is performed during a routine physical.
3. **Are you circumcised? If not, have you had any difficulty keeping this area clean?**	▶ If the patient is having problems with maintaining hygiene of the area, patient teaching may be necessary.
4. **Do you have any genital or body piercings? If so, are you aware of any problems or changes at the piercing site(s)?**	▶ Common complications of genital piercings include scar tissue formation and infection (Dalke, Fein, Jenkins, Caso, & Salgado, 2013).
5. **Are you and your partner using contraception?** • If so, what kind? • Are you using it consistently?	▶ This helps to determine knowledge of the product being used and practice of contraception.

Evidence-Based Practice

Screening for Testicular Cancer

Testicular cancer accounts for about 1% of cancers overall in men and is the most common malignancy in males between ages 15 and 35. The prognosis with treatment is excellent in these germ cell cancers (National Cancer Institute [NCI], n.d.; Siegel, Miller, & Jemal, 2017; Stevenson & Lowrance, 2015). Testicular self-examination is recommended by some, though there is no general recommendation to perform regular screening or self-exam for asymptomatic men (American Cancer Society [ACS], 2016b; National Cancer Institute [NCI], 2018). For those seeking information on how to do a testicular self-exam, the following information can be provided:

• Hold your penis out of the way and examine each testicle separately.

• Hold your testicle between your thumbs and fingers with both hands and roll it gently between your fingers.

• Look and feel for any hard lumps or nodules (smooth rounded masses) or any change in the size, shape, or consistency of your testicles.

It is normal for one testicle to be slightly larger than the other, and for one to hang lower than the other. You should also be aware that each normal testicle has a small, coiled tube called the epididymis that can feel like a small bump on the upper or middle outer side of the testis. Normal testicles also contain blood vessels, supporting tissues, and tubes that carry sperm. Some men may confuse these with abnormal lumps (ACS, 2016b).

Evidence-Based Practice
Prostate Cancer Screening

The American Cancer Society recommends that men partner with their medical provider to determine whether and how often to receive prostate cancer screening (American Cancer Society [ACS], 2016a). Guidelines now put the emphasis of recommendations for prostate cancer screening on informed decision making based on patients' preferences (Halbert et al., 2017). This discussion should take place at the following ages for men with average, high, and very high risk:

- Age 50 for men at average risk who are expected to live at least 10 more years
- Age 45 for men at high risk: African Americans and men with a first-degree relative diagnosed with prostate cancer before age 65 (Halbert et al., 2017)
- Age 40 for men at very high risk: men with more than one first-degree relative diagnosed with prostate cancer before age 65

Prostate cancer screenings include blood testing for prostate-specific antigen (PSA) and the digital rectal exam (DRE). Results of the screening can help the patient and provider decide the course of future screening or treatments (ACS, 2016a).

Focused Interview Questions	Rationales and Evidence
6. Would you like to know more about the use of birth control?	▶ This is a very important question to ask adolescents who shy away from talking about sexual practices but have verbalized that they are sexually active.
7. How do you protect yourself from sexually transmitted diseases, including HIV?	▶ Abstinence is the only 100% effective protection against STDs. Latex condoms offer significant protection, especially when treated with spermicide; however, they are not 100% effective (CDC, 2017a; Mayo Clinic, 2017c).
8. Do you drink alcohol? If so, how many drinks per week do you consume?	▶ Chronic alcoholism has been linked to impotence (Cioe, Anderson, & Stein, 2013). Additionally, intake of alcoholic beverages can contribute to an individual "taking chances," such as failing to use condoms, and can impact fertility.
9. Do you use recreational drugs? If so, what type and how much?	▶ Taken in sufficient amounts, some drugs, such as marijuana and opiates, may decrease libido and lead to impotence (Cioe et al., 2013). Drug use may also contribute to failure to use protection against STDs.

Questions Related to the Environment

Questions related to the internal environment include all of the previous questions and those associated with internal or physiologic responses. Questions regarding the external environment include those related to home, work, or social environments.

The following questions deal with substances and irritants found in the physical environment of the patient. The physical environment includes the indoor and outdoor environments of the home and workplace, those encountered for social engagements, and any encountered during travel.

1. Have you been exposed to lead, chemicals, or toxins in the environment?	▶ Lead exposure may result in decreased libido and sperm abnormalities (Karavolos, Stewart, Evbuomwan, McEleny, & Aird, 2013).
2. Do you use protective equipment when engaged in work or athletic activities?	▶ The use of protective equipment, including athletic supports and cups, reduces the incidence of testicular damage.
3. Do you know if your mother or grandmother received diethylstilbestrol (DES) treatment during pregnancy?	▶ Some reports indicate that sons or grandsons of women who received DES have higher-than-average rates of genitourinary problems, such as hypospadias, infertility, and undescended or enlarged testicles. They may be at risk for testicular cancer and have low sperm counts (Kalfa, Paris, Soyer-Gobillard, Daures, & Sultan, 2011). Physician referral is indicated if the patient's response is "yes."

Patient-Centered Interaction

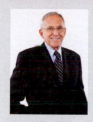

Source: manley099/Getty Images.

Mr. Edward O'Reilly, age 71, comes to the Urgi-Medi Center at 8:00 p.m. accompanied by his son. He tells the clerk at the reception desk that he needs to see Nurse Jack, stating, "I haven't passed my water since yesterday afternoon." His son tells the clerk his father called him about 5:00 p.m. just as he was leaving work, screaming, "I can't go! I'm going to burst. I have a lot of pressure down there." Mr. O'Reilly is observed pacing in the reception area waiting for the nurse. His chart indicates he came to the center 2 weeks ago with a similar complaint. At that time a diagnosis of benign prostatic hypertrophy was made, along with a recommendation for a transurethral resection of the prostate (TURP). The patient was obviously uncomfortable and was quickly escorted to an examination room. During the walk to the room the nurse began to question the patient. The following is an excerpt from the focused interview.

Interview

Nurse: Good evening, Mr. O'Reilly. I see by the report you are having trouble voiding again.

Mr. O'Reilly: Oh, I'm glad you are here tonight. I can't talk to Ms. Pat about my problem.

Nurse: Tell me about the problem.

Mr. O'Reilly: I have not passed any water since yesterday afternoon, not even a few drops. I have to go really bad. The pressure down there really hurts. I need the tube again.

Nurse: The last time you were able to pass your water, did you have trouble starting the stream?

Mr. O'Reilly: Oh, yes. That's been getting worse. I need to push very hard to start, and then I leak when I'm finished.

Nurse: You leak?

Mr. O'Reilly: Yes, I'm like my grandson; I always have wet briefs. I leak, and it never stops. I'm so embarrassed.

Nurse: When was the last time you tried to pass your water?

Mr. O'Reilly: I didn't sleep much last night. I'm always trying. I tried before I left the house—nothing—and then when I was waiting for you, and nothing. Nothing. Don't you understand me?

Analysis

The patient was clearly uncomfortable and was quickly brought to an examination room. In this clinical example, the nurse used several strategies while assisting the patient to the room. First, the patient's request to see a male nurse was honored. The nurse used open-ended statements and reflection and sought clarification as needed. The nurse also used terminology used by the patient (e.g., pass water) to put the patient at ease.

Objective Data—Physical Assessment

Assessment Techniques and Findings

Physical assessment of the urinary system includes the use of inspection, palpation, percussion, and auscultation. The skills are used to gather information about the function of the urinary system. Knowledge of normal parameters and expected findings is essential in determining the meaning of the data as the nurse performs the physical assessment.

Assessment of the patient's psychosocial health, self-care habits, family, culture, and environment is an important part of the focused interview. The nurse must keep these findings in mind when conducting the physical assessment. The nurse also must have a thorough understanding of the constituents of a healthy reproductive system and be able to consider the relationship of other body systems to the reproductive system.

Assessment of the urinary system is incorporated into assessment of the abdomen and reproductive systems. Urinary function is interdependent with other body systems. In addition, psychosocial and developmental factors impact the function of the urinary system.

Many factors, including psychosocial health, self-care habits, family, culture, and environment, impact reproductive health. Therefore, the nurse must consider these factors while conducting the interview and physical assessment. The nurse must have a thorough understanding of the constituents of a healthy reproductive system and consider the relationship of other body systems to the reproductive system.

Throughout the physical assessment, the nurse will assess and evaluate the occasional ambiguous cues of actual and potential reproductive disease and the variety of contributors to the development of pathology. The nurse documents and communicates the findings to the other members of the healthcare team. The nurse also has a key role in teaching the patient how to establish and maintain reproductive wellness.

To be efficient in gathering data, nurses need to understand their own feelings and comfort about various aspects of sexuality. They must put aside personal beliefs and values about sexual practices and focus in a nonjudgmental manner on gathering data to determine the health status of the patient.

It is essential to create an atmosphere that facilitates open communication and comfort for the patient. Patients commonly experience anxiety, fear, and embarrassment when asked for information about a topic that, in most patients' minds, is very personal. These emotions may be expressed either verbally or nonverbally. The nurse should approach the patient in as non-threatening a manner as possible and assure the patient that the information provided and the results of the physical assessment will remain confidential.

EQUIPMENT

- Examination gown and drape
- Clean, nonsterile examination gloves
- Stethoscope
- Specimen container

Techniques and Normal Findings	Abnormal Findings and Special Considerations

MALE URINARY SYSTEM

General Survey

A quick survey of the patient enables the nurse to identify any immediate problem as well as the patient's ability to participate in the assessment.

1. **Instruct the patient.**
   - Explain that you will be looking, listening, touching, and tapping on parts of the abdomen. Tell the patient you will explain each procedure as it occurs. Tell the patient to report any discomfort and that you will stop the examination if the procedure is uncomfortable.

2. **Position the patient.**
   - Begin the examination with the patient in a supine position with the abdomen exposed from the nipple line to the pubis (see Figure 21.7 ■).

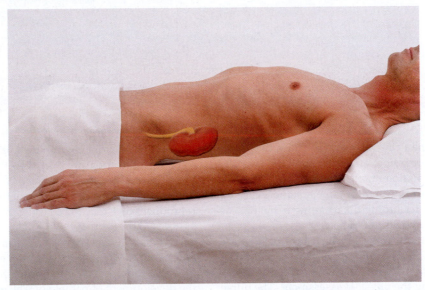

Figure 21.7 Position the patient.

3. **Assess the general appearance.**
   - Assess the patient's general appearance, and inspect the patient's skin for color, hydration status, scales, masses, indentations, or scars.

   - The patient should not show signs of acute distress and should be mentally alert and oriented.

▶ Patients with kidney disorders frequently look tired and complain of fatigue. If a kidney disorder is suspected, it is important to look for signs of circulatory overload (pulmonary edema) or peripheral edema (puffy face or fingers) or indications of pruritus (scratch marks on the skin).

▶ Elevated nitrogenous wastes (azotemia) in the blood contribute to mental confusion.

Techniques and Normal Findings	Abnormal Findings and Special Considerations

4. Inspect the abdomen for color, contour, symmetry, and distention.

- It may be helpful to stand at the foot of the examination table and inspect the abdomen from there (see Figure 21.8 ■).

▶ A distended bladder may be visible in the suprapubic area, indicating the need to void and perhaps the inability to do so.

▶ The increased adipose tissue in the abdomen of the obese patient may inhibit visualization of underlying structures.

▶ Inspection of the skin of the abdomen may provide clues about health history. Striae or stretch marks may signal a previous weight loss; scars indicate injury or surgery; and bruising or skin trauma provides clues about current health.

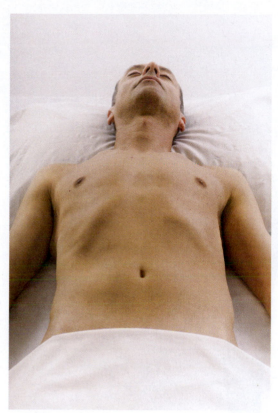

Figure 21.8 Inspecting the patient from the foot of the bed.

- Note that visual inspection of the suprapubic area may confirm the presence or absence of a distended bladder.
- Normally, the patient's abdomen is not distended, is relatively symmetric, and is free of bruises, masses, and swellings. (A complete discussion of abdominal assessment is provided in Chapter 20. ∞)

5. Auscultate the right and left renal arteries to assess circulatory sounds.

- Gently place the bell of the stethoscope over the extended midclavicular line (MCL) on either side of the abdominal aorta, which is located above the level of the umbilicus (see Figure 21.9 ■).
- Be sure to auscultate both the right and left sides, and over the epigastric and umbilical areas.
- In most cases, no sounds are heard; however, an upper abdominal bruit, a swishing or murmurlike sound, is occasionally heard in young adults and is considered normal. On a thin adult, renal artery pulsation may be auscultated.

▶ Many diseases may contribute to abdominal distention. These include renal conditions such as polycystic kidney disease; enlarged kidneys, as seen in acute pyelonephritis; ascites (accumulation of fluid) because of hepatic disease; and displacement of abdominal organs. Pressure from the abdominal contents on the diaphragm may alter the patient's breathing pattern.

▶ Presence of a bruit may indicate narrowing or obstruction of a blood vessel.

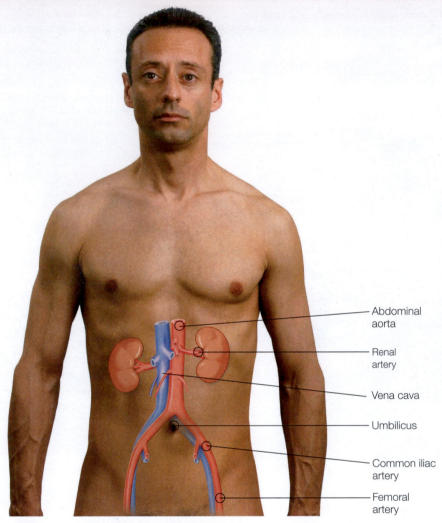

Abdominal
aorta

Renal
artery

Vena cava

Umbilicus

Common iliac
artery

Femoral
artery

Figure 21.9 Auscultating the renal arteries.

6. **For patients with a urinary catheter, inspect the catheter for signs of infection, correct placement, and urinary outflow.**
   - Patients with limited mobility, such as patients with paralysis, recent surgery, or a fractured hip, will likely use an indwelling catheter or undergo intermittent catheterization.
   - Inspect the urine and urethral meatus for signs of infection, irritation, tenderness, and cleanliness.
   - Inspect the collection bag for fullness, and empty if needed; also inspect the bag and tubing for possible obstructions.
   - Inspect the bag for correct placement on the leg and ensure that the bag is lower than the bladder at all times.
   - Record urine outflow and fluid intake to ensure that the urinary drainage system is working properly.

▶ Because of the high risk of infection, the need for a catheter should be assessed at every interaction. Signs of infection include hematuria, foul-smelling or cloudy urine, and lower back pain.

▶ Improper drainage of the catheter may result in urinary backflow into the bladder, which is a major cause of infection.

The Kidneys and Flanks

1. **Position the patient.**
   - Place the patient in a sitting position facing away from you with the patient's back exposed.

2. **Inspect the left and right costovertebral angles for color and symmetry.**
   - The color should be consistent with the rest of the back.

3. **Inspect the flanks (the side areas between the hips and the ribs) for color and symmetry.**
   - The costovertebral angles and flanks should be symmetric and even in color.

▶ A protrusion or elevation over a costovertebral angle occurs when the kidney is grossly enlarged or when a mass is present. This finding must be carefully correlated to other diagnostic cues as the assessment proceeds. If ecchymosis is present (Grey Turner's sign), there may be other signs of trauma, such as blunt, penetrating wounds or lacerations.

ALERT!
- *Do not percuss or palpate the patient who reports pain or discomfort in the pelvic region.*
- *Do not percuss or palpate the kidney if a tumor of the kidney is suspected, such as a neuroblastoma or Wilms tumor.*
- *Palpation increases intra-abdominal pressure, which may contribute to intraperitoneal spreading of this neuroblastoma.*
- *Deep palpation should be performed only by experienced practitioners.*

| **Techniques and Normal Findings** | **Abnormal Findings and Special Considerations** |

4. Gently palpate the area over the left costovertebral angle (see Figure 21.10 ■).
- Watch the reaction and ask the patient to describe any sensation the palpation causes. Normally, the patient expresses no discomfort.

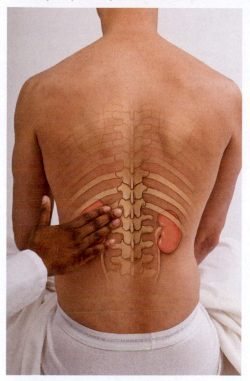

Figure 21.10 Palpating the costovertebral angle.

5. Use blunt or indirect percussion to further assess the kidneys.
- Place your left palm flat over the left costovertebral angle.
- Thump the back of your left hand with the ulnar surface of your right fist, causing a gentle thud over the costovertebral angle (see Figure 21.11 ■).

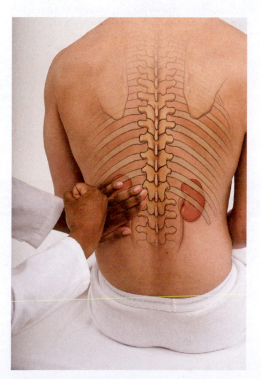

Figure 21.11 Blunt percussion.

▶ Pain, discomfort, or tenderness from an enlarged or diseased kidney may occur over the costovertebral angle, flank, and abdomen. When questioned, the patient complains of a dull, steady ache. This type of pain is associated with polycystic formation, pyelonephritis, and other disorders that cause kidney enlargement. In the patient with polycystic kidney disease, a sharp, sudden, intermittent pain may mean that a cyst in the kidney has ruptured. If the costovertebral angle is tender, red, and warm, and if the patient is experiencing chills, fever, nausea, and vomiting, the underlying kidney could be inflamed or infected.

▶ The pain caused by calculi (stones) in the kidney or upper ureter is unique and different in character, severity, and duration than that caused by kidney enlargement. This pain occurs as calculi travel from the kidney to the ureters and the urinary bladder.

Some patients experience no pain, and others feel excruciating pain. A stationary stone causes a dull, aching pain. As stones travel down the urinary tract, spasms occur. These spasms produce sharp, intermittent, colicky pain (often accompanied by chills, fever, nausea, and vomiting) that radiates from the flanks to the lower quadrants of the abdomen and, in some cases, the upper thigh and scrotum.

▶ If the patient reports severe pain, hematuria (blood in the urine) or **oliguria** (diminished volume of urine), and nausea and vomiting, it is important to be alert for hydroureter, a frequent complication that occurs when a renal calculus moves into the ureter. The calculus blocks and dilates the ureter, causing spasms and severe pain. Hydroureter can lead to shock, infection, and impaired renal function. If the nurse suspects hydroureter or obstruction at any point in the urinary tract, medical collaboration must be sought immediately.

▶ Pain or discomfort during and after blunt percussion suggests kidney disease. This finding is correlated with other assessment findings.

Techniques and Normal Findings	Abnormal Findings and Special Considerations

6. **Repeat the procedure on the right side. Ask the patient to describe the sensation as you examine each side.**
   - The patient should feel no pain or tenderness with pressure or percussion.

Appendix C: Advanced Skills *Appendix C provides step-by-step instructions on palpation of the kidneys.*

The Urinary Bladder

1. **Palpate the bladder to determine symmetry, location, size, and sensation.**
   - Use light palpation over the lower portion of the abdomen. The abdomen should be soft.
   - Use deep palpation to locate the fundus (base) of the bladder, approximately 5 to 7 cm (2 to 2.5 in.) below the umbilicus in the lower abdomen. Once you have located the fundus of the bladder, continue to palpate, outlining the shape and contour (see Figure 21.12 ■). Bimanual palpation may be required in the obese patient.

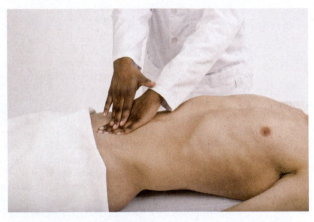

Figure 21.12 Palpating the bladder.

   - Slide your fingers over the surface of the bladder and continue palpating to determine smoothness and continuity.

   - The surface of the bladder should feel smooth and uninterrupted. An empty bladder is usually not palpable. When the bladder is moderately full, it should be firm, smooth, symmetric, and nontender. As the bladder fills, the fundus can reach the level of the umbilicus. A full bladder is firm and buoyant.

   ▶ A distended bladder feels smooth, round, and taut. An asymmetric contour or nodular surface suggests abnormal growth that should be correlated with other findings.

   ▶ In males with urethral obstruction because of hypertrophy or hyperplasia of the prostate, the bladder is enlarged.

2. **Percuss the bladder to determine its location and degree of fullness.**
   - Begin with indirect percussion in the midline of the abdomen at the level of the umbilicus.
   - Move your fingers downward as you continue to percuss toward the suprapubic area. Continue percussing downward until tympanic tones change to dull tones. A full bladder produces a dull sound. The point at which tympanic tones cease is the upper margin of the bladder.

   ▶ Bladder scanning or bedside bladder ultrasonography is a safe, noninvasive technique to assess bladder fullness in suspected urinary retention.

Techniques and Normal Findings	Abnormal Findings and Special Considerations

MALE REPRODUCTIVE SYSTEM

Inspection

1. **Instruct the patient.**
   - Have the patient empty his bladder and bowel before the examination.
   - Explain to the patient that you will be looking at and touching his genitals and pubic area. Tell him that the assessment should not cause physical discomfort. However, he must tell you of pain or discomfort at any point during the examination.
   - Reassure the patient that anxiety and embarrassment are normal. Explain that relaxation and focusing on instructions will make the assessment easier. If the patient experiences an erection during the examination, explain that this is normal and has no sexual connotation.

Techniques and Normal Findings	Abnormal Findings and Special Considerations

2. Position the patient.
- The patient stands in front of the examiner for the first part of the assessment.

3. Position yourself on a stool, sitting in front of the patient.

4. Inspect the pubic hair.
- Observe the pubic hair for normal distribution, amount, texture, and cleanliness (see Figure 21.13 ■).

▶ The amount, distribution, and texture of pubic hair vary according to the patient's age and race. Absent or extremely sparse hair in the pubic area may be indicative of sexual underdevelopment. The pubic hair of elderly males may be gray and thinning. Typical development pattern for presence of pubic hair is shown in Figure 21.14

▶ The nurse may note an absence of pubic hair due to removal by shaving or other grooming techniques. In the United States pubic hair grooming is increasingly common among men, with higher rates among younger men (Gaither et al., 2017).

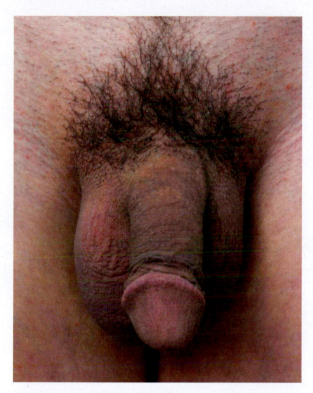

Figure 21.13 Inspecting the male pubic hair.

- Confirm that pubic hair is distributed heavily at the symphysis pubis in a diamond- or triangular-shaped pattern, thinning out as it extends toward the umbilicus. The hair will thin as it reaches the inner thigh area and over the scrotum. Hair should be absent on the penis.
- If the patient has complained of itching in his pubic area, comb through the pubic hair with two or three fingers.
- Confirm the absence of small bluish gray spots, or nits (eggs), at the base of the pubic hairs.

▶ These signs indicate the presence of crabs or pubic lice. Marks may be visible from persistent scratching to relieve the intense itching that crabs cause.

Techniques and Normal Findings	Abnormal Findings and Special Considerations

5. Inspect the penis.

- Inspect the penis size, pigmentation, glans, location of the dorsal vein, and the urethral meatus.
- Start by confirming that the penis size is appropriate for the stage of development of the patient. In adult males, penis size varies.
- Note the pigmentation of the penis.

▶ Penis size varies according to the developmental stage of the patient (see Figure 21.14 ■). The penis appears small in obese males because of the development of a pad of fat at the base of the penis.

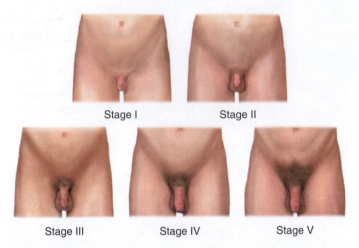

Stage I Stage II

Stage III Stage IV Stage V

Figure 21.14 The Tanner stages of male pubic hair and external genital development with sexual maturation. Stage I, Preadolescent, hair present is no different than that on the abdomen. Testes, scrotum, and penis are the same size and shape as in a young child. Stage II, pubic hair is slightly pigmented, longer, straight, often still downy, usually at base of penis, sometimes on scrotum; enlargement of scrotum and testes. Stage III, pubic hair is dark, definitely pigmented, curly pubic hair appears around base of penis; enlargement of penis, especially in length, further enlargement of testes, descent of scrotum. Stage IV, pubic hair is definitely adult in type but not in extent, spreads no further than inguinal fold. Continued enlargement of penis and sculpturing of glans, increased pigmentation of scrotum. Stage V, hair spreads to medial surface of thighs in adult distribution. Adult stage, scrotum ample, penis reaching nearly to bottom of scrotum.

- Pigmentation should be evenly distributed over the penis. The color depends on the patient's race but will be slightly darker than the color of the skin over the rest of his body.
- Assess the looseness of the skin over the shaft of the penis. The skin should be loose over the flaccid penis.
- Confirm that the dorsal vein is midline on the shaft.
- Inspect the glans penis. It should be smooth and free of lesions or discharge. No redness or inflammation should be present. **Smegma**, a white, cheesy substance, may be present. This finding is considered normal.

▶ Pigmentation of the penis of males with lighter complexions ranges from pink to light brown. In dark-skinned patients, the penis is light to dark brown.

▶ Urethral discharge (see Figure 21.15 ■) or lesions may indicate the presence of infective diseases such as *herpes, genital warts, gonorrhea,* or *syphilis,* or it may indicate cancer. If discharge is present, the substance should be cultured. Consistency, color, and odor are noted.

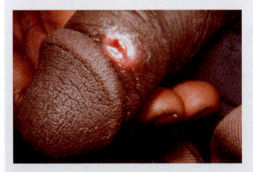

Figure 21.15 Syphilitic chancre.
Source: BSIP SA/Alamy Stock Photo.

| **Techniques and Normal Findings** | **Abnormal Findings and Special Considerations** |

- If the patient is uncircumcised, either ask the patient to pull the foreskin back or do so yourself. To retract the foreskin, gently pull the skin down over the penile shaft from the side of the glans using the thumb and first two fingers or forefinger (see Figure 21.16 ■).

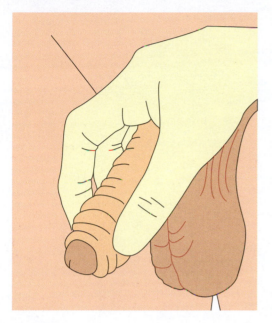

Figure 21.16 Retracting the foreskin.

- Gently move the foreskin back into place over the glans. The foreskin should move smoothly.

6. **Assess the position of the urinary meatus.**
   - The meatus should be located in the center of the tip of the penis (see Figure 21.17 ■).

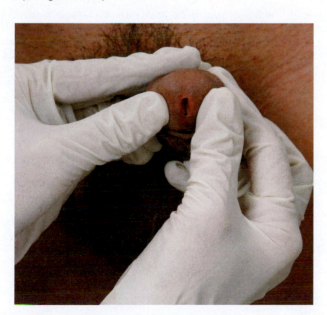

Figure 21.17 Assessing the position of the urinary meatus.

▶ **Phimosis** is a condition in which the foreskin is so tight that it cannot be retracted.

▶ Paraphimosis describes a condition in which the foreskin, once retracted, becomes so tight that it cannot be moved back over the glans.

▶ Immediate assistance must be sought if the foreskin cannot be retracted. Prolonged constriction of the vessels can obstruct blood flow and lead to tissue damage or necrosis.

▶ In rare cases, the urinary meatus is located on the upper side of the glans (**epispadias**) or the underside of the glans (*hypospadias*). These conditions are usually corrected surgically shortly after birth.

▶ A pinpoint appearance of the urinary meatus is indicative of **urethral stricture**.

Techniques and Normal Findings	Abnormal Findings and Special Considerations

7. Inspect the scrotum.

- Ask the patient to hold his penis up so that the scrotum is fully exposed (see Figure 21.18 ■). Optionally, you may hold the penis up by letting it rest on the back of your nondominant hand.

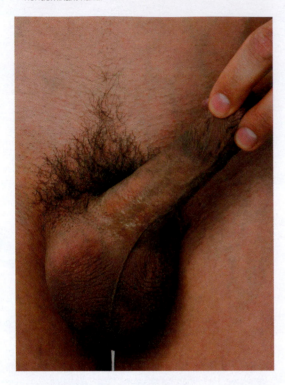

Figure 21.18 Inspecting the scrotum.

- While the patient is standing, observe the shape of the scrotum and how it hangs unsupported. It should be pear shaped, with the left side hanging lower than the right.

- Inspect the front and back of the scrotum. The skin should be wrinkled, loosely fitting over its internal structures. Note any swelling, redness, distended veins, and lesions. If swelling is present, note if it is unilateral or bilateral.

▶ An appearance of flatness could suggest testicular abnormality. Elderly males may have a pendulous, sagging scrotal sac.

▶ Scrotal swelling and inflammation could suggest problems such as **orchitis** (inflammation of the testicles), *epididymitis* (inflammation of the epididymis), *scrotal edema* (an accumulation of fluid in the scrotum), *scrotal hernia*, or *testicular torsion* (twisting of the testicle onto the spermatic cord). Swelling and inflammation may also be seen in renal, cardiovascular, and other systemic disorders. Edema of the genitalia can occur in obesity as a result of increased pressure on the groin from the enlarged abdomen.

8. Inspect the inguinal area.

- The inguinal area should be flat. This may be difficult to confirm if the patient is overweight. Even in the presence of adipose tissue, the contour of the inguinal area should be consistent with the rest of the body. Lymph nodes are present in this location, but not normally visible.
- Inspect both the right and left inguinal areas with the patient breathing normally.
- Have the patient hold his breath and bear down as if having a bowel movement.
- Observe for any evidence of lumps or masses. The contour of the inguinal areas should remain even.

▶ Masses or lumps may be related to the presence of an inguinal hernia or cancer within the reproductive, abdominal, urinary, lymphatic, and other systems.

Techniques and Normal Findings	Abnormal Findings and Special Considerations

9. Inspect the perianal area.

- Reposition the patient. Ask the patient to turn and face the table and bend over at the waist. The patient can rest his arms on the table (see Figure 21.19 ■).

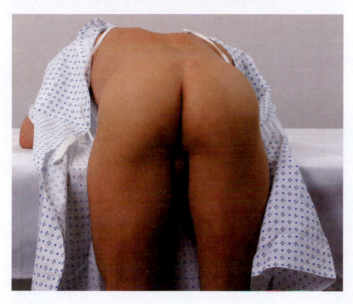

Figure 21.19 Positioning the client for assessment of internal structures.

- If the patient is unable to tolerate this position, he may lie on his left side on the examination table with both knees flexed.
- Inspect the sacrococcygeal and perianal areas. The skin should be smooth and without lesions.

▶ Tufts of hair or dimpling at the sacrococcygeal area are associated with pilonidal cysts. Rashes, redness, excoriation, or inflammation in the perianal area can signal infection or parasitic infestation. Obese males may have fecal incontinence because of pressure from the enlarged abdomen on the bowel and sphincter. This may result in rashes, excoriation, or lesions.

10. Inspect the anus.

- Spread the buttocks apart. Visualize the anus. The skin is darker and coarse. The area should be free of lesions.
- Ask the patient to bear down. The tissue stretches, but there are no bulges or discharge.

▶ Lesions may include skin tags, warts, hemorrhoids, or fissures.

▶ Fistulas, fissures, internal hemorrhoids, or rectal prolapse are more easily detected when the patient bears down.

Palpation

1. Palpate the penis.

- Place the glans between your thumb and forefinger (see Figure 21.20 ■).
- Gently compress the glans, allowing the meatus to gape open. The meatus should be pink, patent, and free of discharge.

▶ The patient may be hesitant to verbalize pain when palpation is performed. It is important to watch for nonverbal facial and body gestures.

▶ A *urethral stricture* is suspected if the meatus is only about the size of a pinpoint.

▶ Signs of *urethritis* include redness and edema around the glans and foreskin, eversion of urethral mucosa, and drainage. If urethritis is suspected, the patient should be asked if he experiences itching and tenderness around the meatus and painful urination. If drainage is present, observe for color, consistency, odor, and amount. Obtain a specimen if indicated. Suspect a gonococcal infection (gonorrhea) if the drainage is profuse and thick, purulent, and greenish yellow (see Figure 21.15).

▶ Consider inflammation or infection higher up in the urinary tract if redness, edema, and discharge are visible around the urethral opening, because the mucous membrane in the urethra is continuous with the mucous membrane in the rest of the tract.

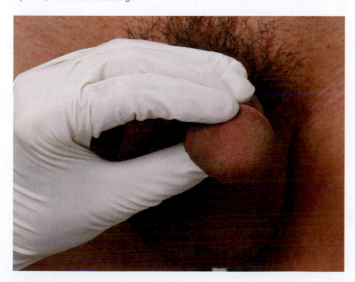

Figure 21.20 Palpating the penis.

Techniques and Normal Findings	Abnormal Findings and Special Considerations

- Note any discharge or tenderness.

- Continue gentle palpation and compression up the entire shaft of the penis.

2. Palpate the scrotum.
- Ask the patient to hold his penis up to expose the scrotum.
- Gently palpate the left and then the right scrotal sacs (see Figure 21.21 ■). Each scrotal sac should be nontender, soft, and boggy. The structures within the sacs should move easily with your palpation.
- Note any tenderness, swelling, masses, lesions, or nodules.

▶ Note characteristics of any abnormal findings. Culture any discharge.

▶ Be alert for any lesions, masses, swelling, or nodules.

▶ Assess shape, size, consistency, location, and mobility of any masses. If the patient expresses pain, lift the scrotum. If the pain is relieved, the patient may have epididymitis (inflammation of the epididymis).

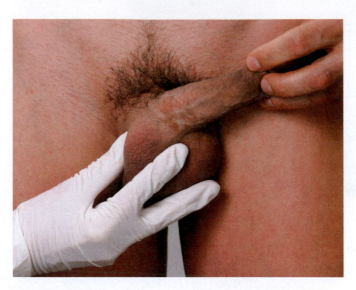

Figure 21.21 Palpating the scrotum.

3. Palpate the testes.
- Be sure that your hands are warm.
- Approach each testis from the bottom of the scrotal sac and gently rotate it between your thumb and fingertips (see Figure 21.22 ■). Each testis should be nontender, oval shaped, walnut sized, smooth, elastic, and solid.

▶ The **cremasteric reflex** may cause the testicles to migrate upward temporarily. Cold hands, a cold room, or the stimulus of touch could cause this response. To prevent this reflexive action when examining a child, have him sit tailor style. Gentle pressure over the canal with the nondominant hand can reduce this response.

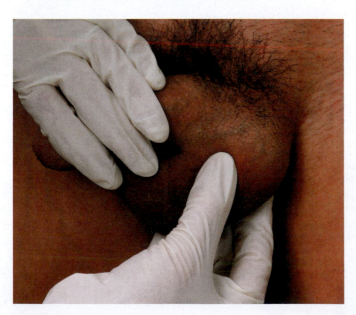

Figure 21.22 Palpating the testes.

Techniques and Normal Findings	Abnormal Findings and Special Considerations

Techniques and Normal Findings

4. Palpate the epididymis.
- Slide your fingertips around to the posterior side of each testicle to find the epididymis, a small, crescent-shaped structure.

5. Palpate the spermatic cord.
- Slide your fingers up just above the testicle, feeling for a vertical, ropelike structure about 3 mm (0.12 in.) wide.
- Gently grasp the cord between your thumb and index finger (see Figure 21.23 ■).
- Do not squeeze or pinch. Trace the cord up to the external inguinal ring using a gentle rotating motion.
- The cord should feel thin, smooth, nontender to palpation, and resilient.

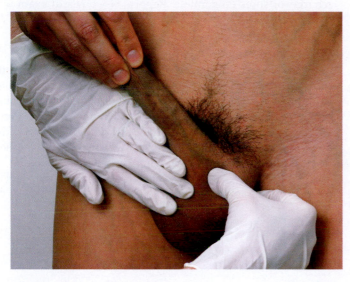

Figure 21.23 Palpating the spermatic cord.

6. Palpate the inguinal lymph chain.
- Using the pads of your first three fingers, palpate the inguinal lymph nodes.
- Confirm that the nodes are nonpalpable and the area is nontender (Figure 21.24 ■).
- Occasionally some of the inguinal lymph nodes are palpable. They are usually less than 0.5 cm (0.197 in.) in size, spongy, movable, and nontender.

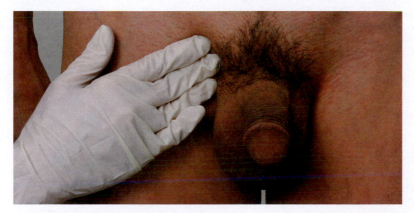

Figure 21.24 Palpating the inguinal lymph nodes.

7. Palpate the sacrococcygeal and perianal areas.
- The areas should be nontender and without palpable masses.

Abnormal Findings and Special Considerations

▶ In some patients, the epididymis may be palpated on the front surface of each testis.

▶ A cord that is hard, beaded, or nodular could indicate the presence of a varicosity or varicocele. A **varicocele** is a distended cord and is a common cause of male infertility. Upon palpation, it may feel like a bag of worms.

▶ It is important to assess if a node is larger than 0.5 cm (0.197 in.) or if multiple nodes are present. Tenderness in this area suggests infection of the scrotum, penis, or groin area.

▶ Tenderness, mass, or inflammation may indicate pilonidal cyst, anal abscess, fissure, or pruritus.

Appendix C: Advanced Skills *Appendix C provides step-by-step instructions on trans-illumination of the scrotum, palpation of the male inguinal region, and palpation of the prostate gland.*

Documenting Your Findings

Documentation of assessment data—subjective and objective—must be accurate, professional, complete, and confidential. When documenting the information from the focused assessment of each body system, the nurse should use measurements where appropriate to ensure accuracy, use medical terminology rather than jargon, include all pertinent information, and avoid language that could identify the patient. The information in the documentation should make it clear what questions were asked and use language to indicate whether it is the patient's response or the nurse's findings. For patient responses, the documentation will say "denies," "states," or "reports," whereas the nurse's findings will simply list the findings as fact, or say "no" along with the condition. For example: patient reports "urine is clear and yellow with no odor" and the nurse found "no pain with suprapubic palpation; no CVA tenderness." The following is an example of normal results for the male genitourinary system.

Sample Documentation: Male Genitourinary System Health Assessment

Focused History (Subjective Data)

This is information from the Review of Systems (ROS) and other pertinent history that is or could be related to the patient's urinary and reproductive systems.

Reports last urinalysis was "normal." Denies personal or family history of kidney disease and urinary problems. Denies urgency, frequency, or other difficulties with urination. Denies history of exposure to environmental toxins. Denies high blood pressure, diabetes, kidney stones, or infection. Reports satisfaction with sexual performance. Reports using condoms with intercourse for contraception. Denies history of smoking, recreational drug use. Reports drinking two or three 12 oz beers 2 days/week. Denies history of STIs, pain, discharge, or sores on genitals. Reports last physical exam was 6 months ago.

Physical Assessment (Objective Data)

Skin is light Caucasian with no lesions; abdomen flat, smooth, no pain on palpation to suprapubic area. Renal arteries with no bruit. No CVA tenderness, flanks symmetric with no discoloration. Pubic hair is evenly distributed, Tanner stage 6. Penis smooth, meatus patent, not circumcised with mobile foreskin. Testes palpable bilaterally, L side lower than R, no masses, erythema, or lesions. Inguinal lymph nodes nonpalpable.

Abnormal Findings of the Male Urinary System

Common alterations of the urinary system include bladder cancer, kidney and urinary tract infections, calculi, tumors, renal failure, and changes in urinary elimination. Each of these alterations is discussed as follows.

Bladder Cancer

Seen later in life, bladder cancer occurs more frequently in males than in females. A history of smoking has been linked to this disease. In some cases, the patient who experiences bladder cancer is asymptomatic.

If signs and symptoms are present:

Subjective findings:
- Flank pain
- Dysuria

Objective findings:
- Hematuria
- Frequent urination
- Edema in lower extremities
- Pelvic mass

Glomerulonephritis

This condition is an inflammation of the glomerulus.

Subjective findings:
- Fatigue
- Changes in urinary patterns

Objective findings
- Hypertension
- Generalized edema
- Hematuria
- Proteinuria

Renal Calculi

Calculi are stones that block the urinary tract. They are usually composed of calcium, struvite, or a combination of magnesium, ammonium, phosphate, and uric acid (see Figure 21.25 ■).

Subjective findings:
- Radiating pain that is variable in location and severity
- Ureteral spasms
- Nausea
- Dysuria
- Increased urinary urgency

Objective findings:
- Vomiting
- Increased urinary frequency
- Gross hematuria

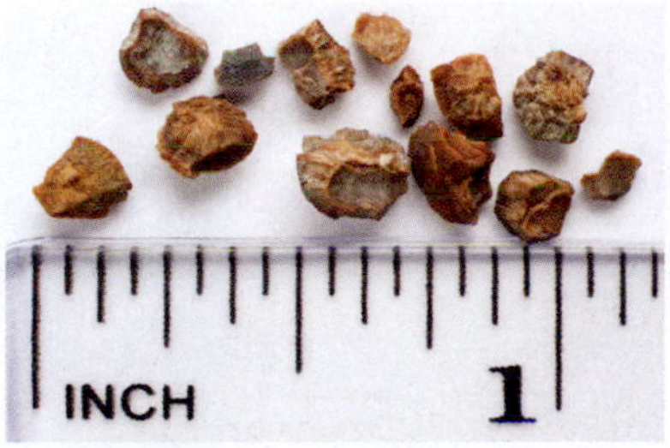

Figure 21.25 Kidney stones.
Source: piotr_malczyk/iStock/Getty Images.

Renal Tumor

Renal tumors may be either benign or malignant, with malignant being more common. Research has shown that there is an association between renal tumors and smoking.

Subjective findings:
- Flank pain
- Lethargy

Objective findings:
- Hematuria
- Weight loss
- Palpable flank mass

Renal Failure

Renal failure may be acute or it may progress to a chronic state. Acute renal failure that does not progress to a chronic state includes three stages: oliguria, diuresis, and recovery. Signs and symptoms of uremia, which is the hallmark of chronic renal failure, may include anorexia, nausea, vomiting, altered mentation, uremic frost, weight loss, fatigue, and edema.

Subjective findings:
- Anorexia
- Nausea
- Pruritus
- Fatigue

Objective findings
- Fluid retention
- Electrolyte imbalances (such as hyperkalemia and hyperphosphatemia)
- Vomiting
- Uremia
- Changes in mentation

Urinary Tract Infection

Bacteria cause urinary tract infections (UTIs). The bladder is the most common site of the infection, which results in inflammation of the bladder (cystitis); however, infection may include the kidneys. UTIs are common with catheter use for urinary retention or incontinence. Therefore, patients with catheters should be assessed regularly for UTIs. Patients may be asymptomatic.

Subjective findings:
- Increased urinary urgency
- Dysuria
- Suprapubic or lower back pain

Objective findings
- Increased urinary frequency
- Hematuria
- Cloudy, foul-smelling urine

Changes in Urinary Elimination

The following are examples of alterations in urinary elimination:

- **Dysreflexia** affects patients with spinal cord injuries at level T7 or higher. Bladder distention causes a sympathetic response that can trigger a potentially life-threatening hypertensive crisis.

- **Incontinence** is the inability to retain urine. If this is the patient's problem, the nurse must determine which of the five types of incontinence is present:

  - *Functional incontinence* occurs when the patient is unable to reach the toilet in time because of environmental, psychosocial, or physical factors.

  - *Reflex incontinence* occurs in patients with spinal cord damage when urine is involuntarily lost.

  - *Stress incontinence*, involuntary urination, occurs when intra-abdominal pressure is increased during coughing, sneezing, or straining. Aging changes may also contribute to stress incontinence.

  - *Urge incontinence* may be caused by consuming a significant volume of fluids over a relatively short period. Urge incontinence may also be because of diminished bladder capacity.

  - *Total incontinence* is related to a neurologic condition.

- **Urinary retention** is a chronic state in which the patient cannot empty the bladder. In most cases, the patient voids small amounts of overflow urine when the bladder reaches its greatest capacity.

Abnormal Findings of the Male Reproductive System

Abnormal findings of the male reproductive system include direct, indirect, and femoral hernias, as previously discussed (see Table 21.1). In addition, reproductive dysfunction may involve disorders of the penis (Table 21.3), abnormalities of the scrotum (Table 21.4), and problems in the perianal area (Table 21.5). These conditions are described on the following pages.

Table 21.3 Abnormalities of the Penis

Hypospadias

The congenital displacement of the meatus to the inferior surface of the penis, most commonly near the tip of the penis. The opening may also appear in the midline or base of the penis, or behind the scrotum.

Peyronie Disease

Hard plaques are found along the dorsum and are palpable under the skin that result in pain and bending of the penis during erection.

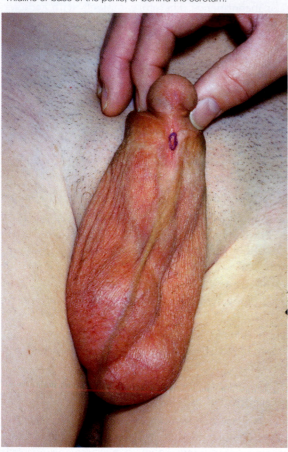

Hypospadias.
Source: Centers for Disease Control and Prevention.

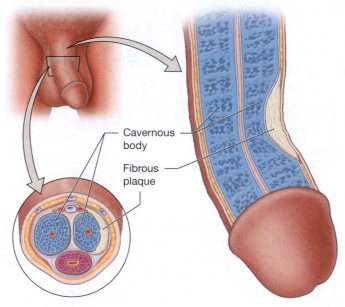

Peyronie disease.

(continued)

Table 21.3 Abnormalities of the Penis (continued)

Carcinoma

Carcinoma of the penis usually occurs in the glans. It appears as a reddened nodule growth, or an ulcerlike lesion.

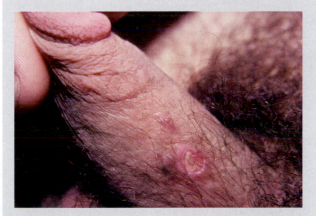

Carcinoma.
Source: Custom Medical Stock Photo/Alamy Stock Photo.

Genital Warts

A sexually transmitted disease that is caused by human papillomavirus (HPV), genital warts are rapidly growing papular lesions.

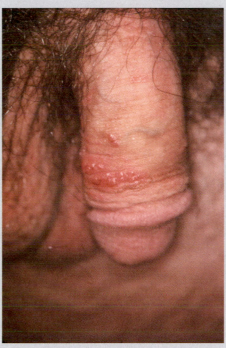

Genital warts.
Source: Dr. M.F. Rein/Centers for Disease Control and Prevention (CDC).

Syphilitic Chancre

These nontender lesions appear as round or oval reddened ulcers. A chancre often is the first symptom of primary syphilis, a sexually transmitted disease. Lymphadenopathy is present.

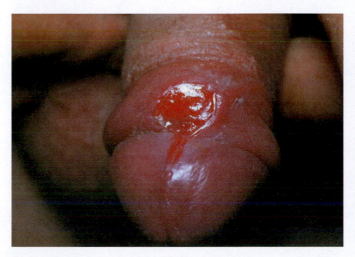

Syphilitic chancre.
Source: SPL/Science Source.

Genital Herpes

A sexually transmitted disease caused by the herpes simplex virus (HSV), these painful, small vesicles appear in clusters on any part of the surface of the penis. The area around the vesicles is erythematous.

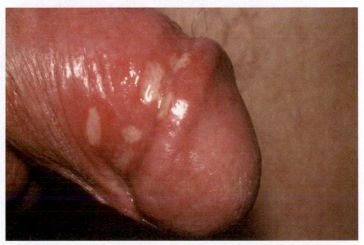

Genital herpes.
Source: Biophoto Associates/Science Source.

Table 21.4 Abnormalities of the Scrotum

Hydrocele
A fluid-filled, nontender mass that occurs within the tunica vaginalis.

Scrotal Hernia
An indirect inguinal hernia located within the scrotum.

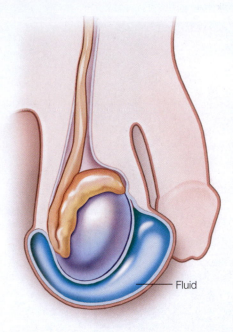

Hydrocele.

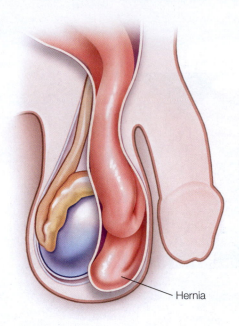

Scrotal hernia.

Testicular Tumor
A painless nodule on the testes. As it grows, the entire testicle seems to be overtaken.

Orchitis
This inflammatory process results in painful, tender, and swollen testes.

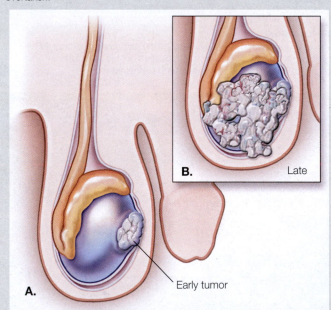

Testicular tumor. A. Early. B. Late.

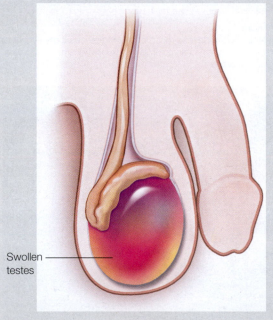

Orchitis.

(continued)

Table 21.4 Abnormalities of the Scrotum (continued)

Epididymitis

The epididymis is inflamed and tender. This condition, which can occur in adult males of any age, is most commonly caused by a bacterial infection.

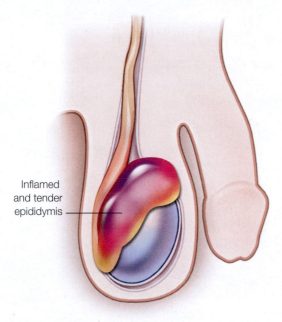

Inflamed and tender epididymis

Epididymitis.

Torsion of the Spermatic Cord

Torsion occurs with the greatest frequency in adolescents. The twisting of the testicle or the spermatic cord creates edema and pain, requiring immediate surgical intervention.

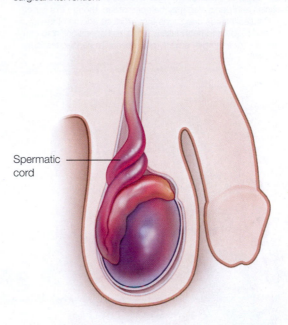

Spermatic cord

Torsion of the spermatic cord.

Small Testes

Testes are considered small when they are less than 2 cm (0.78 in.) long. Atrophy may occur in liver disease, in orchitis, and with estrogen administration.

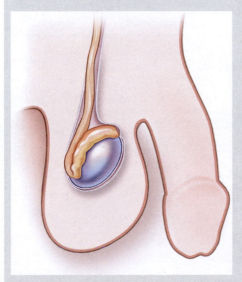

Small testes.

Cryptorchidism

Absence of a testicle in the scrotal sac. This condition may result from an undescended testicle.

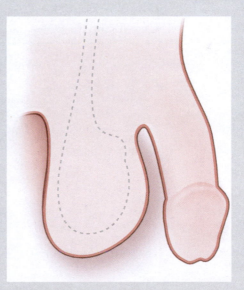

Cryptorchidism.

(continued)

Table 21.4 Abnormalities of the Scrotum (continued)

Scrotal Edema

Edema of the scrotum is seen in conditions causing edema of the lower body, including renal disease and heart failure. Scrotal edema, which may or may not be painful, can occur in males of any age. The edema may be unilateral or bilateral. The testicles and penis also may be edematous, though this is not always the case. Causes include conditions that produce edema of the lower body, such as renal disease and heart failure. Localized conditions also can cause scrotal edema—for example, epididymitis, testicular cancer, testicular torsion, and hydrocele.

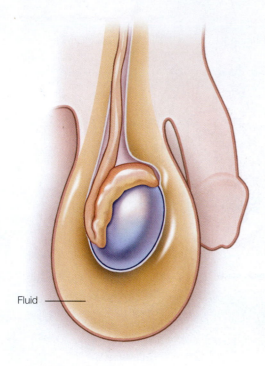

Fluid

Scrotal edema.

Table 21.5 Abnormalities of the Perianal Area

Pilonidal Cyst

Seen as dimpling in the sacrococcygeal area at the midline. An opening is visible and may reveal a tuft of hair. Usually asymptomatic, these cysts may become acutely abscessed or drain chronically.

Anal Fissure

Tears or splits in the anal mucosa that are usually seen in the posterior anal area and most frequently associated with the passage of hard stools or prolonged diarrhea. They are most common in young infants.

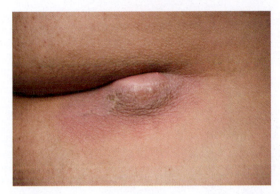

Pilonidal cyst.
Source: Alan Nissa/Shutterstock.

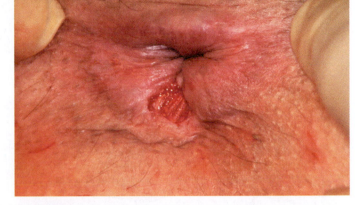

Anal fissure.
Source: BSIP SA/Alamy Stock Photo.

Hemorrhoids (Internal)

Varicosities of the hemorrhoidal veins of the anus or lower rectum.

Internally, they occur in the venous plexus superior to the mucocutaneous junction of the anus and are rarely painful. Identified by bright red bleeding that is unmixed with stool.

Hemorrhoids (External)

External hemorrhoids occur in the inferior venous plexus inferior to the mucocutaneous junction. They rarely bleed but cause anal irritation and create difficulty with cleansing the area.

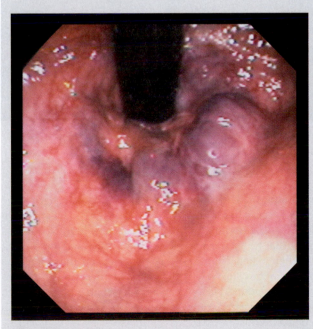

Hemorrhoids, internal.
Source: David M. Martin, M.D./Science Source.

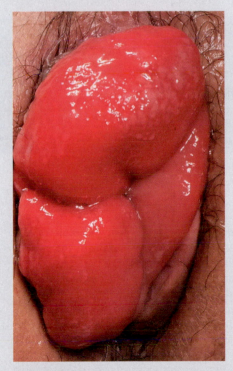

Hemorrhoids, external.
Source: Casa nayafana/Shutterstock.

(continued)

Table 21.5 Abnormalities of the Perianal Area (continued)

Perianal Perirectal Abscess
Painful and tender abscesses with perianal erythema; generally caused by infection of an anal gland. Can lead to fistulas (openings between the anal canal and outside skin).

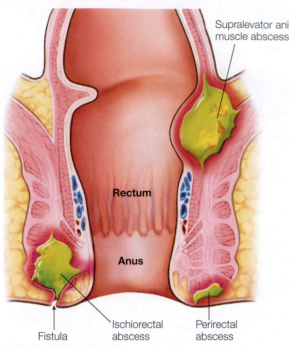

Perianal perirectal abscess.

Prolapse of the Rectum
Occurs when the rectal mucosa, with or without the muscle, protrudes through the anus. In mucosal prolapse, a round or oval pink protrusion is seen outside the anus. When the muscular wall is involved, a large red protrusion is visible.

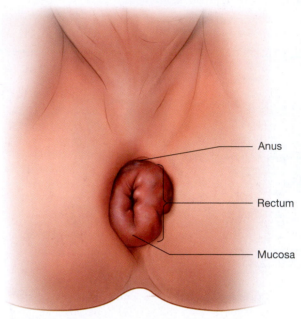

Prolapse of the rectum.

Application Through Critical Thinking

CASE STUDY

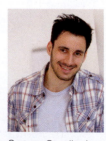

Source: Goodluz/ Shutterstock.

James Lewis is a 24-year-old male who is seen in the clinic for "pain in the groin." During the interview the patient states, "I have a soreness in my groin area on both sides." Mr. Lewis denies any trauma to the area, states he has neither done any heavy lifting nor been involved in athletic activities or "working out." He reports that he is in good health. He does not take any medications except vitamins and, occasionally, some nonaspirin product for a headache. He denies nausea, vomiting, diarrhea, or fever. He has no pain in his legs or back. He tells the nurse his appetite is okay but he is tired. He thinks his fatigue is because he has been "a little

worried about this problem and really having a hard time deciding to come in for help."

When asked about the onset of the problem, Mr. Lewis explains that he "started feeling some achiness about a week ago." When asked if he has ever experienced these feelings before, he replies "no." He is then asked to describe or discuss any other symptoms. He looks away, shifts in his chair, and then says, "Well, I have had some burning when I pass urine, and it's kind of cloudy."

When asked if he has ever had a problem like this before, he replies, "Yes, about two months ago." With further questioning, the nurse learns that Mr. Lewis was diagnosed with gonorrhea and treated with an injection and pills he was supposed to take for a week. He says he was not supposed to have sex until he finished the pills. When asked if he followed the prescribed treatment, he reluctantly responds that he finished all but a couple of the pills and did have sex with one of his girlfriends about 4 or 5 days after he got the injection.

Mr. Lewis tells the nurse he did not inform his girlfriends of his problem and that he generally avoids condoms because "I've known these girls for a long time."

The physical assessment yields the following information: BP 128/86, P 96, RR 20, T 98.6. His color is pale, and the skin is moist and warm. External genitalia are intact, without lesions or erythema. There is lymphadenopathy in bilateral groin areas. Compression of the glans yields milky discharge. A smear of urethral discharge is obtained.

The nurse knows that Mr. Lewis's original gonococcal infection was treated with an injection, most likely ceftriaxone. The nurse also knows that chlamydia is present in almost half of the patients with gonorrhea and is treated with a 7-day regimen of oral antibiotics. Between 40% and 60% of patients with gonorrhea have lymphadenopathy.

Based on the data, the nurse suspects that Mr. Lewis has a reinfection with gonorrhea and may have a concomitant chlamydial infection.

The nurse recommends single-injection treatment for gonorrhea and a new oral regimen for chlamydia. A urine specimen will be obtained and submitted with the urethral discharge smear. The patient will be scheduled for a follow-up phone conference about the laboratory results in 48 hours and a return visit in 7 days. The nurse conducts an information, education, and advice session before discharge from the clinic.

SAMPLE DOCUMENTATION

The following is sample documentation for James Lewis.

SUBJECTIVE DATA: Seeking care for "pain in groin." Pain in groin bilateral. Denies trauma, heavy lifting, athletic activity, or "working out." Reports he is in "good health." Takes no medications except vitamins and nonaspirin product for a headache. Denies nausea, vomiting, diarrhea, or fever. No pain in back or legs. Reports "okay" appetite. Reports fatigue. "Became a little worried about this problem and decided to come in for help." Achiness 1 week ago. Burning on urination, cloudy urine. Gonorrhea diagnosis 2 months ago, treated with injection and oral meds. Did not complete prescription and had intercourse "four or five days after injection." Did not inform partners of diagnosis, generally avoids condoms.

OBJECTIVE DATA: VS: BP 128/86, P 96, RR 20, T 98.6°F. Color pale, skin moist and warm. External genitalia intact, no lesions or erythema. Lymphadenopathy bilateral groin. Milky discharge on compression of glans. Culture and urine sample to lab.

CRITICAL THINKING QUESTIONS

1. Describe the critical thinking process as applied by the nurse to direct the care of this patient.

2. What additional data should the nurse seek when conducting the health assessment for this patient?

3. What data informed the nurse of a need to provide education for the patient?

4. What data will the nurse seek upon the return visit with Mr. Lewis?

REFERENCES

Agarwal, A., Aitken, R. J., & Alvarez, J. G. (Eds.). (2012). *Studies on men's health and fertility.* New York, NY: Humana Press.

American Cancer Society. (2016a). *American Cancer Society recommendations for prostate cancer early detection.* Retrieved from https://www.cancer.org/cancer/prostate-cancer/early-detection/acs-recommendations.html

American Cancer Society. (2016b). *Can testicular cancer be found early?* Retrieved from https://www.cancer.org/cancer/testicular-cancer/detection-diagnosis-staging/detection.html

American Cancer Society. (2018). *Bladder cancer risk factors.* Retrieved from https://www.cancer.org/cancer/bladder-cancer/causes-risks-prevention/risk-factors.html

Asokan, S., Narasimhan, M., & Rajagopalan, V. (2017). Cutaneous manifestations in chronic renal failure patients on hemodialysis and medical management. *International Journal of Research in Dermatology, 3*(1), 24–32. doi:10.18203/issn.2455-4529.IntJResDermatol20170432

Berman, A., Snyder, S. J., & Frandsen, G. (2016). *Kozier & Erb's fundamentals of nursing: Concepts, process, and practice* (10th ed.). Hoboken, NJ: Pearson.

Byun, J. S., Lyu, S. W., Seok, H. H., Kim, W. J., Shim, S. H., & Bak, C. W. (2013). Sexual dysfunctions induced by stress of timed intercourse and medical treatment. *British Journal of Urology International, 111*(4b), E227–E234.

Cek, M., Sturdza, L., & Pilatz, A. (2017). Acute and chronic epididymitis. *European Urology Supplements, 16,* 124–131. doi:10.1016/j.eursup.2017.01.003

Centers for Disease Control and Prevention (CDC). (2017a). *Condom effectiveness.* Retrieved from https://www.cdc.gov/condomeffectiveness/index.html

Centers for Disease Control and Prevention (CDC). (2017b). *Genital herpes–CDC fact sheet.* Retrieved from http://www.cdc.gov/std/herpes/stdfact-herpes-detailed.htm

Centers for Disease Control and Prevention (CDC). (2018). *Diabetes, high blood pressure raise kidney risk.* Retrieved from http://www.cdc.gov/features/worldkidneyday

Cioe, P. A., Anderson, B. J., & Stein, M. D. (2013). Change in symptoms of erectile dysfunction in depressed men initiating buprenorphine therapy. *Journal of Substance Abuse Treatment, 45*(5), 451–456. http://dx.doi.org/10.1016/j.jsat.2013.06.004

Dalke, K. A., Fein, L., Jenkins, L. C., Caso, J. R., & Salgado, C. J. (2013). Complications of genital piercings. *Anaplastology, 2*(122). doi:10.4172/2161-1173.1000122

Dellis, A., Mitsogiannis, I., & Mitsikostas, D. D. (2017). Neurogenic bladder in multiple sclerosis. *Hellenic Urology, 29*(2), 34–40. Retrieved from http://www.hellenicurology.com/index.php/Hellenic-Urology/article/view/169/130

Devarajan, P. (2017). *Oliguria.* Retrieved from https://emedicine.medscape.com/article/983156-overview

Frederick, D. A., Lever, J., Gillespie, B. J., & Garcia, J. R. (2017). What keeps passion alive? Sexual satisfaction is associated with sexual communication, mood setting, sexual variety, oral sex, orgasm, and sex frequency in national U. S. study. *Journal of Sex Research, 54*(2), 186–201. doi:10.1080/00224499.2015.1137854

Gaither, T. W., Awad, M. A., Osterberg, E. C., Rowen, T. S., Shindel, A. W., & Breyer, B. N. (2017). Prevalence and motivation: Pubic hair grooming among men in the United States. *American Journal of Men's Health, 11*(3), 620-640. doi:10.1177/1557988316661315

Halbert, C. H., Gattoni-Celli, S., Savage, S., Prasad, S. M., Kittles, R., Briggs, V., . . . Johnson, J. C. (2017). Ever and annual use of prostate cancer screening in African American men. *American Journal of Men's Health, 11*(1), 99–107. doi:10.1177/1557988315596225

Holloway, V., & Wylie, K. (2015). Sex drive and sexual desire. *Current Opinion in Psychiatry, 28*(6), 424–429. doi:10.1097/YCO.0000000000000199

Johns Hopkins Medicine. (n.d.). *Male factor infertility: What is infertility?* Retrieved from https://www.hopkinsmedicine.org/healthlibrary/conditions/mens_health/male_factor_infertility_85,P01484

Kalfa, N., Paris, F., Soyer-Gobillard, M., Daures, J., & Sultan, C. (2011). Prevalence of hypospadias in grandsons of women exposed to diethylstilbestrol during pregnancy: A multigenerational national cohort study. *Fertility and Sterility, 95*(8), 2574–2577. doi:10.1016/j.fertnstert.2011.02.047

Karavolos, S., Stewart, J., Evbuomwan, I., McEleny, K., & Aird, I. (2013). Assessment of the infertile male. *The Obstetrician & Gynaecologist, 15*(1), 1–9. doi:10.1111/j.1744–4667.2012.00145.x

Klein, J. W. (2014). Common anal problems. *Medical Clinics of North America, 98*(3), 609–623. doi:10.1016/j.mcna.2014.01.011

MacDonald, S., Colaco, M., & Terlecki, R. (2017). Waves of change: National trends in surgical management of male stress incontinence. *Urology, 108*, 175–179. doi:10.1016/j.urology.2017.04.055

Marieb, E. N., & Keller, S. M. (2018). *Essentials of human anatomy and physiology* (12th ed.). Redwood City, CA: Benjamin Cummings/Pearson Education.

Mayo Clinic. (2016). *Getting pregnant: How to get pregnant.* Retrieved from https://www.mayoclinic.org/healthy-lifestyle/getting-pregnant/in-depth/art-20047611

Mayo Clinic. (2017a). *Peyronie's disease.* Retrieved from https://www.mayoclinic.org/diseases-conditions/peyronies-disease/symptoms-causes/syc-20353468

Mayo Clinic. (2017b). *Premature ejaculation: Symptoms & causes.* Retrieved from https://www.mayoclinic.org/diseases-conditions/premature-ejaculation/symptoms-causes/syc-20354900

Mayo Clinic. (2017c). *Sexually transmitted diseases (STDs): Risk factors.* Retrieved from https://www.mayoclinic.org/diseases-conditions/sexually-transmitted-diseases-stds/symptoms-causes/syc-20351240

Mayo Clinic. (2017d). *Urinary tract infection (UTI).* Retrieved from https://www.mayoclinic.org/diseases-conditions/urinary-tract-infection/symptoms-causes/syc-20353447

Mayo Clinic. (2018). *Hydrocele: Symptoms & causes.* Retrieved from https://www.mayoclinic.org/diseases-conditions/hydrocele/symptoms-causes/syc-20363969

National Cancer Institute. (n.d.). *Cancer stat facts: Testicular cancer.* Retrieved from https://seer.cancer.gov/statfacts/html/testis.html

National Cancer Institute. (2018). *Testicular cancer screening (PDQ®) health professional version: Description of the evidence.* Retrieved from https://www.cancer.gov/types/testicular/hp/testicular-screening-pdq#section/_6

National Institute of Diabetes and Digestive and Kidney Diseases (NIDDKD). (2014). *Urinary retention.* Retrieved from https://www.niddk.nih.gov/health-information/urologic-diseases/urinary-retention

National Institute on Drug Abuse. (2017). *Medical consequences of drug misuse: Kidney damage.* Retrieved from https://www.drugabuse.gov/publications/health-consequences-drug-misuse/kidney-damage

National Kidney Foundation. (2017). *Genetics and kidney disease.* Retrieved from https://www.kidney.org/news/kidneyCare/winter10/Genetics

Office of Minority Health. (2014). *Diabetes data and statistics.* Retrieved from https://minorityhealth.hhs.gov/omh/content.aspx?ID=2913

O'Lone, E., Connors, M., Masson, P., Wu, S., Kelly, P. J., Gillespie, D., . . . Webster, A. C. (2016). Cognition in people with end-stage kidney disease treated with hemodialysis: A systematic review and meta-analysis. *American Journal of Kidney Diseases, 67*(6), 925–935. doi:10.1053/j.ajkd.2015.12.028

Ozkanli, S., Girgin, B., Kosemetin, D., & Zemheri, E. (2014). Case report – Hemangioma of the urinary bladder. *Science Journal of Clinical Medicine, 3*(1), 15–16. doi:10.11648/j.sjcm.20140301.14

Rodriguez-Iturbe, B., & Haas, M. (2016, Feb. 10). Poststreptococcal glomerulonephritis. In J. J. Feretti, D. L. Stevens, & V. A. Fischetti (eds.), *Streptococcus pyogenes: Basic biology to clinical manifestations* [Internet]. Oklahoma City, OK: University of Oklahoma Health Sciences Center. Retrieved from https://www.ncbi.nlm.nih.gov/books/NBK333429

Shamaskin-Garroway, A. M., Giordano, N., & Blakley, L. (2017). Addressing elder sexual abuse: The critical role for integrated care. *Translational Issues in Psychological Science, 3*(4), 410–422. doi:10.1037/tps0000145

Shaw, D., Graeme, L., Pierre, D., Elizabeth, W., & Kelvin, C. (2012). Pharmacovigilance of herbal medicine. *Journal of Ethnopharmacology, 140*(3), 513–518. doi:10.1016/j.jep.2012.01.051

Siegel, R. L., Miller, K. D., & Jemal, A. (2017). Cancer statistics, 2017. *CA: A Cancer Journal for Clinicians, 67*(7), 7–30. doi:10.3322/caac.21387

Sise, M. E., Lo, G. C., Goldstein, R. H., Allegretti, A. S., & Masia, R. (2017). Case 12-2017: A 34-year-old man with nephropathy. *The New England Journal of Medicine, 376*(16), 1575–1585. doi:10.1056/NEJMcpc1616395

Spector, R. (2017). *Cultural diversity in health and illness.* New York, NY: Pearson.

Stevenson, S. M., & Lowrance, W. T. (2015). Epidemiology and diagnosis of testis cancer. *Urologic Clinics of North America, 42*(3), 269–275. doi:10.1016/j.ucl.2015.04.001

Tang, Y. H., Yeung, V. H. W., Chu, P. S. K., & Man, C. W. (2017). A 55-year old man with right testicular pain: Too old for torsion? *Urology Case Reports, 11,* 74–75. doi:10.1016/j.eucr.2016.11.023

Wingate, J. T., Erickson, B. A., Murphy, G., Smith, T. G., Breyer, B. N., Boelzke, B. B., & TURNS. (2018). Multicenter analysis of patient reported outcomes following artificial urinary sphincter placement for male stress urinary incontinence. *The Journal of Urology, 199*(3), 785–790. doi:10.1016/j.juro.2017.09.089

World Health Organization. (2018). *Sexual and reproductive health: Infertility definitions and terminology.* Retrieved from http://www.who.int/reproductivehealth/topics/infertility/definitions/en

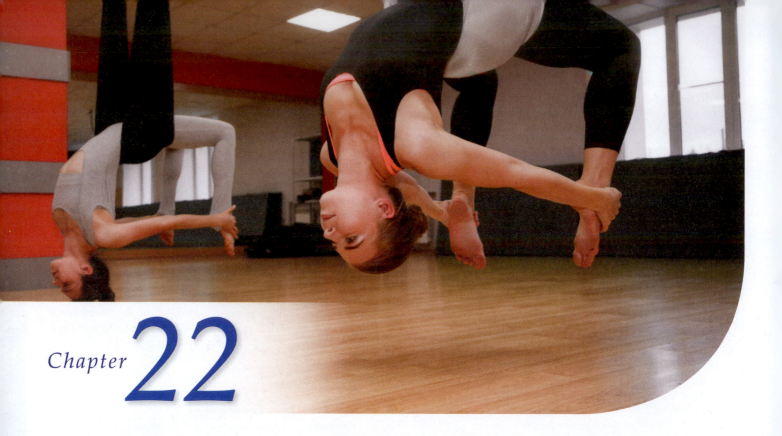

Chapter 22

Female Genitourinary System

LEARNING OUTCOMES

Upon completion of this chapter, you will be able to:

1. Describe the anatomy and physiology of the female genitourinary system.

2. Identify anatomic, physiologic, developmental, psychosocial, and cultural variations that guide assessment of the female genitourinary system.

3. Determine questions about the female genitourinary system to use for the focused interview.

4. Outline the techniques for assessment of the female genitourinary system.

5. Generate the appropriate documentation to describe the assessment of the female genitourinary system.

6. Identify abnormal findings in the physical assessment of the female genitourinary system.

KEY TERMS

anus, 494	cystocele, 516	introitus, 492	prolapsed uterus, 516
azotemia, 499	dysreflexia, 518	kidneys, 489	rectocele, 516
Bartholin's glands, 492	femoral hernia, 494	labia, 491	ureters, 490
calculi, 517	genital warts, 514	medulla, 489	urethra, 490
cervical os, 493	glomeruli, 489	nocturia, 497	urinary retention, 518
cervix, 493	hematuria, 499	oliguria, 511	urinary system, 489
clitoris, 493	hymen, 515	ovaries, 494	uterine tubes, 494
cortex, 489	incontinence, 518	paraurethral glands, 492	uterus, 493
costovertebral angle (CVA), 491	inguinal hernia, 494	perineum, 491	vagina, 493

MEDICAL LANGUAGE

-cele	Suffix meaning "hernia"	**hyster-**	Prefix meaning "uterus," "womb"
cyst-	Prefix meaning "urinary bladder," "cyst," "sac of fluid"	**nephr-**	Prefix meaning "kidney"
		-rrhea	Suffix meaning "flow," "discharge"
-ectomy	Suffix meaning "removal," "excision," "resection"	**-uria**	Suffix meaning "urine," "condition of urine"

Introduction

The female genitourinary system includes the urinary and reproductive systems. These systems are often described together because of their close proximity within the body. The urinary system eliminates liquid waste from the body in the form of urine. The female reproductive system provides for both human reproduction and sexual gratification.

Female Genitourinary System Anatomy and Physiology Review

The anatomy and physiology of the female genitourinary system is described in the following sections.

Urinary Anatomy and Physiology

The **urinary system** is composed of the kidneys, renal vasculature (blood vessels), ureters, urinary bladder, and urethra. The organs of the urinary system are distributed among the retroperitoneal space, abdomen, and genitals. The **glomeruli** (tufts of capillaries) of the kidneys filter more than 1 liter (L) of fluid each minute. As a result, wastes, toxins, and foreign matter are removed from the blood. The urinary system acts through the kidneys to prevent the accumulation of nitrogenous wastes, promotes fluid and electrolyte balance, assists in maintenance of blood pressure, and contributes to *erythropoiesis* (development of mature red blood cells).

Kidneys The **kidneys** are bean-shaped organs located in the retroperitoneal space on either side of the vertebral column. Extending from the level of the 12th thoracic vertebra to the 3rd lumbar vertebra, the upper portion of the kidneys is protected by the lower rib cage (Marieb & Keller, 2018). The right kidney is displaced downward by the liver and sits slightly lower than the left kidney. A layer of fat cushions each kidney, and the kidney itself is surrounded by tissue called the renal capsule (see Figure 22.1A ■ and Figure 22.1B ■). The renal fascia connects the kidney and fatty layer to the posterior wall of the abdomen. Each adult kidney weighs approximately 150 g (5 oz) and is 11 to 13 cm (4 to 5 in.) long, 5 to 7 cm (2 to 3 in.) wide, and 2.5 to 3 cm (1 in.) thick. The lateral surface of the kidney is convex. The medial surface is concave and contains the hilus, a vertical cleft that opens into a space within the kidney referred to as the renal sinus. The ureters, renal blood vessels, nerves, and lymphatic vessels pass through the hilus into the renal sinus. The superior part of the kidney is referred to as the upper pole, whereas the inferior surface is called the lower pole.

The inner portion of the kidney is called the *renal medulla*. The renal **medulla** is composed of structures called pyramids and calyces. The pyramids are wedgelike structures made up of bundles of urine-collecting tubules. At their apex, the pyramids have papillae that are enclosed by cuplike structures called calyces. The calyces collect urine and transport it into the renal pelvis, which is the funnel-shaped superior end of the ureter (see Figure 22.2 ■).

The outer portion of each kidney is called the renal **cortex**. It is composed of over 1 million nephrons, which form urine. The first part of each nephron is the renal corpuscle, which consists of a tuft of capillaries called a glomerulus. These glomeruli begin the filtration of the blood. Larger blood components, such as red blood cells and larger proteins, are separated from most of the fluid, which passes into the glomerular capsule (or Bowman's capsule). The filtrate then moves into a proximal convoluted tubule, then into the loop of Henle, and finally into a distal convoluted tubule, from which it is collected as urine by a collecting tubule. Along the way, some of the filtrate is resorbed along with electrolytes and chemicals such as glucose, potassium, phosphate, and sodium. Each collecting tubule guides the urine from several nephrons out into the renal pyramids and calyces and from there through the renal pelvis and into the ureters.

The major functions of the kidneys are the following:

- Eliminating nitrogenous waste products, toxins, excess ions, and drugs through urine
- Regulating volume and chemical makeup of the blood
- Maintaining balance between water and salts and acids and bases
- Producing renin, an enzyme that assists in the regulation of blood pressure
- Producing erythropoietin, a hormone that stimulates production of red blood cells in the bone marrow
- Assisting in the metabolism of vitamin D

Renal Arteries The kidneys require a tremendous amount of oxygen and nutrients and receive about 25% of the cardiac output. Although not part of the urinary system, an extensive network of arteries intertwines within the renal network. These arteries include renal arteries, arcuate arteries, interlobular arteries, afferent arteries, and efferent arterioles. The vasa recta are looping capillaries that connect with the juxtamedullary

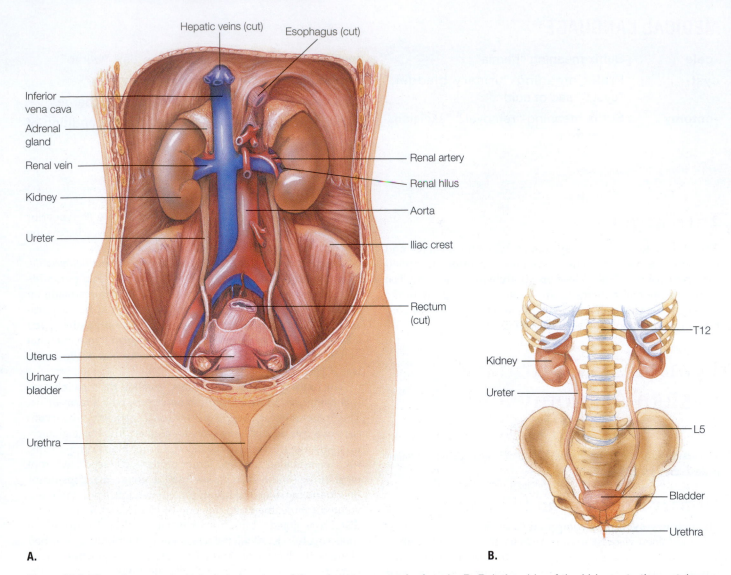

Figure 22.1 The urinary system. A. Anterior view of the urinary organs of a female. B. Relationship of the kidneys to the vertebrae.

nephrons and continue into the medulla alongside the loop of Henle. The vasa recta help to concentrate urine. The major function of the renal arteries is providing a rich supply of blood (approximately 1,200 mL per minute when an individual is at rest) to the kidneys.

Ureters The **ureters** are mucus-lined narrow tubes approximately 25 to 30 cm (10 to 12 in.) in length and 6 to 12 mm (0.25 to 0.5 in.) in diameter (Marieb & Keller, 2018). The major function of the ureters is transporting urine from the kidney to the urinary bladder. As the ureter leaves the kidney, it travels downward behind the peritoneum to the posterior wall of the urinary bladder. The middle layer of the ureters contains smooth muscle that is stimulated by transmission of electric impulses from the autonomic nervous system. Their peristaltic action propels urine downward to the urinary bladder. The major function of the ureters is transporting urine from the kidney to the urinary bladder.

Urinary Bladder The urinary bladder is a hollow, muscular, collapsible pouch that acts as a reservoir for urine (Marieb & Keller, 2018). It lies on the pelvic floor in the retroperitoneal

space. The bladder is composed of two parts: (1) the rounded muscular sac made up of the detrusor muscle and (2) the portion between the body of the bladder and the urethra, known as the neck. In females, the bladder lies anterior to the vagina and uterus. The detrusor muscle allows the bladder to expand as it fills with urine and to contract to release urine to the outside of the body during micturition (voiding). When empty, the bladder collapses upon itself, forming a thick-walled, pyramidal organ that lies low in the pelvis behind the symphysis pubis. As urine accumulates, the fundus, the superior wall of the bladder, ascends in the abdominal cavity and assumes a rounded shape that is palpable. When moderately filled (500 mL), the bladder is approximately 12.5 cm (5 in.) long. When larger amounts of urine are present, the bladder becomes distended and rises above the symphysis pubis.

The major functions of the urinary bladder are the following:

- Storing urine temporarily
- Contracting to release urine during micturition

Urethra The **urethra** is a mucus-lined tube that transports urine from the urinary bladder to the exterior (Marieb & Keller,

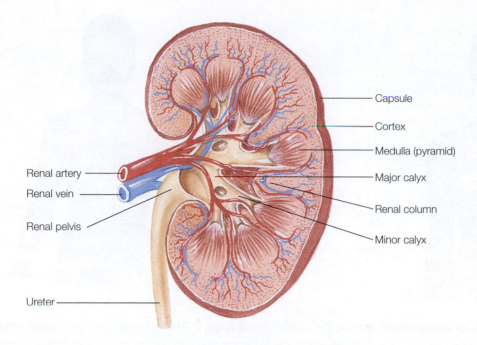

Figure 22.2 Internal anatomy of the kidney.

2018). In females, the urethra is approximately 3 to 4 cm (1.5 in.) long and lies along the anterior wall of the vagina. The female urethra terminates in the external urethral orifice or meatus, which lies between the clitoris and the vagina. Because the female urethra is short and its meatus lies close to the anus, it can become contaminated with bacteria more readily than the male urethra. The major function of the urethra is providing a passage for the elimination of urine.

Landmarks During assessment of the urinary system, the nurse uses three landmarks to locate and palpate the kidneys and urinary bladder. These landmarks are the costovertebral angle, the rectus abdominis muscle, and the symphysis pubis. The **costovertebral angle (CVA)** is the area on the lower back formed by the vertebral column and the downward curve of the last posterior rib, as depicted in Figure 22.3A ■. It is an important anatomic landmark because the lower poles of the kidney and ureter lie below this surface. The rectus abdominis muscles are a longitudinal pair of muscles that extend from the pubis to the rib cage on either side of the midline, as illustrated in Figure 22.3B ■. These muscles are used as guidelines for positioning the hands when palpating the kidneys through the abdominal wall. The symphysis pubis is the joint formed by the cartilaginous union of the two pubic bones at the midline of the body (see Figure 22.3B). The bladder is cradled under the symphysis pubis. When the bladder is full, the nurse is able to palpate it as it rises above the symphysis pubis.

Female Reproductive Anatomy and Physiology

The female reproductive system is unique in that it experiences cyclic changes in direct response to hormonal levels of estrogen and progesterone during the childbearing years. The uterus changes throughout the ovarian cycle during which the

ova (eggs) are prepared for fertilization with sperm (Marieb & Keller, 2018). During the menstrual cycle, the uterine lining is prepared for the development of a fetus. The onset of menopause represents the end of the childbearing years.

Unlike the male reproductive system, the female reproductive tract is completely separate from the urinary tract. However, structures of the two tracts lie within close proximity.

The functions of the female reproductive system include the following:

- Manufacturing and protecting ova for fertilization
- Transporting the fertilized ovum for implantation and embryonic/fetal development
- Regulating hormonal production and secretion of several sex hormones
- Providing sexual stimulation and pleasure

External Genitalia and Perineum Female external genitalia include the mons pubis, labia majora, labia minora, greater vestibular glands, and clitoris (Marieb & Keller, 2018). The area encompassing the structures of the external genitalia as well as the anus makes a diamond shape known as the **perineum**.

MONS PUBIS The mons pubis is the mound of adipose tissue overlying the symphysis pubis (see Figure 22.4 ■). In the mature woman, it is thickly covered with hair and provides protection to the underlying reproductive structures.

LABIA MAJORA AND LABIA MINORA The **labia** are a dual set of liplike structures lying on either side of the vagina (see Figure 22.4). The exterior labia majora are two thick, elongated pads of tissue that become fuller toward the center. An extension of the external skin surface, the labia majora are covered with coarse hair extending from the mons pubis. The enclosed labia minora are two thin, elongated pads of tissue that overlie the

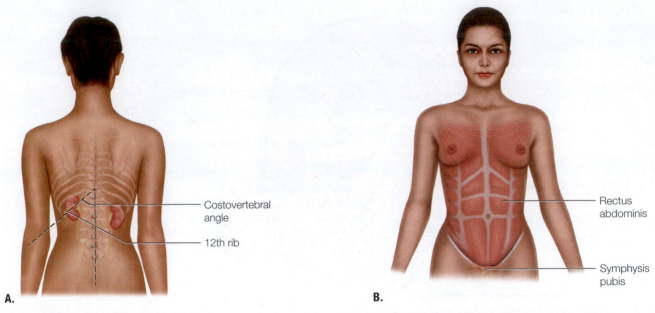

Figure 22.3 Landmarks for urinary assessment: A. The costovertebral angle. B. The rectus abdominis muscles and the symphysis pubis.

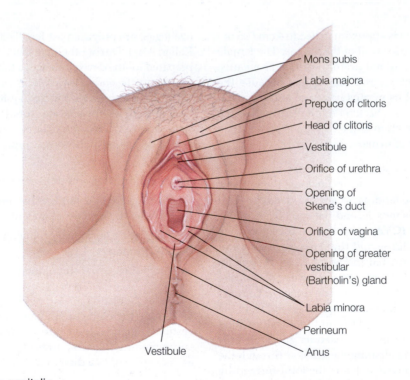

Figure 22.4 External female genitalia.

vaginal and urethral openings as well as several glandular openings. Anteriorly, the labia minora join to form the prepuce, which covers the clitoris. Posteriorly, the labia join to form the *fourchette* (small fold of membrane). The labia minora border an almond-shaped area of tissue known as the *vestibule*. It extends from the clitoris to the fourchette. The urethral meatus, vaginal opening (**introitus**), Skene's glands, and Bartholin's glands lie within the vestibule. The major function of the labia is providing protection

from infection and physical injury to the urethra and vagina and, ultimately, other urinary and reproductive structures.

SKENE'S GLANDS AND BARTHOLIN'S GLANDS The Skene's glands, also called **paraurethral glands**, are located just posterior to the urethra (see Figure 22.4). They open into the urethra and secrete a fluid that lubricates the vaginal vestibule during sexual intercourse. The **Bartholin's glands**, or greater vestibular glands, are located posteriorly at the base of the vestibule and produce mucus, which is released into the vestibule. This mucus actively promotes sperm motility and viability.

CLITORIS Located at the anterior of the vestibule is the **clitoris**, a small, elongated mound of erectile tissue (see Figure 22.4). As the labia minora merge together anteriorly, a small hoodlike covering is formed that lies over the top of the clitoris. The clitoris is homologous with the penis. It is permeated with numerous nerve fibers responsive to touch. When stimulated, the clitoris becomes erect as its underlying corpus cavernosa become vasocongested. The major function of the clitoris is serving as the primary organ of sexual stimulation.

Internal Reproductive Organs

The internal female reproductive organs are the vagina, uterus, cervix, uterine (fallopian) tubes, and ovaries. These organs are described in the following paragraphs.

VAGINA The **vagina** is a long, tubular, muscular canal (approximately 9 to 15 cm [3.5 to 5.9 in.] in length) that extends from the vestibule to the cervix at the inferior end of the uterus (see Figure 22.5A ■). The muscularity of the vaginal wall and its thick, transverse rugae (ridges) allow it to dilate widely to accommodate the erect penis and, during childbirth, the head of the fetus. At the point of juncture with the cervix, a continuous circular cleft called the *fornix* is formed. The major functions of the vagina are serving as the female organ of copulation, the birth canal, and the channel for the exit of menstrual flow.

UTERUS The **uterus** is a pear-shaped, hollow, muscular organ that is located centrally in the pelvis between the neck of the bladder and the rectal wall (see Figure 22.5A). The body of the uterus is about 4 cm (1.56 in.) wide and 6 to 8 cm (2.34 to 3.12 in.) in length. Its walls are 2 to 2.5 cm (0.78 to 0.94 in.) thick and are composed of serosal, muscular, and mucosal layers. Anatomically, the uterus is divided into three segments. These segments are the fundus, the corpus, and the cervix. The **cervix** projects into the vagina about 2.5 cm and is about 2.5 cm (0.98 in.) round. A small central canal connects the vagina to the inside of the uterus. The *external* **cervical os** is the inferior opening (the vaginal end of the canal), and the *internal cervical os* opens directly into the uterine chamber. The uterus has two pairs of adnexal, or accessory, structures: the uterine (fallopian) tubes and the ovaries.

The uterus is easily moved within the pelvic cavity, but its basic position is secured with several ligaments that attach it to the pelvic floor. The ligaments also prevent the uterus from

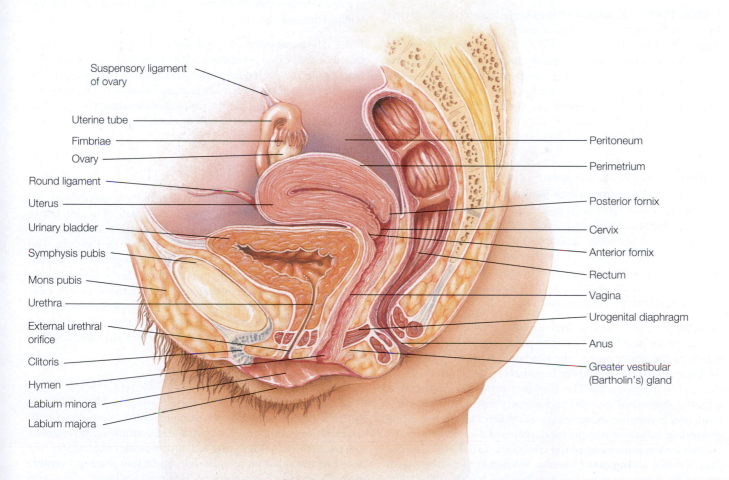

Figure 22.5A Internal organs of the female reproductive system within the pelvis.

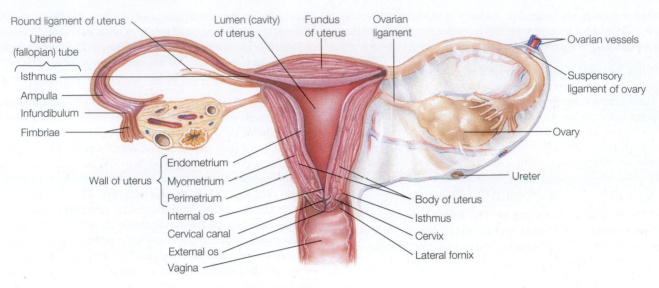

Figure 22.5B Cross-section of the anterior view of the female pelvis.

dropping into the vaginal canal. The major functions of the uterus are serving as the site of implantation of the fertilized ovum and as a protective sac for the developing embryo and fetus.

UTERINE TUBES The **uterine tubes** (or fallopian tubes) are two ducts on either side of the fundus of the uterus (see Figure 22.5B ■). They are about 7 to 10 cm (2.75 to 3.9 in.) in length and extend from the uterus almost to the ovaries. An ovum released by an ovary travels to the uterus within the uterine tubes. Normally fertilization takes place within the uterine tubes. The major functions of the uterine (fallopian) tubes include serving as the site of fertilization and providing a passageway for unfertilized and fertilized ova to travel to the uterus.

OVARIES Lying close to the distal end of either side of the uterine tubes are the **ovaries** (see Figure 22.5B). These almond-shaped glandular structures produce ova as well as estrogen and progesterone. They are about 3 cm (1.17 in.) long and 2 cm (0.78 in.) wide. The ovarian ligaments and suspensory ligaments hold the ovaries in place. The ovaries become fully developed after puberty and atrophy after menopause. The major functions of the ovaries are producing ova for fertilization by sperm and producing estrogen and progesterone.

Inguinal Region The inguinal areas, often referred to as the groin, are located laterally to the pubic region over the iliac region or the upper part of the hip bone. Within this area are the inguinal ligaments and the inguinal canals, which lie above the inguinal ligaments. The inguinal canals are associated with the abdominal muscles and actually represent a potential weak link in the abdominopelvic wall. When a separation of the abdominal muscle exists, the weak points of these canals afford an area for the protrusion of the intestine into the groin region. This is called an **inguinal hernia**. Women are less likely than men to develop an inguinal hernia (Brookes & Hawn, 2018). The femoral hernia is another type of hernia occurring in the groin area, and it is more common in women than men. A **femoral hernia** is a bulging over the area of the femoral artery in the groin caused by a weakening or tear in the abdominal wall.

Inguinal and femoral hernias can be confused, leading to the need for a good understanding of these types of hernias and thorough examination. Table 21.1 (see Chapter 21) describes types, characteristics, and signs and symptoms of inguinal and femoral hernias. ∞

Anus The **anus** is the terminal end of the gastrointestinal system. The anal canal is between 2 and 4 cm (0.78 to 1.57 in.) long, opens onto the perineum at the midpoint of the gluteal folds, and has internal and external muscles. The external muscles are skeletal muscles, which form the part of the anal sphincter that voluntarily controls evacuation of stool. Mucosa of the anus is moist, darkly pigmented, and hairless.

Special Considerations

Throughout the assessment process, the nurse gathers subjective and objective data reflecting the patient's state of health. Using critical thinking and the nursing process, the nurse identifies many factors to be considered when collecting the data. The subjective and objective data gathered throughout the assessment process inform the nurse about the patient's state of health. A variety of factors, including age, developmental level, race, ethnicity, work history, living conditions, socioeconomics, and emotional well-being, influence health and must be considered during assessment. The impact of these factors is discussed in the following sections.

Health Promotion Considerations

The American College of Obstetricians and Gynecologists (ACOG) (2017c) recommends annual well-woman visits for all women beginning around age 13 and continuing throughout the adult lifespan. Visits provide opportunities not only for history and examination but also for counseling about preventive care. Guidelines for screening, laboratory testing, evaluation and counseling, and immunizations vary by age, personal and family medical history, and other risk factors.

Cervical cancer is most often diagnosed in women ages 35 to 44 (American Cancer Society [ACS], 2018c). It can frequently be found early, or it can be completely prevented through screening (ACS, 2018a). Although it used to be one of the most common causes of death from cancer in women in the United States, early detection through screening has reduced cervical cancer deaths significantly, and it is now one of the most treatable types of all cancers (ACS, 2018c). According to the most recent Centers for Disease Control and Prevention (CDC) (2017a) data from 2010 to 2014, the human papilloma virus (HPV) is the most common cause of cervical cancer in the United States, as well as for some cancers of the vagina, vulva, penis, anus, and oropharynx. Screening for cervical cancer is recommended for women ages 21 to 65 and is done by performing cervical cytology (i.e., Pap smear or Pap test) and, for some women, HPV testing (ACOG, 2017a). These screening guidelines are followed for women who are at average risk for cervical cancer. For women who fall outside of the "average risk" criteria, such as those who have had abnormal Pap smears and those who are infected with the human immunodeficiency virus (HIV), healthcare providers will follow specific guidelines for these situations. Guidelines for cervical cancer screening in women of average risk are as follows:

- 21–29 years: Pap test alone every 3 years
- 30–65 years: Pap test and HPV test every 5 years (preferred), *or* Pap test alone every 3 years
- > 65 years: Stop screening if no history of moderate or severe abnormal cervical cells or cervical cancer *and* have had either three negative Pap test results in a row or two negative co-test results in a row within the past 10 years, with the most recent test performed within the past 5 years

Although research has shown that infections can be transmitted sexually even when the partners are using a latex condom, its use significantly lowers the incidence of transmission (CDC, 2017b). A history of HPV and more than four sexual partners in a lifetime increases a woman's risk for cervical cancer. HPV vaccines have been designed to prevent the most common types of HPV infection and are proven to be almost 100% effective in protecting against cervical precancers and genital warts (CDC, 2016). Since the introduction of the HPV vaccine in 2006, vaccine-type HPV infection rates have decreased by 64% in the United States and even more so in countries such as Australia where there is a higher rate of vaccination. CDC's Advisory Committee on Immunization Practices (ACIP) recommends routine two-dose vaccination of girls and boys ages 11 and 12. This two-dose vaccination series can be given any time between ages 9 and 14. If vaccinating individuals 15 years or older, a three-dose series is recommended (CDC, 2016). It is recommended that women through age 26 and men through age 21 can still receive the vaccine if they did not complete the series at a younger age.

Updated guidelines no longer recommend annual pelvic examinations or screening for ovarian cancer (ACOG, 2017b). However, women are encouraged to be aware of changes within their own bodies and to discuss them with their obstetrician-gynecologist (OB-GYN) or other healthcare provider who will determine if the symptoms may be associated with ovarian cancer and if further examination and testing are needed.

Lifespan Considerations

A patient's age and developmental stage have a tremendous influence on the female reproductive system. Growth and development are dynamic processes that cause changes over time.

Data collection and interpretation of these findings in relation to expected values are important. Details about differences in the assessment of the female genitourinary system are noted in Chapter 25, Chapter 26, and Chapter 27. ∞

Psychosocial Considerations

It is important to consider psychosocial factors and their impacts on the urinary and reproductive systems.

Urinary System Patients suffering from incontinence are at increased risk for social isolation, self-esteem disturbance, and other psychosocial problems (Institute on Aging, 2017). Increasing body mass index (BMI) has been associated with stress and urge incontinence (Palma et al., 2014). In addition, the increased weight of adipose tissue in obesity impacts the function of the muscles of the bladder and rectal sphincters, possibly resulting in incontinence. Urinary tract infections (UTIs) in women may also result from sexual trauma, sexual intercourse with a new partner, or coital frequency. The nurse should consider the possibility of sexual abuse in a child or adolescent who presents with a UTI.

Female Reproductive System Fatigue, depression, and stress can decrease sexual desire in a woman of any age (Mayo Clinic, 2018a). Grief over the loss of a relationship, whether because of separation, divorce, or death, can have long-term effects on a patient's willingness to seek new relationships. Feelings of betrayal—for example, when a partner becomes intimate with another person—can have the same effect.

Past or recent trauma, as from childhood abuse, physical assault, and sexual assault, whether or not penetration occurred, may have a significant impact on a woman's ability to enjoy a sexual relationship (Mayo Clinic, 2018a). This may be true even if the trauma is unremembered.

Some women may fear sexual intimacy because of an altered body image related to their weight, body type, breast size, or other factors (Mayo Clinic, 2018a). Reproductive surgeries can affect a woman's self-image and sexual expression. For example, patients who have had a hysterectomy may feel free from the worry of unwanted pregnancy and experience an increase in sexual desire, or they may feel less feminine than before the surgery and withdraw from sexual relationships.

Cultural and Environmental Considerations

When considering the influence of culture on a patient's healthcare practices, the nurse must be open-minded and sensitive to the specific values and beliefs of the patient without passing judgment. It is important to note, however, that not all individuals adhere to the norms, values, and practices of their culture. Consideration for the patient's privacy and modesty is essential when obtaining subjective and objective data regarding urinary elimination. Though not every patient is embarrassed by these components of assessment, many individuals experience considerable uneasiness. It is essential to afford the patient as much privacy and dignity as possible. Some individuals will not disrobe or allow a physical examination by anyone of the opposite sex. Other patients will not allow a sample of their body fluids to be taken and examined by strangers.

Patients with hypertension or diabetes mellitus are especially vulnerable to kidney damage if they do not follow a strict medication and diet regimen (Nasari & Rafieian-Kopaei, 2015). Higher rates of hypertension and diabetes mellitus are experienced by Hispanics and African Americans (Office of Minority Health [OMH], 2016); however, these conditions are not limited to these populations. The nurse can help all patients maintain optimal health by providing information on diet, prevention of hypertension, and the importance of compliance with medication regimens.

Information obtained during the focused interview may identify whether the patient is taking herbs or using other treatments that are a part of cultural traditions. The nurse should obtain information that is as complete as possible about the herbal remedies.

Some cultures and religions have specific beliefs or encourage specific behaviors related to sexual practices. For example, many religions forbid premarital sex. Likewise, among certain cultures, female genital mutilation (FGM) is a common practice (Population Reference Bureau, 2014). Believed to affect as many as 140 million women worldwide, FGM involves partial or total excision of the external female genitalia for nonmedical reasons. FGM constitutes a breach of human rights law. In many parts of the world—including Africa, where FGM is commonly performed—FGM is illegal. FGM also is prevalent in Asia and the Middle East. When assessing patients, the nurse should be aware of the individual's potential cultural practices, while avoiding making assumptions about the patient's beliefs or experiences.

Environmental influences also can significantly impact sexual and reproductive health. Sexual dysfunction can result from sexual, physical, or verbal abuse among family members. Negative reactions to an individual's sexual orientation and lifestyle choices from family, friends, and others, including healthcare providers may impact the individual's ability to find a sexual partner and maintain a satisfying sexual relationship. In addition, discrimination and fear of stigmatization by healthcare providers may cause delay or complete avoidance for seeking preventative medical help (Mirza & Rooney, 2018). This can have a negative emotional and physical impact, especially among female adolescents.

Women who work in the microelectronics industry (i.e., high-speed electronics, such as circuit boards) may be exposed to arsenic, glycol ethers, lead, and radiation. These substances have been linked to birth defects and spontaneous abortions. Lead is also still present in some homes. Exposure to vinyl chloride (used in construction and building materials) may increase the risk for stillbirths and premature births. Exposure to high concentrations of halogenated hydrocarbons, such as polychlorinated biphenyls (PCBs), found in plastics manufacturing and in the electrical industries, is associated with low birth weight, spontaneous abortion, hyperpigmentation of infants, and microcephaly (abnormally small head size). Oncology nurses exposed to antineoplastic drugs may have spontaneous abortions, fetal anomalies, changes in the regularity of their menstrual cycle, or even cessation of their menstrual cycle.

Maintaining the cleanliness of the female genitalia requires daily washing and changing of underclothes. Douching is not only unnecessary, but it may even be harmful as it has been shown to promote irritation, rashes, and infection in some women. The likelihood of rashes or infections can be reduced by keeping the genitals dry by changing sweaty underclothes after physical exercise, changing into dry clothes immediately after bathing or swimming, and changing an infant's diaper immediately after it is wet.

Other important points of note during history and physical exam include the following:

- A history of STDs in children may indicate sexual abuse.
- The risk for cervical cancer is increased in those women who participate in early (before age 18) and frequent sexual activity and have a history of many sexual partners.
- Obesity is a risk factor for uterine cancer.

Subjective Data—Health History

Health assessment of the female genitourinary system includes gathering subjective and objective data. Subjective data collection occurs during the patient interview, before the actual physical assessment. The nurse uses a variety of communication techniques to elicit general and specific information about the health of the female genitourinary system.

Focused Interview

Subjective data gathered during the focused interview of the female genitourinary system concerns data related to the structures and functions of this system. The nurse should be prepared to observe the patient and listen for cues related to the function of this body system. Open-ended and closed questions are used to obtain information. Often a number of follow-up questions or requests for descriptions are required to clarify data or gather missing information. Follow-up questions are aimed at identifying the source of problems, duration of difficulties, measures to alleviate problems, and clues about the patient's knowledge of her own health.

Information about the urinary system, genital areas, reproduction, and sexual activity is generally considered very private. The nurse must be sensitive to the patient's need for privacy and carefully explain that all information is confidential. A conversational approach with the use of open-ended statements is often helpful in a situation that can cause anxiety and embarrassment. The patient's terminology about body parts and functions should guide the nurse's questions.

The focused interview guides the physical assessment of the female genitourinary system. The information is always considered in relation to normal parameters and expectations about the health of the system. Therefore, the nurse must consider age, gender, race, culture, environment, health practices, past and concurrent problems, and therapies when framing questions and using techniques to elicit information. In order to address all of the factors when conducting a focused interview, categories of questions related to status and function of the reproductive system have been developed. These categories include general questions that are asked of all patients; those addressing illness and infection; questions related to symptoms, pain, and behaviors; those related to habits or practices; questions that are specific to patients according to age; and questions that address environmental concerns. One approach to elicit information about symptoms is the OLD-CART & ICE method as described in Chapter 5. ∞ See Figure 5.3.

The nurse must consider the patient's ability to participate in the focused interview and physical assessment of the genitourinary system. If a patient is experiencing pain, urgency, incontinence, or anxiety that accompanies any of these problems, attention must focus on relief of these symptoms. Abnormal vaginal discharge, pelvic pain, inflammation, infection, and suspicion of contracting an STD are some of the more frequent problems that the woman reports.

Focused Interview Questions	Rationales and Evidence

The following section provides sample questions and follow-up questions in each of the categories previously mentioned. A rationale for questions is provided. The list of questions is not all-inclusive but rather represents the types of questions required in a thorough focused interview related to the urinary system. The follow-up bulleted questions are asked to seek clarification with additional information from the patient to enhance the subjective database.

FEMALE URINARY SYSTEM

General Questions

1. **What are your normal patterns when you urinate?**
   - How often do you urinate each day?
   - How much do you pass each time you urinate? (Note: The nurse may use terms familiar to the patient, such as *pass water*, when asking about urination.)

   ▶ Many factors influence the number of times and amount that a patient voids. Among these are size of the bladder, amount of fluid intake, type of fluid or solid intake, medications, amount of perspiration, and the patient's temperature. The adult may void five or six times per day in amounts averaging 100 mL to 400 mL. For adults, daily urine output typically averages 1,500 mL (Berman, Snyder, & Frandsen, 2016). However, adults may urinate as much as 2 L of fluid. At a minimum, the adult patient should produce urine at a rate of 30 mL/ hour. The child may void more frequently in smaller amounts. The key point is to determine the patient's normal patterns and to identify excess or insufficient urine output.

2. **Have you noticed any change from your normal urination patterns?**
   - Have you noticed any changes in your pattern recently?
   - Have you had any of these changes: urinating more often, urinating less often, urinating more fluid, or urinating less fluid?

   ▶ Changes in urinary elimination patterns can sometimes signal fluid retention, which may indicate heart failure, kidney failure, or improper nutritional intake. Other considerations include obstructions, infections, and endocrine alterations (Devarajan, 2014).

3. **When you urinate, do you feel you are able to empty your bladder completely?**
   - If not, describe your feeling.

   ▶ The feeling of being unable to empty the bladder may indicate that the patient is retaining urine or developing increased residual urine, which may contribute to the development of infection (Moore & Spence, 2014).

4. **Are you always able to control when you are going to urinate?**
   - If not, do you have to hurry to the bathroom as soon as you feel the urge to urinate?
   - When you feel the urge to urinate, are you able to get to the toilet?
   - Have you ever had an "accident" and wet yourself?
   - Have you ever urinated by accident when you have coughed, sneezed, or lifted a heavy object?

   ▶ Urgency and stress incontinence may be caused by an infection, an inflammatory process, or the loss of muscle control over urination (e.g., after the vaginal birth of a child or vaginal hysterectomy) (Forsgren et al., 2012).

5. **Do you ever have to get up at night to urinate?**
   - If so, can you describe why?
   - Is there any predictable pattern?
   - How many times per night?
   - Describe your fluid intake for a day.

   ▶ **Nocturia** (nighttime urination) may indicate the presence of aging changes in the older adult, cardiovascular changes, diuretic therapy, or habit. Nocturia can be influenced by the amount and timing of fluid intake.

6. **If you have urinary problems, have they caused you embarrassment or anxiety?**
   - Have your urinary problems affected your social, personal, or sexual relationships?

   ▶ These are important considerations because they may affect patients' abilities to function in other parts of their lives.

7. **Has anyone in your family had a kidney disease or urinary problem?**
   - If so, when did they have it?
   - How was it treated?
   - Do they still have it?

   ▶ A family history of kidney disease may signify a genetic predisposition to the development of renal disorders in some individuals (National Kidney Foundation, 2017).

8. **Have you had a recent urinalysis or blood work evaluating your kidneys?**
   - If so, do you know the results?

   ▶ It is valuable for patients to know the results of laboratory work and to provide the healthcare professional with their impression of the results.

Focused Interview Questions	Rationales and Evidence

Questions Related to Illness or Infection

1. Have you ever been diagnosed with a disease of the kidney or bladder?
- When were you diagnosed with the problem?
- What treatment was prescribed for the problem?
- Was the treatment helpful?
- What kinds of things do you do to help with the problem?
- Has the problem ever recurred (acute)?
- How are you managing the disease now (chronic)?

▶ The patient has an opportunity to provide information about specific urinary illnesses. If a diagnosed illness is identified, follow-up about the date of diagnosis, treatment, and outcomes is required. Data about each illness identified by the patient are essential to an accurate health assessment. Illnesses can be classified as acute or chronic, and follow-up regarding each classification will differ.

2. *Alternative to question 1:* List possible illnesses of the urinary system, such as renal calculi, nephrosis, and renal failure, and ask the patient to respond "yes" or "no" as each is stated.

▶ This is a comprehensive and easy way to elicit information about all diagnoses. Follow-up would be carried out for each identified diagnosis as in question 1.

3. Do you now have or have you had an infection in the urinary system?
- When were you diagnosed with the infection?
- What treatment was prescribed for the problem?
- Was the treatment helpful?
- What kinds of things do you do to help with the problem?
- Has the problem ever recurred (acute)?
- How are you managing the infection now (chronic)?

▶ If an infection is identified, follow-up about the date of infection, treatment, and outcomes is required. Data about each infection identified by the patient are essential to an accurate health assessment. Infections can be classified as acute or chronic, and follow-up regarding each classification will differ.

4. *Alternative to question 3:* List possible urinary system infections, such as cystitis, pyelonephritis, and prostatitis, and ask the patient to respond "yes" or "no" as each is stated.

▶ This is a comprehensive and easy way to elicit information about all urinary system infections. Follow-up would be carried out for each identified infection as in question 2.

5. Have you ever had surgery on the urinary system?
- If so, describe the procedure. How long ago did you have it done? Is the problem corrected?
- If not, describe it.
- Has anyone in your family ever had surgery on the urinary system?
- If so, please describe the procedures.
- How long ago was the surgery?
- Is the problem corrected?
- If not, describe it.

▶ Previous surgeries help provide insight as to the patient's history of urological problems. Some urinary problems, such as overflow incontinence, are more common among patients who have had urological surgery (Urology Care Foundation, 2018).

6. Do you have any of these problems: high blood pressure, diabetes, frequent bladder infections, kidney stones?
- If so, how has the problem been treated?
- Describe any associated symptoms.
- Do you still have problems with this condition?
- Do you have any idea what causes this problem?

▶ High blood pressure may contribute to the development of renal disease (CDC, 2018). Diabetes may significantly contribute to the development of renal disease (CDC, 2018). Infections may be caused by inadequate fluid intake, inadequate hygiene, and structural anomalies (Berman et al., 2016). In some patients this is an infrequent situation; in others it is a common malady. Kidney stones may be an isolated event or a recurring condition. Parathyroid disorders and any condition that causes an increase in calcium may contribute to the formation of kidney stones (National Institute of Diabetes and Digestive and Kidney Diseases, 2012).

7. Do you have any of these neurologic diseases: multiple sclerosis, Parkinson disease, spinal cord injury, or stroke?
- If so, which one?
- When was it diagnosed?
- How are you being treated?

▶ These conditions contribute to the retention and stasis of urine, thus placing the patient at risk for chronic urinary infections (Moore & Spence, 2014).

8. Do you have any type of cardiovascular disease?
- If so, what was the diagnosis?
- When was it diagnosed?
- How are you being treated?

▶ Hypertension in particular may significantly contribute to the development of renal failure (CDC, 2018).

9. Have you had influenza, a skin infection, a respiratory tract infection, or other infection recently?
- If so, what was it?
- What medication did the physician prescribe?
- Did you take all of the medication?
- Is this a recurrent problem?

▶ If the infection was untreated, the patient may be at risk for developing a renal infection (Wong & Stevens, 2013).

Questions Related to Symptoms, Pain, and Behaviors

When gathering information about symptoms, many questions are required to elicit details and descriptions that assist in the analysis of the data. Discrimination is made in relation to the significance of a symptom, in relation to specific diseases or problems, and in relation to potential follow-up examination or referral. One rationale may be provided for a group of questions in this category.

The following questions refer to specific symptoms and behaviors associated with the urinary system. For each symptom, questions and follow-up are required. The details to be elicited are the characteristics of the symptom; the onset, duration, and frequency of the symptom; the treatment or remedy for the symptom, including over-the-counter (OTC) and home remedies; the determination if diagnosis has been sought; the effect of treatments; and family history associated with a symptom or illness.

Focused Interview Questions	Rationales and Evidence

Questions Related to Symptoms

1. Have you noticed any changes in the quality of the urine?
- If so, describe the change.
- Has your urine been cloudy?
- Does it have an odor?
- Has the color changed?
- If there has been a color change, what is it?
- Does the color change happen each time you urinate?
- Is there a pattern?
- Can you predict the color change?

▶ Color changes offer clues to the presence of infection, kidney stones, or neoplasm. The quantity of urine may indicate the presence of renal failure or may reflect hydration status (Berman, 2016).

2. If the urine is bloody (hematuria), the nurse should ask these questions:
- Have you fallen recently?
- Do you experience burning when the blood is present? Have you seen clots in the urine?
- Have you noticed any stones or other material in the urine?
- Have you noticed any granular material on the toilet paper after you wipe?

▶ The patient may offer valuable information about the source and characteristics of bleeding, because this symptom is present in a wide variety of conditions. Hematuria is a serious finding and warrants additional follow-up (Berman et al., 2016).

3. Is your urine foamy and amber in color?

▶ This finding may indicate the presence of kidney dysfunction or other illnesses (Stöppler, 2012).

4. Have you had any weight gain recently?
- If so, describe it.
- Are you retaining fluid?
- Are your rings, clothing, or shoes becoming tighter?
- Has this change been gradual or did it come on suddenly?

▶ This may alert the nurse to the presence of hypertension, associated heart failure, or endocrine problems. These ultimately affect the renal circulation and function of the kidneys.

5. Have you noticed any discharge from the urethra?
- If so, describe the color, odor, amount, and frequency.
- When did it start?
- Is this a recurrent problem? If so, what was the diagnosis?
- How was it treated?
- Did you follow the treatment as prescribed by the physician?

▶ Discharge signals the potential presence of an infective process.

6. Have you noticed any redness or other discoloration in the urethral area? If so, describe the characteristics.

▶ Redness may indicate the presence of inflammation, irritation, or infection.

7. Has your skin changed recently?
- Describe the change.
- Has the color changed?
- Is it itchy all the time?

▶ Patients with chronic renal failure have itchy skin (pruritus), and lichenification (a thickening of the skin) may develop (Adigun, Badu, Berner, & Oladele, 2015).

8. Have you recently had nausea, vomiting, diarrhea, or chills?
- If so, which one? Describe it.
- How was it treated?
- Has it recurred?

▶ These conditions may indicate the presence of infection or recurring infection.

9. Have you had any shortness of breath or difficulty breathing lately? If so, describe it.

▶ This may alert the nurse to the presence of hypertension and associated heart failure. These ultimately affect the renal circulation and function of the kidneys.

10. Do you have difficulty concentrating, reading, or remembering things?

▶ Difficulty remembering may be associated with **azotemia** (a buildup of wastes in the bloodstream because of renal dysfunction) (Toor, Liptzin, & Fischel, 2013). There are many conditions that contribute to memory disturbances.

Questions Related to Pain

When assessing pain, the nurse needs to gather information about the characteristics of the pain, which include quality, severity, location, duration, predictability, onset, relief, and radiation.

1. Do you ever have pain, burning, or other discomfort before, during, or after urination?
- If so, describe the discomfort, location, and timing.
- Do you have symptoms all of the time or some of the time?
- Is the discomfort predictable? For instance, is it related to time of the day or to certain foods or beverages?
- Do you feel it after sexual intercourse?

▶ Painful urination may indicate the presence of an infective process (Berman et al., 2016).

Focused Interview Questions	Rationales and Evidence

2. Do you have any pain or discomfort in your back, sides, or abdomen?
- If so, show me where the pain or discomfort is located.
- Describe the pain.
- What aggravates or alleviates the symptoms?

▶ Back or abdominal pain often accompanies renal disease (Berman et al., 2016).

3. Have you noticed any pain or discomfort when your urine is bloody?
- If so, describe the type, location, and timing of the discomfort.

▶ Hematuria without pain is often associated with bladder cancer (Ozkanli, Girgin, Kosemetin, & Zemheri, 2014).

Questions Related to Behaviors

1. Describe your diet.
- Describe what you have eaten and drunk over the last week.
- How is your appetite?
- On a typical day, how much do you eat and drink?
- Do you drink alcoholic beverages?
- How many glasses of water do you drink each day?
- Are there any foods or beverages that bother you?
- Do any foods or beverages cause you discomfort either before or upon urination?
- Do any foods or beverages cause you to feel bloated or gassy?
- Do any foods or beverages affect the color, clarity, or smell of your urine?
- How much salt do you use?
- Do you retain fluid after consuming certain foods or beverages?

▶ Questions such as these may provide information regarding the patient's hydration status, potential allergic reaction to foods, and retention of fluid.

2. Do you smoke, or are you exposed to passive smoke?
- If so, what is the source (cigarette, cigar, pipe)?
- For how long?
- How many packs per day?

▶ Smoking has been linked to hypertension, which over time may contribute to the development of renal failure. A history of smoking also significantly increases an individual's risk for developing bladder cancer (ACS, 2018b).

3. Do you use any recreational drugs?
- If so, describe the type, amount, and frequency.
- How long have you been using these drugs?

▶ Abuse of certain drugs over time may lead to kidney failure (National Institute on Drug Abuse [NIDA], 2017), potential for inadequate nutrition and hydration, and susceptibility to infection.

4. How often do you have intercourse?
- Do you urinate after intercourse?
- Are you aware of any sexual partners who may have sexually transmitted diseases?

▶ Some patients may have a tendency to develop UTIs if they do not urinate after intercourse (University of Maryland Medical Center [UMMC], 2013).

5. How do you cleanse yourself after urination or bowel movement?
- Do you use bubble bath?
- Do you use sprays, powders, or feminine hygiene products?

▶ Cleansing materials such as bubble bath, sprays, and powders may increase the incidence of UTIs. Improper cleansing methods after elimination may also lead to infection (UMMC, 2013).

Questions Related to Age and Pregnancy

The focused interview must reflect the anatomic and physiologic differences in the urinary system that exist along the age span as well as during pregnancy. Specific questions related to the urinary system for each of these groups are provided in Chapter 25, Chapter 26, and Chapter 27. ∞

Questions Related to the Environment

Environment refers to both the internal and external environments. Questions related to the internal environment include all of the previous questions and those associated with internal or physiologic responses. Questions regarding the external environment include those related to home, work, or social environments.

Internal Environment

1. What medications do you currently take?
- What medications have you been taking over the last several months?
- Describe the type, the dose, and the reason why you are taking the medication.
- How often do you take it? Every day, as needed, or only when you remember?

▶ It is important to know the patient's compliance with the medication regimen. If the patient has not completed a regimen of antibiotic therapy to clear a UTI, kidney infection, or sexually transmitted disease, the infection may persist (Wong & Stevens, 2013).

2. Do you take any vitamins, protein powders, or dietary supplements?
- If so, which ones?
- How much do you take?
- How many days a week do you take it?
- How many times a day?
- Why do you take it?

▶ Excessive ingestion of certain nutritional supplements or herbal agents may contribute to the development of renal disorders (Shaw, Graeme, Pierre, Elizabeth, & Kelvin, 2012).

Focused Interview Questions	Rationales and Evidence

External Environment

The following questions deal with substances and irritants found in the physical environment of the patient. The physical environment includes the indoor and outdoor environments of the home and workplace, those encountered for social engagements, and any encountered during travel.

1. **Do you live in an environment or work in an industry that exposes you to toxic chemicals?**

2. **Have you traveled recently to a foreign country or any unfamiliar place?**

▶ These may contribute to the development of cancer of the urinary system (ACS, 2018b).

Focused Interview Questions	Rationales and Evidence

FEMALE REPRODUCTIVE SYSTEM

General Questions

1. **Do you have any concerns about your reproductive health? Have you had concerns in the past? If so, please tell me about those concerns.**

   ▶ This question may prompt the patient to discuss any concerns about reproductive health.

2. **How old were you when you had your first menstrual period?**

   ▶ Onset of menses is influenced by a variety of factors including percentage of body fat. Menarche (onset of menstruation) between ages 11 and 14 indicates normal development. Late onset is associated with endocrine problems (Lee, Oh, Yoon, & Choi, 2012).

3. **What was the first day of your last menstrual period?**

   ▶ This establishes a pattern for the patient and has significance for physical assessment in relation to physical changes that occur at points throughout the cycle.

4. **How many days does your cycle usually last?**
   - Is this consistent with each period?
   - How many days does bleeding occur?

   ▶ A cycle is defined as the first day of one period to the first day of the next. These questions establish the pattern for the patient.

5. **Describe your menstrual flow.**
   - Is this consistent for each period?
   - How many tampons or pads do you use each day?
   - For how many days?

   ▶ Clotting and excessive bleeding warrant additional follow-up. Any uterine bleeding that the patient views as unusual warrants additional follow-up. The patient's assessment of her menstrual flow is subjective. Generally, an excessively heavy flow is characterized by use of more than one pad or tampon per hour (Mayo Clinic, 2017).

6. **How do you usually feel during your period? Is this a pattern for you?**

   ▶ This may provide clues as to whether discomfort is occurring. Dysmenorrhea (painful or difficult menstruation) is a common gynecologic disorder (Ju, Jones, & Mishra, 2014).

7. **How do you usually feel just before your period?**
   - Has this gotten worse or better?
   - Do you use any self-care remedies?

   ▶ Premenstrual syndrome (PMS) presents with a variety of signs and symptoms including irritability, headache, cramping, and breast engorgement. PMS usually occurs a few days before menstruation. Typically, sudden relief occurs with the onset of full menstrual flow.

8. **Do you take any medications for cramps?**
   - If so, what do you take and how much?
   - If not, how do you relieve your cramps?

9. **Are you sexually active?**

   ▶ The patient may feel pressured to be in a sexual relationship. These pressures may be external (expectations of family, friends, or work associates) or internal (fear of being viewed by others as less than desirable or not of an accepted sexual orientation, fear of being alone, or fear of not being loved and accepted).

Focused Interview Questions	Rationales and Evidence

10. Are there any obstacles to your ability to achieve sexual satisfaction?

▶ Causes of inability to achieve sexual satisfaction include fear of acquiring an STD; fear of being unable to satisfy the partner; fear of pregnancy; confusion regarding sexual preference; unwillingness to participate in sexual activities enjoyed by the partner; job stress; financial considerations; crowded living conditions; loss of partner; attraction to or sexual involvement with individuals the partner does not know about; criticism of sexual performance by the partner; or history of sexual trauma.

11. Have you noticed a change in your sex drive recently?

▶ This may be indicative of some physical or psychologic problems that need follow-up.

12. If the patient answers "yes" to question 11:
- Can you associate the change with anything in particular?

▶ Often patients can relate a decrease in sex drive with stress, illness, drug therapy, or some other factor (Mayo Clinic, 2018a; Nippoldt, 2017).

13. Do you use contraceptives?
- Which type of contraceptives do you use?
- How long have you been using contraceptives?
- Do you take oral contraceptives for a reason other than preventing pregnancy?
- Have you ever had any adverse effects from using contraceptives?

▶ This question provides information about the patient's knowledge about contraception, at-risk behaviors, and specific contraceptive devices or medications.

▶ In addition to preventing pregnancy, some women take oral contraceptives to regulate hormones and menstrual flow or to control symptoms of diseases such as polycystic ovarian syndrome. Discussing contraception use may provide insight into the patient's medical history.

14. Have you ever been pregnant? If so, how many times?

15. Did you have any problems during pregnancy, the birth, or postpartum?
- If the patient answers "yes": Describe the problem(s).

▶ Questions 14 through 16 provide information about significant obstetric history, which impacts current status and anticipated physical findings.

16. Was birth vaginal or by cesarean section?

17. Have you ever had a miscarriage?
- What were you told was the cause?
- Was surgery required?
- Have you ever had an abortion?
- At how many weeks, and by what method?
- How has it been emotionally since the abortion or miscarriage?

▶ Strong emotions often accompany the issue of termination of a pregnancy by either spontaneous or surgical abortion. The nurse may want to follow up.

18. Do you have children?
- If so, how many?

19. Have you tried to have children?
- If the patient answers "yes": How long have you been trying to conceive?
- If the patient indicates inability to conceive after 1 year: How often do you and your partner have intercourse?

▶ The couple is not considered potentially infertile unless they have been unable to conceive for a year (World Health Organization [WHO], 2018).

▶ For couples attempting to have a child, it is important to engage in intercourse routinely, such as two to three times a week (Mayo Clinic, 2016). Although nurses do not treat infertility, they may be involved in teaching the patient about certain measures that may be helpful, such as temperature tracking to determine the optimal time for intercourse. Concerns about infertility can produce great anxiety and depression for many women.

20. Have you ever sought professional help for fertility problems?
- If so, describe this experience.

▶ The patient can explain and describe specific diagnostic procedures and treatments for infertility as well as the emotional response to the processes and procedures.

21. Has an inability to conceive placed a strain on your relationship with your partner?
- How has this problem affected your relationship?
- How are you feeling about this?

▶ Specific questions enable the patient to affirm or deny relationship problems, to discuss changes in the relationship, and to discuss feelings about the partnership.

Questions Related to Illness or Infection

1. Do you now have or have you ever had an illness associated with the female reproductive system?
- When were you diagnosed with the problem?
- What was the treatment for the illness?
- Was the treatment helpful?
- What kinds of things do you do to help with the problem?
- Has the problem ever recurred?
- How are you managing the problem now?

▶ This allows the patient to provide her own perceptions about problems with her reproductive system.

Focused Interview Questions	Rationales and Evidence

2. ***Alternative to question 1:*** List common problems with the reproductive system such as dysmenorrhea, uterine fibroids, and uterine, ovarian, or vulvar cancer. Ask the patient to respond "yes" or "no" as each is stated.

▶ This is a comprehensive and easy way to elicit information about illnesses associated with the female reproductive system. Follow-up would be carried out for each identified diagnosis as in question 1.

3. **Do you now have or have you ever had an infection of the reproductive system?**
   - When were you diagnosed with the infection?
   - What treatment was prescribed for the problem?
   - Was the treatment helpful?
   - What kinds of things do you do to help with the problem?
   - Has the problem ever recurred (acute)?
   - How are you managing the infection now (chronic)?

▶ If an infection is identified, follow-up about the date of infection, treatment, and outcomes is required. Data about each infection identified by the patient are essential to an accurate health assessment. Infections can be classified as acute or chronic, and follow-up regarding each classification will differ.

4. ***Alternative to question 3:*** List possible infections, such as vaginitis, cystitis, and pelvic inflammatory disease (PID), and ask the patient to respond "yes" or "no" as each is stated.

▶ This is a comprehensive and easy way to elicit information about all reproductive system infections. Follow-up would be carried out for each identified infection as in question 3.

5. **Have you ever had any surgery of the reproductive system?**
   - If so, what was it? When? Where?
   - What was the outcome?

6. **Have you ever had an abnormal Pap smear?**
   - If so, how long ago was this?
   - What treatment, if any, did you receive?
   - Have you had follow-up Pap smears? When? What were the results?

▶ Questions 5 and 6 provide information about patient knowledge in regard to pathologies and treatments. This establishes variations in expected findings in a physical examination.

7. **Have you ever had an STD such as herpes, gonorrhea, syphilis, HPV, or chlamydia?**
   - *If the patient answers "yes":* Was it treated?
   - Did you inform your partner?
   - Was your partner treated?
   - Did you have sexual relations with your partner while you were infected?
   - *If the patient answers "yes":* Did you use condoms?
   - What treatment did you receive?

▶ Serious, sometimes fatal, complications can develop if treatment is delayed. STDs can be detected only by testing. If untreated, STDs can cause sterility and problems with the reproductive and other body systems (CDC, 2017d).

8. **Are you aware of having had any exposure to HIV?**
   - *If the patient answers "yes":* Describe the situation and how you believe you were exposed.
   - What are your views on sexual relations and the potential for acquiring HIV?

▶ The incidence of HIV is still greatly on the rise. Despite the wide availability of information on the risks and methods of protection for sexually active individuals, many women continue to have unprotected sex.

9. **Have you ever been tested for HIV?**
   - *If the patient answers "yes":* On one occasion or routinely?
   - What were the results of the test?

Questions Related to Symptoms, Pain, and Behaviors

When gathering information about symptoms, many questions are required to elicit details and descriptions that assist in the analysis of the data. Discrimination is made in relation to the significance of a symptom, in relation to specific diseases or problems, and in relation to potential follow-up examination or referral. One rationale may be provided for a group of questions in this category.

The following questions refer to specific symptoms and behaviors associated with the female reproductive system. For each symptom, questions and follow-up are required. The details to be elicited are the characteristics of the symptom; the onset, duration, and frequency of the symptom; the treatment or remedy for the symptom, including over-the-counter and home remedies; the determination if diagnosis has been sought; the effect of treatments; and family history associated with a symptom or illness.

Questions Related to Symptoms

1. **Have you noticed any rashes, blisters, ulcers, sores, or warts on your genital area or surrounding areas?**

▶ Rashes may occur with yeast infections, which are the most common female genital infection. Yeast infections generally produce redness, pruritus (itching), and cottage cheese–like discharge. Herpes infection causes small painful ulcerations, whereas syphilitic chancres are not painful. In the older patient, a raised, reddened lesion may indicate carcinoma of the vulva. Reddened lesions that eventually weep and form crusts characterize contact dermatitis. Venereal warts are cauliflower shaped (Osborn, Wraa, Watson, & Holleran, 2013).

Focused Interview Questions	Rationales and Evidence
2. Have you felt any lumps or masses in your genital area or surrounding areas? • If so, describe the mass. Exactly where is it? • About what size? • Is it soft or hard? • Is it movable? • When did you first notice the mass? • Is it painful? • Have you noticed any change in it since it developed? • Have you used any remedies, such as ice, heat, or creams?	▶ Sebaceous cysts can be noted in the labial area. A lump created by an abscess of the Bartholin's gland causes localized pain. An abscess of the Bartholin's gland may indicate the presence of gonorrhea (Kessous et al., 2013).
3. Have you noticed any swelling or redness of your genitals?	▶ Vulvovaginitis may cause edema in the genital and perineal area, including the vulva. Redness and swelling may indicate an alteration in health, such as an abscess of the Bartholin's gland, which may be caused by gonorrhea. Bruising may indicate sexual trauma.
4. Have you noticed any changes in the appearance of your vaginal opening? • Have you felt any pressure from your vagina? • Have you felt bulging or masses from within your vagina?	▶ Uterine prolapse may be so severe that the uterus protrudes into and at times out of the vagina. Surgery may be indicated.
5. Have you experienced any itching in your labia or vaginal area? • If so, when did it start? • Has it been treated and, if so, how? • Have there been any associated urinary symptoms?	▶ Crab lice, atrophic vaginitis, candidiasis, and contact dermatitis may cause intense itching.
6. Have you noticed any discharge from your vagina? • If so, what color is it? • Is there any odor to it? • Is it a small, moderate, or large amount? • When did you first notice the discharge?	▶ Vaginal discharge is a typical complaint of patients with vaginitis. The most common presenting symptom in women with STDs is vaginal discharge; however, the patient may have no symptoms (Xu et al., 2013).
7. Have you had any vaginal bleeding outside the time of your normal menstrual period?	▶ Abnormal bleeding may be related to hormonal influences and may be easily corrected. Conditions such as uterine fibroids and several forms of cancer can also cause abnormal bleeding patterns (Permanente Medical Group, 2018).
8. If the patient answers "yes" to question 7: • When did it occur? How much bleeding was there?	▶ The nurse should obtain quantitative data by asking whether panties were saturated or how many pads or tampons were saturated in 24 hours. A calendar should be used to determine the number of days since the patient's last menstrual period.
9. Have you had any problems in and around your rectal area, such as pain, itching, burning, or bleeding? • When did the problem begin? • Do you know the cause of the problem? • Have you sought health care for the problem? • Was a diagnosis made? • What treatment was prescribed? • What do you do to help with the problem? • Has the treatment helped?	▶ Pain, itching, bleeding, or burning may indicate the presence of abuse; infection; irritation; or injury to the anus, rectum, or perineum. Rectal bleeding, pain, and irritation may result from passing hard stools, from hemorrhoids, or from injuries. Fungal infection may result in pruritus or irritation of the perianal area (Osborn et al., 2013).
	▶ When symptoms in the perianal area are associated with hemorrhoids or hard stool, follow-up would include questions about diet, exercise, and bowel habits.
	▶ Irritation or injury to the perianal area can occur as a result of sexual practices or sexual abuse involving anal intercourse. Sensitive questioning about these topics is required when sexual activity is described or when sexual abuse is suspected or disclosed.
Questions Related to Pain **1. Do you have any pain, tenderness, or soreness in your pelvic area?** • If so, describe the pain. • Is it dull? Sharp? Radiating? Intermittent? Continuous? • When did it start? • Are you having any pain in the area now? • What lessens the pain or makes it worse? • Do you have associated symptoms of headache, vomiting, or diarrhea?	▶ Common causes of gynecologic pain include infection, menstrual difficulties, endometriosis (abnormal condition involving the endometrial lining of the uterus), ectopic pregnancy (fetus implanted in abnormal location), threatened abortion, pelvic masses, uterine fibroids, and ovarian cancer (Osborn et al., 2013).

Focused Interview Questions	**Rationales and Evidence**

Questions Related to Behaviors

1. **How often do you get physical examinations?**

▶ Screening for problems of the genitourinary system is typically performed during routine physical or gynecologic examinations.

2. **Do you use tampons?**
   - If so, how frequently do you change the tampons?
   - Are you aware of the risk for toxic shock syndrome with the use of tampons?
   - Are you aware of the signs of toxic shock?

▶ Tampons, when not used cautiously (e.g., lack of frequent changes), have been linked with toxic shock syndrome (MacPhee et al., 2013).

3. **What kinds of products do you use for hygiene in the genital area?**

▶ Use of soap, sprays, powders, and douche products can irritate the tissues of the reproductive system. Some studies suggest that females who have used talc in the genital area for many years may be at increased risk of developing ovarian cancer.

4. ***If the patient is sexually active:*** Are you in a mutually monogamous relationship? If not, how many sexual partners have you or your partner had over the last year? Do you or your partner regularly use protection during sexual intercourse?

▶ Sexual activity with many different partners increases the risk of acquiring STDs and, possibly, certain gynecologic cancers.

▶ Use of protection (e.g., male or female condoms) can reduce the risk of acquiring STDs.

5. **Are you able to be sexually aroused?**
   - Has this ability changed over time or recently?

▶ A variety of factors may interfere with a woman's ability to be sexually aroused. These factors include prescribed or illicit drug use, disorders of the nervous or endocrine systems, stress, and fear (e.g., of intimacy, inability to satisfy a partner, acquiring an STD, or becoming pregnant).

6. **Are you satisfied with your sexual experiences?**
   - *If the patient expresses dissatisfaction:* Are you able to achieve orgasm?
   - Have you noticed a change in your ability to have an orgasm?

▶ A variety of factors may interfere with a woman's ability to experience orgasm.

7. **Are you using contraception?**
   - If so, what kind?
   - Are you using it consistently?

▶ This provides information about knowledge of contraception in general and regarding the products indicated by the patient.

8. **Would you like to know more about the use of birth control?**

▶ This is a very important question to ask adolescents who shy away from talking about sexual practices but have verbalized that they are sexually active.

9. **How do you protect yourself from sexually transmitted diseases, including HIV?**

▶ Abstinence is the only 100% effective protection against STDs. Latex condoms offer significant protection, especially when treated with spermicide; however, they are not 100% effective (CDC, 2013).

Questions Related to Age and Pregnancy

The focused interview must reflect the anatomic and physiologic differences in the female reproductive system that exist along the age span as well as during pregnancy. Specific questions related to the female reproductive system for each of these groups are provided in Chapter 25, Chapter 26, and Chapter 27. ∞

Questions Related to the Environment

Environment refers to both the internal and external environments. Questions related to the internal environment include all of the previous questions and those associated with internal or physiologic responses. Questions regarding the external environment include those related to home, work, or social environments.

Internal Environment

1. **Do you know if your mother received diethylstilbestrol (DES) treatment during pregnancy with you?**

▶ Studies indicate that daughters of mothers who received DES during pregnancy have a significantly higher number of reproductive tract problems, including cervical cancer, infertility, and ectopic pregnancy (Laronda, Unno, Butler, & Kurita, 2012). This may have some bearing on the current problem. If the patient answers "yes" to this question, the nurse should refer her to a physician.

2. **Do you drink alcohol? How many drinks per week?**

▶ Intake of alcoholic beverages can contribute to an individual taking chances, such as failing to ask the partner to use condoms.

3. **Do you use illicit drugs? If so, what type and how much?**

▶ Taken in sufficient amounts, some drugs, such as marijuana and opiates, may decrease libido. Drug use may also contribute to failure to use protection against STDs.

Focused Interview Questions	Rationales and Evidence

External Environment

The following questions deal with substances and irritants found in the physical environment of the patient. The physical environment includes the indoor and outdoor environments of the home and the workplace, those encountered for social engagements, and any encountered during travel.

1. Do your family and friends support your relationship with your sexual partner?

2. Are you able to talk to your partner about your sexual needs?
   • Does your partner accept your needs and help you fulfill them?
   • Are you able to do the same for your partner?

3. Some patients come to a healthcare provider to discuss sexual abuse.
   • Have you ever been forced to have sexual intercourse or other sexual contact against your will?
   • Have you ever been molested or raped?
   • *If the patient answers "yes"*: When was this?
   • Who abused you?
   • What was the experience?
   • What was done about the situation and for you?

▶ The patient's family and friends can influence the patient's sexual relationship in a variety of ways. The patient may feel tension if the partner is not accepted.

▶ The ability to openly discuss sexual needs and preferences fosters strong and lasting relationships.

Patient-Centered Interaction

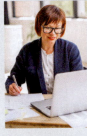

Source: Olena Kachmar/123RF.

Ms. Angela Carbone, age 55, comes to the Medi-Center at 10:30 a.m. with the chief complaint of left back pain. She has some nausea but denies vomiting. She complains of dysuria and gross hematuria and indicates she had a kidney stone on the right side several years ago. The following is an excerpt from the focused interview with Ms. Carbone.

Interview

Nurse: Good morning. Ms. Carbone. Are you having pain now?

Ms. Carbone: Yes, I am.

Nurse: On a scale of zero to ten with ten being the highest, how do you rate your pain?

Ms. Carbone: Now it is about four, but I'm afraid it will become ten or twelve like the last time.

Nurse: I need to ask you some questions to get information from you. Will you be able to talk to me for a few minutes?

Ms. Carbone: I think so! I'll try. I'll let you know if I can't sit any more.

Nurse: Tell me about the pain.

Ms. Carbone: I have back pain on my left side, right here (pointing to the left costovertebral area). It feels like it moves down my back but not all the time. It really hurts and is getting worse each day.

Nurse: When did the pain start?

Ms. Carbone: It started about five days ago. That's when I noticed my urine was darker than usual.

Nurse: Did you do anything to help reduce the pain?

Ms. Carbone: Not really. At first I thought I slept funny. Then my urine got darker. I tried to drink three glasses of water a day, but I became nauseated and had to stop drinking.

Nurse: Earlier you commented that you are afraid the pain will become ten or twelve like the last time. Tell me more.

Ms. Carbone: I had a kidney stone about three years ago on my right side. Now the pain is similar on the left side.

Analysis

The nurse immediately asked Ms. Carbone about her current pain status to determine her ability to participate in the interview. Throughout the interview, the nurse used open-ended questions and leading statements. These statements encouraged verbalization by the patient to explore and describe actions and feelings in detail. The open-ended questions and leading statements permitted the patient to provide detail, thereby eliminating the need for multiple closed questions.

Objective Data—Physical Assessment

Assessment Techniques and Findings

Physical assessment of the urinary and reproductive systems follows an organized pattern. Knowledge of normal or expected findings is essential in determining the meaning of the data as the nurse conducts the physical assessment. In addition, assessment of the patient's psychosocial health, self-care habits, family, culture, and environment should be considered during the physical examination. Before proceeding, it may be helpful to practice the techniques of physical assessment of this system. In addition, health records and results of laboratory and diagnostic tests are important secondary sources to be reviewed and included in the data-gathering process (see Table 22.1).

Examination of the urinary system is often incorporated into the assessment of the abdomen and begins with a survey of the patient's general appearance followed by inspection of the abdomen. The renal arteries are auscultated, and then the costovertebral angles and flank areas are inspected, palpated, and percussed. The kidneys are palpated. Bladder fullness is determined by palpation and percussion of the lower abdomen. Physical assessment of the female reproductive system begins with inspection of the external genitalia and perianal area. The physical assessment of the female reproductive system beyond what is described here is considered an advanced level skill and is discussed in Appendix C. ∞

During the physical assessment, the nurse will assess and evaluate the occasional ambiguous cues of actual and potential disease of the genitourinary system and the variety of contributors to the development of pathology. The nurse documents and

Table 22.1 Potential Secondary Sources for Patient Data Related to the Female Genitourinary System

LABORATORY TESTS FOR THE FEMALE URINARY SYSTEM	NORMAL VALUES
Blood Chemistry	
Albumin	3.5–5 g/dL
Ammonia	15–45 mcg/dL
Blood Urea Nitrogen (BUN)	6–23 mg/dL
Creatinine	Female 0.6–1.1 mg/dL
Urinalysis	
Color	Yellow-straw
Specific Gravity	1.005–1.030
pH	5–8
Glucose	Negative
Sodium	10–40 mEq/L
Potassium	<8 mEq/L
Chloride	25–40 mEq/L
Protein	negative–trace
Osmolality	500–800 mOsm/L
Urine Culture, Colony Count, Sensitivity	Varies
Diagnostic Tests	
Angiography	
Computed Tomography (CT)	
Cystoscopy	
Cystourethography	
Intravenous Urography	
Magnetic Resonance Imaging (MRI)	
Radionuclide Scanning	
Tissue and Cell Sampling—Kidney Biopsy	
Ultrasonography	
Urine Cytology	

(continued)

Table 22.1 Potential Secondary Sources for Patient Data Related to the Female Genitourinary System (continued)

LABORATORY TESTS FOR THE FEMALE REPRODUCTIVE SYSTEM	NORMAL VALUES
Follicle Stimulating Hormone (FSH)	Before puberty: 0–4 mIU/mL
	During puberty: 0.3–10 mIU/mL
	Women who are menstruating: 4.7–21.5 mIU/mL
	Postmenopausal: 25.8–134.8 mIU/mL
	Pregnant women: too low to measure
Luteinizing Hormone (LH)	5–25 International units/L
Progesterone	Female (preovulation): less than 1 ng/mL
	Female (midcycle): 5 to 20 ng/mL
	Postmenopausal: less than 1 ng/mL
Estradiol	Female (premenopausal): 30–300 pg/mL
	Female (postmenopausal): <15 pg/mL
Pap Smear	Normal
Serum Studies for STDs	
Diagnostic Tests	
Endometrial Biopsy	
Hysterosalpingogram	
Hysteroscopy	
Laparoscopy	
Pelvic/Transvaginal Ultrasonography	

communicates the findings to the other members of the healthcare team. Additionally, the nurse has a key role in teaching the patient how to establish and maintain reproductive wellness. Throughout assessment of the female reproductive system, the nurse considers not only the function of the reproductive system but also the patient's sexual fulfillment on both a physical and psychologic basis.

To be efficient in gathering data, nurses need to understand their own feelings and comfort about various aspects of sexuality. They must put aside personal beliefs and values about sexual practices and focus in a nonjudgmental manner on gathering data to determine the health status of the patient.

It is essential to create an atmosphere that facilitates open communication and comfort for the patient. Patients commonly experience anxiety, fear, and embarrassment when asked for information about a topic that, in most patients' minds, is very personal. These emotions may be expressed either verbally or nonverbally. The nurse should approach the patient in as nonthreatening a manner as possible and assure the patient that the information provided and the results of the physical assessment will remain confidential.

EQUIPMENT

- Examination gown and drape
- Clean, nonsterile examination gloves
- Handheld mirror
- Stethoscope

HELPFUL HINTS

- Provide a warm, private environment.
- Have the patient void and empty bowels before the assessment.
- Use appropriate draping to maintain the patient's dignity.
- Determine if the patient has had this kind of assessment before. If not, sharing booklets with diagrams are helpful before proceeding.
- It is helpful to show the patient pictures of equipment, slides, and the bimanual assessment.
- Use an unhurried, deliberate manner and ask the patient how she is doing as the assessment proceeds.
- Explore and remedy cultural or language issues at the onset of the interaction.
- Use Standard Precautions.

Techniques and Normal Findings	Abnormal Findings and Special Considerations

FEMALE URINARY SYSTEM

General Survey

A quick survey of the patient enables the nurse to identify any immediate problem as well as the patient's ability to participate in the assessment.

1. **Instruct the patient.**
   - Explain that you will be looking, listening, touching, and tapping on parts of the abdomen. Tell the patient you will explain each procedure as it occurs. Tell the patient to report any discomfort and that you will stop the examination if the procedure is uncomfortable.

2. **Position the patient.**
   - Begin the examination with the patient in a supine position with the abdomen exposed from the nipple line to the pubis (see Figure 22.6 ■).

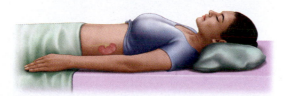

Figure 22.6 Position the patient.

3. **Assess the general appearance.**
   - Assess the general appearance and inspect the patient's skin for color, hydration status, scales, masses, indentations, or scars.
   - The patient should not show signs of acute distress and should be mentally alert and oriented.

   ▶ Patients with kidney disorders frequently look tired and complain of fatigue. If a kidney disorder is suspected, it is important to look for signs of circulatory overload (pulmonary edema) or peripheral edema (puffy face or fingers) or indications of pruritus (scratch marks on the skin).

4. **Inspect the abdomen for color, contour, symmetry, and distention.**
   - It may be helpful to stand at the foot of the examination table and inspect the abdomen from there (see Figure 22.7 ■).
   - Note that visual inspection of the suprapubic area may confirm the presence or absence of a distended bladder.

   ▶ Elevated nitrogenous wastes (azotemia) in the blood contribute to mental confusion.

   ▶ A distended bladder may be visible in the suprapubic area, indicating the need to void and perhaps the inability to do so.

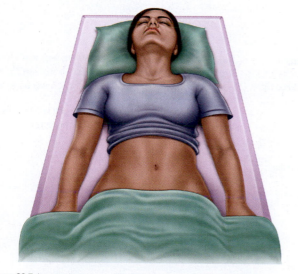

Figure 22.7 Inspecting the abdomen from the foot of the bed.

Techniques and Normal Findings	Abnormal Findings and Special Considerations

- Normally, the patient's abdomen is not distended, is relatively symmetric, and is free of bruises, masses, and swellings. (A complete discussion of abdominal assessment is provided in Chapter 20). ∞

5. Auscultate the right and left renal arteries to assess circulatory sounds.
- Gently place the bell of the stethoscope over the extended midclavicular line (MCL) on either side of the abdominal aorta, which is located above the level of the umbilicus (see Figure 22.8 ■).
- Be sure to auscultate both the right and left sides, and over the epigastric and umbilical areas.
- In most cases, no sounds are heard; however, an upper abdominal bruit, a swishing or murmurlike sound, is occasionally heard in young adults and is considered normal. On a thin adult, renal artery pulsation may be auscultated.

▶ Many diseases may contribute to abdominal distention. These include renal conditions such as polycystic kidney disease; enlarged kidneys, as seen in acute pyelonephritis; ascites (accumulation of fluid) because of hepatic disease; and displacement of abdominal organs. Pressure from the abdominal contents on the diaphragm may alter the patient's breathing pattern.

▶ Presence of a bruit may indicate narrowing or obstruction of a blood vessel.

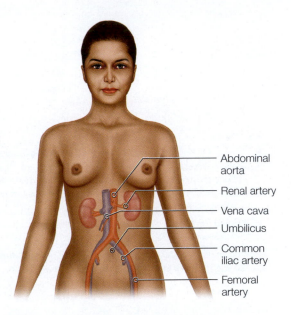

Abdominal aorta
Renal artery
Vena cava
Umbilicus
Common iliac artery
Femoral artery

Figure 22.8 Auscultation sites for identification of bruits.

6. For patients with a urinary catheter, inspect the catheter for signs of infection, correct placement, and urinary outflow.
- Patients with limited mobility, such as patients with paralysis, recent surgery, or a fractured hip, will likely use an indwelling catheter or undergo intermittent catheterization.
- Inspect the urine and urethral meatus for signs of infection, irritation, tenderness, and cleanliness.
- Inspect the collection bag for fullness, and empty it if needed; also, inspect the bag and tubing for possible obstructions.
- Inspect the bag for correct placement on the leg, and ensure that the bag is lower than the bladder at all times.
- Record urine outflow and fluid intake to ensure that the urinary drainage system is working properly.

▶ Because of the high risk of infection, the need for a catheter should be assessed at every interaction. Signs of infection include hematuria, foul-smelling or cloudy urine, and lower back pain.

▶ Improper drainage of the catheter may result in urinary backflow into the bladder, which is a major cause of infection.

The Female Kidneys and Flanks

1. Position the patient.
- Place the patient in a sitting position facing away from you with the patient's back exposed.

2. Inspect the left and right costovertebral angles for color and symmetry.
- The color should be consistent with the rest of the back.

3. Inspect the flanks (the side areas between the hips and the ribs) for color and symmetry.
- The costovertebral angles and flanks should be symmetric and even in color.

▶ A protrusion or elevation over a costovertebral angle occurs when the kidney is grossly enlarged or when a mass is present.

▶ This finding must be carefully correlated to other diagnostic cues as the assessment proceeds. If ecchymosis is present (Grey Turner's sign), there may be other signs of trauma, such as blunt, penetrating wounds or lacerations.

Techniques and Normal Findings	**Abnormal Findings and Special Considerations**

▶ Pain, discomfort, or tenderness from an enlarged or diseased kidney may occur over the costovertebral angle, flank, and abdomen. When questioned, the patient complains of a dull, steady ache. This type of pain is associated with polycystic formation, pyelonephritis, and other disorders that cause kidney enlargement. In the patient with polycystic kidney disease, a sharp, sudden, intermittent pain may mean that a cyst in the kidney has ruptured. If the costovertebral angle is tender, red, and warm, and if the patient is experiencing chills, fever, nausea, and vomiting, the underlying kidney could be inflamed or infected.

ALERT! *Do not percuss or palpate the patient who reports pain or discomfort in the pelvic region. Do not percuss or palpate the kidney if a tumor of the kidney is suspected, such as a neuroblastoma or Wilms' tumor. Palpation increases intra-abdominal pressure, which may contribute to intraperitoneal spreading of this neuroblastoma. Deep palpation should be performed only by experienced practitioners.*

4. **Gently palpate the area over the left costovertebral angle (see Figure 22.9 ■).**
  • Watch the reaction, and ask the patient to describe any sensation the palpation causes. Normally, the patient expresses no discomfort.

▶ The pain caused by calculi (stones) in the kidney or upper ureter is unique and different in character, severity, and duration than that caused by kidney enlargement. This pain occurs as calculi travel from the kidney to the ureters and the urinary bladder.

▶ Some patients experience no pain, and others feel excruciating pain. A stationary stone causes a dull, aching pain. As stones travel down the urinary tract, spasms occur. These spasms produce sharp, intermittent, colicky pain (often accompanied by chills, fever, nausea, and vomiting) that radiates from the flanks to the lower quadrants of the abdomen and, in some cases, the upper thigh and scrotum or labium.

▶ If the patient reports severe pain, hematuria (blood in the urine) or **oliguria** (diminished volume of urine), and nausea and vomiting, it is important to be alert for hydroureter, a frequent complication that occurs when a renal calculus moves into the ureter. The calculus blocks and dilates the ureter, causing spasms and severe pain. Hydroureter can lead to shock, infection, and impaired renal function. If the nurse suspects hydroureter or obstruction at any point in the urinary tract, medical collaboration must be sought immediately.

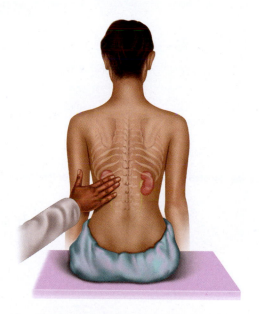

Figure 22.9 Palpating the costovertebral angle.

Techniques and Normal Findings	Abnormal Findings and Special Considerations

5. Use blunt or indirect percussion to further assess the kidneys.
- Place your left palm flat over the left costovertebral angle.
- Thump the back of your left hand with the ulnar surface of your right fist, causing a gentle thud over the costovertebral angle (see Figure 22.10 ■).

▶ Pain or discomfort during and after blunt percussion suggests kidney disease. This finding is correlated with other assessment findings.

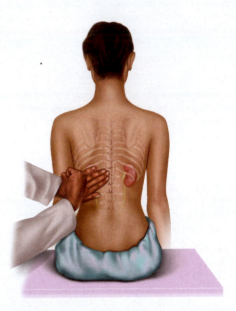

Figure 22.10 Blunt percussion over the left costovertebral angle.

6. Repeat the procedure on the right side. Ask the patient to describe the sensation as you examine each side.
- The patient should feel no pain or tenderness with pressure or percussion.

Appendix C: Advanced Skills *Appendix C provides step-by-step instructions on palpation of the kidneys.*

The Female Urinary Bladder

1. Palpate the bladder to determine symmetry, location, size, and sensation.
- Use light palpation over the lower portion of the abdomen. The abdomen should be soft.
- Use deep palpation to locate the fundus (base) of the bladder, approximately 5 to 7 cm (2 to 2.5 in.) below the umbilicus in the lower abdomen. Once you have located the fundus of the bladder, continue to palpate, outlining the shape and contour (see Figure 22.11 ■). Bimanual palpation may be required in the obese patient.

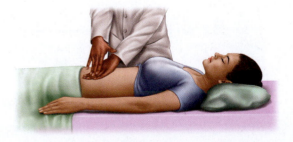

Figure 22.11 Palpating the bladder.

Techniques and Normal Findings	Abnormal Findings and Special Considerations
• Slide your fingers over the surface of the bladder and continue palpating to determine smoothness and continuity. • The surface of the bladder should feel smooth and uninterrupted. An empty bladder is usually not palpable. When the bladder is moderately full, it should be firm, smooth, symmetric, and nontender. As the bladder fills, the fundus can reach the level of the umbilicus. A full bladder is firm and buoyant.	▶ A distended bladder feels smooth, round, and taut. An asymmetric contour or nodular surface suggests abnormal growth that should be correlated with other findings.
2. Percuss the bladder to determine its location and degree of fullness. • Begin with indirect percussion in the midline of the abdomen at the level of the umbilicus. • Move your fingers downward as you continue to percuss toward the suprapubic area. Continue percussing downward until tympanic tones change to dull tones. A full bladder produces a dull sound. The point at which tympanic tones cease is the upper margin of the bladder. • Some practitioners conclude the assessment of the urinary system with the inspection and palpation of the urethral meatus. Other practitioners consider these structures with the assessment of the genitalia.	▶ Bladder scanning or bedside bladder ultrasonography is a safe, noninvasive technique to assess bladder fullness in suspected urinary retention.

FEMALE REPRODUCTIVE SYSTEM

Inspection

1. Instruct the patient.
- Explain to the patient that you will be looking at and touching her external genital area. Tell her that it should not cause discomfort, but if pain occurs she should tell you and you will stop. Explain that deep breathing is a good way to relax during the examination.
- Tell the patient you will provide instructions and explanations at each point in the assessment.

2. Position the patient.
- Ask the patient to lie down on the examination table.
- Assist her into the lithotomy position (supine with knees and hips flexed so that feet rest flat on the examination table), and then have her slide her hips as close to the end of the table as possible.
- Place her feet in the stirrups (see Figure 22.12 ■).

▶ In the obese patient, the presence of large thighs and extra adipose tissue in the perineal area may require having an assistant to hold thighs apart or to move extra tissue during the examination. It may be necessary to raise the hips and increase flexion of the hips to visualize genital structures.

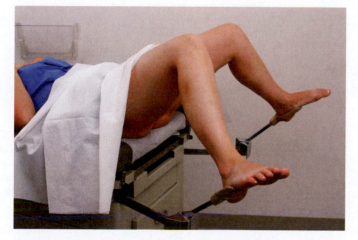

Figure 22.12 Positioning the patient.

Techniques and Normal Findings	Abnormal Findings and Special Considerations

3. Inspect the pubic hair.

- Confirm that the hair grows in an inverted triangle and is scattered heavily over the mons pubis. It should become sparse over the labia majora, perineum, and inner thighs (see Figure 22.13 ■).

▶ A sparse hair pattern may be indicative of delayed puberty. It is also a common and normal finding in women of Asian ancestry. The elderly patient's pubic hair will become sparse, scattered, and gray.

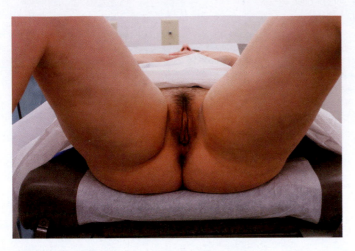

Figure 22.13 Inspecting the pubic hair.

- If the patient has complained of itching in the pubic area, comb through the pubic hair with two or three fingers.
- Confirm the absence of small, bluish gray spots, or nits (eggs), at the base of the pubic hairs.

▶ These signs indicate pubic lice (crabs). Marks may be visible from persistent scratching to relieve the intense itching caused by the lice.

4. Inspect the labia majora.

- Confirm that the labia majora are fuller and rounder in the center of the structure and that the skin is smooth and intact.
- Compare the right and left labia majora for symmetry.
- Observe for any lesions, warts, vesicles, rashes, or ulcerations. If you notice drainage, note the color, distribution, location, and characteristics.

▶ The labia majora of older women may be thinner and wrinkled.

▶ These findings may signal a variety of conditions. *Contact dermatitis* appears as a red rash with associated lesions that are weepy and crusty. There often are scratches because of intense itching.

▶ **Genital warts** are raised, moist, cauliflower-shaped papules.

▶ The herpes simplex virus (HSV) may produce red, painful vesicles accompanied by localized swelling of the genitals and surrounding areas. Genital herpes is usually caused by herpes simplex virus type 2 (HSV-2).

- Remember to change gloves as needed during the exam to prevent cross-contamination. Also remember to culture any abnormal discharge.

- Confirm the absence of any swelling or inflammation in the area of the labia majora.

▶ Swelling over red, inflamed skin that is tender and warm to palpation may indicate an abscess in the Bartholin's gland. The abscess may be caused by gonorrhea. Labia and other structures in the perineum may be edematous in the obese patient as a result of pressure in the groin from the enlarged abdomen.

5. Inspect the labia minora.

- Confirm that the labia minora are smooth, pink, and moist.
- Observe for any redness or swelling. Note any bruising or tearing of the skin.

6. Inspect the clitoris.

- Place your right or left hand over the labia majora and separate these structures with your thumb and index finger.
- The clitoris should be midline, about 1 cm (0.39 in.) in length, with more fullness in the center. It also should be smooth.
- Observe for any redness, lesions, or tears in the tissue.

▶ An elongated clitoris may signal elevated levels of testosterone and warrants further investigation and referral to a physician.

Techniques and Normal Findings	**Abnormal Findings and Special Considerations**

7. Inspect the urethral orifice.

- Confirm that the urethral opening is midline, pink, smooth, slitlike, and patent (see Figure 22.14 ■).

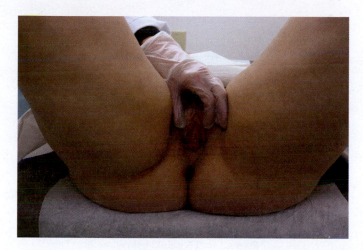

Figure 22.14 Inspection of the urethra.

- Ask the patient to cough. No urine should leak from the urethral opening.

- Inspect for any redness, inflammation, or discharge.

▶ Urine leakage indicates stress incontinence and weakening of the pelvic musculature.

▶ These symptoms indicate urinary tract infection. Pressure of the enlarged abdomen in the obese patient may lead to urinary incontinence, resulting in redness and excoriation.

8. Inspect the vaginal opening, perineum, and anal area.

- Confirm that the vaginal opening or introitus is pink and round. It may be either smooth or irregular.
- Locate the **hymen** (a thin layer of skin within the vagina). It may be present in women who have never had sexual intercourse; however, certain activities, including tampon usage or vigorous exercise, may result in hymen rupture despite the absence of sexual activity (Hegazy & Al-Rukban, 2012).
- Inspect for tears, bruising, or lacerations.

▶ Tears, bruising, or lacerations could be because of forceful, consensual sex or rape. Additional follow-up is needed after examination. It is important not to ask any questions that the patient may interpret as probing or threatening during the physical assessment.

- The perineum (the space between the vaginal opening and anal area) should be smooth and firm.
- Scars from episiotomy procedures may be observed in parous women. These are normal.
- The anus should be intact, moist, and darkly pigmented. There should be no lesions.

▶ Fecal incontinence is common in the obese patient because of increased abdominal pressure on the bowel and anal sphincter. This may result in redness or excoriation.

- Have the patient bear down.

▶ Thin, fragile perineal tissues indicate atrophy. Tears and fissures may indicate trauma.

Techniques and Normal Findings	Abnormal Findings and Special Considerations

- Inspect for any protrusions from the vagina.

▶ A **prolapsed uterus** may protrude right at the vaginal wall with straining, or it may hang outside of the vaginal wall with any straining (see Figure 22.15 ■).

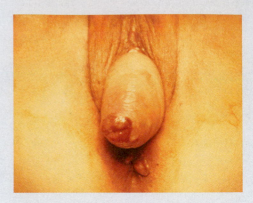

Figure 22.15 Prolapsed uterus.
Source: DELALANDE/BSIP SA/Alamy Stock Photo.

▶ A **cystocele** is a hernia that is formed when the urinary bladder is pushed into the anterior vaginal wall.

▶ A **rectocele** is a hernia that is formed when the rectum pushes into the posterior vaginal wall.

Appendix C: Advanced Skills *Appendix C provides step-by-step instructions on the inspection of the female pelvis with a speculum, obtaining a PAP smear and gonorrhea culture, and bimanual palpation.*

Documenting Your Findings

Documentation of assessment data—subjective and objective—must be accurate, professional, complete, and confidential. When documenting the information from the focused assessment of each body system, the nurse should use measurements where appropriate to ensure accuracy, use medical terminology rather than jargon, include all pertinent information, and avoid language that could identify the patient. The information in the documentation should make it clear what questions were asked and should use language to indicate whether it is the patient's response or the nurse's findings. For patient responses the documentation will say "denies," "states," or "reports," whereas the nurse's findings will simply list the findings as fact, or will note "no" along with the condition—for example, patient reports "urine is clear and yellow with no odor" and the nurse found "no pain with suprapubic palpation; no CVA tenderness." See an example of normal results for the female genitourinary system below.

Urinary System

Skin is moist and supple with pink undertones. The abdomen is symmetric and free of lesions, bruises, and swelling. The renal arteries are without bruits. The costovertebral angle and flanks are symmetric, even in color, and nontender to palpation and percussion. The kidneys are not enlarged; they are rounded, smooth, firm, and nontender. The bladder is nonpalpable, and percussion reveals tympany above the symphysis pubis.

Female Reproductive System

Pubic hair is distributed in an even, inverted triangular pattern over the mons pubis. Hair distribution is less dense over the labia, perineum, and inner thighs. The labia majora are symmetric, smooth, and without lesions. The labia minora are smooth, pink, and moist. The clitoris is smooth, midline, and about 1 cm (0.39 in.) in length. The urethra is slitlike, midline, smooth, pink, and patent. The vaginal opening is pink and round. On bearing down, there is no urine leakage at the meatus or protrusions from the vagina. The perineum is smooth and firm. The anus is intact, moist, darkly pigmented, and without lesions.

Abnormal Findings of the Female Urinary System

Common alterations of the urinary system include bladder cancer, kidney and urinary tract infections, calculi, tumors, renal failure, and changes in urinary elimination. Each of these alterations is discussed in Table 22.2.

Table 22.2 Abnormal Findings of the Female Urinary System

Bladder Cancer

Seen later in life, bladder cancer occurs more frequently in men than in women. A history of smoking has been linked to this disease. In some cases, the patient who experiences bladder cancer is asymptomatic.
If signs and symptoms are present:

Subjective findings:
- Flank pain
- Dysuria

Objective findings:
- Hematuria
- Frequent urination
- Edema in lower extremities
- Pelvic mass

Glomerulonephritis

This condition is an inflammation of the glomerulus.

Subjective findings:
- Fatigue
- Changes in urinary patterns

Objective findings:
- Hypertension
- Generalized edema
- Hematuria
- Proteinuria

Renal Calculi

Calculi are stones that block the urinary tract. They are usually composed of calcium, struvite, or a combination of magnesium, ammonium, phosphate, and uric acid.

Subjective findings:
- Radiating pain that is variable in location and severity
- Ureteral spasms
- Nausea
- Dysuria
- Increased urinary urgency

Objective findings:
- Vomiting
- Increased urinary frequency
- Gross hematuria

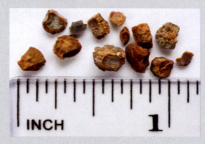

Renal calculi.
Source: piotr_malczyk/iStock/Getty Images.

Renal Tumor

Renal tumors may be either benign or malignant, with malignant being more common. Research has shown that there is an association with renal tumors and smoking.

Subjective findings:
- Flank pain
- Lethargy

Objective findings:
- Hematuria
- Weight loss
- Palpable flank mass

Renal Failure

Renal failure may be acute or may progress to a chronic state. Acute renal failure that does not progress to a chronic state includes three stages: oliguria, diuresis, and recovery. Signs and symptoms of uremia, which is the hallmark of chronic renal failure, may include anorexia, nausea, vomiting, altered mentation, uremic frost, weight loss, fatigue, and edema.

Subjective findings:
- Anorexia
- Nausea
- Pruritus
- Fatigue

Objective findings:
- Fluid retention
- Electrolyte imbalances (such as hyperkalemia and hyperphosphatemia)
- Vomiting
- Uremia
- Changes in mentation

Urinary Tract Infection

Bacteria cause urinary tract infections (UTIs). The bladder is the most common site of the infection, which results in inflammation of the bladder (cystitis); however, infection may include the kidneys. UTIs are common with catheter use for urinary retention or incontinence. Therefore, patients with catheters should be assessed regularly for UTIs. Patients may be asymptomatic.

Subjective findings:
- Increased urinary urgency
- Dysuria
- Suprapubic or lower back pain

Objective findings:
- Increased urinary frequency
- Hematuria
- Cloudy, foul-smelling urine

Changes in Urinary Elimination

The following are examples of alterations in urinary elimination:

Dysreflexia affects patients with spinal cord injuries at level T7 or higher. Bladder distention causes a sympathetic response that can trigger a potentially life-threatening hypertensive crisis.

Incontinence is the inability to retain urine. If this is the patient's problem, the nurse must determine which of the five types of incontinence is present.
- *Functional incontinence* occurs when the patient is unable to reach the toilet in time because of environmental, psychosocial, or physical factors.
- *Reflex incontinence* occurs in patients with spinal cord damage when urine is involuntarily lost.
- *Stress incontinence* (involuntary urination) occurs when intra-abdominal pressure is increased during coughing, sneezing, or straining. Aging changes may also contribute to stress incontinence.
- *Urge incontinence* may be caused by consuming a significant volume of fluids over a relatively short period. Urge incontinence may also be because of diminished bladder capacity.
- *Total incontinence* is related to a neurologic condition.

Urinary retention is a chronic state in which the patient cannot empty the bladder. In most cases, the patient voids small amounts of overflow urine when the bladder reaches its greatest capacity.

Abnormal Findings of the Female Reproductive System

Abnormal findings from assessment of the female genitourinary system include but are not limited to problems with the external genitalia, perianal area, cervix, internal reproductive organs, and inflammatory processes. Problems in the perianal area are described in this chapter. Abnormal findings of the external genitalia are depicted and described in Table 22.3. Abnormal findings of the cervix are illustrated and described in Table 22.4. Common inflammatory processes in the female reproductive system are depicted and described in Table 22.5. Abnormal findings of the perianal area are described and illustrated in Table 22.6.

Table 22.3 Abnormal Findings of the Female External Genitalia

Pediculosis Pubis

Nits and lice are on and around roots of pubic hair and cause itching. The area is reddened and excoriated.

Herpes Simplex

A sexually transmitted disease caused by the herpes simplex virus (HSV), these small vesicles appear on the genitalia and may spread to the inner thigh. Ulcers are painful and may rupture. The virus may be dormant for long periods.

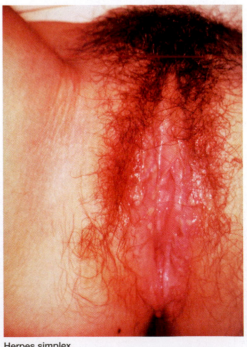

Herpes simplex.
Source: Lester V. Bergman/Corbis NX/Getty Images.

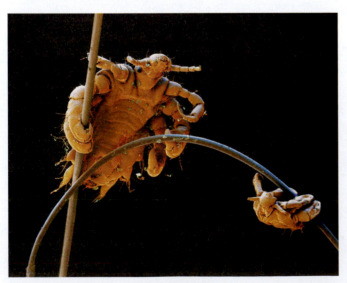

Pediculosis pubis (crab lice, magnification 40X).

(continued)

Table 22.3 Abnormal Findings of the Female External Genitalia (continued)

Syphilitic Lesion

A nontender solitary papule that gradually changes to a draining ulcer. A rash of syphilitic lesions typically develops during the second stage of symptoms associated with syphilis. In most cases, the first stage of syphilis presents as a single chancre (CDC, 2017e).

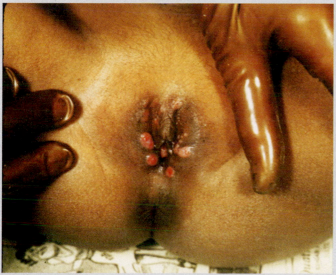

Syphilitic lesions.
Source: Centers for Disease Control and Prevention (CDC)

Human Papillomavirus (HPV)

Infection with this sexually transmitted disease causes wartlike, painless growths that appear in clusters. These are seen on the vulva, inner vagina, cervix, or anal area.

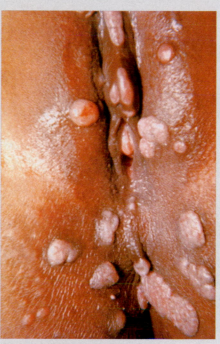

Human papillomavirus (genital warts).
Source: Centers for Disease Control and Prevention (CDC)

Abscess of Bartholin's Gland

The Bartholin's gland may become obstructed, causing fluid to back up and form a cyst. Cysts range in size from 1 cm to 3 cm or larger. If infected, a cyst develops into an abscess that includes labial edema and erythema with a palpable mass. There is purulent drainage from the duct.

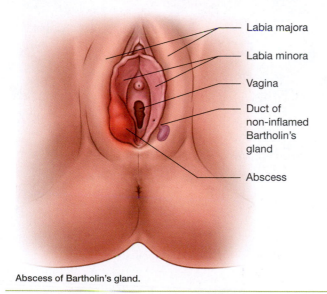

Labia majora

Labia minora

Vagina

Duct of non-inflamed Bartholin's gland

Abscess

Abscess of Bartholin's gland.

Table 22.4 Abnormal Findings of the Cervix

Cyanosis

Cyanosis of the cervix is associated with hypoxic conditions such as congestive heart failure (CHF). Blue coloring of the cervix is normal in pregnancy.

Diethylstilbestrol (DES) Syndrome

Abnormalities of the cervix arise in women who had prenatal exposure to DES. Epithelial abnormalities occur as granular patchiness extending from the cervix to the vaginal walls.

Carcinoma

Ulcerations with vaginal discharge, postmenopausal bleeding or spotting, or bleeding between menstrual periods are characteristics of cervical carcinoma. Diagnosis is confirmed by Pap smear.

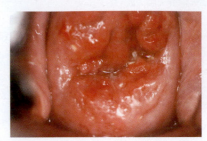

Cervical carcinoma.
Source: Centers for Disease Control and Prevention (CDC)

Erosion

Inflammation and erosion are visible on the surface of the cervix. It is difficult to distinguish erosion from carcinoma without a biopsy.

Polyp

A soft, fingerlike growth extends from the cervical os. A polyp is usually bright red and may bleed. Polyps are usually benign.

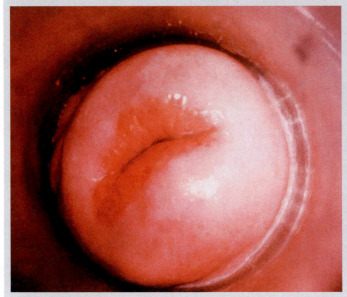

Erosion of the cervix.
Source: Centers for Disease Control and Prevention (CDC)

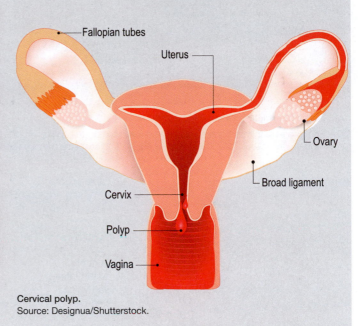

Cervical polyp.
Source: Designua/Shutterstock.

Table 22.5 Common Inflammatory Processes in the Female Reproductive System

Atrophic Vaginitis

Estrogen deficiency in postmenopausal women results in dryness, itching, and burning sensations in the vagina. The vaginal mucosa may appear pale with mucousy discharge.

Chlamydia

A sexually transmitted disease (STD) that is often asymptomatic, characterized by purulent discharge with tenderness to movement of the cervix. Chlamydia can cause sterility if untreated.

Pelvic Inflammatory Disease (PID)

An infection of a woman's reproductive organs. PID may cause lower abdominal pain, fever, malodorous discharge from the vagina, painful intercourse or urination, or irregular menstrual bleeding (CDC, 2017c).

Candidiasis

Alteration of the pH of the vagina or antibiotic use predispose women to this condition. The vulva and vagina are erythematous. Thick, cottage cheese-like white discharge is seen.

Gonorrhea

This sexually transmitted disease is caused by a bacterial infection. One may see vaginal discharge or bleeding and abscesses in Bartholin's or Skene's glands; generally asymptomatic.

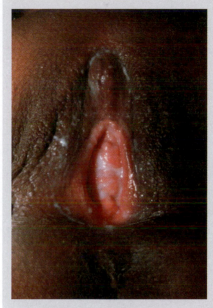

Candidiasis (yeast infection).
Source: Aubert/Science Source.

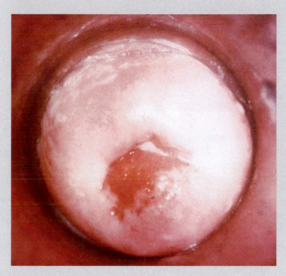

Gonorrhea.
Source: Centers for Disease Control and Prevention (CDC)

Trichomoniasis

This is a sexually transmitted disease that causes painful urination, vulvular itching, and purulent vaginal discharge. The vagina and vulva are reddened, and the discharge is yellow and foul smelling.

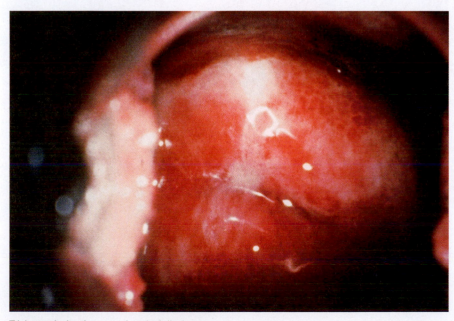

Trichomoniasis, close-up of vaginal discharge.
Source: PR BOUREE/BSIP SA/Alamy Stock Photo.

Table 22.6 Abnormalities of the Perianal Area

Pilonidal Cyst

Seen as dimpling in the sacrococcygeal area at the midline. An opening is visible and may reveal a tuft of hair. Usually asymptomatic, these cysts may become acutely abscessed or drain chronically.

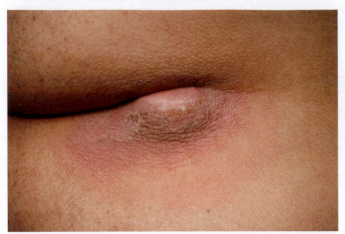

Pilonidal cyst.

Source: Alan Nissa/Shutterstock.

Anal Fissure

Tears or splits in the anal mucosa that are usually seen in the posterior anal area and most frequently associated with the passage of hard stools or prolonged diarrhea. They are most common in young infants.

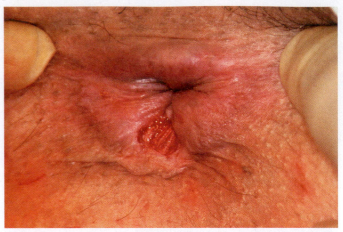

Anal fissure.

Source: BSIP SA/Alamy Stock Photo.

Hemorrhoids (Internal)

Varicosities of the hemorrhoidal veins of the anus or lower rectum. Internally, they occur in the venous plexus superior to the mucocutaneous junction of the anus and are rarely painful. Identified by bright red bleeding that is unmixed with stool.

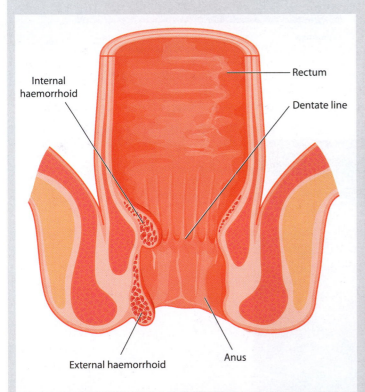

Hemorrhoids, internal.

Source: Blamb/Shutterstock.

Hemorrhoids (External)

Varicosities of the hemorrhoidal veins of the anus or lower rectum. Externally, they occur in the inferior venous plexus inferior to the mucocutaneous junction. Rarely bleed. Cause anal irritation and create difficulty with cleansing the area.

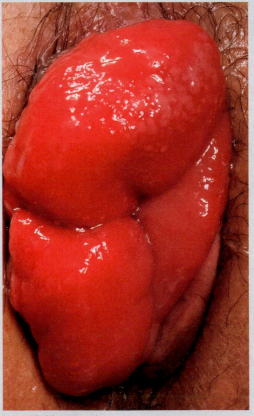

Hemorrhoids, external.

Source: Casa nayafana/Shutterstock.

(continued)

Table 22.6 Abnormalities of the Perianal Area (continued)

Perianal Perirectal Abscess

Painful and tender abscesses with perianal erythema; generally caused by infection of an anal gland. Can lead to fistulas (openings between the anal canal and outside skin).

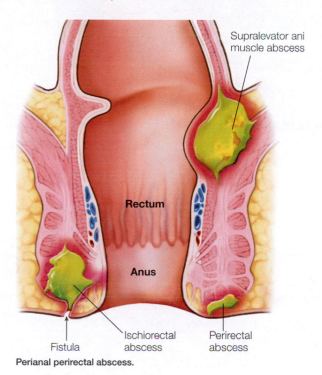

Perianal perirectal abscess.

Prolapse of the Rectum

Occurs when the rectal mucosa, with or without the muscle, protrudes through the anus. In mucosal prolapse, a round or oval pink protrusion is seen outside the anus. When the muscular wall is involved, a large red protrusion is visible.

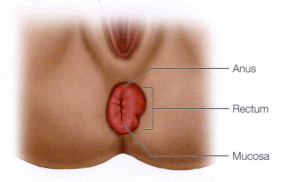

Prolapse of the rectum.

Disorders of the Female Internal Reproductive Organs

Abnormal findings of the internal reproductive organs include myomas/fibroids, ovarian cancer, and ovarian cysts and are described as follows.

MYOMAS/FIBROIDS

Myomas, or uterine fibroids, are tumors that consist of smooth muscle tissue. They may form in several locations, including the uterine cavity or the uterine muscles (see Figure 22.16 ■). Although the exact cause is unknown, estrogen is believed to influence their development (Osborn et al., 2013). Some patients who experience this disorder will be asymptomatic.

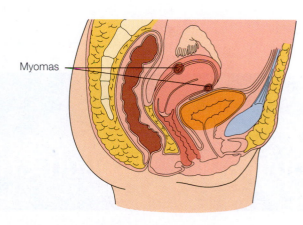

Figure 22.16 Myomas/fibroids.

Subjective findings:
- Abdominal pain
- Constipation
- Frequent urination
- Excessive menstrual bleeding

Objective findings:
- Uterine enlargement
- Abdominal distention
- Intestinal obstruction

OVARIAN CANCER

Ovarian cancer (see Figure 22.17 ■) is a type of cancer that begins in the cells of the ovaries and includes the epithelial and germ cells. Although this form of cancer may occur in women of any age, it is most common among women who are ages 50 to 60. Factors that increase the risk for development of ovarian cancer include estrogen hormone replacement therapy, smoking, and never being pregnant (Mayo Clinic, 2018b). In early stages, patients who experience ovarian cancer may be asymptomatic.

Subjective findings:
- Abdominal pressure or cramping
- Unexplained weight loss
- Changes in bowel habits
- Loss of appetite
- Pain in the calves or lower back

Objective findings:
- Abdominal bloating
- Ascites
- Abnormal vaginal bleeding

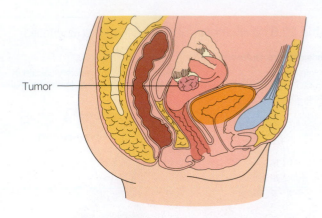

Figure 22.17 Ovarian cancer.

OVARIAN CYSTS

Ovarian cysts are nonmalignant vesicles that may develop at any point between puberty and menopause. These fluid-filled sacs form within the ovary or on the ovarian surface (see Figure 22.18 ■). Some patients who experience ovarian cysts may be asymptomatic.

Subjective findings:
- Pelvic pain
- Lower back pain
- Pain during intercourse

Objective findings:
- Abdominal distention
- Vomiting
- Increased urination
- Menstrual irregularities

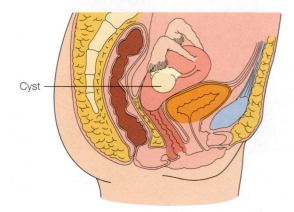

Figure 22.18 Ovarian cysts.

Application Through Critical Thinking

CASE STUDY

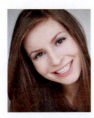

Source: Miroslava Levina / Shutterstock

Jessica Johnson, a 24-year-old Caucasian female, arrives in the clinic with lower abdominal pain and nausea. She states, "I've had this throbbing pain for three days, and it kept getting worse." She further states, "I haven't been able to eat. I feel awful. You have to do something for the pain."

The nurse explains that more information is needed so that the proper treatment can be initiated. In further interview, the following information is obtained. Ms. Johnson's last menstrual period was 1 week ago, and she had more cramping than usual. She has had brownish, thick vaginal discharge on and off since then. She has had some itchiness in the vaginal area and burning when she voids. She states she has to go to the bathroom all the time: "All I did was pee little bits, until this pain got to me. I have hardly gone since last night."

When asked about the pain, Ms. Johnson says it is mostly 8 on a scale of 1 to 10 and getting pretty constant. "Nothing I do helps, except it helps a little if I curl up and hold still."

Physical assessment reveals a thin, pale female.

VS: BP 108/64, P 92, RR 20, T 101.4°F.

Skin is hot, dry, poor turgor.

Mucous membranes dry. Posture—abdominal guarding.

Abdomen BS × 4, tender in RLQ & LLQ to palpation. Vulvar pruritus, thick purulent vaginal drainage, pain upon cervical and uterine movement.

Cultures from vaginal secretions obtained   To lab

Blood drawn for CBC   To lab

Urine specimen obtained—clear, yellow   To lab

The patient's clinic record reveals that she has been sexually active since age 16. She has had multiple partners and one abortion. She has been treated for an STD three times, most recently 2 months before this visit. The patient is on birth control pills. She has no allergies to medications, and no family history of cardiovascular, abdominal, neurologic, urologic, endocrine, or reproductive disease.

Interpretation of the data suggests a diagnosis of PID. The options are outpatient treatment with antibiotics and education about limitations in activity and sexual practices, or inpatient treatment with intravenous fluids, antibiotics, analgesia, and bed rest.

Because Ms. Johnson is acutely ill, with pain and dehydration, she is admitted to the acute care facility with a diagnosis of PID.

SAMPLE DOCUMENTATION

The following is sample documentation for Jessica Johnson.

SUBJECTIVE DATA: Throbbing abdominal pain for 3 days and getting worse. Rated 8 on scale of 1 to 10 with slight relief when "curled up and still." Nausea, unable to eat. LMP 1 week ago with increased cramping. Brownish thick vaginal discharge. Vaginal itchiness. Urgent, burning urination of small amounts until past 12 hours. Sexually active with history of multiple partners, recent STD. No family history of disease, no allergies to medication.

OBJECTIVE DATA: Thin, pale female. Dry mucous membranes, skin hot, dry, poor turgor. Abdominal guarding, BS present × 4, tender RLQ, LLQ to light palpation. Vulvar pruritus, purulent vaginal discharge, adnexal tenderness with vaginal and bimanual examination.

CRITICAL THINKING QUESTIONS

1. What clusters of information suggest the diagnosis of PID?
2. What additional information is required to develop a plan of care for Jessica Johnson?
3. What would discharge planning for Ms. Johnson include?
4. What environmental considerations should you screen for in a young woman of childbearing age during the patient interview?

REFERENCES

Adigun, M., Badu, L. A., Berner, N. M., & Oladele, A. A. (2015). *Uremic pruritis review.* Retrieved from https://www.uspharmacist.com/article/uremic-pruritus-review

American Cancer Society (ACS). (2018a). *About cervical cancer.* Retrieved from https://www.cancer.org/cancer/cervical-cancer/about.html

American Cancer Society (ACS). (2018b). *Bladder cancer risk factors.* Retrieved from https://www.cancer.org/cancer/bladder-cancer/causes-risks-prevention/risk-factors.html

American Cancer Society (ACS). (2018c). *Key statistics for cervical cancer.* Retrieved from https://www.cancer.org/cancer/cervical-cancer/about/key-statistics.html

The American College of Obstetricians and Gynecologists (ACOG). (2017a). *Cervical cancer screening.* Retrieved from https://www.acog.org/Patients/FAQs/Cervical-Cancer-Screening

The American College of Obstetricians and Gynecologists (ACOG). (2017b). *Ovarian cancer.* Retrieved from https://www.acog.org/Patients/FAQs/Ovarian-Cancer

The American College of Obstetricians and Gynecologists (ACOG). (2017c). *Well-woman recommendations.* Retrieved from https://www.acog.org/About-ACOG/ACOG-Departments/Annual-Womens-Health-Care/Well-Woman-Recommendations

Berman, A., Snyder, S. J., & Frandsen, G. (2016). *Kozier and Erb's fundamentals of nursing: Concepts, process, and practice* (10th ed.). Hoboken, NJ: Pearson Education, Inc.

Brookes, D. C., & Hawn, M. (2018). *Classification, clinical features, and diagnosis of inguinal and femoral hernias in adults.* Retrieved from https://www.uptodate.com/contents/classification-clinical-features-and-diagnosis-of-inguinal-and-femoral-hernias-in-adults

Centers for Disease Control and Prevention (CDC). (2013). *Condoms and STDs: Fact sheet for public health personnel.* Retrieved from http://www.cdc.gov/condomeffectiveness/docs/condoms_and_stds.pdf

Centers for Disease Control and Prevention (CDC). (2016). *Human papillomavirus: Questions and answers.* Retrieved from https://www.cdc.gov/hpv/parents/questions-answers.html

Centers for Disease Control and Prevention (CDC). (2017a). *Cancers associated with human papillomavirus, United States—2010–2014. USCS data brief, no. 1.* Atlanta, GA: Centers for Disease Control and Prevention. Retrieved from https://www.cdc.gov/cancer/hpv/pdf/USCS-DataBrief-No1-December2017-508.pdf

Centers for Disease Control and Prevention (CDC). (2017b). *Condom effectiveness.* Retrieved from https://www.cdc.gov/condomeffectiveness/index.html

Centers for Disease Control and Prevention (CDC). (2017c). *Pelvic inflammatory disease (PID)*. Retrieved from http://www.cdc.gov/std/pid/stdfact-pid.htm

Centers for Disease Control and Prevention (CDC). (2017d). *Sexually transmitted diseases (STDs): STDs & infertility.* Retrieved from http://www.cdc.gov/STD/infertility/default.htm

Centers for Disease Control and Prevention (CDC). (2017e). *Syphilis: CDC fact sheet.* Retrieved from http://www.cdc.gov/std/syphilis/stdfact-syphilis-detailed.htm

Centers for Disease Control and Prevention (CDC). (2018). *Get tested for chronic kidney disease.* Retrieved from http://www.cdc.gov/features/worldkidneyday

Devarajan, P. (2014). *Oliguria*. Retrieved from http://emedicine.medscape.com/article/983156-overview#aw2aab6b2b2

Forsgren, C., Lundholm, C., Johansson, A. L., Cnattingius, S., Zetterström, J., & Altman, D. (2012). Vaginal hysterectomy and risk of pelvic organ prolapse and stress urinary incontinence surgery. *International Urogynecology Journal, 23*(1), 43–48. doi:10.1007/s00192-011-1523-z

Hegazy, A. A., & Al-Rukban, M. O. (2012). Hymen: Facts and conceptions. *The Health, 3*(4), 109–115.

Institute on Aging. (2017). *The physical—and psychological—effects of urinary incontinence on older adults* [Blog post]. Retrieved from https://blog.ioaging.org/medical-concerns/physical-psychological-effects-urinary-incontinence-older-adults

Ju, H., Jones, M., & Mishra, G. (2014). The prevalence and risk factors of dysmenorrhea. *Epidemiologic Reviews, 36*(1), 104–113. doi:10.1093/epirev/mxt009

Kessous, R., Aricha-Tamir, B., Sheizaf, B., Steiner, N., Moran-Gilad, J., & Weintraub, A. Y. (2013). Clinical and microbiological characteristics of Bartholin gland abscesses. *Obstetrics & Gynecology, 122*(4), 794–799. doi:10.1097/AOG.0b013e3182a5f0de

Laronda, M. M., Unno, K., Butler, L. M., & Kurita, T. (2012). The development of cervical and vaginal adenosis as a result of diethylstilbestrol exposure in utero. *Differentiation, 84*(3), 252–260. doi:10.1016/j.diff.2012.05.004

Lee, D. Y., Oh, Y. K., Yoon, B. K., & Choi, D. (2012). Prevalence of hyperprolactinemia in adolescents and young women with menstruation-related problems. *American Journal of Obstetrics and Gynecology, 206*(3), 213.e1–213.e5. doi:10.1016/j.ajog.2011.12.010

MacPhee, R. A., Miller, W. L., Gloor, G. B., McCormick, J. K., Hammond, J. A., Burton, J. P., & Reid, G. (2013). Influence of the vaginal microbiota on toxic shock syndrome toxin 1 production by Staphylococcus aureus. *Applied and Environmental Microbiology, 79*(6), 1835–1842. doi:10.1128/AEM.02908-12

Marieb, E. N., & Keller, S. M. (2018). *Essentials of human anatomy and physiology* (12th ed.). New York, NY: Pearson.

Mayo Clinic. (2016). *Getting pregnant: How to get pregnant.* Retrieved from http://www.mayoclinic.org/healthy-living/getting-pregnant/in-depth/how-to-get-pregnant/art-20047611

Mayo Clinic. (2017). *Menorrhagia (heavy menstrual bleeding): Symptoms.* Retrieved from http://www.mayoclinic.org/diseases-conditions/menorrhagia/basics/symptoms/con-20021959

Mayo Clinic. (2018a). *Low sex drive in women.* Retrieved from https://www.mayoclinic.org/diseases-conditions/low-sex-drive-in-women/symptoms-causes/syc-20374554

Mayo Clinic. (2018b). *Ovarian cancer: Risk factors.* Retrieved from http://www.mayoclinic.org/diseases-conditions/ovarian-cancer/basics/risk-factors/con-20028096

Mirza, S. A., & Rooney, C. (2018). Discrimination prevents LGBTQ people from accessing health care. *Center for American Progress.* Retrieved from https://www.americanprogress.org/issues/lgbt/news/2018/01/18/445130/discrimination-prevents-lgbtq-people-accessing-health-care/

Moore, K., & Spence, K. (2014). Urinary tract infection. *Hospital Medicine Clinics, 3*(1), e93–e110. doi:10.1016/j.ehmc.2013.09.003

Nasari, H., & Rafieian-Kopaei, M. (2015). Diabetes mellitus and renal failure: Prevention and management. *Journal of Research in Medical Sciences, 20*(11), 1112–1120. doi:10.4103/1735-1995.172845

National Institute of Diabetes and Digestive and Kidney Diseases. (2012). Primary hyperparathyroidism. Retrieved from https://www.niddk.nih.gov/health-information/endocrine-diseases/primary-hyperparathyroidism

National Institute on Drug Abuse (NIDA). (2017). *Medical consequences of drug abuse: Kidney damage.* Retrieved from http://www.drugabuse.gov/publications/medical-consequences-drug-abuse/kidney-damage

National Kidney Foundation. (2017). *Genetics and kidney disease.* Retrieved from https://www.kidney.org/news/kidneyCare/winter10/Genetics

Nippoldt, T. B. (2017). *Is loss of sex drive normal as a man gets older?* Retrieved from https://www.mayoclinic.org/healthy-lifestyle/sexual-health/expert-answers/loss-of-sex-drive/faq-20058237

Office of Minority Health (OMH). (2016). *Diabetes data and statistics.* Retrieved from https://minorityhealth.hhs.gov/omh/content.aspx?ID=2913

Osborn, K. S., Wraa, C. E., Watson, A., & Holleran, R. S. (2013). *Medical-surgical nursing: Preparation for practice* (2nd ed.). Upper Saddle River, NJ: Pearson.

Ozkanli, S., Girgin, B., Kosemetin, D., & Zemheri, E. (2014). Case report – Hemangioma of the urinary bladder. *Science, 3*(1), 15–16. doi:10.11648/j.sjcm.20140301.14

Palma, T., Raimondi, M., Souto, S., Fozzatti, C., Palma, P., & Riccetto, C. (2014). Correlation between body mass index and overactive bladder symptoms in pre-menopausal women. *Revista Da Associacao Medica Brasileira, 60*(2), 111–117. doi:10.1590/1806-9282.60.02.007

Permanente Medical Group. (2018). Abnormal vaginal bleeding (irregular periods) in adults. Retrieved from https://mydoctor.kaiserpermanente.org/ncal/mdo/presentation/conditions/condition_viewall_page.jsp?condition=Condition_Abnormal_Vaginal_Bleeding_in_Adults_-_Ob_Gyn.xml

Population Reference Bureau. (2014). *Female genital mutilation/cutting: Data and trends.* Retrieved from https://assets.prb.org/pdf14/fgm-wallchart2014.pdf

Shaw, D., Graeme, L., Pierre, D., Elizabeth, W., & Kelvin, C. (2012). Pharmacovigilance of herbal medicine. *Journal of Ethnopharmacology, 140*(3), 513–518. doi:10.1016/j.jep.2012.01.051

Stöppler, M. C. (2012). *Cloudy urine.* Retrieved from http://www.medicinenet.com/cloudy_urine/symptoms.htm

Toor, R., Liptzin, B., & Fischel, S. V. (2013). Hospitalized, elderly, and delirious: What should you do for these patients? *Current Psychiatry, 12*(8), 10–18. Retrieved from https://www.mdedge.com/sites/default/files/Document/September-2017/010_0813CP_Liptzin_Cov_FINAL.pdf

University of Maryland Medical Center (UMMC). (2013). *Urinary tract infection.* Retrieved from http://umm.edu/health/medical/reports/articles/urinary-tract-infection

Urology Care Foundation. (2018). *What is urinary incontinence?* Retrieved from https://www.urologyhealth.org/urologic-conditions/urinary-incontinence

Wong, C. J., & Stevens, D. L. (2013). Serious Group A Streptococcal infections. *Medical Clinics of North America, 97*(4), 721–736. doi:10.1016/j.mcna.2013.03.003

World Health Organization (WHO). (2018). *Sexual and reproductive health: Infertility definitions and terminology.* Retrieved from http://www.who.int/reproductivehealth/topics/infertility/definitions/en

Xu, F., Stoner, B. P., Taylor, S. N., Mena, L., Martin, D. H., Powell, S., & Markowitz, L. E. (2013). "Testing-only" visits: An assessment of missed diagnoses in patients attending sexually transmitted disease clinics. *Sexually Transmitted Diseases, 40*(1), 64–69. doi:10.1097/OLQ.0b013e31826f32f3

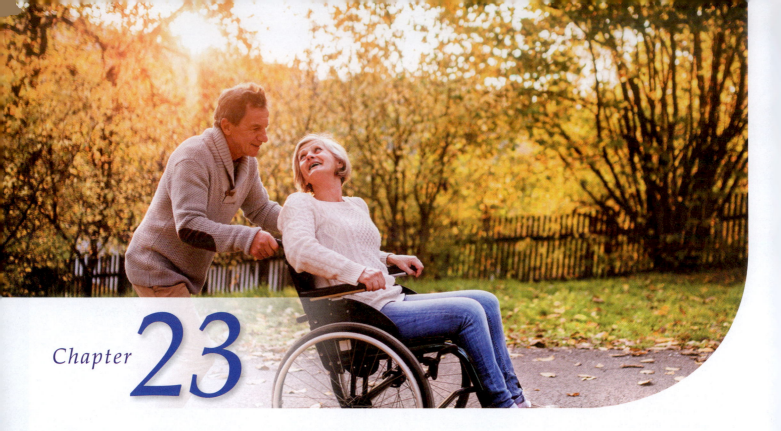

Chapter 23

Musculoskeletal System

LEARNING OUTCOMES

Upon completion of this chapter, you will be able to:

1. Describe the anatomy and physiology of the musculoskeletal system.

2. Identify the anatomic, physiologic, developmental, psychosocial, and cultural variations that guide assessment of the musculoskeletal system.

3. Determine which questions about the musculoskeletal system to use for the focused interview.

4. Outline the techniques for assessment of the musculoskeletal system.

5. Generate the appropriate documentation to describe the assessment of the musculoskeletal system.

6. Identify abnormal findings in the physical assessment of the musculoskeletal system.

KEY TERMS

MEDICAL LANGUAGE

ab- Prefix meaning "away from"

ad- Prefix meaning "toward"

arthr- Prefix meaning "joint"

circum- Prefix meaning "around"

dorsi- Prefix meaning "back"

hyper- Prefix meaning "high," "elevated," "above normal"

osteo- Prefix meaning "bone"

Introduction

The primary function of the musculoskeletal system is to provide structure and movement for the human body. The 206 bones of the musculoskeletal system and accompanying skeletal muscles allow the body to stand erect and move, and they support and protect body organs. This system produces red blood cells, stores fat and minerals, and generates body heat.

A thorough assessment of the musculoskeletal system provides data relevant to activity, exercise, nutrition, and metabolism. The physical assessment of the musculoskeletal system is extensive, requiring a head-to-toe approach because it extends throughout the body. Musculoskeletal assessment could be combined with assessment of other body systems to obtain data reflecting the patient's total health status, because every other body system is affected by or affects this body system. For example, should the patient have difficulty moving a specific part of the body, the nurse will need to collect data that are useful in determining whether the origin of the problem is neurologic or musculoskeletal. Bone density and curvatures vary widely among people of different cultural groups. Working conditions that require heavy lifting, repetitive motions, or substantial physical activity present potential risks to this system. Participation in hobbies and athletic activities can contribute to wear-and-tear damage to joints and create risks for trauma to bones, muscles, and joints.

Anatomy and Physiology Review

The musculoskeletal system consists of the bones, skeletal muscles, and joints. A thorough discussion of these anatomic structures is included in the following sections.

Bones

The bones support and provide a framework for the soft tissues and organs of the body. They are classified according to shape and composition. Bone shapes include *long bones* (e.g., femur, humerus); *short bones* (e.g., carpals, tarsals); *flat bones* (e.g., the parietal bone of the skull, the sternum, ribs); and *irregular bones* (e.g., vertebrae, hip bones) as shown in Figure 23.1 ■. Bones are

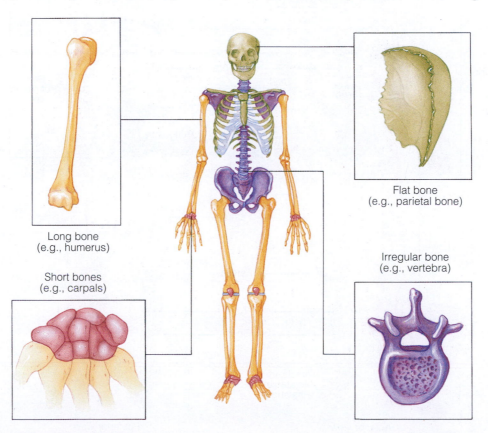

Long bone
(e.g., humerus)

Short bones
(e.g., carpals)

Flat bone
(e.g., parietal bone)

Irregular bone
(e.g., vertebra)

Figure 23.1 Classification of bones according to shape.

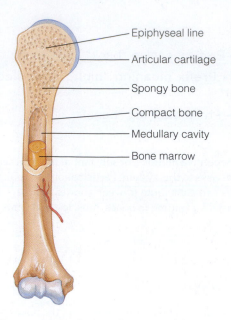

Epiphyseal line

Articular cartilage

Spongy bone

Compact bone

Medullary cavity

Bone marrow

Figure 23.2 Composition of a long bone.

composed of osseous tissue that is arranged in either a dense, smooth, compact structure or a cancellous, spongy structure with many small open spaces (see Figure 23.2 ■). The bones of the human skeleton are illustrated in Figure 23.3 ■.

The major functions of the bones include providing a framework for the body, protecting structures, acting as levers for movement, storing fat and minerals, and producing blood cells.

Skeletal Muscles

A skeletal muscle is composed of hundreds of thousands of elongated muscle cells or fibers arranged in striated bands that attach to skeletal bones (see Figure 23.4 ■). Although some skeletal muscles react by reflex, most skeletal muscles are voluntary and are under an individual's conscious control. Figure 23.5 ■ illustrates the muscles of the human body. The major functions of the skeletal muscles include providing for movement, maintaining posture, and generating body heat.

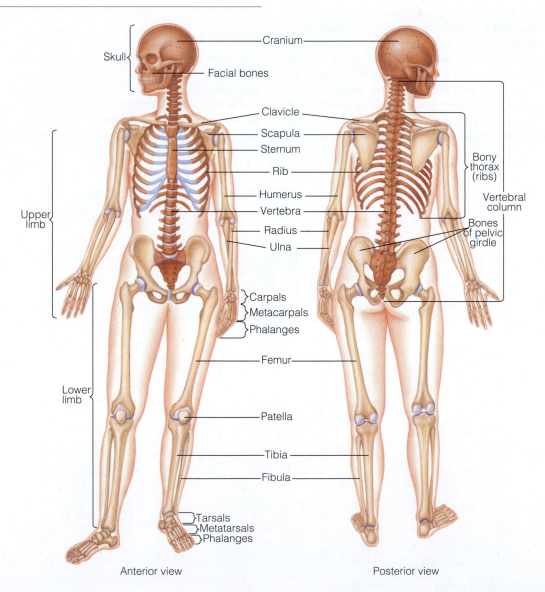

Skull
Cranium
Facial bones
Clavicle
Scapula
Sternum
Rib
Humerus
Vertebra
Radius
Ulna
Carpals
Metacarpals
Phalanges
Femur
Patella
Tibia
Fibula
Tarsals
Metatarsals
Phalanges
Upper limb
Lower limb
Bony thorax (ribs)
Vertebral column
Bones of pelvic girdle

Anterior view   Posterior view

Figure 23.3 Bones of the human skeleton.

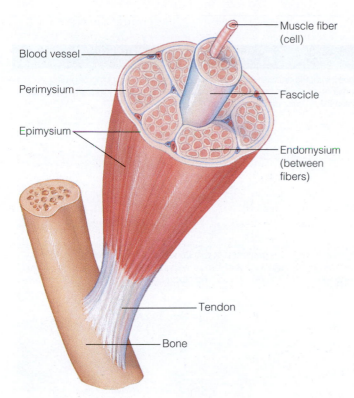

Figure 23.4 Composition of a skeletal muscle.

Joints

A **joint** (or *articulation*) is the point where two or more bones in the body meet. Joints may be classified structurally as fibrous, cartilaginous, or synovial. Bones joined by fibrous tissue, such as the sutures joining the bones of the skull, are called **fibrous joints**. Bones joined by cartilage, such as the vertebrae, are called **cartilaginous joints**. Bones separated by a fluid-filled joint cavity are called **synovial joints**. The structure of synovial joints allows tremendous freedom of movement, and all joints of the limbs are synovial joints. Most synovial joints are reinforced and strengthened by a system of *ligaments*, which are bands of flexible tissue that attach bone to bone. Some ligaments are protected from friction by small, synovial fluid–filled sacs called **bursae**. **Tendons** are tough fibrous bands that attach muscle to bone or attach muscle to muscle. Tendons, subjected to continuous friction, develop fluid-filled bursae called *tendon sheaths* to protect the joint from damage.

During the assessment of the musculoskeletal system, the nurse assesses the joint, its range of motion (ROM), and its surrounding structures of muscles, ligaments, tendons, and bursae. Table 23.1 describes the classification of synovial joints, and Table 23.2 describes the movements of the joints. A description of selected joints to be examined during the physical assessment of the musculoskeletal system follows. Information about

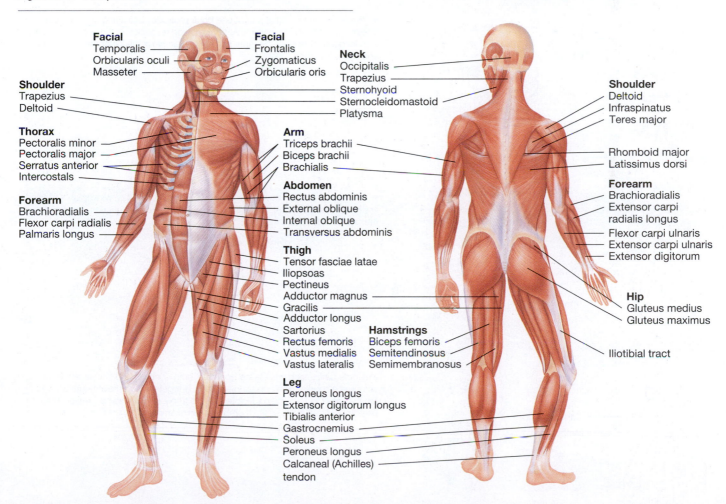

Figure 23.5 Anterior and posterior views of the muscles of the human body.

Table 23.1 Classification of Synovial Joints

TYPE OF JOINT

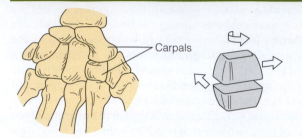

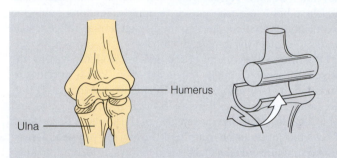

A. Plane joint

In *plane joints*, the articular surfaces are flat, allowing only slipping or gliding movements. Examples include the intercarpal and intertarsal joints and the joints between the articular processes of the ribs.

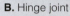

B. Hinge joint

In *hinge joints*, a convex projection of one bone fits into a concave depression in another. Motion is similar to that of a mechanical hinge. These joints permit flexion and extension only. Examples include the elbow and knee joints.

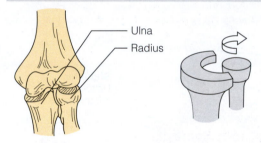

C. Pivot joint

In *pivot joints*, the rounded end of one bone protrudes into a ring of bone (and possibly ligaments). The only movement allowed is rotation of the bone around its own long axis or against the other bone. An example is the joint between the atlas and axis of the neck.

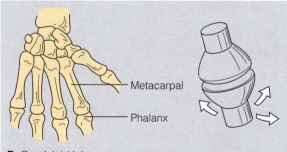

D. Condyloid joint

In *condyloid joints*, the oval surfaces of two bones fit together. Movements allowed are flexion and extension, abduction, adduction, and circumduction. An example is the radiocarpal (wrist) joints.

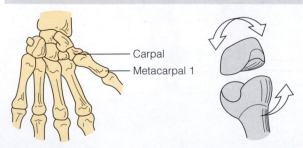

E. Saddle joint

In *saddle joints*, each articulating bone has both concave and convex areas (resembling a saddle). The opposing surfaces fit together. The movements allowed are the same as for condyloid joints, but the freedom of motion is greater. The carpometacarpal joints of the thumbs are an example.

(continued)

Table 23.1 Classification of Synovial Joints (*continued*)

TYPE OF JOINT

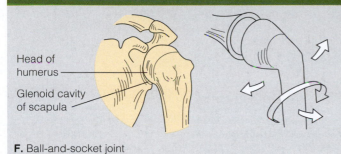

Head of humerus
Glenoid cavity of scapula

F. Ball-and-socket joint

In *ball-and-socket joints*, the ball-shaped head of one bone fits into the concave socket of another. These joints allow movement in all axes and planes, including rotation. The shoulder and hip joints are the only examples in the body.

Table 23.2 Joint Movement

TYPE OF MOVEMENT

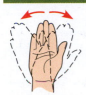

Gliding movements are the simplest type of joint movements. One flat bone surface glides or slips over another similar surface. The bones are merely displaced in relation to one another.

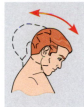

Flexion is a bending movement that decreases the angle of the joint and brings the articulating bones closer together. **Extension** increases the angle between the articulating bones. **Hyperextension** is a bending of a joint beyond 180 degrees.

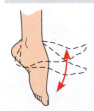

Flexion of the ankle so that the superior aspect of the foot approaches the shin is called **dorsiflexion**. Extension of the ankle (pointing the toes) is called **plantar flexion**.

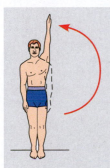

Abduction is movement of a limb away from the midline or median plane of the body, along the frontal plane. When the term is used to describe movement of the fingers or toes, it means spreading them apart. **Adduction** is the movement of a limb toward the body midline. Bringing the fingers close together is adduction.

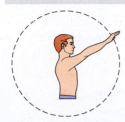

Circumduction is the movement in which the limb describes a cone in space: The distal end of the limb moves in a circle, whereas the joint itself moves only slightly in the joint cavity.

(continued)

Table 23.2 Joint Movement (*continued*)

TYPE OF MOVEMENT	
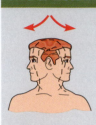	**Rotation** is the turning movement of a bone around its own long axis. Rotation may occur toward the body midline or away from it.
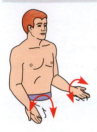	The terms **supination** and **pronation** refer only to the movements of the radius around the ulna. Movement of the forearm so that the palm faces anteriorly or superiorly is called *supination*. In *pronation*, the palm moves to face posteriorly or inferiorly.
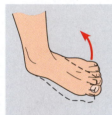	The terms **inversion** and **eversion** refer to movements of the foot. In *inversion*, the sole of the foot is turned medially. In *eversion*, the sole faces laterally.
	**Protraction** is a nonangular anterior movement in a transverse plane. **Retraction** is a nonangular posterior movement in a transverse plane.
	**Elevation** is a lifting or moving superiorly along a frontal plane. When the elevated part is moved downward to its original position, the movement is called **depression**. Shrugging the shoulders and chewing are examples of alternating elevation and depression.
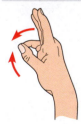	**Opposition** is only allowed at the saddle joint of the thumb between metacarpal 1 and the carpals. It is the movement of touching the thumb to the tips of the other fingers of the same hand.

terminology used to describe anatomic planes and positions is provided in Chapter 1, Table 1.1. ∞

Temporomandibular Joint The temporomandibular joint (TMJ) permits articulation between the mandible and the temporal bone of the skull (see Figure 23.6 ■). Lying just anterior to the external auditory meatus, at the level of the tragus of the ear, the temporomandibular joint allows an individual to speak and chew. Temporomandibular joint movements include the following:

- Opening and closing of the lower jaw
- Protraction and retraction of the lower jaw
- Side-to-side movement of the lower jaw

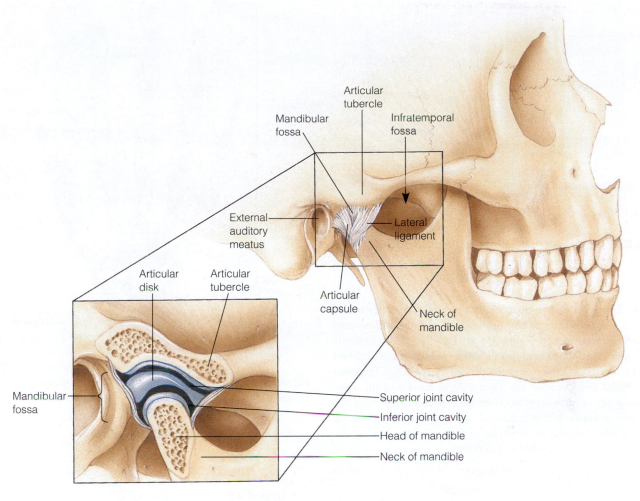

Figure 23.6 Temporomandibular joint. The enlargement shows a sagittal section through the joint.

Shoulder The shoulder joint is a ball-and-socket joint in which the head of the humerus articulates in the shallow glenoid cavity of the scapula (see Table 23.1). The shoulder is supported by the rotator cuff, a sturdy network of tendons and muscles, as well as a series of ligaments (see Figure 23.7 ■). The major landmarks of the shoulder include the scapula, the acromion process, the greater tubercle of the humerus, and the coracoid process. The subacromial bursa, which allows the arm to abduct smoothly and with ease, lies just below the acromion process. Movements of the shoulder include the following:

- Abduction (180 degrees)
- Adduction (50 degrees)
- Horizontal forward flexion (180 degrees)
- Horizontal backward extension (50 degrees)
- Circumduction (360 degrees)
- External rotation (90 degrees)
- Internal rotation (90 degrees)

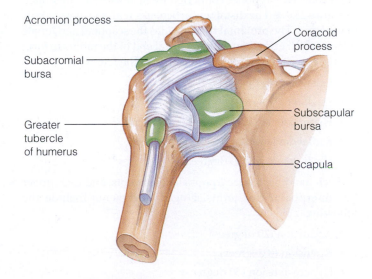

Figure 23.7 Shoulder joint.

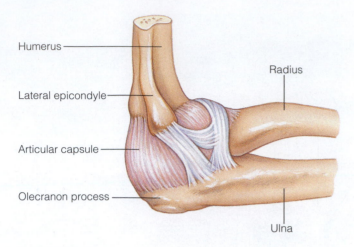

Humerus

Radius

Lateral epicondyle

Articular capsule

Olecranon process

Ulna

Figure 23.8 Elbow joint. Lateral view of the right elbow.

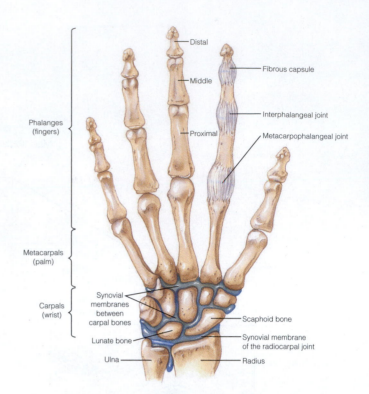

Distal

Fibrous capsule

Middle

Phalanges (fingers)

Interphalangeal joint

Proximal

Metacarpophalangeal joint

Metacarpals (palm)

Carpals (wrist)

Synovial membranes between carpal bones

Scaphoid bone

Lunate bone

Synovial membrane of the radiocarpal joint

Ulna

Radius

Figure 23.9 Bones of the wrist, hand, and phalanges.

Elbow The elbow is a hinge joint that allows articulation between the humerus of the upper arm and the radius and ulna of the forearm (see Figure 23.8 ■). Landmarks include the lateral and medial epicondyles on either side of the distal end of the humerus and the olecranon process of the ulna. The olecranon bursa sits between the olecranon process and the skin. The ulnar nerve travels between the medial epicondyle and the olecranon process. When inflamed, the synovial membrane is palpable between the epicondyles and the olecranon process. Elbow movements include the following:

- Flexion of the forearm (160 degrees)
- Extension of the forearm (160 degrees)
- Supination of the forearm and hand (90 degrees)
- Pronation of the forearm and hand (90 degrees)

Wrist and Hand The wrist (or *carpus*) consists of two rows of eight short carpal bones connected by ligaments, as illustrated in Figure 23.9 ■. The distal row articulates with the metacarpals of the hand. The proximal row includes the scaphoid and lunate bones, which articulate with the distal end of the radius to form the wrist joint. Wrist movements include the following:

- Extension (70 degrees)
- Flexion (90 degrees)
- Hyperextension (30 degrees)
- Radial deviation (20 degrees)
- Ulnar deviation (55 degrees)

Each hand has metacarpophalangeal joints, and each finger has interphalangeal joints. Finger movements include the following:

- Abduction (20 degrees)
- Extension (0 degrees)
- Hyperextension (30 degrees)
- Flexion (90 degrees)
- Circumduction (360 degrees)

Thumb movements include the following:

- Extension
- Flexion (80 degrees)
- Opposition

Hip The hip joint is a ball-and-socket joint composed of the rounded head of the femur as it fits deep into the **acetabulum**, a rounded cavity on the right and left lateral sides of the pelvic bone (see Figure 23.10 ■). Although not as mobile as the shoulder, the hip is surrounded by a system of cartilage, ligaments, tendons, and muscles that contribute to its strength and stability. Landmarks include the iliac crest (not shown), the greater trochanter of the femur, and the anterior inferior iliac spine. Hip movements include the following:

- Extension (90 degrees)
- Hyperextension (15 degrees)
- Flexion with knee flexed (120 degrees)
- Flexion with knee extended (90 degrees)
- Internal rotation (40 degrees)
- External rotation (45 degrees)
- Abduction (45 degrees)
- Adduction (30 degrees)

Knee The knee is a complex joint consisting of the patella (kneecap), femur, and tibia (see Figure 23.11 ■). It is supported and stabilized by the cruciate and collateral ligaments, which have a stabilizing effect on the knee and prevent dislocation.

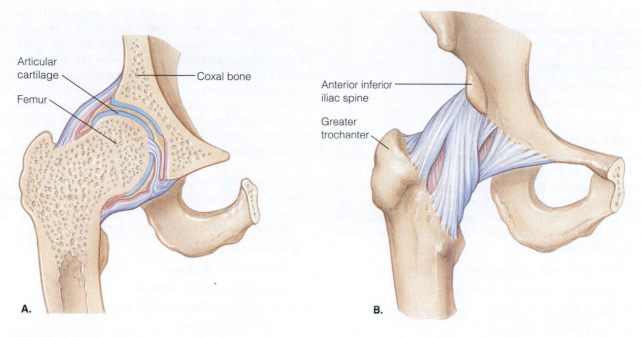

Figure 23.10 Hip joint. A. Cross-section. B. Anterior view.

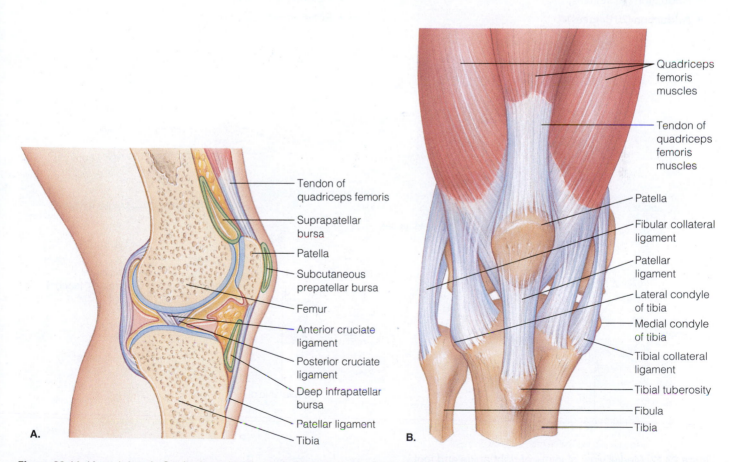

Figure 23.11 Knee joint. A. Sagittal section through the right knee. B. Anterior view.

The landmarks of the knee include the tibial tuberosity and the medial and lateral condyles of the tibia. Knee movements include the following:

- Extension (0 degrees)
- Flexion (130 degrees)
- Hyperextension (15 degrees)

Ankle and Foot   The ankle is a hinge joint that accommodates articulation between the tibia, fibula, and *talus*, a large, posterior tarsal of the foot (see Figure 23.12 ■). The **calcaneus** (heel bone) is just inferior to the talus. It is stabilized by a set of taut ligaments that are anchored from bony prominences at the distal ends of the tibia and fibula (the lateral and medial malleoli), which extend and attach to the foot. Movements of the ankle and foot include the following:

- Dorsiflexion of ankle (20 degrees)
- Plantar flexion of ankle (45 degrees)
- Inversion of foot (30 degrees)
- Eversion of foot (20 degrees)

Movements of the toes include the following:

- Extension (0 degrees)
- Flexion (0 degrees)
- Abduction (10 degrees)
- Adduction (20 degrees)

Spine   The spine is composed of 26 irregular bones called vertebrae (see Figure 23.13 ■). There are 7 *cervical vertebrae*, which support the base of the skull and the neck. All 12 of the *thoracic vertebrae* articulate with the ribs. The 5 *lumbar vertebrae* support the lower back. They are heavier and denser than the other vertebrae, reflecting their weight-bearing function. The *sacrum* shapes the posterior wall of the pelvis, offering strength and stability. The *coccyx* is a small, triangular tailbone at the base of the spine.

Viewed laterally, the spine has cervical and lumbar concavities and a thoracic convexity. As a person bends forward, the normal concavity should flatten, and there should be a single convex C-shaped curve. Figure 23.5 shows the main muscles of the neck and the spine.

Movements of the neck include the following:

- Flexion (45 degrees)
- Extension (55 degrees)
- Hyperextension (10 degrees)
- Lateral flexion (bending) (40 degrees)
- Rotation (70 degrees)

Movements of the spine include the following:

- Lateral flexion (35 degrees)
- Extension (30 degrees)
- Flexion (90 degrees)
- Rotation (30 degrees)

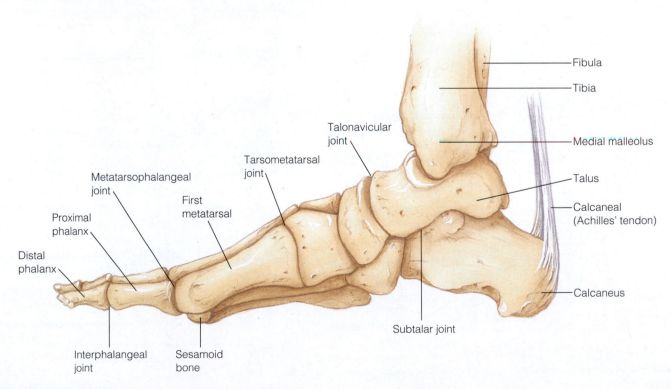

Figure 23.12 Medial view of joints of right ankle and foot.

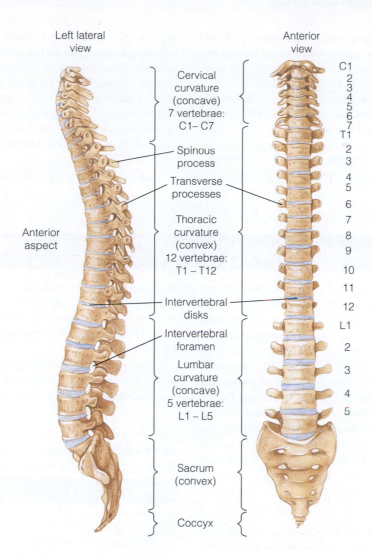

Left lateral view

Anterior view

Cervical curvature (concave) 7 vertebrae: C1– C7

C1
2
3
4
5
6
7

Spinous process

T1
2
3

Transverse processes

4
5

6

Anterior aspect

7

Thoracic curvature (convex) 12 vertebrae: T1 – T12

8

9

10

11

Intervertebral disks

12

L1

Intervertebral foramen

2

Lumbar curvature (concave) 5 vertebrae: L1 – L5

3

4

5

Sacrum (convex)

Coccyx

Figure 23.13 The spine.

Special Considerations

A variety of factors or special considerations contribute to health status. Among these are age, developmental level, race, ethnicity, work history, living conditions, socioeconomics, and emotional well-being. The following sections describe special considerations to include when gathering subjective and objective data.

Health Promotion Considerations

Objectives related to musculoskeletal health include prevention of illness and disability because of disorders including arthritis, osteoporosis, and chronic back conditions.

Lifespan Considerations

Growth and development are dynamic processes that describe change over time. The collection of data and the interpretation of findings in relation to normative values are important. Accurate interpretation of findings requires knowledge of the variations in anatomy and physiology that occur with growth and development. Specific variations in the musculoskeletal system across the lifespan are described in the following sections. See Chapter 25, Chapter 26, and Chapter 27 for more lifespan considerations. ∞

Cultural and Environmental Considerations

The bone density of people of African ancestry is significantly higher than that of people of other ethnicities (May, Pettifor, Norris, Ramsay, & Lombard, 2013). Asians typically have lower bone density than people of European descent (Kruger et al., 2013). The risk for developing osteoporosis is greater for women, and Asians and Caucasians tend to experience a higher incidence of osteoporosis than do African Americans (Mayo Clinic, 2016a, 2016b). The curvature of long bones varies widely among cultural groups and seems to be related to genetics and body weight. Weight also impacts the incidence of lower back problems; obesity is linked to an increased risk for lumbar back pain (Wasser, Vasilopoulos, Zdziarski, & Vincent 2017).

The number and distribution of vertebrae vary. Although 24 vertebrae is the average (present in about 85% to 90% of all people), 23 or 25 vertebrae are not uncommon.

Certain working conditions present potential risks to the musculoskeletal system. Workers required to lift heavy objects may strain and injure their back. Jobs requiring substantial physical activity, such as those of construction workers, firefighters, or athletes, increase the likelihood of musculoskeletal injuries such as sprains, strains, and fractures. Frequent repetitive movements may lead to misuse disorders such as carpal tunnel syndrome, pitcher's elbow, or vertebral degeneration. Musculoskeletal injuries may also arise when individuals sit for long periods at desks with poor ergonomic design.

Subjective Data—Health History

Health assessment of the musculoskeletal system includes gathering subjective and objective data. Subjective data collection occurs during the patient interview, before the physical assessment. During the interview, various communication techniques are used to elicit general and specific information about the status of the patient's musculoskeletal system and ability to function. Health records, the results of laboratory tests, X-rays, and imaging reports are important secondary sources to be included in the data-gathering process. During the physical assessment of the musculoskeletal system, the techniques of inspection and palpation will be used to gather objective data. See Table 23.3 for information on potential secondary sources of patient data.

Focused Interview

The focused interview for the musculoskeletal system concerns data related to the structures and functions of that system. Subjective data are gathered during the focused interview. The nurse must be prepared to observe the patient and to listen for cues related to the function of the musculoskeletal system. The nurse may use open-ended and closed questions to obtain information. A number of follow-up questions or requests for descriptions may be required to clarify data or gather missing information. Follow-up questions are intended to identify the sources of problems, duration of difficulties, and measures used to alleviate or manage problems. They also provide clues about the patient's knowledge of his or her own health.

The focused interview guides the physical assessment of the musculoskeletal system. The information is always considered in relation to norms and expectations about musculoskeletal function. Therefore, the nurse must consider age, gender, race, culture, environment, health practices, past and concurrent problems, and therapies when framing questions and using techniques to elicit information. In order to address all of the factors when conducting a focused interview, categories of questions related to the status and function of the musculoskeletal system have been developed. These categories include general questions that are asked of all patients; those addressing illness and infection; questions related to symptoms, pain, and behaviors; those related to habits or practices; questions that are specific to patients according to age or pregnancy, and questions that address environmental concerns. One approach to elicit information about symptoms is the OLDCART & ICE method, described in Chapter 5. See Figure 5.3. ∞

The nurse must consider the patient's ability to participate in the focused interview and physical assessment of the musculoskeletal system. Illness, discomfort, and disease may

Table 23.3 Potential Secondary Sources for Patient Data Related to the Musculoskeletal System

LABORATORY TESTS	NORMAL VALUES
Calcium	8.9–10.3 mg/dL
Phosphorus	2.5–4.5 mg/dL
AST/SGOT	Males 8–48 Units/L Females 8–43 Units/L
Alkaline Phosphatase (ALP)	44–147 Units/L
Aldolase	< 7.7 Units/L
Creatinine Phosphokinase (CPK)	Males 52–336 Units/L Females 38–176 Units/L
Erythrocyte Sedimentation Rate (ESR)	Males < 23 mm/hr Females < 29 mm/hr
Rheumatoid Factor	< 15 IU/mL
Antinuclear Antibodies (ANA)	negative
Diagnostic Tests	
Arthroscopy	
Bone Density Scan	
Bone Scan	
Computed Tomography (CT)	
Joint Aspiration	
Magnetic Resonance Imaging (MRI)	
Myelography	
X-ray	

affect the ability to participate in the interview. Participation in the focused interview may be influenced by the ability to communicate in the same language. Language barriers interfere with the accuracy of data collection and cause anxiety in the patient and examiner. A nurse may have to use a translator in conducting interviews and during the physical assessment. If the patient is experiencing acute pain, recent injury, or anxiety, attention must be focused on relief of discomfort and relief of symptoms before proceeding with the in-depth interview.

Focused Interview Questions	Rationales and Evidence

The following section provides sample questions and bulleted follow-up questions in each of the categories previously mentioned. A rationale for each of the questions is provided. The list of questions is not all-inclusive but represents the types of questions required in a comprehensive focused interview related to the musculoskeletal system. As these questions are asked, the subjective data obtained help to identify strengths or risks associated with the musculoskeletal system.

General Questions

1. **Describe your mobility today, 2 months ago, and 2 years ago.**

▶ This gives patients the opportunity to provide their own perceptions about mobility.

2. **Are you able to carry out all of your regular activities?**
   - Describe the change in your activity.
   - Do you know what is causing the problem?
   - What do you do about the problem?
   - How long has this been happening?
   - Have you discussed this with a healthcare professional?

▶ Musculoskeletal problems affect activities of daily living (ADLs) because of pain or decreased mobility.

3. **Do you have any chronic diseases such as diabetes mellitus, chronic obstructive pulmonary disease (COPD), hypothyroidism, sickle cell anemia, lupus, or rheumatoid arthritis?**
   - If so, describe the disease and its progression, treatment, and effects on daily activities.

▶ When a musculoskeletal disorder occurs in conjunction with a chronic disease, there can be a greater impact on physical health (van der Zee-Neuen et al., 2016). In COPD, musculoskeletal changes may lead to exercise limitation and disability (Heneghan, Abab, Jackman, & Balanos, 2015).

4. **Please describe any musculoskeletal problems of any family member.**
   - What is the disease or problem?
   - Who in the family has had the problem?
   - When was it diagnosed?
   - Describe the treatment.
   - How effective has the treatment been?

▶ Some conditions, such as rheumatoid arthritis, are genetic or familial and recur in a family (Mayo Clinic, 2017).

Questions Related to Illness, Infection, or Injury

1. **Have you ever been diagnosed with a musculoskeletal illness?**
   - When were you diagnosed with the problem?
   - What treatment was prescribed for the problem?
   - Was the treatment helpful?
   - What kinds of things do you do to help with the problem?
   - Has the problem ever recurred (acute)?
   - How are you managing the disease now (chronic)?

▶ The patient has an opportunity to provide information about a specific illness. If a diagnosed illness is identified, follow-up about the date of diagnosis, treatment, and outcomes is required. Data about each illness identified by the patient are essential to an accurate health assessment. Illnesses can be classified as acute or chronic, and follow-up regarding each classification will differ.

2. *Alternative to question 1:* List possible musculoskeletal illnesses, such as arthritis, myalgia, and lupus, and ask the patient to respond "yes" or "no" as each is stated.

▶ This is a comprehensive and easy way to elicit information about all musculoskeletal diagnoses. Follow-up would be carried out for each identified diagnosis as in question 1.

3. **Have you ever had an infection in your bones, muscles, or joints?**
   - When were you diagnosed with the infection?
   - When did the problem begin?
   - What treatment was prescribed?
   - Was the treatment helpful?
   - What do you do to help the problem?
   - Has the problem ever recurred (acute)?
   - How are you managing the problem now (chronic)?

▶ Osteomyelitis, an infection of the bone, frequently recurs in patients with a history of previous infections (MedlinePlus, 2018).

Focused Interview Questions	Rationales and Evidence
4. Have you had any fractures (broken bones)? If so, tell me about the frequency, cause, injuries, treatment, and present problems with daily activities.	▶ Older adults who have osteoporosis and osteomalacia (adult vitamin D deficiency) are prone to develop multiple fractures of the bone (Weycker et al., 2013). Physical abuse should be considered when an individual has a history of frequent fractures; however, disease or hereditary illness can predispose fractures.
5. Have you ever experienced any penetrating wounds (punctures from a nail or sharp object, stabbing, or gunshot)? If so, please describe them.	▶ Penetrating wounds may be a causative factor for osteomyelitis (Izadi et al., 2013). Follow-up for questions 4 and 5 would follow the format for questions 1 and 3.

Questions Related to Symptoms, Pain, and Behaviors

When gathering information about symptoms, many questions are required to elicit details and descriptions that assist in the analysis of the data. Discrimination is made in relation to the significance of a symptom, in relation to specific diseases or problems, and in relation to potential follow-up examination or referral. One rationale may be provided for a group of questions in this category.

The following questions refer to specific symptoms and behaviors associated with the musculoskeletal system. For each symptom, questions and follow-up are required. The details to be elicited are the characteristics of the symptom; the onset, duration, and frequency of the symptom; the treatment or remedy for the symptom, including over-the-counter and home remedies; the determination if diagnosis has been sought; the effect of treatments; and family history associated with a symptom or illness.

1. Tell me about any swelling, heat, redness, or stiffness you have had in your muscles or joints.

   ▶ Swelling, heat, redness, and stiffness are associated with disorders of the musculoskeletal system such as arthritis or sprains (Mayo Clinic, 2017).

2. How long have you had the symptom?

   ▶ Determining the duration of symptoms is helpful in identifying the significance of the symptoms in relation to specific diseases and problems.

3. Do you know what causes the symptom?

4. Does the symptom differ at different times of day?

   ▶ Questions 3 through 9 elicit information about the need for diagnosis, referral, or continued evaluation of the symptom; information about the patient's knowledge about a current diagnosis or underlying problems; and the patient's response to intervention.

5. Have you sought treatment?

6. When was the treatment sought?

7. What happened when you sought treatment?

8. Was something prescribed or recommended?

9. What was the effect of the remedy?

10. Do you now use, or have you ever used, over-the-counter (OTC) or home remedies for the symptom?

    ▶ Questions 10 through 13 elicit information about drugs and substances that may relieve symptoms or provide comfort. Some substances may mask symptoms, interfere with the effect of prescribed medication, or harm the patient.

11. What are the OTC or home remedies that you use?

12. How often do you use them?

13. How much of them do you use?

14. Do you experience constipation or abdominal distention?

    ▶ These diagnostic cues commonly occur in patients who have decreased mobility, atrophy of the abdominal muscles, or spinal deformity.

15. Do you have difficulty breathing? If so, describe.

    ▶ Spinal deformities, osteoporosis, and any other condition that restricts trunk movement may interfere with normal breathing movements.

Questions Related to Pain

1. Please describe any pain you experience in your bones, muscles, or joints
   - How would you rate the pain on a scale of 0 to 10, with 10 being the worst?
   - When did the pain begin?
   - What were you doing when the pain began?
   - What activities increase the pain?
   - What activities seem to decrease or eliminate the pain?
   - Does this pain radiate from one place to another?
   - Do you experience any unusual sensations along with the pain?

   ▶ These questions help determine if the pain has a sudden or gradual onset. Also, certain activities, such as lifting heavy objects, can strain ligaments and vertebrae in the back, causing acute pain. Weight-bearing activities may increase the pain if the patient has degenerative disease of the hip, knee, and vertebrae. The pain from hiatal hernia and from cardiac, gallbladder, and pleural conditions may be referred to the shoulder. Lumbosacral nerve root irritation may cause pain to be felt in the leg. (See Figure 11.5 for an illustration of common sites of referred pain.) Sensations of burning, tingling, or prickling (paresthesia) may accompany compression of nerves or blood vessels in that body region.

Focused Interview Questions	Rationales and Evidence

2. What do you do to relieve the pain?

3. Is that treatment effective?

▶ Questions 2 and 3 are intended to determine if the patient has selected a treatment based on past experience, knowledge of musculoskeletal illness, or use of complementary and alternative medicine and its effectiveness.

Questions Related to Behaviors

1. **Do you smoke?**
   - If so, how much?
   - How much caffeine do you consume each day?
   - How many cups of coffee, tea, or cola?
   - How much alcohol do you drink?

▶ Smoking, caffeine consumption, and alcohol consumption increase the patient's risk for osteoporosis (Mayo Clinic, 2016a, 2016b).

2. **Tell me about your exercise program.**

▶ A sedentary lifestyle leads to muscle weakness, contributes to poor coordination skills, and predisposes postmenopausal females to osteoporosis (Pervaiz, Cabezas, Downes, Santoni, & Frankle, 2013).

Questions Related to Age and Pregnancy

The focused interview must reflect the anatomic and physiologic differences in the musculoskeletal system that exist along the age span as well as during pregnancy. Specific questions related to the musculoskeletal system for each of these groups are provided in Chapter 25, Chapter 26, and Chapter 27. ∞

Questions Related to the Environment

Environment refers to both the internal and external environments. Questions related to the internal environment include all of the previous questions and those associated with internal or physiologic responses. Questions regarding the external environment include those related to home, work, or social environments.

Internal Environment

1. **Describe your typical daily diet.**
   - Do you have problems eating or drinking dairy products?
   - If so, describe the problems you experience.

▶ Protein deficiency interferes with bone growth and muscle tone; calcium deficiency predisposes an individual to low bone density, resulting in osteoporosis; and vitamin C deficiency inhibits bone and tissue healing (Osborn et al., 2013). Patients with intolerance to milk products frequently ingest low amounts of calcium, leading to musculoskeletal problems such as osteoporosis.

2. **Have you had any recent gain or loss in weight?**
   - If so, how much weight?

▶ Increased weight puts added stress on the musculoskeletal system. New weight loss (e.g., in those having had gastric bypass surgery) increases the risk for osteoporosis (Chicoski, 2018).

3. **Are you currently taking any medications, such as steroids, estrogen, muscle relaxants, or any other drugs?**

▶ These drugs may cause a variety of symptoms such as weakness, swelling, and increased muscle size that could affect the musculoskeletal system (Wilson, Shannon, & Shields, 2018).

External Environment

1. **How much sunlight do you get each day?**

▶ Twenty minutes of sunshine each day helps the body manufacture vitamin D. Vitamin D deficiency can lead to osteomalacia (Osborn et al., 2013).

2. **What kind of work do you do?**
   - Do you work on a computer?
   - What are your typical workplace lifting requirements?

▶ Frequent repetitive movements may lead to misuse syndromes such as carpal tunnel syndrome, an inflammation of the tissues of the wrist that causes pressure on the median nerve. Work that requires heavy lifting or twisting may lead to lower back problems.

3. **Describe your hobbies or athletic activities.**

▶ Participation in athletic or sports activities can predispose the individual to trauma or wear-and-tear injuries. Sitting for long periods and repetitive motion, such as in sewing, crocheting, and woodworking, can cause musculoskeletal damage.

Patient-Centered Interaction

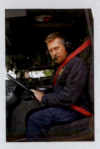

Mr. Alexander French, a 49-year-old truck driver, returns to the pain clinic at 10:30 a.m. accompanied by his wife. His health history includes having been diagnosed with a herniated intervertebral disk at L4–L5 about 10 months ago. At that time, he declined surgery and selected the alternative method of treatment, which included wearing a back brace and home exercises to help strengthen his back muscles. Now his chief complaint is back pain radiating to his left leg. The following is an excerpt from the focused interview.

Source: Flashon Studio/Shutterstock.

Interview

Nurse: Good morning, Mr. French. I see by your report you are having back pain again. Your last visit was about three months ago for a routine follow-up with no pain.

Mr. French: Yes, that is correct.

Nurse: First, we need to determine your pain level right now and find a comfortable position for you.

Mr. French: Right now my pain is about four on a scale of zero to ten, and it sometimes shoots down my left leg. It was higher at home, but I took my pills before coming here. That's why my wife drove and is here with me. I will be able to sit for a while. When I can't sit any longer, I will tell you.

Nurse: I need more information about the cause, actions you have taken to decrease the pain, and activities since your last visit. Where shall we begin?

Mr. French: I'll start with the cause. I was outside Saturday after it stopped snowing, and I shoveled our front walk. Then I helped the children build a big snowman. I was tired and had a backache that evening, but I tried to ignore it.

Nurse: You ignored it?

Mr. French: I should have taken the medicine right away. I should have had my brace on when I was shoveling and building the snowman with the children.

Nurse: You weren't wearing your back brace?

Mr. French: That's right. I wear it every day to work. I never forget because I move heavy boxes from the truck. I had been feeling so good, no problems, and the snow was not heavy. I guess when I lifted the second snowball for the snowman, that did me in though.

Analysis

Several techniques were used to obtain subjective data from the patient. The nurse first clarified the reason for the visit and then determined the patient's pain level and position for comfort. Using open-ended statements and listening to the patient, the nurse encouraged the patient to focus on details of the topics being discussed. However, the nurse introduced several thoughts and questions at one time. This could have hindered the communication process during the interview.

Objective Data—Physical Assessment

EQUIPMENT
- Examination gown
- Clean, nonsterile examination gloves
- Examination light
- Skin marking pen
- Goniometer
- Tape measure

Assessment Techniques and Findings

Physical assessment of the musculoskeletal system requires the use of inspection and palpation. During each of the procedures, the nurse is gathering data related to the patient's skeleton, joints, musculature, strength, and mobility. Knowledge of normal or expected findings is essential in determining the meaning of the data as the nurse conducts the physical assessment.

Both adults and children who are preschool age and older have erect posture, an even gait, and symmetry in size and shape of muscles. A healthy individual is capable of active and complete ROM in all joints. Joints are nonswollen and nontender. Muscle strength is equal bilaterally, and the movements against resistance are smooth and symmetric. The spine is midline and cervical; thoracic and lumbar curves are present. The extremities are of equal length. The arm span is equal to height, and the distance from head to pubis is equal to the distance from pubis to toes.

Physical assessment of the musculoskeletal system follows an organized pattern. It begins with a patient survey and proceeds in a cephalocaudal direction to include inspection, palpation, assessment of ROM of each joint, and assessment of muscle size, symmetry, and strength.

HELPFUL HINTS

- Age and agility influence the patient's ability to participate in the assessment.
- It is often more helpful to demonstrate the movements you expect of the patient during this assessment than to use easily misunderstood verbal instructions. A Simon Says approach works well, especially with children.
- When assessing ROM, do not push the joint beyond its normal range.

- Stop when the patient expresses discomfort.
- Measure the joint angle with a goniometer when ROM appears limited.
- Use an orderly approach: head to toe, proximal to distal, compare the sides of the body for symmetry.
- The musculoskeletal assessment may be exhausting for some patients. Provide rest periods or schedule two sessions.
- Use Standard Precautions.

Techniques and Normal Findings	Abnormal Findings and Special Considerations

Survey

A quick survey of the patient enables the nurse to identify any immediate problems and to determine the patient's ability to participate in the assessment.

Inspect the overall appearance, posture, and position of the patient. Observe for deformities, inflammation, and immobility (see Figure 23.14 ■).

▶ If a patient is experiencing pain or inflammation, these issues must be addressed first. The complete assessment of the musculoskeletal system may have to be delayed until acute problems are attended to. Limited strength and mobility must be considered throughout the assessment.

▶ The posture and position of body parts in obese patients is often the first indication of underlying problems with bones or ligaments. *Valgum* (knock knees) and *genu varum* (bowlegs) abnormalities suggest cartilage loss in obese patients.

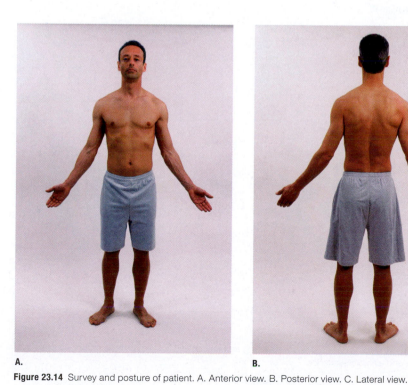
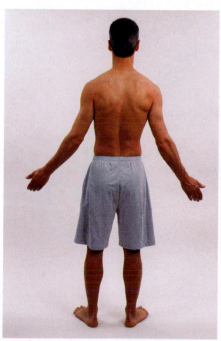
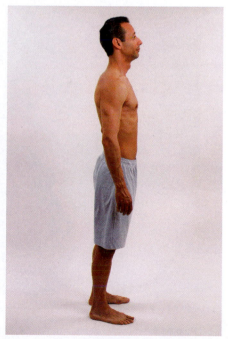

A. B. C.

Figure 23.14 Survey and posture of patient. A. Anterior view. B. Posterior view. C. Lateral view.

Techniques and Normal Findings	Abnormal Findings and Special Considerations

Assessment of the Joints

1. **Position the patient.**
   - The patient should be in a sitting position and wearing an examination gown.

2. **Instruct the patient.**
   - Explain that you will be touching the patient for the purpose of assessing bones, muscles, and joints and that you will ask the patient to move different parts of the body to determine the mobility of the joints.
   - Explain that part of the assessment will require the patient to move against the resistance you provide. It is helpful to demonstrate or describe the movements expected of the patient for one joint and to apply resistance as the patient repeats the expected movement. Then explain that each joint will be assessed in a similar manner with the same amount of resistance and that you will provide direction with each examination.
   - Explain that the assessment should not cause discomfort, and tell the patient to inform you of pain, discomfort, or difficulty with any assessment. Explain that you will provide assistance or support when necessary and can provide rest periods throughout the assessment.
   - Muscle strength should be equal bilaterally, and the patient should be able to fully resist the opposing force you apply during testing. Table 23.4 provides a scale for rating muscle strength.

3. **Inspect the temporomandibular joint (TMJ) on both sides.**
   - The joints should be symmetric and not swollen or painful.

4. **Palpate the temporomandibular joints.**
   - Place the finger pads of your index and middle fingers in front of the tragus of each ear. Ask the patient to open and close the mouth while you palpate the temporomandibular joints (see Figure 23.15 ■).
   - As the patient's mouth opens, your fingers should glide into a shallow depression of the joints. Confirm the smooth motion of the mandible.
   - The joint may audibly and palpably click as the mouth opens. This is normal.

▶ Palpation of the ankle, knee, hip, shoulder, and back is difficult in the obese patient because of increased subcutaneous fat.

▶ An enlarged or swollen joint shows as a rounded protuberance.

▶ Discomfort, swelling, crackling sounds, and limited movement of the jaw are unexpected findings that require further evaluation for dental or neurologic problems or TMJ syndrome.

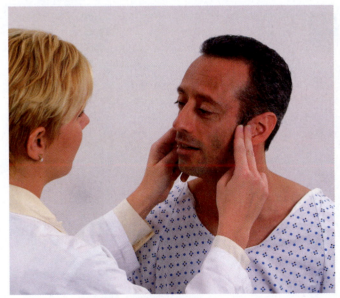

Figure 23.15 Palpating the temporomandibular joints.

5. **Palpate the muscles of the jaw.**
   - Instruct the patient to clench the teeth as you palpate the masseter and temporalis muscles. Confirm that the muscles are symmetric, firm, and nontender.

6. **Test for ROM of the temporomandibular joints.**
   - Ask the patient to open the mouth as wide as possible. Confirm that the mouth opens with ease to as much as 3 to 6 cm (1.17 to 2.34 in.) between the upper and lower incisors.
   - With the mouth slightly open, ask the patient to push out the lower jaw, and then return the lower jaw to a neutral position. The jaw should protrude and retract with ease.
   - Ask the patient to move the lower jaw from side to side. Confirm that the jaw moves laterally from 1 to 2 cm (0.39 to 0.78 in.) without deviation or dislocation.
   - Ask the patient to close the mouth. The mouth should close completely without pain or discomfort.

▶ Swelling and tenderness suggest arthritis and myofascial pain syndrome.

▶ TMJ dysfunction should be suspected if facial pain and limited jaw movement accompany clicking sounds as the jaw opens and closes.

Techniques and Normal Findings	**Abnormal Findings and Special Considerations**

7. **Test for muscle strength and for motor function of cranial nerve V.**
   - Instruct the patient to repeat the movements in step 6 as you provide opposing force. The patient should be able to perform the movements against your resistance. The strength of the muscles on both sides of the jaw should be equal.
   - For more detailed testing of cranial nerve V, including sensory function, see Chapter 24. ∞

Shoulders

1. **With the patient facing you, inspect both shoulders.**
   - Compare the shape and size of the shoulders, clavicles, and scapula. Confirm that they are symmetric and similar in size both anteriorly and posteriorly.

   ▶ Swelling, deformity, atrophy, and misalignment, combined with limited motion, pain, and crepitus (a grating sound caused by bone fragments in joints), suggest degenerative joint disease, traumatized joints (strains, sprains), or inflammatory conditions (rheumatoid arthritis, bursitis, or tendinitis).

2. **Palpate the shoulders and surrounding structures.**
   - Begin palpating at the sternoclavicular joint; then move laterally along the clavicle to the acromioclavicular joint.
   - Palpate downward into the subacromial area and the greater tubercle of the humerus.
   - Confirm that these areas are firm and nontender, the shoulders are symmetric, and the scapulae are level and symmetric.

   ▶ Shoulder pain without palpation or movement may result from insufficient circulation to the myocardium. This cue, known as *referred pain*, can be a precursor to a myocardial infarction (heart attack). If the patient exhibits other symptoms such as chest pain, indigestion, and cardiovascular changes, medical assistance must be obtained immediately.

3. **Test the ROM of the shoulders.**
   - Instruct the patient to use both arms for the following maneuvers:
     - Shrug the shoulders by flexing them forward and upward.
     - With the elbows extended, raise the arms forward and upward in an arc. The patient should demonstrate a forward flexion of 180 degrees.
     - Return the arms to the sides. Keeping the elbows extended, move the arms backward as far as possible (see Figure 23.16 ■).

   ▶ If the patient expresses discomfort, it is important to determine if the pain is referred. Conditions that increase intra-abdominal pressure, such as hiatal hernia and gastrointestinal disease, may cause pain in the shoulder area. Whenever limitation or increase in ROM is assessed, the goniometer should be used to precisely measure the angle.

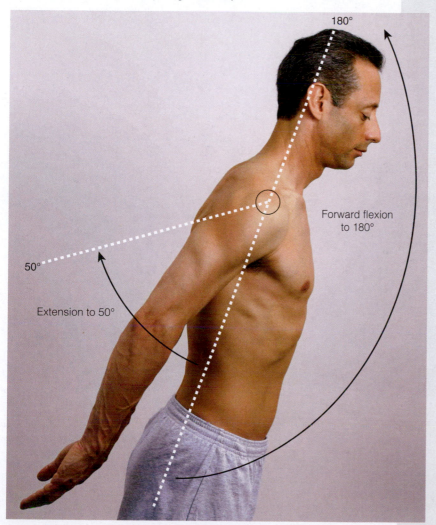

Figure 23.16 Flexion and extension of the shoulders.

- The patient should demonstrate an extension of as much as 50 degrees.
- Ask the patient to clasp his or her hands on the back as high above the waist as possible (internal rotation; see Figure 23.17 ■).

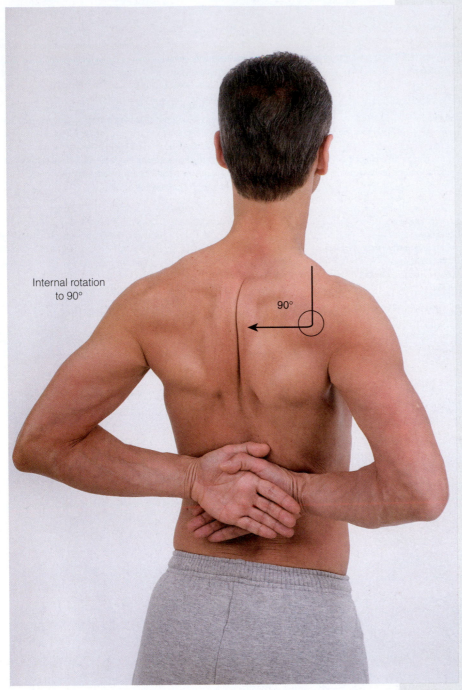

Figure 23.17 Internal rotation of the shoulders.

Techniques and Normal Findings	Abnormal Findings and Special Considerations

- Ask the patient to clasp his or her hands behind the head (external rotation; see Figure 23.18 ■).

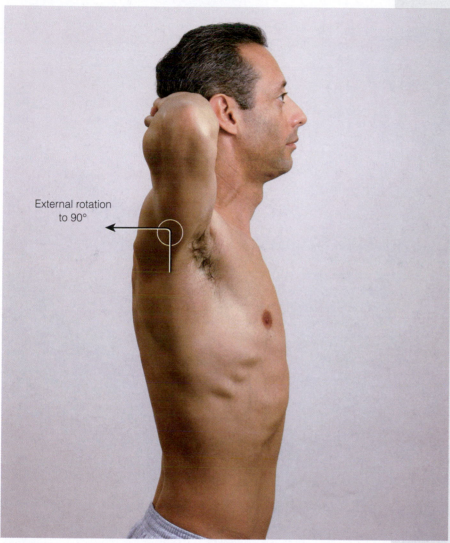

External rotation to 90°

Figure 23.18 External rotation of the shoulders.

- With elbows extended, ask the patient to swing the arms out to the sides in arcs, touching the palms together above the head. The patient should demonstrate abduction of 180 degrees.

▶ In rotator cuff tears, the patient is unable to perform abduction without lifting or shrugging the shoulder. This sign is accompanied by pain, tenderness, and muscle atrophy.

- With the elbows extended, ask the patient to swing each arm toward the midline of the body (see Figure 23.19 ■).
- The patient should demonstrate adduction of as much as 50 degrees.

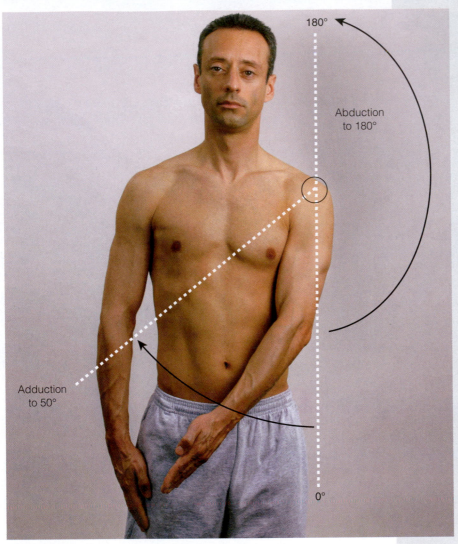

Figure 23.19 Abduction and adduction of the shoulder.

Techniques and Normal Findings	Abnormal Findings and Special Considerations

4. Test for strength of the shoulder muscles.
- Instruct the patient to repeat the movements in step 3 as you provide opposing force. The patient should be able to perform the movements against your resistance. The strength of the shoulder muscles on both sides should be equal.
- Muscle strength is rated on a scale of 0 to 5, with 0 representing absence of strength and 5 indicating maximum or normal strength. Table 23.4 includes information about rating muscle strength.

▶ Full resistance during the shoulder shrug indicates adequate cranial nerve XI (spinal accessory) function. See Chapter 26 for more details. ∞

Table 23.4 Rating Muscle Strength

RATING	DESCRIPTION OF FUNCTION	CLASSIFICATION
5	Full ROM against gravity with full resistance	Normal
4	Full ROM against gravity with moderate resistance	Good
3	Full ROM with gravity	Fair
2	Full ROM without gravity (passive motion)	Poor
1	Palpable muscle contraction but no movement	Trace
0	No muscle contraction	Zero

Elbows

1. Support the patient's arm and inspect the lateral and medial aspects of the elbow.
- The elbows should be symmetric.

2. Palpate the lateral and medial aspects of the olecranon process.
- Use your thumb and middle fingers to palpate the grooves on either side of the olecranon process.
- The joint should be free of pain, thickening, swelling, or tenderness.

▶ Swelling, deformity, or malalignment requires further evaluation. If there is a **subluxation** (partial dislocation), the elbow looks deformed, and the forearm is misaligned.

▶ In the presence of inflammation, the grooves feel soft and spongy, and the surrounding tissue may be red, hot, and painful.

▶ Inflammatory conditions of the elbow include arthritis, bursitis, and epicondylitis. *Rheumatoid arthritis* may result in nodules in the olecranon bursa or along the extensor surface of the ulna. Nodules are firm, nontender, and not attached to the overlying skin. *Lateral epicondylitis* (tennis elbow) results from constant, repetitive movements of the wrist or forearm. Pain occurs when the patient attempts to extend the wrist against resistance. *Medial epicondylitis* (pitcher's or golfer's elbow) results from constant, repetitive flexion of the wrist. Pain occurs when the patient attempts to flex the wrist against resistance.

Techniques and Normal Findings	Abnormal Findings and Special Considerations

3. Test the ROM of each elbow.

- Instruct the patient to perform the following movements:
  - Bend the elbow by bringing the forearm forward and touching the fingers to the shoulder (see Figure 23.20 ■). The elbow should flex to 160 degrees.
  - Straighten the elbow. The lower arm should form a straight line with the upper arm. The elbow in a neutral position is at 0 degrees of extension. The elbow should extend to 0 degrees.
  - Holding the arm straight out, turn the palm upward facing the ceiling, then downward facing the floor (see Figure 23.22 ■). The elbow should supinate and pronate to 90 degrees.

▶ To use the goniometer, begin with the joint in a neutral position and then flex the joint as far as possible. Measure the angle with the goniometer. Fully extend the joint and measure the angle with the goniometer. Compare the goniometer measurements to the expected degree of flexion and extension. See Figure 23.21 ■ for an example.

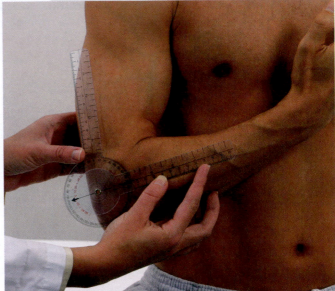

Figure 23.21 Goniometer measure of joint range of motion.

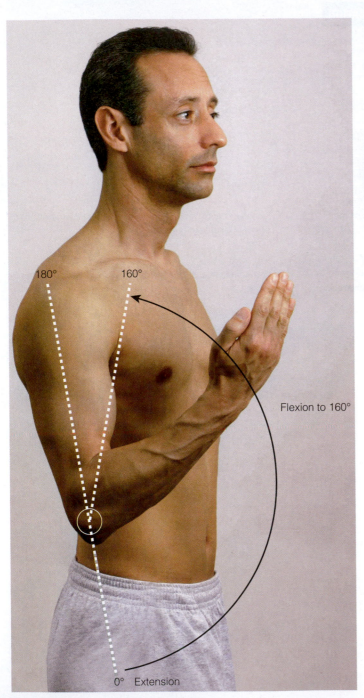

180°   160°

Flexion to 160°

0°   Extension

Figure 23.20 Flexion and extension of the elbow.

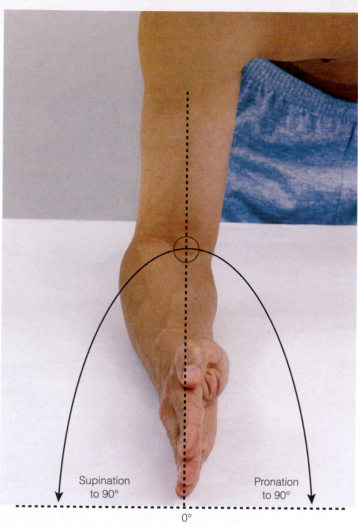

Supination
to 90°

Pronation
to 90°

0°

Figure 23.22 Supination and pronation of the elbow.

- The patient should be able to put each elbow through the normal ROM without difficulty or discomfort.

4. **Test for muscle strength.**
   - Stabilize the patient's elbow with your nondominant hand while holding the wrist with your dominant hand.
   - Instruct the patient to flex the elbow while you apply opposing resistance (see Figure 23.23 ■).
   - Instruct the patient to extend the elbow against resistance.
   - The patient should be able to perform these movements. The strength of the muscles associated with flexion and extension of each elbow should be equal. Muscle strength is measured by testing against the strength of the examiner as resistance is applied.

Techniques and Normal Findings	Abnormal Findings and Special Considerations

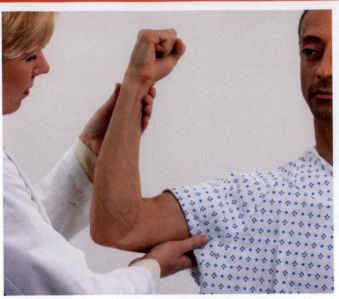

Figure 23.23 Testing muscle strength using opposing force.

Wrists and Hands

1. **Inspect the wrists and dorsum of the hands for size, shape, symmetry, and color.**
   - The wrists and hands should be symmetric and free from swelling and deformity. The color should be similar to that of the rest of the body. The ends of either the ulna or radius may protrude further in some individuals.

2. **Inspect the palms of the hands.**
   - There is a rounded protuberance over the thenar eminence (the area proximal to the thumb).

3. **Palpate the wrists and hands for temperature and texture.**
   - The temperature of the wrists and hands should be warm and similar to the rest of the body. The skin should be smooth and free of cuts. The skin around the interphalangeal joints may have a rougher texture.

▶ Redness, swelling, or deformity in the joints requires further evaluation. It is important to note any nodules on the hands or wrists or atrophy of the surrounding muscles. In acute rheumatoid arthritis, the wrist, proximal interphalangeal, and metacarpophalangeal joints are likely to be swollen, tender, and stiff. As the disease progresses, the proximal interphalangeal joints deviate toward the ulnar side of the hand; the interosseous muscles atrophy; and rheumatoid nodules form, giving the rheumatic hand its characteristic appearance.

▶ Carpal tunnel syndrome is a nerve disorder in which an inflammation of tissues in the wrist causes pressure on the median nerve (which innervates the hand). Thenar atrophy is a common finding associated with carpal tunnel syndrome; however, some atrophy of the thenar eminence occurs with aging.

Techniques and Normal Findings	**Abnormal Findings and Special Considerations**

4. Palpate each joint of the wrists and hands.
- Move your thumbs from side to side gently but firmly over the dorsum, with your fingers resting beneath the area you are palpating (see Figure 23.24A and Figure 23.24B ■). As you palpate, make sure you keep the patient's wrist straight.

- To palpate the interphalangeal joints, pinch them gently between your thumb and index finger (see Figure 23.24C ■). All joints should be firm and nontender with no swelling.
- As you palpate, note the temperature of the patient's hand.

▶ A ganglion is a typically painless, round, fluid-filled mass that arises from the tendon sheaths on the dorsum of the wrist and hand. It may require surgery. Ganglia that are more prevalent when the wrist is flexed do not interfere with ROM or function.

▶ A cool temperature in the extremities may indicate compromised vascular function, which may in turn influence muscle strength.

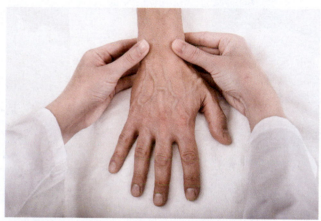

Figure 23.24A Palpating the wrist.

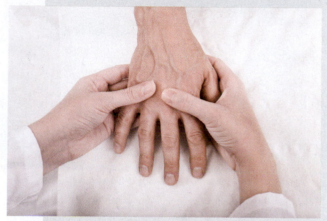

Figure 23.24B Palpating the hand.

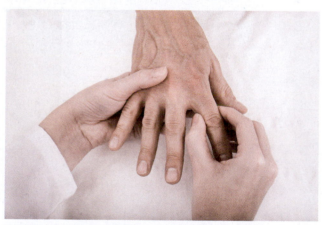

Figure 23.24C Palpating the fingers.

5. Test the ROM of the wrist.
- Instruct the patient to perform the following movements:
  - Straighten the hand (extension).
  - Using the wrist as a pivot point, bring the fingers backward as far as possible, and then bend the wrist downward (see Figure 23.25 ■). The wrist should hyperextend to 70 degrees and flex to 90 degrees.

Techniques and Normal Findings	Abnormal Findings and Special Considerations

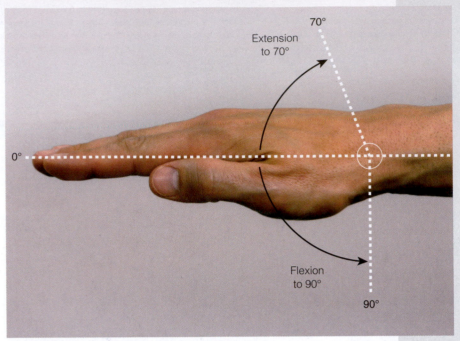

Figure 23.25 Hyperextension and flexion of the wrist.

- Turn the palms down; move the hand laterally toward the fifth finger, then medially toward the thumb (see Figure 23.26 ■). Be sure the movement is from the wrist and not the elbow. Ulnar deviation should reach as much as 55 degrees, and radial deviation should reach as much as 20 degrees.

▶ Abnormalities of wrist flexion or extension may be related to arthritis or other musculoskeletal conditions. Unusual sensations when performing these motions, such as numbness or tingling in the fingers, may be suggestive of carpal tunnel syndrome or other disorders. Abnormalities should be reported to the primary care provider for further evaluation.

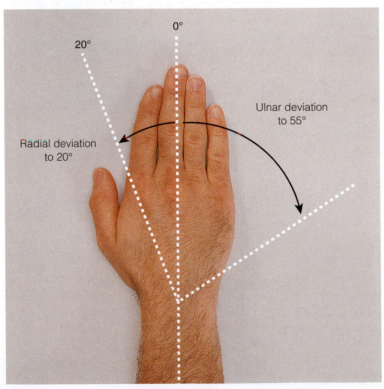

Figure 23.26 Ulnar and radial deviation of the wrist.

Techniques and Normal Findings	**Abnormal Findings and Special Considerations**

- Press the thumbs over the medial nerve, which runs down the middle of the underside of the wrist to perform the Durkan's test (carpal tunnel compression test). Hold the pressure for 30 seconds, looking for pain or numbness to appear with carpal tunnel.

- Bend the wrists downward and press the backs of both hands together (*Phalen's test*; see Figure 23.27 ■). This causes flexion of the wrists to 90 degrees. Normally patients experience no symptoms with this maneuver.

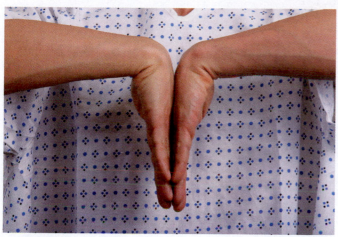

Figure 23.27 Phalen's test.

▶ The Durkan's test or carpal compression test has been found to be more sensitive (90%) and more specific (87%) in making a diagnosis than the Phalen's test (70% for sensitivity and 83% for specificity) or Tinel's test (50% for sensitivity and 77% for specificity) (Calandruccio & Thompson, 2018).

▶ When a Phalen's test is performed on individuals with carpal tunnel syndrome, 80% experience pain, tingling, and numbness that radiates to the arm, shoulder, neck, or chest within 60 seconds.

▶ If carpal tunnel syndrome is suspected, it is important to check for Tinel's sign by percussing lightly over the median nerve in each wrist. If carpal tunnel syndrome is present, the patient feels numbness, tingling, and pain along the median nerve (Figure 23.28 ■).

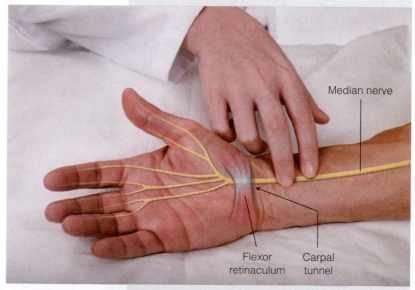

Median nerve

Flexor retinaculum

Carpal tunnel

Figure 23.28 Tinel's sign.

6. **Test the ROM of the hands and fingers.**
   Instruct the patient to perform the following movements:
   - Make a tight fist with each hand with the fingers folded into the palm and the thumb across the knuckles (thumb flexion).
   - Open the fist and stretch the fingers (extension).

- Point the fingers downward toward the forearm, and then back as far as possible (see Figure 23.29 ■). Fingers should flex to 90 degrees and hyperextend to as much as 30 degrees.

▶ In *Dupuytren's contracture*, the patient is unable to extend the fingers. This is a progressive, painless, inherited disorder that causes severe flexion in the affected fingers, is usually bilateral, and is more common in middle-aged and older males.

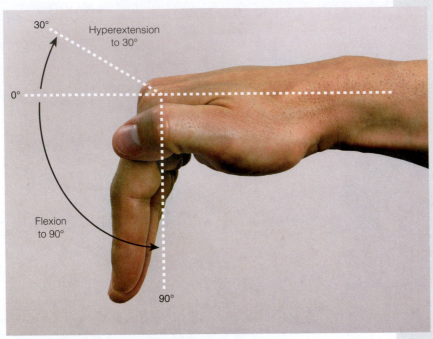

Figure 23.29 Flexion and extension of the fingers.

- Spread the fingers far apart, then back together. Fingers should abduct to 20 degrees and should adduct fully (to touch).
- Move the thumb toward the ulnar side of the hand and then away from the hand as far as possible.
- Touch the thumb to the tip of each of the fingers and to the base of the little finger.

7. **Test for muscle strength of the wrist.**
   - Place the patient's arm on a table with his or her palm facing up.
   - Stabilize the patient's forearm with one hand while holding the patient's hand with your other hand.
   - Instruct the patient to flex the wrist while you apply opposing resistance (see Figure 23.30 ■). The patient should be able to provide full resistance.

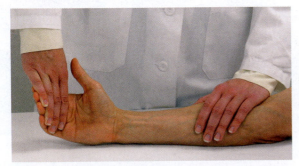

Figure 23.30 Testing the muscle strength of the wrist.

8. **Test for muscle strength of the fingers.**
   - Ask the patient to spread his or her fingers, after which you try to force the fingers together.
   - Ask the patient to touch his or her little finger with the thumb while you place resistance on the thumb in order to prevent the movement.

▶ Patients with carpal tunnel syndrome manifest weakness when attempting opposition of the thumb.

Techniques and Normal Findings	Abnormal Findings and Special Considerations

Hips

1. **With the patient in a supine position, inspect the position of each hip and leg.**
   - The legs should be slightly apart and the toes should point toward the ceiling. The legs should be of equal length.

2. **Palpate each hip joint and the upper thighs.**
   - The hip joints are firm, stable, and nontender.

3. **Test the ROM of the hips.**

▶ External rotation of the lower leg and foot is a classic sign of a fractured femur. Shortening of a limb is associated with hip fracture.

▶ Pain, tenderness, swelling, deformity, limited motion (especially limited internal rotation), and crepitus are diagnostic cues that signal inflammatory or degenerative joint diseases in the hip. A fractured femur should be suspected if the joint is unstable and deformed.

ALERT! *Do not ask patients who have undergone hip replacement to perform these movements without permission of the physician; these motions can dislocate the prosthesis.*

- Instruct the patient to perform the straight leg raise (SLR) test.
- Raise one leg straight off the bed or table (see Figure 23.31 ■). The other leg should remain flat on the bed. Hip flexion with straight knee should reach 90 degrees. Return the leg to its original position and repeat this maneuver with the other leg.

▶ In the patient with a herniated disk, the straight leg raise test may produce the *Lasègue's sign*, which includes back and leg pain along the course of the sciatic nerve. Presence of the Lasègue's sign is nonspecific and may be indicative of a variety of conditions; as such, follow-up evaluation is required to confirm sciatic nerve involvement (Yamin, Musharraf, Rehman, & Aziz, 2016).

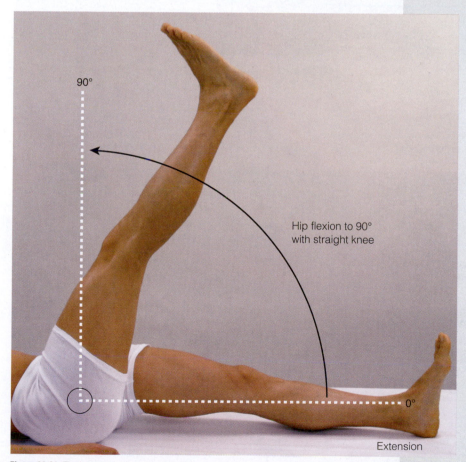

90°

Hip flexion to 90°
with straight knee

0°

Extension

Figure 23.31 Flexion of the hip with straight knee.

Techniques and Normal Findings	Abnormal Findings and Special Considerations

- Raise the leg with the knee flexed toward the chest as far as it will go (see Figure 23.32 ■). Hip flexion with flexed knee should reach 120 degrees. Return the leg to its original position.

▶ Abnormalities of hip flexion and rotation may be reflective of numerous musculoskeletal conditions, including arthritis, inguinal hernia, and spinal and joint disorders (Mayo Clinic, 2018). Abnormalities should be reported to the primary care provider for further evaluation.

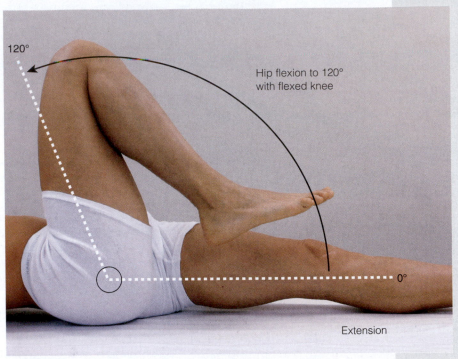

Hip flexion to 120°
with flexed knee

Extension

Figure 23.32 Flexion of the hip with flexed knee.

- Move the foot away from the midline as the knee moves toward the midline (see Figure 23.33 ■). Internal hip rotation should reach 40 degrees.

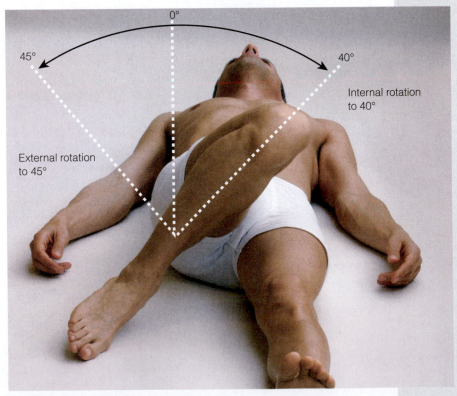

Internal rotation to 40°

External rotation to 45°

Figure 23.33 Internal and external hip rotation.

Techniques and Normal Findings	Abnormal Findings and Special Considerations

Techniques and Normal Findings

- Move the foot toward the midline as the knee moves away from the midline. External hip rotation should reach 45 degrees.
- Move the leg away from the midline (see Figure 23.34 ■), then as far as possible toward the midline. Abduction should reach 45 degrees. Adduction should reach 30 degrees.

Abnormal Findings and Special Considerations

▶ Abnormalities of hip abduction or adduction may be indicative of various injuries, including tearing of the acetabular labrum, which is a ring of cartilage that covers the outer rim of the socket of the hip joint. Injury to this structure may be caused by repetitive motions of hip abduction or adduction, which occur when playing certain sports, such as golf and soccer. Musculoskeletal disorders such as **developmental dysplasia of the hip (DDH)** also are associated with acetabular labrum tears (Mayo Clinic, 2018). Abnormalities should be reported to the primary care provider for further evaluation.

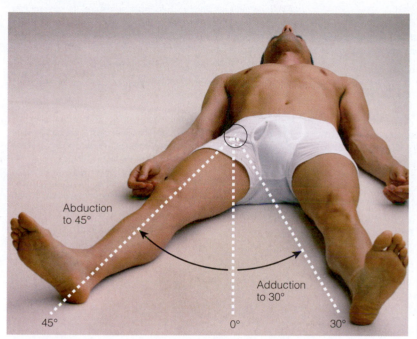

Figure 23.34 Abduction and adduction of the hip.

- Assist the patient to turn onto his or her abdomen. An alternative position could be side lying. With the patient's knee extended, ask the patient to raise each leg backward and up as far as possible (see Figure 23.35 ■). Hips should hyperextend to 15 degrees. (You may also perform this test later, during assessment of the spine, with the patient standing.)

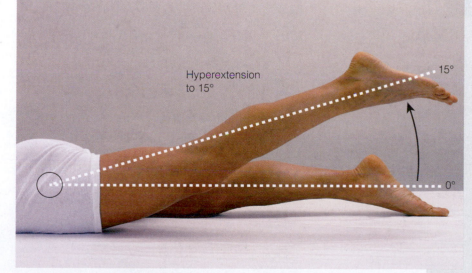

Figure 23.35 Hyperextension of the hip.

Techniques and Normal Findings	Abnormal Findings and Special Considerations

4. **Test for muscle strength of the hips.**
   - Assist the patient in returning to the supine position.
   - Press your hands on the patient's thighs and ask the patient to raise his or her hip.
   - Place your hands outside the patient's knees and ask the patient to spread both legs against your resistance.
   - Place your hands between the patient's knees, and ask the patient to bring the legs together against your resistance.

Knees

1. **Inspect the knees.**
   - With the patient in the sitting position, inspect the knees.
   - The patella should be centrally located in each knee. The normal depressions along each side of the patella should be sharp and distinct. The skin color should be similar to that of the surrounding areas.

2. **Inspect the quadriceps muscle in the anterior thigh.**
   - The muscles should be symmetric.

3. **Palpate the knee.**
   - Using your thumb, index finger, and middle finger, begin palpating approximately 10 cm (3.9 in.) above the patella with your thumb, index, and middle fingers (see Figure 23.36 ■). Palpate downward, evaluating each area.
   - The quadriceps muscle and surrounding soft tissue should be firm and nontender. The suprapatellar bursa is usually not palpable.

▶ Swelling and signs of fluid in the knee and its surrounding structures require further evaluation. Fluid accumulates in the suprapatellar bursa, the prepatellar bursa, and other areas adjacent to the patella when there is inflammation, trauma, or degenerative joint disease.

▶ Atrophy in the quadriceps muscles occurs with disuse or chronic disorders.

▶ Any pain, swelling, thickening, or heat should be noted while palpating the knee. These diagnostic cues occur when the synovium is inflamed. Painless swelling frequently occurs in degenerative joint disease. A painful, localized area of swelling, heat, and redness in the knee is caused by the inflammation of the bursa (bursitis)—for example, *prepatellar bursitis* (housemaid's knee).

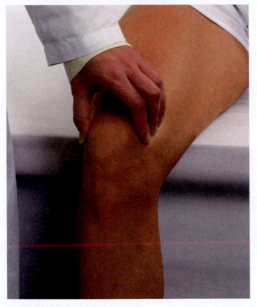

Figure 23.36 Palpating the knee.

4. **Test the ROM of each knee.**
   - Instruct the patient to bend each knee against the chest as far as possible (flexion) (see Figure 23.37 ■), and then to return the knee to its extended position.

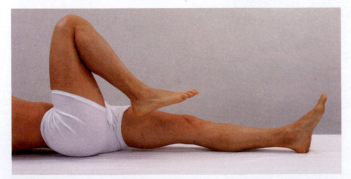

Figure 23.37 Flexion of the knee.

Techniques and Normal Findings	Abnormal Findings and Special Considerations

5. Test for muscle strength.
- Instruct the patient to flex each knee while you apply opposing force.
- Now instruct the patient to extend the knee again.
- The patient should be able to perform the movement against resistance.
- The strength of the muscles in both knees should be equal.

6. Inspect the knee while the patient is standing.
- Ask the patient to stand erect. If the patient is unsteady, allow the patient to hold onto the back of a chair.
- The knees should be in alignment with the thighs and ankles.
- Ask the patient to walk at a comfortable pace with a relaxed gait.

▶ Look for *genu varum*, *genu valgum*, or *genu recurvatum*.

Appendix C: Advanced Skills *Appendix C provides step-by-step instructions on testing for the bulge sign and ballottement.*

Ankles and Feet

1. Inspect the ankles and feet with the patient sitting, standing, and walking.
- The color of the ankles and feet should be similar to that of the rest of the body. They should be symmetric, and the skin should be unbroken. The feet and toes should be in alignment with the long axis of the lower leg. No swelling should be present, and the patient's weight should fall on the middle of the foot.

▶ The following abnormalities require further evaluation:

- *Gouty arthritis:* The metatarsophalangeal joint of the great toe is swollen, hot, red, and extremely painful.

- ***Hallux valgus*** *(bunion):* The great toe deviates laterally from the midline, crowding the other toes. The metatarsophalangeal joint and bursa become enlarged and inflamed, causing a bunion.

- *Hammertoe:* There is flexion of the proximal interphalangeal joint of a toe, and the distal metatarsophalangeal joint hyperextends. A callus or corn frequently occurs on the surface of the flexed joint from external pressure.

- *Pes planus (flatfoot):* The arch of the foot is flattened, sometimes coming in contact with the floor. The deformity may be noticeable only when an individual is standing and bearing weight on the foot.

2. Palpate the ankles.
- Grasp the heel of the foot with the fingers of both hands while palpating the anterior and lateral aspects of the ankle with your thumbs (see Figure 23.38 ■).
- The ankle joints should be firm, stable, and nontender.

▶ Pain or discomfort on palpation and movement frequently indicates degenerative joint disease.

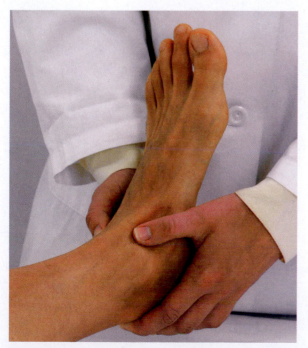

Figure 23.38 Palpating the ankle.

Techniques and Normal Findings	Abnormal Findings and Special Considerations

3. Palpate the length of the calcaneal (Achilles) tendon at the posterior ankle.
- The calcaneal tendon should be free of pain, tenderness, and nodules.

▶ Pain and tenderness along the tendon may indicate tendinitis or bursitis. Small nodules sometimes occur in patients with rheumatoid arthritis.

4. Palpate the metatarsophalangeal joints just below the ball of the foot.
- The metatarsophalangeal joints should be nontender.

▶ Pain and discomfort with this maneuver suggest early involvement of rheumatoid arthritis. Acute inflammation of the first metatarsophalangeal joint suggests gout.

5. Deeply palpate each metatarsophalangeal joint.
- The joints should be firm and nontender.

▶ Pain, swelling, or tenderness may be associated with inflammation or degenerative joint disease.

6. Test the ROM of the ankles and feet.
- Instruct the patient to perform the following movements:
  - Point the foot toward the nose. Dorsiflexion should reach 20 degrees.
  - Point the foot toward the floor. Plantar flexion should reach 45 degrees.
  - Point the sole of the foot outward and then inward. The ankle should evert to 20 degrees and invert to 30 degrees (see Figure 23.39 ■).
  - Curl the toes downward (flexion).
  - Spread the toes as far as possible (abduction), and then bring the toes together (adduction).

▶ Limited ROM and painful movement of the foot and ankle without signs of inflammation suggest degenerative joint disease.

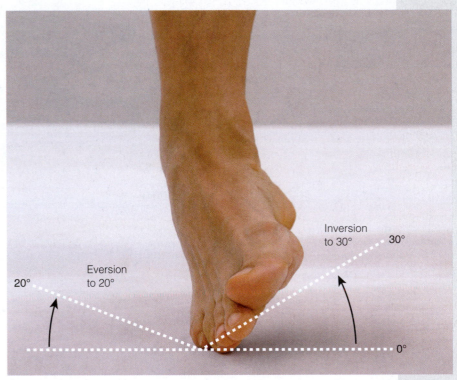

Figure 23.39 Eversion and inversion of the ankles.

7. Test muscle strength of the ankle.
- Ask the patient to perform dorsiflexion and plantar flexion against your resistance.

8. Test muscle strength of the foot.
- Ask the patient to flex and extend the toes against your resistance.

9. Palpate each interphalangeal joint.

▶ Pain, swelling, or tenderness may be associated with inflammation or degenerative joint disease.

- As you did for the hand, note the temperature of the extremity. Confirm that it is similar to the temperature of the rest of the patient's body.

▶ A temperature in the lower extremities that is significantly cooler than the rest of the body may indicate vascular insufficiency, which in turn may lead to musculoskeletal abnormalities.

Spine

1. **Inspect the spine.**
   - With the patient in a standing position, move around the patient's body to check the position and alignment of the spine from all sides. Confirm that the cervical and lumbar curves are concave and that the thoracic curve is convex (see Figure 23.40A ■).
   - Imagine a vertical line falling from the level of T1 to the gluteal cleft. Confirm that the spine is straight (see Figure 23.40B ■).

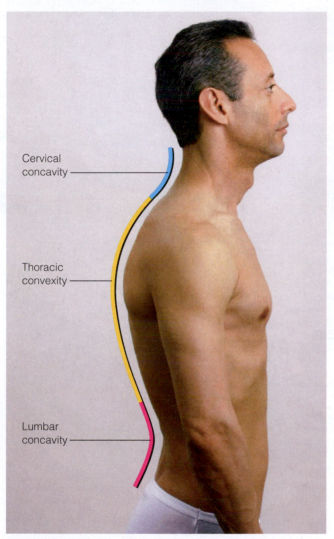

Figure 23.40A Lateral view of spine.

Cervical concavity

Thoracic convexity

Lumbar concavity

▶ Lack of symmetry of the scapulae may indicate thoracic surgery. A scapula may appear higher if a lung has been removed on that side. In addition, the following abnormalities require further evaluation:

- *Kyphosis*: An exaggerated thoracic dorsal curve that causes asymmetry between the sides of the posterior thorax.

- *Lordosis*: An exaggerated lumbar curve that compensates for pregnancy, obesity, or other skeletal changes.

- *Flattened lumbar curve:* A reduced lumbar concavity frequently occurs when spasms affect the lumbar muscles.

- *List:* The spine leans to the left or right. A plumb line drawn from T1 does not fall between the gluteal cleft. This condition may occur with spasms in the paravertebral muscles or a herniated disk.

Techniques and Normal Findings	Abnormal Findings and Special Considerations

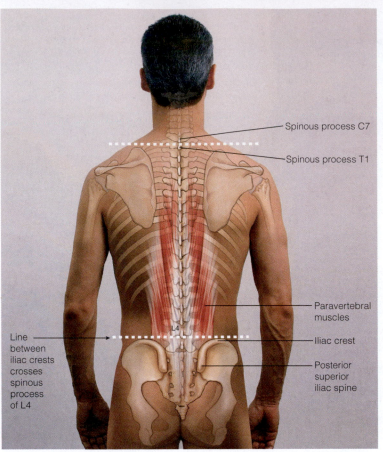

Figure 23.40B Posterior view of spine.

- Imagine a horizontal line across the top of the scapulae. Confirm that the scapulae are level and symmetric (see Figure 23.40B). Similarly, check that the heights of the iliac crests and the gluteal folds are level (see Figure 23.40B). Ask the patient to bend forward, and assess the alignment of the vertebrae.

2. **Palpate each vertebral process with your thumb.**
   - The vertebral processes should be aligned, uniform in size, firm, stable, and nontender.

3. **Palpate the muscles on both sides of the neck and back.**
   - The neck muscles should be fully developed and symmetric, firm, smooth, and nontender.

- *Scoliosis*: The spine curves to the right or left, causing an exaggerated thoracic convexity on that side. The body compensates, and a plumb line dropped from T1 falls between the gluteal cleft. Unequal leg length may contribute to scoliosis; therefore, if scoliosis is suspected, it is necessary to measure the patient's leg length. With the patient supine, measure the distance from the anterior superior iliac spine to the medial malleolus, crossing the tape measure at the medial side of the knee (Figure 23.41 ■). Spinal abnormalities are depicted in Table 25.7.

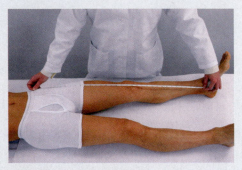

Figure 23.41 Measuring leg length.

▶ A *compression fracture* should be considered if the patient is elderly, complains of pain and tenderness in the back, and has restricted back movement. T8 and L3 are the most common sites for compression fractures.

▶ *Muscle spasms* feel like hardened or knotlike formations. When they occur, the patient may complain of pain and restricted movement. Muscle spasms may be associated with TMJ dysfunction or with *spasmodic torticollis*, a disorder in which the spasms cause the head to be pulled to one side.

Techniques and Normal Findings	Abnormal Findings and Special Considerations

4. **Test the ROM of the cervical spine.**
   - Instruct the patient to perform the following movements:
     - Touch the chest with the chin (flexion).
     - Look up toward the ceiling (hyperextension).
     - Attempt to touch each shoulder with the ear on that side, keeping the shoulder level (lateral bending or flexion).
     - Turn the head to face each shoulder as far as possible (rotation).

5. **Test the ROM of the thoracic and lumbar spine.**
   - Sit or stand behind the standing patient. Stabilize the pelvis with your hands and ask the patient to bend sideways to the right and to the left. Right and left lateral flexion should reach 35 degrees (see Figure 23.42 ■).

▶ Limited ROM, crepitation, or pain with movement in the joint requires further evaluation. If the patient complains of sharp pain that begins in the lower back and radiates down the leg, perform the straight leg raise (SLR) test as shown in Figure 23.31. If the patient reports pain when performing the SLR test, additional clues as to the origin of the pain may be identified by adding foot dorsiflexion, which may increase the sensation of pain (Magee, 2014). Record the distribution and severity of the pain and the degree of leg elevation at the time the pain occurs. Also record whether dorsiflexion increases the pain. Pain with straight leg raising may indicate a herniated disk.

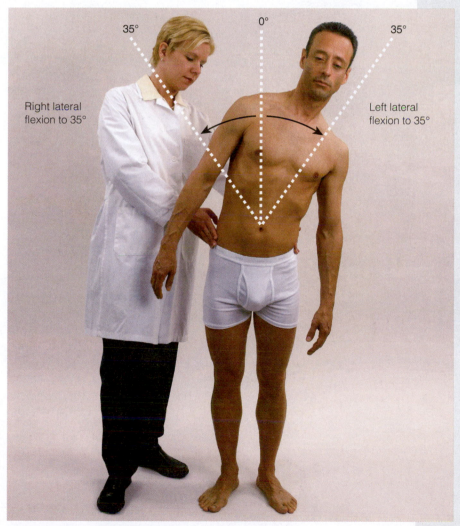

Figure 23.42 Lateral flexion of the spine.

Techniques and Normal Findings	Abnormal Findings and Special Considerations

- Ask the patient to bend forward and touch the toes (flexion). Confirm that the lumbar concavity disappears with this movement and that the back assumes a single C-shaped convexity (see Figure 23.43 ■).

▶ If the forward bend test reveals unevenness in the height of the posterior rib cage or the scapulae, scoliosis may be present. Abnormalities should be reported to the primary care provider for further evaluation.

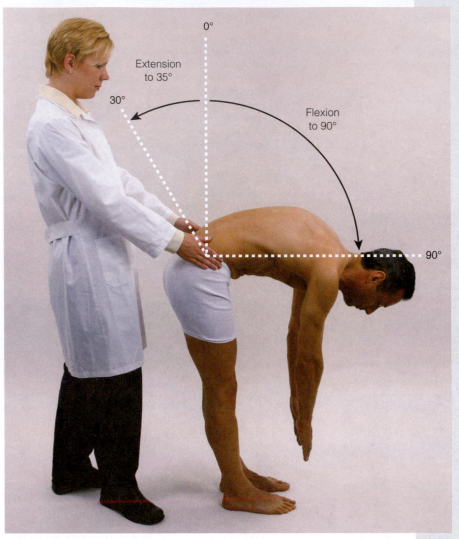

Figure 23.43 Forward flexion of the spine.

Techniques and Normal Findings	Abnormal Findings and Special Considerations

- Ask the patient to bend backward as far as is comfortable. Hyperextension should reach 30 degrees.
- Ask the patient to twist the shoulders to the left and to the right. Rotation should reach 30 degrees (see Figure 23.44 ■).

▶ Pain during spinal rotation or decreased mobility during this maneuver may be indicative of various disorders, including degenerative joint disease of the spine or damage to one or more of the intervertebral disks. Abnormalities should be reported to the primary care provider for further evaluation.

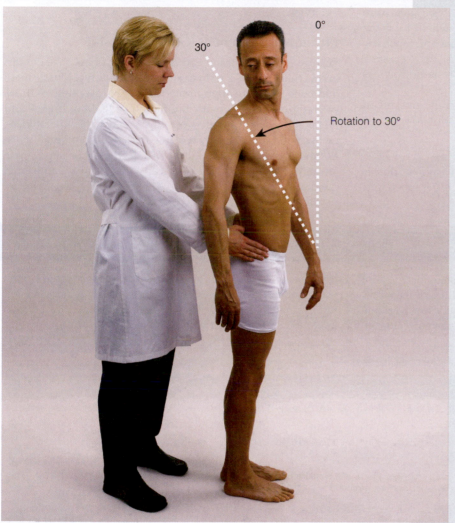

Figure 23.44 Rotation of the spine.

Documenting Your Findings

Documentation of assessment data—subjective and objective—must be accurate, professional, complete, and confidential. When documenting the information from the focused assessment of each body system, the nurse should use measurements where appropriate to ensure accuracy, use medical terminology rather than jargon, include all pertinent information, and avoid language that could identify the patient. The information in the documentation should make it clear what questions were asked, and the language used should indicate whether it is the patient's response or the nurse's findings. For patient responses, the documentation will say "denies," "states," or "reports," whereas the nurse's findings will simply list the findings as fact or say "no" along with the condition.

An example of normal results for the musculoskeletal system follows.

Focused History (Subjective Data)

Patient reports generalized joint pain and weakness that is worse in the hands and feet bilaterally. Pain is described as a dull ache with a pain score of 3 on a 0–10 scale. Reports stiffness in all joints with movement that is worse in the mornings, occurs on most days, and is often worse with activity. Takes Motrin 400 mg twice daily as needed. Patient reports no difficulty in performing ADLs. Denies swelling or redness in joints. No history of bone or muscle pain, deformities, fractures, or falls in the past. Walks three times a week approximately 1–2 miles.

Physical Assessment (Objective Data)

Posture erect, gait steady and even. No use of assistive devices at this time. Scoliosis test negative upon bending. Muscle mass and bone structure appropriate for age. No swelling, redness, or crepitus noted in joints. Limitation in ROM of fingers and feet with muscle strength = 4/5. ROM of TMJ, neck, shoulders, elbow, wrist, spine, hip, knees and ankle within normal limits. ROM in hands, fingers, ankles with decreased flexion Muscle strength of deltoid, biceps, triceps, wrist, hip, hamstring, quadriceps and ankle = 4/5.

Abnormal Findings

Abnormal findings of the musculoskeletal system include joint disorders, inflammatory disorders, abnormalities of the spine, and trauma-induced disorders. Table 23.5 provides an overview of common inflammatory diseases that affect the musculoskeletal system. Table 23.6 summarizes several of the most common traumatic musculoskeletal injuries. A general review of common spinal abnormalities is provided in Table 23.7. Common joint disorders are described in Table 23.8.

Table 23.5 Overview of Inflammatory Musculoskeletal Diseases

DISEASE	DESCRIPTION
Osteoarthritis (OA)	In OA the joint cartilage erodes, resulting in pain and stiffness. Disability is associated with osteoarthritic changes in the spine, knees, and hips.
Rheumatoid Arthritis (RA)	Inflammation of the synovium of the joint occurs in RA. The inflammation leads to pain, swelling, damage to the joint, and loss of function. RA affects the hands and feet symmetrically.
Juvenile Rheumatoid Arthritis (JRA)	This form of arthritis occurs in children before age 16 and can affect any body part. Inflammation causes pain, swelling, stiffness, and loss of function of joints. Symptoms may include fever and skin rash.
Systemic Lupus Erythematosus (SLE)	SLE is an autoimmune disease. The autoimmune response results in inflammation and damage to joints and other organs, including the kidneys, lungs, blood vessels, and heart.
Scleroderma	In scleroderma there is an overproduction of collagen in the skin or organs, which results in damage to the skin, blood vessels, and joints. Typically, the skin becomes hard and tight.
Fibromyalgia	Fibromyalgia is a chronic disease that is characterized by pain in the muscles and soft tissues that support and surround joints. Pain is experienced in tender points of the head, neck, shoulders, and hips.
Ankylosing Spondylitis (AS)	AS is a chronic inflammatory disease of the spine. It occurs more frequently in males than in females. Fusion of the spine results in stiffness and inflexibility. This disorder may also affect the hips.
Gout	Gout is a type of arthritis caused by uric acid crystal deposits in the joints. The uric acid deposits (**tophi**) cause inflammation, pain, and swelling in the joint.
Infectious Arthritis	Infectious arthritis refers to joint inflammatory processes that occur as a result of bacterial or viral infection. Infectious arthritis can occur as parvovirus arthritis, as gonococcal arthritis, or in Lyme disease.
Psoriatic Arthritis (PsA)	PsA may occur in individuals with psoriasis, a skin disease. Joint inflammation occurs in the fingers and toes and, occasionally, in the spine.
Bursitis	Bursitis refers to inflammation of the bursae (fluid-filled sacs) that surround joints. The pain of bursitis may limit ROM of the affected area.
Tendinitis	Overuse or inflammatory processes can result in tendinitis. The inflammation of the tendon results in pain and limitation in movement.
Polymyositis	Polymyositis refers to inflammation and weakness in skeletal muscles. This disease can affect the entire body and result in disability.

Table 23.6 Traumatic Musculoskeletal Injuries

DISORDER	DESCRIPTION
Dislocation	A displacement of the bone from its usual anatomic location in the joint.
Joint Sprain	A stretching or tearing of the capsule or ligament of a joint because of forced movement beyond the joint's normal range.
Fracture	A partial or complete break in the continuity of the bone from trauma.
Muscle Strain	A partial muscle tear resulting from overstretching or overuse of the muscle.

Table 23.7 Common Spinal Abnormalities

Kyphosis

An exaggeration of the normal convex curve of the thoracic spine that may result from congenital abnormality, rheumatic conditions, compression fractures, or other disease processes, including syphilis, tuberculosis, and rickets. Severe kyphosis may occur with aging because of other contributing factors, such as degenerative joint disease, poor posture, or hormonal changes.

Scoliosis

A lateral curvature of the spine that may occur congenitally, or as a result of disease, injury, habitual improper posture, unequal leg length, weakening of musculature, or chronic head tilting in visual disorders.

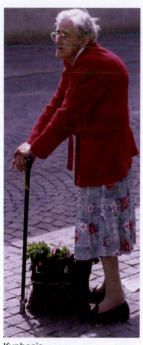

Kyphosis.
Source: Bengt-Göran Carlsson/Nordicphotos/Alamy Stock Photo.

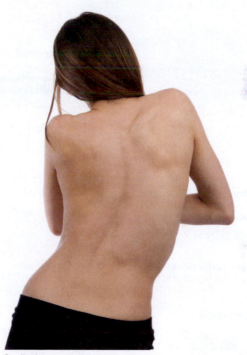

Scoliosis.
Source: Dmitry Lobanov/123RF.

(continued)

Table 23.7 Common Spinal Abnormalities (continued)

Lordosis

An exaggeration of the normal lumbar curve. Lordosis occurs in pregnancy and in obesity to compensate for the protuberance of the abdomen. Benign juvenile lordosis occurs congenitally. Other conditions such as spondylolisthesis may also aid in the formation of lordosis later in life.

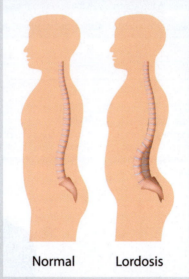

Normal   Lordosis

Benign juvenile lordosis.
Source: Alila Medical Media/Shutterstock.

Table 23.8 Common Joint Disorders

Temporomandibular Joint Syndrome

Inflammation or trauma can result in temporomandibular joint (TMJ) syndrome.

Findings include swelling and crepitus or pain in the TM joint, especially on movement such as opening and closing the mouth.

Rotator Cuff Tear

Arises from repeated impingement, injury, or falls. Impaired abduction of the glenohumeral joint occurs with a complete tear of the supraspinatus tendon.

Findings include muscle atrophy of the infraspinatus and supraspinatus, tenderness, and pain.

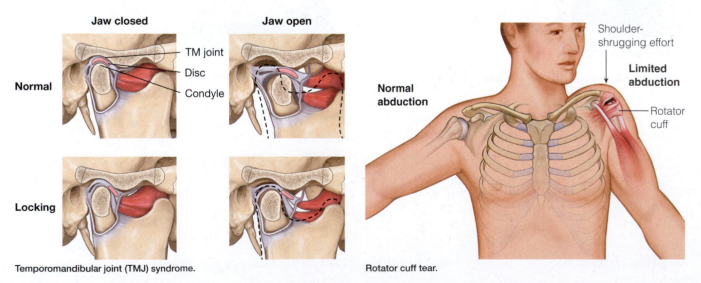

Temporomandibular joint (TMJ) syndrome.

Rotator cuff tear.

(continued)

Table 23.8 Common Joint Disorders (continued)

Olecranon Bursitis

Inflammation of the olecranon bursa at the bony prominence of the elbow that may be caused by trauma or inflammation from rheumatoid or gouty arthritis. Bursitis can develop in a variety of body regions.

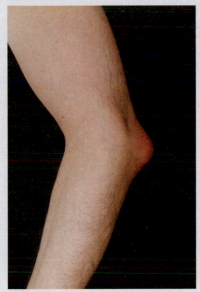

Olecranon bursitis.
Source: joseelias/123RF.

Joint Effusion

Inflammatory joint disease results in fluid in the joint capsule, causing joint effusion. Joint effusion produces distention of the tissue around the inflamed joint.

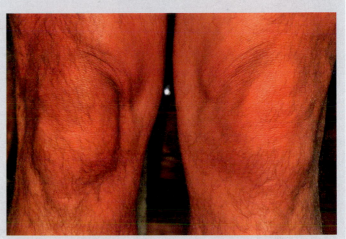

Joint effusion of the knee.
Source: mountainpix/Shutterstock.

Rheumatoid Nodules

Firm, nontender subcutaneous nodules that often are seen distal to the olecranon bursa in the hands and fingers.

Rheumatoid nodules may occur along the extensor surface of the ulna.

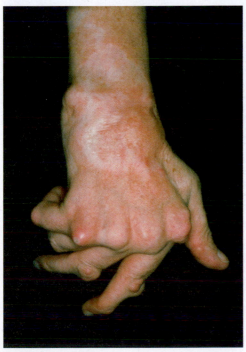

Rheumatoid nodules.

Carpal Tunnel Syndrome

Chronic repetitive motion results in compression of the median nerve, which lies inside the carpal tunnel. Decreased motor function leads to atrophy of the thenar eminence. Findings in carpal tunnel syndrome include pain, numbness, and positive Phalen's test.

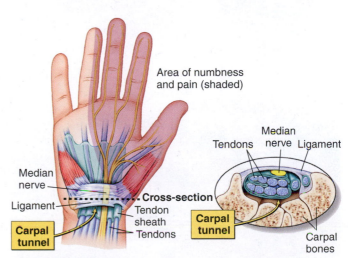

Carpal tunnel syndrome.

(continued)

Table 23.8 Common Joint Disorders (continued)

Dupuytren's Contracture

Flexion contracture of the fingers is a result of hyperplasia of the fascia of the palmar surface of the hand. Impaired ROM is a hallmark of contractures. Dupuytren's contracture may be inherited or occur with diabetes or alcoholic cirrhosis.

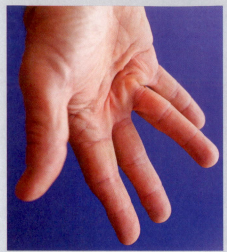

Dupuytren's contracture.
Source: fineart/123RF.

Ulnar Deviation

In RA the chronic inflammation of the metacarpophalangeal and interphalangeal joints leads to ulnar deviation. RA can lead to a number of musculoskeletal deformities, the most common of which affect the hands and feet.

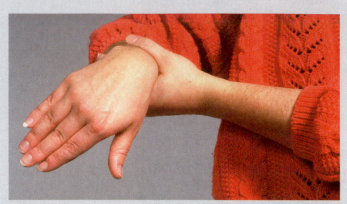

Ulnar deviation.

Swan-Neck and Boutonnière Deformities

Flexion contractures associated with rheumatoid arthritis. *Swan-neck contractures* refer to hyperextension of the proximal interphalangeal joints with fixed flexion of the distal interphalangeal joints. *Boutonniére deformities* involve proximal interphalangeal joint flexion in conjunction with distal interphalangeal joint hyperextension.

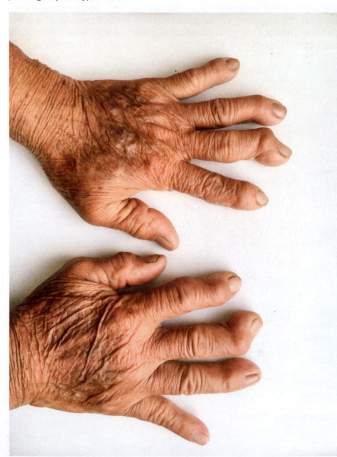

Swan-neck and boutonnière deformities.
Source: chatuphot/Shutterstock.

Osteoarthritis

OA is associated with the development of Bouchard's and Heberden's nodes, which are hard nodules over the proximal and distal interphalangeal joints.

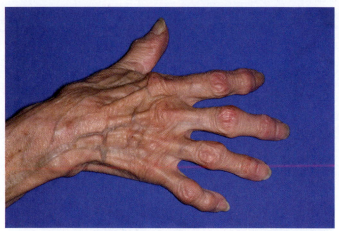

Heberden's nodes are found in the distal interphalangeal joints.
Source: Scott Camazine/Alamy Stock Photo.

(continued)

Table 23.8 Common Joint Disorders (continued)

Rheumatoid Arthritis

RA results in symmetric fusiform swelling in the soft tissue around the proximal interphalangeal joints. Other symptoms may include pain, fatigue, and morning joint stiffness.

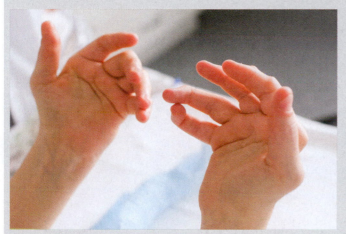

Rheumatoid arthritis.
Source: BURGER/Phanie/Alamy Stock Photo.

Synovitis

Refers to inflammation of the synovium, which is the tissue that lines the joints. In the knee, effusion within the synovium results in distention of the suprapatellar area and the lateral aspects of the knee.

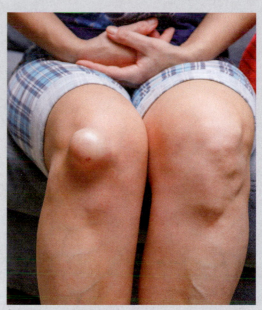

Synovitis.
Source: dziewul/123RF.

Gout

Altered purine metabolism results in inflammation of the joints. Usually seen in the metatarsophalangeal joint of the first toe, gout is manifested in erythema, pain, and edema. Hard nodules (tophi) may appear over the joint.

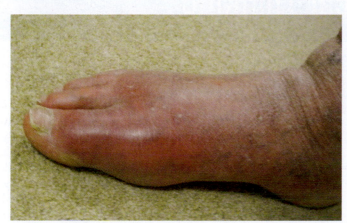

Gout.
Source: David Cole/Alamy Stock Photo.

Hallux Valgus (Bunion)

A bunion is a thickening and inflammation of the bone or the bursa of the joint of the great toe that produces lateral displacement of the toe with marked joint enlargement. The big toe may turn toward the second toe. The tissues around the joint may be swollen and tender.

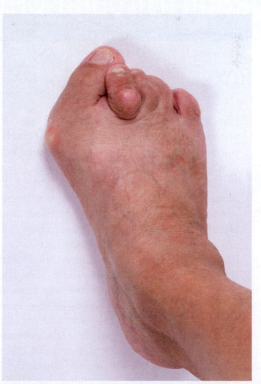

Hallux valgus (bunion); also note the hammertoe of the second digit.
Source: Julio Rivalta/123RF.

(continued)

Table 23.8 Common Joint Disorders (continued)

Hammertoe

Hammertoe is caused by an imbalance of the muscle and ligament around the toe joint. It may be the result of trauma or genetic factors. This condition also may be caused by wearing certain types of footwear, including narrow-toed shoes, high heels, or shoes that are too small. The middle toe joint becomes fixed in a flexed position. Without treatment, this condition will progressively worsen.

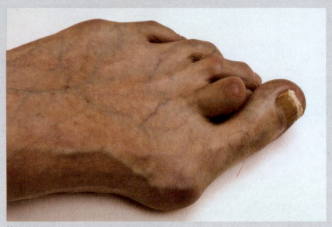

Hammertoe.
Source: Pavel Kocur/Alamy Stock Photo.

Application Through Critical Thinking

CASE STUDY

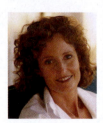

Source: Ryan McVay/Getty Images.

Mrs. Rhonda Barber is a 43-year-old teacher. She visits the clinic for assessment of swelling and stiffness all over, especially in her hands.

The health history reveals that for several months Mrs. Barber has had some stiffness in her joints when awakening from sleep and after long periods of physical activity "like housework." She became "alarmed" when her hands were "hot, red, and swollen" and that she "could hardly move them." She has had no recent illness but has "felt weak and tired" and has not had much of an appetite lately. She reports no family history of musculoskeletal disease. She reports that she has had regular physical examinations, including blood work, and that nothing has been abnormal. Her last exam was 6 months ago. She takes no prescribed medications but has been using Advil and Aleve for the stiffness with moderate relief. She states that she is concerned about her hands because she must write on the board and correct papers. She also fears that "if something is really wrong and I don't get relief, I won't be able to care for my family or myself for that matter."

Physical assessment reveals a well-developed female 5'3" tall, weighing 120 lb. Her skin is pale and warm. Her gait is steady. She has normal ROM in the upper and lower extremities. ROM of her wrists, hands, and fingers is limited. The joints of her fingers are erythematous, hot, and edematous bilaterally. Her joints are tender to touch and painful upon movement. Pain is 6 to 7 on a scale of 0 to 10.

The nurse suspects that Mrs. Barber may have rheumatoid arthritis. The nurse will obtain laboratory tests and X-rays.

SAMPLE DOCUMENTATION

The following is a sample documentation from assessment of Rhonda Barber.

SUBJECTIVE DATA For several months, stiffness in joints on waking and after long periods of physical activity. "Alarmed" when hands were hot, red, swollen, and could hardly move them. No recent illness. Weak, tired, and loss of appetite lately. No family history of musculoskeletal disease. Regular physical examinations with normal results and normal "blood work." Last examination 6 months ago. No prescribed medications. Advil and Aleve for stiffness—moderate relief. Concerned about ability to work as teacher and "if something is really wrong," about ability to care for family.

OBJECTIVE DATA Well-developed 43-year-old female. 5′3″, 120 lb. Skin pale, warm. Gait steady. Full ROM all extremities except hands and fingers. Joints of fingers erythematous, hot, edematous bilaterally, tender to touch, and painful on movement. Pain 6 to 7 on scale of 0 to 10.

CRITICAL THINKING QUESTIONS

1. Describe the thoughts and actions of the nurse that led to the suspicion of rheumatoid arthritis.

2. What information would help in developing a plan of care for Mrs. Barber?

3. How would the nurse discriminate between findings for rheumatoid arthritis and osteoarthritis?

4. As Mrs. Barber ages, what additional age-related changes will she need to be concerned about?

5. What are some strategies that would help Mrs. Barber get through the physical exam portion?

REFERENCES

Calandruccio, J. H., & Thompson, N. B. (2018). Carpal tunnel syndrome making evidence-based treatment decisions. *Orthopedic Clinics of North America, 49*, 223–229.

Chicoski, A., (2018). Caring for the orthopaedic patient with a history of bariatric surgery. *Orthopaedic Nursing, 37*(2), 106–112.

Heneghan, N., Adab, P., Jackman, S., & Balanos, G. (2015). Musculoskeletal dysfunction in chronic obstructive pulmonary disease (COPD): An observational study. *International Journal of Therapy and Rehabilitation, 22*(3), 119–128.

Izadi, M., Sadat, S. E., Zamani, M. M., Mousavi, S. A., Jafari, N. J., Fard, M. M., . . . Talakoob, H. (2013). Trauma induced chronic osteomyelitis: Specimens from sinus tract or bone? *Galen Medical Journal, 2*(4), 146–151.

Kruger, M. C., Todd, J. M., Schollum, L. M., Kuhn-Sherlock, B., McLean, D. W., & Wylie, K. (2013). Bone health comparison in seven Asian countries using calcaneal ultrasound. *BMC Musculoskeletal Disorders, 14*(1), 81.

Magee, D. J. (2014). *Orthopedic physical assessment* (6th ed.). St. Louis, MO: Elsevier.

May, A., Pettifor, J. M., Norris, S. A., Ramsay, M., & Lombard, Z. (2013). Genetic factors influencing bone mineral content in a black South African population. *Journal of Bone and Mineral Metabolism, 31*(6), 708–716.

Mayo Clinic. (2016a). *Osteoporosis: Definition*. Retrieved from http://www.mayoclinic.org/diseases-conditions/osteoporosis/basics/definition/con-20019924

Mayo Clinic (2016b). *Osteoporosis*. Retrieved from https://www.mayoclinic.org/diseases-conditions/osteoporosis/symptoms-causes/syc-20351968

Mayo Clinic (2017). *Rheumatoid arthritis*. Retrieved from https://www.mayoclinic.org/diseases-conditions/rheumatoid-arthritis/symptoms-causes/syc-20353648

Mayo Clinic (2018) *Hip pain*. Retrieved from https://www.mayoclinic.org/symptoms/hip-pain/basics/causes/sym-20050684

MedlinePlus. (2018). *Osteomyelitis*. Retrieved from http://www.nlm.nih.gov/medlineplus/ency/article/000437.htm

Osborn, K. S., Wraa, C. E., Watson, A., & Holleran, R. S. (2013). *Medical-surgical nursing: Preparation for practice* (2nd ed.). Upper Saddle River, NJ: Pearson.

Pervaiz, K., Cabezas, A., Downes, K., Santoni, B. G., & Frankle, M. A. (2013). Osteoporosis and shoulder osteoarthritis: Incidence, risk factors, and surgical implications. *Journal of Shoulder and Elbow Surgery, 22*(3), e1–e8.

van der Zee-Neuen, A., Putrik, P., Ramiro, S., Keszei, A., de Bie, R., Chorus, A., & Boonen, A. (2016). Impact of chronic diseases and multimorbidity on health and health care costs: The additional role of musculoskeletal disorders. *Arthritis Care and Research, 68*(12), 1823–1831.

Wasser, J. G., Vasilopoulos, T., Zdziarski, L. A., & Vincent, H. K. (2017). Exercise benefits for chronic low back pain in overweight and obese individuals. *PM&R Journal of Injury, Function & Rehabilitation, 9*(2), 181–192.

Weycker, D., Lamerato, L., Schooley, S., Macarios, D., Woodworth, T. S., Yurgin, N., & Oster, G. (2013). Adherence with bisphosphonate therapy and change in bone mineral density among women with osteoporosis or osteopenia in clinical practice. *Osteoporosis International, 24*(4), 1483–1489.

Wilson, B. A., Shannon, M. T., & Shields, K. M. (2018). *Pearson nurse's drug guide*. Upper Saddle River, NJ: Pearson.

Yamin, F., Musharraf, H., Rehman, A. U., & Aziz, S. (2016.) Efficacy of sciatic nerve mobilization in lumbar radiculopathy due to prolapsed intervertebral disc. *Indian Journal of Physiotherapy and Occupational Therapy, 10*(1), 37–41.

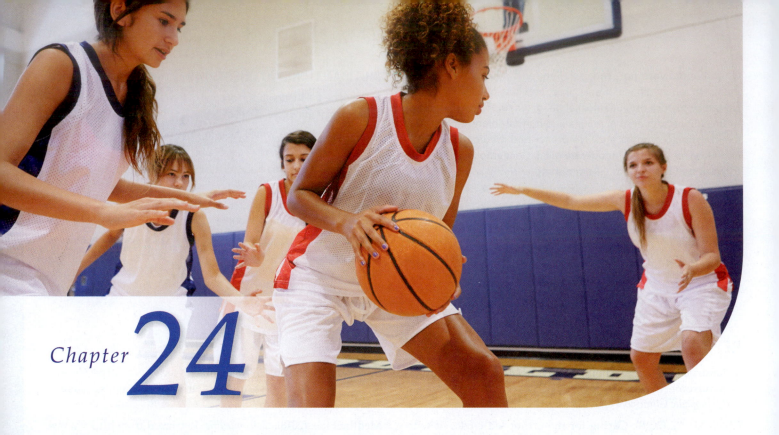

Chapter 24

Neurologic System

LEARNING OUTCOMES

Upon completion of this chapter, you will be able to:

1. Describe the anatomy and physiology of the neurologic system.

2. Identify the anatomic, physiologic, developmental, psychosocial, and cultural variations that guide assessment of the neurologic system.

3. Determine which questions about the neurologic system to use for the focused interview.

4. Outline the techniques for assessment of the neurologic system.

5. Generate the appropriate documentation to describe the assessment of the neurologic system.

6. Identify abnormal findings in the physical assessment of the neurologic system.

KEY TERMS

MEDICAL LANGUAGE

extra-	Prefix meaning "outside"	**ophthalm-**	Prefix meaning "eye"
-graphy	Suffix meaning "process of recording"	**-opia**	Suffix meaning "vision condition"
-itis	Suffix meaning "inflammation"	**photo-**	Prefix meaning "light"

Introduction

The complex integration, coordination, and regulation of body systems, and, ultimately, all body functions, are achieved through the mechanics of the nervous system. The intricate nature of the nervous system permits the individual to perform all physiologic functions, perform all activities of daily living, function in society, and maintain a degree of independence. A threat to any aspect of neurologic function is a threat to the whole person. A neurologic deficit could alter self-concept, produce anxiety related to decreased function and loss of self-control, and restrict the patient's mobility. Thus, it is essential to assess the psychosocial health status of a patient experiencing a neurologic deficit.

A thorough neurologic assessment gives the nurse detailed data regarding the patient's health status and self-care practices. It is imperative to develop and refine assessment skills regarding the wellness and normal parameters of the neurologic functions in the body. The nurse needs to foster a keen discriminatory skill concerning the subtle changes that could be occurring in the patient. Neurologic assessment is an integral aspect of the patient's health and must be carefully considered when conducting a thorough health assessment.

Anatomy and Physiology Review

The neurologic system, a highly integrated and complex system, is divided into two principal parts: the central nervous system (CNS) and the peripheral nervous system (PNS). The **central nervous system** consists of the brain and the spinal cord, whereas the cranial nerves and the spinal nerves make up the **peripheral nervous system**. The two systems work together to receive an impulse, interpret it, and initiate a response, enabling the individual to maintain a high level of adaptation and homeostasis. The nervous system is responsible for control of cognitive function and both voluntary and involuntary actions.

The basic cell of the nervous system is the *neuron*. This highly specialized cell sends impulses throughout the body. Many of the nerve fibers that have a large diameter or are long in length are covered with a *myelin sheath*. This white, fatty cover helps to protect the neuron while increasing the delivery of a nerve impulse, hence the term *white matter of the nervous system*.

Central Nervous System

The central nervous system (CNS) includes the brain and spinal cord. These structures are described in the following sections.

Brain The brain is the largest portion of the central nervous system. It is covered and protected by the meninges, the cerebrospinal fluid, and the bony structure of the skull. The **meninges** are three connective tissue membranes that cover, protect, and nourish the central nervous system. The cerebrospinal fluid also helps to nourish the central nervous system; however, its primary function is to cushion the brain and prevent injury to the brain tissue. The brain is made up of the cerebrum, diencephalon, cerebellum, and brainstem (see Figure 24.1 ■).

CEREBRUM The **cerebrum** is the largest portion of the brain. The outermost layer of the cerebrum, the *cerebral cortex*, is composed of gray matter. Responsible for all conscious behavior, the cerebral cortex enables the individual to perceive, remember, communicate, and initiate voluntary movements. The cerebrum consists of the frontal, parietal, occipital, and temporal lobes. The lobes of the cerebrum are illustrated in Figure 24.2 ■.

The frontal lobe of the cerebrum helps control voluntary skeletal movement, speech, emotions, and intellectual activities. The prefrontal cortex of the frontal lobe controls intellect, complex

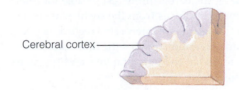

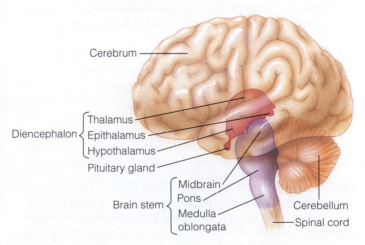

Figure 24.1 Regions of the brain.

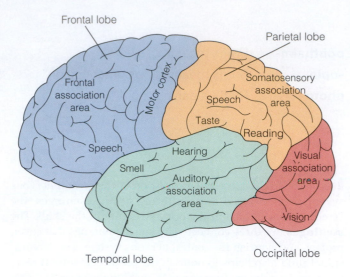

Figure 24.2 Lobes of the cerebrum.

learning abilities, judgment, reasoning, concern for others, and creation of abstract ideas.

The parietal lobe of the cerebrum is responsible for conscious awareness of sensation and somatosensory stimuli, including temperature, pain, shapes, and two-point discrimination—for example, the ability to sense a round versus square object placed in the hand or hot versus cold materials against the skin.

The visual cortex, located in the occipital lobe, receives stimuli from the retina and interprets the visual stimuli in relation to past experiences.

The temporal lobe of the cerebrum is responsible for interpreting auditory stimuli. Impulses from the cochlea are transmitted to the temporal lobe and are interpreted regarding pitch, rhythm, loudness, and perception of what the individual hears. The olfactory cortex is also in the temporal lobe and transmits impulses related to smell.

DIENCEPHALON   The diencephalon is composed of the thalamus, hypothalamus, and epithalamus. The **thalamus** is the gateway to the cerebral cortex. All input channeled to the cerebral cortex is processed by the thalamus.

The hypothalamus, an autonomic control center, influences activities such as blood pressure, heart rate, force of heart contraction, digestive motility, respiratory rate and depth, and perception of pain, pleasure, and fear. Regulation of body temperature, food intake, water balance, and sleep cycles are also regulated by the hypothalamus.

The epithalamus helps control moods and sleep cycles. It contains the choroid plexus, where the cerebrospinal fluid is formed.

CEREBELLUM   The **cerebellum** is located below the cerebrum and behind the brainstem. It coordinates stimuli from the cerebral cortex to provide precise timing for skeletal muscle coordination and smooth movements. The cerebellum also assists with maintaining equilibrium and muscle tone. The cerebellum receives information about the body position from the inner ear and then sends impulses to the muscles, whose contraction maintains or restores balance.

BRAINSTEM   The **brainstem** contains the midbrain, pons, and medulla oblongata. Located between the cerebrum and the spinal cord, the brainstem connects pathways between the higher and lower structures. Of the 12 pairs of cranial nerves, 10 originate in the brainstem. As an autonomic control center, the brainstem influences blood pressure by controlling vasoconstriction. It also regulates respiratory rate, depth, and rhythm as well as vomiting, hiccupping, swallowing, coughing, and sneezing.

Spinal Cord   The **spinal cord** is a continuation of the medulla oblongata. About 42 cm (17 in.) in length, it passes through the skull at the foramen magnum and continues through the vertebral column to the first and second lumbar vertebrae. The meninges, cerebrospinal fluid, and bony vertebrae protect the spinal cord. The spinal cord has the ability to transmit sensory impulses to and motor impulses from the brain via the ascending and descending pathways. It also mediates stretch reflexes and reflexes for defecation and urination. Some reflex activity takes place within the spinal cord; however, for this activity to be useful, the brain must interpret it.

Reflexes

Reflexes are stimulus–response activities of the body. They are fast, predictable, unlearned, innate, and involuntary reactions to stimuli. The individual is aware of the results of the reflex activity and not the activity itself. The reflex activity may be simple and take place at the level of the spinal cord, with interpretation at the cerebral level. For example, if the tendon of the knee is sharply stimulated with a reflex hammer, the impulse follows the afferent nerve fibers. A synapse occurs in the spinal cord, and the impulse is transmitted to the efferent nerve fibers, leading to an additional synapse and stimulation of muscle fibers. As the muscle fibers contract, the lower leg moves, causing the knee-jerk reaction. The individual is aware of the reflex after the lower leg moves and the brain has interpreted the activity. Figure 24.3 ■ illustrates two simple reflex arcs.

Peripheral Nervous System

The peripheral nervous system (PNS) includes the 12 pairs of cranial nerves, which take impulses to and from the brain, and the paired spinal nerves, which transmit impulses to and from the spinal cord. They are described in the following paragraphs.

Cranial Nerves   The 12 pairs of cranial nerves originate in the brain and serve various parts of the head and neck (see Figure 24.4 ■). The first 2 pairs originate in the anterior brain, and the remaining 10 pairs originate in the brainstem. The vagus nerve is the only cranial nerve to serve a muscle and body region below the neck. The cranial nerves are numbered using Roman numerals and many times are discussed by number rather than by name. Composition of the cranial nerve fibers varies, producing sensory nerves, motor nerves, and mixed nerves. A summary of the names, numbers, functions, and activities of the cranial nerves is presented in Table 24.1.

Spinal Nerves   The spinal cord supplies the body with 31 pairs of spinal nerves that are named according to the vertebral level of origin as shown in Figure 24.5 ■.

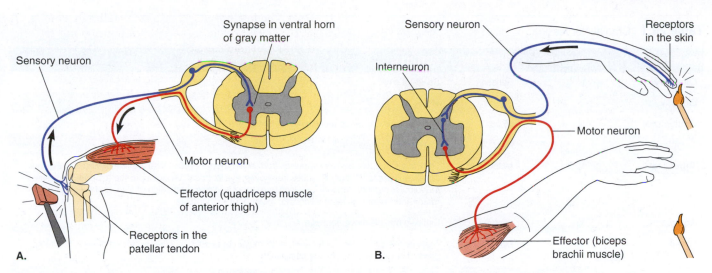

Figure 24.3 Two simple reflex arcs. A. In the two-neuron reflex arc, the stimulus is transferred from the sensory neuron directly to the motor neuron at the point of synapse in the spinal cord. B. In the three-neuron reflex arc, the stimulus travels from the sensory neuron to an interneuron in the spinal cord, and then to the motor neuron. (Sensory nerves are shown in blue, motor nerves in red.)

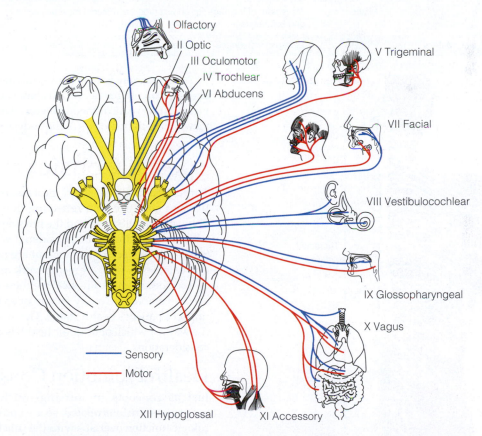

Figure 24.4 Cranial nerves and their target regions. (Sensory nerves are shown in blue, motor nerves in red.)

There are 8 pairs of cervical nerves, 12 pairs of thoracic nerves, 5 pairs of lumbar nerves, 5 pairs of sacral nerves, and 1 pair of coccygeal nerves. At the cervical level, the nerves exit superior to the vertebra except for the eighth cervical nerve. This nerve exits inferior to the seventh cervical vertebra. All remaining descending nerves exit the spinal cord and vertebral column inferior to the same-numbered vertebrae. Spinal nerves are all classified as mixed nerves because they contain motor and sensory pathways that produce motor and sensory activities. Each pair of nerves is responsible for a particular area of the body. The nerves provide some overlap of body segments they serve. This overlap is more complete on the trunk than on the extremities.

Table 24.1 Cranial Nerves

NAME	NUMBER	FUNCTION	ACTIVITY
Olfactory	I	Sensory	Sense of smell
Optic	II	Sensory	Vision
Oculomotor	III	Motor	Pupillary reflex, extrinsic muscle movement of eye
Trochlear	IV	Motor	Eye-muscle movement
Trigeminal	V	Mixed	*Ophthalmic branch:* Sensory impulses from scalp, upper eyelid, nose, cornea, and lacrimal gland *Maxillary branch:* Sensory impulses from lower eyelid, nasal cavity, upper teeth, upper lip, palate *Mandibular branch:* Sensory impulses from tongue, lower teeth, skin of chin, and lower lip; motor action includes teeth clenching, movement of mandible
Abducens	VI	Mixed	Extrinsic muscle movement of eye
Facial	VII	Mixed	Taste (anterior two thirds of tongue); facial movements such as smiling, closing of eyes, frowning; production of tears and salivary stimulation
Vestibulocochlear	VIII	Sensory	*Vestibular branch:* Sense of balance or equilibrium *Cochlear branch:* Sense of hearing
Glossopharyngeal	IX	Mixed	Produces the gag and swallowing reflexes; taste (posterior third of the tongue)
Vagus	X	Mixed	Innervates muscles of throat and mouth for swallowing and talking; other branches responsible for baroreceptors and chemoreceptor activity
Accessory	XI	Motor	Movement of the trapezius and sternocleidomastoid muscles; some movement of larynx, pharynx, and soft palate
Hypoglossal	XII	Motor	Movement of tongue for swallowing; movement of food during chewing, and speech

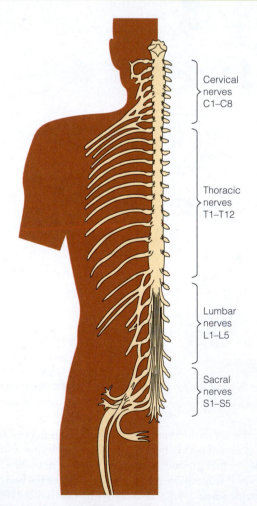

Cervical nerves C1–C8

Thoracic nerves T1–T12

Lumbar nerves L1–L5

Sacral nerves S1–S5

Figure 24.5 Spinal nerves.

A **dermatome** is an area of skin innervated by the cutaneous branch of one spinal nerve. All spinal nerves except the first cervical (C1) serve a cutaneous region. The anterior and posterior views of the dermatomes of the body are shown in Figure 24.6 ■.

Special Considerations

Throughout the assessment process, the nurse gathers subjective and objective data reflecting the patient's state of health. Using critical thinking and the nursing process, the nurse identifies many factors to be considered when collecting the data. Some of these factors include but are not limited to age, developmental level, race, ethnicity, work history, living conditions, and socioeconomics. Physical wellness and emotional wellness are also among the many factors or special considerations that impact a patient's health status. The following sections describe the ways in which neurologic health is affected by these special considerations.

Health Promotion Considerations

Just as concepts in nursing—such as oxygenation and perfusion—are interrelated, so are body systems. As such, neurologic function overlaps with the function of many other body systems, such as vision, hearing, and smell. Alterations in neurologic health also include disorders of central and peripheral nervous system function, such as various forms of dementia and motor nerve disorders.

Because factors such as diet, alcohol intake, smoking, and other health practices can influence neurologic health, the nurse must consider the patient's self-care practices when assessing the patient's neurologic system. A healthy diet, exercise, and rest help ensure optimum neurologic functions. Alcohol causes neurologic impairments ranging from mild sedation to severe

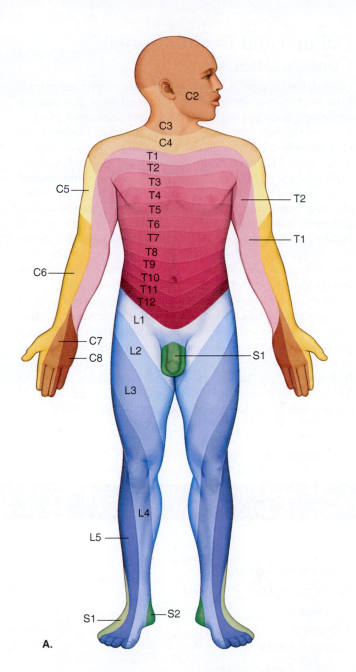

A.

Figure 24.6A Dermatomes of body, anterior view.

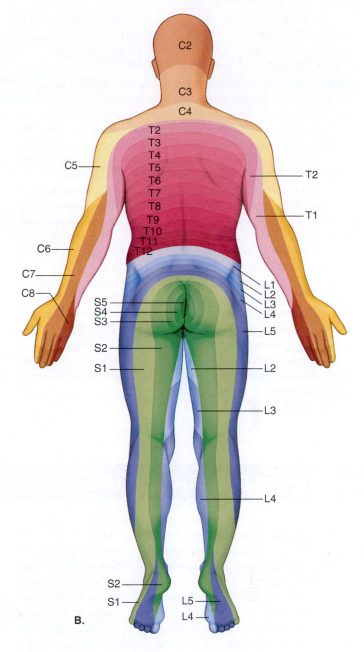

B.

Figure 24.6B Dermatomes of body, posterior view.

motor deficits. Caffeine is a mild stimulant that may cause restlessness, tremors, and insomnia.

Factors relating to the patient's occupation, environment, and genetic background also contribute to neurologic health. A variety of home, work, and environmental factors may cause neurologic impairments. For example, lead-based paint in older homes may cause lead poisoning and encephalopathy in children.

Lifespan Considerations

Growth and development are dynamic processes that describe change over time. The following discussion presents specific variations for different age groups across the lifespan. The structures and functions of the neurologic system undergo change as a result of normal growth and development. Accurate interpretation of subjective and objective data from assessment of the neurologic system is dependent on knowledge of expected variations.

The nervous system is immature at birth. Many reflexes that are present in the newborn begin to disappear as the system matures. The older adult experiences a decrease in neurologic function; the senses diminish, as do reactions to stimuli. Degeneration of the nervous system may lead to a variety of psychosocial problems, such as social isolation, lowered self-esteem, stress, anxiety, and ineffective coping. Expected variations in the neurologic system for different age groups are discussed in Chapter 25, Chapter 26, and Chapter 27. ∞

Psychosocial Considerations

Changes in nervous system functioning may alter an individual's ability to control body movements, speech, and elimination patterns and to engage in activities of daily living. Inevitably, these changes will affect the individual's psychosocial health. Patients' self-esteem may suffer as they suddenly or progressively become unable to carry out the roles they previously assumed in their family and society. Another common psychosocial problem associated with neurologic disorders is social isolation. For example, an individual in the first stage of Alzheimer disease will decline invitations to social functions because the individual feels anxious and confused in unfamiliar surroundings. Such problems indicate a need for improved coping strategies and increased support systems.

As stresses accumulate, an individual becomes increasingly susceptible to neurologic problems, such as forgetfulness, confusion, inability to concentrate, sleeplessness, and tremors. For example, a college senior who is studying for examinations, who is writing applications for graduate school, and who has just broken up with his or her significant other might experience one or all of these symptoms. Chronic stress may also contribute to clinical depression in some patients.

Cultural and Environmental Considerations

Huntington disease is a genetically transferred neurologic disorder. However, the genetic link to most other degenerative neurologic disorders, such as Alzheimer disease, multiple sclerosis, myasthenia gravis, and others, is unclear. The incidence of Alzheimer disease is higher among individuals of African American and Hispanic descent (Alzheimer's Association, 2018).

Research is also inconclusive on the effects of environmental toxins on the development of degenerative neurologic disorders. However, some research indicates that toxins such as carbon monoxide, manganese, and mercury may cause some cases of Parkinson disease (Polito, Greco, & Seripa, 2016). Peripheral neuropathy (damage to the peripheral nerves) occurs more often among farm workers exposed to the organophosphates in many insecticides (Ross, McManus, Harrison, & Mason, 2013).

Lead poisoning also causes peripheral neuropathy and encephalopathy (Rao, Vengamma, Naveen, & Naveen, 2014). Although not as common as in the past, the risk for lead poisoning still remains high among preschool children who live in old apartments or houses in which walls are painted with lead-based paints. Lead poisoning not only affects those who live in low-cost, inner-city dwellings, but it also may occur in wealthy families living in restored older homes.

Subjective Data—Health History

Health assessment of the neurologic system includes gathering subjective and objective data. Subjective data are collected during the patient interview, before the physical assessment. During the interview, various communication techniques are used to elicit general and specific information about the status of the patient's neurologic system and ability to function. Health records, results of laboratory tests, X-rays, and imaging reports are important secondary sources to be included in the data-gathering process. During the physical assessment, the techniques of inspection and palpation, as well as techniques and methods specific to neurologic function, will be used. See Table 24.2 for further information on potential secondary sources of patient data.

Oral glucose tolerance test

Antibodies to nerve components (e.g., anti-myelin-associated glycoprotein [anti-MAG] antibody)

Antibodies related to celiac disease

Lyme disease

HIV/AIDS

Hepatitis C and B

Analysis of cerebrospinal fluid

Genetic testing for neurologic disease

Diagnostic Tests

Angiography

Carotid ultrasonography

Computed tomography (CT)

Discography electromyography (EMG)

Electroencephalography (EEG)

Evoked potentials

Fluoroscopy

Lumbar puncture

Magnetic resonance imaging (MRI)

Neurosonography

Positron emission tomography (PET)

X-ray of the skull

Table 24.2 Potential Secondary Sources for Patient Data Related to the Neurologic System

LABORATORY TESTS
Blood Tests
Blood tests are used to detect hemorrhage, blood vessel disease, and autoimmune diseases; to monitor therapeutic drug levels; and to detect toxins. These blood tests may include:
Vitamin B_{12} and folate levels
Thyroid, liver, and kidney functions
Vasculitis evaluation

Focused Interview

The focused interview for the neurologic system concerns data related to the functions of this body system. Subjective data are collected during the focused interview. The nurse must be prepared to observe the patient and to listen for cues related to the function of the neurologic system. The nurse may use open-ended and closed questions to obtain information. A number of follow-up questions or requests for descriptions may be required to clarify data or gather missing information. Follow-up questions are intended to identify the sources of problems, duration of difficulties, measures to alleviate or manage problems, and clues about the patient's knowledge of his or her own health.

The focused interview guides the physical assessment of the neurologic system. The information is always considered in relation to norms and expectations of neurologic function. Therefore, the nurse must consider age, gender, race, culture, environment, health practices, past and concurrent problems, and therapies when framing questions and using techniques to elicit information. In order to address all of the factors when conducting a focused interview, categories of questions related to the status and function of the neurologic system have been developed. These categories include general questions that are asked of all patients; those addressing illness and infection; questions related to symptoms, pain, and behaviors; those related to habits or practices; questions that are specific for patients according to age and pregnancy; and questions that address environmental concerns. One approach to elicit information about symptoms is the OLDCART & ICE method, described in Chapter 5 (see Figure 5.3). ∞

The nurse must consider the patient's ability to participate in the focused interview and physical assessment of the neurologic system. Participation in the focused interview is influenced by the ability to communicate in the same language. Language barriers interfere with the accuracy of the data and cause anxiety in the patient. The nurse may have to use a translator when conducting an interview and the physical assessment. If the patient is experiencing pain, recent injury, or anxiety, attention must focus on relief of symptoms or discomfort before proceeding with an in-depth interview.

Focused Interview Questions	Rationales and Evidence

The following section provides sample questions and bulleted follow-up questions in each of the previously mentioned categories. A rationale for each question is provided. The list of questions is not all-inclusive but, rather, represents the types of questions required in a comprehensive focused interview related to the neurologic system. As these questions are asked, the subjective data obtained help to identify patient strengths or risks associated with the neurologic system.

General Questions

1. Please complete this sentence: "After I get out of bed in the morning, a typical day in my life includes _____."

   ▶ The nurse is asking the patient to describe activities of daily living (ADLs). If these data have been obtained in another area of the assessment, the nurse should alter the lead statement accordingly. The patient usually perceives this opening as nonthreatening. It places a focus on activities, self-care practices, and the patient's level of wellness. The nurse can then employ therapeutic communication skills to seek clarification and encourage the patient to relate all of the activities of the day.

2. Explain what brings you here today.

   ▶ This open-ended statement allows the patient to state what is important. It increases the patient's control in what may be a stressful situation, thereby producing a less threatening environment. Based on the patient's response, the nurse should adjust the sequence of questions to explore the patient's concern.

3. Have you had a change in your ability to carry out your daily activities?
   * Describe the change.
   * Do you know what is causing the change?
   * What do you do about the problem?
   * How long has this been happening?
   * Have you discussed this with your healthcare provider?

   ▶ Neurologic problems can interfere with the ability to carry out ADLs.

4. Do you have any chronic disease such as diabetes or hypertension?

   ▶ Chronic diseases such as diabetes and hypertension can predispose patients to neurologic problems (National Institute of Diabetes and Digestive and Kidney Diseases (NIDDK), 2017).

5. Do any members of your family now have, or have they ever had, a neurologic problem or disease?
   * What is the disease or problem?
   * Who in the family has the problem?
   * When was it diagnosed?
   * How has it been treated?
   * How effective has the treatment been?

   ▶ Some conditions are familial and recur in families. For example, certain forms of Alzheimer disease and amyotrophic lateral sclerosis (ALS, or Lou Gehrig disease), both of which are discussed later in this chapter, are familial conditions (University of Michigan Health Systems, n.d.).

Focused Interview Questions	Rationales and Evidence

Questions Related to Illness, Infection, or Injury

1. **Have you ever been diagnosed with a neurologic illness, meningitis, for example?**
   - When were you diagnosed with the problem?
   - What treatment was prescribed for the problem?
   - What kinds of things do you do to help with the problem?
   - Has the problem ever recurred (acute)?
   - How are you managing the disease now (chronic)?

2. *Alternative to question 1:* List possible neurologic illnesses such as stroke, paresis, epilepsy, multiple sclerosis, and myasthenia gravis and ask the patient to respond "yes" or "no" as each is stated.

3. **Have you ever had an infection of the neurologic system? Follow-up would be the same as in question number 1.**

4. **An alternative to question 3 is to list neurologic infections such as poliomyelitis, meningitis, and encephalitis and ask the patient to state "yes" or "no" as each is stated. The rationale is the same as in question 2.**

5. **Have you ever had an injury to your head or back?**
   - If so, please explain what happened.
   - When did this happen?
   - What treatments did you receive?
   - As a result of this injury, what problems do you have today? Follow-up would be the same as in question 1.

▶ The patient has the opportunity to provide information about a specific illness. If a diagnosed illness is identified, follow-up about the date of diagnosis, treatment, and outcomes is required. Data about each illness identified by the patient are essential to an accurate health assessment. Illnesses can be classified as acute or chronic, and follow-up regarding each classification will differ.

▶ This is a comprehensive and easy way to elicit information about all neurologic diagnoses. Follow-up would be carried out for each identified diagnosis as in question 1.

▶ The medical history being developed should include past incidents and residual deficits.

Questions Related to Symptoms, Pain, and Behaviors

When gathering information about symptoms, many questions are required to elicit details and descriptions that assist in analysis of the data. Discrimination is made in relation to the significance of a symptom, in relation to specific diseases or problems, and in relation to the potential need for follow-up examination or referral.

The following questions refer to specific symptoms associated with the neurologic system. For each symptom, questions and follow-up are required. The details to be elicited are the characteristics of the symptom; the treatment or remedy for the symptom, including over-the-counter (OTC) and home remedies; the determination if diagnosis has been sought; the effects of treatments; and family history associated with a symptom.

Questions Related to Symptoms

1. **Do you have fainting spells?**
   - Describe your fainting.

2. **Do you have a history of seizures or convulsions?**
   - If so, when did you have your first episode?
   - What happens to you immediately before the seizure?
   - What have you been told about what your body does during the seizure?
   - How do you feel after the seizure?
   - What medications do you take?
   - Do you take your medications regularly?
   - When was the last time you had a seizure?

3. **Has your vision changed in any way?**
   - Do you ever see two objects when you know there is just one?
   - Are you able to see off to the sides without turning your head?
   - When you go from a bright room to a darker room, do your eyes adjust to the change rapidly?

4. **What changes, if any, have you noticed in your hearing?**
   - Have you noticed any ringing in the ears?

5. **Have you noticed any change with your ability to smell or taste?**

6. **Describe your balance.**
   - Are you steady on your feet?
   - Are you able to perform daily activities without difficulty?
   - Is one leg stronger than the other?
   - Do you notice any tremors?
   - Could you bend down to pick up a straight pin and stand up again?
   - Do you drop things easily?
   - Do you find yourself being very clumsy—tripping, spilling things, and knocking things over?
   - If so, how long have the symptoms been present?
   - Are the symptoms continuous?
   - Are they getting worse? What do you do to control or limit the symptoms?

▶ Fainting or loss of consciousness can be associated with neurologic problems (van Dijk & Wieling, 2013).

▶ The patient should be encouraged to identify the type of seizure(s): partial, complex, or mixed. The questions focus on an aura, muscular activity, postictal period, and use of medications. Lifestyle changes are important, because these individuals must be cautioned regarding driving and the use of dangerous equipment (Berman & Snyder, 2016).

▶ Changes in vision may indicate problems with the cranial nerves, a brain tumor, increased intracranial pressure, or ocular disease (Osborn, Wraa, Watson, & Holleran, 2013).

▶ Changes in hearing and ringing in the ears (tinnitus) may indicate a problem with the eighth cranial nerve, auditory functions, or aspirin toxicity (Mayo Clinic, 2018).

▶ A change in the ability to smell or taste may also indicate a problem with cranial nerve function (Berman & Snyder, 2016).

▶ All of these questions relate to activities of the cerebellum.

Focused Interview Questions	**Rationales and Evidence**

7. Do you have numbness or tingling in any part of your body?
- How long have you had this?
- Do you know what causes it?
- Have you sought treatment?
- What do you do to relieve the problem?

▶ Numbness or tingling may result from neurologic changes alone or as a result of systemic or circulatory disease (Berman & Snyder, 2016).

Questions Related to Pain

1. Are you having any pain?
- If so, where is it?
- When did the pain begin?
- Is the pain constant or intermittent?
- What relieves or decreases the pain?
- What increases the pain?
- Does the pain interfere with your daily activities?
- How would you describe the pain: sharp, dull, acute, burning, stabbing, stinging?
- On a scale of 0 to 10, with 10 being highest, how would you rate the pain?

▶ Pain, a completely subjective experience, can be acute or chronic. Understanding the patient's view of the pain will help the nurse understand the physiological cause of the pain and will help guide treatment.

2. Do you get headaches?
- If so, describe them.
- Where are they located?
- Are they always in the same area?
- How often do they occur?
- Are you able to function with these headaches?
- What do you think causes your headaches?
- What do you do to help relieve the pain?
- Does this remedy work?
- On a scale of 0 to 10, rate the severity of your headaches.

▶ The nurse is obtaining a medical history to determine if headaches are migraines, tension, cluster, unilateral, bilateral, or associated with other disease. (Refer to Chapter 13 ∞ for more information on headaches.)

Questions Related to Behaviors

1. Do you now use or have you ever used recreational drugs or alcohol?
- What was the drug or substance?
- When did you use it?
- How long have you used it?
- Have you experienced problems as a result of this drug?
- How much alcohol do you consume?
- For how long?

▶ *Recreational drugs* is a common term used to imply illegal substances. This category could include heroin, cocaine, marijuana, ketamine, oxycodone, and other substances. Use of social drugs and alcohol can create risk for neurologic symptoms or disorders that may be temporary or have long-term consequences.

2. Describe your memory.
- Do you need to make a list or write things down so you won't forget?
- Do you lose things easily?
- What did you do today before you came here?

▶ Memory loss is indicative of some neurologic or psychiatric disease such as Alzheimer, depression, or stroke. The nurse is developing a baseline regarding the patient's memory and the ability to recall recent and distant events.

Questions Related to Age and Pregnancy

The focused interview must reflect the anatomic and physiologic differences in the neurologic system that exist along the age span as well as during pregnancy. Specific questions related to the neurologic system for each of these groups are provided in Chapter 25, Chapter 26, and Chapter 27. ∞

Questions Related to the Environment

Environment refers to both the internal and external environments. Questions related to the internal environment include all of the previous questions and those associated with internal or physiologic responses. Questions related to the external environment include those related to home, work, or social environments.

Internal Environment

1. Describe your daily diet.
- Do you have problems eating or drinking certain products?

▶ The diet provides nutrients and electrolytes responsible for neuromuscular activity and electrical activity in the nervous system.

2. Are you currently taking any medications?
- What are the medications?
- Do you use prescribed, OTC, herbal, or culturally derived medications?
- Do you use home remedies?

▶ Medications alone can cause neurologic problems. The interaction of medications, herbs, or other products may alter or affect the absorption or effects of prescribed medications (Wilson, Shannon, & Shields, 2018).

Focused Interview Questions | Rationales and Evidence

External Environment

1. **Are you now or have you ever been exposed to environmental hazards such as insecticides, organic solvents, lead, toxic wastes, or other pollutants?**
   - If so, which one, when, and for what period of time were you exposed?
   - What treatment did you seek?
   - Are you left with any problems because of the exposure?

▶ Such exposure could contribute to neurologic deficits and neoplastic activity in the body (Ross et al., 2013).

Patient-Centered Interaction

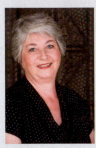

Mrs. Roberta Andoli, age 59, reports to her primary care provider with the chief complaint of weakness of the right side of her face. Her right eye is tearing and she has noticed some drooling. All of the symptoms have developed within the last 3 days. A tentative diagnosis of Bell's palsy is made. The following is an excerpt taken from the focused interview.

Source: Sean Nel/Shutterstock.

Interview

Nurse: Good afternoon, Mrs. Andoli. I would like to talk with you about your reason for coming today.

Mrs. Andoli: My face didn't feel right when I got up today. I can't explain it.

Nurse: Did you notice anything else about your face?

Mrs. Andoli: When I washed my face this morning, I noticed the crease by my nose was gone. When I brushed my teeth, the water and toothpaste were dripping out the right side of my mouth. I could not keep the water in on that side.

Nurse: Did you have breakfast this morning?

Mrs. Andoli: Oh yes, I had one cup of tea and cereal with milk, my usual breakfast.

Nurse: Did the tea or cereal milk drip out of your mouth?

Mrs. Andoli: Oh yes, I could have used a bib. I had trouble swallowing, and my cereal didn't taste right. I don't know why. My milk was not sour or anything.

Nurse: What other changes have you noticed?

Mrs. Andoli: When I went to put on eye makeup today, I noticed my right eye was funny.

Nurse: I'm not sure I know what funny means.

Mrs. Andoli: My right eye seemed to be open wider than my left eye this morning. I usually line my eyelids, but I didn't this morning. My bottom lid is turned. I don't know what I did. Gee, I'm really a mess.

Analysis

During the interview, the nurse used several strategies to obtain specific subjective data from the patient. The nurse built on the first statement made by the patient describing feelings of the face. Clarification was sought. Open-ended statements were used to elicit greater information.

Objective Data—Physical Assessment

Assessment Techniques and Findings

Physical assessment of the neurologic system requires the use of inspection, palpation, auscultation, and special equipment and procedures to test the functions of the system. During each part of the assessment, the nurse is gathering objective data related to the functioning of the patient's central and peripheral nervous systems. The assessment begins with evaluation of the patient's mental status and includes cranial nerves, motor and sensory function, balance, and reflexes. Knowledge of normal or expected findings is essential in interpretation of the data.

Adults and children who are preschool age or older have erect posture and a smooth gait. Facial expressions correspond to the content and topic of discussion. The speech is clear, and vocabulary and word choice are appropriate to age and experience. Adults are well groomed, clean, and attired appropriately for the season and setting. The adult is oriented to person, place, and time and can respond to questions and directions. The adult demonstrates intact short- and long-term memory, is capable of abstract thinking, and can perform calculations. Children should also be able to respond to increasingly difficult questions based on their age. For

EQUIPMENT

- Examination gown
- Clean, nonsterile examination gloves
- Cotton wisp
- Percussion hammer
- Tuning fork
- Sterile cotton balls
- Penlight
- Ophthalmoscope
- Stethoscope
- Tongue blade
- Applicator
- Hot and cold water in test tubes
- Objects to touch, such as coins, paper clips, or safety pins
- Substances to smell, such as vanilla, mint, and coffee
- Substances to taste, such as sugar, salt, lemon, and grape

HELPFUL HINTS

- Data gathering begins with the initial nurse–patient interaction. As nurses meet patients, they make assessments regarding their general appearance, personal hygiene, and ability to walk and sit down. These activities are related to cerebral function.
- Physical assessment of the neurologic system proceeds in a cephalocaudal and distal-to-proximal pattern and includes comparison of corresponding body parts.
- Several assessments may occur at one time. For example, asking the patient to smile tests cranial nerve VII. The ability to follow directions and initiate voluntary movements tests hearing (cranial nerve VIII) and the functions of the cerebral cortex.
- Provide specific information about what is expected of the patient. Demonstrate movements.
- Explain and demonstrate the purposes and uses of the equipment.
- Use Standard Precautions.

adults and children, the cranial nerves are intact. Motor function is intact, and movements are coordinated and smooth. Sensory function is demonstrated in the ability to identify touch, pain, heat, and cold; to sense vibrations; to identify objects; and to discriminate between place and points of touch on the body. The response to testing of reflexes is 2+ on a scale of 0 to 4+. Carotid arteries are without bruits.

Physical assessment of the neurologic system follows an organized pattern. It begins with assessment of the patient's mental status and proceeds to assessment of cranial nerves, motor and sensory function, reflexes, and auscultation of carotid arteries. Assessment proceeds in a cephalocaudal manner. The nurse tests distal to proximal and moves from gross function to fine function, always comparing corresponding body parts. More than one technique can be used to assess one function.

Techniques and Normal Findings	Abnormal Findings and Special Considerations

Mental Status

The nurse assesses the mental status of the patient when meeting the patient for the first time. This process begins with taking the health history and continues with each patient contact.

▶ A variety of tools are available to conduct mental status assessment. These tools are described in Table 24.3.

Table 24.3 Tools for Assessment of Mental Status

TOOL	ASSESSMENT
Mini-Mental State Examination (MMSE)	Cognitive status—conducted via interview
Addenbrooke's Cognitive Examination	Detects early dementia
Confusion Assessment Method (CAM)	Tests for delirium
Telephone Interview for Cognitive Status (TICS)	Similar to MMSE, cognitive function assessed via telephone interview
Cornell Scale for Depression in Dementia	Assessment of behavioral problems
Dementia Symptoms Scale	Assessment of behavioral problems
Psychogeriatric Dependency Rating Scale	Assessment of behavioral problems
Hopkins Competency Assessment Test	Assessment of ability to make decisions about healthcare
General Health Questionnaire	Assessment of emotional disturbance in those with normal cognitive ability
Hamilton Depression Rating Scale	Assessment of depression in patients with impaired cognition
Short Portable Mental Status Questionnaire (SPMSQ)	Assessment of organic brain deficit

Evidence-Based Practice

Caffeine and Dementia Testing

Neuropsychologic tests, such as the Folstein Mini-Mental Screening Exam (MMSE) used in the diagnosis of dementia, have been shown to be influenced by the time of day of the screening and the use of caffeine by the patient (Borella, Ludwig, Dirk & de Ribaupierre, 2010; Lesk, Honey, & de Jager, 2009; Schmidt, Collette, Cajochen, & Peigneux, 2007; Walters & Lesk, 2015). Older adults' peak performance with the MMSE is generally in the morning, with studies showing a decline in their results when taken in the afternoon and evening (Borella et al., 2010; Schmidt et al., 2007). Consuming caffeine equal to one medium-size coffee also led to a decrease in performance on the MMSE in older adults (Lesk et al., 2009; Walters & Lesk, 2015). These findings indicate the need to be aware of these factors when performing the MMSE on an older adult to ensure accurate results.

Techniques and Normal Findings   **Abnormal Findings and Special Considerations**

1. **Instruct the patient.**
   - Explain to the patient that you will be conducting a variety of tests. Tell the patient that you will provide instructions before beginning each examination. Explain that moving about and changing position during the examination will be required.
   - Provide reassurance that the tests will not cause discomfort; however, also emphasize that the patient must inform you of problems if they arise during any part of the assessment.
   - Identify the types of equipment you will use and describe the purpose in relation to neurologic function.
   - Tell the patient that you will begin the assessment with some general questions about the present and past. Then you will ask the patient to respond to number and word questions.

2. **Position the patient.**
   - The patient should be sitting on the examination table wearing an examination gown (see Figure 24.7 ■).

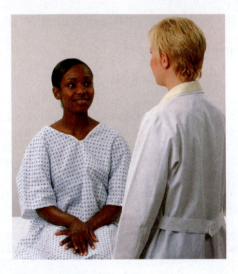

Figure 24.7 Positioning the patient.

3. **Observe the patient.**
   - Look at the patient and note hygiene, grooming, posture, body language, facial expressions, speech, and ability to follow directions.

   ▶ Inadequate self-care, flatness of affect, and inability to follow directions may be associated with mental illnesses, such as depression or schizophrenia, or with neurologic abnormalities, such as organic brain syndrome. Abnormal facial expressions or body language also may be reflective of neurologic or psychiatric disorders.

4. **Note the patient's speech and language abilities.**
   - Throughout the assessment, note the patient's rate of speech, ability to pronounce words, tone of voice, loudness or softness (volume) of voice, and ability to speak smoothly and clearly.
   - Assess the patient's choice of words, ability to respond to questions, and ease with which a response is made.

   ▶ Changes in speech could reflect anxiety, Parkinson disease, depression, or dysphasia (difficulty speaking).

5. **Assess the patient's sensorium and orientation.**
   - Determine the patient's orientation to person, place, time, and date. Ask the patient his or her name, current location, and day and date. Orientation × 1 indicates awareness of who they are (person). Orientation × 2 shows awareness of person and location (place) and Orientation × 3 reveals his or her ability to answer correctly about person, place, and time. Grade the level of alertness on a scale from full alertness to coma.

   ▶ Neurologic disease can produce a sliding or changing degree of alertness. Change in the level of consciousness may be related to cortical or brainstem disease. A stroke, seizure, or hypoglycemia could also contribute to a change in the level of consciousness (LOC).

6. **Assess the patient's memory.**
   - Ask for the patient's date of birth, names and ages of any children or grandchildren, educational history with dates and events, work history with dates, and job descriptions. Ask questions for which the responses can be verified.

   ▶ Loss of long-term memory may indicate cerebral cortex damage, which occurs in Alzheimer disease.

7. **Assess the patient's ability to calculate problems.**
   - Start with a simple problem, such as 4 + 3, 8 ÷ 2, and 15 − 4.

   ▶ Inability to calculate simple problems may indicate the presence of organic brain disease, or it may simply indicate lack of exposure to mathematical concepts, nervousness, or an incomplete understanding of the examiner's language. In an otherwise unremarkable assessment, a poor response to calculations should not be considered an abnormal finding.

- Progress to more difficult problems, such as $(10 + 4) - 8$, or ask the patient to start with 100 and subtract 7 ($100 - 7 = 93$, $93 - 7 = 86$, $86 - 7 = 79$, and so on).
- Remember to use problems that are appropriate for the patient's developmental, educational, and intellectual levels.
- Asking the patient to calculate change from one dollar for the purchase of items costing 25, 39, and 89 cents is a quick test of calculation.

8. **Assess the patient's ability to think abstractly.**
   - Ask the patient to identify similarities and differences between two objects or topics, such as wood and coal, king and president, orange and apple, and pear and celery. Quote a proverb and ask the patient to explain its meaning, for example:
     ◦ "Don't count your chickens before they hatch."
     ◦ "The empty barrel makes the most noise."
     ◦ "Don't put all your eggs in one basket."
   - Be aware that age and culture influence the ability to explain American proverbs and slang terms.

▶ Responses made by the patient may reflect lack of education, mental retardation, or dementia. Patients with personality disorders and patients with disorders such as schizophrenia or depression may make bizarre responses.

9. **Assess the patient's mood and emotional state.**
   - Observe the patient's body language, facial expressions, and communication technique. The facial expression and tone of voice should be congruent with the content and context of the communication.

   - Ask if the patient generally feels this way or if he or she has experienced a change, and if so, over what period of time.
   - Ask the patient if it is possible to identify an event or incident that fostered the change in mood or emotional state.
   - The patient's mood and emotions should reflect the current situation or response to events that trigger mood change or call for an emotional response (e.g., a change in health status, a loss, or a stressful event).

▶ Lack of congruence of facial expression and tone of voice with the content and context of communication may occur with neurologic problems, emotional disturbance, or a psychogenic disorder such as schizophrenia or depression.

▶ Lack of emotional response, lack of change in facial expression, and flat tone of voice can indicate problems with mood or emotional responses. Other abnormal findings in relation to mood and emotional state include anxiety, depression, fear, anger, overconfidence, ambivalence, euphoria, impatience, and irritability. Mood disorders include bipolar disorder, anxiety disorders, and major depression.

10. **Assess perceptions and thought processes.**
    - Listen to the patient's statements. Statements should be logical and relevant. The patient should complete his or her thoughts.
    - Assessment of perception includes determining the patient's awareness of reality.

▶ Disturbed thought processes can indicate neurologic dysfunction or mental disorder.

▶ Disturbances in sense of reality can include hallucination and illusion. These are associated with mental disturbances as seen in schizophrenia.

11. **Assess the patient's ability to make judgments.**
    - Determine if the patient is able to evaluate situations and to decide on a realistic course of action. For example, ask the patient about future plans related to employment.
    - The plans should reflect the reality of the patient's health, psychologic stability, and family situation and obligations. The patient's responses should reflect an ability to think abstractly.

▶ Impaired judgment can occur in emotional disturbances, schizophrenia, and neurologic dysfunction.

Cranial Nerves

1. **Instruct the patient.**
   - Tell the patient that you will be testing special nerves and the senses of smell, vision, taste, and hearing. Explain that several of the tests will require the patient to close both eyes. You will be asking the patient to make changes in facial expression. Occasionally, you will touch the patient with your hands while using different types of equipment during each test.

2. **Test the olfactory nerve (cranial nerve I).**
   - If you suspect the patient's nares are obstructed with mucus, ask the patient to blow his or her nose.

▶ **Anosmia,** the absence of the sense of smell, may be because of cranial nerve dysfunction, colds, rhinitis, or zinc deficiency, or it may be genetic. A unilateral change in this sense may be indicative of a brain tumor.

Techniques and Normal Findings	Abnormal Findings and Special Considerations

- Ask the patient to close both eyes and then apply gentle pressure to the external surface of one naris with his or her index finger. If necessary, the nurse could occlude the patient's naris. Place a familiar odor under the open naris (see Figure 24.8 ■).
- Ask the patient to sniff and identify the odor. Use coffee, peppermint, or other scents that are familiar to the patient. Repeat with the other naris.

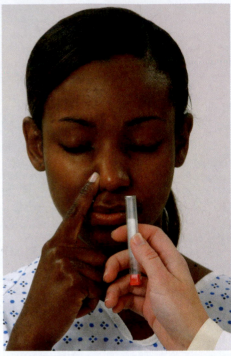

Figure 24.8 Olfactory nerve assessment.

3. **Test the optic nerve (cranial nerve II).**
   - Test near vision by asking the patient to read from a magazine, newspaper, or prepared card. Observe closeness or distance of page to face. Also note the position of the head.
   - Use the Snellen chart to test distant vision (see Figure 14.8 ∞). Color vision may be tested using Ishihara cards, which feature colored dot patterns that contain embedded symbols or numbers.

   - Use the ophthalmoscope to inspect the fundus of the eye. Locate the optic disc and describe the color and shape.
   - See Chapter 14 ∞ for a detailed description of the techniques for all of these activities.

4. **Test the oculomotor, trochlear, and abducens nerves (cranial nerves III, IV, and VI).**
   - Test the six cardinal points of gaze.
   - Test direct and consensual pupillary reaction to light (cranial nerve III).
   - Test convergence and accommodation of the eyes.
   - These three tests are described in detail in Chapter 14. ∞

▶ Pathologic conditions of the optic nerve include retrobulbar neuritis, papilledema, and optic atrophy. **Retrobulbar neuritis** is an inflammatory process of the optic nerve behind the eyeball. Multiple sclerosis is the most common cause.

▶ Inability to distinguish symbols or numbers on one or more of the Ishihara cards is reflective of impaired color vision (MedlinePlus, 2017).

▶ **Papilledema** (or *choked disc*) is a swelling of the optic nerve as it enters the retina. A symptom of increased intracranial pressure, papilledema can be indicative of brain tumors or intracranial hemorrhage.

▶ Immediate medical attention is required if intracranial hemorrhage is suspected.

▶ **Optic atrophy** produces a change in the color of the optic disc and decreased visual acuity. It can be a symptom of multiple sclerosis or brain tumor.

▶ Pathologic conditions include nystagmus, strabismus, diplopia, or ptosis of the upper lid. **Nystagmus** is the constant involuntary movement of the eyeball. A lack of muscular coordination, *strabismus*, causes deviation of one or both eyes.

▶ **Diplopia** is double vision. A dropped lid, or *ptosis* of the lid, is usually related to weakness of the muscles.

5. **Explain the procedure for testing the trigeminal nerve.**
   - Show the patient the cotton wisp. Touch the patient's arm with the wisp and explain that the wisp will feel like that when a body part is touched. Ask the patient to close both eyes.
   - Touch the arm with the wisp. Ask the patient to say "Now" when the wisp is felt. Explain that further tests with the wisp will be carried out with the eyes closed, and "Now" is to be stated when the wisp is felt.
   - Show the patient the broken tongue blade. Explain that while you touch the arm with the rounded end the sensation is dull and with the broken end the sensation is sharp.
   - Tell the patient that both eyes must be closed during several tests with the tongue blade.
   - The patient is expected to identify each touch or sensation as sharp or dull.
   - Discard the tongue blade at the completion of the examination.

6. **Test the trigeminal nerve (cranial nerve V).**
   - Test the sensory function.
   - Ask the patient to close both eyes.
   - Touch the patient's face, forehead, and chin with a cotton wisp (see Figure 24.9 ■).
   - Direct the patient to say "Now" every time the cotton wisp is felt. Repeat the test using sharp and dull stimuli.

▶ Document any loss of sensation, pain, or noted fasciculations (fine rapid muscle movements).

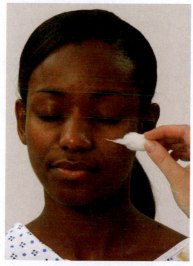

Figure 24.9 Testing sensory function of the trigeminal nerve.

   - Be random with the stimulation. Do *not* establish a pattern when testing.
   - Test the motor function of the nerve. Ask the patient to clench the teeth tightly. Bilaterally palpate the masseter and temporalis muscles, noting muscle strength (see Figure 24.10 ■).
   - Ask the patient to open and close the mouth several times. Observe for symmetry of movement of the mandible without deviation from midline.

▶ Muscle pain, spasms, and deviation of the mandible with movement can indicate myofascial pain dysfunction.

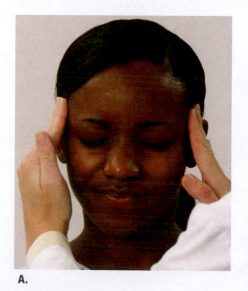
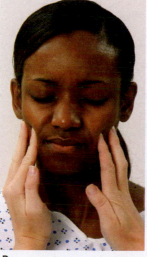

A.   **B.**

Figure 24.10 Testing muscle strength. A. Temporalis muscles. B. Masseter muscles.

Techniques and Normal Findings	Abnormal Findings and Special Considerations

7. **Test the facial nerve (cranial nerve VII).**
   - Test the motor activity of the nerve.
   - Ask the patient to perform several functions, such as the following: smile, show your teeth, close both eyes, puff your cheeks, frown, and raise your eyebrows (see Figure 24.11 ■).

▶ Asymmetry or muscle weakness may indicate nerve damage. Muscle weakness includes drooping of the eyelid and changes in the nasolabial folds.

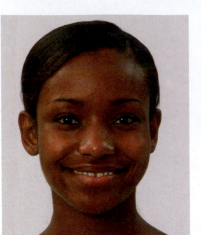

A.

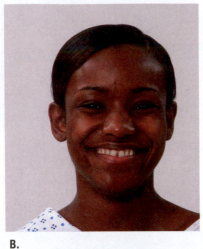

B.

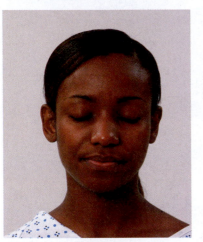

C.

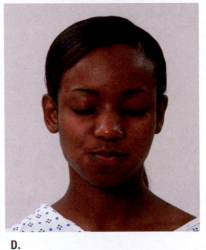

D.

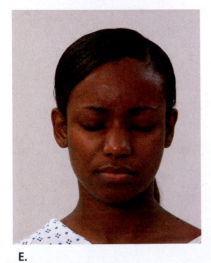

E.

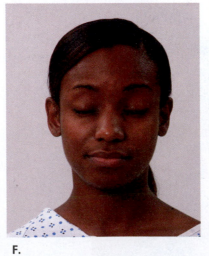

F.

Figure 24.11 Testing motor function of cranial nerve VII. A. Smile. B. Show teeth. C. Close both eyes. D. Puff cheeks. E. Frown. F. Raise eyebrows.

Techniques and Normal Findings	Abnormal Findings and Special Considerations

- Look for symmetry of facial movements.
- Test the muscle strength of the upper face.
- Ask the patient to close both eyes tightly and keep them closed.
- Try to open the eyes by retracting the upper and lower lids simultaneously and bilaterally (see Figure 24.12 ■).

▶ Inability to perform motor tasks could be the result of a lower or upper motor neuron disease.

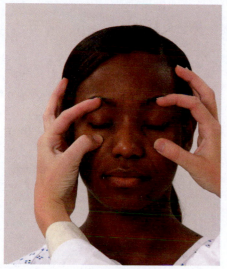

Figure 24.12 Testing the strength of the facial muscles.

- Test the muscle strength of the lower face:
  - ○ Ask the patient to puff the cheeks.
  - ○ Apply pressure to the cheeks, attempting to force the air out of the lips.
- Test the sense of taste:
  - ○ Moisten three applicators and dab one in each of the samples of sugar, salt, and lemon.
  - ○ Touch the patient's tongue with one applicator at a time and ask the patient to identify the taste.
  - ○ Water may be needed to rinse the mouth between tests.
- Test the corneal reflex:
  - ○ This may have been tested with the trigeminal nerve assessment (see Figure 24.9). Cranial nerve VII regulates the motor response of this reflex.

8. **Test the vestibulocochlear nerve (cranial nerve VIII).**
   - Test the auditory branch of the nerve by performing the Weber test. This test uses the tuning fork and provides lateralization of the sound.
   - Perform the Rinne test. This compares bone conduction of sound with air conduction. Both the Rinne and Weber tests are described in detail in Chapter 15. ∞
   - Romberg's test assesses coordination and equilibrium. It is discussed later in this chapter and in Chapter 15. ∞

▶ Tinnitus and deafness are deficits associated with the cochlear or auditory branch of the nerve.

9. **Test the glossopharyngeal and vagus nerves (cranial nerves IX and X).**
   - Test motor activity:
     - Ask the patient to open the mouth.
     - Depress the patient's tongue with the tongue blade.
     - Ask the patient to say "aah."
   - Observe the movement of the soft palate and uvula (see Figure 24.13 ■). Normally, the soft palate rises and the uvula remains in the midline.

▶ Unilateral palate and uvula movement indicate disease of the nerve on the opposite side.

▶ Bifid uvula, a condition in which the uvula is split into two segments, occurs in approximately 1% of the general population. Although this condition usually is benign, in rare cases it may be linked to serious genetic disorders, including cleft palate (Liberty et al., 2014).

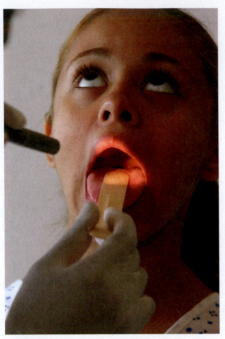

Figure 24.13 Testing cranial nerves IX and X.

   - Test the gag reflex. This tests the sensory aspect of cranial nerve IX and the motor activity of cranial nerve X.

▶ Patients with a diminished or absent gag reflex have an increased potential for aspiration and need medical evaluation.

   - Inform the patient that you are going to place an applicator in the mouth and lightly touch the throat.
   - Touch the posterior wall of the pharynx with the applicator.
   - Observe pharyngeal movement.
   - Test the motor activity of the pharynx:
     - Ask the patient to drink a small amount of water and note the ease or difficulty of swallowing.
     - Note the quality of the voice or hoarseness when speaking.

▶ **Dysphagia**, difficulty with swallowing, could be related to cranial nerve disease.

▶ Vocal changes could be indicative of lesions, paralysis, or other conditions.

10. **Test the accessory nerve (cranial nerve XI).**
   - Test the trapezius muscle:
     - Ask the patient to shrug the shoulders.
     - Observe the equality of the shoulders, symmetry of action, and lack of fasciculations (see Figure 24.14 ■).

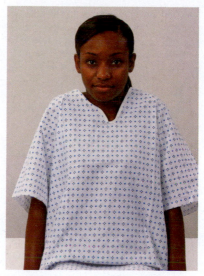

Figure 24.14 Trapezius muscle movement.

   - Test the sternocleidomastoid muscle:
     - Ask the patient to turn the head to the right and then to the left (see Figure 24.15 ■).

▶ Abnormal findings include muscle weakness, muscle atrophy, fasciculations, uneven shoulders, and the inability to raise the chin following flexion.

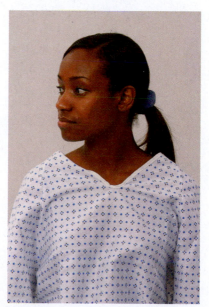

Figure 24.15 **Sternocleidomastoid muscle movement.**

   - Ask the patient to try to touch the right ear to the right shoulder without raising the shoulder.
   - Repeat with the left shoulder.
   - Observe ease of movement and degree of range of motion.

|

- Test trapezius muscle strength;
  - Have the patient shrug the shoulders while you resist with your hands (see Figure 24.16 ■).

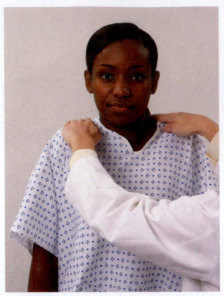

Figure 24.16 Testing the strength of the trapezius muscle against resistance.

- Test sternocleidomastoid muscle strength:
  - Ask the patient to turn the head to the left to meet your hand.
  - Attempt to return the patient's head to midline position (see Figure 24.17 ■).
  - Repeat the preceding steps with the patient turning to the right side.

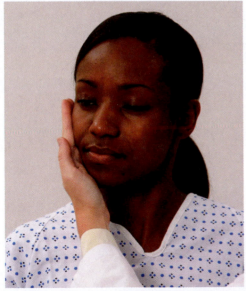

Figure 24.17 Testing the strength of the sternocleidomastoid muscle against resistance.

11. **Test the hypoglossal nerve (cranial nerve XII).**
  - Test the movement of the tongue:
    - Ask the patient to protrude the tongue.
    - Ask the patient to retract the tongue.
    - Ask the patient to protrude the tongue and move it to the right and then to the left.
    - Note ease of movement and equality of movement (see Figure 24.18 ■).

▶ Note atrophy, tremors, and paralysis. An ipsilateral paralysis will demonstrate deviation and atrophy of the involved side.

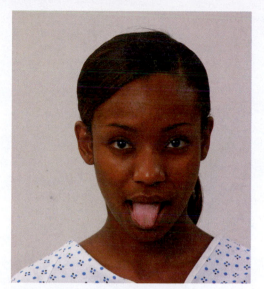

Figure 24.18A Protruding movement of tongue.

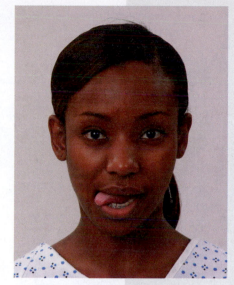

Figure 24.18B Lateralization of tongue.

- Test the strength of the tongue:
  - Ask the patient to push against the inside of the cheek with the tip of the tongue.
  - Provide resistance by pressing one or two fingers against the patient's outer cheek (see Figure 24.19 ■).
  - Repeat on the other side.

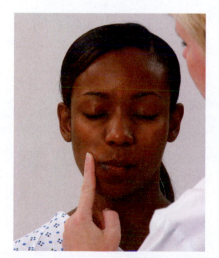

Figure 24.19 Testing the strength of the tongue.

Motor Function

Motor function requires the integrated efforts of the musculoskeletal and the neurologic systems. Assessment of the musculoskeletal system is discussed in detail in Chapter 23. ∞ The neurologic aspect of motor function is directly related to activities of the cerebellum, which is responsible for coordination, smoothness of movement, and equilibrium. All of the following tests focus on activities of the cerebellum.

Techniques and Normal Findings	Abnormal Findings and Special Considerations

ALERT! *Be ready to support and protect the patient to prevent an accident, injury, or fall.*

1. **Assess the patient's gait and balance.**
   - Ask the patient to walk across the room and return (see Figure 24.20 ■).
   - Ask the patient to walk heel to toe (or tandem) by placing the heel of the left foot in front of the toes of the right foot, then the heel of the right foot in front of the toes of the left foot. Be sure the patient is looking straight ahead and not at the floor. Continue this pattern for several yards (see Figure 24.21 ■).

▶ A change in gait could be indicative of drug or alcohol intoxication, motor neuron weakness, or muscle weakness.

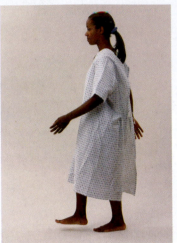

Figure 24.20 Evaluation of gait.

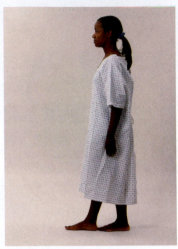

Figure 24.21 Heel-to-toe walk.

   - Ask the patient to walk on his or her toes.
   - Ask the patient to walk on the heels. Observe the patient's posture. Does the posture demonstrate stiffness or relaxation? Note the equality of steps taken, the pace of walking, the position and coordination of arms when walking, and the ability to maintain balance during all of these activities.

2. **Perform Romberg's test.**
   - **Romberg's test** assesses coordination and equilibrium (cranial nerve VIII).
   - Ask the patient to stand with feet together and arms at the sides. The patient's eyes are open.
   - Stand next to the patient to prevent falls. Observe for swaying.
   - Ask the patient to close both eyes without changing position.
   - Observe for swaying while the patient's eyes are closed. Swaying normally increases slightly when the eyes are closed (see Figure 24.22 ■).

▶ A positive Romberg sign occurs when swaying greatly increases or the patient experiences difficulty maintaining his or her balance. This may indicate disease of the posterior column of the spinal cord.

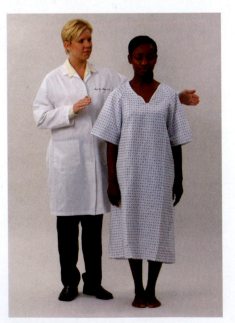

Figure 24.22 Romberg's test for balance.

3. **Perform the finger-to-nose test.**
    - The finger-to-nose test also assesses coordination and equilibrium. It is sometimes called the pass-point test.
    - Ask the patient to resume a sitting position.
    - Ask the patient to extend both arms from the sides of the body.
    - Ask the patient to keep both eyes open.
    - Ask the patient to touch the tip of the nose with the right index finger, and then return the right arm to an extended position.
    - Ask the patient to touch the tip of the nose with the left index finger, and then return the left arm to an extended position.
    - Repeat the procedure several times.
    - Ask the patient to close both eyes and repeat the alternating movements (see Figure 24.23 ■).

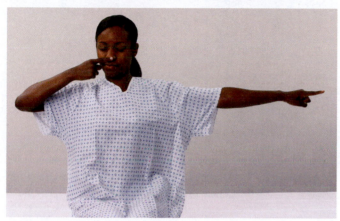

Figure 24.23 Finger-to-nose test.

- Observe the movement of the arms, the smoothness of the movement, and the point of contact of the finger. Does the finger touch the nose, or is another part of the face touched?
- *An alternative:* Have the patient touch the nose with the index finger and then touch the finger of the nurse (see Figure 24.24 ■).

▶ With the eyes closed, the patient with cerebellar disease will reach beyond the tip of the nose because the sense of position is affected.

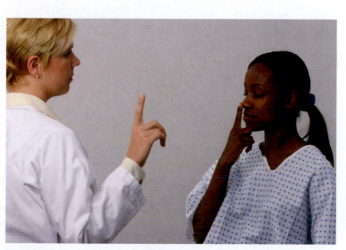

Figure 24.24 Alternative for finger-to-nose test.

4. Assess the patient's ability to perform a rapid alternating action.
- Ask the patient to sit with the hands placed palms down on the thighs (see Figure 24.25A ■).
- Ask the patient to turn the hands palms up (see Figure 24.25B ■).

▶ Inability to perform this task could indicate upper motor neuron weakness.

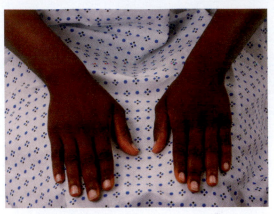

Figure 24.25A Testing rapid alternating movement, palms down.

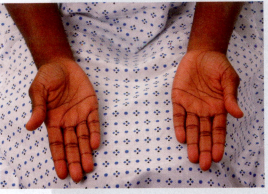

Figure 24.25B Testing rapid alternating movement, palms up.

- Ask the patient to return the hands to a palms-down position.
- Ask the patient to alternate the movements at a faster pace. If you suspect any deficit, test one side at a time.
- Observe the rhythm, rate, and smoothness of the movements.
- Figure 24.26 ■ demonstrates the finger-to-finger test, which is an alternative method to assess coordination.
- Ask the patient to touch the thumb to each finger in sequence with increasing pace.

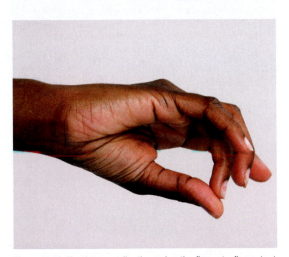

Figure 24.26 Testing coordination using the finger-to-finger test.

5. Ask the patient to perform the heel-to-shin test.
- Assist the patient to a supine position.
- Ask the patient to place the heel of the right foot below the left knee.
- Ask the patient to slide the right heel along the shin bone to the ankle.
- Ask the patient to repeat the procedure, reversing the legs (see Figure 24.27 ■).
- Observe the smoothness of the action. The patient should be able to move the heel in a straight line so that it does not fall off the lower leg.

▶ Inability to perform this test could indicate disease of the posterior spinal tract.

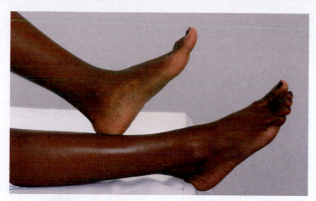

Figure 24.27 Heel-to-shin test.

Sensory Function

This part of the physical assessment evaluates the patient's response to a variety of stimuli. This assessment tests the peripheral nerves, the sensory tracts, and the cortical level of discrimination. A variety of stimuli are used, including light touch, hot/cold, sharp/dull, and vibration. Stereognosis, graphesthesia, and two-point discrimination are also assessed. Each of these assessments is described in the following sections.

Remember, always ask the patient to describe the stimulus and the location. Do not suggest the type of stimulus or location. Tell the patient to keep both eyes closed during testing. To promote full patient understanding and cooperation, you may have to demonstrate what you will be doing and what you expect the patient to do while using a cotton wisp, the uncovered end of an applicator, or a tongue blade. Specific dermatomes are tested as you assess corresponding locations.

ALERT! *The patient may tire during these procedures. If this happens, stop the assessment and continue at a later time. Be sure to test corresponding body parts. Take a distal-to-proximal approach along the extremities. When the patient describes sensations accurately at a distal point, it is usually not necessary to proceed to a more proximal point. If a deficit is detected at a distal point, then it becomes imperative to proceed to proximal points while attempting to map the specific area of the deficit. Repeat testing to determine accuracy in areas of deficits.*

1. **Assess the patient's ability to identify light touch.**
   - Using a cotton wisp, touch various parts of the body, including feet, hands, arms, legs, abdomen, and face (see Figure 24.28 ■).
   - Touch at random locations and use random time intervals.
   - Ask the patient to say "Yes" or "Now" when the stimulus is perceived. Be sure to test corresponding dermatomes.

▶ **Anesthesia** is the inability to perceive the sense of touch. **Hyperesthesia** is an increased sensation, whereas **hypoesthesia** is a decreased but not absent sensation.

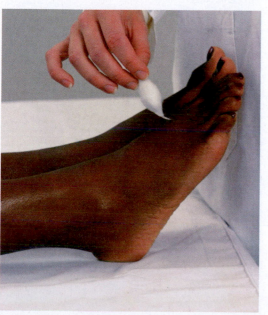

Figure 24.28 Evaluation of light touch.

Techniques and Normal Findings	Abnormal Findings and Special Considerations

2. **Assess the patient's ability to distinguish the difference between sharp and dull.**
   - Ask the patient to say "Sharp" or "Dull" when something sharp or dull is felt on the skin.
   - Touch the patient with the uncovered end of an applicator or the irregular edge of a broken tongue blade. The sharp edge is used to identify pain, whereas the dull edge is a repeat of step 1 (see Figure 24.29A ■).
   - Now touch the patient with the cotton end of the applicator or the smooth edge of a tongue blade (see Figure 24.29B ■).
   - Alternate between sharp and dull stimulation.
   - Touch the patient using random locations, random time intervals, and alternating patterns.
   - Be sure to test corresponding body parts. This tests specific dermatomes.
   - Discard the applicator or tongue blade.

▶ The absence of pain sensation is called **analgesia**. Decreased pain sensation is called **hypoalgesia**. These conditions may result from neurologic disease or circulatory problems such as peripheral vascular disease.

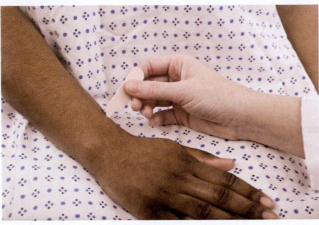

Figure 24.29A Testing the patient's ability to identify sharp sensations.

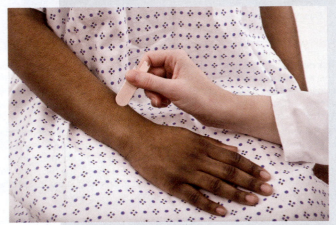

Figure 24.29B Testing the patient's ability to identify dull sensations.

3. **Assess the patient's ability to distinguish temperature.**
   - Perform this test only if the patient demonstrates an absence or decrease in pain sensation.
   - Randomly touch the patient with test tubes containing warm and cold water.
   - Ask the patient to describe the temperature.
   - Be sure to test corresponding body parts.

4. **Assess the patient's ability to feel vibrations.**
   - Set a tuning fork in motion and place it on bony parts of the body, such as the toe, ankle, knee, iliac crest, spinal process, finger, sternum, wrist, or elbow (see Figure 24.30 ■).
   - Ask the patient to say "Now" when the vibration is perceived and "Stop" when it is no longer felt.
   - If the patient's perception is accurate when you test the most distal aspects (toe, ankle, finger, and wrist), end the test at this time.
   - Proceed to proximal points if distal perception is diminished.

▶ If an area of decreased or absent sensation is assessed, attempt to map the region to determine if it is associated with a dermatome or peripheral sensory nerve pattern. Diminished sensation may indicate peripheral nerve, polyneuropathy, or CNS involvement.

▶ The inability to perceive vibration may indicate neuropathy. This may be associated with aging, diabetes, intoxication, or posterior column disease.

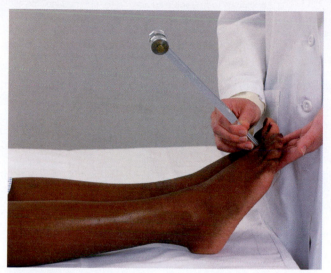

Figure 24.30A Testing the patient's ability to feel vibrations, the toe.

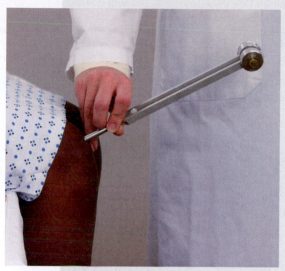

Figure 24.30B Testing the patient's ability to feel vibrations, the knee.

5. **Test stereognosis, the ability to identify an object without seeing it.**
   - Direct the patient to close both eyes. Place a closed safety pin in the patient's right hand and ask the patient to identify it.
   - Place a different object, such as a key, in the left hand, and ask the patient to identify it.
   - Place a coin in the right hand and ask the patient to identify it (see Figure 24.31 ■).
   - Place a different coin in the left hand and ask the patient to identify it.
   - The objects you use must be familiar and safe to hold (no sharp objects).
   - Test each object independently.

▶ Inability to identify a familiar object could indicate cortical disease.

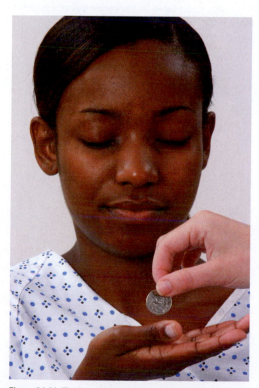

Figure 24.31 Testing stereognosis using a coin.

Techniques and Normal Findings	Abnormal Findings and Special Considerations

6. **Test graphesthesia, the ability to perceive writing on the skin.**
   - Direct the patient to keep both eyes closed.
   - Using the noncotton end of an applicator or the base of a pen, scribe a number such as 3 into the palm of the patient's right hand (see Figure 24.32 ■).
   - Be sure the number faces the patient.
   - Ask the patient to identify the number.
   - Repeat in the left hand using a different number such as 5 or 2.
   - Ask the patient to identify the number.

▶ Inability to perceive a number on the skin may indicate cortical disease.

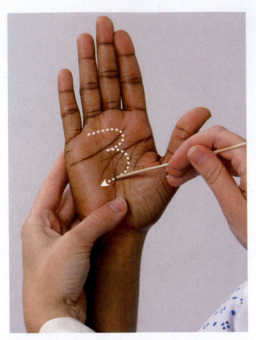

Figure 24.32 Testing graphesthesia.

7. **Assess the patient's ability to discriminate between two points.**
   - Using the unpadded end of two applicators, simultaneously touch the patient with the two stimuli over a given area (see Figure 24.33 ■).
   - Vary the distance between the two points according to the body region being stimulated.

▶ An inability to perceive two separate points within normal distances may indicate cortical disease.

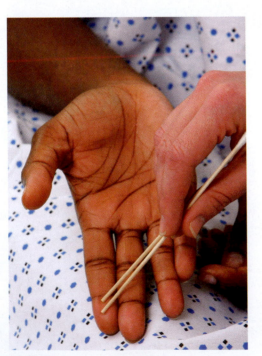

Figure 24.33 Two-point discrimination.

Techniques and Normal Findings	**Abnormal Findings and Special Considerations**

The more distal the location, the more sensitive the discrimination.

- Normally, the patient is able to perceive two discrete points at the following distances and locations:

Fingertips	0.3 to 0.6 cm (0.12 to 0.24 in.)
Hands and feet	1.5 to 2 cm (0.59 to 0.78 in.)
Lower leg	4 cm (1.56 in.)

- Ask the patient to say "Now" when the two discrete points of stimulus are first perceived.
- Note the smallest distance between the points at which the patient can perceive two distinct stimuli.
- Discard the applicators.

8. **Assess topognosis, the ability of the patient to identify an area of the body that has been touched.**
   - This need not be a separate test. Include it in any of the previous steps by asking the patient to identify what part of the body was involved. Also ask the patient to point to the area you touched.

9. **Assess kinesthesia, the position sense of joint movement.**
   - Ask the patient to close both eyes. Grasp the great toe. Move the joint into dorsiflexion, plantar flexion, and abduction.
   - Ask the patient to identify the movement (see Figure 24.34 ■).

▶ Inability of the patient to identify a touched area demonstrates sensory or cortical disease.

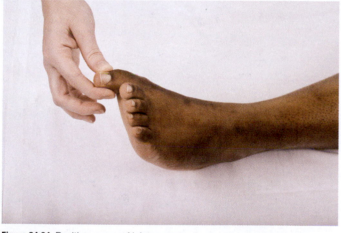

Figure 24.34 Position sense of joint movement.

Reflexes

Reflex testing is usually the last part of the neurologic assessment. The patient is usually in a sitting position; however, you can use a supine position if the patient's physical condition so requires. Position the patient's limbs properly to stretch the muscle partially.

Proper use of the reflex hammer requires practice. Hold the handle of the reflex hammer in your dominant hand between your thumb and index finger. Use your wrist, not your hand or arm, to generate the striking motion. Proper wrist action will provide a brisk, direct, smooth arc for stimulation with the flat or pointed end of the hammer. Stimulate the reflex arc with a brisk tap to the tendon, not the muscle. Through continued practice and experience, you will learn the amount of force to use. Strong force will cause pain, and too little force will not stimulate the arc. After striking the tendon, remove the reflex hammer immediately.

Evaluate the response on a scale from 0 to 4+:

0	no response
1+	diminished
2+	normal
3+	brisk, above normal
4+	hyperactive

▶ Neuromuscular disease, spinal cord injury, or lower motor neuron disease may cause absent or diminished (hypoactive) reflexes.

▶ Hyperactive reflexes may indicate upper motor neuron disease.

▶ **Clonus**, rhythmically alternating flexion and extension, confirms upper motor neuron disease.

Before concluding that a reflex is absent or diminished, repeat the test. Encourage the patient to relax. You might need to help the patient adjust his position or you might need to strike the tendon with slightly more force. It may be necessary to distract the attention of the patient to achieve muscle relaxation. Distraction, which involves simultaneously performing an isometric activity of a distant muscle group, helps relax the muscle that is being tested and enhances the reflex. For example, ask the patient to pull on his hands (isometric activity) while testing the reflexes of the leg (see Figure 24.35 ■).

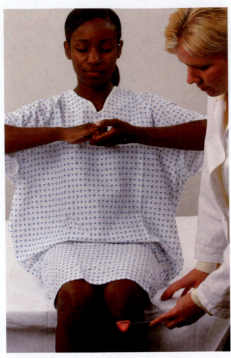

Figure 24.35 Testing the patellar reflex using a distraction technique.

1. **Assess the biceps reflex (C5, C6).**
   - Support the patient's lower arm with your nondominant hand and arm. The arm must be slightly flexed at the elbow with palm up.
   - Compress the biceps tendon with the thumb of your nondominant hand.
   - Using the pointed side of a reflex hammer, briskly tap your thumb (see Figure 24.36 ■).
   - Look for contraction of the biceps muscle and slight flexion of the forearm.

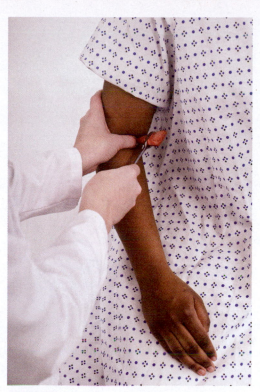

Figure 24.36 Testing the biceps reflex.

2. **Assess the triceps reflex (C6, C7).**
   - Support the patient's elbow with your nondominant hand.
   - Sharply percuss the tendon just above the olecranon process with the pointed end of the reflex hammer (see Figure 24.37 ■).
   - Observe contraction of the triceps muscle with extension of the lower arm.

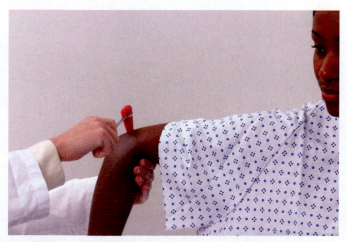

Figure 24.37 Testing the triceps reflex.

3. **Assess the brachioradialis reflex (C5, C6).**
   - Position the patient's arm so the elbow is flexed and the hand is resting on the patient's lap with the palm in a semi-pronating position.
   - Using the flat end of the reflex hammer, briskly strike the tendon toward the radius about 2 or 3 inches above the wrist (see Figure 24.38 ■).
   - Observe flexion of the lower arm and supination of the hand.

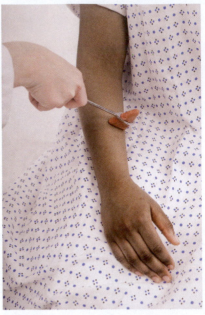

Figure 24.38 Testing the brachioradialis reflex.

4. **Assess the patellar (knee) reflex (L2, L3, L4).**
   - Palpate the patella to locate the patellar tendon inferior to the patella.
   - Briskly strike the tendon with the flat end of the reflex hammer (see Figure 24.39 ■).
   - Note extension of lower leg and contraction of the quadriceps muscle.

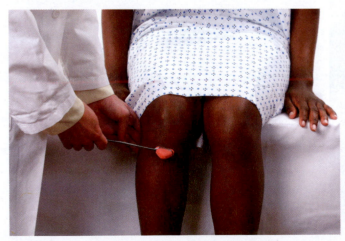

Figure 24.39A Testing the patellar reflex, patient in a sitting position.

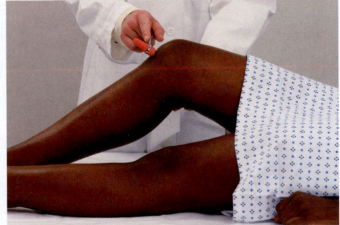

Figure 24.39B Testing the patellar reflex, patient in a supine position.

5. **Assess the Achilles tendon (ankle) reflex (S1).**
   - Flex the leg at the knee.
   - Dorsiflex the foot of the leg being examined.
   - Hold the foot lightly in the nondominant hand.
   - Strike the Achilles tendon with the flat end of the reflex hammer (see Figure 24.40 ■).
   - Observe plantar flexion of the foot; the heel will "jump" from your hand.

▶ Occasionally, the response is not obtained. Distraction such as that depicted in Figure 24.35 may be required.

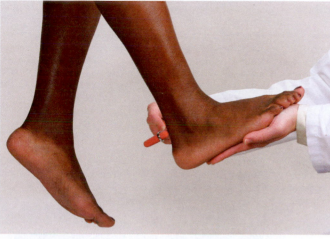

Figure 24.40A Testing the Achilles tendon reflex, patient in a sitting position.

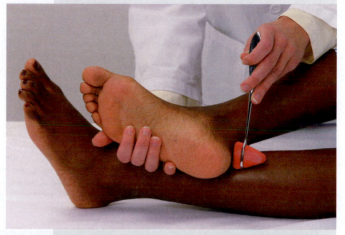

Figure 24.40B Testing the Achilles tendon reflex, patient in a supine position.

6. **Assess the plantar reflex (L5, S1).**
   - Position the leg with a slight degree of external rotation at the hip.
   - Stimulate the sole of the foot from the heel to the ball of the foot on the lateral aspect. Continue the stimulation across the ball of the foot to the big toe.
   - Observe for plantar flexion, in which the toes curl toward the sole of the foot (see Figure 24.41 ■). It may be necessary to hold the patient's ankle to prevent movement.

▶ A **Babinski response** is the fanning of the toes with the great toe pointing toward the dorsum of the foot (see Figure 24.42 ■). This is called dorsiflexion of the toe and is considered an abnormal response in the adult. It may indicate upper motor neuron disease.

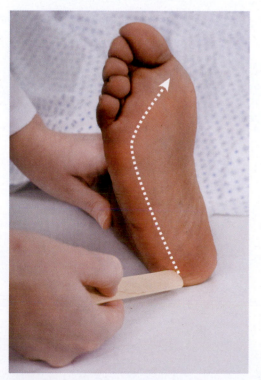

Figure 24.41 Testing the plantar reflex.

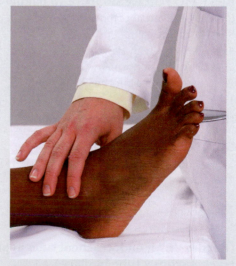

Figure 24.42 A Babinski response in an adult is an abnormal finding.

▶ A positive Babinski response is considered a normal response in the child until about 2 years of age (see Chapter 26, Table 26.1 ∞).

Techniques and Normal Findings	Abnormal Findings and Special Considerations

Appendix C: Advanced Skills *Appendix C provides step-by-step instructions on testing abdominal reflexes.*

Additional Assessment Techniques

Meningeal Assessment

- Ask the patient to flex the neck by bringing the chin down to touch the chest.
- Observe the degree of range of motion and the absence or presence of pain. The patient should be able to flex the neck about 45 degrees without pain.
- When the patient complains of pain and has decreased neck flexion, you will observe for *Brudzinski's sign.* With the patient in a supine position, assist the patient with neck flexion. Observe the legs. Brudzinski's sign is positive when neck flexion causes flexion of the legs and thighs.

▶ A positive Brudzinski's sign may be indicative of irritation or inflammation of the meningeal membranes, as in meningitis. **Nuchal rigidity** (severe neck stiffness) is a hallmark of meningitis.

Use of the Glasgow Coma Scale

The *Glasgow Coma Scale* assesses the level of consciousness of the individual on a continuum from alertness to coma (see Figure 24.43 ■). The scale tests three body functions: verbal response, motor response, and eye response. A maximum total score of 15 indicates the person is alert, responsive, and oriented. A total score of 3, the lowest achievable score, indicates a nonresponsive comatose individual.

▶ **Syncope** is a brief loss of consciousness and is usually sudden. **Coma** is a more prolonged state with pronounced and persistent changes. A patient experiencing any loss of consciousness needs immediate medical interventions.

▶ The Glasgow Coma Scale has limitations. For example, a patient with an endotracheal tube or tracheostomy cannot verbally communicate. As a result, the score is carried out according to each individual component of the scale. The verbal response score would then indicate intubation or tracheostomy. In addition, the motor response scale is invalid in a patient with a spinal cord injury, and eye opening may be impossible to assess in those individuals with severe orbital injury.

GLASGOW COMA SCALE

BEST EYE-OPENING RESPONSE

4 = Spontaneously
3 = To speech
2 = To pain
1 = No response

(Record "C" if eyes closed by swelling)

BEST MOTOR RESPONSE to painful stimuli

6 = Obeys verbal command
5 = Localizes pain
4 = Flexion—withdrawal
3 = Flexion—abnormal
2 = Extension—abnormal
1 = No response

(Record best upper limb response)

BEST VERBAL RESPONSE

5 = Oriented × 3
4 = Conversation—confused
3 = Speech—inappropriate
2 = Sounds—incomprehensible
1 = No response

(Record "E" if endotracheal tube in place, "T" if tracheostomy tube in place)

Figure 24.43 Glasgow Coma Scale.

Documenting Your Findings

Documentation of assessment data—subjective and objective—must be accurate, professional, complete, and confidential.

Focused History (Subjective Data)

This is information from Review of Systems (ROS) and other pertinent history information that is or could be related to the patient's neurologic function.

Patient reports a change in coordination and balance. States difficulty in climbing stairs and doing usual stretching exercise routine. Denies history of head injury, seizures, migraines, or other neurologic illnesses. States no change in vision, hearing, taste, smell, sensation, or memory.

Physical Assessment (Objective Data)

Grooming and hygiene appropriate, posture erect, body language and facial expressions appropriate. Able to follow directions, complete calculations accurately, speech and language clear, abstract thinking and judgment intact. Oriented × 3. CN I–X11 intact. Positive Babinski. Unable to complete tandem walk or standing on one foot without losing balance. Upper extremity coordination and RAM intact. Sensation intact to light touch, sharp/dull, temperature, vibration, stereognosis.

Abnormal Findings

Problems commonly associated with the neurologic system include changes in motor function, including gait and movement; seizures; spinal cord injury; traumatic brain injury; infections; degenerative disorders; and cranial nerve dysfunction. These conditions are described next and in Table 24.4 and Table 24.5.

Table 24.4 Problems with Motor Function

GAIT	MOVEMENT
Ataxic Gait A walk characterized by a wide base, uneven steps, feet slapping, and a tendency to sway. This type of walk is associated with posterior column disease or decreased proprioception regarding extremities. Seen in multiple sclerosis and drug or alcohol intoxication.	**Fasciculation** Commonly called a twitch, this is an involuntary, local, visible muscular contraction. It is not significant when it occurs in tired muscles. It can be associated with motor neuron disease.
Scissors Gait A walk characterized by spastic lower limbs and movement in a stiff, jerky manner. The knees come together; the legs cross in front of one another; and the legs are abducted as the individual takes short, progressive, slow steps. This is seen in individuals with multiple sclerosis.	**Tic** Commonly called a *habit*, a tic is usually psychogenic in nature. The involuntary spasmodic movement of the muscle is seen in a muscle under voluntary control, usually in the face, neck, or shoulders, and increases during stress. Tourette's syndrome is a neurologic disorder characterized by involuntary movements and vocalizations called tics.
Steppage Gait Sometimes called the "foot drop" walk. The individual flexes and raises the knee to a higher-than-usual level, yielding a flopping of the foot when walking. This usually is indicative of lower motor neuron disease. Seen in individuals with alcoholic neuritis and progressive muscular atrophy.	**Tremor** A rhythmic or alternating involuntary movement from the contraction of opposing muscle groups. Tremors vary in degree and are seen in Parkinson disease, multiple sclerosis, uremia (a form of kidney failure), and alcohol intoxication.
Festination Gait Referred to as the "Parkinson walk." The individual has stooped posture, takes short steps, and turns stiffly. There is a slow start to the walk and frequent, accelerated steps. This gait is associated with basal ganglia disease.	**Athetoid Movement** A continuous, involuntary, repetitive, slow, "wormlike," arrhythmic muscular movement. The muscles are in a state of hypotoxicity, producing a distortion to the limb. This movement is seen in cerebral palsy.
Dystonia Similar to athetoid movements, dystonia involves larger muscle groups. The twisting movements yield a grotesque change to the individual's posture. Torticollis, or wryneck, is an example of dystonia. Primary dystonia is unrelated to any illness and accounts for almost 50% of all cases. Secondary dystonia can result from trauma, tumor, strokes, or toxins.	**Myoclonus** A continual, rapid, short spasm involving a muscle, part of a muscle, or even a group of muscles. Frequently occurs in an extremity as the individual is falling asleep. Myoclonus is also seen in seizure disorders.

Table 24.5 Problems Associated with Dysfunction of Cranial Nerves

CRANIAL NERVE		DYSFUNCTION
I	Olfactory	Unilateral or bilateral anosmia
II	Optic	Optic atrophy, papilledema, amblyopia, field defects
III	Oculomotor	Diplopia, ptosis of lid, dilated pupil, inability to focus on close objects
IV	Trochlear	Convergent strabismus, diplopia
V	Trigeminal	Tic douloureux, loss of facial sensation, decreased ability to chew, loss of corneal reflex, decreased blinking
VI	Abducens	Diplopia, strabismus
VII	Facial	Bell's palsy, decreased ability to distinguish tastes
VIII	Vestibulocochlear	Tinnitus, vertigo, deafness
IX	Glossopharyngeal	Loss of "gag" reflex, loss of taste, difficulty swallowing
X	Vagus	Loss of voice, impaired voice, difficulty swallowing
XI	Accessory	Difficulty with shrugging of shoulders, inability to turn head to left and right
XII	Hypoglossal	Difficulty with speech and swallowing, inability to protrude tongue

Seizures

Seizures are sudden, rapid, and excessive discharges of electrical energy in the brain. They are usually centered in the cerebral cortex. Some seizure disorders stem from neurologic problems that occur before or during birth, or they can develop secondary to childhood fevers. In children and adults, seizures can result from a variety of factors, including trauma, infections, cerebrovascular disease, environmental toxins, drug overdose, and withdrawal from alcohol, sedatives, or antidepressants. *Epilepsy* is a chronic seizure disorder.

Spinal Cord Injuries

The spinal cord extends from the medulla oblongata of the brainstem. As it continues down the back, the cervical, thoracic, and lumbar vertebrae protect it. Spinal cord injuries result from trauma to the vertebrae, which causes dislocation fractures that in turn compress or transect the spinal cord. The most common causes of this type of trauma are automobile and motorcycle accidents, sports accidents such as football and diving accidents, and penetrating injuries such as stab wounds and gunshots. Generally speaking, the higher the level of the injury, the greater the loss of neurologic function. Injuries to the cervical region are the most common and the most devastating.

TRAUMATIC BRAIN INJURY

Traumatic brain injury (TBI) is an acquired brain injury in which damage to the brain results from a sudden, forceful impact to the brain. TBI commonly results from motor vehicle accidents, sports injuries, blasts, and other accidents. It may also occur during violence such as a gunshot wound or blow to the head or during abuse. Depending on the extent and location of the damage, symptoms can be mild, moderate, or severe.

Subjective findings:
- Headache
- Confusion
- Dizziness
- Fatigue
- Sensory problems (e.g., blurred vision, tinnitus, bad taste in mouth, light or sound sensitivity)
- Cognitive problems (e.g., inability to concentrate, mood swings, depression, aggression, etc.)

Objective findings:
- Vomiting
- Seizures
- Unconsciousness
- Slurred speech
- Dilation of pupils (National Institute of Neurological Disorders and Stroke [NINDS], 2018)

Infections of the Neurologic System

Infections of the neurologic system include meningitis, myelitis, brain abscess, and Lyme disease. Each of these is described in the following paragraphs.

MENINGITIS

Meningitis is caused by a virus or bacteria that infects the coverings, or meninges, of the brain or spinal cord. Meningitis may result from a penetrating wound, fractured skull, or upper respiratory infection, or it may occur secondary to facial or cranial surgery.

In some cases, meningitis may spread to the underlying brain tissues, causing encephalitis. *Encephalitis* is defined as an inflammation of the tissue of the brain. It usually results from a virus, which may be transmitted by ticks or mosquitoes, or it may result from a childhood illness such as chickenpox or the measles.

Subjective findings:
- Headache or stiff neck
- Nausea
- Photophobia
- Confusion

Objective findings:
- Fever
- Irritability
- Vomiting
- Seizures
- Coma (Centers for Disease Control and Prevention [CDC], 2018)

MYELITIS

Myelitis is an inflammation of the spinal cord. Poliomyelitis and herpes zoster infection are two common causes. It may develop after an infection such as measles or gonorrhea, or it may follow vaccination for rabies.

Subjective findings:
- Lower neck or back pain
- Muscle weakness
- Abnormal sensations such as numbness, tingling, or burning

Objective findings:
- Paralysis
- Urinary retention
- Loss of bowel control (Mayo Foundation for Medical Education and Research, 2014)

BRAIN ABSCESS

A brain abscess is usually the result of a systemic infection. It is marked by an accumulation of pus in the brain cells. Most brain abscesses develop secondary to a primary infection. Others result from skull fractures or penetrating injuries, such as a gunshot wound.

Subjective findings:
- Headache
- Stiff neck
- Nausea or vomiting

Objective findings:
- Fever
- Seizures
- Papilledema
- Focal neurologic deficits or hemiparesis
- Altered level of consciousness (Miranda, Castellar-Leones, Elzain, & Moscote-Salazar, 2013)

LYME DISEASE

Lyme disease is an infection caused by a spirochete transmitted by a bite from an infected tick that lives on deer. If untreated, Lyme disease may cause neurologic disorders including, but not limited to, Bell's palsy, visual disturbances, and nerve damage in the extremities.

Subjective findings:
- Arthritis
- Headache or neck stiffness
- Flulike symptoms (fatigue, chills, fever, joint aches)
- Dizziness
- Heart palpitations (Centers for Disease Control [CDC], 2016)

Objective findings:
- Bull's-eye rash (erythema migrans)
- Swollen lymph nodes
- Fever (CDC, 2016)

Degenerative Neurologic Disorders

Degenerative neurologic disorders include Alzheimer disease, amyotrophic lateral sclerosis, Huntington disease, multiple sclerosis, myasthenia gravis, and Parkinson disease. These are discussed in the following paragraphs.

ALZHEIMER DISEASE

Alzheimer disease is a progressive degenerative disease of the brain that leads to dementia. Although it is more common in people over age 65, its onset may occur as early as middle adulthood.

Subjective findings:
- Memory loss, particularly of recent events
- Hallucinations
- Paranoid fantasies (in later stage of disease)

Objective findings:
- Shortened attention span
- Confusion
- Disorientation
- Wandering

AMYOTROPHIC LATERAL SCLEROSIS

Amyotrophic lateral sclerosis (ALS), commonly known as Lou Gehrig disease, is a chronic degenerative disease involving the cerebral cortex and the motor neurons in the spinal cord. The result is a progressive wasting of skeletal muscles that eventually leads to death. Although the cause is unknown, research has implicated viral infection. Certain forms of ALS are familial (University of Michigan Health Systems, n.d.).

Subjective findings:
- Muscle weakness
- Muscle cramping
- Shortness of breath

Objective findings:
- Muscle fasciculations (twitching)
- Difficulty speaking (dysphonia)
- Impaired movement of limbs

HUNTINGTON DISEASE

Huntington disease is an inherited disorder characterized by uncontrollable jerking movements, called *chorea*, which literally means "dance." It typically progresses to mental deterioration and, ultimately, death. Symptoms usually first appear in early middle age; thus, those with Huntington disease often have had children before they know they have the disorder.

Subjective findings:
- Difficulty with reasoning
- Difficulty swallowing (dysphagia)
- Disinhibition

Objective findings:
- Muscle rigidity
- Choreiform movements (involuntary, irregular, jerking movements)
- Slow movements (bradykinesia)

MULTIPLE SCLEROSIS

Multiple sclerosis is the deterioration of the protective sheaths, composed of myelin, of the nerve tracts in the brain and spinal cord. The first attack usually occurs between the ages of 20 and 40. Some individuals experience repeated attacks that progress in severity. In these individuals, permanent disability with progressive neuromuscular deficits develops.

Subjective findings:
- Blurred vision
- Transient tingling sensations
- Numbness
- Weakness (sometimes limited to one limb or one side of the body)

Objective findings:
- Slurred speech
- Wide, uneven gait (ataxia)
- Tremors

MYASTHENIA GRAVIS

Myasthenia gravis is a chronic neuromuscular disorder involving increasing weakness of voluntary muscles with activity and some abatement of symptoms with rest. Onset is gradual and usually occurs in adolescence or young adulthood. The precise etiology is unknown, but it is believed that myasthenia gravis is an *autoimmune* disorder—that is, the individual's immune system attacks the individual's own normal cells rather than foreign pathogens.

Subjective findings:
- Diplopia (double vision)
- Dysphagia (difficulty swallowing)
- Difficulty speaking (dyphasia)

Objective findings:
- Ptosis (drooping eyelids)
- Flat affect
- Weak, monotone voice

PARKINSON DISEASE

Parkinson disease is a degeneration of the basal nuclei of the brain, which are collections of nerve cell bodies deep within the white matter of the cerebrum. These nuclei are responsible for initiating and stopping voluntary movement. Although the precise etiology is unknown, research indicates that environmental toxins, such as carbon monoxide or certain metals, may cause some cases of Parkinson disease. It may also result from previous encephalitis.

Subjective findings:
- Difficulty speaking (dysphasia)
- Decrease in unconscious movements, such as blinking
- Impaired sense of balance
- Muscle pain

Objective findings:
- Slowed movements (bradykinesia)
- Muscle rigidity
- Rhythmic shaking of the hands
- Pill-rolling tremor of the forefinger and thumb
- Masklike facial expression

Application Through Critical Thinking

CASE STUDY

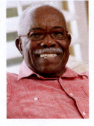

Source: Cathy Yeulet/123RF.

Mr. John Phelps, age 65, is an African American male who comes to the community health clinic. He and his wife, Helen, recently celebrated their 40th wedding anniversary. He has a 35-year-old daughter, a 32-year-old son, and three grandchildren. Mr. Phelps retired 4 months ago from a busy accounting firm where he worked as a certified public accountant (CPA) for 25 years. He and his wife have been planning their retirement and are looking forward to traveling across the country to visit family.

Mr. Phelps's chief complaint is tremors that seem to be getting worse over the past few months. He noticed the tremors about 6 months ago and thought they were related to fatigue because the office was very busy and he was working late hours. He anticipated that the tremors would stop after he retired and became rested. Mrs. Phelps indicates that her husband's handwriting has become small and almost illegible and that she had to write several checks for him last week. She also comments that her husband seems depressed about his recent retirement, because he has a "blank look" on his face and his speech is slow. Mari Chung, RN, conducts a focused interview and then proceeds with the physical assessment. She gathers the following objective and subjective data:

- Mood swings
- Tremors, movement of thumb and index finger in a circular fashion
- Shuffling gait, falls easily
- Constipation
- Fatigue
- Loss of 10 lb
- Drooling
- Speaks in a monotone; voice slow, weak, and soft
- Rigidity during passive range of motion (ROM)
- Jerky movements
- Muscle pain and soreness
- Decrease in corneal response
- Posture not erect, forward flexion
- Unable to perform finger-to-nose test and rapid alternating movement
- Difficulty standing from sitting position without assistance

Ms. Chung consults with the clinic physician. After further evaluation, Mr. Phelps is admitted to the neurologic unit of the community hospital with a diagnosis of Parkinson disease.

SAMPLE DOCUMENTATION

The following is sample documentation from the health assessment of John Phelps.

SUBJECTIVE DATA Complains of tremors, getting worse over 6 months. He has had some change in his moods, has lost some weight, and is constipated frequently. He has occasional drooling. Experiences muscle pain and soreness. Requires assistance to get up from a chair and falls easily. Wife states writing increasingly illegible. She reports he has become depressed, has a "blank look," and has slow speech.

OBJECTIVE DATA Posture not erect—favored flexion, shuffling gait, jerky movements. Voice monotone, slow, weak, soft. Decreased corneal response. Rigidity during passive ROM. Unable to perform finger-to-nose and rapid alternating movement tests. Drooling. Weight loss 10 lbs. in past three months.

CRITICAL THINKING QUESTIONS

1. What data were considered in the medical diagnosis of Parkinson disease?

2. What additional data would be required to confirm a diagnosis of Parkinson disease?

3. What are the nursing considerations for Mr. Phelps?

4. What psychosocial considerations should the nurse be aware of when assessing Mr. Phelps?

5. What environmental considerations should the nurse screen for in this case?

REFERENCES

Alzheimer's Association (2018). *Risk factors.* Retrieved from https://www.alz.org/alzheimers_disease_causes_risk_factors.asp

Berman, A., & Snyder, S. (2016). *Kozier and Erb's fundamentals of nursing: Concepts, process, and practice* (10th ed.). Upper Saddle River, NJ: Prentice Hall.

Borella, E., Ludwig, C., Dirk, J., & de Ribaupierre, A. (2010). The influence of time of testing on interference, working memory, processing speed, and vocabulary: Age differences in adulthood. *Experimental Aging Research, 37*(1), 76–107. doi:10.1080/0361073X.2011.536744

Centers for Disease Control and Prevention (CDC). (2016). Signs and symptoms of Lyme disease. Retrieved from http://www.cdc.gov/lyme/signs_symptoms/index.html

Centers for Disease Control and Prevention (CDC). (2018). Meningitis. Retrieved from http://www.cdc.gov/meningitis/index.html

Lesk, V. E., Honey, T. E. M., & de Jager, C. A. (2009). The effect of recent consumption of caffeine-containing foodstuffs on neuropsychological tests in the elderly. *Dementia and Geriatric Cognitive Disorders, 27*, 322–328. http://dx.doi.org/10.1159/000207445

Liberty, G., Shaul, C., Anteby, E. Y., Zohav, E., Cohen, S. M., Boldes, R., & Yagel, S. (2014). OP28. 05: 2D and 3D ultrasound imaging of the fetal normal and bifid uvula. *Ultrasound in Obstetrics & Gynecology, 44*(S1), 152.

Mayo Clinic. (2018). *Tinnitus.* Retrieved from https://www.mayoclinic.org/diseases-conditions/tinnitus/symptoms-causes/syc-20350156

Mayo Foundation for Medical Education and Research. (2014). *Rochester test catalog: 2014 online test catalog.* Available at http://www.mayomedicallaboratories.com/test-catalog

MedlinePlus. (2017). *Color vision test.* Retrieved from https://medlineplus.gov/ency/article/003387.htm

Miranda, H. A., Castellar-Leones, S. M., Elzain, M. A., & Moscote-Salazar, L. R. (2013). Brain abscess: Current management. *Journal of Neurosciences in Rural Practice, 4*(Suppl 1), S67–S81.

National Institute of Diabetes and Digestive and Kidney Diseases (NIDDK). (2017). *Diabetes, heart disease, and stroke.* Retrieved from https://www.niddk.nih.gov/health-information/diabetes/overview/preventing-problems/heart-disease-stroke

National Institute of Neurological Disorders and Stroke (NINDS). (2018). *Traumatic brain injury fact sheet.* Retrieved from https://www.ninds.nih.gov/Disorders/All-Disorders/Traumatic-Brain-Injury-Information-Page

Osborn, K. S., Wraa, C. E., Watson, A., & Holleran, R. S. (2013). *Medical-surgical nursing: Preparation for practice* (2nd ed.). Upper Saddle River, NJ: Pearson.

Polito, L., Greco, A., & Seripa, D. (2016). Genetic profile, environmental exposure, and their interaction in Parkinson's disease. *Parkinson's Disease,* 1–9. http://dx.doi.org/10.1155/2016/6465793

Rao, J. B., Vengamma, B., Naveen, T., & Naveen, V. (2014). Lead encephalopathy in adults. *Journal of Neurosciences in Rural Practice, 5*(2), 161–163.

Ross, S. M., McManus, I. C., Harrison, V., & Mason, O. (2013). Neurobehavioral problems following low-level exposure to organophosphate pesticides: A systematic and meta-analytic review. *Critical Reviews in Toxicology, 43*(1), 21–44.

Schmidt, C., Collette, F., Cajochen, C., & Peigneux, P. (2007). A time to think: Circadian rhythms in human cognition. *Cognitive Neuropsychology, 24,* 755–789. http://dx.doi.org/10.1080/02643290701754158

University of Michigan Health Systems. (n.d.). *Genetic disorders: Neurogenetics.* Retrieved from http://www.uofmhealth.org/medical-services/neurogenetics

van Dijk, J. G., & Wieling, W. (2013). Pathophysiological basis of syncope and neurological conditions that mimic syncope. *Progress in Cardiovascular Diseases, 55*(4), 345–356.

Walters, E. R., & Lesk, V., E. (2015). Time of day and caffeine influence some neuropsychological tests in the elderly. *Psychological Assessment, 27*(1), 161–168. http://dx.doi.org/10.1037/a0038213

Wilson, B. A., Shannon, M. T., & Shields, K. M. (2018). *Pearson nurse's drug guide.* Upper Saddle River, NJ: Pearson.

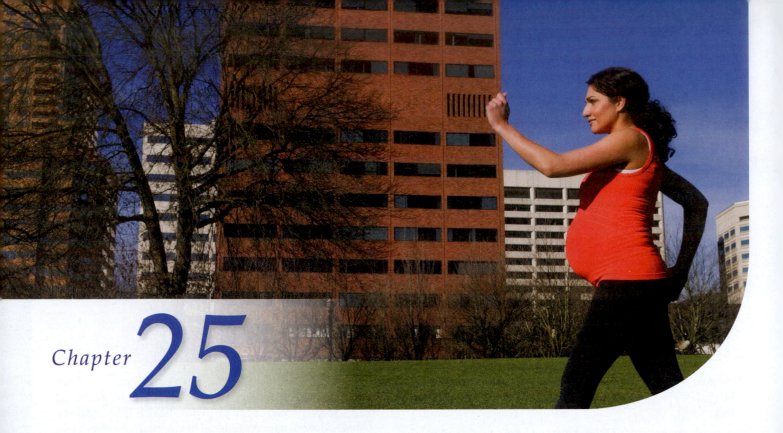

Chapter 25

The Pregnant Woman

LEARNING OUTCOMES

Upon completion of the chapter, you will be able to:

1. Describe the anatomy and physiology of the pregnant woman.

2. Identify the anatomic, physiologic, developmental, psychosocial, and cultural variations that guide assessment of the pregnant woman.

3. Determine questions about the pregnant woman to use for the focused interview.

4. Outline the techniques for assessment of the pregnant woman.

5. Generate the appropriate documentation to describe the assessment of the pregnant woman.

6. Identify abnormal findings in the physical assessment of the pregnant woman.

KEY TERMS

MEDICAL LANGUAGE

a-, an-	Prefix meaning "no," "not," "without"	**macro-**	Prefix meaning "large"
gravida	Root word meaning "pregnant woman"	**mast-**	Prefix meaning "breast"
hyper-	Prefix meaning "high," "elevated," "above normal"	**-uria**	Suffix meaning "urine," "condition of urine"
hypo-	Prefix meaning "below," "deficient"		

Introduction

Through the actions of the nurse, pregnancy and the postpartum period offer a unique opportunity for health promotion, disease prevention, and changes in lifestyle behaviors. For the vast majority of childbearing women, pregnancy and postpartum are normal processes that can be enhanced through education, healthcare, and supportive intervention. Changes in personal lifestyle behaviors and healthcare can influence not only the course of the pregnancy and the health of mother and child but also the future health behaviors of the entire family. Knowledge of variations in body systems during the three trimesters of pregnancy and postpartum periods will enable the nurse to differentiate normal from abnormal changes. The risk for and development of many pathologic conditions in pregnancy and postpartum can be ascertained and prevented by a careful, thorough interview. Past medical, obstetric, gynecologic, family, genetic, and social history will influence the focus of the physical assessment and teaching. Knowledge of lifestyle and health practices, nutrition and exercise history, environmental exposures, and current symptoms will also guide assessment and teaching.

The physical assessment also provides an opportunity for patient education and clarification of misperceptions. Cultural, familial, and personal beliefs can be discussed as appropriate during the history taking and physical assessment. Whether the nurse is perceived as kind and personal or cold and bureaucratic, as knowledgeable and helpful or ill-informed and ineffective, will influence the patient's willingness and ability to implement health recommendations. This life transition is also an opportunity for sharing much joy and excitement with childbearing families. The nurse can influence a whole generation through caring, as well as accurate and appropriate assessment and intervention (see Figure 25.1 ■).

Anatomy and Physiology Review

In order to implement programs of maternal–infant care to promote health, the nurse must understand the adaptations that occur in the female body during pregnancy and postpartum. The anatomic and physiologic changes during the 40 weeks of pregnancy serve three important functions:

- Maintain normal maternal physiologic function
- Meet maternal metabolic needs as the woman adapts to the pregnancy
- Meet the growth and development needs of the fetus

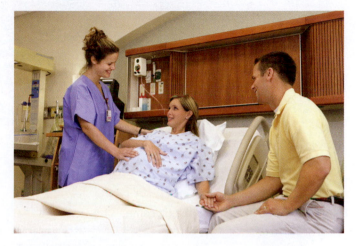

Figure 25.1 Nurse with pregnant patient and partner.
Source: Jupiterimages/Getty Images.

An assessment of the changes in each body system during pregnancy and postpartum will enable the nurse to interpret findings in the interview and assessment.

The Placenta

The physiologic and anatomic changes in pregnancy occur because of the hormones secreted by the fetus and placenta and the mechanical effects of the growing fetus. The human **placenta** is a unique organ that promotes and provides for fetal growth and development. Its functions include metabolism, transport of gases and nutrients to and removal of waste from embryonic blood, and secretion of hormones (Marieb & Keller, 2018). It develops from the fertilized ovum but generally also includes the maternal uterine lining at the site of implantation. The placenta is an ovoid organ that weighs approximately one-sixth the weight of the fetus and covers one-third of the inner surface area of the uterus at term. Implantation of the fertilized egg, called a *blastocyst*, in the endometrium or lining of the uterus begins 6 days after fertilization. The umbilical blood vessels and placenta develop. Two arteries and a vein exit the fetus at the umbilicus, forming the umbilical cord, and insert in the center of the placenta (see Figure 25.2 ■). The fetal vessels branch out into treelike chorionic villi where the fetal capillaries are the sites of exchange between the maternal and fetal circulations. The fetal and maternal circulations are kept essentially separate by the placental membrane covering the villi. The exchange of nutrients from the maternal to the fetal circulation takes place here, as does passage of waste products such as carbon dioxide and uric acid from the fetal to maternal circulation. The placenta,

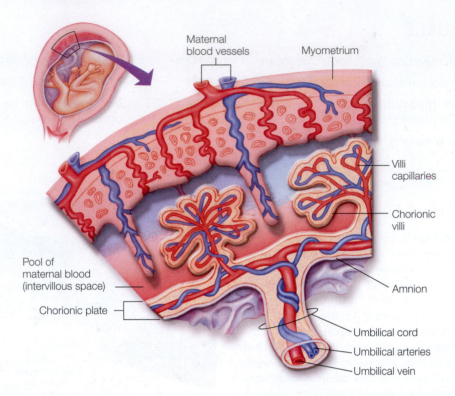

Figure 25.2 Cross-section of the placenta.

in conjunction with the fetus and maternal uterine lining, also produces hormones, including human chorionic gonadotropin (hCG), estrogen, progesterone, relaxin, prolactin, and others.

Fetal Development

Pregnancy is divided into three trimesters, each lasting approximately 13 weeks (3 months in lay terms). The age of the developing human can be referred to in weeks beyond fertilization (as used in discussion of fetal development) or in weeks from the last normal menstrual period, more commonly known as **gestational age**.

The first 2 weeks after fertilization are the early embryo stage. From 2 to 8 weeks after fertilization, the **embryo** is in the stage of *organogenesis* (Marieb & Keller, 2018). During this period, a **teratogen**—an agent such as a virus, a drug, a chemical, or radiation that causes malformation of an embryo or **fetus**—may be present and induce major congenital anomalies. After the completion of 8 weeks until birth, the developing human is referred to as the fetus (see Figure 25.3 ■).

By the end of the first trimester, all major systems have formed. **Viability**, the point at which the fetus can survive outside the uterus, may occur as early as 22 weeks or at the weight of 500 g. During the fetal period the body grows, and differentiation of tissues, organs, and systems occurs.

Although fetal movement can be detected as early as 7 weeks through diagnostic techniques, **quickening**, the fluttery initial sensations of fetal movement perceived by the mother, usually occurs at approximately 18 weeks, possibly earlier in women who have given birth before.

The fetal heart begins beating at 22 days. During assessment, the fetal heartbeat can be heard via Doppler starting between 7 and 12 weeks of pregnancy, and with a **fetoscope**,

a specialized stethoscope for listening to fetal heart sounds, beginning at approximately 18 weeks of gestation. The *uterine souffle*, the sound of the uterine arteries, which is synchronous with the maternal pulse, may be heard, as may the *funic souffle*, the sound of the umbilical vessels that is synchronous with the fetal heartbeat.

Fetal circulation before birth has three shunts that enable the fetus to maximize oxygenation from the maternal circulation because lungs are not yet functional for oxygen exchange. Oxygenated blood from the placenta is carried via the umbilical vein to the fetus, entering at the umbilicus. The fetal liver is partially bypassed by the **ductus venosus**, so that highly oxygenated blood continues on to the heart. More highly oxygenated blood flows into the second shunt, the **foramen ovale**, which connects the fetal right atrium to the fetal left atrium. The other half of the blood continues to the right ventricle. The more highly oxygenated blood from the umbilical vein continues to the left ventricle and is shunted across the **ductus arteriosus** into the descending aorta. In this way, only a small part of the blood flow enters the pulmonary bed. The oxygenated blood then perfuses the rest of the fetal body and returns to the placenta via the umbilical arteries (see Figure 25.4 ■).

Reproductive System Changes

In addition to the fetus and placenta, extensive changes occur in the reproductive organs. The uterus, cervix, fallopian tubes, and vagina undergo massive changes in size and function.

Uterus The uterus is profoundly transformed in pregnancy. The crisscross muscle fibers of the body of the uterus increase in size and number because of the effects of progesterone and estrogen. The uterus increases in size from 70 grams (2.5 oz) to

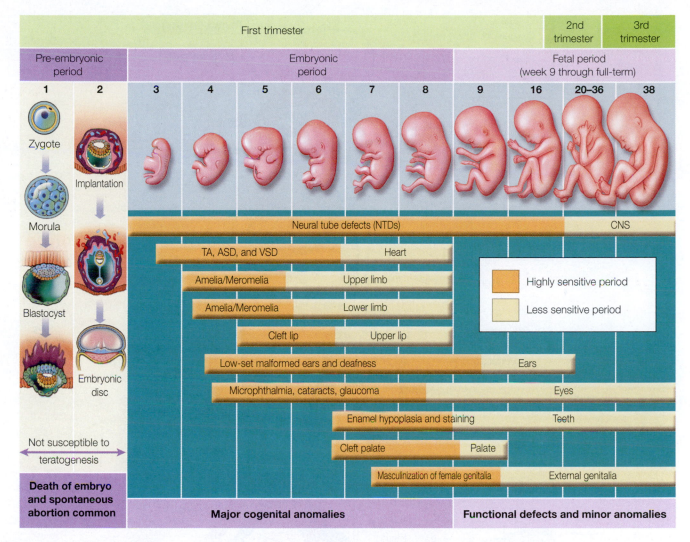

Figure 25.3 Fetal development.

1000 grams (2.2 lb); from 7.5 cm (3 in.) long, 5 cm (2 in.) wide, and 2.5 cm (1 in.) deep to 25 cm (10 in.) long, 20 cm (8 in.) wide, and 22.5 cm (9 in.) deep; and its capacity increases from 10 mL to 5000 mL. During the second and third trimesters, the growing fetus also mechanically expands the uterus.

Early in pregnancy the uterus retains its nonpregnant pear shape but becomes more globular by 12 weeks. Bimanual palpation is used to assess the size of the uterus during the early weeks. The early sizes can be compared with fruits: 6 weeks, a lemon; 8 weeks, a small orange; 10 weeks, a large orange; and 12 weeks, a grapefruit. The growing uterus can be palpated abdominally by about 10 to 12 weeks, at which time the top of the uterus, or **fundus**, is slightly above the symphysis pubis. Women begin to "show" externally at approximately 14 to 16 weeks, later for a **primigravida**, a woman who is pregnant for the first time, and earlier for a **multigravida**, a woman who has been pregnant two or more times. At 16 weeks, the fundus is halfway between the symphysis and umbilicus. Between 20 and 22 weeks, the fundus reaches the umbilicus. Fundal height increases until 38 weeks. The distance from the symphysis pubis to the fundus is measured with a measuring tape to assess fetal growth and dating in pregnancy. **McDonald's rule** for estimating fetal growth states that after

20 weeks in pregnancy, the weeks of gestation approximately equal the **fundal height** in centimeters (see Figure 25.5 ■). Between 38 and 40 weeks **lightening**, or the descent of the fetal head into the pelvis, occurs, and the fundal height drops slightly.

The decidua, or lining of the uterus, becomes four times thicker during pregnancy. Amenorrhea, or the absence of menstruation, is one of the first signs that pregnancy has occurred. Throughout pregnancy the uterus softens, as does the region that connects the body of the uterus and cervix, referred to as **Hegar's sign**. **Piskacek's sign** is the irregular shape of the uterus because of the implantation of the ovum. The contractility of the uterus increases because of the action of estrogen. **Braxton-Hicks contractions**, painless and unpredictable contractions of the uterus that do not dilate the cervix, start in the first trimester, are palpable to the nurse by the second trimester, and are felt by the mother usually starting in the third trimester. **Ballottement**, a technique of palpation, where the examiner's hand is used to push against the uterus and detect the presence or position of a fetus by its return impact, can be elicited after about 20 weeks because the **amniotic fluid**, a clear, slightly yellowish liquid that surrounds the fetus, is greater in comparison to the still small fetus.

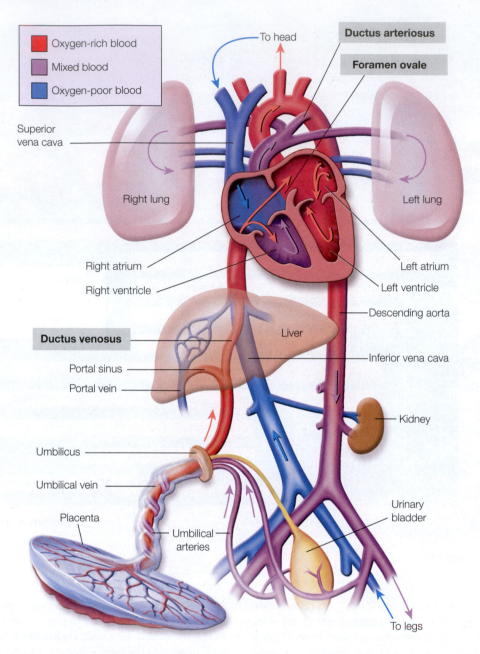

Figure 25.4 Fetal circulation.

Cervix and Vagina   The cervix, or opening of the uterus, develops a protective **mucous plug** during pregnancy, because of the action of progesterone, which also causes **leukorrhea**, a profuse, nonodorous, nonpainful vaginal discharge that protects against infection. Increased glycogen in vaginal cells predisposes the mother to yeast infections in pregnancy. **Goodell's sign** is the softening of the cervix starting at about 6 weeks. At the same time, increased vascularity causes the cervix and vagina to appear bluish (**Chadwick's sign**). Because of these changes, the cervix is more friable and may bleed slightly with sexual intercourse or vaginal examination. Near the end of pregnancy, cervical **ripening**, or softening, and **effacement**, or thinning, occur in preparation for labor. Progressive **dilation**, or opening of the cervix, does not usually occur until the onset of active labor. Externally, the labia majora, labia minora, clitoris, and vaginal introitus enlarge because of hypertrophy and increased vascularity.

Changes in Breasts

Often, one of the first symptoms in pregnancy is breast tenderness, enlargement, and tingling, which is noticeable at 4 to 6 weeks of gestation. These changes are caused by the growth of the alveoli and ductal system and the deposition of fat in the breasts under the influence of estrogen and progesterone. The nipple and the **areola**, the pink circle around the nipple, darken in color in pregnancy, and the sebaceous glands on the areola, **Montgomery's glands (tubercles)**, enlarge and produce a secretion that protects and lubricates the nipples. With the doubling of the blood flow to the breasts, the vascular network above the breasts enlarges and becomes more visible.

Colostrum, a yellowish specialized form of early breast milk high in protein, fat soluble vitamins, minerals, and immunoglobulin, is produced starting in the second trimester and is replaced by transitional milk about 2 to 4 days after the birth of the baby (see Figure 25.6 ■). Production of mature milk begins about 2 weeks postpartum.

Respiratory System Changes

Mechanical and biochemical changes during pregnancy allow the respiratory needs of both mother and fetus to be met. The ligaments of the thorax relax, and the horizontal diameter expands. The enlarging uterus lifts the diaphragm up 4 cm (1.034 in.), the

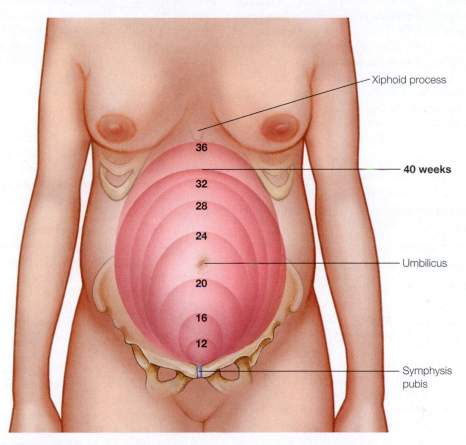

Figure 25.5 Fundal height in pregnancy.

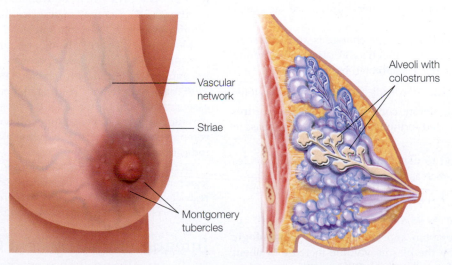

Figure 25.6 Breast changes in pregnancy.

transverse diameter of the chest increases, the ribs flare, and the subcostal angle increases. At rest, the diaphragm rises into the chest to accommodate the fetus, and respirations are diaphragmatic. Shortness of breath and dyspnea, especially in the last trimester, are common as the maternal and fetal demand for oxygen increases. Throughout pregnancy, the total oxygen consumption can increase by 20% and the maternal respiratory rate increases approximately two breaths per minute. Maternal hyperventilation occurs because of an increase in minute ventilation, which is the total volume of air that is inhaled and exhaled in a 1-minute period. The pregnant woman may report great fatigue, particularly in the first trimester, because of these changes. Hyperventilation may occur, and rales in the base of the lung may be heard as a result of compression by the growing uterus. The increasing hormonal levels of progesterone and relaxin allow these changes in the thorax.

The respiratory-stimulating properties of progesterone contribute to the following:

- An increase in respiratory rate of about two breaths per minute and vital capacity, and decrease in residual volume leading to dyspnea, particularly in late pregnancy
- A lowered threshold for carbon dioxide, contributing to a sense of dyspnea
- Decreased airway resistance
- Increased tidal volume and inspiratory capacity
- Decreased expiratory volume

Cardiovascular and Hematologic System Changes

During pregnancy, a woman's body undergoes phenomenal adaptations, especially in the cardiovascular system. Usually these adaptations do not place her life at risk; however, if preexisting cardiovascular or other disease is present, her health may be significantly compromised. The heart is displaced to the left and upward, and the apex is pushed laterally and to the left. This anatomic shift may be seen when examining the electrical axis on the 12-lead ECG of a pregnant patient. The axis is rotated to the left. The physical strength of the woman's abdominal muscles, the shape of the fetus, the gestational age, and the structural anatomy of the uterus influence the extent of this shift.

The most significant hematologic change is an increase in blood and plasma volume of as much as 30% to 50% beginning at 6 to 8 weeks. This change is facilitated by three factors:

- The increased progesterone leads to decreased venous tone.
- The increased progesterone combined with increased estrogen results in increased sodium retention and an increase in total body water.
- The shunt of blood to uteroplacental circulation provides physical space for increased plasma volume.

Other hematologic changes include the following:

- A 25% to 33% increase in red blood cells (RBCs)
- Decrease in hemoglobin and hematocrit, or **physiologic anemia**, caused by the plasma volume increase of about 50% outpacing the increase in RBCs, with a converse decrease in plasma albumin

- Gradual increase in reticulocytes
- Increased white blood cells (WBCs)
- Hypercoagulable state caused by increased activity of most coagulation factors and decreased activities of factors that inhibit coagulation

The upward displacement of the diaphragm by the growing uterus shifts the heart upward and to the left. Most pregnant women will have increased loudness of the S1 sound. Systolic murmurs are usually heard. Because of increased blood flow, a murmur over the mammary vessels, the **mammary souffle**, is occasionally heard. The heart rate gradually increases by 10 to 20 beats per minute (beats/min) over the course of the pregnancy.

Dilation of surface veins, together with the low resistance of the uteroplacental circulation, increases the venous return to the heart. Stroke volume increases 30%. Because of the substantial increase in volume and the resultant increased workload, the heart may appear as much as 10% larger on chest radiography. Systolic blood pressure may decrease by 2 to 3 mmHg, and diastolic blood pressure by 5 to 10 mmHg during the first half of the pregnancy. These values return to their previous levels as the pregnancy progresses.

There may be a slight increase in resting pulse by about 10 to 15 beats/min, although not every patient experiences this increase. Because of the increased volume, preexisting murmurs may become louder. Murmurs may even be auscultated for the first time. Systolic murmurs are the most common (90% incidence), whereas diastolic murmurs occur less frequently (20% incidence). Heart tones may also change. The S1 may split, and a prominent S3 may be heard.

The position of the patient may influence the cardiovascular dynamic state. Cardiac output may decrease when she lies on her back because of compression of the vena cava and aorta. The brachial pressure is highest when the patient is sitting, then decreases when she is supine. Pressure is lowest when she is in the lateral recumbent position. The changes in hemodynamics can cause orthostatic stress when the pregnant woman changes position from sitting to standing or lying to sitting. **Supine hypotension syndrome**, also known as the vena cava syndrome, occurs when pressure from the pregnant uterus compresses the aorta and the inferior vena cava when the woman is in the supine position (Figure 25.7 ■). She may experience dizziness, syncope, and a significant drop in heart rate and blood pressure.

Monitoring a patient's blood pressure and the pattern of the pressures is crucial. Unless a pregnant woman has preexisting uncontrolled hypertension, her blood pressure should be below 140/90; a blood pressure reading higher than this needs further assessment and monitoring. If the pregnant woman does have chronic hypertension, a significant increase in blood pressure compared with her normal baseline blood pressure may be an indication of preeclampsia.

Decreased peripheral resistance leads to increased filling in the legs, but the pressure of the growing uterus on the femoral veins restricts venous return, leading to increased dependent edema and varicosities in the legs, vulva, and rectum (hemorrhoids).

Integumentary System Changes

Hormonal and mechanical factors cause the integumentary changes seen with pregnancy. Categories of change include

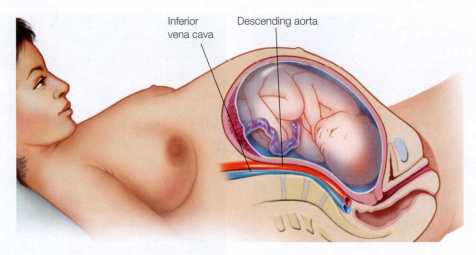

Inferior vena cava

Descending aorta

Figure 25.7 Supine hypotension in pregnancy. The weight of the uterus compresses the vena cava, trapping blood in the lower extremities.

alterations in pigmentation, connective tissue, vascular system, secretory glands, skin, hair, and pruritus (itching). The changes are not usually pathologic but are a source of concern to expectant mothers.

Alterations in pigmentation, the most common integumentary changes in pregnancy, are caused by the increase in estrogen and progesterone early in pregnancy and, later in pregnancy, by the increase in placental hormones and melanocyte-stimulating hormone, as well as others. Any areas of pigmentation in the body will usually become darker for women of all skin colors, including the areolae, axillae, perineum, and inner thighs. The *linea alba*, a tendinous line that extends midline from the symphysis pubis to the xiphoid, darkens with the progression of the fundus up through the abdomen and becomes the **linea nigra**. *Melasma*, also called chloasma or the "mask of pregnancy," occurs in a butterfly pattern over the forehead, nose, and cheeks. There is a strong genetic predisposition for this condition, and it is also seen with the use of combined oral contraceptive pills. Freckles, nevi, and scars may also darken in pregnancy.

A change in connective tissue is **striae gravidarum**, also known as stretch marks: pinkish-purplish streaks that are depressions in the skin. Caused by the stretching of the collagen in skin, they develop in the second half of pregnancy and fade to silver in the postpartum; unlike most integumentary changes, they do not resolve completely after pregnancy. They may develop in the lower abdomen, breasts, thighs, and buttocks.

Vascular alterations that affect the integumentary system are spider angiomas or nevi and palmar erythema. Spider angiomas or nevi are arterioles dilated at the center, with branches radiating outward, appearing on the face, neck, and arms. They fade after pregnancy but do not usually disappear. They often occur with palmar erythema, a reddening or mottling of the palms or fleshy side of the fingers, which occurs after the first trimester, has a genetic predisposition, and regresses by the first week after birth.

Alterations in secretory glands in pregnancy include a decrease in apocrine sweat gland activity in the axillae, abdomen, and genitalia. The eccrine sweat glands in the palms, soles, and forehead increase in activity because of increases

in thyroid and metabolic activity, allowing for dissipation of increased heat. Some women experience a "glow" in their skin during pregnancy, and some experience an increase in acne due to increased sebaceous gland activity.

A skin change that sometimes occurs in the second half of pregnancy is the development of soft, pedunculated, flesh-colored or pigmented skin tags. Although a common occurrence in the general population, elevated hormones may cause an increase in the formation. They occur on the sides of the face and neck, on the upper axillae, between and under the breasts, and in the groin, often where skin rubs against clothing or skin rubs against skin. These may or may not have to be removed after childbirth.

Because of the hormonal influence of estrogen in pregnancy, more hairs enter the growth phase. Some women experience mild hirsutism and report thicker hair. Consequently, more than the usual number of hairs reach maturity and fall out in the postpartum period during months 1 to 5. Usually all hair regrows by 6 to 15 months postpartum. Occasionally nails become soft or more brittle.

Pruritus is common in the abdomen in the third trimester, and if severe must be distinguished from rare dermatologic disorders in pregnancy such as cholestasis of pregnancy, pruritic urticarial papules and plaques of pregnancy (PUPPP), herpes gestationis, and prurigo of pregnancy. Figure 25.8 ■ depicts some of the common integumentary changes in pregnancy, including striae, linea nigra, melasma, and spider angioma.

Changes in the Eyes, Ears, Nose, Throat, and Mouth

Pregnant women may complain of dry eyes and may discontinue wearing contact lenses during pregnancy. The pregnant woman may also describe visual changes because of shifting fluid in the cornea. These symptoms are usually not significant and disappear after childbirth. Changes in eyesight, such as refraction changes requiring a new prescription for glasses or contact lenses, blurriness, or distorted vision, can occur because of temporary changes in the shape of the eye during the last trimester of pregnancy and the first 6 weeks postpartum.

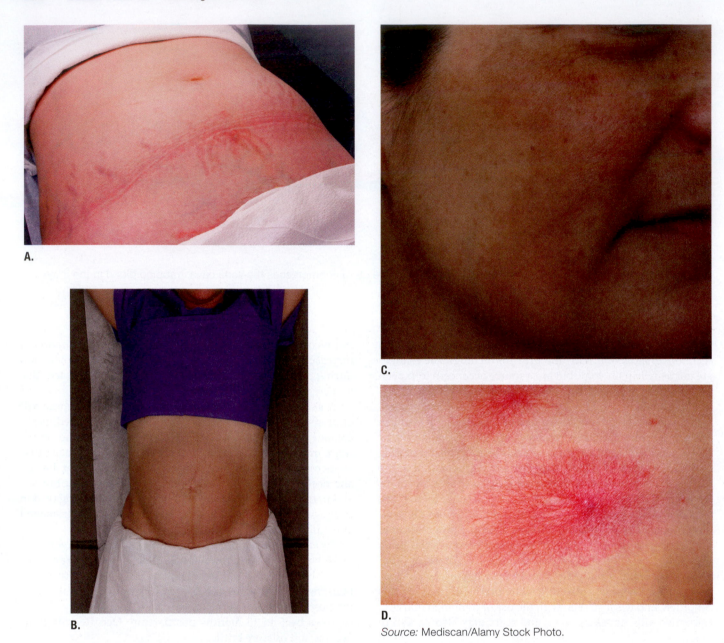

A.

B.

C.

D.

Source: Mediscan/Alamy Stock Photo.

Figure 25.8 Integumentary changes in pregnancy. A. Striae. B. Linea nigra. C. Melasma. D. Spider angioma.

An increase in estrogen increases vascularity throughout the body in pregnancy. Increased vascularity of the middle ear may cause a feeling of fullness or earaches. Increased blood flow (hyperemia) to the sinuses can cause rhinitis and epistaxis. The sense of smell is heightened in pregnancy. Edema of the vocal cords may cause hoarseness or deepening of the voice. Hyperemia of the throat can lead to an increase in snoring. In the mouth, small blood vessels and connective tissue increase. Gingivitis or inflammation of the gums occurs in many women. This leads to bleeding and discomfort with brushing and eating. Occasionally a hyperplastic overgrowth forms a mass on the gums called epulis, which bleeds easily and recedes after birth.

Gastrointestinal System Changes

Nausea and vomiting are common beginning at 4 to 6 weeks and usually resolve by 12 weeks of gestation. The exact cause is unknown, although hormonal and psychologic factors have been implicated. Other gastrointestinal changes occur during the second and third trimesters. *Ptyalism*, an increase in saliva production, may occasionally occur with nausea and vomiting. The pregnant woman may also report **pica**, an abnormal craving for and ingestion of nonnutritive substances such as starch, dirt, or ice. Mechanical pressure from the growing uterus contributes to displacement of the small intestine and reduces motility. The increased secretion of progesterone further reduces motility because of decreased gastric tone and increased smooth muscle relaxation; thus, the emptying time of the stomach and bowel is prolonged, and constipation and increased flatulence are common. Progesterone's relaxing effect on smooth muscle also accounts for the prolonged emptying time of the gallbladder, and gallstone formation may result. *Pyrosis*, or heartburn, the regurgitation of the acidic contents of the stomach into the esophagus, is related to the enlarging uterus displacing the stomach upward and to the relaxation of the esophageal sphincter. Hemorrhoids are another common finding in the third trimester, resulting from the increasing size of the uterus creating pressure on the pelvic veins. If the mother is constipated, the pressure on the venous structures from straining to move the bowels can also lead to hemorrhoids.

Nutritional demands of the pregnancy and fetus increase the maternal requirements. Each day, the mother requires an increased intake of 300 calories and 15 g or more of protein. Most nutrient requirements increase from 20% to 100%. The recommended weight gain for women of average weight is 25 to 35 lb, 28 to 40 lb if underweight, 15 to 25 lb if overweight, and 11 to 20 lb if obese.

Urinary System Changes

The growing uterus causes displacement of the ureters and kidneys, especially on the right side. A slower flow of urine through the ureters causes physiologic **hydronephrosis** and **hydroureter**. Estrogen causes increased bladder vascularity, predisposing the mucosa to bleed more easily. Urinary frequency occurs in the first trimester as the uterus grows and puts pressure on the bladder. Relief from frequency occurs after the uterus moves out of the pelvis, only to return in the third trimester when the enlarged uterus again presses on the bladder. In the postpartum period, edema and hyperemia of the bladder mucosa cause decreased sensation and contribute to overdistention of the bladder. Incomplete emptying of the bladder often accompanies this condition, increasing the patient's susceptibility to urinary tract infection (UTI).

The functional changes in the urinary system include the following:

- Increased renal blood flow by 35% to 60%
- Increased glomerular filtration rate by as much as 50% above prepregnancy levels
- Decreased reabsorption of filtered glucose in the renal tubules, contributing to glycosuria
- Increased tubular reabsorption of sodium, promoting necessary retention of fluid
- **Glycosuria** (glucose in urine) resulting from impaired tubular reabsorption of glucose in normal pregnancy
- Decreased bladder tone because of the effects of progesterone on smooth muscle, and increased capacity
- Dilation of ureters, leading to increased risk of urinary tract infection
- Nocturia, increased urination at night, because of dependent edema resolving while recumbent

Musculoskeletal Changes

Anatomic changes in the musculoskeletal system result from the influence of hormones, growth of the fetus, and maternal weight gain. Round ligaments, which attach to the uterus just under the fallopian tubes and insert in the groin, may cause sharp, shooting lower abdominal and groin pain in early pregnancy as the uterus enlarges. As pregnancy advances, the growing uterus tilts the pelvis forward, increasing the lumbosacral curve and creating a gradual lordosis (exaggeration of the lumbar spinal curve). The woman's center of gravity shifts forward, and she shifts her weight farther back on her lower extremities (see Figure 25.9 ■). This shift strains the lower spine, causing stretching of the broad ligament attaching the uterus to the sacrum, which may cause back pain (see Figure 25.10 ■). The enlarging breasts pull the shoulders forward, and the patient may assume a stoop-shouldered stance. The pelvic joints and ligaments are relaxed by progesterone and relaxin. The rectus abdominis muscles that run vertically down the midline of the abdomen may separate during the third trimester. This is called **diastasis recti abdominis** and may allow the abdominal contents to protrude (see Figure 25.11 ■).

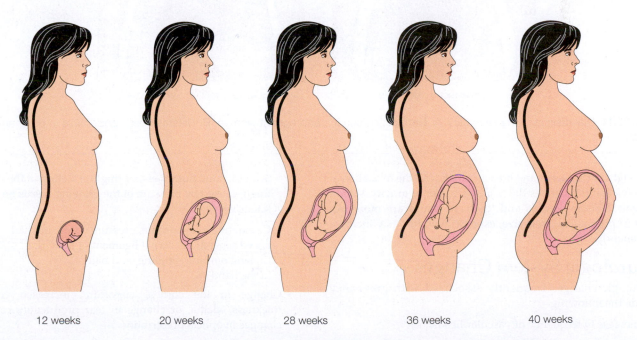

| 12 weeks | 20 weeks | 28 weeks | 36 weeks | 40 weeks |

Figure 25.9 Postural changes with pregnancy, demonstrating lordosis of the spine as pregnancy progresses.

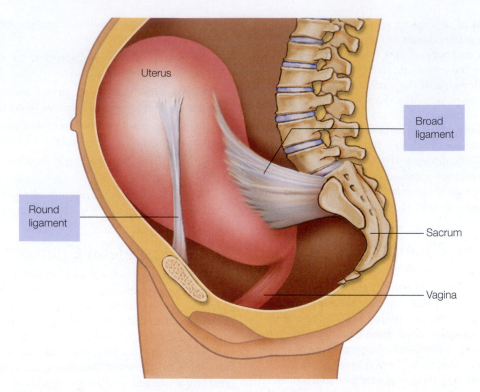

Figure 25.10 Round and broad ligaments.

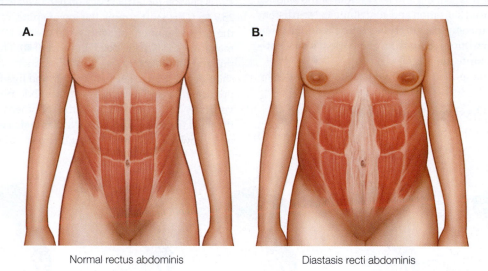

Normal rectus abdominis

Diastasis recti abdominis

Figure 25.11 Diastasis recti in pregnancy. A. Normal position in nonpregnant woman. B. Diastasis recti abdominis in pregnant woman.

The weight of the uterus and breasts, along with the relaxation of the pelvic joints, changes the patient's center of gravity, stance, and gait. Muscle cramps and ligament injury are more frequent in pregnancy. Shoe size, especially width, may increase permanently.

Neurologic System Changes

Neurologic changes frequently associated with pregnancy include the following:

- Increase in frequency of vascular headaches
- Entrapment neuropathies because of mechanical pressures in the peripheral nervous system such as

  ○ Sciatica, pain, numbness, or tingling feeling in the thigh, caused by pressure of the growing uterus on the sciatic nerve
  ○ Carpal tunnel syndrome, pressure on the median nerve beneath the carpal ligament of the wrist, causing burning, tingling, and pain in the hand

- Change in the corneal curvature, increased corneal thickness/edema, or change in tear production, causing changes in optical prescription
- Increased total sleep time and insomnia in first and third trimesters

- Leg cramps, which may be caused by inadequate intake of calcium
- Dizziness and light-headedness, which may be associated with supine hypotension syndrome and vasomotor instability

Endocrine System Changes

Changes in the endocrine system facilitate the metabolic functions that maintain maternal and fetal health throughout the pregnancy. Human chorionic gonadotropin (hCG), the hormone that is detected by pregnancy tests, is secreted by tissue surrounding the embryo soon after implantation. It serves as a messenger to the corpus luteum to maintain progesterone and estrogen production until the placenta starts to produce these hormones at approximately 5 weeks. It also may be involved in the suppression of maternal immunologic rejection of the fetal tissue.

The fetus and placenta become additional sites for synthesis and metabolism of hormones. The pituitary, thyroid, parathyroid, and adrenal glands enlarge because of estrogen stimulation and increased vascularity. Increases in the production of thyroid hormones, particularly T_3 and T_4, increase the basal metabolic rate (BMR), cardiac output, vasodilation, heart rate, and heat intolerance. The BMR may increase by eightfold.

Changes also occur in the metabolism of protein, glucose, and fats because of the increasing production of human placental lactogen (hPL) by the placenta. Throughout pregnancy, protein is metabolized more efficiently to meet fetal needs. In the second trimester, insulin production increases in response to the rising glucose levels and falls to nonpregnant levels at the end of pregnancy. In addition, the mother's body tissues develop a decreased sensitivity to insulin, sometimes referred to as the diabetogenic state of pregnancy. This ensures an adequate supply of glucose, which the fetus requires in large amounts. A disruption in this delicate homeostatic balance results in gestational diabetes mellitus (GDM). A form of glucose sparing, accelerated starvation, causes the metabolism of fats stored in pregnancy, which makes more glucose available to the fetus but puts pregnant women at greater risk of ketosis; in addition, ketones are harmful to the fetal brain. Pregnant women are also at increased risk of lipolysis during pregnancy secondary to hypoglycemia or prolonged fasting.

After birth, *oxytocin*, secreted by the posterior pituitary, stimulates uterine contractions and causes milk ejection in the mammary glands. Prolactin, secreted by the anterior pituitary, increases production of breast milk after the birth.

Special Considerations

Although pregnancy is considered a healthy state, the mother requires extra care to ensure a healthy pregnancy for both the mother and the infant. Factors such as previous pregnancies and miscarriages, presence of sexually transmitted infections, chronic maternal conditions, and maternal nutrition all contribute to potential complications in pregnancy. In addition, sexually active women who do not want to be pregnant are a growing concern and may require additional education and counseling to help prevent unwanted pregnancies and help the mother adapt emotionally to the realities of pregnancy and childbirth.

Developmental Considerations

Although traditionally most women who are pregnant are between the ages of 20 and 34, a significant number of younger adolescents (ages 19 and under) and women of advanced maternal age (considered to be ages 35 and above) become pregnant.

Adolescent Females Adolescent pregnancies have declined over the past several decades. In 2016, close to 210,000 babies were born to young women ages 15 to 19 (Hamilton, Martin, Osterman, Driscoll, & Rossen, 2017). It is important to teach adolescents about abstinence, safe sex, and contraception. Once the adolescent has become pregnant, nursing care must include substantial emotional counseling and support in addition to the typical nursing responsibilities. Options for care and support of the infant must be discussed, including who will care for the infant while the mother is in school, who will provide financial support for the infant's needs, the potential role of the baby's father in providing support, and the possibility of giving up the baby for adoption.

Older Women Because many women are getting married later or choosing to wait to have children, pregnancies in older women have become more common. Although many women over age 35 give birth to healthy babies, complications are more common in pregnant women of this age group. Women over age 35 may take longer to become pregnant, and the use of in vitro fertilization increases the chance of having a multiple pregnancy. Women over age 35 are more likely to develop complications such as gestational diabetes and high blood pressure. These conditions can lead to fetal complications such as being large for gestational age, placental problems, and infant death because of preeclampsia. Women over age 35 may also be at risk for giving birth to a low-birth-weight baby or giving birth prematurely. They are also more likely than younger women to need a cesarean section (C-section), and the risk of pregnancy loss is higher. Additionally, older women are at higher risk of giving birth to an infant with chromosomal abnormalities such as trisomy 21, which causes Down syndrome (National Down Syndrome Society, 2018). Therefore, nursing care of older women should include discussions about potential complications associated with age, options for genetic testing, and the importance of testing for gestational diabetes and high blood pressure.

The Postpartum Woman

The critical role of the nurse in assisting patients through the maternity cycle continues after the birth with postpartum assessment.

Anatomy and Physiology Review During the postpartum period, the reproductive organs return to the nonpregnant state through the process of involution. Immediately after the birth of the placenta, the uterine fundus is located midway between the symphysis pubis and the umbilicus. The fundus rises to the umbilicus by 12 hours later, and it decreases approximately 1 cm or fingerbreadth per day until it is nonpalpable externally by 10 days. The contracted uterus is firm, preventing postpartum hemorrhage through ligation of the uterine arteries by the contraction. The uterus is longer and wider in mothers who have a C-section and shorter in mothers who breastfeed.

The uterine lining or endometrium returns to the nonpregnant state through the process of a postpartum vaginal discharge called lochia. The initial *lochia rubra* contains blood from the placental site, amniotic membrane, cells from the decidua basalis, vernix and lanugo from the infant's skin, and meconium. It is dark red, has a fleshy odor, and lasts anywhere from 2 days to 18 days. Next, the discharge becomes pinkish and is called *lochia serosa*. It is composed of blood, placental site exudates, erythrocytes, leukocytes, cervical mucus, microorganisms, and decidua and lasts approximately a week. Finally, the discharge becomes whitish-yellow, *lochia alba*, and is composed of leukocytes, mucus, bacteria, epithelial cells, and decidua. Most women will have vaginal discharge from 10 days to 5 or 6 weeks.

The cervix closes over the next 2 weeks, and the vagina regains its folds or rugae. Decreased lubrication and lacerations or surgical incisions to the perineum cause discomfort. Gastric motility slows during labor and resumes afterward. Bowel movements usually restart after 2 to 3 days postpartum. Hemorrhoids may have occurred during pregnancy because of increased pelvic pressure or pushing during childbirth. The urethra may be bruised, swollen, or damaged by childbirth or episiotomy.

The hormones estrogen and progesterone, secreted by the placenta, decrease rapidly after birth. Prolactin, which controls milk production, increases after birth, causing milk production to occur within 2 to 3 days after birth. Oxytocin acts on the smooth muscle of the uterus, causing contractions needed for uterine involution. Oxytocin also stimulates the muscle cells surrounding the breast alveoli, causing them to eject milk into the ducts during breastfeeding. In non-breastfeeding mothers, menses return at 6 to 10 weeks postpartum. In lactating mothers, menses usually do not return for 12 or more weeks; with exclusive breastfeeding and introduction of solid foods after 6 months, amenorrhea may last a year or more. In lactating mothers, 80% of first menses are preceded by anovulatory cycles because of the action of prolactin. These hormonal swings, combined with role changes and exhaustion, contribute to emotional fragility, expressed as "baby blues."

After birth, breasts become fuller and larger when breast milk production occurs as a part of lactation (Smith, 2016). Fullness can turn into engorgement in some women resulting in increased breast size and tender, hard breasts. The non-breastfeeding mother may experience breast engorgement when the transitional milk starts to be produced by postpartum days 2 to 4 and is not emptied by a suckling baby. The breastfeeding mother who puts the baby to breast soon after birth breastfeeds frequently as demanded by their infants typically does not experience breast engorgement. Engorgement should be relieved to avoid further engorgement or the potential for plugged ducts and mastitis, an infection of the breast tissue. Applying cold compresses, wearing a supportive bra, nursing frequently (if breastfeeding), and expressing or pumping of milk can be used to relieve engorgement.

In the circulatory system, it may take up to 6 weeks for slowed blood velocity and relaxed veins to return to the nonpregnant state, so a risk of thromboembolism remains during the postpartum period. In the renal system, diuresis occurs on days 2 to 5, and decreased bladder tone and urinary retention can be worsened by birth trauma.

The BUBBLESHE Head-to-Toe Postpartum Assessment

With all the physiologic changes occurring in the postpartum period, a thorough postpartum assessment plays an important role in healthcare. The mnemonic BUBBLESHE can be used to remember the steps in assessing a postpartum patient.

B Breast

U Uterus

B Bowel

B Bladder

L Lochia

E Episiotomy/perineum

S Support system

H Homans sign and extremities

E Emotional state

In preparation for the postpartum assessment, the nurse gathers the following supplies: lab coat, stethoscope, black ink pen, and penlight. Before entering the room, it is important to review the data needed to fill out the assessment flow sheet (e.g., data on pain, urinary tract infection [UTI] symptoms, voiding, stooling, flatus, bleeding, support system, bonding, etc.) as well as the physical assessment. Establishing a good rapport with the patient is important, along with the physical assessment. The nurse should project caring and confidence and use eye contact. Throughout all aspects of the assessment, the nurse must be sure to maintain the patient's privacy and dignity.

Assess the vital signs, and auscultate the lungs, the heart, and the abdomen. Inspect the IV/saline lock site. Examine the patient's breasts, palpate for costovertebral angle tenderness, and palpate the fundus to determine the height and firmness. Assess the surgical incision for the woman who gave birth by C-section.

Inspect the lower extremities for vascular changes and assess for signs and symptoms of deep vein thrombosis and edema. Place the patient in a lateral position to inspect the perineum for an episiotomy and the rectum for any tears. The acronym REEDA (redness, ecchymosis, edema, discharge, and approximation) is useful for assessing wound healing or the presence of inflammation or infection.

Psychosocial Considerations

A woman's adaptation to pregnancy will depend heavily on her development within a social environment. For many women, the support of a boyfriend, husband, partner, or other family member is essential to their ability to cope with the physical and emotional changes they are experiencing. This support system is especially important for women who undergo postpartum depression. The socioeconomic status of the pregnant woman also contributes to her health during pregnancy, because mothers without access to regular healthcare during pregnancy will not have adequate care if complications occur before, during, or after birth.

Cultural and Environmental Considerations

At the time of pregnancy and birth, women in all stages of acculturation to the mainstream culture will hear the call of their roots. Culturally competent nurses will know specifics about individual cultural groups so as not to stereotype patients but to gain a perspective on what issues might pertain to the individual. Beliefs about pregnancy, childbirth, the postpartum period, and care of the newborn may vary among different groups of individuals from various cultures, races, and ethnicities. Sources of diversity within groups include timing of immigration, urban or rural origin, socioeconomic status, educational level, religion, strength of ethnic identity, family style, and personal characteristics.

Subjective Data—Health History

The role of the nurse in assessment of the pregnant woman includes collecting subjective data from the focused interview.

Focused Interview

At the first prenatal visit, a very thorough interview is conducted. Important information that may dramatically affect the health of the fetus and mother can be obtained; the quality of the relationship with the patient for the entire pregnancy is begun. The environment for the interview should be comfortable, quiet, private, and relaxing.

For the purposes of identification, statistics, billing, and record keeping, collect the demographic information listed in Box 25.1 for each pregnant patient. For discussion of cultural considerations related to the patient interview, see Chapter 3. ∞

Box 25.1 Demographic Information

- Complete name and nickname (knowing a nickname helps during stressful situations such as labor)
- Address
- Date of birth (screens for age-related complications)
- Race or ethnicity (screens for race/ethnicity-related genetic disorders)
- Occupation, hours worked per week, activities at work (screens for occupational hazards to the mother and fetus)
- Marital or relationship status (patient's support system)
- Baby's father's name (patient's support system); partner's name, if that is a different person (patient's support system)
- Emergency contact and phone number
- People residing in same residence as patient (patient's support system)
- Religion (relates to maternity care, such as attitudes toward blood products)
- Number of years of school completed (assists in the development of the teaching plan)

Focused Interview Questions	Rationales and Evidence

The following sections provide sample questions for each of the categories identified above. A rationale and evidence for each of the questions is provided. The list of questions is not comprehensive but represents the type of questions required in a comprehensive prenatal focused interview.

Questions Related to Confirmation of Pregnancy

Before the provision of a prenatal interview and physical assessment, it must be ensured that the patient is indeed pregnant. Pregnancy can be determined through urine and serum pregnancy tests as well as signs and symptoms of pregnancy.

Urine pregnancy tests look for the beta subunit of hCG and can be accurate 7 days after implantation, or they can indicate pregnancy before a missed menstrual period. These tests produce results in 1 to 5 minutes and are 99% accurate. Serum pregnancy tests may indicate pregnancy as soon as 7 to 9 days after ovulation, or just after implantation. This test can be qualitative, with a value of positive or negative, or quantitative, with a level of hCG reported. Serum progesterone can also be obtained if necessary; nonviable pregnancies have lower levels than normal pregnancies.

Presumptive signs of pregnancy are symptoms that the patient reports which may have multiple causes other than pregnancy. These presumptive signs include amenorrhea, breast tenderness, nausea and vomiting, frequent urination, quickening, or the patient's perception of fetal movement, skin changes, and fatigue. Probable signs are elicited by the nurse and have few causes other than pregnancy. Probable signs include positive pregnancy test, abdominal enlargement, Piskacek's sign, Hegar's sign, Goodell's sign, Chadwick's sign, and Braxton-Hicks contractions. Positive signs of pregnancy have no possible explanation other than pregnancy. These include hearing the fetal heart with Doppler, fetoscope, or ultrasound; fetal movements verified by the examiner; and visualization of the fetus via ultrasound or radiology.

Questions Related to Menstrual History

1. **When was the date of your last menstrual period?**

▶ The estimated date of birth (EDB), also known as the estimated date of delivery (EDD), estimated date of confinement (EDC), or due date, is usually calculated by using the first day of the last menstrual period (LMP), which may also be useful in estimating gestational age (American Pregnancy Association [APA], 2018b).

Focused Interview Questions	Rationales and Evidence
2. Do you know the date you ovulated?	▶ This can help determine the due date.
3. Do you know the date you conceived?	▶ This also can assist in dating the pregnancy.
4. Were you using any methods of contraception at the time you conceived?	▶ Although oral contraceptive pills have not shown any adverse effects on pregnancy, their use does affect the timing of ovulation. An intrauterine device (IUD) in place at the time of conception can cause complications in the pregnancy (Magee Women's Hospital, 2018).
5. Describe your usual menstrual cycle.	▶ The typical menstrual cycle is 28 days in length. Prolonged, shortened, or irregular menstrual cycles affect the EDB. If the LMP was not normal for the patient, it may have been implantation bleeding or a menstrual dysfunction. Some prenatal charts ask for last *normal* menstrual period (LNMP) to assist in dating the pregnancy.
6. Have you had any cramping, bleeding, or spotting since your LMP?	▶ Cramping, bleeding, or spotting may indicate a problem with the pregnancy and could potentially lead to miscarriage (American Pregnancy Association [APA], 2018a).
7. How old were you when you first menstruated?	▶ The number of years since **menarche**, or age of the first menstrual period, helps determine physical maturity of the patient.

Calculating Estimated Date of Birth and Gestational Weeks

A pregnancy lasts approximately 266 days from conception, or 280 days from the LMP, based on a 28-day cycle. **Nägele's rule** can be used to compute the EDB based on the LMP (Box 25.2). To use this approximate guide to determine the due date, 7 days are added to the day of the month of the first day of the LMP, 3 is subtracted from the number of the month (12 is added to the month number if the LMP occurs in January, February, or March), and the year of the due date is the year of the LMP, plus 1 year if January 1 is passed during the pregnancy.

A gestational wheel is a two-layer round computational device, usually made of laminated paper, that also can be used to compute the EDB and weeks of gestation. Each day of the month in the year has a line on the outer wheel, and each day of the week of the pregnancy has a line on the inner wheel. Zero weeks and days indicate the LMP, and exactly 40 weeks indicates the EDB on the inner wheel. If the zero or LMP line on the inner wheel is aligned with the date of the LMP on the outer wheel, the EDB can be found by determining which date lines up with exactly 40 weeks. If the LMP or EDB is correctly lined up with its date on the outer wheel, the current date on the outer wheel will line up with the gestational age (e.g., 36 weeks and 4 days, often recorded as 36.4 or 36 4/7, based on a 7-day week).

The third way that the EDB can be determined is through the use of ultrasound (Doppler, or sonograms) in the first half of pregnancy. The EDB should be shared as soon as it is determined with the patient, along with its degree of certainty. The fact that a due date actually is the middle day of a month straddling the due date by 2 weeks on each side should be emphasized (±2 weeks of the date determined).

Box 25.2 Using Nägele's Rule to Compute an Estimated Date of Birth (EDB)

EXAMPLE: LMP = January 29, 2018
Rule = first day of LMP + 7, number of month − 3 (year of LMP + 1 if January 1 is passed during pregnancy)

Jan 29

30	Day 1	Month Dec = 12th month
31	2	Jan = 13 (if LMP is in January, February, or March, add 12 to month to prevent negative number)
Feb 1	3	Feb = 14
2	4	14 − 3 = 11 = November
3	5	
4	6	
5	7	

Due date = November 5, 2018

Focused Interview Questions	Rationales and Evidence

Questions Related to Current Obstetric and Gynecologic History

1. Have you experienced any discomfort or unusual occurrences since your LMP?

▶ The patient's response allows the nurse to evaluate whether the symptoms reported are expected or if they suggest development of a complication. The patient will most likely report subjective signs of pregnancy, such as absence of menstrual periods, nausea, vomiting, breast tenderness, fatigue, abdominal enlargement, or urinary frequency. Patient teaching and other nursing interventions can also be identified.

Questions Related to Reaction to Pregnancy

1. Was this pregnancy planned?

▶ Pregnancy usually causes ambivalent feelings whether it was planned or not (Patel, Laz, & Beronson, 2015; Yoo, Guzzo, & Hayford, 2014). If the pregnancy was unplanned, the nurse needs to assess the mother's desire to maintain the pregnancy and explain available options.

2. How do you feel about this pregnancy? How do your family and partner (if applicable) feel about the pregnancy?

▶ This discussion can strengthen the relationship between the nurse and the patient and provide important cues to the home environment of the patient.

Questions Related to Past Obstetric History

1. Have you been pregnant before? If so, how many times?

▶ Certain risk factors can be present for women, depending on number of prior pregnancies beyond 20 weeks gestation. Teaching needs are also affected by the patient's previous experiences.

2. Have you had any spontaneous or induced abortions?
   • If so, how far along in weeks were you?
   • Did you have any follow-up such as a D&C (dilation and curettage procedure)?

▶ Approximately 10% to 25% of pregnancies end in miscarriage (American Pregnancy Association [APA], 2017c), and 1% of pregnancies end in stillbirth (Centers for Disease Control and Prevention [CDC], 2017). Although many women do not experience a recurrent miscarriage, about 1% will have two or more (Mayo Clinic Staff, 2016). There is also some risk of recurrent stillbirth (Lamont, Jones, & Bhattacharya, 2015; Malcova et al., 2018). It is important to know if testing has been conducted to determine causes of pregnancy loss and the results. Surgical procedures such as D&C may cause trauma to the cervix and potentially interfere with cervical dilation and effacement during labor (Stovall, 2017).

3. Describe any previous pregnancies, including the length of the pregnancy, the length of labor, problems during pregnancy, medications taken during pregnancy, prenatal care received, type of birth, and your perception of the experience.

▶ Discussion of the patient's previous pregnancies helps the nurse anticipate needs and complications of the current pregnancy.

4. Describe your birth experience, including labor or childbirth complications, the infant's condition at birth, the infant's weight, and whether the infant required additional treatment or special care after birth.

▶ Reviewing the patient's previous birth experience(s) helps to anticipate needs and complications of the current pregnancy and to assess the patient's current knowledge base and the success with which the patient integrated the previous birth experience into her life experiences. An example of a previous complication that would impact the current pregnancy is group B *Streptococcus* (GBS) colonization. If a patient has a history of GBS colonization of the vagina in a previous pregnancy, her baby has a risk for early- and late-onset infection related to serious morbidity and mortality, so she will need to be treated in labor with antibiotics (Morgan & Cooper, 2018).

5. Do you attend or plan to attend prenatal education classes?

▶ Assessment of prenatal education provides information on the patient's current knowledge base and attitude toward education for self-care.

6. What are your expectations for this pregnancy?

▶ Identification of the patient's desires helps the nurse provide guidance in formulating the birth plan for the present pregnancy.

Questions Related to Past Gynecologic History

1. When was your most recent Pap smear, and what was the result?

▶ Abnormal Pap smears must be followed up during pregnancy as at any time.

2. At what age did you become sexually active?

▶ This influences risk for certain conditions.

Focused Interview Questions	Rationales and Evidence
3. What is your current number of sexual partners?	▶ This addresses risk for sexually transmitted infections.
4. How would you describe your sexual orientation: heterosexual, bisexual, lesbian, or other orientation?	▶ This addresses risk for sexually transmitted infections.
5. What types of safer sex methods do you use, and how often do you use them?	▶ This determines how much teaching in this area is required.
6. What methods of birth control have you used in the past? How satisfied were you with each method?	▶ This will influence teaching on this topic later in the pregnancy.
7. Have you ever had a sexually transmitted infection (STI)? • What was the treatment? • Were your partners treated and notified?	▶ Untreated STIs can cause complications in pregnancy (WebMD, 2017b).
8. Were you exposed to diethylstilbestrol (DES) while your mother was pregnant with you?	▶ Women with exposure to DES, given from the 1940s to 1970s to prevent miscarriage, may have uterine anomalies and increase risk for certain cancers (e.g., breast cancer, cervical cancer) (Centers for Disease Control and Prevention [CDC], n.d.).
9. Have you had any problems with or surgeries on your breasts, vagina, fallopian tubes, ovaries, or urinary tract?	▶ Problems in the genitourinary system may impact pregnancy. Fibroids will affect the measurement of fundal height during pregnancy (Tobah, 2017). Some types of vaginitis, particularly bacterial vaginosis, can cause preterm labor (March of Dimes, 2018). ▶ Surgery on the breasts may impact the ability to breastfeed.
10. Have you ever been a victim of sexual assault? Did you receive any care afterward?	▶ It is important to understand that this is a sensitive topic and should be approached in a compassionate, supportive manner by healthcare providers. Discussing a sexual assault experience may be traumatic for the patient and trigger negative feelings (Sachs & Chapman, 2017). Pregnancy resulting from rape can be very traumatic and can influence a patient's psychologic adaptation to pregnancy (Coleman, 2015; Cybulska, 2013).
11. Do you have a history of infertility?	▶ Many causes of previous infertility can impact the current pregnancy. For example, pelvic inflammatory disease increases a patient's risk of an ectopic pregnancy (Mayo Clinic, 2018b).

Questions Related to Past Medical/Surgical History and Family History

1. Have you or any members of your family or your partner's family had any of the following conditions:	▶ The nurse needs to assess the family medical history to identify and investigate risk factors thoroughly. ▶ Preexisting maternal conditions may increase maternal and fetal risk. ▶ Previous corrective surgery may impact the course and/or outcome of the pregnancy.
• Hypertension	▶ Hypertension during pregnancy predisposes women to many risk factors, including diminished placental blood flow, placental abruption, intrauterine growth restriction (IUGR), injury to organs, premature birth, and future cardiovascular disease (Mayo Clinic Staff, 2018). Family history of hypertension poses a significant risk for preeclampsia in pregnant women (Endeshaw et al., 2016).
• Heart disease/congenital heart disease	▶ More women with congenital heart disease are surviving into childbearing age, thus adding cardiac risk to their pregnancy (Warnes & Krasuski, n.d.).
• Asthma	▶ Hormone changes can have an effect on the lungs of pregnant women. In some cases, those with asthma may find their symptoms improve, although others have a more difficult time controlling their asthma (WebMD, 2017a). The nurse should ask if asthma is well controlled and how stable medication levels have been and should note which medications are currently being used. If asthma symptoms are not controlled, it can affect the amount of oxygen that can be transported to the fetus.

Focused Interview Questions	Rationales and Evidence
• Kidney or gallbladder problems	▶ Previous occurrences of urinary tract infection may increase risk for asymptomatic bacteriuria, the presence of bacteria in the urine without the usual cystitis symptoms of urinary frequency, burning upon urination, and flank pain. Asymptomatic bacteriuria may lead to pyelonephritis (kidney infection) (Hooton & Gupta, 2017). UTIs in pregnancy are associated with preterm labor and low birth weight (Johnson & Kim, 2017). Gallbladder problems may be exacerbated in pregnancy.
• Diabetes mellitus	▶ Pregestational diabetes (diabetes that was present before the pregnancy) can cause problems for the mother and her fetus (Stanford Children's Health, 2018). Maternal complications, especially in those with poorly controlled blood glucose levels, may include more frequent insulin injections, ketoacidosis, and the potential for blood vessel damage and changes to the retina. Fetal complications can include certain birth defects, delayed lung maturation, larger-size baby (which can create problems during childbirth), and hypoglycemia after birth.
• Blood or bleeding disorders	▶ Anemia can increase risk for preterm birth and infection in the postpartum period (Friel, 2017). Pregnant women with sickle cell disease and thalassemia are at risk for poor maternal and fetal outcome. Those with sickle cell disease may experience an increase in maternal and perinatal mortality. Some women may have a thrombophilia disorder, which encompasses a variety of blood clotting disorders and can cause problems during pregnancy such as IUGR, placental insufficiency, preeclampsia, premature birth, miscarriage, and still birth (March of Dimes, 2014).
• Hepatitis	▶ The hepatitis virus can be transmitted to the fetus (American College of Obstetricians and Gynecologists [ACOG], 2013). In many cases, a pregnant woman may not know she has contracted the virus. All pregnant women are tested for hepatitis B. Babies born to mothers infected with hepatitis B should have the first dose of the hepatitis B immunization along with hepatitis B immunoglobulin (HBIG) administered within a few hours of birth. Women with hepatitis C face less risk of passing on the virus to their babies; however, it is recommended that the infant be tested at 18 months of age. Other forms of hepatitis can cause problems with the mother and fetus, as well.
• Cancer	▶ A diagnosis of cancer before or while pregnant lends to unique challenges in the care of the pregnant woman (American Society of Clinical Oncology, 2018). Considerations for continuation or beginning treatment of cancer during pregnancy must be taken. Breast cancer is the most commonly diagnosed cancer during pregnancy. Another point to consider is that if cancer of the cervix was treated with cone biopsy, the patient is at risk for preterm labor (Castanon et al., 2014).
• Infectious diseases such as HIV	▶ Transmission of HIV to the newborn can be dramatically reduced by treatment before and after childbirth (U.S. Department of Health and Human Services, 2017).
• Tuberculosis (TB)	▶ TB treatment in pregnancy decreases neonatal mortality and morbidity (Centers for Disease Control and Prevention [CDC], 2014b).
• Chickenpox	▶ If the patient does not report a history of varicella (chickenpox) and is not immune by blood test, she is susceptible to infection during pregnancy. Chickenpox, or varicella, can cause abnormalities in the fetus if contracted between 8 and 20 weeks in pregnancy (Tobah, 2015). Varicella-zoster immune globulin can be given to pregnant women within 10 days of exposure to chickenpox to reduce the severity of symptoms, although it is unclear if this treatment helps the developing fetus.
• Allergies	▶ Allergies are identified in the prenatal period in case medications are recommended during the perinatal period. The nurse should note the type of reaction.

Focused Interview Questions	Rationales and Evidence

2. What medications have you taken since your LMP?

▶ This will help identify any teratogenic exposures as well as medications for illnesses and symptoms. Drugs in pregnancy are rated in risk categories A, B, C, D, and X (Box 25.3).

Box 25.3 Drugs in Pregnancy: Risk Categories

A: Adequate and well-controlled studies in pregnant women have not shown an increased risk of fetal abnormalities. Example drugs: folic acid, levothyroxine.

B: Animal studies have revealed no evidence of harm to the fetus; however, there are no adequate and well-controlled studies in pregnant women, or animal studies have shown an adverse effect, but adequate and well-controlled studies in pregnant women have failed to demonstrate a risk to the fetus. Example drugs: acetaminophen, chlorpheniramine, pseudoephedrine, loperamide, aluminum hydroxide/magnesium hydroxide, amoxicillin, ondansetron, metformin, insulin.

C: Animal studies have shown an adverse effect and there are no adequate and well-controlled studies in pregnant women, or no animal studies have been conducted and there are no adequate and well-controlled studies in pregnant women. Example drugs: guaifenesin, dextromethorphan, calcium carbonate, fluconazole, albuterol, sertraline, fluoxetine.

D: Adequate well-controlled or observational studies in pregnant women have demonstrated a risk to the fetus. However, the benefits of therapy may outweigh the potential risk. Example drugs: aspirin, paroxetine, lithium, phenytoin.

X: Adequate well-controlled or observational studies in animals or pregnant women have demonstrated positive evidence of fetal abnormalities. The use of the product is contraindicated in women who are or who may become pregnant. Example drugs: isotretinoin, thalidomide.

---

3. Have you ever had a blood transfusion?

▶ This will help identify increased risk for abnormal antibody reactions or bloodborne pathogens.

4. What infections and immunizations have you had?

▶ Some infections, including chickenpox and rubella, can cause birth defects (March of Dimes, 2013; Tobah, 2015). Babies born to mothers infected with hepatitis B should have the first dose of the hepatitis B immunization along with hepatitis B immunoglobulin (HBIG) administered within a few hours of birth (ACOG, 2013). Prior immunizations and exposures affect the patient's risk for contracting certain infections during pregnancy.

5. Have you had any surgeries such as:
- Breast reduction/augmentation

▶ Breastfeeding is usually possible following breast reduction or augmentation surgeries (Cleveland Clinic, 2018); however, the amount of milk produced may be lower.

- Back

▶ Thoracic or lumbar spinal surgery that has scarred, distorted, or obliterated the epidural space will not allow the use of an epidural for either analgesia or anesthesia.

- Hip

▶ Hip surgery may impact the ability of the patient to use stirrups in the lithotomy position.

- Bariatric

▶ Bariatric surgery is either restrictive or restrictive/malabsorptive. This can cause nutritional deficiencies (American College of Obstetricians and Gynecologists [ACOG], 2017b). These women will still need to consume about 1,500 calories each day, necessitating dietary counseling. These women also need to be checked regularly for nutrient deficiencies, particularly folic acid, calcium, iron, and vitamin B_{12}. There is a trend for increased risk of small-for-gestational-age infants. Previous bariatric surgery is not an indication for childbirth via cesarean section (Consumer Guide to Bariatric Surgery, 2018).

- Uterine

▶ Women who have undergone uterine surgery for conditions such as fibroids or malformations of the uterus, endometriosis, dilation and curettage (D&C), or prior C-section may experience scarring and adhesions leading to infertility or pregnancy loss (USC Fertility, 2018).

Focused Interview Questions	Rationales and Evidence

- Other prior surgeries

▶ Any previous surgeries should be discussed in regard to the impact they may have on pregnancy and subsequent childbirth.

Questions Related to Body Systems

In addition to the review of systems questions normally asked in each body system when taking an adult history, there are special considerations for the pregnant woman that must be considered related to certain body systems. For each body system, the nurse should discuss benign as well as worrisome changes in pregnancy.

Questions Related to Integumentary System

1. What changes have you noticed in your skin since you became pregnant?

▶ The hormonal changes of pregnancy may cause various benign changes in skin pigmentation, moisture, texture, and vascularity that are entirely normal.

2. Do you use any topical medications for problems with the skin, hair, or nails?

▶ Topical medications that can result in birth defects include Retin-A for acne, antifungal agents, and minoxidil for hair growth.

3. Do you use topical medications for other problems? If so, identify the medications.

▶ Many medications that are absorbed through the skin may reach the baby through the bloodstream. Some of these medications may harm the developing fetus. Among the medications are antibiotics, steroids, and medications for muscle pain.

4. Have your nails changed? If so, what are the changes?

▶ Nail changes in pregnancy include brittleness, formation of grooves, or onycholysis (separation of the nail from the nail bed).

Questions Related to Head, Neck, and Lymphatics

1. Do you have frequent headaches?

▶ Headaches are common during the first trimester, but it is important to rule out other possible complications of pregnancy such as preeclampsia.

2. Have you noticed changes in the skin on your face? If yes, what changes have occurred?

▶ Increasing hormonal changes can result in melasma or chloasma, which are pigmented areas on the face. In addition, the hormonal changes cause increased secretions of oils from the skin's sebaceous glands, which may result in acne.

3. Do you have a history of thyroid disease? If yes, what is the disease and treatment?

▶ Thyroid diseases can result in problems with the developing fetus (National Institute of Diabetes and Digestive and Kidney Diseases [NIDDKD], 2017). Existing thyroid problems require careful monitoring of medications.

Questions Related to Eyes

1. Have you had any changes in your eyesight during your pregnancy?

▶ Visual complaints should be referred to an ophthalmologist.

Questions Related to Ear, Nose, Throat, and Mouth

1. Have you ever experienced a ringing in your ears?

▶ Ringing in the ears during pregnancy may occur with hypertension associated with preeclampsia (a serious condition that can threaten maternal and fetal health).

2. Have you experienced an earache or a feeling of fullness in your ears?

▶ Changes in estrogen produce increased vascularity throughout the systems of the body during pregnancy. The vascularity may cause a feeling of fullness or an aching in the ears.

3. Have you had nosebleeds during your pregnancy? If so, how often?

▶ During pregnancy, increased circulatory blood flow leads to swelling of mucous membranes, including those in the nasal passages. Swollen mucous membranes are more susceptible to bleeding.

Questions Related to Lungs and Thorax

1. Do you experience any shortness of breath or dyspnea?
   - When does it occur?
   - How long have you experienced this?
   - Have you sought a remedy?

▶ The enlarged uterus elevates the diaphragm and can decrease lung expansion, which may result in shortness of breath (Tan & Tan, 2013).

Questions Related to Breasts and Axillae

1. What changes in your breasts have you noticed since your last examination?

▶ The breasts continue to change throughout pregnancy. Some expected changes are increased size, sense of fullness or tingling, prominent veins, darkened areolae, and a more erect nipple. A thick, yellowish discharge (colostrum) may be expressed from the breasts in the final weeks of pregnancy. The patient should be reassured that all these signs are normal.

Focused Interview Questions	Rationales and Evidence

Questions Related to Cardiovascular System

1. Do you have any history of heart disease?

▶ The changes of pregnancy can place the patient with preexisting heart disease at risk.

2. Have you had any problems with high blood pressure during this pregnancy?
   - Do you have a history of high blood pressure?

▶ Hypertension is a symptom of preeclampsia and places the mother and infant at risk (Preeclampsia Foundation, 2016).

3. Have you observed any swelling in your face and hands?
   - Have you experienced headaches or dizziness?v

▶ Swelling can indicate a preeclamptic condition. Headaches and dizziness are associated with hypertension and preeclampsia. Preeclampsia can also be accompanied by visual changes, nausea or vomiting, and/or pain in the abdomen, shoulder, or lower back (Preeclampsia Foundation, 2016).

Questions Related to Peripheral Vascular System

1. Have you had your blood pressure monitored?

▶ Monitoring can reduce risks for pregnancy-induced hypertension.

2. Are you experiencing swelling of the face, hands, wrists, fingers, legs, ankles, or feet?

▶ Edema in the lower extremities is common in pregnancy, especially at the end of the day and into the third trimester.

Questions Related to Abdomen

1. Are you experiencing any nausea or vomiting?

▶ Nausea is common during early pregnancy and may be because of changing hormone levels and changes in carbohydrate metabolism. Fatigue is also a factor. Vomiting is less common. If it occurs more than once a day or for a prolonged period, the patient should be referred to a physician.

2. Are you experiencing any elimination problems, such as constipation?

▶ A number of factors increase the likelihood of constipation during pregnancy. Among these are displacement of the intestines by the growing uterus, bowel sluggishness caused by increased progesterone and steroid metabolism, and the use of oral iron supplements, which are prescribed for many patients during pregnancy.

3. Are you experiencing heartburn or flatulence?

▶ Heartburn (regurgitation of gastric contents into the esophagus) is primarily caused by displacement of the stomach by the enlarging uterus. Flatulence results from decreased gastrointestinal motility, which is common during pregnancy, and from pressure on the large intestine from the growing uterus.

Questions Related to Urinary System

1. Have you noticed any changes in your urinary pattern?

▶ Often, the developing fetus places increasing pressure on the mother's bladder, causing urinary urgency. As a result, the patient voids more often in smaller amounts.

Questions Related to Musculoskeletal System

1. Please describe any back pain you are experiencing.
   - Tell me about the effects of the pain on your daily activities.

▶ Lordosis may occur in the last months of pregnancy along with back pain.

Questions Related to Neurologic System

1. Do you have a history of seizures?
   - Have you had any seizures during this pregnancy or previous pregnancies?
   - If so, how often?

▶ Seizures could indicate neurologic pathology or eclampsia.

2. Are you taking any vitamins or other nutritional supplements?
   - Please describe these.

▶ Prenatal supplements are important to provide for the neurologic health of the growing fetus. For example, vitamin B6 (pyridoxine) is required for nerve myelination, and folic acid has been shown to reduce the incidence of neural tube defects (Centers for Disease Control and Prevention [CDC], 2018).

Questions Related to Genetic Information

In order to obtain information to determine genetic risk factors, the nurse will ask the patient about three generations of her family. This is called a medical family tree or genetic pedigree. These questions refer to her brothers and sisters, her mother and father, her aunts and uncles on both sides, her grandparents and their siblings, all of her children, and all of her cousins on both sides. This information is also needed for the baby's father's family.

Focused Interview Questions	Rationales and Evidence

1. Please tell me the date of birth and, if applicable, death as well as any health problems or diseases for each of these individuals. For those who have died, tell me what the cause was and date of death.

▶ Three generations of medical history are needed to determine recessive as well as dominant genetic diseases.

2. Do you or the baby's father, or anybody in your families, have any of the following conditions?
   - Sickle cell disease or trait
   - Thalassemia
   - Down syndrome
   - Cystic fibrosis
   - Huntington disease
   - Muscular dystrophy
   - Tay-Sachs disease
   - Hemophilia
   - Any other blood or genetic disorders

▶ Sometimes charting the medical family tree will not jog the memory of the patient, but a specific mention of the condition will.

3. What is your ethnic background?

▶ Tay-Sachs occurs more frequently in Ashkenazi Jews, cystic fibrosis trait occurs in 1 in 29 northern European Caucasians, and the sickle cell trait occurs in 1 in 8 African Americans.

Questions Related to Lifestyle and Social Health Practices

1. How much do you smoke per day? Does anyone in your household smoke?

▶ Smoking doubles the risk of a low-birth-weight baby and increases the risk of ectopic pregnancy or placental complications (March of Dimes, 2015). It also increases the infant's risk of sudden infant death syndrome (SIDS), asthma, and autism after birth. Secondhand smoke exposure also may contribute to low birth weight.

2. Since the start of pregnancy, how many alcoholic drinks have you consumed each day?

▶ Any amount of alcohol consumption during pregnancy can cause fetal alcohol syndrome and related disorders composed of physical, neurologic, and behavioral defects in the infant (American Pregnancy Association [APA], 2017b).

3. What recreational drugs have you used since your LMP? This includes marijuana, cocaine, heroin, prescription painkillers, methadone, and so on.

▶ Cocaine and other illicit drugs have been shown to cause placental problems, preterm labor, miscarriage, stillbirth, and multiple fetal defects (March of Dimes, 2016).

4. Have you ever been emotionally or physically abused by your partner or someone important to you?
   - Within the last year, have you been pushed, shoved, slapped, hit, kicked, or otherwise physically hurt by someone?
   - If yes, by whom?
   - Within the last year, have you been forced to have sex?
   - If yes, by whom?
   - Are you afraid of your partner or anyone else?

▶ All pregnant patients should be screened during each trimester for abuse (American College of Obstetricians and Gynecologists (ACOG), 2012). Around 324,000 pregnant women in the United States are abused annually. Abuse can cause miscarriage, fetal trauma, maternal stress, smoking, and drug abuse. Risk factors for abuse in pregnancy include unintended pregnancy, unhappiness with pregnancy, young maternal age, single maternal status, higher parity, late or absent entry to care, and substance abuse. The nurse should notify the physician or midwife of any positive findings and work together to develop a plan of care.

Questions Related to Exercise History and Nutrition

1. What kind of exercise do you currently engage in? How many days per week for how many minutes do you do it?

▶ Exercise is safe and encouraged for most pregnant women (ACOG, 2017b; Centers for Disease Control and Prevention [CDC], 2015). Moderate aerobic activity for 150 minutes each week is recommended. There are some conditions, however, in which exercise is not considered safe such as certain heart and lung diseases, cervical insufficiency, pregnancies with risk for preterm labor, placenta previa, rupture of membranes, preeclampsia, and severe anemia.

▶ Pregnant women should avoid lying on their backs during exercise for long periods of time following the first trimester, and others may be instructed to avoid this type of exercise at all times because of the potential for diminished blood flow that results from the pressure of the growing uterus on the vena cava (APA, 2017a).

Focused Interview Questions	Rationales and Evidence

ALERT! *If a pregnant woman experiences any of the following conditions during exercise, she should stop exercising and call her healthcare provider:*

- ▶ Bleeding from the vagina
- ▶ Difficulty or labored breathing before exercising
- ▶ Dizziness, headache, or chest pain
- ▶ Muscle weakness, calf pain, or swelling

- ▶ Preterm labor symptoms
- ▶ Decreased movement of the fetus
- ▶ Leakage of fluid from the vagina

2. Describe everything you have consumed for the past 24 hours. Include water, vitamins, and supplements.

Table 25.1 Dietary Reference Intakes (DRIs): Estimated Average Requirements of Major Nutrients by Women's Age Groups and in Pregnancy

FEMALE RDA (BY AGE)	14–18	19–30	31–50	51+	PREGNANT
Calcium (mg/d)	1,100	800	800	1,000	800
Protein (g/kg/d)	0.71	0.66	0.66	0.66	0.88
Vitamin E (mg/d)	12	12	12	12	12
Vitamin A (mcg/d)	485	500	500	500	550
Vitamin C (mg/d)	60	60	60	60	70
Thiamin (mg/d)	0.9	0.9	0.9	0.9	1.2
Riboflavin (mg/d)	0.9	0.9	0.9	0.9	1.2
Niacin (mg/d)	11	11	11	11	14
Vitamin B_6 (mg/d)	1.0	1.1	1.1	1.3	1.6
Folate (mcg/d)	330	320	320	320	520
Vitamin B_{12} (mcg/d)	2.0	2.0	2.0	2.0	2.2
Iron (mg/d)	7.9	8.1	8.1	5	22
Zinc (mg/d)	7.3	6.8	6.8	6.8	9.5
Selenium (mcg/d)	45	45	45	45	49

Source: Food and Nutrition Board, Institute of Medicine, National Academies (2011).

▶ Nutritional health plays a primary role in a successful pregnancy. A mother's preconception nutritional status, appropriate weight gain, and adequate nutrition during pregnancy are important contributing factors to the health of a newborn. A comprehensive nutritional history is important when assessing the nutritional health of a pregnant woman. Diet recall and food frequency questionnaires remain important tools to use to assess intake. Assessment of the preconception diet should also be obtained in general detail, as well, because it provides the foundation for nutritional health in early pregnancy and beyond. Table 25.1 outlines daily reference intakes [DRIs] in pregnancy, and Box 25.4 outlines specific data to be assessed when conducting a nutritional history of pregnant and lactating women.

▶ Caffeine is a stimulant found in coffee, tea, chocolate, and many medications. In large quantities it may cause miscarriage or low-birth-weight babies and dehydration for the mother and should be avoided.

▶ Everyone, but especially pregnant women, should practice safe food handling, including hand washing, keeping refrigerator temperature below 5°C (40°F), cleaning the refrigerator regularly, refrigerating and freezing food promptly, and avoiding cross-contamination between cooked and uncooked foods to avoid listeriosis and other foodborne infections (U.S. Department of Agriculture, Food Safety and Inspection Service [FSIS], 2017).

▶ During lactation, the nursing mother requires adequate nutrition to support her own nutritional needs as well as production of sufficient breast milk for her child. In addition to assessing the general nutritional status of the mother, the nurse should assess the number and timing of all feedings; the mother's intake of all fluids, including alcohol and caffeinated beverages; the use of dietary supplements, both prescribed and self-prescribed; the details of any postpregnancy attempts at weight management; and, in the vegan mother, the daily source of vitamin B_{12} because only active intake passes to the child in breast milk.

▶ Some herbal supplements and vitamin supplements can be a problem during pregnancy. As research in herbs in pregnancy is continuing, it is recommended that women check with their healthcare provider before consuming herbal teas and supplements. A partial list of common herbs known to be harmful in pregnancy includes aloe vera, black cohosh, blue cohosh, dong quai, goldenseal, pennyroyal, saw palmetto, yohimbe, passion flower, and Roman chamomile (APA, 2018c). Although most healthcare providers recommend that pregnant patients consume a prenatal vitamin during pregnancy, some vitamin supplements (such as vitamin A) can cause harm if consumed beyond the RDA.

Focused Interview Questions	Rationales and Evidence

Box 25.4 Nutritional History Data for Gestation and Lactation

Assess for Specific Foods and Nutrients
- Folic acid—fortified flour and cereals, orange juice, green leafy vegetables, legumes
- Calcium and vitamin D—dairy, fortified juices, fortified soy products
- Iron—meats, poultry, shellfish, fortified cereals and grains, legumes, dried fruit
- Vitamin B_{12} if vegan—must be synthetic, plant sources not bioavailable
- Vitamin A—dairy, fish, meats
- Fluids, include alcohol and water intake
- Caffeine—coffee, tea, cola and other soda, cocoa, chocolate, over-the-counter (OTC) medications
- Mercury—recommendation is to eat 8 to 12 oz/week of a variety of fish that are lower in mercury, such as salmon, shrimp, pollock, light canned tuna, tilapia, catfish, and cod

Assess for Eating Patterns and Behaviors
- Weight gain with any prior pregnancies
- Restrictive eating, missed meals, dieting attempts
- Cultural beliefs related to food and pregnancy
- Food aversions
- Pica
- Gastrointestinal complaints and any resultant alterations in diet

Assess for Supplement Use
- Prenatal vitamin compliance
- Iron supplement compliance
- Other vitamins—high intake of vitamin A is teratogenic
- Herbs—most untested in pregnant or lactating women
- Remedies for any pregnancy symptoms

ALERT! *Great nutrition is vital to the health of every mother and fetus during pregnancy. The nurse should give the patient a "gold spoon" (plastic, of course) to remind her how valuable every bite is during pregnancy.*

Questions Related to Environmental Exposure

1. **What kind of chemicals are you exposed to in your home and workplace?**

▶ To prevent birth defects and miscarriage, pregnant women should avoid cigarette smoke, lead (in water and paint), carbon monoxide, mercury, pesticides, insect repellents, some oven cleaners, solvents such as alcohol and degreasers, paint, paint thinners, benzene, and formaldehyde. If the pregnant woman must be around these substances, she should minimize her exposure by ensuring good ventilation, wearing protective gear such as a face mask and gloves, and checking with the water or health department about the quality of the drinking water.

2. **Have you been exposed to radiation?**

▶ In general, exposure to radiation from common medical and environmental radiation falling within regulatory limits is not likely to cause harm to the fetus (Centers for Disease Control and Prevention [CDC], 2014a). However, exposure to radiation at levels outside of these limits can cause complications such as fetal growth retardation, reduced mental capacity, or major malformations (e.g., neurologic and motor deficiencies). Potential for miscarriage is also a concern.

Evidence-Based Practice:

Preventing Teenage Pregnancy

Teen pregnancy prevention programs developed by the CDC, Office of Adolescent Health (OAH), and the Office of Population Affairs have produced evidence supporting the effectiveness of preventing teen pregnancies, sexually transmitted infections, or sexual risk behaviors. These programs have been targeted to U.S. communities demonstrating the highest rates of teen pregnancy and birth, with a special focus on African American and Latino or Hispanic adolescents ages 15 to 19 years old (Centers for Disease Control and Prevention [CDC], 2016).

Patient-Centered Interaction

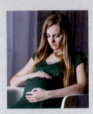

Olu Adams, age 16, presents for a return prenatal visit at 20 weeks gestation. The prenatal record indicates that this is her first pregnancy, she lives with her parents in a nearby apartment building, and she is in 10th grade. Besides her unplanned adolescent pregnancy, the problems identified so far in this pregnancy include a UTI that was treated with antibiotics and a total weight gain of 10 lb; she is 5´7˝ tall and weighed 120 lb at the beginning of the pregnancy.

Source: Katarzyna Bialasiewicz/123RF.

Interview

Nurse: Hi, Ms. Adams. Have a seat and tell me how you have been doing since your last visit.

The nurse leads the patient to a chair in the examination room and pulls up a stool to sit beside the patient. The teenager stares down at her lap.

Ms. Adams: Fine.

Nurse: Have you had any vaginal bleeding, contractions, or pelvic pressure?

The patient shrugs.

Nurse: Any more problems with peeing, like burning, or peeing more frequently than usual?

The patient shakes her head.

Nurse: Is your mom or the baby's father in the waiting room?

Ms. Adams: Nah.

Nurse: Ms. Adams?

Nurse waits for Olu to look up.

Have you felt the baby move yet? It would feel like a little tickle on the middle of your belly.

Ms. Adams: (Face lights up, her voice is louder.) **Yes, I am feeling that! Is it the baby?**

Nurse: Yes, it probably is. Tell me about it.

Ms. Adams: **In the mornings for about the last week I feel something brushing my insides. And I don't feel so sick anymore.**

Nurse: Well, that is certainly good news. Why don't you sit on the exam table and we will listen to the baby's heartbeat and see how much your baby has grown since the last visit?

Ms. Adams: **I hope you can tell me how big the baby is now.**

ALERT! *Research indicates that patients are often not clear on the signs of preterm labor.*
The nurse should discuss the following signs of preterm labor with all patients at every prenatal visit after 20 weeks:

▶ *More than six contractions per hour (This may feel like "the baby balling up," menstrual cramps, backache, or diarrhea.)*
▶ *Leaking fluid, vaginal bleeding, or increased vaginal discharge*
▶ *Pelvic pressure, heaviness, or suprapubic pain*

Analysis

The nurse was appropriate in sitting beside the patient and providing a time away from the examination table for questions. Her initial question about preterm contractions was probably not well understood by a patient of this age and education level. The nurse's question about urinary symptoms was at a more appropriate level, but yes/no questions to teenagers or any uncommunicative patient are not the best choice. The nurse tried to elicit information about the patient's family, but again with a closed question. When the patient became more animated about

quickening, the nurse wisely provided an open-ended question that led to a more productive interchange with the patient. The nurse can now go on to find out what the patient knows about topics that are relevant at this point in pregnancy: symptoms of preterm labor, continuing importance of good nutrition, results of laboratory tests from the previous visit, and fetal development, among other possible topics. During pregnancy, a great deal of teaching is done with the pregnant patient and her family. In order to ensure that all topics are covered, many obstetric practices use a teaching checklist (Table 25.2).

Table 25.2 Pregnancy Teaching Checklist

GESTATIONAL AGE/ TIMING OF VISIT	TEACHING TOPICS	GESTATIONAL AGE/ TIMING OF VISIT	TEACHING TOPICS
Initial prenatal visit	Welcome Types of providers and scope of practice Hours of office/clinic Phone number, after-hours contact number Warning signs in first trimester Schedule of prenatal care and laboratory studies Safe medications in pregnancy Resources: Pregnancy and childbirth classes Nutritional requirements in pregnancy; request 3-day food diary Exercise in pregnancy Discomforts in pregnancy and relief measures Dental care Abuse screen Benefits of breastfeeding Bathing and clothing	Throughout pregnancy	Fetal growth and development Sexuality/partner relationship Traveling while pregnant
		15 to 20 weeks	Second trimester laboratory testing Genetic testing Ultrasound Warning signs in the second trimester Abuse screen
		21 to 34 weeks	Preterm labor signs Preparation for birth Car seats Breastfeeding instructions, if appropriate Home preparation for newborn 28-weeks testing
Second prenatal visit	Explanation of test results Discuss 3-day food diary Psychologic adaptation to pregnancy Body mechanics	35 to 42 weeks	Signs of labor Sibling preparation for birth Abuse screen Breast preparation 36-weeks testing

Objective Data—Physical Assessment

Objective data are obtained from the physical assessment and from secondary sources such as health records, the results of laboratory tests, and radiologic and ultrasound studies. Preparation for the physical assessment includes gathering equipment, positioning, and informing the patient about what will take place during the physical assessment. The room should be warm and private. For prenatal blood tests, a variety of collection tubes and collection equipment will be required and differs for each site.

Anthropometric Measurements

Weight, weight history, and gestational weight-gain pattern and amount are important considerations during pregnancy. Preconception weight, height, and body mass index (BMI) are necessary to determine gestational weight gain goals. The importance of achieving gestational weight gain goals needs to be stressed. Excessive gestational weight gain in some women may result in retained weight after childbirth. In pregnant adolescents, gynecologic age should be determined to assess whether linear growth may still be occurring. **Gynecologic age** is the difference between current age and age at menarche. Young women with a gynecologic age of 3 years or less are considered to still be com-

pleting linear growth and will have competing nutritional needs between their own growth and that of the fetus.

Recent trends in obesity among childbearing women dictated the need to revise weight-gain guidelines for pregnant women. On June 1, 2009, the Institute of Medicine, a division of the National Academy of Sciences, issued new guidelines for weight gain during pregnancy (Institute of Medicine and National Research Council, 2009). These current guidelines are listed in Table 25.3. Weight gain guidelines for other racial and ethnic groups have had insufficient research focus to establish a consensus. For each patient, the nurse should develop individual weight-gain guidelines, with the prevention of excess weight gain an important focus.

During the physical assessment, the nurse can screen for factors for low-weight-gain patterns. Smoking, alcohol consumption, drug use, lack of social support, and depression have all been associated with low weight gain. An adolescent trying to hide a pregnancy may be at risk for low weight gain.

The nurse can also ask questions about the presence of physical symptoms that may be affecting nutritional status. Gastrointestinal discomfort, nausea and vomiting, constipation,

Table 25.3 Gestational Weight Gain Recommendations

BMI (PREPREGNANCY)	TOTAL GAIN FOR A SINGLETON (I.E., ONE BABY) PREGNANCY (LB)	SINGLETON PREGNANCY WEEKLY GAIN FOR SECOND AND THIRD TRIMESTER (LB/WK)	TOTAL GAIN FOR A TWIN PREGNANCY (LB)
Underweight <18.5	28–40	1 (1–1.3)	No recommendation
Normal Weight 18.5–24.9	25–35	1 (0.8–1)	37–54
Overweight 25–29.9	15–25	0.6 (0.5–0.7)	31–50
Obese (includes all classes ≥30)	11–20	0.5 (0.4–0.6)	25–42

Note: Guidelines above are for a singleton pregnancy. Second and third trimester estimates are based on the assumption of a 1.1- to 4.4-lb weight gain in the first trimester.
Source: Institute of Medicine and National Research Council (2009).

and heartburn can occur during pregnancy and alter dietary intake and food tolerance. Follow-up questions should seek information on remedies used to relieve symptoms. Pregnant women with a history of an eating disorder and hyperemesis gravidarum should be screened for current signs of an eating disorder. Box 25.5 outlines physical findings with an eating disorder.

Box 25.5 Clinical Findings Consistent with Eating Disorders

General Eating Disorder Findings
- Body dissatisfaction. Ask: "How do you feel about your weight?" followed by "Have you ever tried to gain or lose weight? Tell me what you did."
- Constipation
- Bloating
- Fatigue

Bulimia/Binge-Purge Behavior
- Bloodshot eyes
- Broken blood vessels on the face
- Swollen parotid glands or "chipmunk cheeks"
- Dental erosion
- Hoarse voice
- Scarring on the dorsal surface of the hand from teeth during purge attempts
- Poor or lacking gag reflex
- Weight fluctuations

Anorexia/Restrictive Eating Behavior
- Cold intolerance
- Lanugo, soft white hair growth on body
- Pedal edema
- Dry skin
- Alopecia
- Bradycardia
- Hypotension
- Amenorrhea in nonpregnant postmenarcheal females
- Loss of strength and muscle tone

Laboratory Measurements

Laboratory assessment of the pregnant woman should routinely include screening for iron deficiency anemia. The increased iron needs during pregnancy put many women at risk for iron deficiency. Hemoglobin and hematocrit decrease until the end of the second trimester because of expansion of blood volume and red cell mass during pregnancy. Pregnancy-specific standards for normal hemoglobin and hematocrit values should be used (Table 25.4).

Assessment for gestational diabetes is performed between weeks 24 and 28. The American College of Obstetricians and Gynecologists (ACOG) supports the recommendations of the National Institute of Diabetes and Digestive and Kidney Diseases (NIDDK) and American Diabetes Association (ADA) for screening of gestational diabetes mellitus (GDM) early in pregnancy if the pregnant woman has a BMI of 25 (or 23 in Asian women) and has at least one of a long list of other factors—such as known impaired glucose metabolism, pregnancy history of GDM, Macrosomia ≥4000 g), or stillbirth—and hypertension

(140/90 mm Hg or being treated for hypertension) (ACOG, 2017a). If the initial screening is negative, the woman should be rescreened between 24 and 28 weeks. A fasting plasma glucose level above 105 mg/dL and a 1-hour glucose greater than 180 mg/dL following ingestion of a 100-g glucose load is considered positive for GDM. Both the nutritional health of the mother and the outcome of the pregnancy can be negatively affected if diet changes are not instituted in women found to have GDM.

Special consideration should be given to screen for plasma lead in women who report pica (the eating of nonfood items or ice) because consumption of earth or clay can be a source of environmental contamination. Pregnant women following a **vegan** diet with no consumption of animal products are at risk for vitamin B_{12} deficiency unless the diet is fortified or supplemented. Plant sources of vitamin B_{12} are not considered biologically available. Women without added synthetic vitamin B_{12} should be assessed for vitamin B_{12} status. Pregnant women with a history of phenylketonuria should have a plasma assay for phenylalanine to screen for elevated levels. Elevated phenylalanine levels are harmful to fetal brain development. In addition, it is helpful to note that an increase in plasma lipid levels is a normal physiological change that occurs during pregnancy (American College of Cardiology, 2018). Unless there are extreme concerns for the patient's cardiovascular health, treatment interventions are not needed.

Assessment Techniques and Findings

The nurse should ask the patient to empty her bladder and should explain how to collect a clean-catch urine specimen. If this is the patient's first gynecologic assessment, the nurse should explain the components and general purposes of the physical assessment to the patient, using pictures and the equipment as necessary, and should ask the patient if she has any special needs or questions about the exam. It is important to provide privacy while the patient puts on the gown with the opening in back and lays a drape across her lap.

For the initial parts of the physical assessment, the patient can be sitting (see Figure 25.12 ■) and later will be assisted to a semi-Fowler position on the examination table. During the pelvic part of the assessment, the patient should be assisted to the lithotomy position (see Figure 25.13 ■). Some patients may need to have this assessment in the side-lying position with top knee bent.

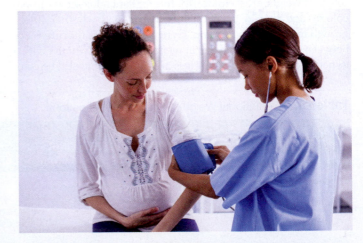

Figure 25.12 Blood pressure measurement in pregnancy.
Source: Wavebreak Media Ltd/123RF.

Table 25.4 Gestational Hemoglobin and Hematocrit References for Anemia

	FIRST AND THIRD TRIMESTERS	SECOND TRIMESTER
Hemoglobin (g/dL)	<11	<10.5
Hematocrit (%)	<33	<32

Source: Centers for Disease Control and Prevention (CDC, 2011).

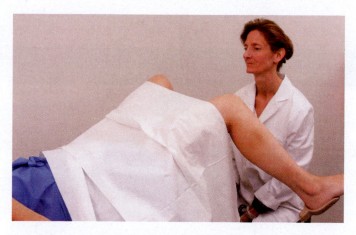

Figure 25.13 Pregnant patient in lithotomy position.

The nurse assists the patient in placing her feet in the stirrups, which should be padded if possible. The legs should be symmetrically and comfortably positioned. The patient can then be instructed to move her buttocks down to the end of the table until about 0.5 inch is hanging over the edge. For the initial part of the pelvic assessment, it is helpful to tell the patient what she will feel before the nurse touches her (e.g., "You will feel me touching your leg," "You will feel me touching your labia," etc.).

It is important to note that there are many elements of the physical exam of a pregnant woman that are more commonly performed by a women's health advanced practice registered nurse (APRN), certified nurse midwife (CNM), obstetrician-gynecologist (OB-GYN) physician, or physician's assistant (PA).

Several types of laboratory tests can be performed during pregnancy. Table 25.5 provides information about these various tests, when they should be performed during pregnancy, the normal and abnormal values, and any patient education that is needed as follow-up.

EQUIPMENT

- Examination gown and drape
- Sphygmomanometer
- Adjustable light source
- High-performance stethoscope
- Centimeter tape measure
- Reflex hammer
- Fetoscope or fetal Doppler and ultrasonic gel
- Urine collection containers
- Urine testing strips
- Perineal cleansing wipes
- Tongue depressor

HELPFUL HINTS

- Ask the patient to empty her bladder before the assessment.
- Explain the purposes and processes of each part of the assessment. Use pictures or diagrams as needed.
- Assist the patient to the sitting, lying, and lithotomy positions.
- Explain what the patient will feel before touching her.
- Be sure to maintain the patient's dignity throughout the assessment.
- The side-lying position may be used to inspect the perineum and rectum of the postpartum patient.
- Use Standard Precautions throughout the assessment.

Table 25.5 Tests in Pregnancy

NAME OF TEST	TIMING OF TEST IN PREGNANCY	NORMAL VALUE	ABNORMAL VALUES	SPECIAL TEACHING
Blood Type, Rh Factor, and Antibody Screen	Initial obstetric (OB) visit and 28 weeks for Rh-negative women	A, B, AB, O, Rh+ or −; no irregular antibodies	Irregular antibodies found	If not her first pregnancy, inquire about previous Rh immune globulin (RhoGAM) administration if Rh−.
Hematocrit	Initial OB visit and 36 weeks	First trimester: 31.0%–41.0% Second trimester: 30.0%–39.0% Third trimester: 28.0%–40.0%	Outside range	Eat iron-rich foods. Report any bleeding.
Hemoglobin	Initial OB visit and 36 weeks	First trimester: 11.6–13.9 g/dL Second trimester: 9.7–14.8 g/dL Third trimester: 9.5–15.0 g/dL	Outside range	Effects of pregnancy on iron needs and possible need for iron supplements.
RBC	Initial OB visit	First trimester: 3.42–4.55 million/mcL Second trimester: 2.81–4.49 million/mcL Third trimester: 2.71–4.43 million/mcL	Outside range	Red cell indices will also be examined to R/O hemoglobinopathies.

(continued)

Table 25.5 Tests in Pregnancy (continued)

NAME OF TEST	TIMING OF TEST IN PREGNANCY	NORMAL VALUE	ABNORMAL VALUES	SPECIAL TEACHING
WBC	Initial OB visit	First trimester: 5,700–13,600/mcL Second trimester: 5,600–14,800/mcL Third trimester: 5,900–16,900/mcL	Outside range	Report signs of infection.
Platelets	Initial OB visit	First trimester: 174–391 billion/L Second trimester: 155–409 billion/L Third trimester: 146–429 billion/L	Outside range	Report abnormal bleeding from gums, bruising.
HIV	Offered at initial OB visit and prn	Negative	Positive, confirmed by further testing: Western blot	Obtain specific informed consent before testing. Advise of dramatic decrease in vertical (mother to child) transmission with medication.
Hepatitis B	Initial OB visit	Negative	Positive	Inform patient of sexual transmissibility. Explain importance of prophylaxis for infant.
Gonorrhea	Initial OB visit; third trimester if high risk	Negative	Positive	Educate patient about infection. Use empathetic listening if test is positive. Stress the importance of compliance and partner treatment.
Chlamydia	Initial OB visit; third trimester if high risk	Negative	Positive	Address STD prevention.
Rubella Titer	Initial OB visit	Immune	Nonimmune	Recommend maternal immunization after birth. Stress the avoidance of pregnancy for 3 months after immunization. Avoid first-trimester exposure to infection because of risk of congenital rubella syndrome.
Tuberculin Skin Testing	Initial OB visit if high risk	Negative	Positive induration >10 mm in non-immunocompromised patient	Educate mother about infection. Teach respiratory precautions. Encourage smoking cessation.
Urinalysis	Every OB visit	Negative	Presence of protein, glucose, ketones, RBCs, WBCs	Urine collected should be a clean-catch mid-stream sample.
Urine Culture	Initial OB visit	Negative	Positive bacteria >100,000 colony-forming units (CFUs)	Wipe from front to back during toileting. Report urgency, flank pain, frequency, burning upon urination.
Papanicolaou Smear	Initial OB visit	Negative	Epithelial cell abnormalities or neoplasms present	Refrain from intercourse or douching 2 to 3 days before test (for accuracy). Discuss individualized schedule of testing.
RPR/VDRL FTA-ABS (Syphilis)	Initial OB visit; third trimester	Nonreactive	Reactive FTA-ABS reports a ratio	Educate about infection stages and treatment; advise compliance and abstinence during treatment; reinforce importance of follow-up.
Multiple Marker Genetic Screen	15 to 20 weeks gestation; first trimester for PAPP-A and Free Beta	No increased risk	Elevated risk	Discuss conditions screened for and limitations of test. Emphasize need for diagnostic testing if screen is positive.
Alpha fetoprotein (AFP) screening test for neural tube defects	16–18 weeks	<40 micrograms/liter	Low-level possible chromosomal abnormalities; elevated levels positive for neural tube defects	Abnormal results necessitate further diagnostic testing for explanation.
Amniocentesis	11–20 weeks Third trimester for fetal lung maturity	No genetic abnormalities L/S ratio >2:1 Positive Phosphatidylglycerol (PG) Positive Phosphatidylinositol (PI)	Genetic abnormalities Ratio <2:1 Negative PG & PI	A risk of <1% pregnancy loss exists; abnormal results will necessitate a decision about pregnancy termination. Normal value will allow safe early birth.

NAME OF TEST	TIMING OF TEST IN PREGNANCY	NORMAL VALUE	ABNORMAL VALUES	SPECIAL TEACHING
Chorionic villus sampling	10–12 weeks	No genetic abnormalities	Genetic abnormalities	Same as amniocentesis; questionable results may require more testing.
50-g Glucose Challenge Test (GCT)	24 to 28 weeks; may be done at initial prenatal visit for patients with increased risk of gestational diabetes mellitus (GDM)	≤140 mg/dL	>140	Not fasting; blood drawn exactly 1 hour after glucose is drunk.
3-Hour GTT (100 g glucose given)	Follow-up to elevated 50 g GCT	Fasting <95 mg/dL 1-hr <180 mg/dL 2-hr <155 mg/dL 3-hr <140 mg/dL	Two or more values met or exceeded	Three days of unrestricted carbohydrates and physical activity; fasting before test; no smoking or caffeine before and during test; inform regarding schedule of blood draws.
Group B *Streptococcus*	Third trimester/35 to 37 weeks	Positive	Negative	Intravenous (IV) antibiotics will be given in active labor to decrease risk of transmission to infant.
Ultrasound	Optional, frequently at 15 to 20 weeks, dependent on rationale	Normal	Abnormal	Patient can decide whether gender of child should be revealed. Some ultrasound studies require vaginal probe. Nuchal translucency test at 11 weeks is to screen for chromosomal abnormalities.

Techniques and Normal Findings

Abnormal Findings and Special Considerations

General Survey

1. **Measure the patient's height and weight.**
   - At the initial exam, take these measurements to establish a baseline. In the first trimester, the patient should gain 4 to 6 lb. The patient should gain 1 lb per week in both the second and the third trimesters, for a total weight gain of about 25 to 35 lb, if she is normal weight at conception.

   ▶ A gain of 6.6 lb or more per month may be associated with a large-for-gestational-age baby or with developing preeclampsia. A gain of less than 2.2 lb per month may cause preterm birth, a small-for-gestational-age infant, or IUGR.

2. **Assess the patient's general appearance and mental status.**
   - Tiredness and ambivalence are normal in early pregnancy. Most women express well-being and energy during the second trimester. During the third trimester, most report increased fatigue and concern regarding the upcoming birth.

   ▶ It is important to watch for signs of depression, such as decreased appetite; persistent feelings of sadness, guilt, or worry; and suicidal thoughts.

3. **Take the patient's vital signs.**
   - The respiratory rate may increase slightly during pregnancy, the heart rate increases, and the blood pressure may drop to below prepregnancy baseline during the second trimester.

   ▶ For women who typically have blood pressure in the normal range, blood pressure should not be greater than 140/90. Elevated blood pressure could be a sign of gestational hypertension or, if accompanied by significant proteinuria, preeclampsia. Note that the pregnant woman's blood pressure should be compared with her blood pressure in a nonpregnant state to determine if she has chronic hypertension or if her elevated blood pressure may be related to gestational hypertension or preeclampsia.

ALERT! *As preeclampsia worsens, multiple systems of the body are affected, producing symptoms such as (from head to toe) the following:*
   - ▶ *Headache unrelieved by acetaminophen*
   - ▶ *Blurred vision, dizziness, or vision changes*
   - ▶ *Dyspnea, or difficulty breathing*
   - ▶ *Epigastric (upper abdominal) pain*
   - ▶ *Nausea, vomiting, or malaise ("I don't feel right")*
   - ▶ *Sudden weight gain or sudden, severe edema of face, hands, and legs*
   - ▶ *Signs noted by healthcare providers include hypertension greater than 140/90, proteinuria ≥0.3 grams in a 24-hour urine specimen or urine dipstick of +1 or higher, oliguria (decreased urine output), hyperreflexia, and abnormal laboratory values such as elevated liver enzymes and uric acid.*

Techniques and Normal Findings	Abnormal Findings and Special Considerations
4. **Test the patient's urine for glucose and protein.** • Occasional mild glycosuria or trace protein can be normal findings in pregnancy.	▶ Persistent glycosuria may indicate gestational diabetes and necessitates follow-up. Greater-than-trace protein may indicate preeclampsia. If the patient has lost weight, it is important to check the urine for ketones, indicating ketoacidosis, which is harmful to the fetus.
5. **Observe the patient's posture.** • Increasing lordosis is a normal adaptation to pregnancy.	
6. **Assist the patient to a sitting position.**	

Skin, Hair, and Nails

1. **Observe the skin, hair, and nails for changes associated with pregnancy.** • These include linea nigra, striae, melasma, spider nevi, palmar erythema, and darkened areola and perineum. Softening and thinning of nails are common. Hair may become thicker in pregnancy.	▶ Bruises may indicate physical abuse. Lesions may indicate infection. Scars along veins may indicate intravenous drug abuse.

Head and Neck

1. **Inspect and palpate the neck.** • Slight thyroid gland enlargement is normal in pregnancy.	▶ Enlarged or tender lymph nodes may indicate infection or cancer. Marked thyroid gland enlargement may indicate hyperthyroidism.

Eyes, Ears, Nose, Mouth, and Throat

1. **Inspect the eyes and ears.** • There are no visible changes associated with pregnancy.	▶ Redness or discharge may indicate infection.
2. **Inspect the nose.** • Increased swelling of nasal mucosa and redness may accompany the increased estrogen of pregnancy.	▶ Epistaxis may occur if the vascular increase is extreme.
3. **Inspect the mouth.** • Hypertrophy of gum tissue is normal.	▶ Epulis nodules, which are formed by hyperplastic tissue overgrowth on the gums, or poor dentition warrant referral to a dentist. Pale gums may indicate anemia. Redness or exudates may indicate infection.
4. **Inspect the throat.** • The throat should appear pink and smooth.	

Thorax and Lungs

1. **Inspect, palpate, percuss, and auscultate the chest.** • Note diaphragmatic expansion and character of respirations. Later in pregnancy, pressure from the growing uterus produces a change from abdominal to thoracic breathing. • Observe for symmetric expansion with no retraction or bulging of the intercostal spaces. Confirm that the lungs are clear in all fields.	▶ Unequal expansion or intercostal retractions are signs of respiratory distress. Rales, rhonchi, wheezes, rubs, and absent or unequal sounds may indicate pulmonary disease.

Heart

1. **Auscultate the heart.** • Confirm that the rhythm is regular and that the rate is from 70 to 90 beats/min. The heart rate in pregnancy increases 10 to 20 beats/min above the baseline. Short systolic murmurs are due to increased blood volume and displacement of the heart.	▶ Irregular rhythm, dyspnea, or markedly decreased activity tolerance may indicate cardiac disease.
2. **Position the patient.** • Assist the patient into a semi-Fowler position for the next portion of the assessment, and pull out the bottom of the table extension so the patient may lie backward on the slightly elevated head rest.	

Breasts and Axillae

1. **Inspect the breasts.** • Normal changes include enlargement, increased venous pattern, enlarged Montgomery tubercles, presence of colostrum after 12 weeks, striae, and darkening of nipple and areola (Figure 25.6).	▶ Flat or inverted nipples can be treated with breast shells in the last month of pregnancy. ▶ Bloody discharge or fixed, unchanging masses or skin retraction could indicate breast cancer.
2. **Palpate the breasts and axillae.** • Breasts are more tender to touch and more nodular during pregnancy.	

Extremities

1. **Inspect and palpate the extremities.** • Varicose veins in the lower extremities are normal with pregnancy. Mild dependent edema of the hands and ankles is common in pregnancy. Inspect and palpate the extremities for raised or tender veins. Palpate for ankle or lower-leg edema.	▶ Raised, hard, tender, warm, painful, or reddened veins may indicate thrombophlebitis. Marked edema may indicate preeclampsia.

Techniques and Normal Findings	Abnormal Findings and Special Considerations

Neurologic System

1. **Percuss the deep tendon reflexes.**
   - Reflexes should be +1 or +2 and bilaterally equal.
   - Refer to Chapter 26 for more details. ∞

▶ Hyperreflexia and clonus are signs of preeclampsia.

Abdomen and Fetal Assessment

1. **Inspect and palpate the abdomen.**
   - The uterus becomes an abdominal organ after 12 weeks in pregnancy. Uterine contractions are palpable after the first trimester. Palpate uterine contractions by laying both hands on the abdomen. The *frequency* of contractions is determined by measuring the interval from the beginning of one contraction to the beginning of the next contraction. Indent the uterus with a finger to measure *intensity* or strength of contractions. The strength can be classified as mild, moderate, or strong. These distinctions can be described by comparing the rigidity of the uterus to the firmness of certain other body features. Mild contractions are comparable to the firmness of the nose, moderate contractions feel like the chin, and strong contractions are as hard and unyielding as the forehead. The *duration* of contractions is measured from the beginning to the end of the contraction.

▶ Liver enlargement is abnormal.

▶ More than five contractions per hour may indicate preterm labor.

2. **Assess fetal growth through fundal height assessment.**
   - Before 20 weeks, fundal height is measured by indicating the number of finger breadths or centimeters above the symphysis pubis or below the umbilicus. Once the uterus rises above the umbilicus, a tape measure is used.
   - The 0 line of the measuring tape is placed at the superior edge of the symphysis pubis.
   - The other hand is placed at the xiphoid with the ulnar surface against the abdomen. When the superior edge of the uterus is encountered by the descending hand, the top of the uterus has been located.
   - The measuring tape is stretched from the top of the symphysis pubis to the fundus. The superior aspect of the tape is held between the middle fingers of the hand that is resting perpendicular to the fundus. The fundal height in centimeters is noted and compared with the weeks of pregnancy. Uterine size in centimeters is approximately equal to the weeks of pregnancy. The uterus should measure within 2 units of the weeks of pregnancy (see Figure 25.14 ■).

▶ If the uterus is more than 2 cm larger or smaller than the weeks of pregnancy, a growth disorder such as IUGR, multiple gestation, amniotic fluid disorders, incorrect dating, fetal malpresentation, or anomalies may be occurring.

▶ An unexpectedly large uterus also may be indicative of macrosomia, a condition in which the newborn is substantially larger than average, characterized by a weight of more than 8 pounds, 13 ounces at birth. Babies born with macrosomia are at greater risk for health disorders, including hyperglycemia and childhood obesity (Mayo Clinic, 2018a).

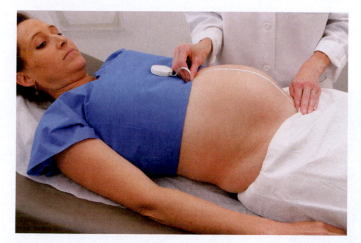

Figure 25.14 Fundal height measurement.

3. **Assess fetal activity.**
   - After 24 weeks, fetal movement is palpable by the examiner. Maternal perception of movement occurs between 16 and 18 weeks in pregnancy.

▶ The *fetal alarm signal* occurs when there is no fetal movement for 8 hours, fewer than 10 movements in 12 hours, a change in the usual pattern of movements, or a sudden increase in violent fetal movements followed by a complete cessation of movement. Immediate evaluation of the fetus should take place.

4. **Assess fetal lie, presentation, and position.**
   - **Leopold's maneuvers** use a specialized palpation of the abdomen sequence to answer a series of questions to determine the position of the fetus in the abdomen and pelvis after 28 weeks gestation.
   - *First Leopold's maneuver: What is in the fundus?* With the patient in a supine position, stand facing her head. Place the ulnar surface of both hands on the fundus, with the fingertips pointing toward the midline. Palpate the shape and firmness of

▶ Leopold's maneuver may be useful in recognizing fetal macrosomia, which increases both the difficulty of vaginal childbirth and the risk of injury to the baby during the birth and process (Mayo Clinic, 2018a).

the contents of the upper uterus. A longitudinal line will find the head or breech in the fundus. A round, firm mass is the fetal head. A soft, irregular mass is the fetal breech. Nothing in the fundus indicates a transverse lie. The fetus can also be oblique, at an oblique angle to the midline (see Figure 25.15 ■).

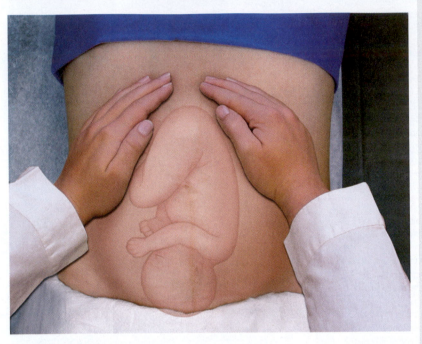

Figure 25.15 First Leopold's maneuver.

- *Second Leopold's maneuver: Where is the fetal back?* Move the hands down the sides of the abdomen along the uterine contour. A smooth, long, firm, continuous outline is found on the side with the fetal back. Irregular, lumpy, moving parts are found on the side with the fetal small parts, or feet and hands. Note whether the back is found on the patient's left or right side; if an indentation about the size of a dinner plate is seen at the midline and movements are at the center of the abdomen, the fetal back may be against the mother's spine (posterior position) (see Figure 25.16 ■).

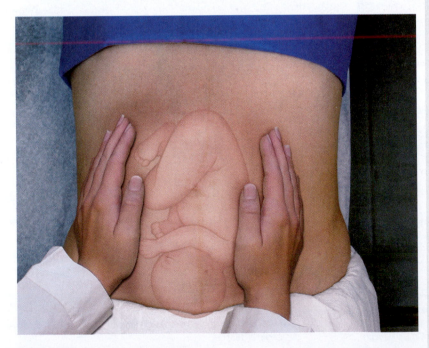

Figure 25.16 Second Leopold's maneuver.

Techniques and Normal Findings	**Abnormal Findings and Special Considerations**

- *Third Leopold's maneuver: What part of the fetus is presenting at the pelvis?* Next, slide your hands down to the area above the symphysis pubis to determine the "presenting" part of the fetus, the part of the fetus entering the pelvic inlet. Palpate the shape and firmness of the presenting part. Use the thumb and third finger of one hand to grasp the presenting part. This may require pressing into the area above the symphysis pubis with some pressure. Try to move the presenting part with one hand and see if the part of the fetus in the fundus moves with it using the other hand. If the breech is presenting, the whole mass of the fetus will move when the presenting part is moved, and it will feel irregular and soft above the symphysis pubis. If a hard, round, independently movable mass is palpated in the pelvis, it is the head (see Figure 25.17 ■).

▶ A face presentation or forehead presentation may delay the progression of labor and lengthen the time before birth (Medline-Plus, 2018). In some cases, cesarean section may be necessary.

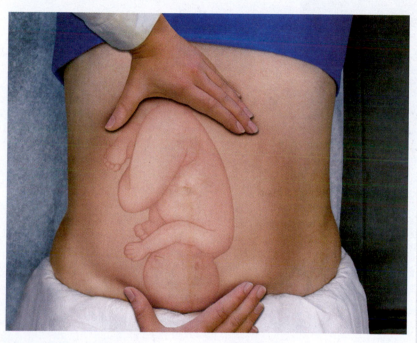

Figure 25.17 Third Leopold's maneuver.

- *Fourth Leopold's maneuver: How deep in the pelvis is the presenting part?* Now, face the patient's feet. Place the ulnar surface of your two hands on each side of the patient's abdomen. Follow the uterine/fetal contour to the pelvic brim. If the fingers come together above the superior edge of the symphysis pubis, the presenting part is floating above the pelvic inlet. If the fingers snap over the brim of the pelvis before coming together, the presenting part has descended into the pelvis. A prominent part on one side is the *cephalic prominence* if the presenting part is the fetal head; this indicates a face presentation if felt on the same side as the back. If a prominence is felt on both sides, the forehead is presenting. If no prominence is felt or the prominence is felt on the same side as the small parts, the fetus is well flexed, with the chin on the chest (flexion) (see Figure 25.18 ■).

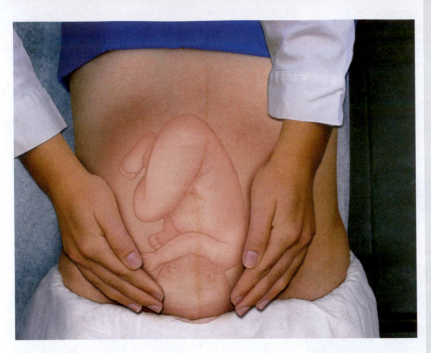

Figure 25.18 Fourth Leopold's maneuver.

- *Fetal position.* The position of the fetus is the relationship of the presenting part to the four quadrants of the maternal pelvis. The fetus can be in the left or right half of the maternal pelvis and in the anterior, posterior, or transverse portion of the pelvis. Three notations are used to designate the fetal position. The first notation is L or R for left or right, indicating in which half of the maternal pelvis the presenting part is found. The second notation is a letter abbreviating the part of the fetus that is presenting at the top of the pelvis. The most common notations for presenting part are O, indicating occiput, or the back of the head in a flexed position; S, indicating sacrum for a breech presentation; Sc, indicating scapula in a transverse lie; and M, indicating mentum or face presentation. The third notation indicates if the presenting part is in the anterior, posterior, or transverse portion of the pelvis. For example, a position of LOA indicates that the presenting part is the occiput, and it is in the left half of the anterior part of the pelvis.

5. **Estimate fetal weight.**
   - Estimating fetal weight by abdominal palpation is only an approximation. It is done in conjunction with fundal height measurement and ultrasound to detect growth abnormalities.
   - Use Leopold's maneuvers to assess fetal size. Experience can be gained by palpating undressed term and preterm infants in the nursery. Compare your estimates with the known weights of the infants.

▶ Large-for-gestational-age (LGA) or small-for-gestational-age (SGA) infants must be further evaluated.

Techniques and Normal Findings	Abnormal Findings and Special Considerations

6. Auscultate fetal heart rate.

- Once the position of the fetus has been determined, the fetal heart tones (FHTs) can be located. They are usually heard loudest over the left scapula of the fetus, so this is the area that should be auscultated (see Figure 25.19 ■).

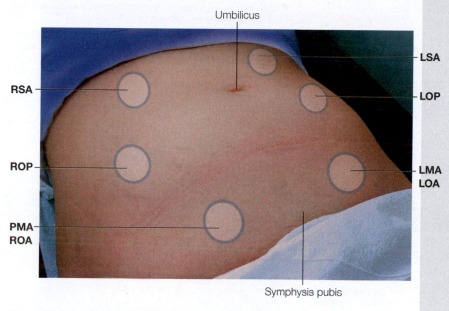

Figure 25.19 Location of fetal heart tones for various fetal positions.

- Place the fetoscope or fetal Doppler in the location where the FHTs are most likely to be heard given the findings of Leopold's maneuvers. Place ultrasonic gel, warmed if possible, on the Doppler before placement on the abdomen.

- Auscultate the FHT for 1 minute.

▶ If the fetal heartbeat is not found by 12 weeks with a fetal Doppler, or 20 weeks with a fetoscope, ultrasound evaluation of the fetal viability may be indicated. Other causes could be incorrect dating of pregnancy or retroverted uterus.

▶ Irregular heartbeats, tachycardia (heart rate above 160 beats/min), bradycardia (heart rate below 120 beats/min, or 110 beats/min in postterm fetuses), or decelerations in fetal heart rate below the baseline should be followed up with electronic fetal monitoring.

7. Assist the patient into the lithotomy position for the next portion of the assessment.

ALERT! *Portions of the external and internal genitalia exam are typically performed by nurses and other practitioners with advanced-level training. However, all nurses working with pregnant women should have an understanding of the techniques in the context of the changes that may occur because of pregnancy and any effects on labor and birth. These techniques are included in this chapter, but they are denoted as advanced level. Some of the advanced techniques are the same for the female reproductive system. They are explained in more detail in Appendix C and include a notation to "See Appendix C."*

Techniques and Normal Findings	Abnormal Findings and Special Considerations

External Genitalia

1. **Inspect the external genitalia.**
   - Normal findings include enlargement of the clitoris and labia, gaping vaginal introitus for multiparas (patients who have given birth before), scars on perineum from previous births, small hemorrhoids, and darkened pigmentation (see Figure 25.20 ■).
   - Ask the patient to bear down, and note any bulges of the vaginal walls or cervix outside the vagina.

▶ Varicosities can occur in the labia and upper thighs. Lesions may indicate sexually transmitted infection. Redness may indicate vaginitis.

▶ The cervix or vaginal walls may protrude from the vagina in cases of uterine, bladder (cystocele), or rectal (rectocele) prolapse. If the cervix is at the introitus, it is graded as a first-degree uterine prolapse. In a second-degree prolapse, the uterus descends through the introitus. In a third-degree prolapse, the entire uterus is outside the vagina.

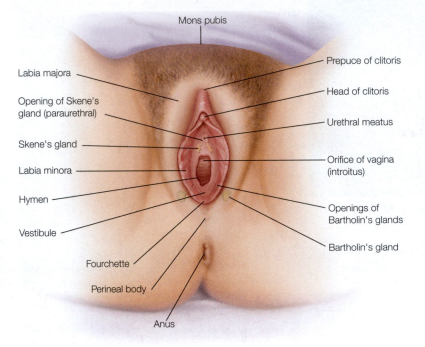

Mons pubis
Prepuce of clitoris
Head of clitoris
Labia majora
Urethral meatus
Opening of Skene's gland (paraurethral)
Skene's gland
Orifice of vagina (introitus)
Labia minora
Hymen
Openings of Bartholin's glands
Vestibule
Bartholin's gland
Fourchette
Perineal body
Anus

Figure 25.20 External female genitalia.

2. **Palpate Bartholin's gland, urethra, and Skene's glands. (Advanced Skill.)**

Appendix C: Advanced Skills *Appendix C provides step-by-step instructions for palpating Bartholin's gland, the urethra, and Skene's glands.*

Inspection of Vagina and Cervix

1. **Observe the vagina.**
   - The vagina may also be bluish in pregnancy. Note the color, consistency, odor, and amount of discharge. Increased whitish, odorless discharge (leukorrhea) is normal in pregnancy.

▶ White, clumping discharge or gray, green, bubbly, fishy-smelling discharge is indication of vaginitis or sexually transmitted infections. The patient may complain of itching, burning, dyspareunia or pain on intercourse, or pelvic pain.

▶ A rough, reddened texture may represent the growth of cells from the internal cervical canal to the outside of the os (ectopy). It is seen in multiparas and women who use oral contraceptives. If the speculum is pushed too deeply into the fornices or corners of the vagina, the internal canal may also appear; this eversion should be eliminated by pulling the speculum back slightly.

2. **Visualize the cervix. (See Appendix C.)**
   - If the cervix is covered with secretions, a Papanicolaou (Pap) smear will be obtained. Use a sponge stick or a large swab to blot the cervix.

Techniques and Normal Findings	**Abnormal Findings and Special Considerations**

Palpation of Pelvis

Advanced Skill: *Some nurses with advanced training assess the size and shape of the pelvis to screen for problems during birth.*

1. **Assess the angle of the pubic arch.**
   - Place the thumbs at the midline of the lower border of the symphysis pubis (see Figure 25.21 ■). Follow the edge of the pubic bone down to the ischial tuberosity. Estimate the angle of the pubic arch. A pubic arch greater than 90 degrees is best for vaginal birth.

▶ An angle less than 90 degrees may be more difficult for a fetus to navigate in labor.

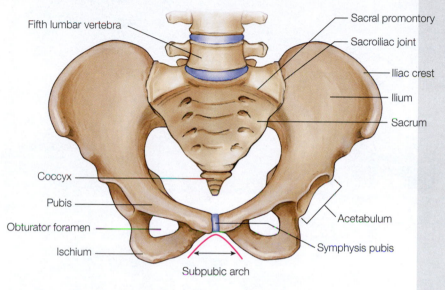

Fifth lumbar vertebra

Sacral promontory

Sacroiliac joint

Iliac crest

Ilium

Sacrum

Coccyx

Pubis

Obturator foramen

Ischium

Acetabulum

Symphysis pubis

Subpubic arch

Figure 25.21 Internal structures of the female pelvis for landmarks.

2. **Lubricate the gloved fingers.**
   - Apply a teaspoon or more of lubricating jelly to the index and middle fingers.

3. **Estimate the angle of the subpubic arch.**
   - Insert the index and middle fingers slightly into the vagina, palmar side up. Keep the fingers separated slightly to prevent pressure on the urethra. Palpate the inner surface of the symphysis pubis. Using both thumbs, externally trace the descending sides of the pubis down to the tuberosities. The symphysis pubis should be at least two finger breadths wide, and parallel to the sacrum, without any abnormal thickening (see Figure 25.22 ■).

▶ An anterior or posterior tilting, or width less than two fingerbreadths, is abnormal.

Techniques and Normal Findings	Abnormal Findings and Special Considerations

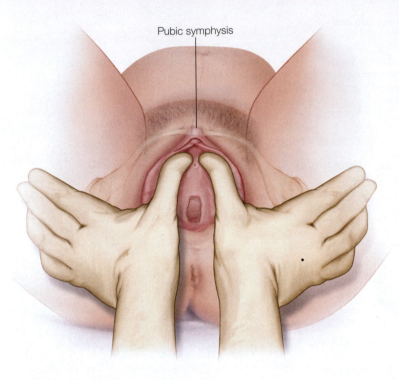

Pubic symphysis

Figure 25.22 Estimation of angle of subpubic arch.

4. **Assess the interspinous diameter.**
   - Turn the fingers to the side and follow the lateral walls of the pelvis to the ischial spine. (As the fingers go deeper into the vagina, ensure that the thumb stays away from the perineum.) Determine if the spine is blunt, flat, or sharp. Sweep your fingers across the pelvis to the opposite ischial spine. Average diameter is approximately 10.5 cm (see Figure 25.23 ■).

▶ A pointy ischial spine can impede labor.

▶ A smaller diameter may indicate a contracted pelvis.

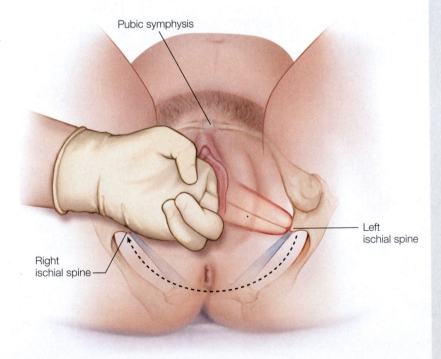

Pubic symphysis

Left ischial spine

Right ischial spine

Figure 25.23 Assessing the interspinous diameter.

Techniques and Normal Findings	**Abnormal Findings and Special Considerations**

5. Assess the curvature of the sacrum.

- Sweep your fingers upward as far as you can reach. Determine if the sacrum is concave, flat, or convex. Note if the coccyx at the posterior end of the sacrum is movable or fixed by pressing down on it.

▶ A hollow sacrum provides more room for the fetus moving through the pelvis.

6. Measure the diagonal conjugate.

- Next, position the fingers in the back of the vagina next to the cervix. Drop your wrist so your fingers are at an upward angle of 45 degrees.
- Reach as far toward the sacrum as you can, and raise your wrist until your hand touches the symphysis pubis. If your fingers reach the sacral promontory, note the distance from the tip of your middle finger touching the sacral promontory to the symphysis pubis. If you cannot reach the sacral promontory, the diagonal conjugate is greater than the length of your examining fingers. The diagonal conjugate is an approximation of the pelvic inlet and should be greater than 11.5 cm (see Figure 25.24 ■).

▶ A diagonal conjugate of less than 11.5 cm may prevent a vaginal birth.

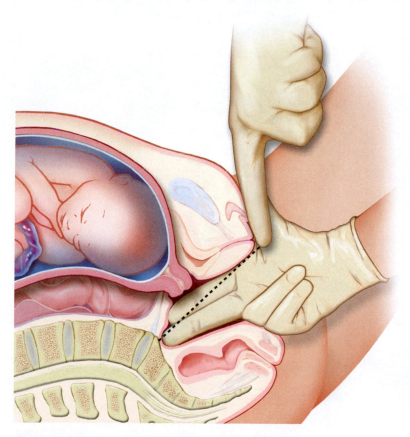

Figure 25.24 Measuring the diagonal conjugate.

Palpation of Cervix, Uterus, Adnexa, and Vagina

1. Assess the cervix.

- Run your fingers around the cervix, and feel the length, width, consistency, and opening. The cervix is usually 1.5 to 2 cm long and 2 to 3 cm wide. In multiparas, the outside of the os may be open up to 2 to 3 cm.

▶ The cervix is softer during pregnancy (Goodell's sign). It becomes even softer and jellylike as the patient approaches labor. The outer opening of the cervix may be open, but the internal os should be closed prior to term, 37 weeks of pregnancy or more. A shortened cervix is also a symptom or predictor of possible preterm labor.

- Assess the texture and position of the cervix. It should be smooth.

▶ Note the roughness of ectopy or any nodules or masses. Nabothian cysts may become infected or be a sign of cervicitis. Normal variations include a retroverted uterus, which will have an anterior cervix, and an anteverted uterus, which will have a posterior cervix.

Techniques and Normal Findings	Abnormal Findings and Special Considerations

- Move the cervix from side to side with your fingers.

2. **Perform bimanual palpation of the uterus. (Advanced Skill)**
   - Place the nondominant hand on the abdomen halfway between the umbilicus and the symphysis pubis. Press the palmar surface of the fingers toward the fingers in the vagina.
   - Insert the fingers of the dominant hand into the vagina. Move the fingers to the sides of the cervix, palmar surfaces upward, and press upward toward the abdomen.
   - Estimate the size, consistency, and shape of the uterus captured between your hands. The uterus softens in pregnancy, and the isthmus, the area between the cervix and the upper body of the uterus, is compressible (Hegar's sign).
   - The uterus will feel about the size of an orange at 10 weeks gestation and a grapefruit at 12 weeks gestation. If the gestation is beyond the first trimester, abdominal fundal height measurement is used (see Figure 25.25 ■).

▶ Cervical motion tenderness (CMT) is a sign of pelvic inflammatory disease and other abnormalities.

▶ If the uterine size is not consistent with what is expected for the gestation, then incorrect dating, multiple gestation, or fibroids are suspected.

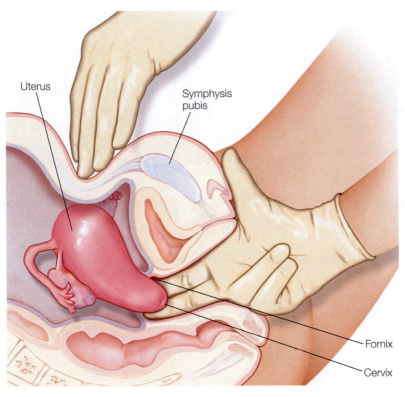

Uterus

Symphysis pubis

Fornix

Cervix

Figure 25.25 Bimanual palpation of the uterus.

3. **Palpate the adnexa. (Advanced Skill)**
   - The fallopian tubes and ovaries, or adnexa, sometimes cannot be palpated, especially after the uterus enters the abdominal cavity as pregnancy progresses.

▶ Any adnexal masses are abnormal and require referral. Bilateral pain is a symptom of pelvic inflammatory disease. During pregnancy an enlarged fallopian tube could indicate ectopic or tubal pregnancy and must be referred to a physician.

4. **Assess vaginal tone. (Advanced Skill)**
   - Withdraw your fingers to just below the cervix, and ask the patient to squeeze her muscles around your fingers as hard and long as she can. Normal strength is demonstrated by a snug squeeze lasting a few seconds and with upward movement. This provides an opportunity to teach the patient about pelvic-floor strengthening exercises.

Techniques and Normal Findings	Abnormal Findings and Special Considerations

5. Measure the intertuberous diameter of the pelvic outlet. (Advanced Skill)

- This part of the pelvic assessment is done at the end of the internal exam. As you gently withdraw your hand, make a fist with your thumb on the downward side, and press it between the ischial tuberosities. A diameter of 11 cm is average, and 8.5 cm or greater usually is adequate. You must know the diameter of your fist to make this determination (see Figure 25.26 ■).

▶ A diameter smaller than 8.5 cm may inhibit fetal descent during expulsion.

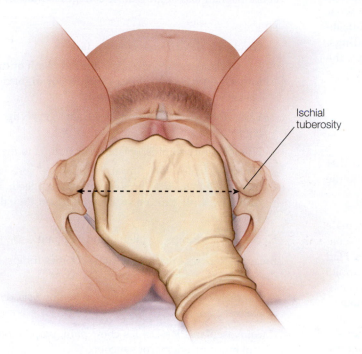

Ischial tuberosity

Figure 25.26 Assessing the pelvic outlet.

Anus and Rectum

1. Inspect the rectum.

▶ Hemorrhoids are commonly noted in pregnancy.

▶ Thrombosed hemorrhoids are tender, swollen, and bluish in color.

▶ *Candida* (yeast), moving trichomonads, or epithelial cells covered with black bacterial spots are abnormal findings.

2. Perform the rectovaginal exam. (See Appendix C.)

- The exam is sometimes deferred, but it enables the nurse to evaluate internal structures more deeply and is especially important if any fistulas are noted in the vagina, or if an early pregnancy is in a retroflexed or retroverted uterus.

3. Conclude the exam.

- Disposable equipment should be placed in a biohazard container. Use the tissue to wipe the patient's perineum, or offer tissues to her to do so. Offer your hand to assist her to the sitting position, and leave the room so she can dress in privacy. Share your findings with her.

Documenting Your Findings

Documentation of assessment data—subjective and objective—must be accurate, professional, complete, and confidential. When documenting the information from the assessment of the pregnant woman, the nurse should use measurements where appropriate to ensure accuracy, use medical terminology rather than jargon, include all pertinent information, and avoid language that could identify the patient. The information in the documentation should make it clear what questions were asked and should use language to indicate whether it is the patient's response or the nurse's findings. When documenting the subjective and objective findings, the nurse should be concise, but as thorough with the data findings as possible.

Sample Documentation: Pregnant Woman

Focused History (Subjective Data)

This information is from the review of systems (ROS) and other pertinent history information that is or could be related to the patient's overall health.

Reason for Visit: Mrs. A.P. is a 25-year-old Caucasian female who came to the women's health clinic today for her first prenatal visit. She is G1P0 @ 9 weeks +2 days by LMP 6/25/18. Had (+) home pregnancy test 3 weeks ago. Reports this is a planned pregnancy with her husband. Reports breast tenderness, increased frequency of urination, fatigue, and mild nausea throughout the day for the past 3 weeks. Denies vomiting, dizziness, headache, edema, or vaginal bleeding/fluid. States she is eating a well-balanced diet and staying hydrated. Continuing exercise by walking daily.

OB Hx: G1P0 No hx of STI.

Allergies: No known allergies.

Past Medical/Surgical Hx:

Medical: No medical hx.
Surgical: Tonsillectomy 1997; Wisdom teeth 2010.

Medications: Prenatal vitamin once daily.

Immunizations: Flu vaccine 10/2017; up to date on all childhood vaccines.

Family Hx:

Mother (50 yo) and Father (54 yo) alive and well. No siblings.
Maternal grandmother—type 2 diabetes, chronic kidney disease, deceased age 79 heart failure.
Maternal grandfather (77 yo)—CAD, type 2 diabetes.
Paternal grandmother and grandfather—deceased; health history unknown.

Social Hx: Patient has been married to her husband for 4 years. She is employed full-time as a banker. Denies having any stressors. Has support from her husband, friends, and parents. She feels safe in her home. Denies consumption of alcohol.

Drank one cup of coffee per day up until she had a positive pregnancy test 3 weeks ago. Denies use of illicit drugs.

Review of Systems (ROS):

General—Patient denies fever, weight loss, or poor appetite.

Skin—Denies lesions, pruritus, changes in texture, rashes, abnormal hair loss or growth, or changes in moles.

HEENT:

Head—Denies dizziness, or headaches.

Eyes—Denies vision changes, double vision or discomfort. Wears corrective lenses mainly for night driving. Last eye exam about a year ago.

Ears—Denies earache, tinnitus, discharge, vertigo, hearing loss.

Nose—Denies rhinitis, epistaxis, or trauma to the nose.

Throat—Denies sore throat, hoarseness, sore tongue, bleeding gums, loose, broken, or decaying teeth. Denies difficulty with pain or swallowing. Last dental exam 1 year ago.

Neck—Denies lumps, swollen glands, or pain.

Breasts—Reports breast tenderness. Denies lumps, nipple discharge.

Respiratory—Denies cough, sputum, hemoptysis, dyspnea, or pleural pain.

Cardiovascular/PV—Denies chest pain, palpitations, history of murmur, edema, or syncope.

Gastrointestinal—Has mild nausea throughout the day for the past 3 weeks. Denies dysphagia, vomiting, dyspepsia, hematemesis, history of ulcers, abdominal pain, changes in stool, or constipation.

Genitourinary—Reports increased frequency of urination. Denies dysuria or hematuria.

Female Reproductive—Prior to pregnancy, regular periods every 28 days w/"medium" 4-day flow. Last Pap 3/2018. Denies vaginal bleeding, discharge, itching, pain.

Neurological—Denies seizures, numbness, tingling, weakness, or pain.

Musculoskeletal: Denies joint pain, redness, stiffness, swelling, decreased range of motion, back or neck pain.

Endocrine—Denies excessive thirst or urination; heat or cold intolerance, changes to skin or hair.

Hematologic—Denies history of blood transfusions, anemia, or clotting disorders.

Sexuality—Active, heterosexual, one partner, no history of STDs.

Psychiatric—Denies depression, hallucinations, or mood swings.

Physical Assessment (Objective Data)

General Survey: The patient is alert, oriented x4, in no acute distress.

Vital Signs: BP 112/70, P 74, Respiratory rate 14; Ht 67", Wt 155 lbs, BMI 24.3.

HEENT: Head is normocephalic and atraumatic. Sinuses are nontender. PERRLA. Nares are patent. Oropharynx clear without lesions.

Neck: Supple without lymphadenopathy. Thyroid without nodules. No thyromegaly.

Heart: Regular rate and rhythm.

Lungs: Clear to auscultation bilaterally.

Abdomen: Soft, nontender, nondistended. Normoactive bowel sounds x4, quadrants.

Extremities: Without cyanosis, clubbing or edema. +2 DTR.

Neurologic: Gross nonfocal. Denies HA, visual disturbances.

Fetus: Bimanual exam presents as approximately 9 wks gestation. FHTs 150s. No fetal movement. US performed: estimated gestational age 9w0d. EDD 4/1/2019.

Abnormal Findings

Disease processes can result in abnormal assessment findings or abnormal laboratory results. Cultural variations may lead to unexpected psychosocial adaptation and behaviors if the nurse is not familiar with cultural groups and sources of variation.

Common Complications in Pregnancy

During pregnancy the role of the nurse is to educate the patient to prevent complications of pregnancy and to assist in the screening process to detect complications, identify risk factors, and effectively implement treatment if complications develop. Table 25.6 describes the common complications of pregnancy.

Common Complications in the Postpartum Period

Several common complications are found during the postpartum period. These complications are discussed in the Evidence-Based Practice: Screening for Depression feature and in Table 25.7.

Table 25.6 Common Complications in Pregnancy

COMPLICATION	DESCRIPTION	SUBJECTIVE DATA	OBJECTIVE DATA
FIRST TRIMESTER			
Spontaneous Abortion	Loss of pregnancy (Lay term is *miscarriage*.)	• Patient complains of low back or abdominal pain.	• Vaginal bleeding accompanied by cramping and loss of fetus, placenta, and membranes through dilated cervix • No heart tones heard when expected • Fundal height less than expected
Ectopic Pregnancy	Implantation of fertilized ovum in fallopian tube or other abnormal location	• Patient complains of pelvic pain. • Bimanual exam reveals tenderness in adnexa.	• Vaginal bleeding • Mass palpated near uterus • Gestational sac smaller than expected size for gestational age
Anemia	Deficiency in iron, folate, or B_{12}	• Patient reports fatigue, lightheadedness, pica, cold intolerance.	• Abnormal iron values in complete blood count (CBC) • Tachycardia
Substance Abuse	Use of illicit drugs, alcohol	• Positive screening questionnaire • Patient reports irregular prenatal care.	• Inappropriate affect • Possibly preterm labor
Molar Pregnancy/Gestational Trophoblastic Disease	Abnormal growth of placental trophoblast	• Patient reports nausea or vomiting. • Patient reports pelvic pressure or pain.	• Vaginal bleeding • Fundal height large for dates • Fetal heart tones not heard at appropriate time
Mood Disorders	Depression	• Patient reports depressed mood, diminished interest in activities, sleep disorders, fatigue, decreased concentration, suicidal ideation.	• Weight changes

Table 25.6 Common Complications in Pregnancy (continued)

COMPLICATION	DESCRIPTION	SUBJECTIVE DATA	OBJECTIVE DATA
SECOND AND THIRD TRIMESTERS			
Premature Dilation of the Cervix	Passive, painless dilation of cervix during second trimester	• History of second-trimester loss	• Short cervix • Abnormal cervical ultrasound findings
Preeclampsia	Multisystem reaction to vasospasm	• Patient reports severe headaches or changes in vision. • Patient reports upper abdominal pain and nausea or vomiting.	• Elevated blood pressure above 140/90 after 20 weeks • Proteinuria >1 dipstick • Pathologic edema of face, hands, and abdomen unresponsive to bed rest
Gestational Diabetes	Glucose intolerance during pregnancy	• Patient reports positive history of gestational diabetes.	• Abnormal glucose tolerance test • Glycosuria
Preterm Labor	Uterine contractions at 20 to 37 weeks that cause cervical change	• Patient reports constant low backache and pelvic or abdominal pressure. • Patient reports change in cervical/vaginal discharge.	• Uterine contractions more frequent than every 10 minutes • Progressive cervical change: effacement >80%, dilation >2 cm • Short cervix • Positive fetal fibronectin or salivary estriol test
Intrauterine Growth Restriction	Fetal growth below norms	• Patient may report feeling that her baby is too small.	• Fundal height less than expected • Weight gain less than recommended
Placental Abnormalities	Abnormal placental implantation including placenta previa, when placenta is implanted over cervix, and abruptio placenta, when placenta detaches from uterus	• Patient reports abdominal pain.	• Vaginal bleeding • Nonreassuring fetal heart rate pattern • Abnormal ultrasound

Table 25.7 Common Complications in the Postpartum Period

COMPLICATION	DESCRIPTION	SUBJECTIVE DATA	OBJECTIVE DATA
Postpartum Hemorrhage	Estimated blood loss (EBL) greater than 500 mL at birth for vaginal birth or greater than 1000 mL after cesarean birth	• Patient reports vaginal bleeding that saturates more than one menstrual pad per hour.	• A 10% decrease in hematocrit between admission and postpartum • Uterine fundus may be relaxed or "boggy," even after circular massage, if caused by uterine atony. • If hemorrhage was caused by lacerations of the genital tract, fundus may be firm with continued bleeding.
Preeclampsia	High blood pressure often accompanied by organ damage	• Patient reports headaches, blurred vision, abdominal pain, dyspnea.	• Elevated blood pressure • Excessive edema in hands or face • Proteinuria greater than +1
Subinvolution of the Uterus	Slower than expected return of the uterus to prepregnant size	• Patient reports continued uterine bleeding. • Patient reports pelvic or back pain. • Patient reports fatigue or malaise.	• Uterine fundus is above expected level. • At 6 weeks postpartum, uterus has not returned to nonpregnant size.
Disseminated Intravascular Coagulation (DIC)	Blood disorder in which clotting proteins become overactive and are depleted rapidly	• Patient reports bruising easily. • Patient reports spontaneous bleeding.	• Bleeding from intravenous (IV) site, gums, or nose • Petechiae • Tachycardia • Diaphoresis • Decreased platelets and abnormal clotting factor values
Endometriosis	Lining of the uterus (endometrium) grows ectopically.	• Patient reports chills. • Patient reports extreme pelvic pain upon fundus assessment. • Patient reports increased or foul-smelling lochia.	• Fever • Tachycardia
Deep Vein Thrombophlebitis	Blood clot forms in a vein, typically in the legs but also in the arms or neck	• Patient reports unilateral pain in lower (or upper) extremity.	• Warmth, redness, or swelling over a vein. • Vein feels cordlike. • Homan's sign may be positive.

COMPLICATION	DESCRIPTION	SUBJECTIVE DATA	OBJECTIVE DATA
Hematoma	A localized collection of blood outside the blood vessels	• Patient reports pain in the perineum.	• Perineum is bulging or bluish.
Mastitis	Infection in the breast tissue	• Patient reports mastalgia (breast pain).	• Unilateral red streaks on breast • Presence of flulike symptoms, including fever

Evidence-Based Practice:

Screening for Depression

Screening for depression in pregnant and postpartum women has been shown to be effective in decreasing symptoms of depression in those with a diagnosis of depression and in the reduction of the prevalence of depression (O'Connor, Rossum, & Henninger, 2016).

Application Through Critical Thinking

CASE STUDY

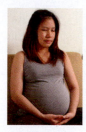

Source: graphixmania/ Shutterstock.

Susan Li, gravida 1, para 1, age 22, is married to a 23-year-old sales clerk who is required to work as much as possible because of family financial problems. Ms. Li has 2 years of college education and was working as a waitress before this pregnancy. She speaks English very well. Her only local family member is her sister, who also works full time. The rest of her family is in China. She gave birth to a 7 lb, 4 oz female infant 24 hours ago. Her blood loss at birth was 400 mL, and her placenta was intact following delivery. A first-degree laceration occurred during birth and was repaired, and a small cluster hemorrhoid developed during the pushing stage of labor. She had an unmedicated birth and breastfed her baby girl right away and two times since for approximately 5 minutes each time. No family members have been to see her since the birth.

COMPLETE DOCUMENTATION

POSTPARTUM ASSESSMENT

Birth: 5/16/2018 09:05

Incision Type: Abdomen intact

Blood Type: B+ Rubella: Nonimmune

Newborn: Female, in room, breastfeeding

Vital Signs: T-97.6, P-74, R-12, BP-104/74

Pain: Intensity 5/10, Location-perineal, Management-heat/ cold, pharmaceuticals

Activity: Out of bed independently

Gastrointestinal: Diet-regular, Fluid Intake-550 ml

Breasts: Smooth, even pigmentation, no redness or warmth, Milk tension-filling, Nipples-supple, intact

Lungs: Clear to bases bilaterally

Reproductive:

Fundus (consistency, height, position): FF U-1
Lochia (type, amount): rubra, small
Incision: N/A
Redness: Ecchymosis+
Edema: +
Approximation: +
Discharge: -
Dressing: N/A

Elimination: UTI sx-None; Voiding-350 cc; Bowel (sounds, flatus, stool): +++

Extremities: Edema-none noted

Psychosocial:

Rest/sleep: adequate
Bonding: +
Adaptation: Taking in
Social Work Consult: yes

CRITICAL THINKING QUESTIONS

1. What should the nurse's priority assessments for Susan be during this postpartum assessment exam at 24 hours after birth?

2. Susan complains that her stitches and hemorrhoids are painful at the level of 7 on a 10-point pain scale. Describe the recommended nursing assessment and relief measures.

3. At 5 weeks postpartum, Susan's sister brings her to the clinic nurse. Susan tells the nurse she feels hopeless and overwhelmed and has been irritable and anxious for the past 3 weeks. What should the nurse's action be?

4. What psychosocial consideration are applicable to this situation?

REFERENCES

American College of Cardiology. (2018). *Dyslipidemia in pregnancy.* Retrieved from https://www.acc.org/latest-in-cardiology/articles/2014/07/18/16/08/dyslipidemia-in-pregnancy

American College of Obstetricians and Gynecologists (ACOG). (2012). *Committee opinion: Intimate partner violence.* Retrieved from https://www.acog.org/Clinical-Guidance-and-Publications/Committee-Opinions/Committee-on-Health-Care-for-Underserved-Women/Intimate-Partner-Violence

American College of Obstetricians and Gynecologists (ACOG). (2013). *Hepatitis B and hepatitis C in pregnancy.* Retrieved from https://www.acog.org/Patients/FAQs/Hepatitis-B-and-Hepatitis-C-in-Pregnancy

American College of Obstetricians and Gynecologists. (2017a). Gestational diabetes mellitus. *ACOG Practice Bulletin, 180,* 1–15.

American College of Obstetricians and Gynecologists (ACOG). (2017b). *Obesity and pregnancy.* Retrieved from https://www.acog.org/Patients/FAQs/Obesity-and-Pregnancy

American Pregnancy Association (APA). (2017a). *Exercise in pregnancy.* Retrieved from http://americanpregnancy.org/pregnancy-health/exercise-and-pregnancy

American Pregnancy Association (APA). (2017b). *Fetal alcohol syndrome (FAS); Fetal alcohol spectrum disorders (FASD).* Retrieved from http://americanpregnancy.org/pregnancy-complications/fetal-alcohol-syndrome

American Pregnancy Association (APA). (2017c). *Miscarriage: Signs, symptoms, treatment, and prevention.* Retrieved from http://americanpregnancy.org/pregnancy-complications/miscarriage

American Pregnancy Association (APA). (2018a). *Bleeding during pregnancy.* Retrieved from http://americanpregnancy.org/pregnancy-complications/bleeding-during-pregnancy

American Pregnancy Association (APA). (2018b). *Calculating conception.* Retrieved from http://americanpregnancy.org/while-pregnant/calculating-conception-due-date

American Pregnancy Association (APA). (2018c). *Herbs and pregnancy.* Retrieved from http://americanpregnancy.org/pregnancy-health/herbs-and-pregnancy

American Society of Clinical Oncology. (2018). *Cancer during pregnancy.* Retrieved from https://www.cancer.net/navigating-cancer-care/dating-sex-and-reproduction/cancer-during-pregnancy

Castanon, A., Landy, R., Brocklehurst, P., Evans, H., Peebles, D., Singh, N., … Sasieni, P. (2014). Risk of preterm delivery with increasing depth of excision for cervical intraepithelial neoplasia in England: Nested case-control study. *British Medical Journal, 349.* doi:10.1136/bmj.g6223

Centers for Disease Control and Prevention (CDC). (n.d.) *About DES.* Retrieved from http://www.cdc.gov/des/consumers/about/index.html

Centers for Disease Control and Prevention (CDC). (2011). *What is PedNSS/PNSS? PNSS health indicators.* Retrieved from http://www.cdc.gov/pednss/what_is/pnss_health_indicators.htm

Centers for Disease Control and Prevention (CDC). (2014a). *Radiation and pregnancy: A fact sheet for clinicians.* Retrieved from https://emergency.cdc.gov/radiation/prenatalphysician.asp

Centers for Disease Control and Prevention (CDC). (2014b). *Tuberculosis and pregnancy.* Retrieved from https://www.cdc.gov/tb/topic/populations/pregnancy/default.htm

Centers for Disease Control and Prevention (CDC). (2015). *Physical activity: Healthy pregnant or postpartum women.* Retrieved from https://www.cdc.gov/physicalactivity/basics/pregnancy/index.htm

Centers for Disease Control and Prevention (CDC). (2016). *Evidence-based teen prevention programs.* Retrieved from https://www.cdc.gov/teenpregnancy/practitioner-tools-resources/evidence-based-programs.html

Centers for Disease Control and Prevention (CDC). (2017). *Facts about stillbirth.* Retrieved from https://www.cdc.gov/ncbddd/stillbirth/facts.html

Centers for Disease Control and Prevention (CDC). (2018). *Folic acid.* Retrieved from http://www.cdc.gov/ncbddd/folicacid/index.html

Cleveland Clinic. (2018). *Breastfeeding after breast or nipple surgery*. Retrieved from https://my.clevelandclinic.org/health/articles/15585-breastfeeding-after-breast-or-nipple-surgery

Coleman, G. D. (2015). Pregnancy after rape. *International Journal of Women's Health and Wellness, 1*(1). Retrieved from https://clinmedjournals.org/articles/ijwhw/international-journal-of-womens-health-and-wellness-ijwhw-1-004.pdf

Consumer Guide to Bariatric Surgery. (2018). *Pregnancy after bariatric surgery*. Retrieved from http://www.yourbariatricsurgeryguide.com/pregnancy

Cybulska, B. (2013). Immediate medical care after sexual assault. *Best Practice and Research Clinical Obstetrics and Gynaecology, 27*(1), 141–149. doi:10.1016/j.bpobgyn.2012.08.013

Endeshaw, M., Abebe, F., Bedimo, M., Asrat, A., Gebeyehu, A., & Keno, A. (2016). Family history of hypertension increases risk of preeclampsia in pregnant women: A case-control study. *Universa Medicina, 35*(3), 181–191. doi:10.18051/UnivMed.2016.v35

Food and Nutrition Board, Institute of Medicine, National Academies. (2011). *Dietary reference intakes (DRIs): Estimated average requirements*. Retrieved from http://iom.edu/Activities/Nutrition/SummaryDRIs/~/media/Files/Activity%20Files/Nutrition/DRIs/1_%20EARs.pdf.

Friel, L A. (2017). *Anemia in pregnancy*. Retrieved from https://www.merckmanuals.com/professional/gynecology-and-obstetrics/pregnancy-complicated-by-disease/anemia-in-pregnancy

Hamilton, B. E., Martin, J. A., Osterman, M. J. K., Driscoll, A. K., & Rossen, L. M. (2017). *Births: Provisional data for 2016. Vital statistics rapid release; no 2*. Hyattsville, MD: National Center for Health Statistics. Retrieved from https://www.cdc.gov/nchs/data/vsrr/report002.pdf

Hooton, T. M., & Gupta, K. (2017). *Urinary tract infections and asymptomatic bacteriuria in pregnancy*. Retrieved from https://www.uptodate.com/contents/urinary-tract-infections-and-asymptomatic-bacteriuria-in-pregnancy

Institute of Medicine and National Research Council. (2009). *Weight gain during pregnancy: Reexamining the guidelines*. Washington, DC: The National Academies Press. Retrieved from https://www.ncbi.nlm.nih.gov/books/NBK32813/pdf/Bookshelf_NBK32813.pdf

Johnson, E. K., & Kim, E. D. (2017). *Urinary tract infections in pregnancy*. Retrieved from https://emedicine.medscape.com/article/452604-overview

Lamont, K., Jones, G. T., & Bhattacharya, S. (2015). Risk of recurrent stillbirth: Systematic review and meta-analysis. *British Medical Journal, 350*. doi:10.1136/bmj.h3080

Magee Women's Hospital. (2018). *Intrauterine devices: Separating fact from fallacy*. Retrieved from https://www.medscape.com/viewarticle/718183_5

Malcova, E., Regan, A., Nassar, N., Raynes-Greenow, C., Leonard, H., Srinivasjois, R., … Pereira, G. (2018). Risk of stillbirth, preterm delivery, and fetal growth restriction following exposure in a previous birth: Systematic review and meta-analysis. *BJOG: An International Journal of Obstetrics and Gynaecology, 125*(2), 183–192. doi:10.1111/1471-0528.14906

March of Dimes. (2013). *Rubella and pregnancy*. Retrieved from https://www.marchofdimes.org/complications/rubella-and-pregnancy.aspx

March of Dimes. (2014). *Thrombophilias*. Retrieved from https://www.marchofdimes.org/complications/thrombophillias.aspx

March of Dimes. (2015). *Smoking during pregnancy*. Retrieved from http://www.marchofdimes.com/pregnancy/smoking-during-pregnancy.aspx

March of Dimes. (2016). *Street drugs and pregnancy*. Retrieved from https://www.marchofdimes.org/pregnancy/street-drugs-and-pregnancy.aspx

March of Dimes. (2018). *Bacterial vaginosis and pregnancy*. Retrieved from https://www.marchofdimes.org/complications/bacterial-vaginosis.aspx

Marieb, E. N., & Keller, S. M. (2018). *Essentials of human anatomy and physiology* (12th ed.). New York, NY: Pearson

Mayo Clinic. (2018a). *Fetal macrosomia: Complications*. Retrieved from https://www.mayoclinic.org/diseases-conditions/fetal-macrosomia/symptoms-causes/syc-20372579

Mayo Clinic. (2018b). *Pelvic inflammatory disease (PID)*. Retrieved from https://www.mayoclinic.org/diseases-conditions/pelvic-inflammatory-disease/symptoms-causes/syc-20352594

Mayo Clinic Staff. (2016). *Pregnancy after miscarriage: What you need to know*. Retrieved from https://www.mayoclinic.org/healthy-lifestyle/getting-pregnant/in-depth/pregnancy-after-miscarriage/art-20044134

Mayo Clinic Staff. (2018). *High blood pressure and pregnancy: Know the facts*. Retrieved from https://www.mayoclinic.org/healthy-lifestyle/pregnancy-week-by-week/in-depth/pregnancy/art-20046098

MedlinePlus. (2018). *Delivery presentations*. Retrieved from http://www.nlm.nih.gov/medlineplus/ency/patientinstructions/000621.htm

Morgan, J. A., & Cooper, D. B. (2018). *StatPearls: Pregnancy, group B Streptococcus*. Retrieved from https://www.ncbi.nlm.nih.gov/books/NBK482443

National Down Syndrome Society. (2018). *What is Down Syndrome?* Retrieved from https://www.ndss.org/about-down-syndrome/down-syndrome/

National Institute of Diabetes and Digestive and Kidney Diseases (NIDDKD). (2017). *Thyroid disease and pregnancy*. Retrieved from https://www.niddk.nih.gov/health-information/endocrine-diseases/pregnancy-thyroid-disease

O'Connor, E., Rossum, R. C., & Henninger, M. (2016). Primary care screening for and treatment of depression in pregnant and postpartum women: Evidence report and systematic review for the US Preventive Services Task Force. *Journal of the American Medical Association, 315*(4), 388–406. doi:10.1001/jama.2015.18948

Patel, P. R., Laz, T. H., & Berenson, A. B. (2015). Patient characteristics associated with pregnancy ambivalence. *Journal of Women's Health, 24*(1), 37–41. doi:10.1089/jwh.2014.4924

Preeclampsia Foundation. (2016). *Signs and symptoms*. Retrieved from https://www.preeclampsia.org/health-information/sign-symptoms

Sachs, C. J., & Chapman, J. (2017). *Sexual assault, history and physical*. Retrieved from https://www.ncbi.nlm.nih.gov/books/NBK448154

Smith, A. (2016). *Engorgement*. Retrieved from https://www.breastfeedingbasics.com/articles/engorgement

Stanford Children's Health. (2018). *Diabetes and pregnancy*. Retrieved from http://www.stanfordchildrens.org/en/topic/default?id=infant-of-diabetic-mother-90-P02354

Stovall, D. W. (2017). *Patient education: Dilation and curettage (D and C) (Beyond the basics)*. Retrieved from https://www.uptodate.com/contents/dilation-and-curettage-d-and-c-beyond-the-basics

Tan, E. K., & Tan, E. L. (2013). Alterations in physiology and anatomy during pregnancy. *Best Practice & Research Clinical Obstetrics & Gynaecology, 27*(6), 791–802. doi:10.1016/j.bpobgyn.2013.08.001

Tobah, Y. B. (2015). *What are the risks associated with chicken pox and pregnancy?* Retrieved from http://www.mayoclinic.org/healthy-living/pregnancy-week-by-week/expert-answers/chickenpox-and-pregnancy/faq-20057886

Tobah, Y. B. (2017). *What's the significance of a fundal height measurement?* Retrieved from https://www.mayoclinic.org/healthy-lifestyle/pregnancy-week-by-week/expert-answers/fundal-height/faq-20057962

U.S. Department of Agriculture, Food Safety and Inspection Service (FSIS). (2017). *Protect your baby and yourself from listeriosis*. Retrieved from http://www.fsis.usda.gov/wps/portal/fsis/topics/food-safety-education/get-answers/food-safety-fact-sheets/foodborne-illness-and-disease/protect-your-baby-and-yourself-from-listeriosis/ct_index

U.S. Department of Health and Human Services. (2017). *Preventing mother-to-child HIV transmission after birth*. Retrieved from https://aidsinfo.nih.gov/understanding-hiv-aids/fact-sheets/24/71/preventing-mother-to-child-transmission-of-hiv-after-birth

USC Fertility. (2018). *Uterine scarring*. Retrieved from http://uscfertility.org/causes-infertility/uterine-scarring

Warnes, C. A., & Krasuski, R. (n.d.). *Pregnancy in women with congenital heart disease*. Retrieved from https://www.achaheart.org/your-heart/health-information/pregnancy-and-chd

WebMD. (2017a). *Asthma and pregnancy: What to know*. Retrieved from https://www.webmd.com/asthma/asthma-pregnancy#1

WebMD. (2017b). *Pregnancy and sexually transmitted diseases*. Retrieved from https://www.webmd.com/baby/pregnancy-sexually-transmitted-diseases#1

Yoo, S. H., Guzzo, K. B., & Hayford, S. R. (2014). Understanding the complexity of ambivalence toward pregnancy: Does it predict inconsistent use of contraception? *Biodemography and Social Biology, 60*(1), 49–66. doi:10.1080/19485565.2014.905193

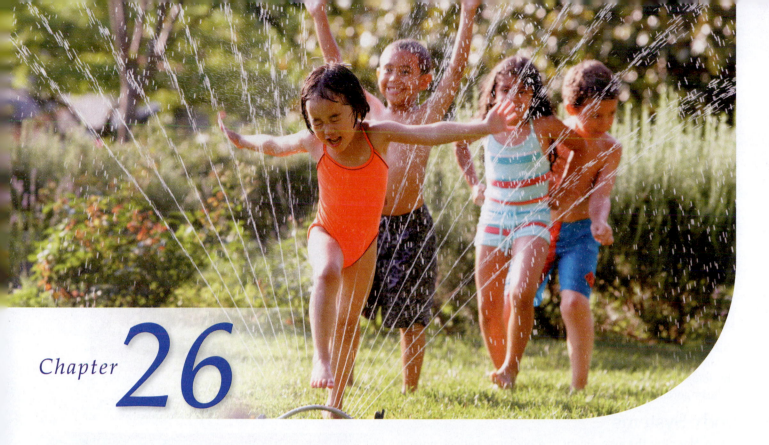

Chapter 26

Infants, Children, and Adolescents

LEARNING OUTCOMES

Upon completion of this chapter, you will be able to:

1. Describe unique aspects of anatomy and physiology of body systems for infants, children, and adolescents.

2. Identify the anatomic, physiologic, developmental, psychosocial, and cultural variations that guide assessment of infants, children, and adolescents.

3. Determine questions about infants, children, and adolescents to use for the focused interview.

4. Outline the techniques for physical assessment of infants, children, and adolescents.

5. Generate the appropriate documentation to describe the assessment findings for infants, children, and adolescents.

6. Identify abnormal findings in the physical assessment of infants, children, and adolescents.

KEY TERMS

epispadias, 674

febrile seizures, 693

gynecomastia, 672

hypospadias, 674

jaundice, 668

labial adhesions, 675

lanugo, 668

milia, 668

nevus flammeus, 668

otitis media, 670

phimosis, 674

thelarche, 672

vellus hair, 668

vernix caseosa, 668

MEDICAL LANGUAGE

a-, an-	Prefix meaning "no," "not," "without"
ante-	Prefix meaning "before," "forward"
cephalo-	Prefix meaning "head"
-genesis	Suffix meaning "production," "development"
gastro-	Prefix meaning "stomach"
-oxia	Suffix meaning "oxygen"
photo-	Prefix meaning "light"

Introduction

The bulk of this textbook focuses on the health and physical assessment of adults. This chapter will shift that focus to the pediatric population: infants, children, and adolescents. Ranging in age from birth to young adulthood, the assessment of infants, children, and adolescents presents a set of unique challenges to the nurse. This chapter will outline the anatomic and physiologic differences, the foundations of child development, along with the psychosocial and cultural variations you will need to perform a comprehensive health history and physical assessment of infants, children, and adolescents.

Anatomy and Physiology Review

This section highlights differences between the normal adult and infants, children, and adolescents in terms of anatomy and physiology. The following sections include descriptions of some of the important differences that will affect assessment findings.

Body Systems

When planning the assessment of a pediatric patient, nurses must be aware of the anatomic and physiologic differences across the lifespan. In infants and children, the developmental, psychosocial, and cultural variations influence the questions and examination at each age and stage of childhood.

Skin, Hair, and Nails

INFANTS At birth, the newborn's skin typically is covered with **vernix caseosa**, a white, cheeselike mixture of sebum and epidermal cells. The skin color of newborns is often bright red for the first 24 hours of life and then fades. Some newborns develop physiologic **jaundice** 3 to 4 days after birth, resulting in a yellowing of the skin, sclera, and mucous membranes. Jaundice can occur within the first 24 hours after birth or as late as 7 days postnatally. Physiologic jaundice is a temporary condition treated with fluids and phototherapy. The skin of dark-skinned newborns normally is not fully pigmented until 2 to 3 months after birth. An infant's skin is very thin, soft, and free of terminal hair.

Many harmless skin markings are common in newborns. For example, they may have areas of tiny white facial papules. These are called **milia** and are due to sebum that collects in the openings of hair follicles (Figure 26.1 ■). Milia usually disappear spontaneously within a few weeks of birth. Vascular markings are also common and may include **nevus flammeus** or "stork bites," which are irregular red or pink patches found most commonly on the back of the neck. Vascular markings disappear spontaneously within a year of birth. The newborn may also have transient mottling or other transient color changes, such as harlequin color change, in which a side-lying infant becomes markedly pink on the lower side and pale on the higher side. Mongolian spots are gray, blue, or purple spots in the sacral and buttocks areas of newborns (Figure 26.2 ■). Mongolian spots occur in about 90% of newborns of African ancestry and in about 80% of newborns of Asian or Native American ancestry and in those with dark or olive skin tones. Mongolian spots fade early in life, usually by 3 years of age. Mongolian spots should not be interpreted as signs of abuse.

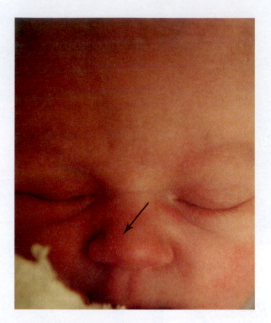

Figure 26.1 Milia.

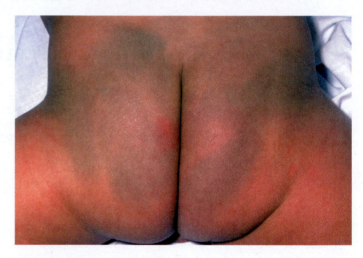

Figure 26.2 Mongolian spots.
Source: Mediscan/Alamy Stock Photo.

Because the subcutaneous fat layer is poorly developed in infants and the eccrine sweat glands do not secrete until after the first few months of life, their temperature regulation is inefficient and absorption of topical medications is increased. The fine, downy hair of the newborn, called **lanugo**, is replaced within a few months by **vellus hair**. Hair growth accelerates throughout childhood.

CHILDREN AND ADOLESCENTS Throughout childhood, the epidermis thickens, pigmentation increases, and more subcutaneous fat is deposited, especially in females during puberty. During adolescence, both the sweat glands and the oil glands increase their production. Increased production of sebum by the oil glands predisposes adolescents to develop acne (Figure 26.3 ■). Increased axillary perspiration occurs as the apocrine glands mature, and body odor may develop for the first time. Pubic and axillary hair appears during adolescence, and males may develop facial and chest hair.

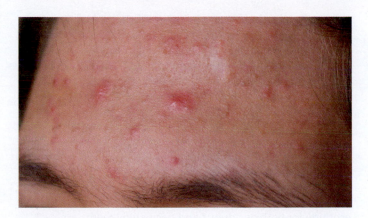

Figure 26.3 Acne.
Source: olavs/Shutterstock.

Head, Neck, and Related Lymphatics

INFANTS An infant's head should be measured at each visit until 2 years of age. The newborn's head is about 34 cm (13 to 14 in.), and this is generally equal to the chest circumference. The shape of the head may indicate *molding,* the shaping of the head by pressure on the bony structures as the head moves through the vaginal canal during childbirth. The degree of molding will be influenced by the presenting part of the head and type of birth. Usually, it takes several days for the head to take on the more normal round shape. Suture lines should be open, as are the fontanels. The anterior fontanel is diamond shaped, and the posterior fontanel is triangular in shape (Figure 26.4■). The fontanels should be firm and even with the skull. Slight pulsations are normal. The posterior fontanel closes at approximately 2 months of age; the anterior fontanel closes between 12 and 18 months of age. The neck of the newborn is short with many skinfolds and begins to lengthen over time. By about 4 months of age, the infant begins to demonstrate control of the head. In toddlers, the head is relatively large and the muscles of the neck are underdeveloped compared with adults. The proportions change throughout the preschool years, and by school age the proportions are similar to those of adults.

The thyroid gland, located in the neck, plays an important role in growth and development. Infants have shorter necks than older children and adults. The thyroid is difficult to palpate on an infant, but it can be accomplished on a child using two or three fingers. Abnormalities in thyroid function are generally detected by assessment of growth and development and through laboratory testing. All U.S. states require newborn screening for congenital hypothyroidism (reduced thyroid function). This screening is conducted through blood testing for thyroid-stimulating hormone levels (Leung, 2018). Ideally, blood samples for this test should be taken when the newborn is 2 to 4 days old.

CHILDREN AND ADOLESCENTS The lymph nodes are present at birth, but differentiation and growth of lymphatic tissue occur primarily between ages 4 and 8 years. As such, preschoolers and school-age children often have "shotty" lymph nodes and slightly enlarged tonsils. (Shotty nodes are noninfected, nontender, slightly enlarged lymph nodes that move when palpated and feel firmer than normal.) Most children under 6 to 7 years have palpable, shotty femoral or cervical lymph nodes. Newborns and infants with a history of internal fetal monitoring during labor often have palpable occipital lymph nodes.

Eyes, Ears, Nose, Mouth, and Throat

INFANTS Babies can see at birth, but the visual acuity of newborns is not as sharp as adults. Children typically have 20/20 vision by the age of 7 years. At birth, the eyes of the neonate should be symmetric. The pupils should be equal and respond to light. The iris is generally brown in dark-skinned neonates, and it is slate gray-blue in light-skinned neonates. By about the third month of age, the color of the eyes begins to change to a more permanent shade. Many times, the eyelids are edematous at birth. Little to no tears are present at birth but begin to appear by the fourth week. Binocular vision (vision in both eyes) begins to develop by 6 weeks of age. Before this time, neonates will fixate on a bright or moving object. An infant who cannot focus on objects at birth needs further evaluation.

The eyes reach adult size by 8 years of age. The *red reflex,* a glowing red color that fills the pupil as light from the

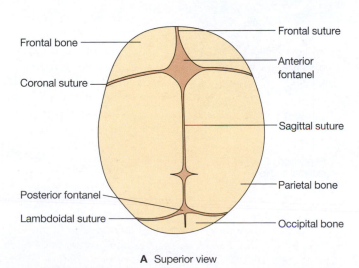

A Superior view

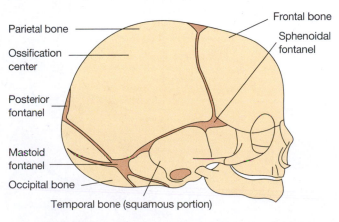

B Lateral view

Figure 26.4 The newborn's skull.

ophthalmoscope reflects off the retina, should be elicited from birth. A whitened red reflex occurs with congenital cataracts. Infants and preschool children with the cancer retinoblastoma often present a history of a diminished red reflex or a "white glow" in the pupil.

The infant's auditory canal is shorter than the adult's and has an upward curve, which persists until about 3 years of age. For children age 3 years and younger, the nurse should pull the earlobe down and back when examining the tympanic membrane with the otoscope, as illustrated in Figure 26.5 ■.

CHILDREN AND ADOLESCENTS Peripheral vision may be assessed by confrontation in children older than 3 years of age. It is important to assess extraocular muscle function as early as possible in young children because delay can lead to permanent visual damage. The corneal light reflex, Hirschberg's test, can be used to determine symmetry of muscle function. Lateral deviations of the eye (disconjugate gaze) are normal findings until 2 months of age (Mansoor, Mansoor, & Ahmed, 2016).

The eustachian tubes of infants, toddlers, and preschoolers are shorter, straighter, and more level than those in older children and adults. This normal variant, in combination with increased frequency of colds and respiratory infections, results in an increased incidence of **otitis media**, or middle ear infections, in children under the age of 4 years. The occurrence of otitis media peaks between 6 and 18 months of age. Children with middle ear infections typically present with fever, decreased appetite, irritability, and the inability to sleep lying down. The tympanic membrane is a vascular tissue that appears red with infection, fever, or any condition that results in skin flushing. Children with red tympanic membranes and no purulent discharge in the middle ear space do not have bacterial otitis media.

The nose of a child is too small to examine with a speculum. The maxillary and ethmoid sinuses are present at birth, but they are proportionately smaller than in adults. The sphenoid sinuses develop before age 5 years and the frontal sinuses by age 10 years. Children rarely have infections of the ethmoid sinuses. The frontal sinuses cause infection only in older school-age and adolescent children. Children under the age of 5 years often have yellow-green nasal discharge during upper respiratory infections because they cannot efficiently clear their nasal passages.

Both sets of teeth develop before birth. Deciduous (baby) teeth begin to erupt between 6 months and 2 years of age. Eruption of permanent teeth begins at around age 6 and continues through adolescence. Salivation begins at 3 months of age. Drooling of saliva occurs for several months until swallowing saliva is learned. Figure 26.6 ■ shows a typical sequence of tooth eruption for both deciduous and permanent teeth.

Because differentiation and growth of lymphatic tissue occur primarily between ages 4 and 8 years, preschoolers and school-age children often have slightly enlarged tonsils. Enlarged, noninfected tonsils are common in children ages 4 to 8 years.

Lungs and Thorax

INFANTS During development, the fetus receives its nutrients and oxygen from its mother. The lungs are nonfunctional, and oxygen is carried in blood from the placenta to the right side of the heart. The majority of this blood passes through the foramen ovale to the left side of the heart, then into the aorta to enter the systemic circulation. The *foramen ovale* is a passageway for blood between the right and left atria. The rest of the blood passes through the pulmonary artery and ductus arteriosus and enters the aorta (Figure 26.7 ■). The *ductus arteriosus* is an opening between the pulmonary artery and the descending aorta.

Inflation of the lungs at birth causes the pulmonary vasculature to dilate. Oxygenation occurs for the first time within the newborn's lungs. The foramen ovale closes shortly after birth because of increased pulmonary vascular return and decreased pressure in the right side of the heart. The ductus arteriosus

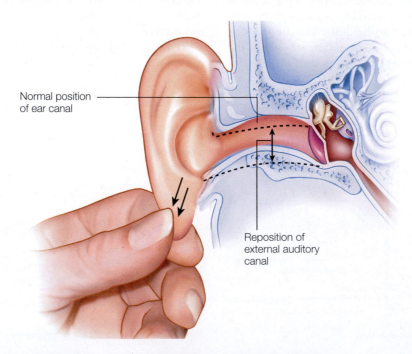

Normal position of ear canal

Reposition of external auditory canal

Figure 26.5 Positioning of external auditory canal for tympanic membrane visualization.

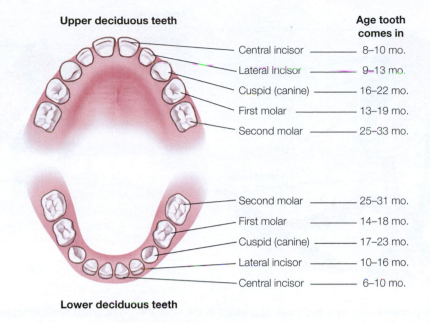

Upper deciduous teeth

	Age tooth comes in
Central incisor	8–10 mo.
Lateral incisor	9–13 mo.
Cuspid (canine)	16–22 mo.
First molar	13–19 mo.
Second molar	25–33 mo.

	Age tooth comes in
Second molar	25–31 mo.
First molar	14–18 mo.
Cuspid (canine)	17–23 mo.
Lateral incisor	10–16 mo.
Central incisor	6–10 mo.

Lower deciduous teeth

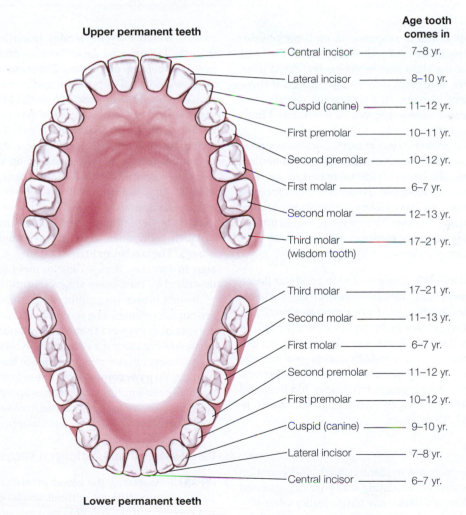

Upper permanent teeth

	Age tooth comes in
Central incisor	7–8 yr.
Lateral incisor	8–10 yr.
Cuspid (canine)	11–12 yr.
First premolar	10–11 yr.
Second premolar	10–12 yr.
First molar	6–7 yr.
Second molar	12–13 yr.
Third molar (wisdom tooth)	17–21 yr.

Third molar	17–21 yr.
Second molar	11–13 yr.
First molar	6–7 yr.
Second premolar	11–12 yr.
First premolar	10–12 yr.
Cuspid (canine)	9–10 yr.
Lateral incisor	7–8 yr.
Central incisor	6–7 yr.

Lower permanent teeth

Figure 26.6 Deciduous and permanent teeth.

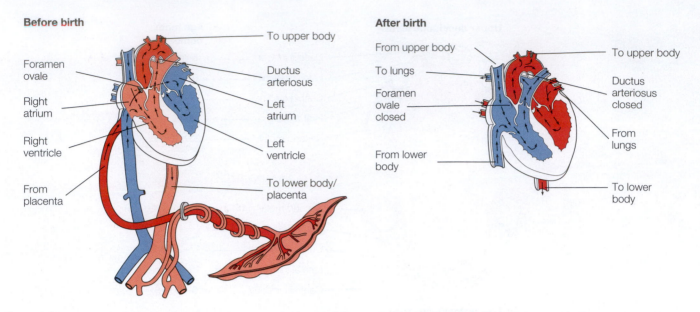

Figure 26.7 Location of the main structures and vessels present in the fetal and postpartal cardiovascular anatomy.

closes within 24 to 48 hours in response to multiple physiologic events, including decreased pulmonary resistance and decreased pressure in the right atrium versus increased pressure in the left atrium. Murmurs may be auscultated if these openings remain patent. However, if a ventricular septal defect is present, the murmur it causes may not be auscultated until week 4 to week 6 after birth.

The infant's arterial pressure rises at birth, and the systemic vascular resistance increases significantly when the umbilical cord is cut. Over time, the left ventricle increases in size and mass as it works to pump blood into the aorta against increasingly elevating systemic vascular resistance. The blood pressure of the full-term infant may average 70/50 mmHg, and 10 mmHg less in both systolic and diastolic readings in the preterm newborn. Weight significantly influences blood pressure.

CHILDREN AND ADOLESCENTS Compared with adults, children have much smaller, more compliant airways until early adolescence. Until that time, children are more prone to airway collapse and blockage. Oxygen needs are higher in small children because their increased metabolic rates result in higher oxygen consumption. It is important to carefully assess and manage children who show signs of dyspnea and respiratory distress. The risk of respiratory failure is greatest in infants, toddlers, and preschoolers, but children of all ages experience respiratory failure much more quickly than adults.

Breasts and Axillae

INFANTS Inverted nipples are evident at birth and common until adolescence. Because of circulating maternal estrogen and prolactin, male and female infants may have a milky white discharge from their nipples that is commonly called "witch's milk." This condition will resolve within 1 to 2 weeks after birth when maternal hormone levels decrease.

CHILDREN AND ADOLESCENTS Breast tissue starts to enlarge in females with the onset of puberty, usually between the ages of 9 and 13. At first there is only a bud around the nipple and

areola, which may be tender initially. The ductile system matures, extensive fat deposits occur, and the areola and nipples grow and become pigmented. These changes are correlated with an increased level of estrogen and progesterone in the body as sexual maturity progresses. Growth of the breasts is not necessarily steady or symmetric. This may be frustrating or embarrassing to some girls. Because a female's primary sexual organs cannot be observed, breast development provides visual confirmation that the adolescent is becoming a woman. For the developing adolescent, her breasts are a visible symbol of her feminine identity and an important part of her body image and self-esteem. The nurse can reassure girls that the rate of breast tissue growth is dependent on changing hormone levels and is uniquely individual, as are the eventual size and shape of the breasts. **Thelarche**, or breast budding, is often the first pubertal sign in females. Breast development follows a clear pattern described by the Tanner stages (Figure 26.8 ■).

Benign breast lumps (fibroadenomas) in adolescent females are not uncommon. The nurse should reassure the girl and her parents or caregivers that no correlation has been established between fibroadenomas and malignant cancers.

Adolescent males may experience temporary breast enlargement, called **gynecomastia**, in one or both breasts. This condition is usually self-limiting and resolves spontaneously. Another concern to adolescent males is transient masses beneath one areola or both. These "breast buds" usually disappear within a year of onset.

Cardiovascular and Peripheral Vascular System

INFANTS Assessing the blood pressure of an infant less than 1 year of age is difficult without special equipment. It is usually not necessary if the infant is moving well and the skin color is good. However, if the infant is lethargic and tires easily during feeding or if the skin becomes cyanotic when the infant cries, the blood pressure should be measured with a Doppler flowmeter. A newborn's blood pressure is much lower than that of an adult and gradually increases with age. The systolic pressure of a newborn is 60 to 76 mmHg; the diastolic pressure is 35 to 55 mmHg.

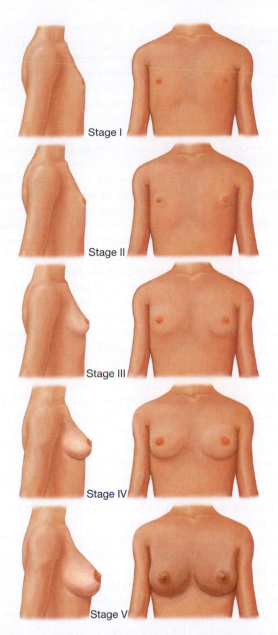

Figure 26.8 Tanner's stages of breast development: I, Preadolescent. Only the nipple is raised above the level of the breast, as in the child. II, Budding stage. Areola increased in diameter and surrounding area slightly elevated. III, Breast and areola enlarged. No contour separation. IV, Areola forms a secondary elevation above that of the breast in half of girls. V, Areola is usually part of the general breast contour and is strongly pigmented. Nipple usually projects.

The heart rate of the newborn initially may be as high as 160 to 180 beats/min. Over the first 6 to 8 hours, it gradually decreases to an average of 115 to 120 beats/min. Stimulation that causes crying, screaming, or coughing may cause the heart rate to rise temporarily to 180 beats/min.

A newborn's cardiovascular system undergoes tremendous changes at birth and during the first several days of life. The infant should be easily aroused and alert. Regardless of the baby's race, the skin should demonstrate perfusion with pink quality in the nail beds, mucous membranes, and conjunctiva.

Precordial bulging and chest deformities, such as pigeon chest and barrel chest, are of concern.

CHILDREN AND ADOLESCENTS All children 3 years and older should have their blood pressure evaluated during their well-child examination. Children younger than 3 years should have their blood pressure evaluated only if they display symptoms of high blood pressure or are at risk for high blood pressure (Moyer & U.S. Preventive Services Task Force, 2013). The cuff should be no larger than two-thirds of the child's arm or smaller than half of the length of the child's arm between the elbow and the shoulder. Pediatric blood pressure cuffs are available.

In young children, the blood pressure should be measured on the thigh to rule out a significant difference between upper- and lower-extremity pressure. Such a difference in pressure could indicate a narrowing (coarctation) of the aorta. In a baby under 1 year of age, the systolic pressure in the thigh should equal that of the arm. A child over 1 year of age will have a systolic pressure in the thigh that is 10 to 40 mmHg higher than that in the arm. The diastolic pressure in the thigh should equal that in the arm.

The pulse increases if the child has a fever. For every degree of fever, the pulse may increase 8 to 10 beats per minute (beats/min). The lymphatic system develops rapidly from birth until puberty and then subsides in adulthood. The presence of enlarged lymph nodes in a child may not indicate illness. However, if an infection is present, the nodes may enlarge considerably.

Abdomen and Gastrointestinal System

INFANTS The abdomen of the newborn and infant is round. The umbilical cord, containing two arteries and one vein, is ligated at birth. The stump dries and ultimately forms the umbilicus. Typically, the umbilical cord will dry and fall off 10 to 14 days after birth.

CHILDREN AND ADOLESCENTS The toddler has a characteristic potbelly appearance as depicted in Figure 26.9 ■. Respirations are abdominal; therefore, movement of the abdomen is seen with breathing. This breathing pattern is evident until about the sixth year, the age at which respirations become thoracic.

Peristaltic waves are usually more visible in infants and children than in adults because the muscle wall of the abdomen is thinner. Children have the tendency to swallow more air than adults when eating, thus creating a greater sound of tympany, a loud, high-pitched, drumlike tone, when percussion is performed. The area of tympany on the right side of the abdomen is smaller because the liver is larger in children.

Congenital defects such as cleft lip, cleft palate, esophageal atresia, pyloric stenosis, and hernias influence the nutritional status, growth, and development of the child and, therefore, must be assessed with care. The size of the abdomen at all ages may be an indication of the nutritional state of the child.

During palpation, the liver edge may be palpable at the right lower costal margin because the thoracic cage of young children is smaller than in older individuals. The lower liver edge is palpable 1 to 2 cm (0.39–0.78 in.) below the costal margin in most infants. Any liver edge that is palpable more than 2 cm below the costal margin indicates hepatomegaly and should be evaluated. If during palpation the nurse detects the presence of tenderness or masses, palpation should be stopped. For example,

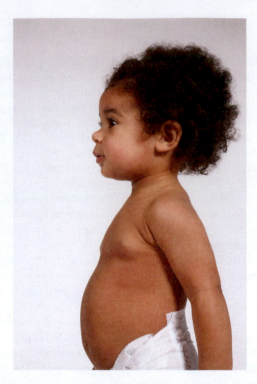

Figure 26.9 Potbelly stance of toddler.
Source: Alex Cao/Photodisc/Getty Images.

a Wilms tumor is a malignancy of the kidney commonly diagnosed in infants and toddlers. The most common presentation of this tumor is parental history of feeling an abdominal mass during bathing or diaper changes. Palpation of the tumor will disseminate the tumor seeds into the abdomen. Children with a suspected Wilms tumor should be referred for immediate evaluation. Other masses that may be palpated in the abdomen include constipation, which may result in a palpable cigar-shaped mass in the left lower quadrant.

Umbilical hernias cause a protrusion at the umbilicus and are visible at birth (Figure 26.10 ■). Umbilical hernias are more common in African American children and among infants who are born prematurely. The majority of umbilical hernias close before 5 years of age. Umbilical hernias require no medical intervention unless they incarcerate, cause symptoms, enlarge, or persist after age 5 years (Troullioud Lucas & Mendez, 2017).

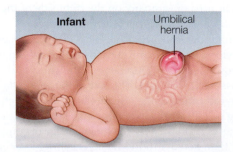

Figure 26.10 Umbilical hernia. Occurs when the abdominal rectus muscle separates or weakens, allowing abdominal structures, usually the intestines, to push through and come close to the skin. More common in children than in adults.

Enlargement of the spleen, or splenomegaly, is often found in patients diagnosed with infectious mononucleosis (Kessenich & Flanagan, 2015). Enlarged spleens are vulnerable to trauma because they no longer fit completely behind the thoracic cage. Careful abdominal assessment is indicated in any child with suspected mononucleosis. Splenomegaly is also a common complication in young children with sickle cell disease (SCD).

Acute gastroenteritis (AGE) is an acute, common diarrhea disease that may or may not be accompanied by vomiting. Additional symptoms include abdominal pain, cramping, and fever. Pertinent history findings include frequency and amount of diarrhea, vomiting, magnitude and duration of fever, and presence and location of abdominal pain. Exposure to infectious substances (e.g., *Salmonella* or *Shigella*) or exhibition of similar symptoms—as well as questions regarding hydration status—are important parts of the history. Abdominal examination may reveal hyperactive bowel sounds. Assessment of hydration status is essential and should include documentation of level of consciousness, presence of thirst, time and amount of last urination, vital signs (heart rate and blood pressure), skin turgor, and capillary perfusion of less than 2 seconds. Fontanels should be assessed, and depressed or sunken fontanels should be further evaluated.

Genitourinary System

INFANTS Renal blood flow increases with a significant allotment to the renal medulla at birth. The glomerular filtration rate also increases at birth compared with the fetal filtration rate and continues to increase until the first or second year of life. The fluid and electrolyte balance in an infant or child is fragile. Illnesses that cause dehydration, loss of fluids, or lack of fluid intake may rapidly lead to metabolic acidosis and fluid imbalance. Serious, chronic dysfunction of this system may impair the child's growth and development.

Minimal genital growth occurs before puberty. The onset of genital development is expected by age 11 in females and age 13 in males. Refer to the Tanner stages shown in Figure 26.11 ■ for males and Figure 26.8 for females.

The male newborn's genitals should be clearly evident and not ambiguous. If there is ambiguity, referral for genetic counseling is indicated. The penis may vary in size but averages about 2.5 cm (0.98 in.) in length and is slender. The urethral meatus should be in the center of the glans. If the opening is located on the underside of the glans, **hypospadias** is present. If the opening is on the superior aspect of the glans, **epispadias** exists. *Chordee*, a tight band of skin, causes bowing of the penis. The penis appears to have a C shape. This is associated with epispadias and hypospadias. The foreskin may be somewhat tight and not retractable until 2 or 3 years of age. By 3 years of age, penile foreskin is retractable in approximately 90% of male children (Modgil, Rai, & Anderson, 2014). If it is still tight after this time, **phimosis** exists. Cultural values and religious beliefs determine whether the family or caregiver circumcises the child. The family must be taught about either maintaining the cleanliness of the uncircumcised penis or caring for the penis in the days following a circumcision.

The male infant's scrotum should be consistent in color with other body parts. It should seem oversized in comparison with the penis. This proportion changes as the infant grows. If the scrotum is enlarged and filled with fluid, a hydrocele may be present. The testes should be palpable and are about 2 cm (0.78 in.)

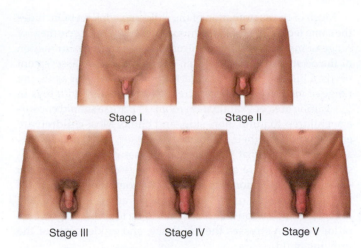

Stage I Stage II

Stage III Stage IV Stage V

Figure 26.11 The Tanner stages of male pubic hair and external genital development with sexual maturation. Stage I, preadolescent, hair present is no different from that on the abdomen. Testes, scrotum, and penis are the same size and shape as in a young child. Stage II, pubic hair is slightly pigmented, longer, straight, often still downy, usually at base of penis, sometimes on scrotum; enlargement of scrotum and testes. Stage III, pubic hair is dark, definitely pigmented, curly pubic hair appears around base of penis; enlargement of penis, especially in length, further enlargement of testes, descent of scrotum. Stage IV, pubic hair is definitely adult in type but not in extent, spreads no further than inguinal fold. Continued enlargement of penis and sculpturing of glans, increased pigmentation of scrotum. Stage V, hair spreads to medial surface of thighs in adult distribution. Adult stage, scrotum ample, penis reaching nearly to bottom of scrotum.

in diameter at birth. Undescended testes (cryptorchidism) is a common finding, especially if the infant is preterm. The testes should descend spontaneously within the first year of life. If both testes do not descend, the male will be infertile and will be at a greater risk for the development of testicular cancer. Enlargement of the testes in adolescence may indicate the presence of a tumor. Testes smaller than 1.5 to 2 cm (0.59 to 0.78 in.) may indicate adrenal hyperplasia.

The female infant's labia majora will be enlarged at birth in response to maternal hormones. The labia majora should cover the labia minora. The urinary meatus and vaginal orifice should be visible. No inflammation should be present. Bloody and mucoid discharge (false menses) is commonly seen in newborns due to exposure to maternal hormones in utero.

Masturbation and exploration of the genitals are usual practices in infants, toddlers, and preschoolers.

CHILDREN AND ADOLESCENTS Children do not have adult bladder capacities (approximately 700 mL) until adolescence. A quick way to estimate a child's bladder capacity is to use the following formula: the child's age (in years) plus or minus 2 oz. For example, a 4-year-old child has a bladder capacity of 2 to 6 oz:

$$\text{Age in years} \pm 2 \text{ oz} = 4 \pm 2 = 2 \text{ to } 6 \text{ oz}$$

On average, children attain bladder sphincter control at approximately age 3 years for females and age $3\frac{1}{2}$ years for males. Bladder training requires bladder sphincter control. Normal urine output for children is at least 1 to 2 mL/kg/hr.

Changes begin to occur at any time from 8 to 13 years of age; most commonly, in females breast changes begin at age 9 and menstruation at age 12. Release of estrogen initiates the changes, which are first demonstrated in the development of breast buds and growth of pubic hair, followed several years later by menstruation. Figure 26.8 describes Tanner's stages of maturation in girls. **Labial adhesions** occur when the labia minora fuse together. They are common in preadolescent females because decreased estrogen levels result in labial and genital atrophy. When present, labial adhesions extend from the posterior fourchette and look like a skin covering of all or part of the introitus. They are of medical concern if there is blockage of urinary flow or if they result in recurrent urinary tract infections.

The female child may experience a precocious puberty. Such children develop the adult female sex characteristics of dense pubic and axillary hair, breasts, and menstrual bleeding before 8 years of age. Early maturation may be caused by a hypothalamic tumor. Further, the early development of sexual characteristics allows for pregnancy before the child is intellectually or emotionally prepared for the experience. Early maturation can also lead to anemia related to menstrual bleeding and to emotional difficulties.

In males, precocious puberty is characterized by the development of adult male characteristics in males under age 10. It includes dense pubic hair, penile enlargement, and enlargement of the testes. Precocious puberty may be idiopathic or caused by a genetic trait, lesions in the pituitary gland or hypothalamus, or testicular tumors. Referral to an endocrinologist may be required for definitive diagnosis.

The onset of puberty in the male child occurs between 10 and 15 years of age. At this time, under the influence of elevating levels of testosterone, the male child begins to develop adult sexual characteristics. The testes and scrotum enlarge. Pubic, facial, and axillary hair develops. The penis begins to elongate, and the testes begin to produce mature sperm. The male child will experience unexpected erections and nocturnal emissions (wet dreams). Open, supportive communication is essential at this time. The nurse can show male children pictures of the sexual maturation of genitals to demonstrate that their development is normal. Figure 26.11 includes Tanner's staging for evaluating sexual maturity. The male child often displays a fascination with his genitals. Males may express curiosity in comparing their genitals with those of other preschool- and school-age children, both male and female.

Musculoskeletal System

INFANTS Fetal positioning and the birth process may cause musculoskeletal anomalies in the infant. These include tibial torsion, a curving apart of the tibias, and metatarsus adductus, a tendency of the forefoot to turn inward. Many such anomalies correct themselves spontaneously as the child grows and walks.

Newborns normally have flat feet; arches develop gradually during the preschool years. Before learning to walk, infants tend to exhibit genu varum (bowlegs). Then, as the child begins to walk, this tendency gradually reverses. By the age of 4 years, most children tend to exhibit genu valgum (knock knees). This condition also resolves spontaneously, usually by late childhood or early adolescence.

The nurse should inspect the newborn's spine. During fetal development and in the early stages of infancy, a baby's spine is C shaped (kyphotic). With development of muscles that allow for lifting of the head and walking, the infant's body weight shifts to the spine. Over time, curvatures in the cervical and lumbar regions develop, forming lordotic curves. Normal development of these curvatures, which produces a slight S shape, continues until growth ceases. Inspection of the spine also includes assessing for tufts of hair, cysts, or masses, which may indicate abnormalities such as spina bifida or a congenital neural tube defect. All known or suspected abnormalities require further evaluation by a primary care provider.

The nurse also palpates the length of the clavicles at each office visit, noting any lumps or irregularities and observing the range of motion of the arms. The clavicle is frequently fractured during birth, and the fracture often goes unnoticed until a callus forms at the fracture site.

The infant is assessed for congenital hip dislocation at every office visit until 1 year of age. Additionally, the Allis sign is used to detect unequal leg length. The nurse is positioned at the child's feet. With the infant supine, the nurse flexes the infant's knees, keeping the femurs aligned, and compares the height of the knees. An uneven height indicates unequal leg length, as depicted in Figure 26.12 ■.

While holding the infant, the nurse's hands should be beneath the infant's axillae. Shoulder muscle strength is present if the infant remains upright between the nurse's hands. Muscle weakness is indicated if the infant begins to slip through the hands.

CHILDREN AND ADOLESCENTS Bone growth is rapid during infancy and continues at a steady rate during childhood until adolescence, at which time both girls and boys experience a growth spurt. Long bones increase in width because of the deposition of new bony tissue around the diaphysis (shaft). Long bones also increase in length because of a proliferation of cartilage at the growth plates at the epiphyses (ends) of the long bones. Longitudinal growth ends at about 21 years of age, when the epiphyses fuse with the diaphysis. Throughout childhood, ligaments are stronger than bones. Therefore, childhood injuries to the long bones and joints tend to result in fractures instead of sprains. Individual muscle fibers grow throughout childhood, but growth is especially increased during the adolescent growth spurt. Muscles vary in size and strength due to genetics, exercise, and diet.

Much of the examination of the child and adolescent includes the same techniques of inspection, palpation, and assessment of range of motion and muscle strength used in the examination of the adult. However, children also have unique assessment needs. Children present wonderful opportunities for assessing range of motion and muscle strength as they play with toys in the waiting area or examination room. The nurse should encourage children to jump, hop, skip, and climb. Most children are eager to show off their abilities.

At each office visit, the nurse should ask children to demonstrate their favorite sitting position. If a child assumes the reverse tailor position (Figure 26.13 ■), common when watching television, the nurse should encourage the child to try other sitting positions. Parents should be told that the reverse tailor position stresses the hip, knee, and ankle joints of the growing child.

The nurse should ask the child to lie supine, then to rise to a standing position. Normally, the child rises without using the arms for support. Generalized muscle weakness may be indicated if the child places the hands on the knees and pushes up the trunk (Gowers sign).

The child's spine is assessed for scoliosis at each office visit. It is also important to inspect the child's shoes for signs of abnormal wear, and assess the child's gait. Before age 3, the gait of the child is normally broad based. After age 3, the child's gait narrows. At each visit, the nurse assesses the range of motion of each arm. Subluxation of the head of the radius occurs commonly when adults dangle children from their hands or remove their clothing forcibly.

The nurse must obtain complete information on any sports activity the child or adolescent engages in, because participation in these can indicate the need for special assessments or preventive teaching, such as the use of helmets and other safety equipment.

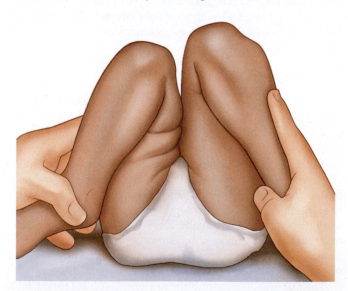

Figure 26.12 Allis sign—demonstration of unequal knee height.

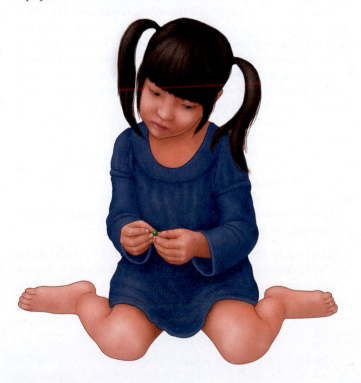

Figure 26.13 Reverse tailor position.

Neurologic System

INFANTS The growth of the nervous system is very rapid during the fetal period. This rate of growth does not continue during infancy. Some research indicates that no neurons are formed after the third trimester of fetal life. It is believed that during infancy the neurons mature, allowing for more complete actions to take place. The cerebral cortex thickens, brain size increases, and myelinization occurs. The maturational advances in the nervous system are responsible for the cephalocaudal and proximal-to-distal refinement of development, control, and movement.

The neonate has several primitive reflexes at birth. These include but are not limited to sucking, stepping, startle (Moro), and the Babinski reflex, in which stimulation of the sole of the foot from the heel toward the toes results in dorsiflexion of the great toe and fanning of other toes. The Babinski reflex and the tonic neck reflex are normal until around 2 years of age (Table 26.1). By about 1 month of age, the reflexes begin to disappear, and the child takes on more controlled and complex activity.

The cry of the newborn helps place the infant on the health–illness continuum. *Strong* and *lusty* are terms used to describe the cry of a healthy newborn. An absent, weak, or catlike or shrill cry usually indicates cerebral disease.

CHILDREN AND ADOLESCENTS Throughout infancy and the early childhood years, it is important to assess the fine and gross motor skills, language, and personal–social skills of the child. The nurse identifies benchmarks or mileposts related to age and level of functioning and compares the child's actual functioning with an anticipated level of functioning. Developmental delays or learning disabilities may be related to, but are not limited to, neurologic conditions such as fetal alcohol syndrome, autism, and attention-deficit/hyperactivity disorder (ADHD).

Table 26.1 Primitive Reflexes of Early Childhood

REFLEX	HOW TO ELICIT	AGE WHEN DISAPPEARS	EXAMPLE
Tonic Neck	Turn the infant's head to one side while the infant is supine. The infant will extend the arm and leg on the side the head is turned to while flexing the opposite arm and leg.	2 to 6 months	
Palmar Grasp	Infant will grasp fingers or objects placed in the palm of the hand.	3 to 4 months	
Plantar Grasp	Infant will curl toes when the base of the toes is touched.	6 to 8 months	

(continued)

Table 26.1 Primitive Reflexes of Early Childhood (*Continued*)

REFLEX	HOW TO ELICIT	AGE WHEN DISAPPEARS	EXAMPLE
Moro (startle)	Infant will extend the arms with the fingers spread and flex the legs in response to loud sounds or if the infant's body drops suddenly.	4 to 6 months	
Rooting	Lightly stroke the infant's cheek. Infant will turn the head with the mouth open toward the stroked side.	3 to 4 months	
Stepping	Infant will flex the leg and take steps if upright with the feet touching a surface.	4 to 5 months	
Babinski	Gently stroke the plantar surface of the foot from heel to toe. Infant will extend and fan the toes and flex the foot.	18 to 24 months	

Special Considerations

Planning care for individuals is dependent upon comprehensive health assessment of health status and all of the factors that impact health. The previous section provided information about the anatomic and physiologic difference in infants, children, and adolescents to consider in health assessment of physical and psychosocial growth and development across the lifespan. Other factors that influence growth and development include family, nutrition, mental health, culture, race, and socioeconomic status. The following discussion provides examples of ways in which these factors impact growth and development.

Health and Wellness: The Family Context

The term *family* refers to a social system made up of two or more individuals living together, who are related by blood, marriage, or agreement. Families today may be identified as nuclear families, extended families, same-sex families, single-parent families, stepfamilies, or single-state families. Families share bonds of affection or love, loyalty, commitment of an emotional or financial nature, continuity, and shared values and rituals. Families help members to develop physically and emotionally by providing for the economic and safety needs of one another. Included in safety needs would be provision of appropriate nutrition to foster physical growth and development as well as objects, interactions, and activities that promote cognitive and emotional well-being. Family members provide support for each other during physical and emotional crises and serve as models for social interaction, all of which impact individual members as they move through the stages of development from infancy to old age.

Nutritional Assessment

Nutrition is essential to physical growth and cognitive development in infants and children. Overnutrition or obesity is a common problem, and the most common approach is to encourage healthy food choices and increase activity levels. Undernutrition or malnutrition may delay or slow a child's growth and development. Healthcare professionals routinely use measures of height and weight in comparison with clinical growth charts to identify rates of growth and weight gain or loss. Slowed growth can be an early indicator of inadequate nutrition or nutritional deficiency. The effects of undernutrition can permanently affect the development of the child. Accurate assessment of nutritional health can help ensure positive outcomes or serve as the necessary foundation for needed nutritional interventions. It is essential for a nurse to have the knowledge and skills to identify nutritionally at-risk children. Further discussion of these concepts is included in Chapter 10. ∞

Mental Health, Substance Use, and Violence Assessment

There has been a marked increase in the number of children accessing mental health services since the mid-1990s. The percentage of youths receiving any outpatient mental health service was 13.3% between 2010 and 2012 (Olfson, Druss, & Marcus, 2015). Early intervention and treatment for conditions such as depression, anxiety, autism, eating disorders, and substance use disorders is shown to improve long-term outcomes. As the number of children with mental health and behavioral health concerns grows, the importance of comprehensive assessment of children is highlighted. The nurse should perform a thorough health history, including questions about a child's emotional and social well-being. An accurate diagnosis requires a comprehensive evaluation by a medical provider and may include data from the use of validated screening tools appropriate for the developmental and chronological age of the patient (Weitzman et al., 2015). For a detailed discussion about substance use and violence assessment, see Chapter 11. ∞

Culture

Growth and development are influenced by cultural factors. For example, perceptions of family roles, in particular those related to childrearing, differ across and within cultures. Family–infant attachment is considered an essential element in psychosocial development that usually occurs in the newborn period. It is important for the nurse to remember that a patient's culture influences the training and discipline of children, the value placed on developing cognitive skills, social interactions outside of the home that promote development, and attitudes toward change, including illness and aging. Further information about culture is included in Chapter 3. ∞

Socioeconomic Status

Socioeconomic status is a major influence on growth and development. Overall, school-age children of low socioeconomic status have been found to have lower height and weight than those in other economic groups. Poverty impacts the ability to meet nutritional needs at all stages of development and increases exposure to environmental elements that influence health status and physical well-being. Socioeconomic status influences values and role expectations and behaviors regarding marriage, family, and gender responsibilities in parenting, education, and occupation. Income, values, and role expectations impact physical and psychosocial development across the age span.

Developmental Considerations

Principles of Growth and Development

Four commonly accepted principles define the orderly, sequential progression of growth and development in all individuals:

1. Growth and development proceed in a cephalocaudal, or head to toe, direction (Figure 26.14 ■). An infant's head grows and becomes functional before the trunk or limbs. A baby's hands are able to grasp before the legs and feet are used purposefully.

2. Growth and development occur in a proximal to distal direction, or from the center of the body outward. A child gains the ability to use the hand as a whole before being able to control individual fingers.

3. Development proceeds from simple to complex or from general to specific. To accomplish an integrated act such as putting something in the mouth, the infant must first learn to reach out to the object, grasp it, move it to the open mouth, and insert it.

4. Differentiated development begins with a generalized response and progresses to a skilled specific response. An infant responds to stimuli with the entire body. An older child responds to specific stimuli with happiness, anger, or fear.

Although the classic theories of human development provide the foundation for nursing assessment, researchers are continuously evolving developmental theories that further define and explain human behavior. Additionally, interpretation of the classic theories broadens as societal changes and advances in technology redefine individuals' relationships, expectations, and goals.

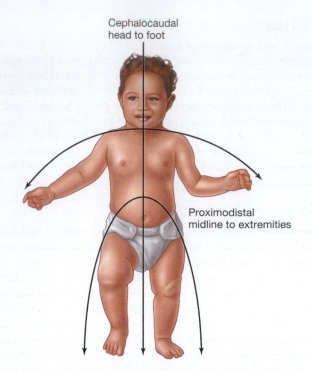

Cephalocaudal
head to foot

Proximodistal
midline to extremities

Figure 26.14 Cephalocaudal growth proceeds in a head-to-toe direction.

Behavior that is widely accepted or even the norm today was often considered unusual or abnormal a generation ago. For instance, the family unit is no longer assumed to be two parents with children but may now consist of a single parent, stepsiblings, half siblings, a surrogate mother, same-sex parents, or other configurations. What are the implications for health and development?

Stages of Development

The most common and traditional approach used by developmental theorists to describe and classify human behavior is according to chronologic age. Theorists attempt to identify meaningful relationships in complex behaviors by reducing them to core problems, tasks, or accomplishments that occur during a defined age range or stage of life. These theories are discussed in the following subsections. The following stages have been delineated to best illustrate the concepts of sequential development. It is important to remember that the ages are somewhat arbitrary. It is the sequence of growth, development, and observed behaviors that is meaningful during nursing assessment.

Infants Through 12 Months Frequent assessments during the first year provide opportunities to monitor the infant's rate of growth and development as well as to compare the infant with the norm for age.

Accurate assessment combining information obtained by history and physical assessment results in early identification of common problems that may easily be resolved with early intervention. Often basic parent education and support remedy problems that, left untreated, could result in significant health problems or disturbed parent–child interactions later.

Toddlers 1–3 Years Although the rate of growth of toddlers decreases, it proceeds in an expected manner. Height and weight continue to follow a percentile, although slight variations are often seen. Because cooperation of the young toddler is unlikely, a health history is often the best way to assess development. Older toddlers are more willing to play with developmental testing materials or explore the environment while in proximity to a caregiver, enabling direct observations of development. Toddlers in a strange or threatening environment may not speak, making language assessment difficult. Listening to the child talk in a playroom or waiting room increases the probability of assessing the toddler's language. Toddlers quickly turn to caregivers for comfort or when confronted with a stranger. Observing the adult–child interaction and listening to how the adult speaks to the child provides information on the quality of the relationship.

Preschoolers 3–5 (or 6) Years Preschoolers' slowed rate of growth is often of concern to caregivers. The nurse can allay anxiety by showing the preschooler's growth chart and discussing caloric expectations. Preschoolers are generally pleasant, cooperative, and talkative. They continue to need the reassurance of a caregiver in view but do not need to return to the caregiver for comfort except in threatening situations. Talking with preschoolers about favorite activities allows the nurse to assess language ability, cognitive ability, and development. The nurse evaluates the child's use of language to express thoughts, sentence structure, and vocabulary.

School-Age Children 6–10 Years The slow, steady growth and changing body proportions of school-age children make them appear thin and gangly. Assessing children's intake of nutrients and calories and reviewing their growth charts reassures parents that their children are not too thin. Older school-age children have an increase in appetite as they enter the prepubertal growth spurt. During the growth spurt, height and weight increase and may normally cross percentiles. School-age children are eager to talk about their hobbies, friends, school, and accomplishments. Increasing neurologic maturity allows them to master activities requiring gross and fine motor control, such as sports, dancing, playing a musical instrument, artistic pursuits, or building things. School-age children enjoy showing off newly acquired skills, and the family displays pride in their children's accomplishments. Adult family members and school-age children communicate openly, with adults setting needed limits. Although peer relationships are becoming more important, the family remains the major influence during most of the school-age years. As children approach adolescence, the relationship with family may become strained as the children are drawn closer to peer groups and seek greater independence.

Adolescents 11–19 Years The pubertal growth spurt requires adolescents to increase their caloric intake dramatically, causing parents concern that they eat constantly but never seem full. Adolescents are at risk for developing eating disorders; feelings surrounding changes in the body should be explored. Adolescents often communicate better with peers and adults outside of the family than with family members. Assessing adolescents with their parents and then one-on-one affords a more complete picture of their relationship and provides adolescents with an opportunity to freely express themselves and discuss concerns. Adolescents are able to hold an adult conversation and are often happy to discuss school, friends, activities, and plans for the future. They tend to be anxious about their bodies and the rapid changes occurring. Often they are unsure if what is happening to them is normal, and they frequently express somatic complaints.

Developmental Theories

Three of the most influential classic theories of development are discussed here to provide a basic framework for nursing assessment. Although no one theory encompasses all aspects of human development, each provides a perspective for understanding, predicting, or guiding behavior.

Cognitive Theory Cognitive theory explores how people learn to think, reason, and use language. Jean Piaget theorized that cognitive development is an orderly, sequential process that occurs in four stages in the growing child. Each stage demonstrates a new way of thinking and behaving. Piaget believed that a child's thinking develops progressively from simple reflex behavior into complex, logical, and abstract thought. All children move through the same stages, in the same order, with each stage providing the foundation for the next. At each stage, the child views the world in increasingly complex terms. Piaget's stages of cognitive development are summarized as follows:

Stage 1: Sensorimotor (Birth to 2 Years). The infant progresses from responding primarily through reflexes to purposeful movement and organized activity. Object permanence (the knowledge that objects continue to exist when not seen) and object recognition are attained.

Stage 2: Preoperational Skills (2 to 7 Years). Highly egocentric, the child is able to view the world only from an individual perspective. The new ability to use mental symbols develops. The child's thinking now incorporates past events and anticipations of the future.

Stage 3: Concrete Operations (7 to 11 Years). During this time period, the child develops symbolic functioning: the ability to make one thing represent a different thing that is not present. The child is able to consider another point of view. Thinking is more logical and systematic.

Stage 4: Formal Operations (11 Years to Adulthood). The child uses rational thinking and deductive reasoning. Thinking in abstract terms is possible. The child is able to deal with hypothetical situations and make logical conclusions after reviewing evidence.

Psychoanalytic Theory Sigmund Freud was an early theorist whose concepts of personality development provided the foundation for the development of many other theories. Freud believed that people are constantly adjusting to environmental changes and that this adjustment creates conflict between outside forces (environment) and inner forces (instincts). The type of conflict varies with an individual's developmental stage, and personality develops through conflict resolution.

Psychoanalytic theory defines the structure of personality as consisting of three parts: id, ego, and superego. The personality at birth consists primarily of the id, which is the source of instinctive and unconscious urges. The ego is the seat of consciousness and mediates between the inner instinctual desires of the id and the outer world. The ego, a minor nucleus at birth, expands and gains mastery over the id. In addition, it is the receiving center for the senses and forms the mechanisms of defense. The superego is the conscience of the personality, acting as a censor of thoughts, feelings, and behavior. The superego begins to form after age 3 or 4 years.

Psychosocial Theory Erikson's psychosocial theory describes eight stages of ego development, but, unlike Freud, Erikson believed the ego is the conscious core of the personality. Erikson's psychosocial theory states that culture and society influence development across the entire lifespan. Erikson viewed life as a sequence of tasks that must be achieved, with each stage presenting a crisis that must be resolved. Each crisis may have a positive or negative outcome, depending on environmental influences and the choices that the individual makes. Crisis resolution may be positive, incomplete, or negative. Task achievement and positive conflict resolution are supportive to the person's ego. Negative resolution adversely influences the individual's ability to achieve the next task. The following are the five stages from birth through adolescence:

Stage 1: (Birth to 1 Year). Trust versus mistrust. The child who develops trust develops hope and drive. Mistrust results in fear, withdrawal, and estrangement.

Stage 2: (1 to 2 Years). Autonomy versus shame and doubt. The child who achieves autonomy develops self-control and willpower. A negative resolution of the crisis results in self-doubt.

Stage 3: (2 to 6 Years). Initiative versus guilt. Initiative leads to purpose and direction, whereas guilt results in lack of self-confidence, pessimism, and feelings of unworthiness.

Stage 4: (6 to 12 Years). Industry versus inferiority. Industry results in the development of competency, creativity, and perseverance. Inferiority creates feelings of hopelessness and a sense of being mediocre or incompetent. Withdrawal from school and peers may result.

Stage 5: (12 to 18 Years). Identity versus role confusion. Achieving ego identity results in the ability to make a career choice and plan for the future. Inferiority creates confusion, uncertainty, indecisiveness, and an inability to make a career choice.

Subjective Data—Health History

Health assessment of the pediatric patient includes the gathering of subjective and objective data. The subjective data are collected during the interview, which is conducted with a parent or caregiver. The professional nurse uses a variety of communication techniques to elicit general and specific information about the health of the child. Health records combine subjective and objective data. The results of labora-tory tests and radiologic studies are important secondary sources of objective data. Physical assessment of the child, during which objective data are collected, includes the techniques of inspection, palpation, percussion, and auscultation. An overview covering the main differences in the observational findings between children and adult patients is described in Chapter 8. ∞

Health History Interview

The interview for assessment of a child's health covers all of the body systems. The nurse will observe the patient and caregiver and listen for cues that relate to the child's health status and function. The nurse may use open-ended and closed questions to obtain information. Follow-up questions or requests for descriptions are required to clarify data or to supply missing information. Follow-up questions are used to identify the source of problems, duration of difficulties, measures to alleviate problems, and cues about the parent or caregiver's knowledge of their children's health.

The health interview guides the physical assessment. The information obtained is considered in relation to norms and expectations about the chronological and developmental age and stage of the child. Therefore, the nurse must consider developmental theories, gender, race, culture, environment, health practices, past and current problems, and therapies when framing questions and using techniques to elicit information. The following interview questions are specific to infants, children, and/or adolescents and are organized by body system. Each section will present focused interview question related to one body system. It is recommended that the nurse incorporate these questions into the overall health interview, which includes the comprehensive questions presented in each chapter. One method to elicit further information about specific symptoms is the OLDCART & ICE method, described in Chapter 5. ∞

Focused Interview Questions	Rationales and Evidence

The following section provides sample questions and bulleted follow-up questions. A rationale for each of the questions is provided. The list of questions is not all-inclusive but represents the types of questions required in a comprehensive health interview related to infants, children, and adolescents. These questions will be used in addition to the appropriate questions from the focused assessment questions in each system chapter.

Skin, Hair, and Nails

1. Does your child have any birthmarks? If so, where are they?

▶ The presence of particular types of birthmarks in infants and young children may be an indication of a genetic disorder and require further investigation (St. John et al., 2016).

2. Has your infant developed an orange hue in the skin?

▶ Ingestion of large amounts of carotene in vegetables such as carrots, sweet potatoes, and squash can cause an orange or yellow hue (Silverberg & Lee-Wong, 2014).

3. Does your child have a rash? If so, what seems to have caused it?

▶ The patient has an opportunity to provide information about specific illnesses. If a diagnosed illness is identified, follow-up about the date of diagnosis, treatment, and outcomes is required. Data about each illness identified by the patient are essential to an accurate health assessment. Illnesses can be classified as acute or chronic, and follow-up regarding each classification will differ.

- Have you introduced any new foods or a different kind of formula into your child's diet?

▶ Many children may have allergic reactions to certain foods; the following eight things cause 90% of food allergies: milk, eggs, peanuts, tree nuts, soy, wheat, fish, and shellfish (WebMD, 2017).

- Is it a diaper rash? If so, how often do you change the child's diaper? How do you clean the child's diaper area? Are you using anything to treat the diaper rash?
- Was the treatment helpful?

▶ Diaper rash is a common condition in infants and may be caused by infrequent changing of diapers or use of particular products such as detergents, lotions, and ointments.

4. Do you use disposable or cloth diapers? If cloth, how do you wash your child's diapers?

5. Does your child have any habits such as pulling or twisting the hair, rubbing the head, or biting the nails?

▶ These habits may signal anxiety or emotional distress. Nail biting may also lead to impaired skin integrity.

Head, Neck, and Related Lymphatics

1. Did you use alcohol or recreational drugs during your pregnancy?

▶ Fetal alcohol syndrome (FAS) causes neurologic disorders, developmental delays, and characteristic head and facial deformities (Popova, Lange, Probst, Gmel, & Rehm, 2017). Use of cocaine, methamphetamines, or opioids during pregnancy can result in a variety of cognitive and physiologic problems in the infant (Forray, 2016).

2. Have you noticed any depression or bulging over your infant's "soft spots" (fontanels)?

▶ A depressed fontanel can indicate dehydration, and a bulging fontanel can indicate an infection (Goldberg, 2013).

Eyes

1. Did the mother have any vaginal infections at the time of birth?

▶ Vaginal infections in the mother can cause eye infections in the newborn (Churchward, Alany, Kirk, Walker, & Snyder, 2017).

2. Did your baby get eye ointment after birth?

3. Does your infant look directly at you? Does your infant follow objects with the eyes?

▶ The infant may have crossed eyes or eyes that move in different directions normally until 2 months of age; then the findings may be associated with weakness of the eye muscles (Varma, Tarczy-Hornoch, & Jiang, 2017).

Focused Interview Questions	Rationales and Evidence
4. Do you have concerns about your child's ability to see? Does your school-age child like to sit at the front of the classroom?	▶ Poor eyesight may necessitate sitting at the front of the room.
5. Has your child had a vision examination? When was the last eye examination? • How often has your child's vision been checked? • By whom? What were the results?	
6. Does your child rub his or her eyes frequently?	▶ Rubbing of the eyes can be associated with infection, allergy, or visual problems. Some children rub their eyes when fatigued.
7. Was your infant born prematurely?	▶ Infants who need oxygen may have damage to the retina (Saugstad, 2018).

Ears, Nose, Mouth, and Throat

Focused Interview Questions	Rationales and Evidence
1. Does your child have recurrent ear infections? • How many ear infections has the child had in the last 6 months? • How were they treated? • Has the child had any ear surgery, such as insertion of ear tubes? • When? • What were the results? • Does the child attend daycare?	▶ Recurrent or chronic ear infections may lead to more serious conditions, including perforation of the tympanic membrane (eardrum). Especially in infants and toddlers, significant periods of hearing impairment can lead to delayed speech development. In rare cases, untreated recurrent ear infections may spread to structures in the skull, including the brain (Mayo Clinic, 2017).
2. Does your child tug at his or her ears?	▶ Tugging at the ears can be an early sign of infection.
3. Does your child respond to loud noises?	▶ A lack of response could indicate hearing loss (Centers for Disease Control and Prevention [CDC], 2015).
4. Have you ever had your child's hearing tested? What were the results?	
5. Has your child had measles, mumps, or any disease with a high fever? • Has the child been treated with any antibiotics such as streptomycin or gentamicin?	▶ Infection-related high fevers or use of certain drugs may cause hearing loss (Shields, Fox, & Liebrecht, 2018).
6. How do you clean your child's ears?	▶ The nurse should ascertain whether the procedure the caregiver uses is harmful, such as cleaning ears with cotton swabs, which may cause impacted cerumen (American Speech-Language-Hearing Association [ASHA], 2015).
7. Does your child put objects into his or her nose?	▶ Foreign objects can cause trauma to nasal tissues.
8. Does your child frequently have drainage from the nose?	▶ Frequent drainage can indicate an infection or allergies.
9. Does your child suck his or her thumb or a pacifier?	
10. When did your child's teeth begin to erupt?	▶ Late eruption of teeth could indicate delayed development.
11. Does your child go to bed with a bottle at night?	▶ Frequent use of a bottle with milk or juice at night can cause decay of teeth.
12. Does your child know how to brush teeth? How often does your child brush his or her teeth?	
13. How often does your child go to the dentist?	▶ Children should begin annual visits to the dentist at the time of the eruption of the first tooth and no later than age 12 months (American Academy of Pediatric Dentistry, 2018).
14. Is your child's drinking water fluoridated?	▶ Fluoride in the water supply helps prevent tooth decay (Iheozor-Ejiofor et al., 2015).

Lungs and Thorax

Focused Interview Questions	Rationales and Evidence
1. Is your child taking solid foods? • When were they started? • What types of foods are taken? • Does the child have difficulty chewing or swallowing?	▶ Introduction of solid foods puts infants at risk for aspiration (Mayo Clinic, 2016).
2. How many colds has your child had in the past 12 months? • What was the course of the cold? • Was any medical care or treatment provided? • What was the effect of the treatment?	▶ Young children may average 6 to 8 colds per year during the cold season; symptoms last an average of 2 weeks (Centers for Disease Control and Prevention [CDC], 2018).
3. Has your child been immunized against respiratory illnesses? • What immunizations did your child have? • When were they given?	▶ This question identifies risk reduction and assists in discrimination of symptoms if and when they occur. Infants are at greater risk for complications from flu and pneumonia.
4. Is your home childproofed regarding small objects and toys?	▶ Reduces the risk for aspiration

Breasts and Axillae

Focused Interview Questions	Rationales and Evidence
1. *For the preadolescent girl:* Have you noticed any changes in the size or shape of your breasts? Tell me about those changes?	▶ Growth of the breasts is not necessarily steady or symmetric. This may be frustrating or embarrassing to girls. The nurse should reassure the patient that her breast development is normal, if appropriate.

Focused Interview Questions	Rationales and Evidence
2. *For boys and girls:* How do you feel about your breasts and the way they are changing?	▶ Breast development provides visual confirmation that the pubescent female is becoming a woman. For the developing pubescent female, her breasts are a visible symbol of her feminine identity and an important part of her body image and self-esteem. Girls should be reassured that the rate of growth of breast tissue depends on changing hormone levels and is uniquely individual, as are the eventual size and shape of the breasts. The nurse can reassure males that breast enlargement is generally temporary and in response to hormonal changes (Berman, Snyder, & Frandsen, 2016).

Cardiovascular and Peripheral Vascular System

1. **What was the pregnancy with this child like?** • During pregnancy, did you have any complications such as fever? If so, what were they? • What was done about them? • How was the infant affected? • How were the infant's complications treated? • Have the interventions helped?	▶ Complications during pregnancy may contribute to malformations in the infant.

Abdomen and Gastrointestinal System

1. **What is the typical stooling pattern for this child?** • Does the child have pain or difficulty with stooling? • Does the child have diarrhea or constipation?	▶ Constipation is one of the most common reasons for parents to take their infant to a medical provider. A detailed history is critical for making a positive diagnosis of constipation (Jiles & Hamrick, 2017).

Genitourinary System

1. **Have you ever been told that your child has a kidney that has failed to grow?**	▶ Renal agenesis may involve one or both kidneys. A genetic factor may be associated with the development of this condition in some cases. Bilateral renal agenesis is invariably fatal. Unilateral renal agenesis may be asymptomatic and is often incidentally diagnosed by abdominal ultrasound or computed tomography (CT) scan secondary to another condition. In infants with unilateral renal agenesis, the remaining kidney may be enlarged, and there is increased risk of problems with the remaining kidney (Westland, Schreuder, Ket, & van Wijk, 2013).
2. **Has your child ever been diagnosed with a kidney disorder?** • What is it called, what were the symptoms, and how was it treated? • Is it still being treated?	▶ Some disorders, such as infections, are easily treated and do not recur; others, such as glomerulonephritis, may be chronic.
3. **Has your child had any hearing problems?**	▶ The ears and kidneys develop at the same time in utero. Congenital deafness may be associated with renal disease (Isaacson, 2018).
4. **Have you noticed any unusual shape or structure in your child's genital anatomy?**	▶ Parents may report abnormally shaped external genitals, as seen in hypospadias and epispadias. In children with exstrophy of the bladder, the lower urinary tract is visible.
5. **Is your child toilet trained?** • Has the child had any problems with involuntary urination? Bedwetting? Daytime accidents? • How were they treated?	▶ *Enuresis* is the medical term for involuntary urination after toilet training has been successful. If it occurs at night, it is termed nocturnal enuresis. This condition may impact the social, mental, and physical well-being of the family and child.
6. **Has your child's urinary output or pattern changed recently?**	▶ There are a variety of contributors to changes in elimination patterns, but renal failure, dehydration, overhydration, diet changes, obstruction, and stress may contribute to a change in normal pattern.
7. **Have you noticed any redness, swelling, or discharge in your child's genital area?** • Has the child complained of itching, burning, swelling, or pain in the genital area?	▶ These may indicate inflammatory processes or infection. These symptoms may indicate the presence of pinworms or infections such as yeast infections (Dennie & Grover, 2013).

Musculoskeletal System

1. **Where you told about any trauma to your infant during labor and birth?** • If so, please describe it.	▶ Traumatic births increase the risk for fractures, especially of the clavicle (Dashe, Roocroft, Bastrom, & Edmonds, 2013).
2. **Did your infant require resuscitation after birth?**	▶ Periods of hypoxia or anoxia can result in decreased muscle tone (Orcesi, 2013).
3. **Have you noticed any deformity of your child's spine or limbs? Any unusual shape of the feet or toes?** • If yes, please describe the condition and treatment.	

Focused Interview Questions	Rationales and Evidence
4. Does your child play any sports or participate on any teams? • What kind of protective equipment is used? • Is there adult supervision?	▶ Sports activities can cause musculoskeletal injuries, especially if played without adequate adult supervision or the use of protective equipment.

Neurologic System

1. Describe the pregnancy with this child. Did it include any health problems or require medications? • Was the pregnancy full term? Preterm? How may weeks of gestation were completed? • Describe the birth of your child, include any complications during labor or birth.	▶ Problems during the antepartal period, including the use of medications, alcohol, or drugs, may affect the neurologic health of the child. Similarly, complications during or shortly after birth may have residual effects (Berman et al., 2016).
2. Has your child ever had a seizure? • If so, how often has this happened? • Describe what happened during the seizure. • Did the child have a fever when the seizure happened?	▶ Febrile seizures are common in infants and toddlers. Seizures without accompanying fever may indicate a seizure disorder such as epilepsy (National Institute of Neurological Disorders and Stroke, 2017).
3. Are you aware of any surfaces in the home that may be painted with lead-based paint? • Have you seen your child eating paint chips or other nonedible items? • Has your child been tested for lead levels in his or her blood?	▶ Lead poisoning may lead to developmental delays, peripheral nerve damage, or brain damage (Grandjean & Landrigan, 2014).
4. How is your child doing in school? • Does the child seem to be able to concentrate on assignments and complete them on time? • Have you ever been told your child has a learning difficulty? • Have you ever been told about any behavioral concerns in daycare, preschool, or school settings? • Describe any assessments or treatments for behavioral issues if present.	▶ Learning and behavioral problems may have a neurologic basis and warrant follow-up.

Patient-Centered Interaction

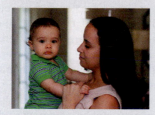

Source: Fotoluminate LLC/Shutterstock.

Mrs. Charlotte and her 3-month-old baby, Anton, are seeing the pediatric primary care provider to ask a few questions about feeding. Anton is exclusively breastfed, sleeps up to 4 hours at a time, and is generally a happy baby. Mrs. Charlotte wants to know how well her baby can see and hear at this age and what he should be able to do. The following is an excerpt from the health history interview.

Interview

Nurse: Hello, Mrs. Charlotte. Hello, Anton. I am going to talk with you today about how Anton is doing.

Mrs. Charlotte: He is doing great, I think. I really don't know if I'm feeding him enough, or if he is getting enough sleep. How can I tell?

Nurse: Why don't you tell me about his feeding routine, as well as the typical number of wet and dirty diapers he has each day?

Mrs. Charlotte: Oh, okay. I breast feed him about every two to three hours during the day and, at night, about every two to four hours—whenever he cries, you know? Each time, I put him to breast for about fifteen to twenty minutes, and then he falls asleep!

Nurse: That sounds just fine! You are attending to his feeding cues—the behaviors he has to tell you he is hungry. Babies can't talk, but we can sure understand what they want, can't we? Also, according to his current weight and length, I can see that he has gained weight and grown, too. These are excellent signs that he's getting enough to eat.

Mrs. Charlotte: What about sleep? Is it okay that he sleeps for four hours at a time? Sometimes I have to wake him up at night to feed him. Oh, and he has lots—like eight or nine—of wet diapers every day, and two or three with stool in them.

Nurse: That is an appropriate number of diapers each day, and it tells us he is well hydrated. It is okay to start to let him sleep a little longer, and let him "tell" you when he's hungry. If you feed him around seven p.m. and again at ten p.m., he may sleep for five or six hours in a row. It is fine for you to start to adjust his feeding schedule a bit.

Mrs. Charlotte: Thank you so much for that information. I am looking forward to getting some more sleep at night!

Analysis

During the interview, the nurse used positive feedback to help Mrs. Charlotte build confidence in her skills. The nurse used open-ended questions to elicit information about feeding, sleeping, and elimination. The nurse made sure her answers were easy to understand, and that the information was accurate for the age and developmental stage of the child.

Objective Data—Physical Assessment

Assessment Techniques and Findings

The approach to physical assessment of children must take into account the age of the child as well as the developmental level. Accurate and complete information from the health history will help the nurse determine what physical assessments are required. In general, the physical examination techniques are the same in children as in adults but may require specialized equipment. For example, vital sign measurements in children may require smaller equipment than what is used for an adult, and children may need the nurse to use simpler language to describe assessments and elicit responses, such as saying "tummy" or "belly" rather than "abdomen." Children may also need additional comfort measures during assessment, such as holding hands with a parent or sitting on a parent's lap; conversation, toys, or television as a distraction; and manipulating or touching the equipment in order to calm fears about unknown objects (Figure 26.15 ■). When possible, children

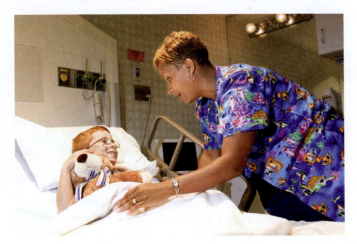

Figure 26.15 Children may need additional comfort measures while hospitalized.

Source: Jupiterimages/Stockbyte/Getty Images.

EQUIPMENT

- Appropriate-size equipment: blood pressure cuff, stethoscope
- Proper size scale for weighing and measuring infants and small children
- Tape measure for head circumference
- Toys or toy medical equipment for distraction
- Adequate seating for parent or caregivers

HELPFUL HINTS

- Sit down to be at eye level with smaller patients.
- Allow child to stay in parent or caregiver's lap if possible.
- Begin with the least invasive procedure and end with the most invasive.
- Build a rapport with parents of toddlers and preschoolers to help build trust.
- Give adolescents privacy and an opportunity to be seen without parents.

should be given an opportunity to make choices about their care, and older children should be given the opportunity to be assessed without parents present. See Chapter 5. Nurses must also consider the cultural or spiritual beliefs of the parents that may affect the assessment and care of children. Some populations may require care by a same-sex provider. Always consult with parents or guardians about assessment procedures before conducting an assessment on children. Determining which adult is the correct person with whom to discuss the child's care may require additional assessment and interviewing. Discussing a parent's observations may also add subjective data to the assessment that will be valuable in providing appropriate care. ∞

The following are specific assessment techniques that differ from the methods used for assessment in adults. These are arranged by body system.

Techniques and Normal Findings	Abnormal Findings and Special Considerations

Skin, Hair, and Nails

Physical assessment of the skin, hair, and nails follows an organized pattern. It begins with a survey and inspection of the skin, followed by palpation of the skin. Inspection and palpation of the hair and nails are then completed. When lesions are present, measurements are used to identify the size of the lesions and the location in relation to accepted landmarks. Also see Chapter 12. ∞

- Infants' skin lacks the ability to contract. Therefore, they cannot shiver and do not perspire, limiting thermal regulation.
- Children's skin texture changes, but perspiration and sebaceous gland function are limited, resulting in dry skin.
- In adolescence, skin texture continues to change. Sebaceous gland activity increases in response to hormonal changes. Eccrine glands increase function, resulting in increased perspiration, especially in response to emotional changes.

▶ Soap and shampoos should be mild, and the skin should be thoroughly rinsed. Patting dry is recommended for sensitive young skin. Further, infants require clothing that is appropriate for the external temperature and environment.

Head, Neck, and Related Lymphatics

In children over 12 to 18 months, the skull should be normocephalic—that is, rounded and symmetric. In children under 12 to 18 months, the cranial bones are not yet fused and the head shape may be misshapen, especially in newborns who underwent a vaginal birth. In all individuals, the frontal parietal and occipital prominences are present and symmetric. The scalp is clear and free of lesions; the hair is evenly distributed. The face is symmetric in shape; the eyes, ears, nose, and mouth are symmetrically placed. The facial movements are smooth and coordinated and demonstrate a variety of expressions. The neck is symmetric without swelling and has full range of motion. Cervical lymph nodes are usually small and palpable in children between the ages of 1 and 11 years. Also see Chapter 13. ∞

Techniques and Normal Findings	Abnormal Findings and Special Considerations

- Assessment of the anterior and posterior fontanels should be done by gently palpating the top and occiput region of the skull.
- In children, the neck is short, making it difficult to assess the lymph nodes or the thyroid.

▶ The anterior fontanel in young infants should measure up to 5 cm; by 18 months it should be closed. The posterior fontanel is often not palpable. A bulging or "tense" fontanel may indicate intracranial swelling; a sunken fontanel may indicate dehydration.

Eyes

Physical assessment of the eyes in children requires the use of inspection, occasionally palpation, and, depending on age, tests of the function of the eyes. The ophthalmoscope is used to assess the internal eye in children. During each of the assessments, the nurse is gathering data related to the patient's vision and the internal and external structures and functions of the eye. Inspection includes looking at the size, shape, and symmetry of the eye, eyelids, eyebrows, and eye movements.

Perform the Cover/Uncover Test

- For cooperative children, you should be sitting at eye level with the patient.
- Ask the patient to fix his gaze on a point directly behind you while you complete the test.
- Cover one eye with a card and observe the uncovered eye, which should remain focused on the designated point.
- Quickly remove the card from the covered eye and observe the other eye for movement; it should focus straight ahead.
- Repeat the procedure with the other eye. (Figure 26.16 ■).

Also see Chapter 14. ∞

▶ If there is a weakness in one of the eye muscles, the fusion reflex is blocked when one eye is covered and the weakness of the eye can be observed.

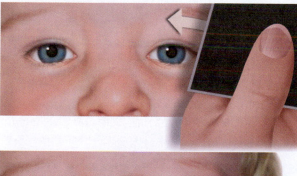

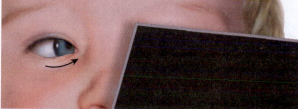

A. Right, or uncovered eye, is weaker.

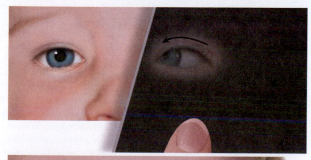

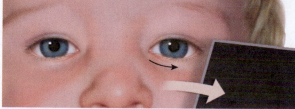

B. Left, or covered eye, is weaker.

Figure 26.16 Cover/uncover test.

Techniques and Normal Findings	Abnormal Findings and Special Considerations

Ears, Nose, Mouth, and Throat

Children normally have binaural hearing, meaning that the brain is capable of simultaneously integrating information that is received from both ears. The ears are symmetric in size, shape, color, and configuration. The external auditory canal is patent and free of drainage. The external ear and mastoid process are free of lesions, and the tragus is movable. Under otoscopic examination, the external ear canal is open, is nontender, and is free of lesions, inflammation, or foreign substances. Cerumen, if present, is soft and in small amounts. The tympanic membrane is flat, gray, and translucent without lesions. The malleolar process and reflected light are visible on the tympanic membrane. During hearing tests, air conduction is longer than bone conduction. Healthy children other than infants are able to maintain balance. The external nose is free of lesions, the nares are patent, and the mucosa of the nasal cavity is dark pink and smooth. The nasal septum is midline, straight, and intact. The sinuses are nontender. The lips are smooth, symmetric, and lesion free. Typically, children begin losing their deciduous teeth by 6 years of age. On average, most children lose their last deciduous tooth at approximately 12 to 13 years of age. Healthy adults and children who are 13 years and older have 32 permanent teeth, including four wisdom teeth, all of which are white with smooth edges. The tongue is mobile, is pink, and has papillae on the dorsum. The oral mucosa is pink, moist, and smooth. The membranes and structures of the throat are pink and moist. The uvula is midline and, like the soft palate, rises when the patient says "aah." Also see Chapter 15. ∞

Lungs and Thorax

Physical assessment of the respiratory system requires the use of inspection, palpation, percussion, and auscultation. During each of the procedures, the nurse is gathering data related to the patient's breathing and level of oxygenation. The nurse inspects skin color, structures of the thoracic cavity, chest configuration, and respiratory rate rhythm and effort. Also see Chapter 16. ∞

Count the Respiratory Rate

- Count the number of respiratory cycles per minute. Newborns have a respiratory rate of 30 to 80, and this rate gradually slows to adult rates by age 17.
- Observe chest movement.

- Observe the muscles of the chest and neck, including the intercostal muscles and sternocleidomastoids.

▶ Infants and children have higher respiratory rates than adults—up to 80 breaths per minute in newborns.

▶ Infants may have an irregular respiratory rate, so count their respirations for 1 full minute.

▶ Intercostal muscle retraction, nasal flaring, and prominent sternocleidomastoids may be seen in respiratory distress.

Breasts and Axillae

Physical assessment of the breasts and axillae requires the use of inspection and palpation. During each of the procedures, the nurse is gathering data related to the breasts and axillae. Inspection includes looking at skin color, structures of the breast, and the appearance of the axillae. Also see Chapter 17. ∞

Cardiovascular and Peripheral Vascular System

Physical assessment of the cardiovascular system requires the use of inspection, palpation, percussion, and auscultation. Physical assessment of the cardiovascular system follows an organized pattern. In infants and children, it begins with inspection of the patient's head and neck, including the eyes, ears, lips, face, skull, and neck vessels. The upper extremities, chest, abdomen, and lower extremities are also inspected. Auscultation includes the heart in five areas with the diaphragm and the bell of the stethoscope. During each of the procedures, the nurse is gathering objective data related to the function of the heart as determined by the heart rate and the quality and characteristics of the heart sounds. In addition, the nurse observes for signs of appropriate cardiac function in relation to oxygen perfusion by assessing skin color and temperature, abnormal pulsations, and the characteristics of the patient's respiratory effort. Also see Chapter 18. ∞

Auscultate the Heart Sounds

- Use the bell and the diaphragm of the stethoscope; if a murmur is heard, the nurse should determine if changing the position of the patient changes the sounds.

▶ The thinner chest wall of children causes heart sounds to seem louder. Infants have a point of maximal impulse (PMI) that is difficult to assess and is located approximately one intercostal space higher than in adults. An S2 split with inspiration may be detected in children under the age of 6. The physiologic S2 split disappears with expiration. Any S2 split that persists throughout the cardiac cycle merits further evaluation. Preadolescents may have a physiologic S3 gallop that results from vibrations during rapid ventricular filling. A detectable innocent, or functional, murmur may be observed in 70% of children sometime during childhood. Any condition that increases metabolism, such as fever or anemia, will make innocent murmurs more pronounced. By definition, innocent murmurs arise from increased blood flow across normal heart structures. Heart murmurs are graded using a scale of 1 to 6. A higher rating is reflective of greater intensity (loudness). For example, a grade 1/6 murmur is very soft and barely audible, whereas a grade 6/6 murmur is very loud.

Abdomen

Physical assessment of the infant or child's abdomen requires the use of inspection, auscultation, and palpation. This order differs from that of physical assessment of other systems. Inspection includes looking at skin color, structures of the abdomen, abdominal contour, pulsations, and abdominal movements. The skin of the abdomen should be consistent with the skin of the rest of the body. The umbilicus should be midline in an abdomen that may be round, flat, convex, or protuberant. The abdomen should be symmetric and free of bulges. Also see Chapter 20. ∞

Techniques and Normal Findings	Abnormal Findings and Special Considerations

Genitourinary System

Physical assessment of the urinary system follows an organized pattern. It begins with a survey of the patient's general appearance followed by inspection of the abdomen. In infants and children, abdominal and genital inspection and palpation of bladder fullness are part of the physical examination. It is important to assess not only the physical development of the male child's sexual organs but also the presence of abnormalities such as infection, tumors, and hernias. Assessment is completed using the same methods as described for the adult male. Also see Chapter 21 and Chapter 22. ∞

> **ALERT!** *The foreskin of uncircumcised males will not retract until the child is between 2 and 4 years old. Do not forcefully retract the foreskin of infants and toddlers. In older children with retractile foreskins, always return the foreskin to the natural position after urethral or glans examination.*

It is essential to assess for sexual molestation with female children. Some signs of sexual molestation are trauma, depression, eating disorders, bruising, swelling, and inflammation in the vaginal, perineal, and anal areas. Foreign bodies commonly cause malodorous, blood-tinged vaginal discharge. The child may appear withdrawn and, in many cases, may deny the experience.

Musculoskeletal System

Physical assessment of the musculoskeletal system requires the use of inspection and palpation. During each of the procedures the nurse is gathering data related to the patient's skeleton, joints, musculature, strength, and mobility. Children who are preschool age and older have erect posture, an even gait, and symmetry in size and shape of muscles. A healthy individual is capable of active and complete range of motion in all joints. Joints are nonswollen and nontender. Muscle strength is equal bilaterally, and the movements against resistance are smooth and symmetric. The spine is midline and cervical; thoracic and lumbar curves are present. The extremities are of equal length. The arm span is equal to height, and the distance from head to pubis is equal to the distance from pubis to toes. Physical assessment of the musculoskeletal system follows an organized pattern. It begins with a patient survey and proceeds in a cephalocaudal direction to include inspection, palpation, assessment of range of motion of each joint, and assessment of muscle size, symmetry, and strength. Also see Chapter 23. ∞

Neurologic System

Children who are preschool age or older have erect posture and a smooth gait. Facial expressions correspond to the content and topic of discussion. The speech is clear, and vocabulary and word choice are appropriate to age and experience. Children should also be able to respond to increasingly difficult questions based on their age. The cranial nerves are intact. Motor function is intact, and movements are coordinated and smooth. Sensory function is demonstrated in the ability to identify touch, pain, heat, and cold; to sense vibrations; to identify objects; and to discriminate between place and points of touch on the body. The response to testing of reflexes is 2+ on a scale of 0 to 4+. Assessment proceeds in a cephalocaudal manner. The nurse tests distal to proximal and moves from gross function to fine function, always comparing corresponding body parts. More than one technique can be used to assess one function. Also see Chapter 24. ∞

For assessment of the primitive reflexes of early childhood, see Table 26.1.

Documenting Your Findings

Documentation of assessment data—subjective and objective—must be accurate, professional, complete, and confidential. When documenting the information from the focused assessment of each body system, the nurse should use measurements where appropriate to ensure accuracy, use medical terminology rather than jargon, include all pertinent information, and avoid language that could identify the patient. The information in the documentation should make it clear what questions were asked and use language to indicate whether it is the patient's response or the nurse's findings. For patient responses, the documentation will say "denies," "states," or "reports," whereas the nurse's findings will simply list the findings as fact, or say "no" along with the condition. For example, the mother of the child states "He eats table food like beans and carrots," and the nurse found "Abdomen is round, soft, and nontender × 4." The following Sample Documentation provides an example of normal results for a portion of the pediatric health and physical assessment.

Sample Documentation: Pediatric Health Assessment

Focused History (Subjective Data)

This is information from Review of Systems (ROS) and other pertinent history information that is or could be related to the patient's overall health.

Mother reports an average of eight wet and two dirty diapers daily. States stool is brown, soft, formed. Denies child's or family history of GI problems. Reports taking no more than 20 oz whole milk daily; eats table food like beans and carrots. Denies use of medications, vitamins, or other supplements for child. Reports last well-child check was at 18 months. States he is up to date on his vaccinations, including flu vaccine in October.

Physical Assessment (Objective Data)

Skin is warm, smooth, elastic, without lesions, and color is consistent with race. Abdomen is round, symmetric; soft and nontender to light and deep palpation × 4. Bladder nonpalpable. Testes are palpable in scrotum bilaterally. Spine straight, no sacral dimple, tufts, or sinuses. Femoral pulses 2+ bilaterally. Full range of motion in all joints, strength 5/5 throughout.

Abnormal Findings

Many examples of abnormal findings are presented in the preceding chapters by body system. The following are selected examples of abnormal findings that are unique to pediatric assessment.

Alterations of the Skin, Hair, and Nails

Some alterations in the skin, hair, and nails in infants, children, and adolescents include skin lesions such as birthmarks or nevi, infection or infestation of the hair, and problems with nails.

BIRTHMARKS AND RASHES

The skin of the newborn will exhibit many changes during the first week of life. Parents are often concerned with the presence of unexpected rashes or lesions. Most newborn birthmarks are benign, and most rashes will resolve (Templet & Lemoine, 2017).

Common Birthmarks:	Description:
• Mongolian spots	• Present at birth, may fade with time, no treatment required.
• Strawberry hemangiomas	• Present at birth, 90% fade by age 10 years. Some cosmetic treatments can be prescribed. Refer to vascular specialist.
• Nevus simplex (These are also known as salmon patches, stork bites, or angel kisses.)	• Present at birth, may fade with time. No treatment required.
• Nevus flammeus (These are also known as port-wine stain.)	• Present at birth, may fade with time. Some cosmetic treatments can be prescribed.

COMMON RASHES

• Erythema toxicum neonatorum (newborn rash)	• Onset in first 3 days of life, usually resolves in a week and may recur.
• Seborrheic dermatitis (cradle cap)	• Onset at 1 month of age, spontaneously resolves with time.

Abnormalities of the Eye

In addition to conditions affecting vision in infants, children, and adolescents, the following are the most common abnormal findings in this age group.

Condition:	Description:
• Conjunctivitis: bacterial or viral infection of the conjunctivae	• Commonly spreads to both eyes; purulent drainage and redness present.
• Lacrimal duct blockage: blocked tear ducts possibly present at birth (WebMD, 2016)	• Usually will open on its own; provide education about massaging the duct to help it open.

Abnormalities of the Head and Neck

Parents often have questions about the shape of the infant's head in the weeks after birth. The following are several common findings.

Common Variations:	Description:
• Molding: shaping of the head from pressure on the bones as the head moves through the vaginal canal during birth	• Present at birth and will take several days for the head to take on the rounded shape.
• Plagiocephaly: asymmetrical flattening of one side of the skull	• Most often caused by placing the infant consistently in one position. Education about repositioning, sometimes physical therapy.
• Torticollis: sometimes called wry neck; a twisting of the neck to one side, causing the head to tilt	• Present at birth, may be due to intrauterine positioning. Treated with physical therapy, occasionally orthopedic referral.

Abnormalities of the Ears, Nose, Mouth, and Throat

A wide range of variations from normal findings are seen in children. The following are several of the most common findings in infants and children.

Condition:	Description:
• Ankyloglossia or "tongue-tie" (Figure 26.17 ■)	• Fixation of the tip of the tongue to the floor of the mouth due to a shortened lingual frenulum. The condition is usually congenital and may be corrected surgically.
	• May interfere with feeding.

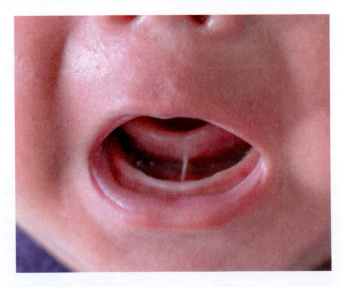

Figure 26.17 Ankyloglossia.
Source: Akkalak Aiempradit/Shutterstock.

Condition:
- Cleft lip and/or palate (Figure 26.18 ■)

Description
- A separation or splitting of the two sides of the upper lip; appears as a gap or narrow opening in the skin of the upper lip. May occur alone or along with cleft palate.
- Careful assessment of feeding needs. Referral to plastic surgery is common.

Subjective Findings:
- Dyspnea, shortness of breath
- Anxiety in children appears as fussiness

Objective Findings:
- Wheezing
- Diminished breath sounds
- Increased respiratory rate
- Accessory muscle use
- Nasal flaring
- Retractions: subcostal, substernal, intracostal
- Decreased oxygen saturation

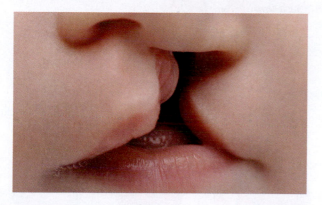

Figure 26.18 Cleft lip.
Source: malost/Shutterstock.

Respiratory Disorders

ASTHMA

A chronic hyper-reactive condition resulting in bronchospasm, mucosal edema, and increased mucus secretion. This condition usually occurs in response to inhaled irritants or allergens. (Figure 26.19 ■.)

Cardiovascular Abnormalities

CONGENITAL HEART DISORDERS

Cardiovascular disease in children can be divided between congenital and acquired, with most of the disease burden being the result of congenital heart defect (CHD). CHDs range in severity from mild to severe, with the most severe defects requiring early surgical intervention (Mayo Clinic, 2018). Mild CHDs include small ventricular and atrial septal defects More severe and complex CHDs are pictured in Table 26.2 and include coarctation of the aorta, patent ductus arteriosus, and tetralogy of Fallot. (see Table 18.7 in Chapter 18.) ∞

Subjective Findings: (depend on the type of defect and may include the following):
- Dyspnea
- Fatigue, sleepiness
- Poor feeding

Objective Findings:
- Tachypnea
- Tachycardia
- Pallor, cyanosis, mottled skin
- Accessory muscle use
- Failure to thrive
- Heart murmur
- Decreased oxygen saturation

Acquired Heart Disease

Several common childhood infectious diseases, if not treated, may cause damage to the heart. Rheumatic heart disease, evidenced by heart valve damage caused by group A *Streptococcus* infection during infancy and childhood is less common in the United States, but it is still a major public health problem in the developing countries (Mirabel et al., 2015). Kawasaki disease is an acute vasculitis of childhood that may lead to coronary artery aneurysms in as many as 25% of cases. Kawasaki disease is thought to be the most common cause of acquired heart disease in children in the developed countries (McCrindle et al., 2017).

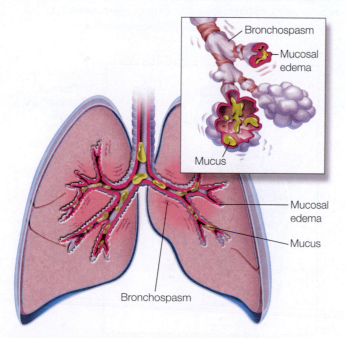

Figure 26.19 Asthma.

Table 26.2 Overview of Congenital Heart Disorders

COARCTATION OF THE AORTA

The aorta is severely narrowed in the region inferior to the left subclavian artery. The narrowing restricts blood flow from the left ventricle into the aorta and out into the systemic circulation, thus contributing to the development of congestive heart failure in the newborn. It can be surgically treated.

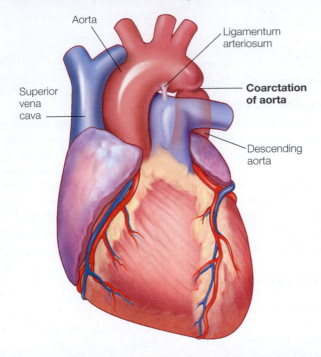

PATENT DUCTUS ARTERIOSUS

Occurs when the ductus arteriosus fails to close completely between 24 and 48 hours after birth. It may be treated medically, through pharmacologic therapy, and surgically.

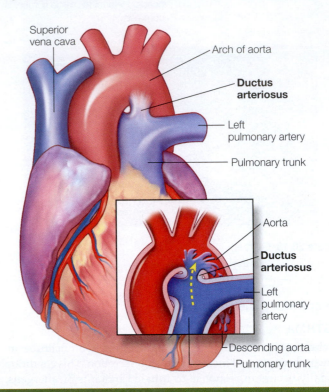

TETRALOGY OF FALLOT

Involves four cardiac defects: pulmonary stenosis, overriding aortic valve, ventricular septal defect, and right ventricular hypertrophy. This condition is life-threatening for the newborn but can be treated surgically.

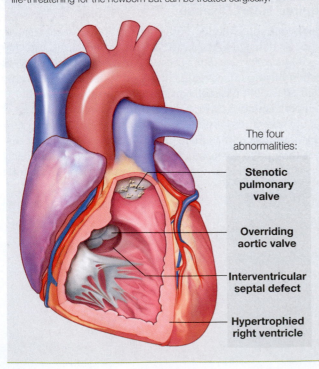

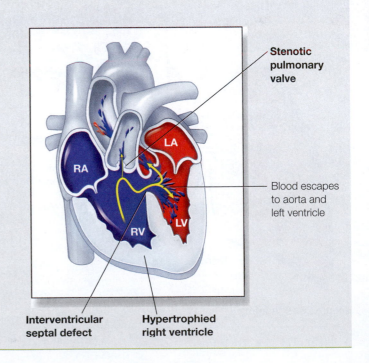

Musculoskeletal System

SCOLIOSIS

The most common form of scoliosis, adolescent idiopathic scoliosis, is a spinal curvature greater than 10 degrees (Figure 26.20 ■). Screening is often done in late childhood and early adolescence. The greater the curvature in late adolescence, the more likely that adult health outcomes may be adversely affected (Dunn et al., 2018).

LORDOSIS

Lordosis is an exaggeration of the normal lumbar curvature of the spine. This condition is common and expected in toddlers due to their normal potbelly stance (Figure 26.9).

Neurologic System

SEIZURE DISORDERS

A seizure is a temporary neurologic event consisting of uncontrolled electrical neuronal discharge in the brain (Berman et al., 2016). Seizures may be caused by trauma before or during birth, infections of the central nervous system, and fevers. In some individuals, the cause is unknown, and these are called idiopathic seizures. **Febrile seizures**, or those caused by fever, are the most common neurological disorder in childhood. This type of seizure is usually benign, and

when a child does not have other risk factors, there is minimal risk of developing a long-term seizure disorder (Renda, Yuksel & Gurer, 2017).

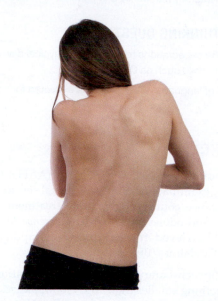

Figure 26.20 Scoliosis.
Source: Dmitry Lobanov/123RF.

Application Through Critical Thinking

CASE STUDY

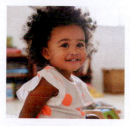

Source: Monkey Business Images/Shutterstock.

Casey is a 2-year-old girl whose mother brought her in for a checkup. Her mother reports that Casey was born at 40 weeks gestation after an uncomplicated pregnancy and vaginal birth. She is pretty sure that Casey has met each developmental milestone at the normal age and does not have any problems that she has identified. Casey has no history of medical problems or diseases other than an occasional "cold," and her immunizations are up-to-date. Casey is a very energetic child and is often running around in the backyard and loves to play in the sandbox and with their dog, Max. The mother states that she is very careful with what she feeds her family and that Casey has good eating habits, although sometimes she throws her food at the dog and laughs. Casey's parents have some good friends whose youngest child is being carefully followed by his pediatrician because of what is thought to be "significant developmental delays." Consequently, Casey's mother is very concerned about developmental milestones and wants her daughter "checked to make sure everything is all right." The mother states that she has read a lot of information on the internet on child development but asks many questions regarding the care and needs of her child. Mom seems very anxious during the visit and very concerned that she may have missed something in Casey's development.

SUBJECTIVE DATA: Mom states Casey does not have any developmental problems. She is an energetic child who loves to run and play outside. States Casey has good eating habits and age-appropriate behavior playing with food. Mom is concerned about developmental milestones r/t friend's daughter with delays. States she is here to have Casey "checked to make sure everything is all right."

OBJECTIVE DATA: Full-term spontaneous vaginal birth. Immunizations up to date, no significant medical or family history. 2-year-old able to run, play, and interact with family and pet.

CRITICAL THINKING QUESTIONS

1. What are the expectations regarding the physical development for a 2-year-old child such as Casey?

2. What level of language development is expected for a toddler?

3. Identify at least two standardized tools that are used to assess physical and psychosocial development across the age span.

4. What are the expectations for cognitive development for a 2-year-old child?

5. How might you validate the mother's assessment that Casey has good eating habits?

REFERENCES

American Academy of Pediatric Dentistry (AAPD). (2018). Periodicity of examination, preventive dental services, anticipatory guidance/counseling, and oral treatment for infants, children, and adolescents. *AAPD Reference Manual, 39*(6), 188–195. Retrieved from http://www.aapd.org/media/Policies_Guidelines/BP_Periodicity.pdf

American Speech-Language-Hearing Association (ASHA). (2015). Nothing smaller than your elbow, please. Audiology Information Series. Retrieved from http://www.asha.org/uploadedFiles/AIS-Earwax.pdf

Berman, A., Snyder, S. J., & Frandsen, G. (2016). *Kozier & Erb's fundamentals of nursing: Concepts, process, and practice* (10th ed.). Hoboken, NJ: Pearson.

Centers for Disease Control and Prevention (CDC). (2015). *Basics about hearing loss in children.* Retrieved from http://www.cdc.gov/ncbddd/hearingloss/facts.html

Centers for Disease Control and Prevention (CDC). (2018). *Common colds: Protect yourself and others.* Retrieved from https://www.cdc.gov/features/rhinoviruses

Churchward, C. P., Alany, R. G., Kirk, R. S., Walker, A. J., & Snyder, L. A. (2017). Prevention of ophthalmia neonatorum caused by *Neisseria gonorrhoeae* using a fatty acid-based formulation. *mBio, 8*(4), e00534-17. doi:10.1128/mBio.00534-17

Dashe, J., Roocroft, J. H., Bastrom, T. P., & Edmonds, E. W. (2013). Spectrum of shoulder injuries in skeletally immature patients. *The Orthopedic Clinics of North America, 44*(4), 541–551. doi:10.1016/j.ocl.2013.06.008

Dennie, J., & Grover, S. R. (2013). Distressing perineal and vaginal pain in prepubescent girls: An aetiology. *Journal of Paediatrics and Child Health, 49*(2), 138–140. doi:10.1111/jpc.12085

Dunn, J., Henrikson, N. B., Morrison, C. C., Blasi, P. R., Nguyen, M., & Lin, J. S. (2018). Screening for adolescent idiopathic scoliosis: Evidence report and systematic review for the US Preventive Services Task Force. *JAMA, 319*(2), 173–187. doi:10.1001/jama.2017.11669

Forray, A. (2016). Substance use during pregnancy. *F1000 Faculty Reviews, 5*, 887. doi:10.12688/f1000research.7645.1

Goldberg, E. M. (2013). Fever and bulging fontanelle mimicking meningitis in an infant diagnosed with benign intracranial hypertension. *Pediatric Emergency Care, 29*(4), 513–514.

Grandjean, P., & Landrigan, P. J. (2014). Neurobehavioural effects of developmental toxicity. *The Lancet Neurology, 13*(3), 330–338. doi:10.1016/S1474-4422(13)70278-3

Iheozor-Ejiofor, Z., Worthington, H. V., Walsh, T., O'Malley, L., Clarkson, J. E., Macey, R., . . . Glenny, A. (2015). Water fluoridation to prevent tooth decay. *Cochrane Database of Systematic Reviews, 6*(CD010856). doi:10.1002/14651858.CD010856.pub2

Isaacson, G. C. (2018). *Congenital anomalies of the ear.* UpToDate. Retrieved from https://www.uptodate.com/contents/congenital-anomalies-of-the-ear#H14

Jiles, K. A., & Hamrick, M. C. (2017). Evaluation and management of pediatric constipation. *Current Treatment Options in Pediatrics, 3*(2), 69-76. doi: 10.1007/s40746-017-0078-8

Kessenich, C. R., & Flanagan, M. (2015). Diagnosis of infectious mononucleosis. *The Nurse Practitioner, 40*(8), 13–16. doi:10.1097/01.NPR.0000469261.28614.88

Leung, A. M. (2018). U.S. newborn screening programs for congenital hypothyroidism vary widely. *Clinical Thyroidology, 30*(2), 88–89. doi:10.1089/ct.2018;30.88-89

Mansoor, N., Mansoor, T., & Ahmed, M. (2016). Eye pathologies in neonates. *International Journal of Ophthalmology, 9*(12), 1832–1838. doi:10.18240/ijo.2016.12.22

Mayo Clinic. (2016). *When's the right time to start feeding a baby solid foods?* Retrieved from https://www.mayoclinic.org/healthy-lifestyle/infant-and-toddler-health/expert-answers/starting-solids/faq-20057889

Mayo Clinic. (2017). *Ear infection (middle ear).* Retrieved from http://www.mayoclinic.org/diseases-conditions/ear-infections/basics/complications/con-20014260

Mayo Clinic. (2018). *Congenital heart defects in children.* Retrieved from https://www.mayoclinic.org/diseases-conditions/congenital-heart-defects-children/symptoms-causes/syc-20350074

McCrindle, B. W., Rowley, A. H., Newburger, J. W., Burns, J. C., Bolger, A. F., Gewitz, M. . . . Pahl, E. (2017). Diagnosis, treatment, and long-term management of Kawasaki disease: A scientific statement for health professionals from the American Heart Association. *Circulation, 135*, e927–e999. doi:10.1161/CIR.0000000000000484

Mirabel, M., Bacquelin, R., Tafflet, M., Robillard, C., Huon, B., Corsenac, P., . . . Marijon, E. (2015). Screening for rheumatic heart disease: Evaluation of a focused cardiac ultrasound approach. *Circulation: Cardiovascular Imaging, 8,* e002324. doi:10.1161/CIRCIMAGING.114.002324

Modgil, V., Rai, S., & Anderson, P. C. B. (2014). Male circumcision: Summary of current clinical practice. *Trends in Urology & Men's Health, 5*(3), 21–24. doi:10.1002/tre.395

Moyer, V. A., on behalf of the U.S. Preventive Services Task Force. (2013). Screening for primary hypertension in children and adolescents: U.S. Preventive Services Task Force recommendation statement. *Annals of Internal Medicine, 159*(9), 613–619. doi:10.7326/0003-4819-159-9-201311050-00725

National Institute of Neurological Disorders and Stroke. (2017). *Febrile seizures information page.* Retrieved from https://www.ninds.nih.gov/Disorders/All-Disorders/Febrile-Seizures-Information-Page

Olfson, M., Druss, B. G., & Marcus, S. C. (2015). Trends in mental health care among children and adolescents. *The New England Journal of Medicine, 372,* 2029–2038. doi:10.1056/NEJMsa1413512

Orcesi, S. (2013). The floppy newborn. *Early Human Development, 89*(S4), S79–S81. doi:10.1016/S0378-3782(13)70110-5

Popova, S., Lange, S., Probst, C., Gmel, G., & Rehm, J. (2017). Estimation of national, regional, and global prevalence of alcohol use during pregnancy and fetal alcohol syndrome: A systematic review and meta-analysis. *The Lancet Global Health, 5,* e290–e299. doi:10.1016/S2214-109X(17)30021-9

Renda, R., Yuksel, D., & Gurer, Y. K. (2017). Evaluation of patients with febrile seizure: Risk factors, recurrence, treatment, and prognosis. *Pediatric Emergency Care,* Published ahead of print. doi:10.1097/PEC.0000000000001173

St. John, J., Summe, H., Csikesz, C., Wiss, K., Hay, B., & Belazarian, L. (2016). Multiple café au lait spots in a group of fair-skinned children without signs or symptoms of neurofibromatosis type 1. *Pediatric Dermatology, 33*(5), 526–529. doi:10.1111/pde.12936

Saugstad, O. D. (2018). Oxygenation of the immature infant: A commentary and recommendations for oxygen saturation targets and alarm limits. *Neonatology, 111,* 69–75. doi:10.1159/000486751

Shields, K., Fox, K., & Liebrecht, C. (2018). *Pearson nurse's drug guide.* Hoboken, NJ: Pearson Education, Inc.

Silverberg, N. B., & Lee-Wong, M. (2014). Generalized yellow discoloration of the skin. *Cutis, 93*(5), E11–E12. Retrieved from https://www.mdedge.com/cutis/article/82284/pigmentation-disorders/generalized-yellow-discoloration-skin

Templet, T., & Lemoine, J. (2017). Benign neonatal skin conditions. *The Journal for Nurse Practitioners, 13*(4), e199–202. doi:10.1016/j.nurpra.2016.09.013

Troullioud Lucas, A. G., & Mendez, M. D. (2017). *Hernia, pediatric umbilical.* Treasure Island, FL: StatPearls Publishing. Retrieved from https://www.ncbi.nlm.nih.gov/books/NBK459294

Varma, R., Tarczy-Hornoch, K., & Jiang, X. (2017). Visual impairment in preschool children in the United States: Demographic and geographic variations from 2015 to 2060. *JAMA Ophthalmology, 135*(6), 610–616. doi:10.1001/jamaophthalmol.2017.1021

WebMD. (2016). *What are blocked tear ducts?* Retrieved from https://www.webmd.com/eye-health/what-are-blocked-tear-ducts#1

WebMD. (2017). *Common food allergy triggers.* Retrieved from https://www.webmd.com/allergies/food-triggers#1

Weitzman, C., Wegner, L., Section on Developmental and Behavioral Pediatrics, Committee on Psychosocial Aspects of Child and Family Health, Council on Early Childhood, & Society for Development and Behavioral Pediatrics. (2015). Promoting optimal development: Screening for behavioral and emotional problems. *Pediatrics, 135*(2), 384–395. doi:10.1542/peds.2014-3716

Westland, R., Schreuder, M. F., Ket, J. C., & van Wijk, J. A. (2013). Unilateral renal agenesis: A systematic review on associated anomalies and renal injury. *Nephrology Dialysis Transplantation, 28*(7), 1844–1855. doi:10.1093/ndt/gft012

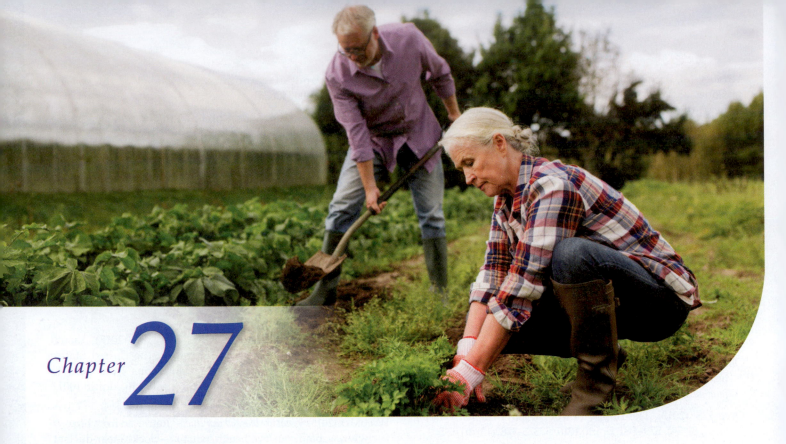

Chapter 27

Older Adults

LEARNING OUTCOMES

Upon completion of this chapter, you will be able to:

1. Describe unique aspects of the anatomy and physiology of body systems in older adults.

2. Identify the anatomic, physiologic, developmental, psychosocial, and cultural variations that guide assessment of older adults.

3. Determine questions about older adults to use for the focused interview.

4. Outline key considerations for physical assessment of older adults.

5. Generate the appropriate documentation to describe the assessment findings for older adults.

6. Identify abnormal findings in the physical assessment of older adults.

KEY TERMS

advance directives, 707
cataract, 700
comprehensive geriatric
   assessment (CGA), 706
Bouchard's nodes, 703
edentulism, 701

functional status, 714
geriatric syndromes, 704
glaucoma, 700
gynecomastia, 710
Heberden's nodes, 703
kyphosis, 703

macular degeneration, 700
menopause, 702
nocturia, 711
orthostatic hypotension, 701
pingueculae, 699
polypharmacy, 705

presbycusis, 700
presbyopia, 699
pterygium, 699
stress incontinence, 711
xanthelasma, 699

MEDICAL LANGUAGE

-ectomy	Suffix meaning "removal," "excision," "resection"
mast-	Prefix meaning "breast"
onycho-	Prefix meaning "nail"

-opia	Suffix meaning "vision condition"
poly-	Prefix meaning "many," "much"
presby-	Prefix meaning "old age"
sclerosis	Root word meaning "hardening"

Introduction

The U.S. population of adults ages 65 and older, also referred to as older adults, has been steadily growing and is expected to continue to increase as Americans are living longer (Office of Disease Prevention and Health Promotion, *Healthy People 2020*, 2018; Ortman, Velkoff, & Hogan, 2014). The different aspects of the geriatric health assessment are outlined throughout this chapter. The nurse should conduct a thorough health assessment in order to effectively collaborate with other members of the multidisciplinary healthcare team to address the unique changes and needs that occur throughout the different stages of the aging process and provide optimum care to the older adult patient.

The health history and physical examination of the older adult follow the same aspects of health assessment that have been outlined throughout this text. However, some important additions must be considered when planning the assessment of the older adult. Nurses must be aware of the anatomic, physiologic, functional, physical, socioenvironmental, and cognitive and other mental health variations unique to this patient population. This chapter will outline these differences, along with the several other considerations needed to perform a comprehensive health history and physical assessment of the older adult.

Anatomy and Physiology Review

Several changes take place in the human body as a person ages (ConsultGeri, n.d.). These changes occur because of alterations at the individual cellular level and of whole organs within different body systems. Changes occur across the lifespan, but age-related changes become more prevalent as a person transitions into and enters the stages of older adulthood (see Box 27.1). Changes are most pronounced in adults who are 85 years and older.

How a person ages is impacted by a variety of factors including genetics and lifestyle behaviors such as nutrition and dietary choices, alcohol use, tobacco use, and illicit drug use, as well as social and environmental factors (ConsultGeri, n.d.). Along with these factors and normal aging, the development of disease is another important consideration. In order to conduct a thorough health assessment, interpret findings, and plan for optimum care, nurses should be able to identify the changes in the normal aging process to distinguish them from abnormal, disease-related changes. Nurses should also recognize that normal changes have the potential to affect older adults' health and functional abilities, increase susceptibility to and mask typical signs and symptoms of certain diseases, and impact treatment response.

Skin, Hair, and Nails

As the skin ages, the epidermis thins and stretches, and collagen and elastin fibers decrease, causing decreased skin elasticity and increased skin wrinkling. The skin becomes slack and may hang loosely on the frame. It may sag, especially beneath the chin and eyes, in the breasts of women, and in the scrotum of men.

The older patient's skin is also more delicate and more susceptible to injury. Decreased production of sebum leads to dryness of both the skin and the hair. The skin may appear especially thin on the dorsal surfaces of the hands and feet and over the bony prominences. Tenting of the skin is common (see Figure 27.1 ■).

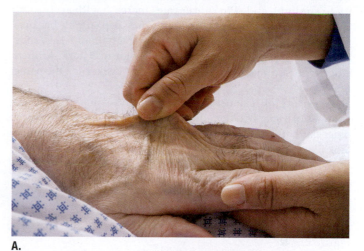

A.

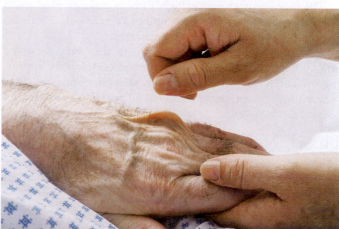

B.

Figure 27.1 Tenting. A. Step one: Nurse's fingers pulling skin; B. Step two: Skin released, remains pulled.

Box 27.1 Older Adult Subpopulations

Young Old: Ages 65–74
Old: Ages 74–84
Old Old: Ages 85+

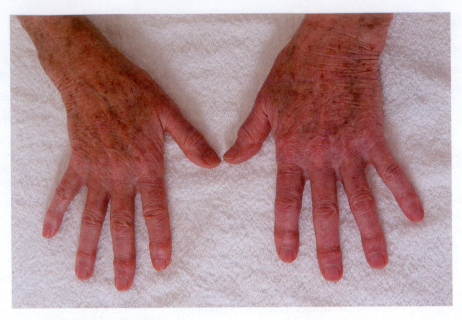

Figure 27.2 Senile lentigines.
Source: CHASSENET/BSIP SA/Alamy Stock Photo.

The sweat glands also decrease their activity, and the older adult perspires less. Decreased melanin production leads to a heightened sensitivity to sunlight, and skin cancer rates increase with age.

Some light-skinned older patients may appear pale because of decreased vascularity in the dermis, even though they may be healthy and well oxygenated. The color of a dark-skinned elderly person may appear dull, gray, or darker for the same reason.

A variety of lesions are common, and some are normal changes of aging in older adults. For example, the skin of many older patients may develop senile lentigines (liver spots), which look like hyperpigmented freckles, most commonly on the backs of the hands and the arms (see Figure 27.2 ■). Cherry angiomas are small, bright red spots common in older adults (see Figure 27.3 ■). They increase in number with age. Cutaneous tags may appear on the neck and upper chest (see Figure 27.4 ■), and cutaneous horns may occur on any part of the face (see Figure 27.5 ■).

The hair becomes increasingly gray as melanin production decreases. Hair thins as the number of active hair follicles decreases. Facial hair may become coarser.

The nails may show little change, or they may show the effects of decreased circulation in the body extremities, appearing thicker, harder, yellowed, oddly shaped, or opaque. They may be brittle and peeling as well as prone to splitting and breaking.

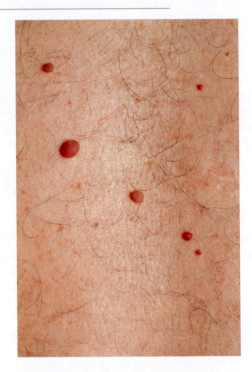

Figure 27.3 Cherry angioma.
Source: whitemay/E+/Getty Images.

Head, Neck, and Related Lymphatics

The older adult loses subcutaneous fat in the face, and the skin's elasticity decreases. This increases the wrinkles in the skin, yielding an older appearance. A decrease in reproductive hormones results in the development of coarse, long eyebrows and nasal hair in men and coarse hair, usually on the chin, in women. Loss of teeth and improperly fitting dentures provide a change to facial expressions and symmetry. Rigidity of the cervical vertebrae is common, causing limited range of motion of the neck. The thyroid gland produces fewer hormones with age. Hypothyroidism is very common in people over age 60, and prevalence increases as one ages (American Thyroid Association [ATA], 2018). Although older adults may not exhibit many of the typical signs and symptoms of thyroid dysfunction, feeling tired, weak, or unwell are common complaints (ATA, 2018). Some symptoms that many people expect with aging, such as weight changes, decreased cognitive function, slowed physical movement, and feeling unwell, may prove to be signs of thyroid disorders.

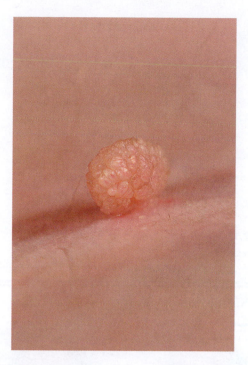

Figure 27.4 Cutaneous tag.
Source: Tetiana Mandziuk/123RF.

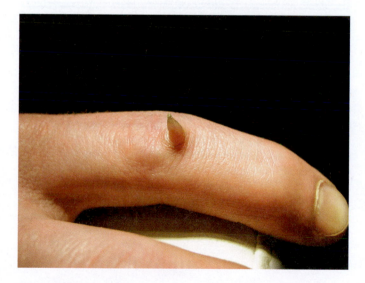

Figure 27.5 Cutaneous horn.
Source: Nau Nau/Shutterstock.

Eyes

Several alterations are associated with normal aging and are not related to vision or eye problems. **Xanthelasma** (Figure 27.6 ■) are soft, yellow plaques on the lids at the inner canthus. These plaques are sometimes associated with cholesterolemia but usually have no pathologic significance because they appear on persons with normal cholesterol counts. **Pingueculae** (Figure 27.7 ■) are yellowish nodules that are thickened areas of the bulbar conjunctiva caused by prolonged exposure to sun, wind, and dust.

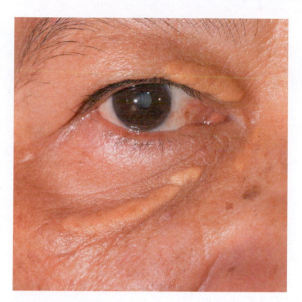

Figure 27.6 Xanthelasma.
Source: ARZTSAMUI/Shutterstock.

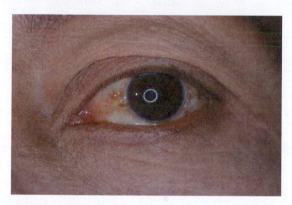

Figure 27.7 Pinguecula.
Source: ARZTSAMUI/Shutterstock.

They may be on either side of the pupil and cause no problems. However, they must be differentiated from **pterygium** (Figure 27.8 ■), opacity of the bulbar conjunctiva that can grow over the cornea and block vision.

By age 45, the lens of the eye loses elasticity, and the ciliary muscles become weaker, resulting in a decreased ability of the lens to change shape to accommodate for near vision. This condition is called **presbyopia**. The loss of fat from the orbit of the eye produces a drooping appearance. The lacrimal glands decrease tear production, and the patient may complain of a burning sensation in the eyes. The cornea of the eye may appear cloudy, and the nurse may detect a light gray or white ring surrounding the iris at the corneal margin because of the deposition of lipids. This common finding, known as arcus senilis (Figure 27.9 ■), does not affect vision. The pupillary light reflex is slower with age, and the pupils may be smaller in size.

Within the eye, the blood vessels are paler in color, and the nurse may detect small, round, yellow dots scattered on the retina. These yellow dots do not interfere with vision. As the patient ages, the lens continues to thicken and yellow, forming a dense area that reduces lens clarity. This condition is the

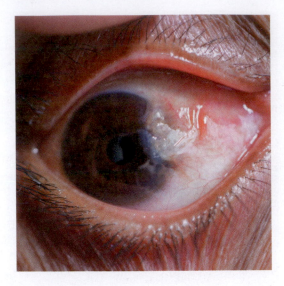

Figure 27.8 Pterygium.
Source: ARZTSAMUI/Shutterstock.

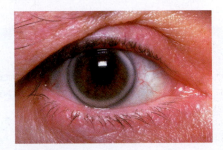

Figure 27.9 Arcus senilis.
Source: Mediscan/Alamy Stock Photo.

Cataract

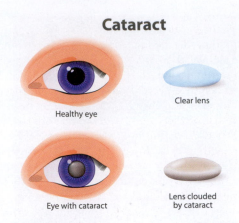

Figure 27.10 Healthy eye versus eye with cataract.
Source: designua/123RF.

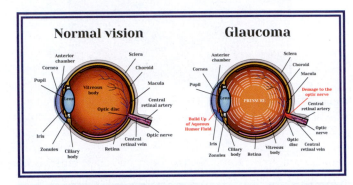

Figure 27.11 Glaucoma.
Source: Mrs_Bazilio/Shutterstock.

beginning of **cataract** formation (Figure 27.10 ■). In the older patient, the ophthalmoscopic examination may reveal **macular degeneration**: narrowed blood vessels with a granular pigment in the macula resulting in a loss of central vision. **Glaucoma** (Figure 27.11 ■), another disease of the eye more commonly diagnosed in older adults, is a group of eye conditions causing optic nerve damage; it is the leading cause of blindness in the United States (Mayo Clinic Staff, 2015).

Ears, Nose, Mouth, and Throat

The older adult may have coarse hairs at the opening of the auditory meatus. The ears may appear more prominent because cartilage formation continues throughout life. The tympanic membrane becomes paler in color and thicker in appearance with aging. Assessment of hearing may reveal a loss of high-frequency tones, which is consistent with aging. Over time, this loss often progresses to lower-frequency sounds as well. Gradual hearing loss with age is called **presbycusis**. Older patients may complain that they do not hear consonants well when listening to normal conversation. This is because of the loss of hair cells in the organ of Corti in the inner ear.

The senses of smell and taste diminish with age because of a decrease in olfactory fibers, taste buds, and saliva production. The lips and buccal mucosa become thinner and less vascular with age. Gums are paler in color. The tongue develops more fissures, and motor function may become impaired, resulting in problems with swallowing. Senile tremors may cause slight protrusion of the tongue. A decreased sense of taste and smell may contribute to a decreased appetite and poor nutrition. Decreased production of saliva also may occur, perhaps because of atrophy of the salivary glands or a side effect of a medication. In some older persons, however, saliva increases, causing cheilitis (also known as angular stomatitis) (Figure 27.12 ■), which manifests as tissue inflammation at the corners of the mouth.

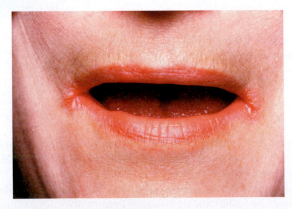

Figure 27.12 Angular stomatitis.
Source: Mediscan/Alamy Stock Photo.

Older adults typically demonstrate gum recession. Tooth loss may occur because of osteoporosis. Partial or complete loss of teeth may also be found, especially in the oldest adults who lived half of their lives before the use of prophylactic fluoride and other modern dental care. In general, however, poor dental health is decreasing; dental care is improving for people of all ages, and the current generation of older adults has lived most of their life drinking fluoridated water and observing modern dental hygiene. Lost teeth may cause the remaining teeth to drift. Ill-fitting dentures can produce oral lesions. **Edentulism**, or complete loss of one's natural teeth, can give the mouth a pursed or sunken look. Individuals with and without teeth should be examined for gingivitis and signs of periodontal disease. This pathology must be differentiated from normal gums that may recede to an extent, making teeth appear longer.

Lungs and Thorax

As individuals age, the respiratory system becomes less efficient. The lungs lose their elasticity, the skeletal muscles begin to weaken, and bones lose their density. As a result, it becomes more difficult for the older adult to expand the thoracic cage and take a deep breath. The diameters of the thoracic cage change. The appearance of a barrel chest and calcification of cartilage contribute to the decrease in the circumference of the chest (thoracic excursion). Thus, the older adult inhales and exhales smaller amounts of air. Weakening of the chest muscles hinders the older adult's ability to cough. Dry mucous membranes, decreased ciliary function, and the inability to cough compromise airway clearance.

The rate of respirations in the older adult is slightly higher than in the middle-aged adult. The older adult has a shallower respiratory cycle because of the decreased vital capacity, which is measured by the amount of air that a person can exhale at once. Auscultatory sounds may be less audible because of the decreased pulmonary function. The trapping of air in the alveoli will produce a sound of hyperresonance upon percussion.

The number of capillaries in the pulmonary tissue decreases, and there is less blood flow available for gas exchange. Normal alveoli enlarge, and their walls become thinner. Because they are less elastic, it becomes more difficult to maintain positive pressure and keep the small airways open. Gas exchange becomes compromised, especially in the bases of the lungs. Alveolar hypoventilation and carbon dioxide retention may occur.

The older person uses more accessory muscles and, therefore, must work harder and use more energy to take in air. Older adults may tire more easily and may need frequent rest periods during the assessment process. Deep mouth breathing during auscultation may increase the fatigue of older adults. As with any patient, the nurse must prevent hyperventilation at this time.

The older adult cannot respond well to stress. Anxiety and physical exertion can cause significant demands on the respiratory system, and infection can have devastating effects. Older adults with a long history of smoking or exposure to environmental pollutants are at increased risk for respiratory diseases. It is important for the older adult to obtain vaccinations against influenza and pneumonia.

Breasts and Axilla

As menopause approaches, there is a decrease in glandular tissue, which is replaced by fatty tissue. The lobular texture of glandular tissue is replaced by a finer, granular texture. Breasts are less firm and tend to be more pendulous. As the suspensory ligaments relax, breast tissue hangs more loosely from the chest wall. The nipples become smaller and flatter and lose some erectile ability. The inframammary ridge thickens and can be palpated more easily.

Cardiovascular System

The heart may stay the same size, enlarge, or atrophy. During normal aging in the absence of disease, the heart walls may thicken to some extent. The left atrium may increase in size over time. Significant enlargement of the left ventricle can be attributed to the influence of hypertension. Aging can also contribute to the loss of ventricular compliance as the cardiac valves and large vessels become more rigid. The aorta may dilate and lengthen.

Physiologically, systolic blood pressure may increase; however, there may be no significant change in resting heart rate. Diastolic filling time and pressure may increase to maintain a cardiac output adequate for physiological needs. Upon auscultation, the older patient may have an S4. In addition, the electrical conduction system may experience a loss of automaticity when the SA node and conducting pathways become fibrotic and lose cellular integrity.

In the healthy older adult, cardiac output may remain stable. Stroke volume may increase just slightly when the patient is at rest. The healthy patient may tolerate exercise well. The healthy older adult may actually show a decreased heart rate, maximum oxygen consumption, and an increase in stroke volume during exercise. A patient who has been physically active most of his or her life may have twice the work capacity of a patient who has not.

Peripheral Vascular System

The aging process causes arteriosclerosis or calcification of the walls of the blood vessels. The arterial walls lose elasticity and become more rigid. This increase in peripheral vascular resistance results in increased blood pressure. Older adults are at increased risk of developing **orthostatic hypotension**, a sudden drop in blood pressure within 3 minutes of moving from a lying to sitting or standing position (Mayo Clinic Staff, 2017d). This can be the result of medications or vascular impairment. The enlargement of calf veins can pose the risk of blood clots in leg veins. However, the amount of circulatory inadequacy at any given age is not predictable. The aging process may not cause any symptoms in some older patients.

Abdomen

The digestive system of the older adult undergoes characteristic changes; however, these may not be as pronounced as changes in other body systems. There is a gradual decrease in secretion of saliva, digestive enzymes, peristalsis, intestinal absorption, and intestinal activity. These changes may lead to indigestion, constipation, and gastroesophageal reflux and could exacerbate any preexisting change or disease. Other changes the nurse should anticipate with this age group are dry mouth, delayed esophageal and gastric emptying, decreased gastric acid production, reduced sensation of defecation, and decreased liver size and hepatic reserve, which can lead to altered drug metabolism.

Urinary System

The effects of aging take their toll on the kidneys. The weight of the kidneys may drop by as much as 30%, particularly in the renal cortex. Renal blood flow and perfusion gradually decrease. The capillary system in the glomeruli atrophies. Although the vasculature in the renal medulla remains relatively well preserved, the arcuate and interlobular arteries may become distorted, resulting in a tortuous configuration. All structures of the renal cortex and the renal medulla experience some degree of decline, especially the nephrons. By ages 75 to 80, a 50% loss of nephrons has occurred; thus, glomerular filtering is decreased. This has major implications for increased susceptibility for drug toxicity in older adults. Atherosclerosis of renal arteries can decrease renal blood flow and may lead to atrophy of the kidneys. Tubular function also diminishes, and urine is not as effectively concentrated as at a younger age; maximum specific gravity may be only 1.024. About 30% to 50% of the glomeruli degenerate because of fibrosis, hyalinization, and fat deposition. All of these factors contribute to the loss of filtration surface area in the glomerular capillary tufts by age 75. Creatinine clearance decreases slowly after age 40, as does the ability to concentrate and dilute urine.

The older patient's decreased sensation of thirst and resultant decreased intake of water relate directly to the body's compensatory response of concentrating urine. However, antidiuretic hormone is not as effective as in a younger patient; thus, concentrations and activity of renin and aldosterone are reduced with advanced age by as much as 30% to 50%. This combination of circumstances places the older patient at risk for hyperkalemia.

The older adult also has a reduced capacity to produce ammonia, which interacts with acids. Reduced ability to clear medications and acids, along with reduced ability to resorb bicarbonate and glucose, make the older patient more susceptible to toxicity related to medications, the effects of respiratory or metabolic acidosis, increased concentrations of glucose in the urine, and the loss of fluids.

Endocrine changes affect size, lubrication, and function of genital structures in both men and women. Decreased hormone production affects both libido and performance. Postmenopausal women experience a decrease in estrogen that affects the strength of the pubic muscles and may lead to urine leakage, reduced acidity in the lower urinary tract, and urinary tract infection (UTI). Diminished bladder elasticity, bladder capacity, and sphincter control also occur as a person ages and can result in problems such as incontinence.

Male Reproductive System

Older men experience changes to the external genitals. Pubic hair thins and grays, the prostate gland enlarges, the size of the penis and testes may diminish, the scrotum hangs lower, and the testes are softer to palpation. Sperm production decreases in middle age; however, older men may remain able to contribute viable sperm and father children throughout their lifespan.

Sexual function and ability change as well. Testosterone production decreases, resulting in diminished libido. Sexual response is often slower and not as intense. Older men may be slower to achieve erection, yet they may be able to maintain the erection longer. Ejaculation can be less forceful and last for a shorter time, and less semen may be ejaculated.

Even though older men can achieve sexual gratification and participate in a satisfying sexual relationship, a decrease in sexual drive may contribute to the patient's withdrawing from sexual experiences and relationships. The following factors are known to influence sexual drive:

- Chronic or acute diseases
- Certain medications
- Loss of spouse or significant other
- Loss of privacy
- Depression
- Fatigue
- Any stressful situation
- Use of alcohol or illicit drugs

Female Reproductive System

Reproductive ability in women usually peaks in the late 20s. Over time, estrogen levels begin to decline. Between ages 46 and 55, menstrual periods become shorter and less frequent until they stop entirely. **Menopause** is said to have occurred when the woman has not experienced a menstrual period in over a year. Other symptoms of menopause include mood changes and unpredictable episodes of sweating or hot flashes.

As women progress into older age, their sexual organs atrophy. Vaginal secretions are not as plentiful, and they may experience pain during intercourse. Intercourse may produce vaginal infections. The clitoris becomes smaller.

Even though older adult women can achieve sexual gratification and participate in a satisfying sexual relationship, a decrease in sexual drive may contribute to the patient's withdrawing from sexual experiences and relationships. Chronic or acute disease, medications, loss of a spouse or significant other, loss of privacy, depression, fatigue, stress, and use of alcohol and illicit drugs are factors known to influence sexual drive.

Musculoskeletal System

As individuals age, physiologic changes take place in the bones, muscles, connective tissues, and joints. These changes may affect the individual's mobility and endurance. Bone changes include decreased calcium absorption and reduced osteoblast production. If the older adult has a chronic illness, such as chronic obstructive lung disease or hyperthyroidism, or takes medications containing glucocorticoids, thyroid hormone preparation, or anticonvulsants, bone strength may be greatly compromised because of decrease in the bone density. Elderly persons who are housebound and immobile or whose dietary intake of calcium and vitamin D is low may also experience reduced bone mass and strength. During aging, bone resorption occurs more rapidly than new bone growth, resulting in the loss of bone density typical of osteoporosis.

The decreased height of the aging adult occurs because of a shortening of the vertebral column. Thinning of the intervertebral disks during middle age and an erosion of individual vertebrae because of osteoporosis contribute to this shortening. There is an average decrease in height of 1 to 2 inches from the 20s through the 70s, and a further decrease in the 80s and 90s because of additional collapse of the vertebrae. **Kyphosis** (Figure 27.13 ■), an exaggerated convexity of the thoracic region of the spine, is common. When the older adult is standing, the nurse may notice a slight flexion of the hips and knees. These changes in the vertebral column may cause a shift in the individual's center of gravity, which in turn may put the older adult at an increased risk for falls.

The size and quantity of muscle fibers tend to decrease by as much as 30% by the 80th year of life. The amount of connective tissue in the muscles increases, and they become fibrous or stringy. Tendons become less elastic. As a result, the older patient experiences a progressive decrease in reaction time, speed of movements, agility, and endurance.

Degeneration of the joints causes thickening and decreased viscosity of the synovial fluid, fragmentation of connective tissue, and scarring and calcification in the joint capsules. In addition, the cartilage becomes frayed, thin, and cracked, allowing the underlying bone to become eroded. Because of these changes, the joints of older people are less shock absorbent and have decreased range of motion and flexibility. These normal degenerative joint

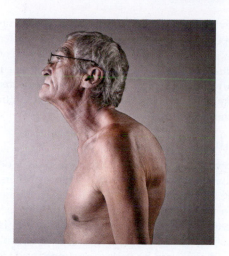

Figure 27.13 Kyphosis.
Source: Ollyy/Shutterstock.

changes that occur from aging and use are referred to as osteoarthrosis. In some individuals, **Heberden's nodes**—hard, typically painless, bony enlargements associated with osteoarthritis—may occur in the distal interphalangeal joints. Others may develop **Bouchard's nodes**, enlargement of proximal interphalangeal joints. Some may develop both types of nodes (Figure 27.14 ■)

The gait of an older patient alters as the bones, muscles, and joints change with advancing age. Both men and women tend to walk slower; some support themselves as they move. Elderly men tend to walk with the head and trunk in a flexed position, using short, high steps, a wide gait, and a smaller arm swing. The bowlegged stance that is observed in older women is because of reduced muscular control, thus altering the normal angle of the hip and leading to increased susceptibility to falls and subsequent fractures.

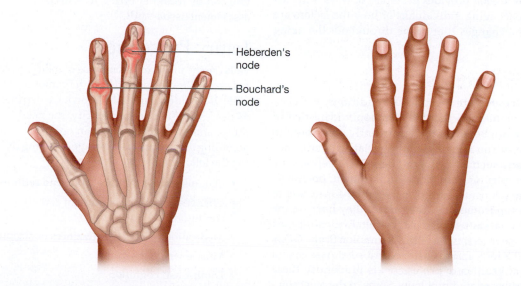

Heberden's node

Bouchard's node

Figure 27.14 Heberden's and Bouchard's nodes.

As individuals age, there is a general decrease in reaction time and speed of performance of tasks. This can affect mobility and safety, especially with unexpected environmental stimuli (e.g., objects on the floor, loose carpeting, or wet surfaces). In addition, any health problem that contributes to decreased physical activity tends to increase the chance of alterations in the health of the musculoskeletal system.

Neurologic System

As the individual ages, many neurologic changes occur. Some of these changes are readily visible, whereas others are internal and are not easily detected. The internal changes could be primary in nature, or secondary to other changes, and could contribute to the aging process. In general, the aging process causes a subtle, slow, but steady decrease in neurologic function. These changes can be more pronounced and troublesome for the individual when they are accompanied by a chronic illness such as heart disease, diabetes, or arthritis. Impulse transmission decreases, as does reaction to stimuli. Reflexes are diminished or disappear, and coordination is not as strong as it once was. Deep tendon reflexes are not as brisk. Coordination and movement may be slower and not as smooth as they were at one time.

The senses—hearing, vision, smell, taste, and touch—become less acute as an individual ages. Taste is not as strong; therefore, the older adult tends to use more seasonings on food. Visual acuity and hearing also begin to diminish.

As muscle mass decreases, the older individual moves and reacts more slowly than during youth. The patient's gait may now include short, shuffling, uncertain, and perhaps unsteady steps. The posture of the older adult demonstrates more flexion than in earlier years.

Special Considerations

During the health assessment of the older adult, the nurse must consider a wide range of issues or conditions related to aging. The following discussion provides examples of ways in which these factors impact aging individuals, or how the factors are influenced by the changes that occur throughout the aging process.

Geriatric Syndromes

Geriatric syndromes are a group of conditions, not classified as a specific disease, that are commonly identified in older adults and are believed to significantly contribute to mortality. Some of the most common geriatric syndromes include conditions such as delirium, dementia, depression, falls, frailty, malnutrition, functional impairment, polypharmacy, and urinary incontinence. It is essential for nurses to recognize these syndromes and the impact they have on the health and functional status of the older adult. Evidence-based assessment tools such as the Geriatric Depression Scale (GDS), the Fulmer SPICES tool, and the Mini Nutritional Assessment (MNA) can assist healthcare professionals to identify these syndromes and their related problems. Some of the most common syndromes will be discussed in the context of other components of this section.

Nutrition

Regular nutritional assessment of the older adult is essential (Wolfram, 2016). Good nutritional health is an important component of ensuring autonomy into older adulthood. Undernutrition can affect quality of life, morbidity, and mortality and is a major cause of frailty (Lucas & Kennedy-Malone, 2014). Skeletal muscle loss, functional decline, altered pharmacokinetics, depressed immune status, and increased risk of institutionalization can all result from malnutrition in the older adult. Further, alterations in sensory perception negatively affect intake. Alterations in sense of smell and taste are intertwined and lead to reduced enjoyment of food. Poor vision can make food preparation difficult or unsafe for the older adult living independently. Additionally, it can be difficult for the older adult with poor vision to discern the location and type of food on the plate when served a meal prepared by others. Reduced hearing can make social dining a challenge and cause some older adults to withdraw from group meals and eat in isolation, a risk factor for poor nutrition.

Quality-of-life issues related to overnutrition are also important in the older population. Being overweight or obese are risk factors for degenerative joint disease and potential functional and mobility problems. Comorbid conditions associated with being overweight, such as diabetes and cardiovascular disease, may require treatment intervention, therapeutic diets, and medications that impact nutritional health.

Poor nutrition occurs along a continuum. In the older adult, changes in nutritional health can go undetected if only strict cutoff values are observed to diagnose nutrition issues. Most general nutritional assessment parameters are applicable to the elderly population, but the nurse should be mindful of any change in nutrition status in the older adult, even when measured values and parameters remain within normal limits. The Mini Nutritional Assessment Short-Form (MNA®-SF) has been validated and is the recommended screening tool for identifying malnutrition, or those at risk for malnutrition, in individuals older than 65 (DiMaria-Ghalili & Amella, 2012). A sample of this tool can be found at https://consultgeri.org/try-this/general-assessment/issue-9.pdf.

Injury Prevention

Falls are the most common cause of injury in older adults (Office of Disease Prevention and Health Promotion, *Healthy People 2020*, 2018). If an older adult falls, it can have detrimental effects, such as decreased functional capacity, the need for surgical procedures, and even death. Falls can occur for a variety of reasons, according to the National Institute on Aging (NIA, 2017d), including the following:

- Diminished eyesight, hearing, and reflexes
- Changes in balance because of certain diseases and conditions
- Medications that cause dizziness or sleepiness
- Muscle weakness
- Diminished cognition
- Issues with balance or gait
- Orthostatic hypotension

- Osteoporosis
- Foot problems (e.g., neuropathy or other painful conditions)
- Unsafe living or community environments
- Ill-fitting or unsafe shoes (e.g., backless or high heel)

Nurses caring for patients in all care settings should follow evidence-based falls protocols and provide education for safety in the living spaces within these facilities. Patients living independently should receive education to prevent falls in the home and general safety. In addition, during the health history interview nurses should be aware of information provided by the older adult that could put the patient at risk for other types of injury. When assessing the patient's fall risk, use a valid and reliable tool, such as the Morse Fall Scale or Tinetti Gait and Balance Assessment.

Pain

Reports in the United States of the prevalence of pain in individuals tends to be higher in the older population, as well as in women and non-Hispanics (Nahin, 2015). In older adults, chronic, or persistent pain is most often an issue with causes ranging from arthritis-related joint pain to pain from cancers (Psychology Today, 2017). Other common causes of pain include injury and surgeries. Pain threshold does not appear to change with aging, although the effect of analgesics may increase because of physiologic changes related to drug metabolism and excretion. In relation to pain, older adults may:

- have multiple conditions presenting with vague symptoms of pain.
- have decreased sensations or perceptions of the pain.
- describe pain differently—that is, as "ache," "hurt," or "discomfort."
- perceive pain as part of the aging process.
- withhold complaints of pain because of fear of the treatment, fear of any lifestyle changes that may be involved, or fear of becoming dependent.
- consider it unacceptable to admit or show pain.

Thorough history and assessment are essential. It is important to spend time with the patient in the assessment of pain, listen carefully, and clarify misconceptions.

For more information about pain assessment, refer to Chapter 9. ∞

Medications

Because older adults may be on multiple medications due to several acute and chronic diseases or conditions, polypharmacy is of concern. **Polypharmacy** is the concurrent use of multiple medications to treat one or more conditions and/or diseases (Ward & Reuben, 2018). Often the medications are being prescribed by a variety of healthcare practitioners who may not be aware of other medications the patient is taking. This practice is of serious concern as it increases the risk for drug-to-drug interactions and adverse drug reactions that could be harmful to the patient. A thorough account of all medications and supplements (prescribed and over the counter), including names, dose, frequency, and reason for use, should be taken during the health history portion of the patient visit so that potential for drug interaction can be assessed.

Depression

Older adults experience many changes in life such as death of a spouse or other loved ones, retirement, and severe illness (National Institute of Mental Health [NIMH], n.d.). Often they are able to find ways to cope and make adjustments, but these events can potentially lead to depression. Depression is not a normal part of the aging process and can lead to other issues and complications. It is important for the nurse to be able to detect signs and symptoms and understand ways to screen for depression in older adults.

The Geriatric Depression Scale: Short Form is an evidence-based, validated screening tool shown to be effective in identifying depression in both healthy and mild to moderately cognitively impaired older adults living in the community as well as in a variety of care settings (Greenberg, 2012). This screening should be incorporated into the comprehensive health assessment of the older adult. A sample of the screening tool can be found at https://consultgeri.org/try-this/general-assessment/issue-4.pdf.

Cognition

Cognitive health is an important component to a healthy brain and to the functional status of the older adult. Some decline in cognitive functioning is an expected part of the aging process. Dementia is a common disorder causing impaired cognition, and incidence of dementia becomes more prevalent as one ages, particularly in individuals 85 year and older (Ward & Reuben, 2018). Individuals can assist in maintenance of cognitive health through self-care behaviors like getting regular checkups and health screenings, managing chronic diseases, decreasing the risk for injury to the brain, limiting alcohol use, quitting smoking, getting the recommended 7 to 8 hours of sleep each night, eating a healthy well-balanced diet, and maintaining activities that promote physical and mental health (National Institute on Aging [NIA], 2017b). However, many factors can accelerate or otherwise contribute to and cause impairments in cognition.

The most common risk factors for cognitive impairment include aging and genetics, both unalterable influences (Mayo Clinic Staff, 2017c). Other risk factors can be altered, such as diabetes, smoking, high blood pressure, high cholesterol, depression, absence of physical exercise, and lack of or infrequent participation in mental or social activities. The nurse should be astute in assessment techniques and other means of identifying impaired cognition in the older adult patient.

The MiniCog™ is an evidence-based, validated screening tool shown to be effective as an initial assessment for identifying persons with dementia (Doerflinger, 2013). It is a quick screening, typically taking only 3 minutes. Patients with a score of 0-2/5 are considered to have a positive screen for dementia, indicating further testing and potential for referral. A score of 3-5/5 is considered a negative screen for dementia. However, the MiniCog is not as sensitive to detecting mild cognitive impairment, and screening may miss individuals who meet this category because their score indicates a negative screen. For that reason, the Montreal Cognitive Assessment (MoCA) is recommended and has been shown to have high validity (Doerflinger, 2012). A sample of the MiniCog™ can be found at https://consultgeri.org/try-this/general-assessment/issue-3.1.pdf, and the MoCA at https://consultgeri.org/try-this/general-assessment/issue-3.2.pdf.

Frailty

Frailty is a condition associated with weakening. When older adults have a compilation of illness or disease states, and other issues related to the dysregulation of several body systems, they are at risk for entering a frail state (Lucas & Kennedy-Malone, 2014). Causes of frailty have been linked to muscle wasting, poor nutrition, inflammation, persistent pain, and multiple comorbid diseases and conditions. Poor psychosocial and lower socioeconomic status are also concerning indicators predisposing older adults to frailty. Frail older adults have a higher potential for complications and incidents such as falls, increased hospitalization, and higher mortality rates.

It is recommended that frail older adults undergo **comprehensive geriatric assessment (CGA)**, a process that assists the interdisciplinary healthcare team to identify concerns and create a comprehensive plan of care related to the medical, psychosocial, and functional capabilities of frail elderly individuals (Ward & Reuben, 2018). High-quality research and meta-analysis show that measurable health improvements in the frail older adult population have been recorded with the use of CGA.

Substance Use and Abuse

Recent research has shown that substance use is on the rise in adults ages 65 and older. It is important to be aware of this evidence and incorporate appropriate questions, screening, and observations when collecting and analyzing objective data from the older adult patient. One major concern is that older adults taking prescription medications may experience adverse reactions when also using or abusing alcohol or other illegal drugs and/or nonprescription medications. Matteson, Lipari, Hays, and van Horn (2017) compiled data from three national data sources and reported the following important information about substance use in older adults:

- Data from 2007 through 2014 National Surveys on Drug Use and Health revealed that on "an average day during the past month, 6.0 million older adults drank alcohol, 132,000 older adults used marijuana, and 4,300 older adults used cocaine." (In Brief section, bullet 2)

- In 2012, there were "14,230 admissions aged 65 or older to substance abuse treatment programs" and "on an average day in 2012, there were 29 admissions to treatment by adults aged 65 or older for alcohol use and 6 admissions to treatment for use of heroin or other opiates." (In Brief section, bullet 3)

- In 2011, "there were 2,056 drug-related ED visits for older adults. Of these, 290 involved illegal drug use, nonmedical use of pharmaceuticals, or use of alcohol combined with other drugs." (In Brief section, bullet 4)

Psychosocial Considerations

People often face many adjustments during life, such as changes in the family structure (e.g., children moving, loss of a spouse), retirement, changing income, illness, transition to a new living environment, awareness of aging bringing mortality closer to reality, and potential for isolation because of decreasing functional activity. It is important for the nurse to determine how the older adult feels about these adjustments and to consider ways to assist them with areas related to particularly challenging adjustments. According to Erik Erikson's psychosocial theory, individuals who enter into the phases of later life are in the final stage of psychosocial development, the ego integrity versus despair stage (McLeod, 2018). In this stage, the older adult reflects on his or her life and considers its meaningfulness. Those who have a sense of fulfillment and satisfaction and feel they have done something meaningful in life are considered to have reached ego integrity. Those who have opposite feelings are thought to experience a sense of despair. In order to support the older adult patient, the nurse should have an awareness of the life changes that have occurred for the patient and determine how the patient may have been affected by them.

Cultural and Environmental Considerations

Culturally competent nurses will know specifics about individual cultural, racial, and ethnic groups so as to not stereotype patients but to gain a perspective on what issues might pertain to the individual. Beliefs about older adulthood may vary among different groups of individuals from various cultures, races, and ethnicities. Sources of diversity within groups include timing of immigration, urban or rural origin, socioeconomic status, educational level, religion, strength of ethnic identity, family style, and personal characteristics. Further information about culture is included in Chapter 3. ∞

Changes in functional ability, cognition, or other situations in the person's life may indicate a need for making suggestions for a more supportive living environment, or potentially making a transition to a different type of living environment (e.g., independent senior living, assisted living, nursing home). A complete assessment of the older adult's living environment is essential for the nurse to include in the health history interview of the older adult. This assessment will help the nurse to identify potential areas of concern related to safety of the patient. In some circumstances, such as home health care, the nurse will have the opportunity to evaluate the home environment and assist in making suggestions for any changes that will improve the living space of the older adult.

Socioeconomic Status Socioeconomic status (SES) is a key component in the quality of life of older adults. It can have a major impact on the environment and health of the older adult. Low SES affects the health of the older adult in a variety of ways (American Psychological Association, 2018). For example, low SES can create barriers to receiving optimal healthcare and has been linked to the development of poor psychologic health, greater risk for functional decline and mortality, and difficulty self-managing chronic illnesses. Health issues in older adults can cause job loss, which leads to low SES and further issues with healthcare.

Elder Abuse Elder abuse can take the form of many different types of mistreatment, including physical abuse, emotional abuse, neglect, abandonment, sexual abuse, financial abuse, and healthcare fraud (National Institute on Aging [NIA], 2016). It can occur no matter what type of environment the older adult is living in. Older adults may be hesitant to report—or will not report—abuse out of fear. The nurse should be aware of signs and symptoms of all forms of elder abuse and neglect so that these may be identified through other subjective and objective data collected throughout the health assessment.

End of Life End-of-life issues can present older adults and their family members with challenging decisions. It is important to discuss these issues with older adults so that their preferences are known. **Advance directives**, written statements of a person's wishes regarding medical treatment, should be discussed with older adults (MedlinePlus, 2016). Ideally, advance directives are in place before the time that an individual will need them. Cultural values can also affect preferences and decisions regarding end of life and should be taken into account when caring for patients with terminal illnesses or assisting with planning for end of life care.

Subjective Data—Health History

Health assessment of the older adult includes the gathering of subjective and objective data. The subjective data are collected during the interview. Ideally, the patient will provide the health history. However, if cognition is impaired, the history may include information from a spouse, partner, child, or other caregiver. The nurse uses a variety of communication techniques to elicit general and specific information about the health of the older adult. Box 27.2 lists that and other information that can make the health history process productive.

Box 27.2 Considerations for Obtaining the Health History of Older Adults

- Encourage patients to come to the visit with a list of concerns.
- Ensure that the room has good lighting, a comfortable temperature, and minimal distractions and noises.
- Sit at eye level, facing the patient.
- Speak clearly.
- Explain the reason for the interview and an overview of what to expect during the entire encounter.
- Try not to interrupt as the patient is discussing his or her concerns.
- Older adults may reminisce while discussing different aspects of the health history. The information provided can be helpful; however, it may extend the length of time spent on this portion of the patient visit.
- Patient stamina should be a consideration for the length of a visit or for scheduling more than one visit to complete the comprehensive history and exam.

- Recognize that some older adults may have sensory changes, such as hearing loss, that can create communication challenges.
- Patients may display other behavior that can affect accuracy of the health history. It is important to be aware of these tendencies and know how to adjust questioning and/or include additional assessment strategies during the physical exam. Patients may:
  - underreport symptoms.
  - have symptoms that are masked by other problems.
  - present with atypical symptoms or have a lack of symptoms for many diseases and acute illnesses.
  - have cognitive impairment.

Focused Interview Questions	Rationales and Evidence

*The following section provides sample questions and bulleted follow-up questions in each of the previously mentioned categories. A rationale for each of the questions is provided. The list of questions is not all-inclusive but represents the types of questions required in a comprehensive focused interview related to older adults. These questions should be asked **in addition to** the questions normally asked during the adult health history interview as outlined throughout this text.*

Questions Related to Body Systems

Integumentary System

1. **What changes have you noticed in your skin in the past few years?**

2. **Does your skin itch?**

▶ The normal changes of aging, such as increased dryness and wrinkling of the skin, may cause distress for some patients.

▶ Pruritus (itching) increases in incidence with age (Berger, Shive, & Harper, 2013). It is usually because of dry skin, which may in turn be caused by excessive bathing or use of harsh skin cleansers.

Focused Interview Questions	Rationales and Evidence
3. Do you experience frequent falls?	▶ Older adults bruise easily (Mayo Clinic Staff, 2017a). Multiple bruises may result from frequent falls.
4. Do you find it difficult to care for your skin, hair, and nails? If so, describe any difficulties you are experiencing.	▶ Older adults with impaired mobility may have difficulty cleansing or grooming their skin, hair, and nails. Some older adults may have trouble reaching down to their feet to groom their toenails.

Head, Neck, and Related Lymphatics

1. Do you carry out safety precautions in your home? When driving or away from home? • Do you have safety rails installed in the bathroom? • Do you keep your floors clear of clutter and rugs that can slip? • Is your home well-lit? • Do you wear your seatbelt while driving? • Do you use an assistive device while walking when away from home?	▶ Older adults are at increased risk for falls (Office of Disease Prevention and Health Promotion, *Healthy People 2020*, 2018). Safety precautions can reduce the risk for falls and injuries to the head and neck.

Eyes

1. Do you experience dryness or burning in your eyes?	▶ Dryness is usually because of the decreased tear production that occurs with aging (American Optometric Association, 2018b).
2. Do you have problems seeing at night?	▶ Night blindness is associated with cataracts and some retinal diseases (Selner, 2016).
3. Do bright lights bother you?	▶ The lens of the eye thickens with aging; therefore, accommodation to light is not as rapid.
4. Are you routinely tested for glaucoma?	▶ Glaucoma is an eye condition commonly diagnosed in older adults (Mayo Clinic Staff, 2015).
5. What was the date of your last eye examination?	▶ Older adults should have annual eye exams to detect and correct common age-related vision changes, as well as any abnormal conditions that may have developed in the eyes (American Optometric Association, 2018a).

Ears, Nose, Mouth, and Throat

1. Do you wear a hearing aid? • If so, is it effective? • How often do you wear your hearing aid? • Do you have any difficulty operating the hearing aid? • How do you clean the hearing aid?	▶ Many older adults have a hearing loss but cannot adjust to using a hearing aid or cannot afford batteries for the hearing aid (Kaiser Health News, 2018). ▶ Some patients periodically forget to clean the tubes of the hearing aid.
2. Are you able to chew all types of food?	▶ If teeth are missing or dentures fit improperly, the patient may not be able to chew meat or certain vegetables, resulting in undernutrition.
3. Do you experience dryness in your mouth?	▶ Certain medications may cause dryness, which may interfere with the patient's appetite or digestion.
4. Do you wear dentures? • If so, do they fit properly?	▶ Ill-fitting dentures can interfere with proper nutrition because of food avoidance and other digestive problems (Gellar & Alter, 2014).
5. When was the date of your last dental exam?	▶ Oral health is important for older adults, and the aging process puts them at risk for certain oral health diseases. Regular dental exam visits at intervals determined by a dentist whose care the older adult is under are recommended (American Dental Association, 2013).

Lungs and Thorax

1. Describe any changes in breathing you have experienced.	▶ Aging changes in the chest, spine, lung tissue, and nervous and immune systems can make older adults more susceptible to lung infections, shortness of breath, diminished oxygen levels, and abnormal breathing patterns such as sleep apnea (MedlinePlus, 2018b).

Focused Interview Questions	Rationales and Evidence

2. Have you had any difficulty performing activities that you once found easy?

3. Do you find that you are more tired than you have been in the past?

4. Have you received any immunization for respiratory illnesses?
   - What immunization did you receive?
   - When was it given?
   - Were there any adverse effects?

▶ Older adults are at greater risk for flu and pneumonia (Centers for Disease Control and Prevention, 2018a).

Breasts and Axillae

Many people have a difficult time talking about something as private as the breasts, and older adults may be even less comfortable with this topic. They may be modest and self-conscious, or they may feel that the nurse is too young to understand. There may also be cultural taboos about such private matters. The nurse should acknowledge that talking about the breasts may be somewhat uncomfortable and should explain that sharing this information will promote the patient's health.

1. Describe your breasts today. How do they differ, if at all, from 3 months ago? From 3 years ago?

▶ This question gives the patient the opportunity to share her perception of her breasts and any changes she has experienced that may be related to breast health. It is important to obtain information from the older patient because the incidence of breast cancer and mortality rates increase with age (American Cancer Society, 2017a).

2. How do you feel about your breasts?

▶ Answers to this question may reveal a body image disturbance, self-esteem disturbance, or dysfunctional grieving (in a woman who has had a mastectomy).

3. Do you have breast implants?

▶ Breast implants do not increase the risk for breast cancer but may create difficulties in visualizing breast tissue on standard mammograms (American Cancer Society [ACS], 2017d).

4. Have you ever had any breast disease such as cancer, fibrocystic breast disease, benign breast disease, or fibroadenoma?

▶ A history of breast cancer poses the risk of a second primary breast cancer (Susan G. Komen Breast Cancer Foundation, 2018b). Both fibroadenoma and the general lumpiness of fibrocystic breast disease need to be differentiated from cancer. Increased risk for breast cancer is associated with some benign breast lesions (Susan G. Komen Breast Cancer Foundation, 2018a)

5. Have you ever had breast surgery?
   - If so, what type and when?
   - How do you feel about it?
   - How has it affected you?
   - Has it affected your sex life? If so, how?

▶ Previous breast surgery has implications for physical and psychologic well-being. Breast surgery includes lumpectomy, mastectomy, breast reconstruction, breast reduction, and breast augmentation.

6. Has your mother or sister had breast cancer?

▶ Having a first-degree relative (mother, sister, or daughter) who has experienced breast cancer approximately doubles a woman's risk for developing the disorder (American Cancer Society [ACS], 2017b).

7. Has one of your grandmothers or an aunt had breast cancer?

▶ Although the risk is higher for women whose first-degree relative has experienced breast cancer, a history of this disorder in a second-degree relative (e.g., grandmother or aunt) also increases the risk (American Society of Clinical Oncology [ASCO], 2017).

8. Has anyone in your family been found to have a genetic mutation linked to breast cancer?

▶ BRCA1 and BRCA2, which are genetic proteins that help repair damaged DNA, are especially important in terms of cancer development. Approximately 72% of women who inherit BRCA1 mutations and 69% who inherit BRCA2 mutations will develop breast cancer by the age of 80 (National Cancer Institute [NCI], 2018).

9. Have you had radiation therapy to the chest area for cancer other than breast cancer?

▶ Radiation to the chest increases the risk for breast cancer (ACS, 2017a).

Focused Interview Questions	Rationales and Evidence
10. Have you noticed any changes in breast characteristics, such as size, symmetry, shape, thickening, lumps, swelling, temperature, color of skin or vessels, or sensations such as tingling or tenderness? • If so, how long have you had them? Please describe them.	▶ Breast self-awareness (becoming familiar with the appearance and feel of one's own breasts) is important, and changes should be reported promptly to a care provider (ACS, 2017a; American College of Obstetricians and Gynecologists [ACOG], 2017). ▶ Pain and tenderness can be caused by fibrocystic breast changes, cancer, or other disorders. A lump may indicate a benign cyst, a fibroadenoma, fatty necrosis, or a malignant tumor (Mayo Clinic Staff, 2018a). Skin irritation may be due to friction from a bra or to pendulous breasts. In older women, decreased estrogen levels may cause the breasts to sag (MedlinePlus, 2018a). ▶ **For males:** **Gynecomastia** (breast enlargement in males) may occur in older men as a result of hormonal changes due to disease or medication such as hormonal treatment for prostate cancer (Mayo Clinic, 2017b). Breast cancer in the male is usually identified as a hard nodule fixed to the nipple and underlying tissue. Nipple discharge may be present. Pseudogynecomastia, an increase in subcutaneous fat, may occur in obese males. On palpation breast tissue is firmer than fat. A mammogram may be required to distinguish enlarged or changed breast tissue from increased subcutaneous fat.
11. Have you ever experienced any trauma or injury to your breasts? • If so, please describe.	▶ Contact sports, automobile accidents, and physical abuse can cause bruising of the breast and tissue changes (Healthline, 2017).
12. Did you breastfeed your children?	▶ Breastfeeding, especially from 1.5 to 2 years, decreases the risk for breast cancer (ACS, 2017a).
13. Have you ever had a mammogram? • If so, when was your most recent one?	▶ Mammography can detect a cancer before it is detectable by palpation (Johns Hopkins Medicine, n.d.). Breast cancer becomes increasingly more common as the population ages; therefore, older women must receive advice and counseling about screening for breast cancer.

Cardiovascular System

1. Have you noticed any change—no matter how subtle—in your ability to concentrate, to remember things, or to perform simple mental tasks such as writing a letter or balancing your checkbook?	▶ In the older adult, a change in mentation may suggest inadequate perfusion and can be seen in patients with myocardial ischemia and infarction or increasingly severe congestive heart failure.
2. Have you experienced reactions to any medications you are currently taking? These may include palpitations, rashes, vision changes, mentation changes, fatigue, or loss of previous sexual desire or function.	▶ Many cardiovascular medications interact with medications for other diseases and may either potentiate or reduce their effects.

Abdomen

1. Are you ever incontinent of feces?	▶ Fecal incontinence is more common in older adults and can be the result of muscle or nerve damage, constipation, diarrhea, loss of rectal storage capacity, rectal surgeries, rectal prolapse, or rectocele (Mayo Clinic Staff, 2018b).

2. How often are you constipated?
  • Do you take laxatives?
  • How often?
  • Which laxative do you take?
	▶ Constipation is a common problem with older adults (Conaway, 2018). Influencing factors include decreased gastrointestinal motility and peristaltic activity; decreased desire to eat; self-limited fluid intake (to decrease frequency of urination); impaired physical mobility; medications such as opioids, anticholinergics, calcium supplements, and NSAIDs; and cognitive disorders. To help relieve the problem, some older patients take OTC laxatives.

3. How many foods containing fiber or roughage do you eat during a typical day?	▶ A diet that is high in fiber is important for older adults for a variety of reasons. It can be particularly helpful for digestive health and prevention of constipation (Bemis, 2013).

Focused Interview Questions	Rationales and Evidence

Urinary System

1. Have you noticed any unusual swelling in your ankles, feet, fingers, or wrists?

▶ Swelling may be indicative of congestive heart failure, kidney disease, or cirrhosis of the liver (Mayo Clinic Staff, 2017b). Associated with the swelling can be weight gain, fatigue, activity intolerance, and shortness of breath.

2. Do you have problems with involuntary leaking of urine?

▶ Incontinence is a more common problem in older adults (National Institute on Aging [NIA], 2017e). Urinary incontinence is related to diminished bladder elasticity, bladder capacity, and sphincter control, as well as to cognitive impairment and sometimes functional impairment. It can cause embarrassment and lead to social isolation, infection, and skin breakdown. Stretching of perineal muscles due to childbirth and obesity further contributes to **stress incontinence** (involuntary leaking of urine caused from stress on the bladder related to pressures such as coughing, sneezing, running, or heavy lifting).

3. Do you notice that you have to urinate more frequently?
4. Have you noticed any changes to the color or odor of your urine?
5. Is there pain with urination?

▶ Urinary elimination becomes a concern as an individual advances in age and significant changes in urinary and bladder function begin to occur (National Institute on Aging 2017a). Changes in men and women include urinary retention leading to increased urinary infections; involuntary bladder contractions resulting in urgency, frequency, and incontinence; decreased bladder capacity causing frequent voiding; and weakening of the urinary sphincters, causing urgency and incontinence.

6. Do you get up frequently at night to urinate?

▶ **Nocturia** (nighttime urination) is another major concern of older persons (National Sleep Foundation, 2018). When an older person is at rest in a horizontal position, the heart is able to pump blood through the kidneys more efficiently, facilitating the excretion of urine. This factor, combined with weakened bladder and urethral muscles, contributes to nocturnal micturition. Other causes of nocturia, such as urinary infection, hyperglycemia, medication use, and stool impactions, should be considered.

7. *For male patients:* Have you noticed difficulty initiating the stream of urine, voiding in small amounts, and feeling the need to void more frequently than in the past?

▶ These symptoms may be due to an enlarged prostate. Benign prostatic hypertrophy (hyperplasia) (BPH) is a common cause of urinary retention and obstruction in men (Urology Care Foundation, 2018). As men age, the prostate gland enlarges, encroaching on the urethra. Prostatic enlargement, which occurs in 95% of all men by age 85, results in problems of urinary retention with frequent overflow voiding, especially during the night. Unrecognized urinary tract obstruction from an enlarged prostate results in damage to the upper urinary tract.

Female Reproductive System

1. Have you or your mother taken diethylstilbestrol (DES)?

▶ A history of DES use is linked with increased risk for breast cancer, clear cell adenocarcinoma, abnormal cells of the cervix and vagina, infertility, and a variety of problems during pregnancy. (American Cancer Society, 2017c).

2. At what age did you go through menopause?
   • Have you had any residual problems?

▶ This information establishes a reference for the onset of physiologic changes that accompany menopause. Women who undergo menopause after age 55 are at greater risk for breast cancer. Postmenopausal weight gain may increase the risk of breast cancer (ACS, 2017a). After menopause, decreased estrogen levels may result in decreased firmness of breast tissue (MedlinePlus, 2018a). The patient should be reassured that this is normal.

3. Have you been treated with hormone therapy during or since menopause?

▶ Combined hormone replacement therapy places patients at increased risk for breast cancer (ACS, 2017a).

Focused Interview Questions	Rationales and Evidence
4. Tell me about physical changes you have noticed since menopause.	▶ It is common for aging females to experience a variety of symptoms, including mood changes and hot flashes. Vaginal dryness causes dyspareunia (painful intercourse) (Office on Women's Health, U.S. Department of Health and Human Services, 2018).
5. Have you had any vaginal bleeding since starting menopause?	▶ Some women assume that postmenopausal bleeding is normal and tend to ignore it. Postmenopausal bleeding may be suggestive of inadequate estrogen therapy and endometrial cancer (Otify, Fuller, Ross, Shaikh, & Johns, 2015). It could also be indicative of serious problems, such as genital tract cancer.

Male Reproductive System

1. Have you had any changes in sexual function?	▶ Some older men may find they need more time to achieve erection or may not be able to keep an erection (Cleveland Clinic Foundation, 2018). These changes are often normal but could be caused by certain diseases, such as heart disease or diabetes, or by the medications used to treat diseases.

Musculoskeletal System and Functional Status

1. Have you noticed any muscle weakness over the past few months? • If so, explain what effect this muscle weakness has on your daily activities.	▶ Muscle weakness is common as a person ages, especially in people with sedentary lifestyles.
2. Have you fallen in the past 6 months? • If so, how many times? • What prompted the fall(s)? • Describe your injuries. • What treatment did you receive? • What effect did your injuries have on your daily activities?	▶ Older adults have an increased rate of falls because of a change in posture that can affect their balance (Office of Disease Prevention and Health Promotion, *Healthy People 2020*, 2018). Loss of balance also may be caused by sensory or motor disorders, inner ear infections, the side effects of certain medications, and other factors.
3. Do you use any walking aids, such as a cane or walker to help you get around? • If so, please describe the aid or show it to me.	▶ These aids help the older adult ambulate, but they can also cause falls, especially if the patient does not use the device properly.
4. *For postmenopausal women:* Do you take calcium supplements?	▶ Calcium supplementation may slow the development of some of the musculoskeletal changes associated with age, such as osteoporosis.
5. Tell me about your typical day.	▶ This can provide insight into the functioning of the older adult's daily routine and can prompt additional probing questions for more clarification or further information.
6. Have your activity levels changed over time?	▶ This question can provide information about declining function.
7. Do you have any trouble with activities such as eating, bathing, dressing, cooking, shopping, and managing finance? • Do you ever need assistance from someone else with these activities?	▶ More specific functional status questions related to activities of daily living (ADLs) and instrumental activities of daily living (IADLs) provide information about the patient's functional status (National Institute on Aging [NIA], 2017c). Any sudden changes could indicate an underlying medical problem.

Neurologic System

1. Do you require more time to perform tasks today than perhaps 2 years ago? 5 years ago? Explain.	▶ Endurance decreases with aging; therefore, more time is required for all activities.
2. When you stand up, do you have trouble starting to walk?	▶ Trouble initiating movement may indicate a variety of conditions in older adults.
3. Do you notice any tremors?	▶ Tremors may indicate motor nerve disease, or they may be attributable to certain medications.
4. What safety features have you added to your home?	▶ Safety precautions, such as handrails, grab bars, night-lights, and nonslip treads, are essential to prevent neurologic trauma from falls and other accidents.

Focused Interview Questions	Rationales and Evidence

Mental Health and Cognition

1. Ask the following two screening questions related to depression (National Institute for Health and Care Excellence, 2018; Ward & Reuben, 2018):
   - During the past month, have you often been bothered by feeling down, depressed, or hopeless?
   - During the past month, have you often been bothered by having little interest or pleasure in doing things?

▶ These two questions can be used as a quick screen during the patient interview (Esiwe et al., 2015; Tsoi, Chan, Hirai, & Wong, 2017). If "Yes" is indicated for one or both of these questions, further screening is warranted. The Geriatric Depression Scale is a more specific screening tool that can be used in the assessment of depression in older adults (Greenberg, 2012). Other cues related to depression in the older adult may become apparent as you ask other questions throughout the health history.

2. Do you have difficulty remembering or concentrating?
   - How often do you have difficulty remembering or concentrating?
   - Can you provide specific examples of times when it's been difficult to remember or concentrate?
   - How concerned are you about not remembering or having difficulty concentrating?

▶ Responses to these questions can provide insight into the cognition of the older adult. In some cases, when family members or other caregivers are present, their input can be helpful. Other cues related to impaired cognition in the older adult may become apparent as you interact with and ask other questions throughout the health assessment.

Patient-Centered Interaction

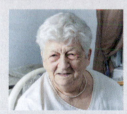

Source: Lopolo/Shutterstock.

Mrs. Schwartz is an 87-year old woman who is seen at the health clinic for reports of generalized fatigue, dizziness, and slight confusion. She has been living alone in a condo for the past 6 months since her husband passed away. Her son comes to check on her at least four times a week and calls on days when he does not visit. Mrs. Schwartz still drives and reports that she does her own shopping, cooking, and other housework. She likes to go to bingo a couple of times a week with her friends, but hasn't been able to make it the past couple of weeks because of her "problem."

Interview

Nurse: Good morning, Mrs. Schwartz. I see by your report you have been feeling pretty tired and have had some confusion.

Mrs. Schwartz: Yes, that's correct.

Nurse: Can you tell me how long this has been going on?

Mrs. Schwartz: It's been about two weeks, but it really started to get worse over the past few days, which is why I called to come in and see you.

Nurse: Have you ever experienced these symptoms before?

Mrs. Schwartz: I can't recall ever having these types of problems before.

Nurse: Is there anything else that has been bothering you lately?

Mrs. Schwartz: Not really. I have been feeling a little anxious and nervous about what's going on with me.

Nurse: Can you tell me a little bit more about the confusion you've been having?

Mrs. Schwartz: It's been little things here and there over the past couple of weeks, but a few days ago I went out to the store and forgot where I parked my car. One of the workers helped me find it. He also helped me turn on my GPS so I could get home. I was so nervous after that, but I didn't want to tell my daughter because I'm afraid she'll take away my keys.

Nurse: Oh my! I bet that was scary for you. Can you tell me about your medical history?

Mrs. Schwartz: I have type 2 diabetes and high blood pressure. I also have had a lot of UTIs in the past.

Nurse: You've had a lot of UTIs. . . . Do you have any burning when going to the bathroom, or have you noticed anything else about your urine?

Mrs. Schwartz: Actually, now that you ask, I did start to notice my pee looked a little cloudy. It wasn't clear like it usually was. I did notice that it kind of smelled different, too.

Analysis

The symptoms that Mrs. Schwarz presents with in this case are vague and could be an indication of a variety of conditions. The nurse built on the first statement made by the patient and was able to ask specific questions as more information was revealed. Open-ended statements were used to elicit greater information.

Objective Data—Physical Assessment

Objective data are obtained from the physical assessment of the older adult. Preparation includes gathering equipment, positioning, and informing the patient about the physical assessment. The room should be warm and private. Objective data are also obtained from secondary sources such as results of laboratory tests and radiologic studies.

EQUIPMENT

The equipment used in the physical examination of the older adult is the same as for other adults across the lifespan. In general you will need the following for a complete head-to-toe exam:

- Cotton balls/wisps and cotton tipped applicators
- Gauze squares
- Gloves
- Measuring tape or ruler
- Penlight or flashlight
- Reflex hammer
- Scale
- Sphygmomanometer
- Stethoscope
- Thermometer
- Tongue blade
- Tuning fork
- Vision chart
- Watch with second hand

For a comprehensive list of equipment related to each body system, see Chapters 12 through 24 of this text. ∞

HELPFUL HINTS

- Additional time may be needed for physical examination of the older adult. Frequent breaks and accommodations may be necessary in positioning for certain parts of the exam. In some cases, a complete history and physical may require two visits.
- Explain what is expected of the patient for each step of the assessment.
- Tell the patient the purpose of each procedure and when and if discomfort will accompany any examination.
- Identify and remedy language or cultural barriers at the outset of the patient interaction.
- Explain to the patient the need to remove any items that would interfere with the assessment, including jewelry, hats, scarves, veils, hairpieces, and wigs.
- Use Standard Precautions.

Key Considerations for Assessment Techniques and Findings for the Older Adult

The sequencing of the comprehensive physical examination of the older adult will follow a head-to-toe format. As noted earlier, the components of the physical examination are the same as described throughout the text in the body system chapters. Therefore, these techniques will not be described in detail in this chapter. The purpose of this section in this chapter is to highlight key differences and considerations that should be taken in the physical examination during a comprehensive health assessment of the older adult. Some overlap within this chapter and the other body systems chapters may be noted as these are aspects of the exam that are considered prevalent across the lifespan of adults, but they may be more prevalent in the older adult. In addition to the typical components of the physical exam, functional assessment of the older adult will be discussed in this section.

Functional Assessment   The functional assessment of the older adult provides the nurse with an opportunity to determine functional capacity, identify existing issues with everyday functioning, and prevent decline in functional status (ConsultGeri, 2012). **Functional status** includes the ability of the individual to safely perform ADLs, IADLs, and advanced activities of daily living (AADLs) (see Table 27.1). Many factors can affect functional status in older adults. Because functional status is considered an important indicator of health or illness state in patients, it is an essential component of the health assessment of the older adult.

Functional status can be evaluated through the use of a variety of validated screening tools. See Table 27.2 for examples and descriptions of these tools. It is important to note that depression and cognition can affect functional status, and use of screening tools for determining depression and impaired cognition, as discussed in other areas of this chapter, should be included in the comprehensive geriatric assessment.

Table 27.1 Activities of Daily Living (ADLs), Instrumental Activities of Daily Living (IADLs), and Advanced Activities of Daily Living (AADLs)

ADLs (Activities People Engage in on a Day-to-Day Basis; Basic Tasks for Self-Care)	IADLs (More Complex Daily Living Skills Needed for Independent Living)	AADLs (Fulfillment of Societal, Family, Recreational, and Occupational Tasks)
■ Grooming ■ Toileting ■ Dressing ■ Bathing ■ Walking ■ Transferring ■ Eating	■ Managing finances ■ Shopping ■ Cooking ■ Handling transportation needs ■ Managing medications ■ Doing housework and laundry ■ Using the phone or other devices for communication	■ Hobbies ■ Exercise ■ Work/occupation responsibilities Note: AADLs differ significantly from one individual to another.

Table 27.2 Screening Tools for the Assessment of Functional Status in the Older Adult

SCREENING TOOL	DESCRIPTION
Fulmer SPICES: An overall assessment tool for older adults	■ Used as an initial screen to alert healthcare providers to the need for additional, more complete screening ■ Can be used in health and frail older adults ■ Assesses commonly occurring problems in older adults **S** = sleep disorders, **P** = problems with eating or feeding, **I** = incontinence, **C** = confusion, **E** = evidence of falls, **S** = skin breakdown A sample of this tool can be found at https://consultgeri.org/try-this/general-assessment/issue-1.pdf. (Fulmer & Wallace, 2012)
Katz Index of Independence in Activities of Daily Living (ADL)	■ Measures patients' abilities to perform ADLs ■ Used to detect problems with performance of ADLs, including the functions of bathing, dressing, toileting, transferring, continence, and feeding ■ Can be used in older adults in a variety of care settings ■ Scoring: 6 = full function, 4 = moderate impairment, 2 = severe functional impairment A sample of this screening tool can be found at https://consultgeri.org/try-this/general-assessment/issue-2.pdf. (Shelky & Wallace, 2012)
The Lawton Instrumental Activities of Daily Living (IADL) Scale	■ Assessment of IADLs ■ Useful for present functioning and identification of improvement or decline over time ■ For use in older adults in community, clinic, or hospital settings; should not be used to assess individuals in long-term-care facilities or other institutions ■ Scores range from 0 (low functioning, dependent) to 8 (high functioning, independent) A sample of this screening tool can be found at https://consultgeri.org/try-this/general-assessment/issue-23.pdf. (Graf, 2013)
Timed Up and Go Test (TUG)	■ Used for assessment of mobility ■ Have patients wear regular footwear and use a walking aid, as needed ■ Ask the patient to rise from a seated position on your cue of "Go" and walk to a marked point in the room 10 feet away, turn around, walk back, and sit down again. ■ Timing starts at "Go." ■ A time of 12 seconds or more indicates that the patient is at risk for falls. A sample of this test can be found at https://www.cdc.gov/steadi/pdf/TUG_Test-print.pdf. (Centers for Disease Control and Prevention [CDC], n.d.)
Vulnerable Elders Scale-13 (VES-13)	■ 13-item screening tool ■ Based on age, self-rated health, and ability to perform functional and physical activities ■ For use with community-dwelling elders ■ Identifies risk for functional decline or death over a 5-year period ■ Administration can be done through self-administration, a nonmedical family member or caregiver, or at an office visit ■ Takes approximately 5 minutes or less to complete A sample of this tool can be found at https://www.rand.org/content/dam/rand/www/external/health/projects/acove/docs/acove_ves13.pdf. (Ward & Reuben, 2018)

General Survey Assessment of general appearance also offers insight into the older adult's overall health status. The dress, grooming, and personal hygiene of an older adult may be affected by limitations in mobility from arthritis, cardiovascular disease, and other disorders, or by a lack of funds.

The gait of an older adult is often slower and the steps shorter. To maintain balance, older adults may hold their arms away from the body or use a cane. The posture of an older adult may look slightly stooped because of a generalized flexion, which also causes the older adult to appear shorter. A loss in height may also be because of thinning or compression of the intervertebral disks.

The behavior of the older adult may be affected by various disorders common to this age group, such as vascular insufficiency and diabetes. In addition, medications may affect the patient's behavior. Some medications may cause the patient to feel anxious, and others may affect the patient's alertness, orientation, or speech. Older adults are likely to have one or more chronic conditions associated with age, such as arthritis, hypertension, or diabetes. As a result, older adults often consume several prescription medications. Overmedication may occur because older adults seek care from multiple healthcare providers without collaboration regarding treatment. Multiple medi-

cations may combine to produce dangerous side effects. Additionally, the schedules for multiple medications may be confusing and result in overmedication, forgotten doses, negative side effects, or ineffectiveness of medication. Therefore, the nurse must conduct a thorough assessment of the patient's medication schedule and history.

Height and Weight The height of older adults may decline somewhat as a result of thinning or compression of the intervertebral disks and a general flexion of the hips and knees. Body weight may decrease because of muscle shrinkage. The older patient may appear thinner, even when properly nourished, because of loss of subcutaneous fat deposits from the face, forearms, and lower legs. At the same time, fat deposits on the abdomen and hips may increase.

Vital Signs Normal ranges for vital signs in older adults include the following:

- Pulse: 60–100
- Respirations: 15–20
- Blood pressure: Less than 120 (systolic), less than 80 (diastolic)
- Temperature: 36.6°C–37.3°C (97.8°F –99.1°F)

Skin, Hair, and Nails

- Check skin carefully for lesions and be able to differentiate normal from abnormal, concerning lesions.

- Check for pressure ulcers, especially in patients who are limited in mobility or reside in long-term-care facilities, are bed or chair bound, or are limited because of recent hospitalization.

- Offer information to older adults regarding the herpes zoster vaccination. This vaccination is recommended for all adults ages 60 and older to prevent shingles (Centers for Disease Control and Prevention [CDC], 2018b).

- Also see Chapter 12. ∞

Head, Neck, and Related Lymphatics

- Care should be taken when examining the range of motion of the neck in older adult patients, and you may need to have the patient perform the movements more slowly.

- Also see Chapter 13. ∞

Eyes

- Examination techniques for testing the eyes such as visual acuity and visual fields can provide some information about abnormal changes but have been found to produce results lower in sensitivity for older adults (Bedsine, 2016). Ensure that patients understand the importance of follow up with an ophthalmologist every 1 to 2 years for a more thorough and accurate eye examination.

- Also see Chapter 14. ∞

Ears, Nose, Mouth, and Throat

- Although presbycusis is common in older adults, conductive sound loss can often occur because of an accumulation of earwax that is drier and becomes more impacted than in a younger person. Any older persons complaining of difficulty in hearing should be checked for outer ear canal blockage and have their ears cleaned before any further testing is performed.

- Also see Chapter 15. ∞

Lungs and Thorax

- Offer information about influenza and pneumonia vaccines, as appropriate.

- Also see Chapter 16. ∞

Breasts

- Note that masses may be easier to palpate because of decreased tissue in this area.

- Gynecomastia may be noted in older men.

- Also see Chapter 17. ∞

Cardiovascular and Peripheral Vascular Systems

- The nurse should assess the older patient in a position that is comfortable and should be careful not to have the patient make any sudden movements, such as suddenly sitting, standing up, or lying down after standing or sitting, because of the potential for orthostatic hypotension.

- The nurse must be mindful of the presence of any other heart sounds beyond S1 and S2 or any change in characteristics of preexisting heart sounds and must inform the patient's physician or other practitioner of any significant findings.

- When evaluating the various arterial pulses, the nurse should keep in mind that the heart rate slows with the aging process. Some persons may normally have a rate of 50 beats/min; however, the patient should be evaluated if the pulse is below 60 beats/min. Likewise, it is common for older patients to manifest irregular pulses often with occasional pauses or extra beats. Any patient with an irregular pulse should be referred for further examination.

- Also see Chapter 18. ∞

Abdomen

- The appearance of the abdomen changes with the aging process. In the older adult, the abdomen may be more rounded or protuberant because of increased adipose tissue distribution, decreased muscle tone, and reduced fibroconnective tissue. The abdomen tends to be softer and more relaxed than in the younger adult. A scaphoid, or sunken in, and flaccid abdomen is seen in the very old with additional fat loss, but this may also be a sign of rapid weight loss accompanying malnutrition or cancer. A distended abdomen is often seen with fluid in the peritoneal cavity (ascites) or excessive gas. Asymmetry may indicate tumors, hernia, constipation, or bowel obstruction. Although the slight up-and-down pulsation from a normal aorta is more readily seen in patients with thin abdominal walls, an aortic aneurysm may be indicated by lateral pulsations or soft, pulsatile masses. Visible tortuous veins on the abdominal wall near the umbilicus, in conjunction with a firm and distended abdomen, may indicate portal hypertension with ascites.

- Bowel sounds may be hypoactive. Borborygmus (stomach growling) may occur because of bleeding or inflammatory bowel disease. High-pitched hyperactive bowel sounds accompanied by colicky pain and distention are signs of small bowel obstruction, which occurs most often in older men. Bruits heard over any of the arteries are signs of stenosis or aneurysms.

- Because of the normally thinner abdominal wall, tympany may be more noticeable, but it should still be within normal ranges. Areas of dullness in the lower left quadrant and sigmoid area are probably related to stool, but it is essential to rule out tumors. Shifting dullness, especially when accompanied by firm dullness, suggests ascites. Dullness above the symphysis pubis could indicate a full bladder.

- Tenderness with moderate distention could be because of flatus but could also indicate irritation of the stomach or bowel. The thinner abdominal wall of the older adult makes it easier to feel the underlying bowel. A soft mass or small firm masses felt in the left lower quadrant may be stool, especially because constipation is common in the elderly. Firmness is associated with fluid or excessive gas, but rigidity is a sign of peritoneal inflammation.

- Distention just above the symphysis pubis may be caused by bladder distention because of prostatic hypertrophy or incomplete emptying.

- If the liver can be palpated below the costal margins, the liver is probably enlarged. Enlargement may reflect passive congestion because of congestive heart failure or liver disease, especially if the liver feels nodular.
- Also see Chapter 20. ∞

Urinary System

- Because the abdominal musculature of older persons tends to be more flaccid than that of younger adults, less pressure is used during deep palpation. The kidneys of the older patient are more difficult to palpate abdominally because the mass of the adrenal cortex decreases with age.
- The nurse should omit blunt percussion in a frail older person. Palpation of the costovertebral angles and flanks can be used instead to reveal any pain or tenderness.
- A digital examination of the prostate gland is generally included as part of the urinary assessment in older men.
- Palpation of the urethra through the anterior vaginal wall is recommended for all older women.
- Also see Chapter 21 and Chapter 22. ∞

Male and Female Reproductive Systems

- Care should be taken with positioning the older adult for certain aspects of the exam. For example, the older female patient may need more assistance with getting her legs into stirrups for a vaginal exam, or an alternative method without the use of stirrups may need to be considered.
- Also see Chapter 21 and Chapter 22. ∞

Musculoskeletal

- Older adults may have limited mobility and range of motion. If so, the patient should be asked to perform exam techniques, such as range of motion of extremities, to the point that does not cause discomfort. This should be considered throughout other parts of the exam where patients may need to change positions or move extremities.
- When testing range of motion, the nurse must be careful not to cause pain, discomfort, or damage to the joint.
- The musculoskeletal exam is conducted at a slower pace when necessary because older patients often have health problems that affect endurance.
- Also see Chapter 23. ∞

Neurologic System

- Include screening such as the GDS, MiniCog™, and MoCA. (See the Special Considerations section for more detail.)
- Also see Chapter 24. ∞

Documenting Your Findings

Documentation of assessment data—subjective and objective—must be accurate, professional, complete, and confidential. When documenting the information from the focused assessment of each body system, the nurse should use measurements where appropriate to ensure accuracy; use medical terminology rather than jargon; include all pertinent information; and avoid language that could identify the patient. The information in the documentation should make it clear what questions were asked and use language to indicate whether it is the patient's response or the nurse's findings.

When documenting the subjective and objective findings of a complete geriatric history and physical examination, the nurse should be concise but as thorough with the data findings as possible. For a sample of the documentation of a comprehensive history and physical for an older adult, see Application Through Critical Thinking at the end of this chapter.

Abnormal Findings

This section includes some selected examples of common abnormal findings in older adults. In addition, Box 27.3 highlights common chronic conditions in older adults. Students should refer to abnormal findings throughout Chapters 12 to 24 for additional information on common abnormal findings related to each body system. ∞

Box 27.3 Common Chronic Conditions in the Older Adult

- Cardiovascular disease
  - Heart failure
  - Ischemic (or coronary) heart disease
  - Hypertension
- Hypercholesterolemia
- Cancer
- Chronic obstructive pulmonary disease (COPD)
  - Chronic Bronchitis
  - Emphysema
- Stroke
- Diabetes mellitus
- Alzheimer disease and other dementias
- Depression
- Arthritis

Sources: National Council on Aging, Healthy Aging Team, 2017; Office of Disease Prevention and Health Promotion, *Healthy People 2020*, 2018).

Onychomycosis

Fungal nail infection most commonly caused by organisms called dermatophytes (Westerberg & Voyak, 2013). More common in older adults because of peripheral vascular disease, immunologic conditions, and diabetes. Seen mostly on toenails and less likely on fingernails (Figure 27.15 ■).

Objective Findings:

- Discoloration
- Thickening
- Separation of nail from nail bed

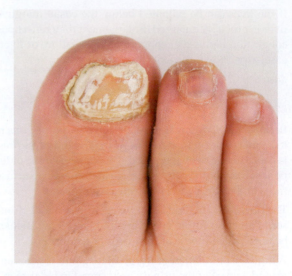

Figure 27.15 Onychomycosis.
Source: Manuel Faba Ortega/123RF.

Onychogryphosis or Ram's Horn Nails

Condition of the nails resulting in overgrowth and hypertrophy that creates a nail that resembles a ram's horn or claw (Kerkar, 2017). More common in older adults because of diminished blood supply to nails occurring with aging. Can also occur because of injury or other trauma to the nail, wearing tight-fitting shoes, infection, poor hygiene. Occurs more often in toenails, generally the fifth toe, and is asymptomatic (Figure 27.16 ■).

Objective Findings:

- Discoloration, yellowish coloring
- Thickening and deformed
- Long nails with ram's horn or clawlike feature

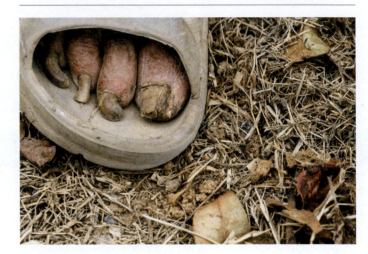

Figure 27.16 Onychogryphosis (ram's horn nails).
Source: PK289/Shutterstock.

Orthostatic Hypotension

Also referred to as postural hypotension; a sudden drop in systolic blood pressure of 20 mmHg or more or diastolic pressure of 10 mmHg within 3 minutes of moving from a lying down to sitting or standing position (Mayo Clinic Staff, 2017d)

Subjective Findings:

- Dizziness
- Blurry vision
- Weakness
- Syncope
- Fainting

Objective Findings:

- Drop in systolic BP of 20 mmHg or drop in diastolic BP of 10 mmHg when going from lying to sitting or standing
- Depends on cause. Could see hypoglycemia, anemia, or irregularities in heart rhythm.

Systolic Murmur

Systolic murmurs become more common as people age, especially because of aortic stenosis. These murmurs are usually best auscultated in the aortic area or base of the heart. Non-physiologic murmurs are not normal findings. An S4 sound is a common finding in older adults who do not have identified cardiovascular disease. In individuals with preexisting heart disease, however, an S4 is a pathologic finding.

Osteoarthritis (OA)

Condition more common in older adults, also known as degenerative joint disease (Arthritis Foundation, n.d.). The most common chronic condition of the joints. Usually results from the breakdown of cartilage, or cushioning between the joint, which is part of wear and tear over time. No specific cause, common risk factors being overweight or obese, injury, overuse of joints, and genetics.

Subjective Findings:

- Stiffness
- Pain

Objective Findings:

- X-ray showing damage and changes related to the condition
- Joint aspiration revealing crystals or other evidence of joint deterioration
- MRI to confirm diagnosis

Osteoporosis

A disease in which bone density and quality diminish (MedlinePlus, 2018c), also known as "porous bone." Bones become more porous and fragile. As a result, bones, especially hips, spine, and wrists, are more prone to breaks and fractures. Most aging adults develop some degree of osteoporosis, but it is more marked in Caucasian women, especially those of Scandinavian ancestry. Other risk factors include being small and thin, family history of osteoporosis, taking certain medications, and having low bone density. Bone loss also occurs in women with low estrogen because of missed periods or following menopause, individuals who are anorexic, those who have low calcium and vitamin D levels, smokers, those who indulge in excessive alcohol intake, and individuals who do not participate in frequent weight-bearing activity (National Institute of Arthritis and Musculoskeletal and Skin Diseases, 2014).

Subjective Findings:
- Pain
- Decrease in height over time

Objective Findings:
- Stooped or hunched posture (kyphosis)
- Bone fracture or break that happens more easily than expected
- Confirmation of loss of bone mineral density from dual-energy x-ray absorptiometry (DXA or DEXA) or bone densitometry

Benign Prostatic Hypertrophy (Hyperplasia) (BPH)

A common condition in older men caused by an enlargement of the prostate beyond the point of natural growth that is part of the aging process (Urology Care Foundation, 2018). As it grows larger, the prostate begins to squeeze the urethra and can cause urinary frequency and nocturia.

Subjective Findings:
- Frequent and urgent sense of urination.
- Nocturia
- Dribbling at the end of urination
- Weak urine stream or starting and stopping in the middle of urination
- Incontinence because of weakened bladder muscles over time

Objective Findings:
- Enlarged prostate palpated on digital rectal examination
- Elevated prostate-specific antigen (PSA) levels

Urinary Incontinence

A common problem in older adults, particularly in women, related to diminished bladder elasticity, bladder capacity, and sphincter control, as well as to cognitive impairment, and sometimes functional impairment (National Institute on Aging [NIA], 2017e). There are different types of urinary incontinence including:

Stress incontinence: leaking of urine caused by pressure put on the bladder.

Subjective Findings:
- Reports of involuntarily leaking small amounts of urine during activities such as running or other types of exercising, laughing, sneezing, or heaving lifting
- Leakage of urine occurring without the feeling, or urge, to urinate

Objective Findings:
- Weakened urethral sphincter, pelvic floor muscles, or both

Urge incontinence: a squeezing, or spasm, of the bladder creates a sudden feeling, or urge, to urinate. This type of incontinence is also referred to as overactive bladder.

Subjective Findings:
- Reports of an uncontrollable urge to urinate followed by loss of urine before reaching a bathroom

Objective Findings:
- Findings on neurological exam (some central nervous system disorders can lead to urge incontinence)
- Diagnostic tests for urinary tract or bladder infections, which can cause temporary urgency
- Results of bladder function tests such as bladder pressure testing, post void residual urine, and urine flow rate

Functional incontinence: loss of urine in individuals who often have normal bladder control, but are experiencing changes in cognition or have functional limitations, such as being able to get to the toilet or having difficulty with buttons and zippers due to arthritis or other disorders.

Subjective Findings:
- Changes in cognition resulting from certain medications, dementia, or mental illness
- Declining functional status related to mobility, leading to an inability to make it to the toilet

Objective Findings:
- Functional impairment
- Impaired mental status

Overflow incontinence: leaking of small amounts of urine due to a bladder that is always full. This type of incontinence can occur more frequently in men who have prostate enlargement, as well as individuals with diabetes and spinal cord injuries.

Subjective Findings:
- Reports of urine leakage (with or without the feeling of needing to urinate)
- Dribbling of urine
- Urinary hesitancy
- Inability to empty bladder

Objective Findings:
- Confirmation of bladder distention
- Post void residual urine > 200 ml
- Enlarged prostate in men
- Uterine or bladder prolapse in women

Alzheimer Disease

A progressive degenerative disease of the brain that leads to dementia (Alzheimer's Association, 2018). More common in people over age 65, but its onset may occur as early as middle adulthood.

Subjective Findings:
- Memory loss, particularly of recent events
- Hallucinations
- Paranoid fantasies (in later stage of disease)

Objective Findings:
- Shortened attention span
- Confusion
- Disorientation
- Wandering

Parkinson Disease

A degeneration of the basal nuclei of the brain, which are collections of nerve cell bodies deep within the white matter of the cerebrum (Parkinson's Foundation, 2018). These nuclei are responsible for initiating and stopping voluntary movement. Although the precise etiology is unknown, research indicates that environmental toxins, such as carbon monoxide or certain metals, may cause some cases of Parkinson disease. It may also result from previous encephalitis. Parkinson disease is most commonly diagnosed in people ages 60 and older.

Subjective Findings:
- Difficulty speaking (dysphasia)
- Decrease in unconscious movements, such as blinking
- Impaired sense of balance
- Muscle pain

Objective Findings:
- Slowed movements (bradykinesia)
- Muscle rigidity
- Shuffling gait
- Rhythmic shaking of the hands
- Pill-rolling tremor of the forefinger and thumb
- Masklike facial expression

Application Through Critical Thinking

CASE STUDY

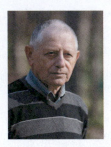

Source: Baevskiy Dmitry/Shutterstock.

Mr. Jones is a 70-year-old Caucasian male who comes to the clinic for a complete history and physical exam. He is a new patient and is accompanied by his adult daughter. He tells you that he has not been to the doctor in about 5 years. He does not have any specific complaints to report but decided to make an appointment because his children keep "pestering" him about some concerns they have noticed lately with his health and memory. Mr. Jones states, "My memory isn't as good as it used to be" and "I've been feeling a little down ever since my wife passed away two years ago" and "I guess it's a good idea for me to get checked out." Mr. Jones's daughter adds that the main reason she and her brother wanted him to be examined is because they have noticed their father isn't getting around as well as he used to and sometimes gets short of breath when working around the house. He has forgotten recently to pay some bills, and a couple of weeks ago even forgot to pick up his granddaughter from school.

SAMPLE DOCUMENTATION

The following is sample documentation from the health history and physical exam of Mr. Jones.

SUBJECTIVE DATA

Reason for Seeking Care: Complete history and physical exam

Medications: Multivitamin (one capsule) every morning, and ibuprofen 600 mg as needed for his joint pain (usually one time during the day, three or four times a week). Denies use of any prescription medications. The last time he saw a doctor, he was told he had high blood pressure and was given instructions on changes in diet, exercise, and taking medication. However, he did not feel sick and decided not to fill the prescription.

Past Medical History: No recent illnesses; reports of high blood pressure 5 years ago but has not followed up to have his BP rechecked.

Past Surgical History: Tonsillectomy at 5 years old

Family History: Mr. Jones is unsure of his family history but knows his father died of a heart attack at age 76. His wife died 2 years ago from breast cancer at age 66. His son (age 48) and daughter (age 43) are in good health and do not have any known medical diseases or conditions.

Psychosocial History: Mr. Jones lives alone in a two-bedroom ranch home. He eats a diet mainly of canned food, frozen meals, or takeout/fast food since his wife passed away because "she was the cook in the family." He denies physical activity other than getting up and walking around the house and working in his garden in the spring and summer. *Caffeine:* Drinks about a 10-cup pot of coffee each day. *Alcohol and Tobacco Use:* Drinks 5 or 6 8-ounce cans of beer each day on the weekends and smokes a pack of cigarettes per day for the past 45 years. *Illicit drugs:* Denies use of illegal substances.

Health Maintenance: Last dental exam 2.5 years ago, eye exam 2.5 years ago. Has not had a hearing exam, EKG, or other screening exams. Has never had immunizations for influenza, pneumonia, or shingles.

REVIEW OF SYSTEMS

General: Feels he is in "pretty good health." Denies fatigue, excessive weight loss, fevers, malaise, chills, or night sweats. Reports a weight gain of about 20 lbs in the past 2 years since his wife passed away, but attributes it to lack of exercise and poor eating habits.

Skin, Hair, and Nails: Denies changes in skin texture, rash, lesions, itching, changes in moles, tendency to bleed or bruise easily, or abnormal hair growth or loss. Denies changes in hair or nails.

HEENT:

Head: Denies head injury, headache, dizziness

Eyes: Wears prescription bifocals, but prescription has not been updated "since my wife died." Denies visual changes, blurred or double vision, discomfort.

Ears: Denies earaches, discharge, vertigo, hearing loss. Reports lately having "a little" difficulty hearing the television or when talking on the phone with his children and grandchildren.

Nose: Denies nasal injury, nosebleeds, or rhinitis. Has seasonal allergies and allergies to cats.

Throat: Denies sore throat, hoarseness, sore/bleeding gums, sore tongue, difficulty swallowing, lose or chipped or decaying teeth, last dental exam 2.5 years ago.

Neck and Related Lymphatics: Denies any lumps, pain on movement, goiters, or swollen glands.

Lungs and Thorax: Cough is present in the morning, but not consistently. Denies coughing up sputum, hemoptysis, pleural pain, or dyspnea.

Breasts: Denies any lumps, pain, or discharge.

Cardiovascular/Peripheral Vascular: Denies chest pain, SOB, heart palpitations, heart murmurs, orthopnea, intermittent claudication, syncope, or EKG.

Abdomen: Denies dysphagia, nausea, vomiting, dyspepsia, hematemesis, history of ulcers, abdominal pain, changes in stool, or rectal issues.

Male Genitourinary: Needs to get up to go to the bathroom during the day and at night more frequently to urinate than he used to. Sometimes the urine seems to stop midstream or he has some "dribbling" at the end of urination. Denies issues with dysuria, incontinence, hematuria, changes in urine color, or renal stones. Denies scrotal masses, pain, discharge, hernia, prostate enlargement or infection, problems with erection or ejaculation. Denies performing testicular self-exams.

Neurological: Denies seizures, weakness, numbness, tingling, pain.

Musculoskeletal: Denies redness, swelling, decreased ROM, and back, neck, or limb pain. Denies pain but reports some stiffness when getting up in the morning and "achiness" in his knees when working in his garden for long periods.

Sexuality: Denies sexual activity since his wife passed away, denies STDs.

Psychiatric: Denies psychiatric disorders, depression, mood swings, delusions, hallucinations. Reports a decline in memory and feeling "down" since the passing of his wife 2 years ago.

OBJECTIVE DATA

General Survey: Mr. Jones is a well-groomed man. He is alert and oriented with clear speech; uses concise and clear responses to questions. He has a steady gait. His skin color is suntanned with pink undertones.

Vital Signs: Blood pressure 148/92, HR 88, RR 18, height 5 feet 9 inches, weight 250 pounds, BMI 36.9.

Skin: Skin is smooth, warm, and dry. Nails are slightly yellow in color, without clubbing or cyanosis, capillary refill < 3 seconds. No rash, petechiae, ecchymosis, or lesions noted. Hair is of normal distribution and average texture with slight male pattern baldness noted.

HEENT:

Head: The skull is normocephalic/atraumatic.

Eyes: Visual acuity left eye 20/50, right eye 20/70. Sclera white, pupils are 4 mm constricting to 2 mm, equally round and reactive to light and accommodations.

Ears: External ears without tenderness, no redness, no pain when pressure applied to tragus. Acuity good to whispered voice.

Nose: Nasal mucosa pink, septum midline. No sinus tenderness.

Throat/Mouth: Oral mucosa pink, dentition good, pharynx without exudates, elevation of uvula.

Neck: Trachea midline, neck supple; thyroid isthmus palpable, lobes not felt.

Lymph Nodes: No preauricular, posterior auricular, tonsillar, submandibular, submental, occipital, superficial cervical, posterior cervical, deep cervical chain, epitrochlear, or supraclavicular nodes felt.

Cardiovascular: S1 and S2. No murmurs or extra sounds.

Thorax/Lungs: Lungs clear bilaterally. Thorax is symmetric with good expansion. There is equal and expected fremitus.

Abdomen: Abdomen is protuberant with active bowel sounds in four quadrants. It is soft and nontender; no palpable masses or hepatosplenomegaly. No costovertebral angle tenderness.

Peripheral Vascular: Extremities are warm and without edema. No stasis changes. Calves are supple and nontender. No carotid bruit or thrill, carotid pulses 2+ bilaterally. No femoral or abdominal bruits. Brachial, radial, femoral, popliteal, dorsalis pedis, and posterior tibial pulses are 2+.

Musculoskeletal: Full range of motion in all joints of upper and lower extremities. Some crepitus can be heard in the knees bilaterally. No evidence of swelling or deformity.

Neurological:

Mental status: Alert and oriented to person, place, and time. Relaxed and cooperative. Thought process coherent. Recent and remote memory intact, calculation and abstract reasoning intact, learning and recall of three words correct.

Motor: Good muscle bulk and tone. Strength 5/5 throughout.

Reflexes: All within normal limits and symmetric.

CRITICAL THINKING QUESTIONS

1. What other subjective and objective data might be important to ask Mr. Jones about regarding his health history?

2. What should the nurse's priority concerns be for Mr. Jones based on the information in this case?

3. Identify at least two evidence-based screening tools that would be important to incorporate into the health assessment of Mr. Jones.

4. What special considerations are applicable to this situation?

REFERENCES

Alzheimer's Association. (2018). *What is Alzheimer's?* Retrieved from https://www.alz.org/alzheimers_disease_what_is_alzheimers.asp

American Cancer Society (ACS). (2017a). *Breast cancer facts and figures: 2017–2018.* Retrieved from https://www.cancer.org/content/dam/cancer-org/research/cancer-facts-and-statistics/breast-cancer-facts-and-figures/breast-cancer-facts-and-figures-2017-2018.pdf

American Cancer Society (ACS). (2017b). *Breast cancer risk factors you cannot change.* Retrieved from https://www.cancer.org/cancer/breast-cancer/risk-and-prevention/breast-cancer-risk-factors-you-cannot-change.html

American Cancer Society (ACS). (2017c). *DES exposure: Questions and answers.* Retrieved from https://www.cancer.org/cancer/cancer-causes/medical-treatments/des-exposure.html

American Cancer Society (ACS). (2017d). *Disproven or controversial breast cancer risk factors.* Retrieved from https://www.cancer.org/cancer/breast-cancer/risk-and-prevention/disproven-or-controversial-breast-cancer-risk-factors.html

American College of Obstetricians and Gynecologists (ACOG). (2017). *Clinical breast examination.* Retrieved from https://www.acog.org/About-ACOG/ACOG-Departments/Annual-Womens-Health-Care/Well-Woman-Recommendations/Clinical-Breast-Examination

American Dental Association. (2013). *American Dental Association statement on regular dental visits.* Retrieved from https://www.ada.org/en/press-room/news-releases/2013-archive/june/american-dental-association-statement-on-regular-dental-visits

American Optometric Association. (2018a). *Adult vision: Over 60 years of age.* Retrieved from https://www.aoa.org/patients-and-public/good-vision-throughout-life/adult-vision-19-to-40-years-of-age/adult-vision-over-60-years-of-age

American Optometric Association. (2018b). *Dry eye.* Retrieved from https://www.aoa.org/patients-and-public/eye-and-vision-problems/glossary-of-eye-and-vision-conditions/dry-eye

American Psychological Association. (2018). *Fact sheet: Age and socioeconomic status.* Retrieved from http://www.apa.org/pi/ses/resources/publications/age.aspx

American Society of Clinical Oncology (ASCO). (2017). *Breast cancer: Risk factors and prevention.* Retrieved from https://www.cancer.net/cancer-types/breast-cancer/risk-factors-and-prevention

American Thyroid Association (ATA). (2018). *Older patients and thyroid disease.* Retrieved from https://www.thyroid.org/thyroid-disease-older-patient

Arthritis Foundation. (n.d.). *Osteoarthritis.* Retrieved from https://www.arthritis.org/about-arthritis/types/osteoarthritis

Bedsine, R. W. (2016). *Evaluation of the elderly patient.* Retrieved from https://www.merckmanuals.com/professional/geriatrics/approach-to-the-geriatric-patient/evaluation-of-the-elderly-patient

Bemis, E. (2013). *The importance of fiber in a senior citizen's diet.* Retrieved from https://www.umh.org/assisted-independent-living-blog/bid/259804/The-Importance-of-Fiber-in-a-Senior-Citizen-s-Diet

Berger, T. G., Shive, M., & Harper, G. M. (2013). Pruritus in the older patient: A clinical review. *Journal of the American Medical Association, 310*(22), 2443-2450. doi:10.1001/jama.2013.282023 Retrieved from https://jamanetwork.com/journals/jama/fullarticle/1788432

Centers for Disease Control and Prevention (CDC). (n.d.). *Assessment: Timed Up and Go (TUG).* Retrieved from https://www.cdc.gov/steadi/pdf/TUG_Test-print.pdf

Centers for Disease Control and Prevention (CDC). (2018a). *What you should know and do this flu season if you are 65 years and older.* Retrieved from https://www.cdc.gov/flu/about/disease/65over.htm

Centers for Disease Control and Prevention (CDC). (2018b). *Zostavax recommendations.* Retrieved from https://www.cdc.gov/vaccines/vpd/shingles/hcp/zostavax/recommendations.html

Cleveland Clinic Foundation. (2018). *Erectile dysfunction.* Retrieved from https://my.clevelandclinic.org/health/diseases/10035-erectile-dysfunction

Conaway, B. (2018). *Aging and digestive health.* Retrieved from https://www.webmd.com/digestive-disorders/features/digestive-health-aging#1

ConsultGeri. (n.d.). *Age-related changes: Overview.* Retrieved from https://consultgeri.org/geriatric-topics/age-related-changes

ConsultGeri. (2012). *Function.* Retrieved from https://consultgeri.org/geriatric-topics/function

Doerflinger, D. M. (2012). *Mental status assessment in older adults: Montreal Cognitive Assessment: MoCA version 7.1 (Original version).* Retrieved from https://consultgeri.org/try-this/general-assessment/issue-3.2.pdf

Doerflinger, D. M. (2013). *Mental status assessment of older adults: The Mini-Cog™.* Retrieved from https://consultgeri.org/try-this/general-assessment/issue-3.1.pdf

DiMaria-Ghalili, R. A., & Amella, E. J. (2012). *Assessing nutrition in older adults.* Retrieved from https://consultgeri.org/try-this/general-assessment/issue-9.pdf

Esiwe, C., Baillon, S., Rajkonwar, A., Lindesay, J., Lo, N., & Dennis, M. (2015). Screening for depression in older adults on an acute medical ward: The validity of NICE guidance in using two questions. *Age and Aging, 44*(5), 771–775. Retrieved from https://academic.oup.com/ageing/article/44/5/771/51792. doi:10.1093/ageing/afv018

Fulmer, T., & Wallace, M. (2012). *Fulmer SPICES: An overall assessment tool for older adults.* Retrieved from https://consultgeri.org/try-this/general-assessment/issue-1.pdf

Gellar, M. C., & Alter, D. (2014). *The impact of dentures on the nutritional health of the elderly.* Retrieved from http://www.jarcp.com/872-the-impact-of-dentures-on-the-nutritional-health-of-the-elderly.html

Graf, C. (2013). *The Lawton Instrumental Activities of Daily Living (IADL) Scale.* Retrieved from https://consultgeri.org/try-this/general-assessment/issue-23.pdf

Greenberg, S. A. (2012). *The Geriatric Depression Scale (GDS).* Retrieved from https://consultgeri.org/try-this/general-assessment/issue-4.pdf

Healthline. (2017). *Traumatic breast injuries: Should you see a doctor?* Retrieved from https://www.healthline.com/health/breast-injury-trauma

Johns Hopkins Medicine. (n.d.). *Mammography.* Retrieved from https://www.hopkinsmedicine.org/healthlibrary/conditions/radiology/mammography_85,P01288

Kaiser Health News. (2018). *Can you hear me now? Senate bill aims to broaden access to hearing services.* Retrieved from https://khn.org/news/can-you-hear-me-now-senate-bill-on-hearing-aids-may-make-the-answer-yes

Kerkar, P. (2017). *Onychogryphosis or ram's horn nails: Causes, signs, symptoms, treatment, prevention.* Retrieved from https://www.epainassist.com/joint-pain/foot-pain/onychogryphosis-or-rams-horn-nails

Lucas, R. W., & Kennedy-Malone, L. (2014). Frailty in the older adult: Will you recognize the signs? *The Nurse Practitioner, 39*(3), 28-34. doi:10.1097/01.NPR.0000443228.72357.96

Matteson, M., Lipari, R. N., Hays, C., & van Horn, S. L. (2017). *A day in the life of older adults: Substance use facts.* Retrieved from https://www.samhsa.gov/data/sites/default/files/report_2792/ShortReport-2792.html

Mayo Clinic Staff. (2015). *Glaucoma.* Retrieved from https://www.mayoclinic.org/diseases-conditions/glaucoma/symptoms-causes/syc-20372839

Mayo Clinic Staff. (2017a). *Easy bruising: Why does it happen?* Retrieved from https://www.mayoclinic.org/healthy-lifestyle/healthy-aging/in-depth/easy-bruising/art-20045762

Mayo Clinic Staff. (2017b). *Edema.* Retrieved from https://www.mayoclinic.org/diseases-conditions/edema/symptoms-causes/syc-20366493

Mayo Clinic Staff. (2017c). *Mild cognitive impairment.* Retrieved from https://www.mayoclinic.org/diseases-conditions/mild-cognitive-impairment/symptoms-causes/syc-20354578

Mayo Clinic Staff. (2017d). *Orthostatic hypotension.* Retrieved from https://www.mayoclinic.org/diseases-conditions/orthostatic-hypotension/symptoms-causes/syc-20352548

Mayo Clinic Staff. (2018a). *Breast lumps.* Retrieved from https://www.mayoclinic.org/symptoms/breast-lumps/basics/causes/sym-20050619

Mayo Clinic Staff. (2018b). *Fecal incontinence.* Retrieved from https://www.mayoclinic.org/diseases-conditions/fecal-incontinence/symptoms-causes/syc-20351397

MedlinePlus. (2016). *Advance directives.* Retrieved from https://medlineplus.gov/advancedirectives.html

MedlinePlus. (2018a). *Aging changes in the breast.* Retrieved from https://medlineplus.gov/ency/article/003999.htm

MedlinePlus. (2018b). *Aging changes in the lungs.* Retrieved from https://medlineplus.gov/ency/article/004011.htm

MedlinePlus. (2018c). *Osteoporosis.* Retrieved from https://medlineplus.gov/osteoporosis.html

McLeod, S. (2018). *Erik Erikson.* Retrieved from https://www.simplypsychology.org/Erik-Erikson.html

Nahin, R. L. (2015). Estimates of pain prevalence and severity in adults: United States, 2012. *The Journal of Pain, 16*(8), 769–780. doi:10.1016/j.jpain.2015.05.002

National Cancer Institute (NCI). (2018). *BRCA mutations: Cancer risk and genetic testing.* Retrieved from https://www.cancer.gov/about-cancer/causes-prevention/genetics/brca-fact-sheet

National Council on Aging, Healthy Aging Team. (2017). *Top 10 chronic conditions in adults 65+ and what you can do to prevent or manage them.* [Blog post] Retrieved from https://www.ncoa.org/blog/10-common-chronic-diseases-prevention-tips

National Institute for Health and Care Excellence. (2018). *Depression in adults: Recognition and care management.* Retrieved from https://www.nice.org.uk/guidance/cg90/chapter/Key-priorities-for-implementation

National Institute of Arthritis and Musculoskeletal and Skin Diseases. (2014). *What is osteoporosis? Fast facts: An easy-to-read series of publications for the public.* Retrieved from https://www.bones.nih.gov/health-info/bone/osteoporosis/osteoporosis-ff

National Institute of Mental Health (NIMH). (n.d.). *Older adults and depression.* Retrieved from https://www.nimh.nih.gov/health/publications/older-adults-and-depression/index.shtml

National Institute on Aging (NIA). (2016). *Elder abuse.* Retrieved from https://www.nia.nih.gov/health/elder-abuse

National Institute on Aging (NIA). (2017a). *Bladder health for older adults.* Retrieved from https://www.nia.nih.gov/health/bladder-health-older-adults

National Institute on Aging (NIA). (2017b). *Cognitive health and older adults.* Retrieved from https://www.nia.nih.gov/health/cognitive-health-and-older-adults

National Institute on Aging (NIA). (2017c). *Obtaining an older patient's medical history.* Retrieved from https://www.nia.nih.gov/health/obtaining-older-patients-medical-history

National Institute on Aging (NIA). (2017d). *Prevent falls and fractures.* Retrieved from https://www.nia.nih.gov/health/prevent-falls-and-fractures

National Institute on Aging (NIA). (2017e). *Urinary incontinence in older adults.* Retrieved from https://www.nia.nih.gov/health/urinary-incontinence-older-adults

National Sleep Foundation. (2018). *Nocturia or frequent urination at night.* Retrieved from https://sleepfoundation.org/sleep-disorders-problems/nocturia

Office of Disease Prevention and Health Promotion, *Healthy People 2020.* (2018). *Older adults.* Retrieved from https://www.healthypeople.gov/2020/topics-objectives/topic/older-adults

Office on Women's Health, U.S. Department of Health and Human Services. (2018). *Menopause symptoms and relief.* Retrieved from https://www.womenshealth.gov/menopause/menopause-symptoms-and-relief

Ortman, J. M., Velkoff, V. A., & Hogan, H. (2014). *An aging nation: The older population in the United States, current population reports, P25-1140.* Washington, DC: U.S. Census Bureau. Retrieved from https://www.census.gov/prod/2014pubs/p25-1140.pdf

Otify, M., Fuller, J., Ross, J., Shaikh, H., & Johns, J. (2015). Endometrial pathology in the postmenopausal woman – an evidence based approach to management. *The Obstetrician and Gynaecologist, 17*(1), 29–38. Retrieved from https://obgyn.onlinelibrary.wiley.com/doi/epdf/10.1111/tog.12150. doi:10.1111/tog.12150

Parkinson's Foundation. (2018). *What is Parkinson's?* Retrieved from http://www.parkinson.org/understanding-parkinsons/what-is-parkinsons

Psychology Today. (2017). *What we know about aging and pain.* Retrieved from https://www.psychologytoday.com/us/blog/evidence-based-living/201704/what-we-know-about-aging-and-pain

Selner, M. (2016). *What causes night blindness?* Retrieved from https://www.healthline.com/symptom/night-blindness

Shelky, M., & Wallace, M. (2012). *Katz Index of Independence in Activities of Daily Living (ADL).* Retrieved from https://consultgeri.org/try-this/general-assessment/issue-2.pdf

Susan G. Komen Breast Cancer Foundation. (2018a). *Facts and statistics.* Retrieved from https://ww5.komen.org/BreastCancer/FactsandStatistics.html

Susan G. Komen Breast Cancer Foundation. (2018b). *Personal history of breast cancer or other cancers.* Retrieved from https://ww5.komen.org/BreastCancer/PersonalHistoryofBreastCancer.html

Tsoi, K. K. F., Chan, J. Y. C., Hirai, H. W., & Wong, S. Y. S. (2017). Comparison of diagnostic performance of Two Question Screen and 15 depression screening instruments for older adults: Systematic review and meta-analysis. *The British Journal of Psychiatry, 210*(4), 255-260. doi: 10.1192/bjp.bp.116.186932

Urology Care Foundation. (2018). *What is benign prostatic hyperplasia (BPH)?* Retrieved from http://www.urologyhealth.org/urologic-conditions/benign-prostatic-hyperplasia-(bph)

Ward, K. T., & Reuben, D. B. (2018). *Comprehensive geriatric assessment.* Retrieved from https://www.uptodate.com/contents/comprehensive-geriatric-assessment

Westerberg, D. P., & Voyak, M. J. (2013). Onychomycosis: Current trends in diagnosis and treatment. *American Family Physician, 88*(11), 762–770. Retrieved from https://www.aafp.org/afp/2013/1201/p762.pdf

Wolfram, T. (2016). *Special nutrient needs of older adults.* Retrieved from https://www.eatright.org/health/wellness/healthy-aging/special-nutrient-needs-of-older-adults

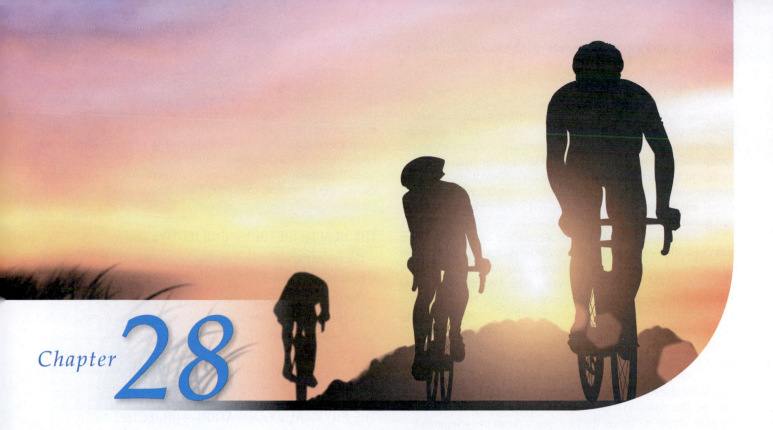

28

Complete Health Assessments: Putting the Pieces Together

LEARNING OUTCOMES

Upon completion of the chapter, you will be able to:

1. Apply knowledge and skills to conduct a general survey and physical assessment of patients in the community setting.

2. Apply knowledge and skills to conduct a general survey and physical assessment of patients in the hospital setting.

3. Outline the data to collect in the rapid assessment.

4. Outline the data to collect in the routine assessment.

5. Identify special considerations that guide assessments in community and hospital settings.

MEDICAL LANGUAGE

bi-	Prefix meaning "two"
esthesia-	Suffix meaning "nervous sensation"
oro-	Prefix meaning "mouth"
post-	Prefix meaning "after," "behind"

Introduction

This chapter is designed to help you perform a complete health assessment in both the community and hospital settings. Conducting a complete health assessment requires effective communication, organization, use of knowledge from the natural and behavioral sciences and nursing, efficient and accurate performance of physical assessment techniques, recognition of verbal and nonverbal patient cues, and the abilities to interpret and document findings.

The nursing process has been recognized as the systematic and cyclic process used by the nurse to plan and provide care for patients. Assessment, the first step of the nursing process, is a dynamic and fluid activity. Analysis of the data gathered in the assessment phase of the nursing process requires critical thinking and application of knowledge about health, illness, and factors that influence a person's response to changes in his or her health status. Only with detailed assessment and accurate analysis of data can nursing care plans be developed to meet the specific needs of the patient. For the student, a complete health assessment may seem difficult and overwhelming. However, it is essential that the data collected is thorough and accurate, so that the resulting plan of care will meet the healthcare needs of each patient.

Applying Health Assessment Skills in a Community Setting

The complete health assessment in a community setting includes the interview, general survey, assessment of vital signs, and physical assessment of body systems. Complete health assessments may be needed for several reasons, including annual physicals, well-child checkups, and sports exams. Complete health assessments may also be necessary when patients have symptoms with an unknown or uncommon cause; the complete health assessment can then be used to help diagnose an acute or chronic condition that requires treatment. Recall that findings are influenced by a number of factors including age, gender, developmental level, genetic makeup, culture, religion, psychologic and emotional status, and the patient's internal and external environments.

The following pages describe one sequence for the complete health assessment. A variety of sequences may be employed. This sequence minimizes the number of position changes for the patient. The complete health assessment should be approached with confidence and a professional demeanor. This important part of professional nursing practice will become easier with practice.

Planning and organization are important steps for a successful assessment. Plan the sequence of steps in a logical fashion. The exam can be performed in many different sequences, so determine an order that feels comfortable. Practice this order until the steps become second nature, gather the necessary equipment, review documentation forms, and have pen and paper or a computer or tablet ready to record data or to write reminders or notes for yourself to clarify points, to prompt follow-up in specific areas, and to help in orderly and concise documentation.

The complete health assessment begins with the first patient encounter. Observations made during your introduction and while settling down for the interview provide data as part of the general survey and may provide cues about the patient. Always begin by introducing yourself, stating the purpose of the complete health assessment, and including assurances regarding the confidentiality of the information. Follow guidelines for patient safety and use Standard Precautions throughout the assessment. In the initial encounter and during the interview, the patient is clothed and sits facing the nurse.

THE HEALTH HISTORY—SUBJECTIVE DATA

Complete the interview (see Figure 28.1 ■).

Include all areas and address cultural and spiritual assessments.

For children, ask about the child's grade level and school.

The data are subjective; document in the patient's own words.

At the completion of the interview, have the patient change into an examination gown. Provide privacy to the patient. Have the patient empty the bladder; if required, provide a container and instructions for collecting a urine specimen.

THE PHYSICAL EXAMINATION—OBJECTIVE DATA
PERFORM HAND HYGIENE

1. **Appearance and Mental Status**

   Compare stated age with appearance.

   Assess level of consciousness.

   Observe body build, height and weight in relation to age, lifestyle, and health.

   Observe facial expression, posture, and position and observe mobility.

   Observe overall hygiene and grooming.

   Note body odor and breath odor.

   Note signs of health or illness (skin color, signs of pain).

   Assess attitude, attentiveness, affect, mood, and appropriateness of responses.

   Listen for quantity, quality, relevance, and organization of speech.

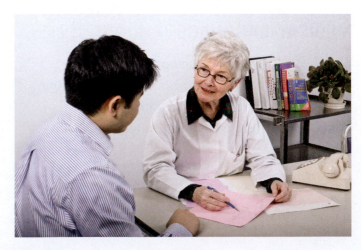

Figure 28.1 The patient participating in the health history.

2. **Measurements**

   Measure height.

   Measure weight (see Figure 28.2 ■).

   Measure skinfold thickness.

   Calculate the body mass index (BMI).

   Assess vision with the Snellen Chart and Jaeger Card (cranial nerve II). For children who cannot read, assess vision using age-appropriate symbols or other available tools.

3. **Vital Signs**

   Assess the radial pulses.

   Count respirations.

   Take the temperature.

   Measure the blood pressure bilaterally.

   Assess for pain. For young children, use a FACES Pain Rating Scale rather than a numerical scale.

4. **Skin, Hair, and Nails**

   Inspect the skin on the face, neck, and upper and lower extremities (other skin areas will be assessed as part of the systems assessment).

   Inspect for color and uniformity of color.

   Inspect and palpate skin.

   Palpate for skin temperature, moisture, turgor, and edema (see Figure 28.3 ■).

   Inspect, palpate, measure, and describe lesions.

   Inspect the hair on the scalp and body.

   Palpate scalp hair for texture and moisture.

   Inspect the fingernails for curvature, angle, and color.

   Palpate the nails for texture and capillary refill.

5. **Head, Neck, and Related Lymphatics**

   Inspect the skull for size, shape, and symmetry.

   Observe facial expressions and symmetry of facial features and movements (cranial nerves V and VII).

   Palpate the skull and lymph nodes of the head and neck (see Figure 28.4 ■).

Palpate the muscles of the face (cranial nerve V).

Assess facial response to sensory stimulation (cranial nerve V).

Inspect the neck for symmetry, pulsations, swelling, or masses.

Assess range of motion and strength of muscles against resistance. Observe as the patient moves the head forward and back and side to side and shrugs the shoulders (cranial nerve XI).

Palpate the trachea.

Palpate the thyroid for symmetry and masses.

Palpate and auscultate the carotid arteries, one at a time (see Figure 28.5 ■).

6. **Eyes**

   Inspect the external eye.

   Inspect the pupils for color, size, shape, and equality.

   Test the visual fields (cranial nerve II).

   Test extraocular movements (cranial nerves III, IV, VI).

   Test pupillary reaction to light and accommodation (cranial nerve III) (see Figure 28.6 ■).

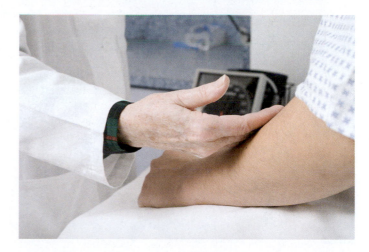

Figure 28.3 Palpating skin moisture.

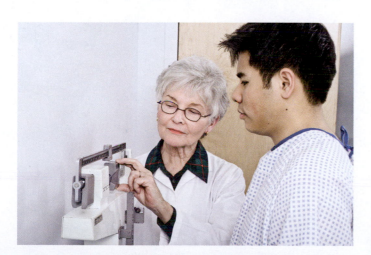

Figure 28.2 Measuring the patient's weight.

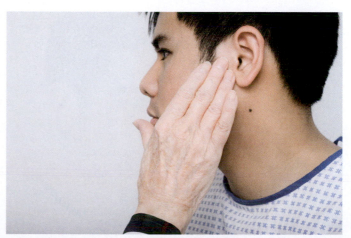

Figure 28.4 Palpating the preauricular lymph nodes.

7. **Ears, Nose, Mouth, and Throat**

Inspect the external ears.

Palpate the auricle and tragus of each ear.

Test hearing using the whisper, Weber, and Rinne tests (cranial nerve VIII).

Assess patency of the nares.

Test sense of smell (cranial nerve I).

Palpate the nose and sinuses.

Palpate the temporal artery.

Palpate the temporomandibular joint (TMJ) as the patient opens and closes the mouth.

Inspect the lips.

Use a penlight to inspect the tongue, palates, buccal mucosa, gums, teeth, the opening to the salivary glands, tonsils, and oropharynx.

Test the sense of taste (cranial nerve VII).

Wearing gloves, palpate the tongue, gums, and floor of the mouth.

Observe the uvula for position and mobility as the patient says "ah," and test the gag reflex (cranial nerves IX, X).

Observe as the patient protrudes the tongue (cranial nerve XII).

8. **The Respiratory System, Breasts, and Axillae**

Inspect the skin of the posterior chest.

Inspect the posterior chest for symmetry, musculoskeletal development, and thoracic configuration.

Observe respiratory excursion.

Auscultate posterior lung sounds.

Palpate and percuss the costovertebral angle for tenderness.

Palpate for thoracic expansion and tactile fremitus.

Inspect and palpate the scapula and spine.

Inspect the skin of the anterior chest.

Inspect the anterior chest for symmetry and musculoskeletal development.

Assess range of motion and movement against resistance of the upper extremities (see Figure 28.7 ■).

Inspect the breasts for symmetry, mobility, masses, dimpling, and nipple retraction. Ask the post-pubescent female to lift arms over her head, press her hands on her hips, and lean forward as you inspect.

Auscultate anterior lung sounds (see Figure 28.8 ■).

Palpate the axillary, supraclavicular, and infraclavicular lymph nodes.

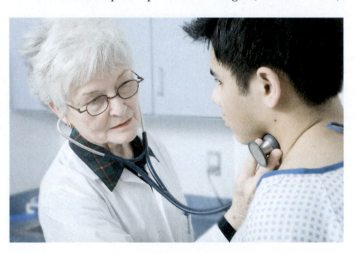

Figure 28.5 Auscultation of the carotid artery.

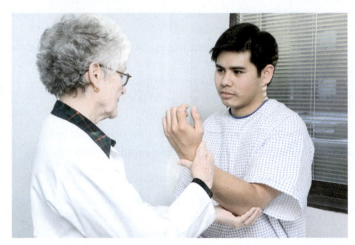

Figure 28.7 Testing movement against resistance.

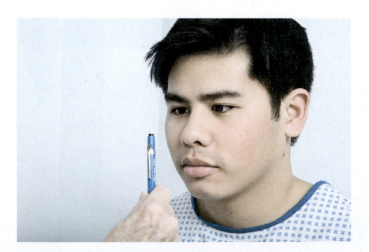

Figure 28.6 Testing for accommodation.

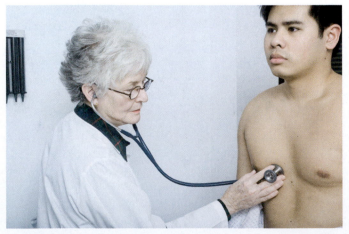

Figure 28.8 Auscultating the anterior thorax.

Palpate the breasts and nipples (see Figure 28.9 ■).

Palpate the anterior chest.

9. The Cardiovascular System

Inspect the neck for jugular pulsations or distention.

Inspect and palpate the chest for pulsations, lifts, or heaves.

Use the bell and diaphragm of the stethoscope to auscultate for heart sounds (Figure 28.10 ■).

At each area of auscultation distinguish the rate, rhythm, and location of S1 and S2 sounds.

Palpate the apical pulse and note the intensity and location.

10. The Abdomen

Inspect the skin of the abdomen.

Inspect the abdomen for symmetry, contour, and movement or pulsation.

Auscultate the abdomen for bowel sounds.

Auscultate the abdomen for vascular sounds.

Palpate to determine if tenderness, masses, or distention are present.

Palpate the inguinal region for pulses, lymph nodes, and presence of hernias.

11. The Musculoskeletal System

Test range of motion and strength in the hips, knees, ankles, and feet (see Figure 28.11 ■).

Assist the patient to a standing position.

Inspect the skin of the posterior legs.

Perform the Romberg test.

Observe as the patient walks in a natural gait.

Observe the patient walking heel to toe.

Observe the patient standing on the right foot, then the left foot with eyes closed.

Observe as the patient performs a shallow knee bend.

Stand behind the patient and observe the spine as the patient touches the toes.

Test range of motion of the spine.

12. The Neurologic System

Assess sensory function. Include light touch, tactile location, pain, temperature, vibratory sense, kinesthetic sensation, and tactile discrimination (see Figure 28.12 ■).

Test position sense.

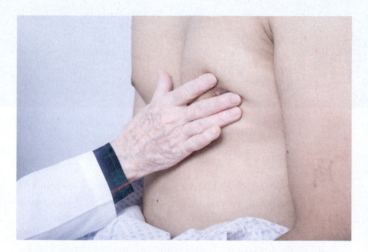

Figure 28.9 Palpating the nipple.

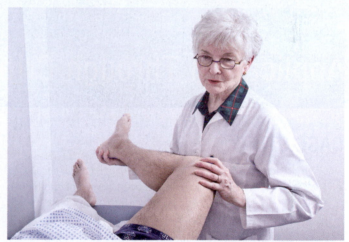

Figure 28.11 Testing range of motion of the lower extremity.

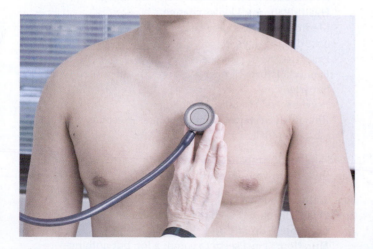

Figure 28.10 Using the bell to auscultate the pulmonic area.

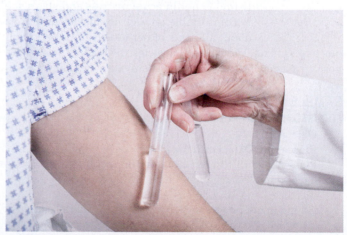

Figure 28.12 Testing temperature sensation.

Test cerebellar function with finger-to-nose test.

Test cerebellar function with heel-shin test.

Test stereognosis and graphesthesia.

Test tendon reflexes bilaterally and compare (see Figure 28.13 ■). Recall that reflexes in newborns will differ from reflexes in children and adults.

13. Completion of Assessment

Complete hand hygiene.

Document findings from the comprehensive health assessment according to agency policy. Include all concepts of patient safety, Standard Precautions, and professional standards in the documentation of assessment data.

Documentation is important; the data documented from the complete assessment establish a baseline for ongoing patient interaction and care.

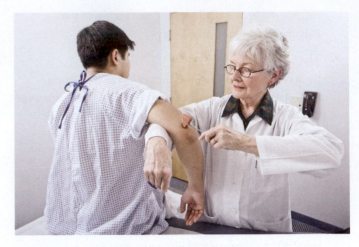

Figure 28.13 Testing the triceps reflex.

Application Through Critical Thinking

CASE STUDY

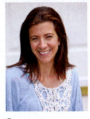

Source: Stuart Monk/ Shutterstock.

Mrs. Amparo Bellisimo arrives at the health center. In her phone call to arrange for a visit, she stated she had abdominal pain and some coughing. Mrs. Bellisimo was last seen at the center 9 months ago for a complete health assessment. In preparation for her assessment, the nurse reviews her health history. Mrs. Bellisimo is not in acute distress and states she is comfortable enough to answer questions about all parts of her health since her previous assessment. The nurse completes the health history and performs a general survey and measurement of vital signs.

SAMPLE DOCUMENTATION
FOCUSED HISTORY (SUBJECTIVE DATA)

Date: March 24

Biographic Data: Unchanged

Present Health/Illness—Reason for Seeking Care: "I have some stomach pain, I have a little cough, I've had diarrhea," and very quietly she states, "I have some itching in my private area, by my vagina. This all started last week. We were on vacation and I got sick. I went to an urgi-center, and they said I had sinusitis and gave me an antibiotic. I had been having pressure in my head, my nose was congested, I had a bad headache and earache. At first I thought I was allergic to something, but it was really uncomfortable and I didn't want to ruin our vacation, so I went to see if I could get medicine. I have been taking the antibiotic for five days and some saline nose drops, but I really feel awful, and now I have to go back to work."

Health Beliefs and Practices: Denies change

Health Patterns: Denies change

Medications: No change except antibiotic 5 days, saline nose drops 5 days

Past History: No change

Family History: Mother was recently diagnosed with hypertension

Psychosocial History: No change

Review of Systems: Denies changes except as noted in reason for visit

Head and Neck Sinusitis—headache, pressure, runny nose, earache—improved since antibiotic

Respiratory Cough

    Onset: "It started with the sinus thing but is worse."

    Location: A throaty and chest cough

    Duration: "I just seem to cough a lot, but nothing comes up."

730

Characteristics: "I have a little clear mucus in my throat in the morning; it's a dry cough."

Aggravating factors: "I don't know—it just comes on sometimes."

Relieving factors: "Being still."

Treatment: "I haven't really done anything. I figured I better see what's what."

Impact on ADLs: "I am okay but really too tired to do much."

Coping strategies: "I'm trying to be calm. My husband has been really good about all of it, and he brought me here."

Emotional impact: "I'm worried that I have something serious, I'm a little nervous."

Abdomen

1. Stomach pain

   Onset: 3 days ago.

   Location: Lower stomach, sometimes one side or the other but right now mostly the left.

   Duration: "It hurts most of the time."

   Characteristics: Sore, achy 3 to 5 on a scale of 0 to 10.

   Aggravating factors: "I'm not sure. It may be with the diarrhea."

   Relieving factors: "When I'm still and not coughing or going to the bathroom, it is okay."

   Treatment: "I really did not know what to do."

   ICE—As above

2. Diarrhea

   Onset: "Four days ago—after I was at the urgi-center."

   Duration: "It was once a day. Now I have had diarrhea about two or three times a day."

   Characteristics: Light brown watery stuff. "Depends on what I eat."

   Aggravating factors: "I really don't know. It seems eating may cause me to go, but not always."

   Relieving factors: "I haven't done anything. It's just happening."

   Treatment: "I haven't taken anything. I was always told to let it out."

   ICE—As above.

Reproductive Vaginal itch, LMP 2 weeks ago

   Onset: 2 days ago

   Location: Vagina and all around

   Duration: "It's itchy almost all the time. It seems to be getting worse."

   Characteristics: Itching and burning

   Aggravating factors: "Nothing really."

   Relieving factors: "It seems a little better after I shower."

   Treatment: "I didn't know what to do."

   ICE—As above

PHYSICAL ASSESSMENT (OBJECTIVE DATA) Mrs. Bellisimo is alert and oriented with clear speech; she uses concise and clear responses to questions. She is fully mobile and has a steady gait. Her skin color is suntanned with pink undertones; she has bluish skin color below the eyes. She is well-groomed and admits to being nervous. She coughed occasionally during the interview and held her abdomen during the cough. The cough was dry, and the episodes were 10 to 20 seconds long.

Vital Signs: Temperature 98.8 oral, BP 118/74, Pulse 88, RR 20. Pain—abdomen 3 to 5 (scale 0 to 10). Height 5′2″ Weight 122 lb. Skin warm and dry.

Mrs. Bellisimo voided and provided a urine specimen as she changed into a gown for the physical assessment.

CRITICAL THINKING QUESTIONS

1. Identify the pattern/approach you would use to conduct the physical assessment of Mrs. Bellisimo.

2. Describe any changes required for any particular body system and the reason for the change.

3. Identify additional information that may be helpful in planning care for Mrs. Bellisimo.

4. What situations require complete health assessments?

5. What factors influence findings in the physical assessment?

Applying Health Assessment Skills in a Hospital Setting

The depth and breadth of assessment of the hospitalized patient vary with both the purpose of the assessment and the health status of the patient. In nonemergent situations, nurses conduct complete (comprehensive) health assessments of patients at the time of admission. When the patient is in distress, or in special circumstances such as following surgery, a more focused and limited assessment is carried out. Routine or ongoing assessments occur throughout the patient's hospital stay. These ongoing assessments include shift-by-shift assessments as well as assessments to ascertain patient response to a treatment or intervention. In practice, each patient encounter includes assessment in relation to current and expected status, change, and progress.

Hospitalized patients undergo frequent assessments; therefore, it is important for the nurse to communicate effectively regarding the type and purpose of the assessment. In addition, the nurse must be sure to have all the required equipment and must be able to use physical assessment techniques with efficiency and competence. Hospitals often have policies to guide the types and frequencies of assessments required in accordance with medical diagnoses or parameters for laboratory findings, monitor readings, patient condition, or administration of medication.

Application of the nursing process is specific for each patient. Integration of assessment data with other knowledge about a patient is essential to planning care. The knowledge base about the patient will include health problems (i.e., current and coexisting medical diagnoses); age; gender; nutritional status; results of laboratory and diagnostic testing; documentation and communication with other members of the healthcare team; medication regimens; and functional capabilities. Additionally, the knowledge base includes psychosocial factors and concerns including, for example, the presence of a support system, knowledge about the health problems, coping abilities, cultural preferences, and spirituality. This knowledge base assists the nurse in making judgments about assessment findings in relation to expected norms in each patient encounter.

The following pages present two types of assessment of the hospitalized patient: a rapid assessment and a routine or initial assessment. Remember to apply all concepts of patient safety, Standard Precautions, and professional standards in each patient encounter, in professional communication, and in documentation of assessment data. Assessment procedures that apply to National Patient Safety Goals are noted throughout and explained in Table 28.1.

The Rapid Assessment

The rapid assessment requires 1 minute or less to complete. This type of assessment is often used as an initial assessment of a group of patients in a nursing assignment. Nurses use the collected data to prioritize their actions and interventions. Beginning students find the rapid assessment of a single patient helpful in reducing anxiety because priorities can be established alone or in collaborative discussion with the faculty, preceptor, or staff. Additionally, documentation of data from the rapid assessment establishes a baseline for ongoing patient interaction and care.

Sequence

Perform hand hygiene (NPSG.07.01.01).

Note isolation precautions, latex allergies, or fall precautions.

Enter the room.

Identify yourself and explain that you will be providing care for a given time period.

Ask the patient's name and identify the patient using at least two patient identifiers, such as wrist band and identification number (NPSG.01.01.01).

Note the location of the patient (bed, chair, bathroom).

If in bed, is it in the lowest position and is the call bell in reach?

Observe for level of consciousness.

Observe for signs of distress.

Table 28.1 Selected Hospital National Patient Safety Goals

NPSG.01.01.01	Use at least two methods of patient identification. For example, use the patient's name *and* date of birth. The patient's room number is not an acceptable means of identification. Verification of the patient's identity ensures that each patient gets the correct medicine and treatment.
NPSG.03.06.01	Confirm the patient's medication regimen with the patient or the patient's primary caregiver. Record and report correct information about the patient's current medication regimen. Review any newly prescribed medications and check for duplications, omissions, and contraindications. Before discharging the patient, provide written instructions for administration of each medication. Make sure the patient or the primary caregiver understands the directions for medication administration. Teach the patient or primary caregiver to bring an up-to-date medication list to every healthcare appointment.
NPSG.06.01.01	Make improvements to ensure that alarms on medical equipment are heard and responded to on time.
NPSG.07.01.01	Use the hand cleaning guidelines from the Centers for Disease Control and Prevention (2018) or the World Health Organization (2009). Set goals for improving hand cleaning. Use the goals to improve hand cleaning.
NPSG.07.04.01	Use proven guidelines to prevent infection of the blood from central lines.
NPSG.07.05.01	Use proven guidelines to prevent infection after surgery.
NPSG.07.06.01	Use proven guidelines to prevent infections of the urinary tract that are caused by catheters.

Source: The Joint Commission (2014).

Observe skin color and respiratory effort.

Observe posture, facial expression, and symmetry.

Observe the patient's response to your introduction.

Observe speech for clarity.

Place a hand on the patient and assess skin temperature.

Note any immediately visible tubes, IV lines, drains, and equipment.

Complete hand hygiene.

Explain that you will return shortly.

Discuss with the faculty, preceptor, or staff, as needed.

Document findings.

The Routine Assessment

The routine assessment is used to gather more in-depth data about a patient for whom care will be provided. Data gathered in the routine assessment will guide the direction of care and inform the nurse about the need for, as well as the type and frequency of, continuing assessment.

1. **Introduction**

   Perform hand hygiene (NPSG.07.01.01).

   Enter the room.

   Identify yourself and explain that you will be providing care for a given length of time.

   Ask the patient's name and identify the patient using at least two patient identifiers, such as wristband and identification number (NPSG.01.01.01; see Figure 28.14 ■).

   Note the patient's location (bed, chair, or bathroom).

   Note that the call light is in reach.

   Note any immediately visible tubes, IV lines, drains, and equipment.

2. **General Appearance**
   Observe the following:
   Level of consciousness
   Respiratory status
   Skin color

   Nutritional status

   Facial expression—symmetry and appropriateness

   Body posture and position; relaxation, comfort, or pain

   Clarity, fluency, quality, and appropriateness of speech

   Hygiene and grooming

   Response to your introduction in relation to hearing and congruence with situation (see Figure 28.15 ■)

3. **Measurement**

   Temperature

   Pulses—radial, dorsalis pedis bilaterally

   Respiration

   Blood pressure (bilaterally if not contraindicated) (see Figure 28.16 ■)

   Pain—use of rating scale. Correlate with administration of pain medication if so indicated (NPSG.03.06.01).

   Measure pulse oximetry.

4. **Respiratory System**

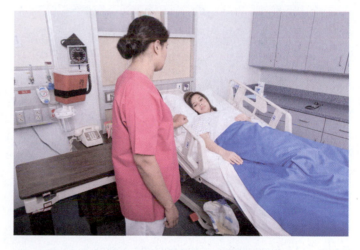

Figure 28.15 The nurse observing the patient in bed.

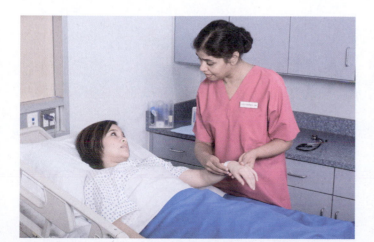

Figure 28.14 The nurse confirms the patient's identification.

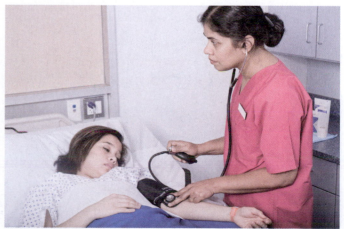

Figure 28.16 The nurse checking vital signs.

Assess respiratory effort.

Implement oxygen therapy—mask, nasal cannula; check placement and flowmeter (NPSG.06.01.01).

Auscultate breath sounds—posterior and anterior. Seek assistance for positioning if required (see Figure 28.17 ■).

Assess for coughing; if productive, assess sputum.

5. **Cardiovascular System**

Auscultate apical pulse for rate and rhythm (see Figure 28.18 ■).

Assess heart sounds in five auscultatory areas.

Assess for capillary refill (see Figure 28.19 ■).

Assess for peripheral edema.

Assess intravenous (IV) site (NPSG.07.04.01); if IV fluid is running, verify that it is the correct solution and rate (NPSG.03.06.01).

6. **Abdomen**

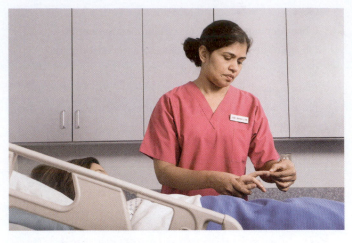

Figure 28.19 Assessment of capillary refill.

Inspect for contour, skin color, and pulsations.

Auscultate bowel sounds.

Palpate all quadrants except when there are reports of abdominal pain, recent surgery, or trauma.

Assess the time of the most recent bowel elimination and/or flatus.

Assess drains, tubes, dressings, when indicated (NPSG.07.05.01; see Figure 28.20 ■).

7. **Genitourinary**

Assess urine output—voiding—frequency and amount, or catheter drainage amount (NPSG.07.06.01).

Assess the color and clarity of urine (see Figure 28.21 ■).

8. **Skin**

Palpate skin temperature, moisture.

Assess skin turgor (see Figure 28.22 ■).

Assess for lesions both anteriorly and posteriorly.

Assess wounds and incision lines if present (NPSG.07.05.01).

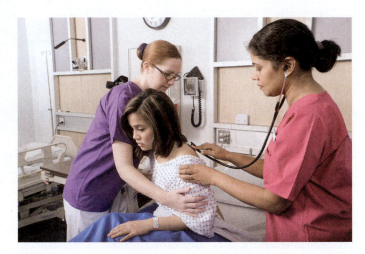

Figure 28.17 Auscultation of the posterior thorax.

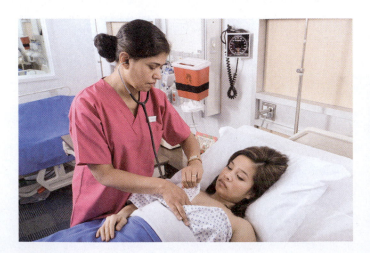

Figure 28.18 Auscultation of the apical pulse.

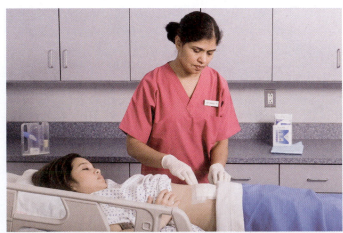

Figure 28.20 Assessment of an abdominal dressing.

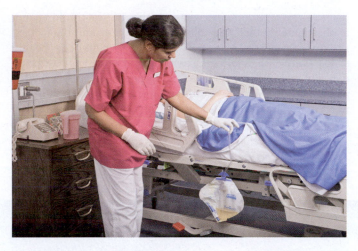

Figure 28.21 Assessment of urinary catheter drainage.

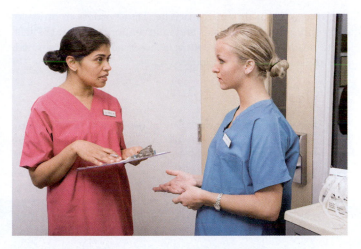

Figure 28.23 Discussion of patient assessment.

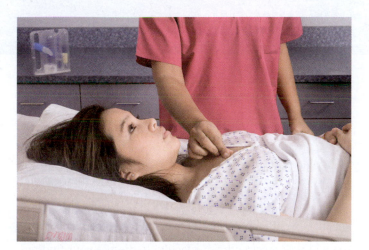

Figure 28.22 Assessment of skin turgor.

Use standardized tools to determine risk for skin problems (scales/questionnaires).

Assess functioning of any devices applied on the skin or used to prevent pressure (NPSG.06.01.01).

9. **Activity**

Assess symmetry and coordination of movements throughout the assessment.

Assess the ability to move self to sitting and standing positions.

Assess for presence of and use of assistive devices.

Use standardized measures to evaluate risk for falls.

Assess the environment for hazards related to mobility, returning the bed to the lowest position. The call light should be within reach.

Complete hand hygiene.

10. **Documentation**

Discuss with the faculty, preceptor, or staff, as needed (see Figure 28.23 ■).

Document findings according to agency policy.

Special Considerations

Some populations of patients require special care when hospitalized, including patients with communication barriers and dying patients.

Patients with communication barriers include patients who do not speak English as their first language (ESL patients) and deaf or hard-of-hearing patients who require communication through American Sign Language. Before assessing these patients, an interpreter should be found who can communicate with the patient to describe assessment procedures and obtain answers to assessment or interview questions. When possible, a staff member should be used as an interpreter. Family members or friends should only be used as interpreters when no other option is available, because some patients and family members may feel that some topics, especially topics related to the genitourinary system, should not be discussed with others in the family. Family members are also more likely than a staff member to change the interpretation of what the patient is saying if they do not agree with the patient's answer or do not want the patient to know specific information about his or her condition. Using an appropriate interpreter can provide emotional care to the patient during assessments and help the provider obtain more accurate assessment information. When assessing these patients, confirm that the patient understands the assessment procedures and questions before beginning the assessment.

Dying patients and their family members also require special care in the hospital. Patients who are dying will require not only physical care but also emotional care. These patients should be treated with respect and allowed to participate in choices about their care as much as possible. Assessments should include interview questions related to the patient's emotional state to determine if counseling or spiritual care is needed. Spending extra time with dying patients to help them feel like they are not alone may provide added comfort during this transition. Nurses should also assess the emotional state of family members and friends who are present to determine if emotional care or information about death, dying, and funeral preparations is needed. This is especially important if the patient is a child or if the death is sudden or unexpected. The nurse should also ask the patient or family about advanced healthcare directives such as living wills or do-not-resuscitate (DNR) orders in order to determine appropriate goals and interventions. Cultural beliefs about death and dying also must be assessed and incorporated into any nursing interventions.

Summary

This chapter presents an overview of different types of health assessments that can be used in the care of patients in both community and hospital settings. The chapter serves as a reminder that analysis of the obtained data requires critical thinking and application of knowledge about health, illness, and the factors that influence a person's response to changes in his or her health status. Only with detailed assessment and accurate analysis of data can nursing care plans be developed to meet the specific needs of the patient. In addition, special considerations are needed when assessing some patients, including those with communication barriers, and dying patients.

Application Through Critical Thinking

CASE STUDY

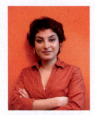

Source: Sergio Azenha/Alamy Stock Photo.

Mrs. Janelle Hoskins is a 34-year-old admitted to the emergency department via ambulance following a bicycle accident. The assessment in the emergency department revealed that Mrs. Hoskins was alert and oriented, stating she had pain "all over" at a level of 8 on a scale of 0 to 10. Further assessment and diagnostic testing revealed a fractured left tibia and fibula, abrasions on both hands, contusions in the chest and abdomen, and a deep laceration on the right lower extremity lateral to the upper border of the patella. Mrs. Hoskins denies any history of acute or chronic illness, takes medication for seasonal allergies, uses oral birth control medication, and takes one ibuprofen for occasional pain or headache. She denies drug or alcohol use and has never been hospitalized.

Mrs. Hoskins was admitted to the hospital and underwent an open reduction–internal fixation (ORIF) of the fracture of the tibia and fibula and closure of the right lower-leg laceration. Her postsurgical treatment plan includes bed rest, use of an incentive spirometer, medication for pain, increasing from a liquid to regular diet as tolerated, intravenous therapy with dextrose in saline at a slow rate, and Foley catheter drainage.

You, a student nurse, were assigned to care for Mrs. Hoskins 26 hours postsurgery. You received information about Mrs. Hoskins and her diagnoses and treatments and had an opportunity to prepare for her care. A brief discussion about her injuries, surgery, and treatments occurred in a preclinical conference.

Your first encounter with Mrs. Hoskins included a rapid assessment. Upon entering the room, you introduced yourself and told Mrs. Hoskins that you would be providing her care. You made some observations. Your findings were as follows:

Mrs. Hoskins was supine in bed; her eyes opened when I entered the room. She nodded to acknowledge my introduction. While checking the identification band, I noticed her hot skin. Her face appeared flushed. Her breathing was shallow. Mrs. Hoskins was supine and held herself in a rigid posture. She had covers over her; the left leg appeared to be elevated on a pillow. An IV was running via a pump, and urine was in the collection bag. Mrs. Hoskins said, "Okay, I'll be here" very quietly when I explained that I would return shortly to begin assessment and care.

You will now meet with your faculty to discuss your findings and proceed with clinical interventions for Mrs. Hoskins.

SAMPLE DOCUMENTATION

SUBJECTIVE DATA Acknowledged your presence by opening eyes, spoke in quiet voice.

OBJECTIVE DATA Supine, face flushed, hot skin to touch, shallow breathing, rigid posture, left leg elevated, IV running, Foley catheter draining.

CRITICAL THINKING QUESTIONS

1. What assessments would you expect to complete in a rapid assessment for Mrs. Hoskins?

2. What is the difference between a rapid assessment and a routine assessment?

3. What information will your faculty expect you to provide about the findings?

4. How will those findings influence your continued assessment of the patient?

5. What further information do you need about findings from your rapid assessment?

Upon your return to Mrs. Hoskins's bedside, you carried out further assessment and documented the findings as follows:

SUBJECTIVE DATA "I feel awful, I am afraid to move, I hurt all over; it hurts to move, to breathe, and even when someone touches me." Asking for pain medication, states "then I can sleep, I am so exhausted. Please don't tell me you have to do anything much, I can't take it." States "I don't want to eat or drink—I'll take one sip of water if you insist." When asked if she had used the incentive spirometer, she replied "that thing—I don't even know what it is or why it is here."

PAIN ASSESSMENT

> **Onset**: "It has been hurting all along."
> **Location**: "Left leg and chest."
> **Duration**: "My leg keeps getting worse, and my chest hurts a lot more than it did during the night."
> **Characteristics**: On a scale of 0 to 10, "Left leg 8, chest 6. It is throbbing and pressure."
> **Aggravating factors**: "Oh, if I try to move, everything hurts, and my chest hurts when I breathe."
> **Relieving factors**: "It seems to help if I stay still. The medication helped a lot."
> **Treatment**: "I had the medication—I don't know when I had it, and I need more now."

Impact on ADLs: "I just don't want to do anything, so don't ask me to."
Coping strategies: "I just keep still, try to sleep, and ask for medication."
Emotional impact: "This pain is wearing me out, I want it to go away, I can't think about anything, and I should be finding out about when I will be able to get out of here—right now, I don't care."

OBJECTIVE DATA Temperature 100.2 oral. BP 128/82, pulse 88, RR 24, shallow. Pulse oximetry 95. Nail bed refill immediate. Auscultation of the lungs is limited to the anterior chest, sounds are distant and difficult to assess. Abdomen is soft with rare bowel sounds. Skin dry with erythema, lips dry. Ecchymosis on chest and abdomen, dressing right lower leg dry and intact, left leg in a cast to thigh. Toes warm bilaterally, no edema.

Foley draining dark yellow urine, 60 mL in collection bag. IV site intact, and dextrose in saline running as ordered. Patient lies still throughout the assessment. Answers questions slowly, grimaces when moving.

REFERENCES

Centers for Disease Control and Prevention (CDC). (2018). *Hand hygiene in healthcare settings.* Retrieved from https://www.cdc.gov/handhygiene/index.html

The Joint Commission. (2014). *Hospital National Patient Safety Goals.* Retrieved from http://www.jointcommission.org/assets/1/6/2014_HAP_NPSG_E.pdf

World Health Organization (WHO). (2009). *WHO guidelines on hand hygiene in health care.* Retrieved from http://www.who.int/gpsc/5may/tools/9789241597906/en

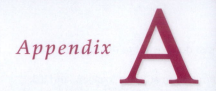
Background

Standard Precautions are to be used during all patient care. The guidelines are based on risk assessment, common-sense behaviors, and use of personal protective equipment to protect healthcare providers from infection and contamination, as well as to prevent the spread of infection to patients.

Guidelines

Use Standard Precautions for the care of all patients. The guidelines, as published by the Centers for Disease Control and Prevention, include detailed instructions and information related to all aspects of patient care and healthcare provider activities. Complete, current, and detailed information is found on the CDC website at https://www.cdc.gov/infectioncontrol/basics/standard-precautions.html. For each of the categories listed, you will find links to resources, training materials, and patient information. The following categories cover all of the activities and behaviors that professional nurses may implement or encounter during the health and physical assessment.

A. Perform Hand Hygiene

B. Use Personal Protective Equipment (PPE) Whenever There Is an Expectation of Possible Exposure to Infectious Materials

C. Follow Respiratory Hygiene/Cough Etiquette Principles

D. Ensure Appropriate Patient Placement

E. Properly Handle and Properly Clean and Disinfect Patient Care Equipment and Instruments/Devices; Clean and Disinfect the Environment Appropriately

F. Handle Textiles and Laundry Carefully

G. Follow Safe Injection Practices/Wear a Surgical Mask When Performing Lumbar Punctures

H. Ensure Healthcare Worker Safety Including Proper Handling of Needles and Other Sharps

More detail regarding the spread of specific contagions is contained in the guidelines for Transmission-Based Precautions found in Appendix B.

Source: Excerpted from *Standard precautions for all patient care.* Centers for Disease Control and Prevention (CDC), 2016. Retrieved from https://www.cdc.gov/infectioncontrol/basics/standard-precautions.html

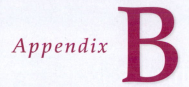
Background

In addition to using Standard Precautions in the care of all patients, patients with certain infectious diseases or presumed exposure to an infectious disease will prompt the healthcare provider to institute Transmission-Based Precautions. Isolating the patient who has been or is presumed to have been exposed to a particular pathogen is a critical step in preventing the spread of infection. Isolation Precautions include specific guidelines for pathogens spread in various ways: through the air, Airborne Precautions; via droplets, Droplet Precautions; and through direct contact with the patient or environment, Contact Precautions. The following categories provide an overview of the particular type of precaution, along with some of the pathogens covered by that method. The nurse must be aware that certain infections require more than one type of precaution. The lists are not all-inclusive, and the nurse must be aware of current precaution guidelines for the particular agency. Complete and detailed information can be found on the CDC website at https://www.cdc.gov/infectioncontrol/basics/transmission-based-precautions.html.

Airborne Precautions

In addition to Standard Precautions, use Airborne Precautions for patients known or suspected to be infected with pathogens transmitted person to person by the airborne route. Common illnesses spread by the airborne route include the following:

- Measles (rubeola)
- Smallpox (variola): also include Contact Precautions
- Varicella (including disseminated zoster)
- Tuberculosis (pulmonary)

Droplet Precautions

In addition to Standard Precautions, use Droplet Precautions for patients known or suspected to be infected with pathogens transmitted by respiratory droplets (i.e., large-particle droplets > 5 μ in size) that are generated by a patient who is coughing, sneezing, or talking. Examples of such illnesses include the following:

- Adenovirus
- Diphtheria (pharyngeal)
- *Haemophilus influenza* Type B (epiglottitis)

- Influenza
- Mumps
- Mycoplasma pneumonia
- Invasive *Neisseria meningitidis* disease, including meningitis, pneumonia, and sepsis
- Parvovirus B19
- Pertussis (whooping cough)
- German measles (rubella)
- Streptococcal (group A) pharyngitis, pneumonia, or scarlet fever in infants and young children

Contact Precautions

In addition to Standard Precautions, use Contact Precautions for patients with known or suspected infections or evidence of syndromes that represent an increased risk for contact transmission. Gastrointestinal, respiratory, skin, or wound infections or colonization with multidrug-resistant bacteria—judged by the infection control program and based on current state, regional, or national recommendations—are of special clinical and epidemiologic significance. Examples of these include the following:

- Bronchiolitis (respiratory syncytial virus)
- *Clostridium difficile*
- Diphtheria, cutaneous
- Draining abscess, major
- Herpes simplex virus (neonatal or mucocutaneous)
- Herpes zoster (varicella zoster, shingles): also include Airborne Precautions
- Major (noncontained) abscesses, cellulitis, or decubiti
- Pediculosis
- Rotavirus
- Scabies
- Staphylococcal furunculosis in infants and young children
- Viral hemorrhagic infections (Ebola, Lassa, or Marburg). Providers caring for patients with or under investigation for Ebola virus in U.S. hospitals should follow Standard, Contact, and Droplet precautions (https://www.cdc.gov/vhf/ebola/clinicians/evd/infection-control.html).

Source: Excerpted from the following: (1) Centers for Disease Control and Prevention. (2007). *Guideline for isolation precautions: Preventing transmission of infectious agents in healthcare settings.* Retrieved from https://www.cdc.gov/infectioncontrol/guidelines/isolation/index.html. (2) Centers for Disease Control and Prevention. (2017). *Type and duration of precautions recommended for selected infections and conditions.* Retrieved from https://www.cdc.gov/infectioncontrol/guidelines/isolation/appendix/type-duration-precautions.html.

Advanced Assessment Techniques

Introduction

Several advanced assessment techniques are shown here for the professional nurse with advanced practice education or for those who may be working in a specialized setting. This appendix includes the step-by-step instructions for gathering the objective data from the physical exam for selected body systems. You should refer to the body system chapter for detailed focused interview questions and anatomy and physiology review. These advanced physical assessment techniques are regularly performed by advanced practice nurses in primary care or specialty care settings. They also may be part of the comprehensive physical assessment completed by the nurse.

Objective Data—Physical Assessment

As for any physical assessment, the professional nurse must ensure that the setting is comfortable for the patient and conducive to gathering the information. For each of the advanced techniques, a list of equipment needed and helpful hints precedes the step-by-step instructions.

Ophthalmoscope Exam of the Fundus of the Eye

Inspecting Fundus with Ophthalmoscope

1. **Instruct the patient.**
   - Explain that you will be using the ophthalmoscope to look into the inner deep part of the eye (fundus) and that the lights in the room will be dimmed. Explain that the patient must stare ahead at a fixed point while you move in front with the ophthalmoscope. Tell the patient to maintain a fixed gaze, as if looking through you. Explain that you will place your hand on the patient's head or shoulder so you both remain stable.

2. **To examine the patient's right eye, hold the ophthalmoscope to your right eye in your right hand with the index finger on the lens wheel.**

3. **Begin with the lens on the 0 diopter. With the light on, place the ophthalmoscope over your right eye (see Figure App C.1 ■).**

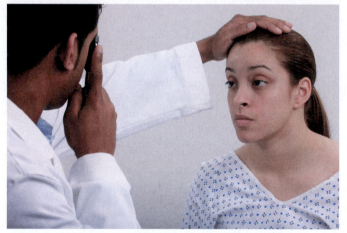

Figure App C.1 Approaching the patient for the ophthalmoscopic exam.

4. **Stand at a slight angle lateral to the patient's line of vision.**

5. **Approach the patient at about a 15-degree angle toward the patient's nose.**

6. **Place your left hand on the patient's shoulder or head.**

7. **Hold the ophthalmoscope against your head, directing the light into the patient's pupil. Keep your other eye open.**

8. **Advance toward the patient.**

9. **As you look into the patient's pupil, you will see the *red reflex*, which is the reflection of the light off the retina.**
   Remember to examine the patient's right eye with your right eye, and the patient's left eye with your left eye. At this point you may need to adjust the lens wheel to bring the ocular structures into focus. Normally, you will see no shadows or dots interrupting the red reflex. If the light strays from the pupil, you will lose the red reflex. Adjust your angle until you see the red reflex again.

10. **Keep advancing toward the patient until the ophthalmoscope is almost touching the patient's eyelashes (see Figure App C.2 ■).**

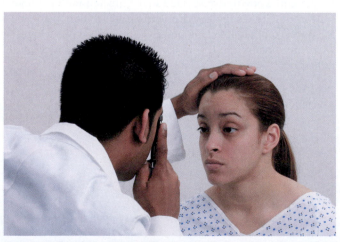

Figure App C.2 Examining the eye using the ophthalmoscope.

Ophthalmoscope Exam of the Fundus of the Eye (*continued*)

11. Rotate the diopter wheel if necessary to bring the ocular fundus into focus (see Figure App C.3 ■).

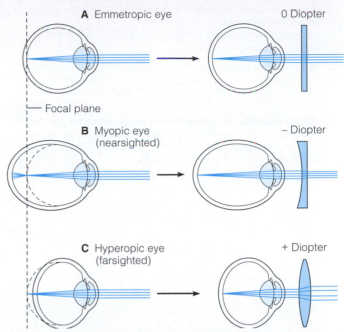

Figure App C.3 Use of diopter to adjust for problems of refraction. A. In the emmetropic (normal) eye, light is focused properly on the retina, and the 0 diopter is used. B. In the myopic eye, light from a distant source converges to a focal point before reaching the retina. Negative diopter numbers are used. C. In the hyperopic eye, light from a near source converges to a focal point past the retina. Positive diopter numbers are used.

12. If the patient's vision is myopic, you will need to rotate the wheel into the minus numbers.

13. If the patient's vision is hyperopic, rotate the wheel into the plus numbers.

14. Begin to look for the optic disc by following the path of the blood vessels. As they grow larger, they lead to the optic disc on the nasal side of the retina (see Figure App C.4 ■).
    The optic disc normally looks like a round or oval yellow-orange depression with a distinct margin. It is the site where the optic nerve and blood vessels exit the eye.

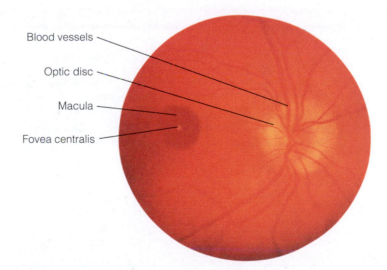

Figure App C.4 The optic disc.

Ophthalmoscope Exam of the Fundus of the Eye (*continued*)

15. **Follow the vessels laterally to a darker circle. This is the macula, or area of central vision.**

    The fovea centralis, a small white spot located in the center of the macula, is the area of sharpest vision.

16. **Systematically inspect these structures.** A crescent shape around the margin of the optic disc is a normal finding. A *scleral crescent* is an absence of pigment in the choroid and is a dull white color. A *pigment crescent,* which is black, is an accumulation of pigment in the choroid.

17. **Use the optic disc as a clock face for documenting the position of a finding and the diameter of the disc (DD) for noting its distance from the optic disc.** For example, "at 2:00, 2 DD from the disc" describes the finding in Figure App C.5 ■.

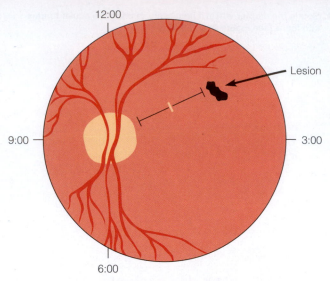

Figure App C.5 Documenting a finding from the ophthalmoscopic examination.

18. **Trace the path of a paired artery and vein from the optic disc to the periphery in the four quadrants of the eyeball.**

19. **Note the number of major vessels, color, width, and any crossing of the vessels.**

Percussion of the Posterior, Anterior, and Lateral Thorax

Percussion of the Posterior Thorax

1. **Visualize the landmarks.**
   - Observe the posterior thorax and visualize the horizontal and vertical lines, the level of the diaphragm, and the fissures of the lungs.

2. **Recall the expected findings.**
   - Percussion allows assessment of underlying structures. The usual sound in the thorax when over lung tissue is resonance, a long, low-pitched hollow sound.

Percussion of the Posterior, Anterior, and Lateral Thorax (*continued*)

3. **Instruct the patient.**
   - Explain to the patient that you will be tapping on the chest in a variety of areas (see Figure App C.6).

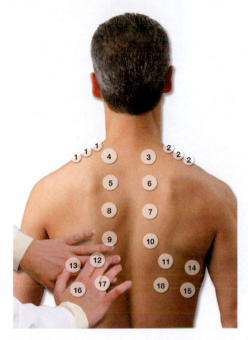

Figure App C.6 Pattern for percussion: Posterior thorax.

   - Tell the patient to breathe normally through this examination. Ask the patient to lean forward and round the shoulders. This position moves the scapulae laterally, permitting more area at the upper vertebral borders, and widens the intercostal spaces for percussion.
   - Position the patient so that your arms are almost fully extended throughout the percussion.

4. **Percuss for movement of the diaphragm (diaphragmatic excursion).**
   - This assessment requires the use of a skin marker and a ruler. The patient remains in the position previously described for percussion. Explain that you will be doing more tapping on the chest and that at two points you will ask the patient to exhale and inhale. Determine the level of the diaphragm during quiet respiration by placing the pleximeter finger above the expected level of diaphragmatic dullness (T7 or T8) at the midscapular line. Percuss in steps downward until dullness replaces resonance on both sides of the chest. Mark those areas. The marks should be at approximately the level of T10.
   - The marks should be parallel.
   - Measure diaphragmatic movement by asking the patient to fully exhale. Starting at the previous skin marking on the left chest, percuss upward from dullness to resonance. Mark that area. Ask the patient to inhale fully and hold it as you begin to percuss from the level of the diaphragm downward, moving from resonance to dullness (see Figure App C.7A). Mark that area and repeat on the right side of the chest. Use the ruler to measure the difference between the marks for exhalation and inhalation (see Figure App C.7B).
   - The distance between the marks should be 3 to 5 cm (1.25 to 2 in.) and even on each side. The right side may be 1 to 2 cm (0.39 to 0.78 in.) higher because of the location of the liver.
   - Anticipate a greater distance on a physically fit patient.

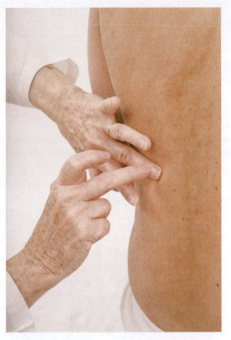

Figure App C.7A Diaphragmatic movement, percussion.

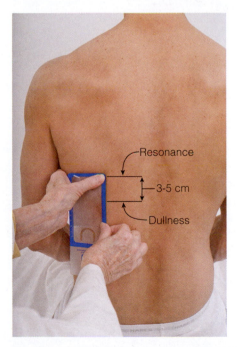

Figure App C.7B Diaphragmatic movement, measurement.

Percussion of the Posterior, Anterior, and Lateral Thorax *(continued)*

Percussion of the Anterior and Lateral Thorax

1. **Visualize the landmarks.**
   - Observe the anterior thorax and visualize the horizontal and vertical lines, the level of the diaphragm, and the lobes of the lungs.

2. **Recall the expected findings.**
   - Percussion allows assessment of underlying structures. The usual sound in the thorax, over the lung tissue, is resonance, which is a low-pitched, hollow sound.

3. **Instruct the patient.**
   - Explain that you will be tapping on the patient's chest in a variety of areas. Tell the patient to breathe normally throughout this examination.

4. **Percuss the lungs.**
   - Begin at the apices of the lungs. Ask the patient to turn the head to the opposite side of percussion to increase the size of the surface required for placing your pleximeter finger and to avoid interference from the clavicle. Move to the chest wall and place the pleximeter in the intercostal space parallel to the ribs during percussion. Percuss the anterior chest from side to side, comparing sounds, in the intercostal spaces. Percuss to the bases and laterally to the midaxillary line (see Figure App C.8).
   - Percussion over bone or organs will yield flat or dull sounds. Avoid percussion over the clavicles, sternum, and ribs. Percussion over the heart will produce dullness to the left of the sternum from the third to fifth intercostal spaces. Percuss the left lung lateral to the midclavicular line. Percussion sounds in the lower left thorax change from resonance to tympany over the gastric air bubble. Percussion sounds in the right lower thorax change from resonance to dullness at the upper liver border.

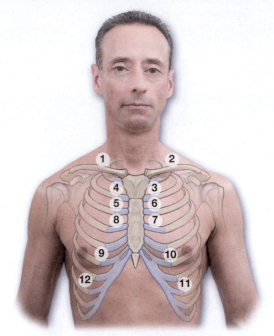

A.

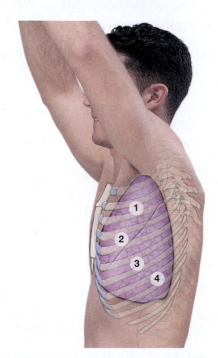

B.

Figure App C.8 Pattern for percussion: A. Anterior thorax. B. Left lateral thorax.

Advanced Assessment of Peripheral Vascular System

Perform Allen's Test

If you suspect an obstruction or insufficiency of an artery in the arm, Allen's test may determine the patency of the radial and ulnar arteries.

- Ask the patient to place the hands on the knees with palms up.
- Compress the radial arteries of both wrists with your thumbs.
- Ask the patient to open and close his or her fist several times.
- While you are still compressing the radial arteries, ask the patient to open his or her hands.
- The palms should become pink immediately, indicating patent ulnar arteries. If normal color does not return, the ulnar arteries may be occluded.
- Next, occlude the ulnar arteries and repeat the same procedure to test the patency of the radial arteries (see Figure App C.9 ■).

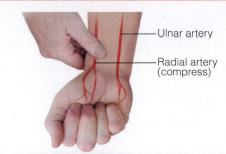

A. Open and close fist

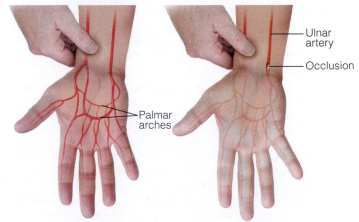

B. Blood returns via ulnar artery   **C. No blood returns**

Figure App C.9 Allen's test.

Percussion of the Abdominal Area

Percussion of the Abdomen

1. **Visualize the landmarks.**
   - Observe the abdomen and visualize the horizontal and vertical lines. Visualize the organs and underlying structures of the abdomen.

2. **Recall the expected findings.**
   - Percussion allows you to assess underlying structures. The normal sounds heard over the abdomen are tympany, a loud hollow sound, and dullness, a short high-pitched sound heard over solid organs and the distended bladder.
   - Hyperresonance is louder than tympany and is heard over air-filled or distended intestines. Flat sounds are short and abrupt and heard over bone. Correct placement of the fingers is important.

3. **Instruct the patient.**
   - Explain that you will be tapping on the patient's abdomen in a variety of areas.
   - Tell the patient to breathe normally through this examination. If muscle tension is detected, ask the patient to take several deep breaths.

4. **Percuss the abdomen.**
   - Place your pleximeter finger on the abdomen during the examination. Start in the right lower quadrant (RLQ) and percuss through all of the remaining quadrants (see Figure App C.10 ■).

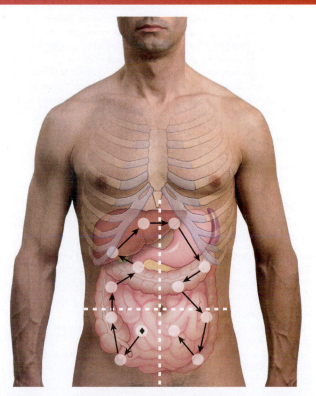

Figure App C.10 Percussion pattern for abdomen.

Percussion of the Abdominal Area *(Continued)*

- Review the technique of percussion in Chapter 7. ∞
- Percussion over the abdomen produces tympany. Tympany is more pronounced over the gastric bubble. Dullness is heard over the liver and spleen.
- Dullness may indicate an enlarged uterus, distended urinary bladder, or ascites. Dullness in the lower left quadrant (LLQ) may indicate the presence of stool in the colon. It is important to ask when the patient last had a bowel movement.

Percussion and Palpation of the Liver and Spleen

Percussion of the Liver

Percuss the liver to determine the upper and lower borders at the anterior axillary line, midclavicular line (MCL), and midsternal line. Measure the distance between marks drawn to identify the borders.

1. **Instruct the patient.**
    - Explain that you will be tapping the patient's abdomen and chest on the right side. Explain that you will be making marks on the abdomen and using a ruler to measure the marks in order to evaluate the size of the liver. Tell the patient to remain relaxed and that there should be no discomfort during this assessment.

2. **Percuss the liver.**
    - Begin percussion at the level of the umbilicus and move toward the rib cage along the extended right MCL (see Figure App C.11 ■).
    - The first sound you should hear is tympany. When the sound changes to dullness, you have identified the lower border of the liver. Mark the point with a skin-marking pen. The lower border is normally at the costal margin. *Tympany often is heard over the lower abdomen due to the presence of gas in the gastrointestinal tract. Dullness below the costal margin suggests liver enlargement or downward displacement due to respiratory disease. Dullness above the fifth or sixth intercostal space could indicate an enlarged liver (hepatomegaly) or displacement upward due to ascites or a mass.*
    - Percuss downward from the fourth intercostal space along the right MCL. The first sound you should hear is resonance because you are over the lung. Percuss downward until the sound changes to dullness. This is the upper border of the liver. Mark the point with a pen. The upper border should be at the level of the sixth intercostal space.
    - Measure the distance between the two points. The distance should be approximately 5 to 10 cm (2 to 4 in.). This distance is called the *liver span.*
    - Percuss along the midsternal line, using the same technique as before. The liver size at the midsternal line should be approximately 4 to 9 cm (1.5 to 3 in.).
    - To determine the movement of the liver with breathing, ask the patient to take a deep breath and hold it. Percuss upward along the extended MCL.
    - The lower liver border should descend about 2.54 cm (1 in.). Remember, liver size is influenced by age, gender, height, and disease process.

Percussion of the Spleen

The spleen is located in the left side of the abdomen. Percussion is conducted to identify enlargement of the organ.

1. **Instruct the patient.**
    - Explain that you will be tapping on the left side of the patient's abdomen to examine the spleen. Tell the patient to continue to relax, taking deep breaths if required.

2. **Percuss the spleen.**
    - Percuss the abdomen on the left side posterior to the midaxillary line (see Figure App C.12 ■).
    - A small area of splenic dullness will usually be heard from the 6th to 10th intercostal spaces.

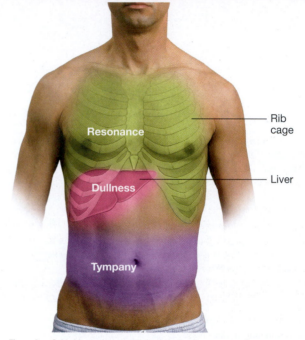

Resonance

Rib cage

Dullness

Liver

Tympany

Figure App C.11 Normal tones elicited during liver percussion.

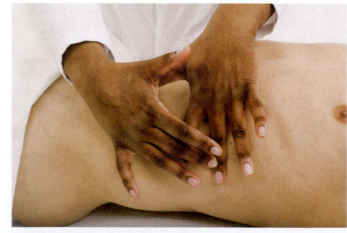

Figure App C.12 Percussing the spleen.

Percussion and Palpation of the Liver and Spleen (*Continued*)

Splenic dullness at the left anterior axillary line indicates splenomegaly, an enlarged spleen. The dull percussion sound is identifiable before an enlarged spleen is palpable. The spleen enlarges anteriorly and inferiorly (see Figure App C.13 ■).

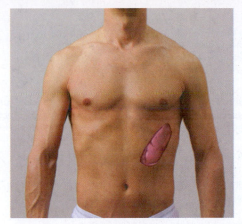

Figure App C.13 Splenic enlargement.

Palpation of the Liver

The liver is palpated to detect enlargement, pain, and consistency.

1. Instruct the patient.
- Explain that you will be using your hands to palpate the patient's liver. Explain that you will place one hand under the ribs in the back and ask the patient to take a deep breath while you apply slight pressure in an upward motion under the ribs on the patient's right side. Instruct the patient to tell you of any pain, and observe the patient for cues of discomfort.

2. Palpate the liver.
- Stand on the right side of the patient. Place your left hand under the lower portion of the ribs (ribs 11 and 12). Tell the patient to relax into your left hand. Lift the rib cage with your left hand.
- Place your right hand into the abdomen using an inward and upward thrust at the costal margin (see Figure App C.14 ■). Ask the patient to take a deep breath. The descent of the diaphragm will cause the liver to descend, and the lower border will meet your right hand.
- Normally, the liver is nonpalpable, except in thin patients. If you feel the lower border of the liver it will be smooth, firm, and nontender.

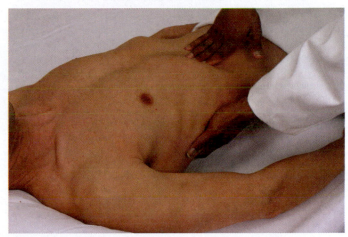

Figure App C.14 Palpating the liver.

Palpation of the Spleen

The spleen is palpated to detect enlargement. Careful palpation is required because the spleen is fragile and sensitive.

1. Instruct the patient.
- Explain that you will be touching the patient with both hands to palpate the spleen. Explain that you will be lifting the patient slightly with your left hand while applying slight pressure with your fingers under the ribs on the left side. Instruct the patient to inform you of any pain or discomfort.

2. Palpate the spleen.
- Stand on the patient's right side. Place your left hand under the lower border of the rib cage on the left side and elevate the rib cage. This moves the spleen anteriorly. Press the fingers of your right hand into the left costal margin area of the patient (see Figure App C.15 ■).
- Ask the patient to take a slow deep breath. As the diaphragm descends, the spleen moves forward to the fingertips of your right hand. The spleen is normally not palpable.

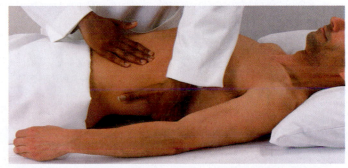

Figure App C.15 Palpating the spleen.

Palpation of the Kidneys

Left Kidney

1. **Attempt to palpate the lower pole of the left kidney.**
   - Although it is not usually palpable, attempt to palpate the lower pole of the kidney for size, contour, consistency, and sensation. Note that the rib cage obscures the upper poles.

> **ALERT!** *Because deep kidney palpation can cause tissue trauma, novice nurses should not attempt either deep palpation or capture of the kidney unless supervised by an experienced nurse or nurse practitioner. Deep kidney palpation should not be done in patients who have had a recent kidney transplant or an abdominal aortic aneurysm.*

   - Position the patient in a supine position. All palpation should be performed from the patient's right side.
   - While standing on the patient's right side, reach over the patient and place your left hand between the posterior rib cage and the iliac crest (the left flank).
   - Place your right hand on the left upper quadrant of the abdomen lateral and parallel to the left rectus muscle just below the costal margin.
   - Instruct the patient to take a deep breath. As the patient inhales, lift the patient's left flank with your left hand and press deeply with your right hand (approximately 4 cm) to attempt to palpate the lower pole of the kidney (see Figure App C.16 ■).

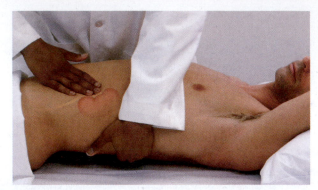

Figure App C.16 Palpating the left kidney.

2. **Attempt to capture the left kidney.**
   - Because of its position deep in the retroperitoneal space, the left kidney is not normally palpable. The capture maneuver may enable you to palpate it. This maneuver is possible because the kidneys descend during inspiration and slide back into their normal position during exhalation.
   - Standing on the patient's right side, place your left hand under the patient's back to elevate the flank as before. Place your right hand on the left upper quadrant of the abdomen lateral and parallel to the left rectus muscle with the fingertips just below the left costal margin. Instruct the patient to take a deep breath and hold it. As the patient inhales, attempt to capture the kidney between your two hands. Ask the patient to exhale slowly and then to briefly hold the breath. At the same time, slowly release the pressure of your fingers.
   - As the patient exhales, you will feel the captured kidney move back into its previous position. The kidney surface should be rounded, smooth, firm, and nontender.

Right Kidney

1. **Attempt to palpate the lower pole of the right kidney.**
   - Standing on the patient's right side, place your left hand under the back parallel to the right 12th rib (about halfway between the costal margin and iliac crest) with your fingertips reaching for the costovertebral angle. Place your right hand on the right upper quadrant of the abdomen lateral to the right rectus muscle and just below the right costal margin.
   - Instruct the patient to take a deep breath. As the patient inhales, lift the flank with your left hand and use deep palpation to feel for the lower pole of the kidney.

2. **Attempt to capture the right kidney.**
   - Place your left hand under the patient's right flank.
   - Place your right hand on the right upper quadrant of the abdomen with the fingertips lateral and parallel to the right rectus muscle just below the right costal margin.
   - Instruct the patient to take a deep breath and hold it. As the patient inhales, attempt to capture the kidney between your two hands.
   - Ask the patient to exhale slowly and then to briefly hold the breath. At the same time, slowly release the pressure of your fingers.
   - As the patient exhales, you will feel the captured kidney move back into its previous position. The kidney surface should be rounded, smooth, firm, and nontender.
   - The lower pole of the right kidney is palpable in some individuals, especially in thin, relaxed females. If palpable, the lower pole of the kidney has a smooth, firm, uninterrupted surface.
   - During the capture maneuver, some patients describe a nonpainful sensation as the kidney slides between the nurse's fingers back into its normal position.

Trans-Illumination of the Scrotum

▶ If a mass is detected during palpation of the scrotum, transillumination may be indicated. While not all nurses will be required to perform this assessment skill, the nurse should be familiar with the basic steps involved, as well as its purpose.

▶ In a darkened room, place a lighted flashlight behind the area in which the abnormal mass was palpated (see Figure App C.17 ▪).

▶ Note that the light shines through the scrotum with a red glow. The testicle shows up as a nontransparent oval structure.

▶ Repeat these steps on the other side and compare the results.
   Light will not penetrate a mass. Masses may indicate testicular tumor, spermatocele (a cyst located in the epididymis), or other conditions.

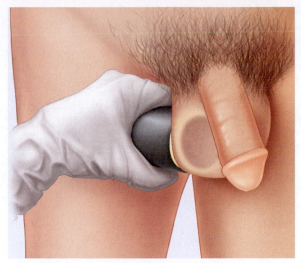

Figure App C.17 Transilluminating the scrotum.

Palpation of the Male Inguinal Region

1. **Palpate the inguinal region.**
   • Start by preparing the patient for palpation in the right inguinal area.
   • Ask the patient to shift his balance so that his weight is on his left leg.
   • Place your right index finger in the upper corner of the right scrotum.
   • Slowly palpate the spermatic cord up and slightly to the patient's left.
   • Allow the patient's scrotal skin to fold over your index finger as you palpate.
   • Proceed until you feel an opening that feels like a triangular slit. This is the external ring of the inguinal canal. Attempt to gently glide your finger into this opening (see Figure App C.18 ▪).

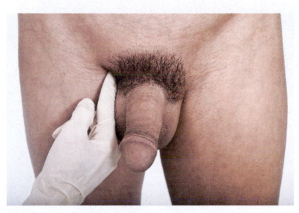

Figure App C.18 Palpating the inguinal canal.

> **ALERT!**   *If you cannot insert your finger with gentle pressure, do not force your finger into the opening.*

• If the opening has admitted your finger, ask the patient to either cough or bear down. An inguinal hernia feels like a bulge or mass.
• Palpate for masses or lumps.
A direct inguinal hernia can be palpated in the area of the external ring of the inguinal ligament. It will be felt either right at the external ring opening or just behind it. An indirect inguinal hernia is more common, especially in younger males. It is located deeper in the inguinal canal than the direct inguinal hernia. It can pass into the scrotum, whereas a direct inguinal hernia rarely protrudes into the scrotum.

> **ALERT!**   *Do not pinch or squeeze any mass, lesion, or other structure.*

• Repeat this procedure by palpating the patient's left inguinal area. Use your left index finger when performing the palpation. It is also possible that a *femoral hernia* may be present. It is more commonly found in the right inguinal area and near the inguinal ligament (see Table 21.1).

> **ALERT!**   *An acute inguinal bulge with tenderness, pain, nausea, or vomiting, may be manifestations of a strangulated hernia, which is a medical emergency and may require surgical intervention. Should a strangulated hernia be suspected, the patient's primary care provider should be notified immediately.*

Trans-Illumination of the Scrotum *(Continued)*

Palpation of the Prostate Gland

1.   Palpate the bulbourethral gland and the prostate gland.
- Lubricate your right index finger with lubricating gel.
- Tell the patient that you are going to insert your finger into his rectum in order to palpate his prostate gland. Explain that the insertion may cause him to feel as if he needs to have a bowel movement. Tell him that this technique should not cause pain but to inform you immediately if it does.
- Place the index finger of your dominant hand against the anal opening (see Figure App C.19 ■). Be sure that your finger is slightly bent and does not form a right angle to the buttocks. If you insert your index finger at a right angle to the buttocks, the patient may experience pain.

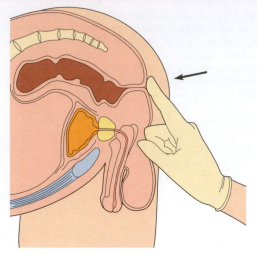

Figure App C.19 Placing the finger against the anal opening.

- Apply gentle pressure as you insert your bent finger into the anus (see Figure App C.20 ■).

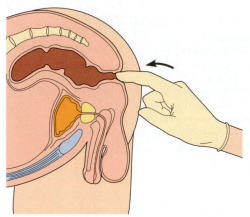

Figure App C.20 Inserting the finger into the anus.

- As the sphincter muscle tightens, stop inserting your finger.
- Resume as the sphincter muscle relaxes.
- Press your right thumb gently against the perianal area.
- Palpate the bulbourethral gland by pressing your index finger gently toward your thumb (see Figure App C.21 ■). This should not cause the patient to feel pain or tenderness. No swelling or masses should be felt.

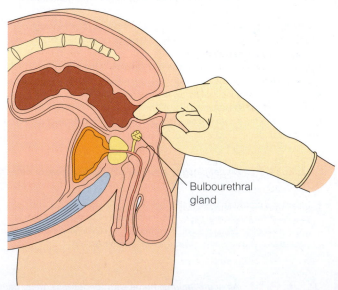

Bulbourethral gland

Figure App C.21 Palpating the bulbourethral gland.

- Release the pressure between your index finger and thumb. Continue to insert your index finger gently.
- Palpate the posterior surface of the prostate gland (see Figure App C.22 ■).
- Confirm that it is smooth, firm, even somewhat rubbery, nontender, and extends out no more than 1 cm (0.39 in.) into the rectal area.
- Remove your finger slowly and gently.
- Remove your gloves.
- Help the patient to a standing position.
- Wash your hands.
- Give the patient tissues to wipe the perianal area.

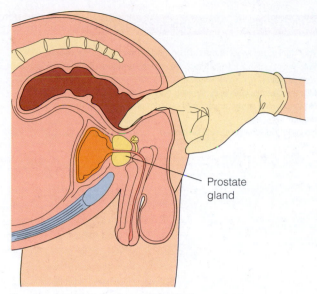

Prostate gland

Figure App C.22 Palpating the prostate gland.

Speculum and Bimanual Examination of the Female Pelvis

Physical assessment of the female genitourinary system includes the techniques of inspection and palpation. Advanced techniques are employed to visualize the vagina and cervix. Upon palpation the vaginal wall is rugated and soft; the Skene's glands and Bartholin's glands are nontender and without discharge. The examination with the speculum reveals a pink, moist, round, and centrally positioned cervix. The cervix is free of lesions with clear, odorless secretions present. Palpation of the cervix reveals it as firm, smooth, and mobile like the tip of the nose. The fornices are smooth and nontender. The uterus is palpated and found tilted upward above the bladder with the cervix tilted forward. Variations in uterine position may be anteverted, midline, or retroverted. During the bimanual exam, when ovaries are palpable, they are smooth, firm, mobile, and almond shaped. They may be slightly tender. The uterine tubes are nonpalpable. The rectovaginal system is thin, smooth, and nontender.

Pelvic Examination

Palpation

1. **Palpate the vaginal walls.**
   - Explain to the patient that you are going to palpate the vaginal walls. Tell her that she will feel you insert a finger into the vagina.
   - Place your left hand above the labia majora and spread the labia minora apart with your thumb and index finger.
   - With your right palm facing toward the ceiling, gently place your right index finger at the vaginal opening. Insert your right index finger gently into the vagina.
   - Gently rotate the right index finger counterclockwise. The vaginal wall should feel rugated, consistent in texture, and soft. Ask the patient to bear down or cough. Note any bulging in this area.

2. **Palpate the urethra and Skene's glands.**
   - Explain to the patient that you are going to palpate her urethra. Tell her that she will again feel pressure against her vaginal wall.
   - Your left hand should still be above the labia majora, and you should still be spreading the labia minora apart with your thumb and index finger.

EQUIPMENT

- Examination gown and examination drape
- Clean, nonsterile examination gloves
- Lubricant
- Pap smear equipment
- Speculum
- Handheld mirror

HELPFUL HINTS

- Provide a warm, private environment.
- Have the patient void and empty bowels before the assessment.
- Use appropriate draping to maintain the patient's dignity.
- Determine if the patient has had this kind of assessment before.
- It is helpful to show the patient pictures of equipment, slides, and the bimanual assessment.
- Use an unhurried, deliberate manner, and ask the patient how she is doing as the assessment proceeds.
- Explore and remedy cultural or language issues at the onset of the interaction.
- Use Standard Precautions.

Speculum and Bimanual Examination of the Female Pelvis (*Continued*)

- Your right index finger should still be inserted in the patient's vagina.
- With your right index finger, apply very gentle pressure upward against the vaginal wall.
- Milk the Skene's glands by stroking outward (see Figure App C.23 ■).
- Now apply the same upward and outward pressure on both sides of the urethra.
- No pain or discharge should be elicited.

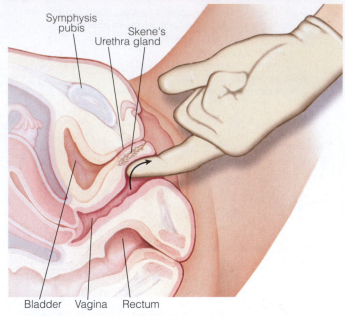

Figure App C.23 Palpating Skene's glands.

3. **Palpate the Bartholin's glands.**
   - With your right index finger still inserted in the patient's vagina, gently squeeze the posterior region of the labia majora between your right index finger and right thumb (see Figure App C.24 ■).
   - Perform this maneuver bilaterally, palpating both Bartholin's glands.
   - No lump or hardness should be felt. No pain response should be elicited. No discharge should be produced.

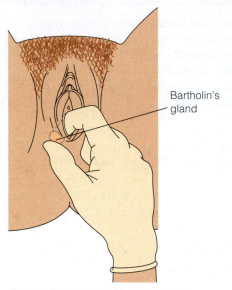

Figure App C.24 Palpating Bartholin's glands.

Inspection with a Speculum

- The speculum should be the proper size for the patient.
  In the obese patient, the sidewalls of the vagina have increased loose connective tissue, resulting in inward collapse of the vaginal walls when using a standard "duckbill" speculum. This examination may require two examiners, one to insert the standard speculum and the second to insert another speculum to open laterally. This permits full visualization of the cervix and enables the examiner to obtain scrapings for slides. This is uncomfortable for the patient.

Speculum and Bimanual Examination of the Female Pelvis (*Continued*)

1. **Hold the speculum in your dominant hand.**
   - Place the index finger on top of the blades, the third finger on the bottom of the blades, and be sure to move the thumb just underneath the thumbscrew before inserting (see Figure App C.25 ■).

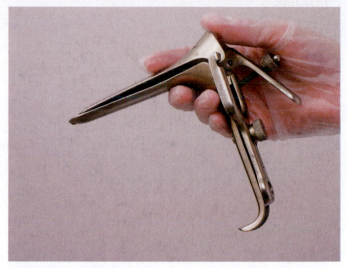

Figure App C.25 Holding the speculum.

2. **Insert the speculum.**
   - Tell the patient that you are going to examine her cervix, and that to do so you are going to insert a speculum. If this is the patient's first vaginal examination, show her the speculum, and briefly demonstrate how you will use it to visualize her cervix. Have a mirror available to share findings with the patient. Also explain that she will feel pressure, first of your fingers, and then of the speculum.
   - With your nondominant hand, place your index and middle fingers on the posterior vaginal opening and apply pressure gently downward.
   - Turn the speculum blades obliquely.
   - Place the blades over your fingers at the vaginal opening and slowly insert the closed speculum at a 45-degree downward angle (see Figure App C.26 ■). This angle matches the downward slope of the vagina when the patient is in the lithotomy position.
   - Ask the patient to bear down as you insert the speculum. It is normal for the patient to tense as the speculum is inserted, and bearing down helps to relax the muscles.
   - Once the speculum is inserted, withdraw your fingers and turn the speculum clockwise until the blades are in a horizontal plane.
   - Advance the blades at a downward 45-degree angle until they are completely inserted.
   - This maneuver should not cause the patient pain.
   - Avoid pinching the labia or pulling on the patient's pubic hair. If insertion of the speculum causes the patient pain, stop immediately and reevaluate your technique.
   - To open the speculum blades, squeeze the speculum handle.
   - Sweep the speculum blades upward until the cervix comes into view.
   - Adjust the speculum blades as needed until the cervix is fully exposed between them. Tighten the thumbscrew to stabilize the spread of the blades.

3. **Visualize the cervix.**
   - Confirm that the cervix is pink, moist, round, and centrally positioned, and that it has a small opening in the center (the os).
   - Note any bluish coloring.
   - Confirm that any secretions are clear or white and without odor.
   - Confirm that the cervix is free from erosions, ulcerations, lacerations, and polyps.

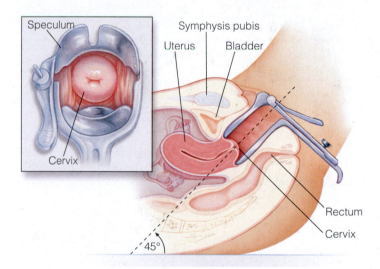

Figure App C.26 Speculum inserted into vagina.

Abnormal Findings of the Cervix

CYANOSIS

Cyanosis of the cervix is associated with hypoxic conditions such as congestive heart failure (CHF). Blue coloring of the cervix is normal in pregnancy.

DIETHYLSTILBESTROL (DES) SYNDROME

Abnormalities of the cervix arise in females who had prenatal exposure to DES. Epithelial abnormalities occur as granular patchiness extending from the cervix to the vaginal walls.

CARCINOMA

Ulcerations with vaginal discharge, postmenopausal bleeding or spotting, or bleeding between menstrual periods are characteristics of cervical carcinoma. Diagnosis is confirmed by Pap smear.

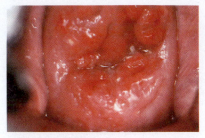

Cervical carcinoma.

EROSION

Inflammation and erosion are visible on the surface of the cervix. It is difficult to distinguish erosion from carcinoma without a biopsy.

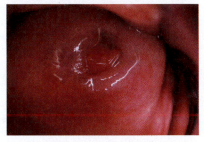

Erosion of the cervix.

POLYP

A soft, fingerlike growth extends from the cervical os. A polyp is usually bright red and may bleed. Polyps are usually benign.

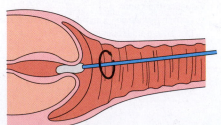

Cervical polyp.
Source: Designua/Shutterstock.

Obtaining the Pap Smear and Gonorrhea Culture

The Pap (Papanicolaou) smear consists of three specimens: an endocervical swab, a cervical scrape, and a vaginal pool sample. Have ready prelabeled slides for specimens, either (a) one labeled endocervical, one labeled vaginal, and one labeled cervical or (b) one slide that has sections for each sample.

1. **Perform an endocervical swab.**
   - Carefully insert a saline-moistened, cotton-tipped applicator or Cytobrush Plus GT into the vagina and into the cervical os.
   - Do not force insertion of the applicator.
   - Rotate the applicator in a complete circle (see Figure App C.27 ■).
   - Roll a thin coat across the slide labeled *endocervical*.
   - Spray fixative on the slide immediately or place it in a container filled with fixative.

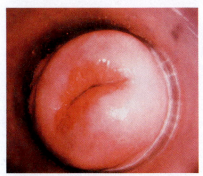

Figure App C.27 The endocervical swab.

Obtaining the Pap Smear and Gonorrhea Culture *(Continued)*

- **Obtain a cervical scrape.**
- Insert the longer end of a bifid spatula into the patient's vagina.
- Advance the fingerlike projection of the bifid end gently into the cervical os.
- Allow the shorter end to rest on the outer ridge of the cervix.
- Rotate the applicator one full 360-degree turn clockwise to scrape cells from the cervix (see Figure App C.28 ■).

If the patient has had a hysterectomy, obtain the scrape from the surgical stump.
- Do not rotate the applicator more than once or turn it in a counterclockwise manner.
- Spread a thin smear across the slide labeled *cervical* from each side of the applicator.
- Spray fixative on the slide immediately or place in a container filled with fixative.

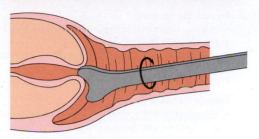

Figure App C.28 The cervical scrape.

2. **Obtain a vaginal pool sample.**
   - Insert the paddle end of the spatula into the vaginal recess area (fornix). Alternatively, you may use a saline-moistened cotton-tipped applicator.
   - Gently rotate the spatula back and forth to obtain a sample (see Figure App C.29 ■).
   - Apply the specimen to the slide labeled *vaginal*.
   - Spray fixative on the slide immediately.

3. **Obtain a gonorrhea culture.**
   - Obtain a gonorrhea culture if the assessment findings indicate.
   - Insert a saline-moistened cotton-tipped applicator into the cervical os.
   - Leave the applicator in place for 20 seconds to allow full saturation of the cotton.
   - Using a Z-shaped pattern, roll a thin coat of the secretions onto a Thayer-Martin culture plate labeled *cervical*.
   Nurses must be sure to check with the laboratory in their institution because techniques and protocols may differ.

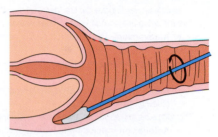

Figure App C.29 The vaginal pool sample.

4. **Remove the speculum.**
   - Gently loosen the thumbscrew on the speculum while holding the handles securely.
   - Slant the speculum from side to side as you slide it from the vaginal canal.
   - While you withdraw the speculum, note that the vaginal mucosa is pink, consistent in texture, rugated, and nontender. Discharge is thin or stringy and clear or opaque.
   - Close the speculum blades before complete removal.

Bimanual Palpation

1. **Stand at the end of the examination table. (The patient remains in the lithotomy position.) Palpate the cervix.**
   - Lubricate the index and middle fingers of your gloved dominant hand.
   - Inform the patient that you are going to palpate her cervix.
   - Place your nondominant hand against the patient's thigh, then insert your lubricated index and middle fingers into her vaginal opening.
   - Proceed downward at a 45-degree angle until you reach the cervix.
   - Keep the other fingers of that hand rounded inward toward the palm, and put the thumb against the mons pubis away from the clitoris.
   - Palpate the cervix. It should feel firm and smooth, somewhat like the tip of a nose (see Figure App C.30 ■).
   - Gently try to move the cervix. It should move easily about 1 to 2 cm (0.39 to 0.78 in.) in either direction.
   If the woman is pregnant, the cervix will be soft. This is a normal finding and is called Goodell's sign.

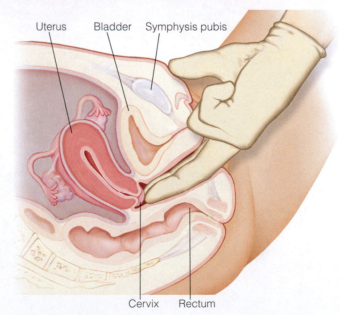

Uterus   Bladder   Symphysis pubis

Cervix   Rectum

Figure App C.30 Palpating the cervix.

Bimanual Palpation (*Continued*)

2. Palpate the fornices.
- Slip your fingers into the vaginal recess areas, called the fornices.
- Palpate around the grooves.
- Confirm that the mucosa of the vagina and cervix in these areas is smooth and nontender.
- Leave your fingers in the anterior fornix when you have checked all sides.

3. Palpate the uterus.
- Place the fingers of your nondominant hand on the patient's abdomen.
- Invaginate the abdomen midway between the umbilicus and the symphysis pubis by pushing with your fingertips downward toward the cervix (see Figure App C.31 ■).
- Palpate the front wall of the uterus with the hand that is inside the vagina.
- As you palpate, note the position of the uterine body to determine that the uterus is in a normal position. When in a normal position, the uterus is tilted slightly upward above the bladder, and the cervix is tilted slightly forward.

The following are normal variations of uterine position:
- **Anteversion**—uterus tilted forward, cervix tilted downward (see Figure App C.32A ■)
- **Midposition**—*uterus lies parallel to tailbone, cervix pointed straight (see Figure App C.32B)*
- **Retroversion**—*uterus tilted backward, cervix tilted upward (see Figure App C.32C).*

The following are abnormal variations of uterine position:
- **Anteflexion**—uterus folded forward at about a 90-degree angle, and cervix tilted downward (see Figure App C.32D)
- **Retroflexion**—*uterus folded backward at about a 90-degree angle, cervix tilted upward (see Figure App C.32E).*
- Move the inner fingers to the posterior fornix, and gently raise the cervix up toward your outer hand.
- Palpate the front and back walls of the uterus as it is sandwiched between the two hands.

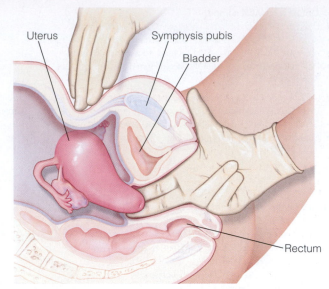

Figure App C.31 Palpating the uterus.

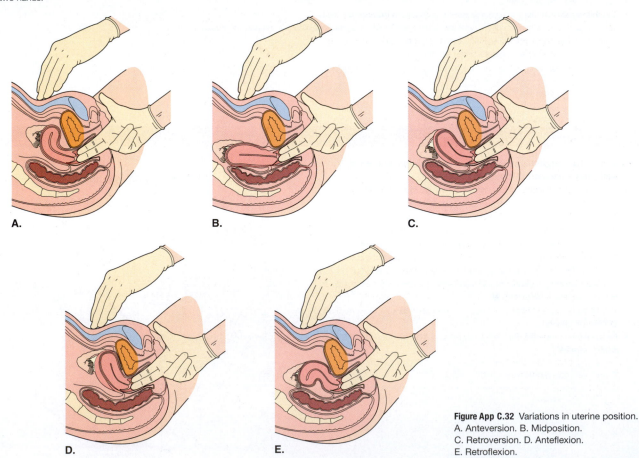

A.

B.

C.

D.

E.

Figure App C.32 Variations in uterine position.
A. Anteversion. B. Midposition.
C. Retroversion. D. Anteflexion.
E. Retroflexion.

Bimanual Palpation (*Continued*)

4. **Palpate the ovaries.**
   - While positioning the outer hand on the left lower abdominal quadrant, slip the vaginal fingers into the left lateral fornix.
   - Push the opposing fingers and hand toward one another, and then use small circular motions to palpate the left ovary with your intravaginal fingers (see Figure App C.33 ■).
   - If you are able to palpate the ovary, it will feel mobile, almond shaped, smooth, firm, and nontender to slightly tender. Often you will be unable to palpate the ovaries, especially the right ovary.
   - Slide your vaginal fingers around to the right lateral fornix and your outer hand to the lower right quadrant to palpate the right ovary.
   - Confirm that the uterine tubes are not palpable.
   - Remove your hand from the vagina and put on new gloves.

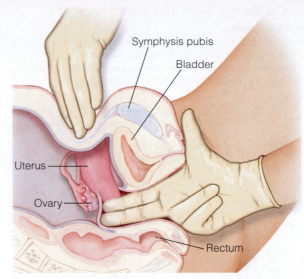

Figure App C.33 Palpating the ovaries.

5. **Perform the rectovaginal exam.**
   - Tell the patient that you are going to insert one finger into her vagina and one finger into her rectum in order to perform a rectovaginal exam. Tell her that this maneuver may make her feel as though she needs to have a bowel movement.
   - Lubricate the gloved index and middle fingers of the dominant hand.
   - Ask the patient to bear down.
   - Touch the patient's thigh with your nondominant hand to prepare her for the insertion.
   - Insert the index finger into the vagina (at a 45-degree downward slope) and the middle finger into the rectum.
   - Compress the rectovaginal septum between your index and middle fingers.
   - Confirm that it is thin, smooth, and nontender.
   - Place your nondominant hand on the patient's abdomen.
   - While maintaining the position of your intravaginal hand, press your outer hand inward and downward on the abdomen over the symphysis pubis.
   - Palpate the posterior side of the uterus with the pad of the rectal finger while continuing to press down on the abdomen (see Figure App C.34 ■).
   - Confirm that the uterine wall is smooth and nontender.
   - If the ovaries are palpable, note that they are normal in size and contour.
   - Remove your fingers from the vagina and rectum slowly and gently.

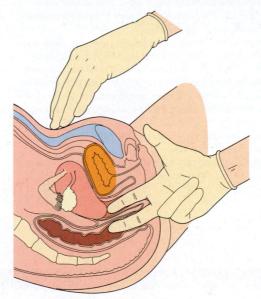

Figure App C.34 Rectovaginal palpation.

6. **Examine the stool.**
   - Remove your gloves.
   - Assist the patient into a comfortable position.
   - Inspect feces remaining on the glove. Feces is normally brown and soft. Test feces for occult blood. Normally the test is negative.
   - Wash your hands.
   - Give the patient tissues to wipe the perineal area. Some patients may need a perineal pad.
   - Inform the patient that she may have a small amount of spotting for a few hours after the speculum examination.

Musculoskeletal Examination Techniques

Test for the Bulge Sign and Ballottement

1. **Test for the bulge sign.**
   - This procedure detects the presence of small amounts of fluid (4 to 8 mL or 0.8 to 1.5 tsp) in the suprapatellar bursa.
   - With the patient in the supine position, use firm pressure to stroke the medial aspect of the knee upward several times, displacing any fluid (see Figure App C.35 ■).
   - Apply pressure to the lateral side of the knee while observing the medial side.
   - Normally no fluid is present.
   - The medial side of the knee bulges if fluid is in the joint.

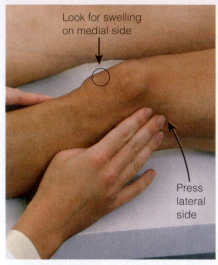

Figure App C.35 Testing for the bulge sign.

2. **Perform ballottement.**
   - Ballottement is a technique used to detect fluid or to examine or detect floating body structures. The nurse displaces body fluid and then palpates the return impact of the body structure.
   - When there are abnormal fluid levels, fluid forced between the patella and femur causes the patella to "float" over the femur. A palpable click is felt when the patella is snapped back against the femur when fluid is present.
   - To detect large amounts of fluid in the suprapatellar bursa, firmly grasp the thigh just above the knee with your thumb and fingers. This action causes any fluid in the suprapatellar bursa to move between the patella and the femur.
   - With the fingers of your left hand, quickly push the patella downward upon the femur (see Figure App C.36 ■).
   - Normally the patella sits firmly over the femur, allowing little or no movement when pressure is exerted over the patella.

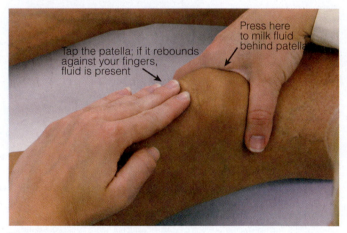

Figure App C.36 Testing for ballottement.

Advanced Neurological Assessment Techniques

Abdominal Reflexes

1. **Assess the abdominal reflexes (T8, T9, T10 for upper and T10, T11, T12 for lower).**
   - Using an applicator or tongue blade, briskly stroke the abdomen from the lateral aspect toward the umbilicus (see Figure App C.37 ■).
   - Observe muscular contraction and movement of the umbilicus toward the stimulus.
   - Repeat this procedure in the other three quadrants of the abdomen.
   Obesity and upper and lower motor neuron pathology can decrease or diminish the response.

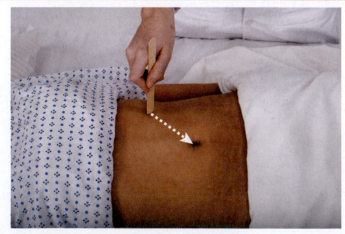

Figure App C.37 Abdominal reflex testing pattern.

Glossary

A

abdomen The largest cavity of the body that contains organs and structures belonging to various systems of the body

abduction Movement of a limb away from the midline or median plane of the body, along the frontal plane

accessory digestive organs The structures connected to the alimentary canal by ducts—the liver, gallbladder, and pancreas—that contribute to the digestive process of foods

accommodation The ability of the eye to automatically adjust clear vision from far to near or a variety of distances

acetabulum A rounded cavity on the right and left lateral sides of the pelvic bone

acini cells Glandular tissue in each breast that produce milk

acromegaly A disorder caused by overproduction of growth hormone by the pituitary gland. The result may be enlargement of the skull and cranial bones; enlargement of the lower jaw; and enlargement of the lips, tongue, hands, and feet

active listening Includes paying attention, showing that you are listening, and offering feedback if appropriate

acute pain Pain that lasts only through the expected recovery period from illness, injury, or surgery, whether it has a sudden or slow onset and regardless of the intensity

adduction The movement of a limb toward the body midline

advance directives Written statements of a person's wishes regarding medical treatment

adventitious sounds Added sounds heard during auscultation of the chest. These sounds are superimposed on normal breath sounds and may indicate underlying airway problems or diseases

air conduction The transmission of sound through the tympanic membrane to the cochlea and auditory nerve

alimentary canal A continuous, hollow, muscular tube, that begins at the mouth and terminates at the anus

alopecia Hair loss caused by an immune-mediated attack on the hair follicles

alopecia areata Sudden patchy or complete loss of body hair for unknown cause. Occurs most often on scalp although it may occur over the entire body

amniotic fluid A clear, slightly yellowish liquid that surrounds the fetus during pregnancy

analgesia The absence of pain sensation

anatomic planes The imaginary lines separating the body into parts

anesthesia The inability to perceive the sense of touch

angle of Louis Also called the sternal angle. A horizontal ridge formed at the point where the manubrium joins the body of the sternum

angular stomatitis A clinical finding of poor nutrition; cracks at the corner of the mouth

anorexia nervosa A complex psychosocial and physiologic problem characterized by a severely restricted intake of nutrients and a low body weight

anosmia The absence of the sense of smell, which may be due to cranial nerve dysfunction, colds, rhinitis, or zinc deficiency, or it may be genetic

anterior triangle A landmark area of the anterior neck bordered by the mandible, the midline of the neck, and the anterior aspect of the sternocleidomastoid muscles

anthropometrics Any scientific measurement of the body

anus The terminal end of the large intestine exiting the body

apical impulse The anatomic point at which the heartbeat is most easily palpated; located at the apex of the heart. Also referred to as point of maximal impulse (PMI)

apocrine glands Glands in the axillary and anogenital regions that are dormant until the onset of puberty and produce a secretion made up of water, salts, fatty acids, and proteins, which is released into hair follicles

aqueous humor A clear, fluidlike substance found in the anterior segment of the eye that helps maintain ocular pressure

areola A circular pigmented field of wrinkled skin containing the nipple

arterial aneurysm A bulging or dilation caused by a weakness in the wall of an artery

arterial insufficiency Inadequate circulation in the arterial system, usually caused by the buildup of fatty plaque or calcification of the arterial wall

arteries Tubular elastic-walled vessels that carry oxygenated blood throughout the body

ascites An abnormal collection of fluid in the peritoneal cavity

assessment The gathering of complete, accurate, and relevant data about the patient

assimilation The adoption and incorporation of characteristics, customs, and values of the dominant culture by those new to that culture

astigmatism A condition in which the refraction of light is spread over a wide area rather than on a distinct point on the retina

atlas The first cervical vertebra, which carries the skull

atelectasis A collapse or impaired inflation of one or more areas of the lung

atrioventricular (AV) node Cluster of specialized cells located between the atria and ventricles that receives electrical impulses from the sinoatrial (SA) node and transmits the electrical impulses to the bundle of His; capable of initiating electrical impulses in the event of SA node failure

atrioventricular (AV) valves Valves that separate the atria from the ventricles within the heart

atrophic papillae A clinical finding of poor nutritional health

attending Giving full attention to verbal and nonverbal messages

auricle The external portion of the ear

auscultation Using a stethoscope to listen to the sounds produced by the body

axillary tail (Tail of Spence) Breast tissue that extends superio-laterally into the axilla

axis The second cervical vertebra (C2), which supports the movement of the head

azotemia A buildup of wastes in the bloodstream due to renal dysfunction

B

Babinski response The fanning of the toes with the great toe pointing toward the dorsum of the foot; considered an abnormal response in the adult that may indicate upper motor neuron disease

ballottement A palpation technique used to detect fluid or examine floating body structures by using the hand to push against the body

Bartholin's glands (Greater vestibular glands) Glands located posteriorly at the base of the vaginal vestibule that produce mucus, which is released into the vestibule and actively promotes sperm motility and viability following intercourse

Bell's palsy A temporary disorder affecting cranial nerve VII and producing a unilateral facial paralysis

binge eating disorder (BED) Characterized by an individual's maladaptive behavior of recurrent binge eating

blepharitis Inflammation of the eyelids

blood pressure Pressure caused by waves of blood as it ebbs and flows within the systemic arteries

Blumberg's sign The experience of sharp, stabbing pain as the compressed area returns to a noncompressed state

bone conduction The transmission of sound through the bones of the skull to the cochlea and auditory nerve

borborygmi Stomach growling; caused by contraction muscles in the stomach and intestines

Bouchard's nodes Enlargement of proximal interphalangeal joints

brainstem Located between the cerebrum and spinal cord, contains the midbrain, pons, and medulla oblongata and connects pathways between the higher and lower structures

Braxton-Hicks contractions Painless and unpredictable contractions of the uterus that do not dilate the cervix

breast self-awareness Becoming familiar with the appearance and feel of one's own breasts

bronchial sounds Loud, high-pitched sounds heard in the upper airways and region of the trachea; expiration is longer in duration than inspiration

bronchophony Auscultation of voice sounds; patient says "ninety-nine" and normal lung sound will be muffled

bronchovesicular sounds Sounds that are medium in loudness and pitch, heard as ausculation moves from the large central airways toward the periphery of the lungs; inspiration and expiration are equal in duration

bruit A group of heart sounds that elicit a loud blowing sound; an abnormal finding, most often associated with a narrowing or stricture of the carotid artery and usually associated with atherosclerotic plaque

bulbourethral glands (Cowper's glands) Small, round glands located below the prostate within the urethral sphincter; just before ejaculation, they secrete a clear mucus into the urethra that lubricates the urethra and increases its alkaline environment

bulimia nervosa An eating disorder characterized by binge eating and purging or another compensatory mechanism to prevent weight gain

bundle branches Expressways of conducting fibers that spread the electrical current through the ventricular myocardial tissue

bundle of His Pathway of cardiac tissue that receives electrical impulses from the atrioventricular (AV) node and transmits the electrical impulses to the ventricles

bursae Small, synovial fluid–filled sacs that protect ligaments from friction

C

calcaneus A tarsal bone of the foot, also known as the heel bone

calculi Stones that block the urinary tract, usually composed of calcium, struvite, or a combination of magnesium, ammonium, phosphate, and uric acid content in water

capillaries The smallest vessels of the circulatory system that exchange gases and nutrients between the arterial and venous systems

cardiac conduction system The heart's conduction system, which can initiate an electrical charge and transmit that charge via cardiac muscle fibers throughout the myocardial tissue

cardiac cycle The events of one complete heartbeat, the contraction and relaxation of the atria and ventricles

cardiac output The amount of blood ejected from the left ventricle over 1 minute

cartilaginous joint Articulation of bones joined by cartilage

cataract A condition in which the lens continues to thicken and yellow, forming a dense area that reduces lens clarity resulting in a loss of central vision

central nervous system (CNS) Nervous system of the body that consists of the brain and the spinal cord

cerebellum Located below the cerebrum and behind the brainstem, it coordinates stimuli from the cerebral cortex to provide precise timing for skeletal muscle coordination and smooth movements; also assists with maintaining equilibrium and muscle tone

cerebrovascular accident (CVA, stroke, brain attack) Interruption or occlusion of cerebral blood flow resulting in impaired delivery of oxygen and nutrients to the brain cells; condition may be fatal; neurologic deficits following CVA may be temporary or permanent, may range from mild to severe

cerebrum The largest portion of the brain, responsible for all conscious behavior

cerumen Yellow-brown wax secreted by glands in the external auditory canal

cervical os The inferior opening; the vaginal end of the canal

cervix Round part of the uterus that projects 2.5 cm into the vagina

Chadwick's sign Vascular congestion that creates a blue-purple blemish or change in cervical coloration

charting Documenting of periodic assessments of hospitalized patients

cheilosis An abnormal condition of the lips characterized by scaling of the surface and by the formation of fissures in the corners of the mouth

choroid The middle layer, the vascular-pigmented layer of the eye

chronic pain Pain that is prolonged, usually recurring or persisting over 6 months or longer, and interferes with functioning

circumduction Movement in which the limb describes a cone in space: while the distal end of the limb moves in a circle, the joint itself moves only slightly in the joint cavity

claudication Pain in the thigh, calf, or buttocks that is caused by arterial insufficiency; may be a sign of peripheral vascular disease

clitoris The primary organ of sexual stimulation in females; the small, elongated mound of erectile tissue located at the anterior of the vaginal vestibule

clonus Rhythmically alternating flexion and extension; confirms upper motor neuron disease

clubbing Flattening of the angle of the nail and enlargement of the tips of the fingers is a sign of oxygen deprivation in the extremities

cochlea A spiraling chamber in the inner ear that contains the receptors for hearing

colostrum A thick, yellowish specialized form of early breast milk that is produced starting in the second trimester and replaced by mature milk during the early days of lactation after the delivery of the baby

coma A prolonged state of unconciousness with pronounced and persistent changes

communication Exchange of information, feelings, thoughts, and ideas

comprehensive geriatric assessment (CGA) A multidisciplinary diagnostic and treatment process that identifies medical, psychosocial, and functional limitations of a frail older person in order to develop a coordinated plan to maximize overall health with aging

concreteness Speaking to the patient in specific terms rather than in vague generalities

confidentiality Protecting information, sharing only to those directly involved in patient care

consensual constriction The simultaneous response of one pupil to the stimuli applied to the other

convergence Movement of the two eyes so that the coordination of an image falls at corresponding points of the two retinas

cornea The clear, transparent part of the sclera that forms the anterior part of the eye, considered to be the window of the eye

cortex The outer portion of each kidney composed of over 1 million nephrons, which form urine

costovertebral angle (CVA) The area on the lower back formed by the vertebral column and the downward curve of the last posterior rib

craniosynostosis A condition that results in cranial deformity due to premature fusion of the cranial bones

cremasteric reflex A reflexive action that may cause the testicles to migrate upward temporarily; cold hands, a cold room, or the stimulus of touch could cause this response

crepitation A crackling, rattling, or grating sound

critical thinking A process of purposeful and creative thinking about resolutions of problems or the development of ways to manage situations

cryptorchidism The failure of one or both testicles to descend through the inguinal canal during the final stages of fetal development

cues Bits of information that hint at the possibility of a health problem

cultural competence The capacity of nurses or health service delivery systems to effectively understand and plan for the needs of a culturally diverse patient or group

culture The nonphysical traits, such as values, beliefs, attitudes, and customs, that are shared by a group of people and passed from one generation to the next

Cushing's syndrome Abnormality where increased adrenal hormone production leads to a rounded "moon" face, ruddy cheeks, prominent jowls, and excess facial hair

cutaneous pain Pain that originates in the skin or subcutaneous tissue

cuticle A fold of epidermal skin along the base of the nail that protects the root and sides of each nail

cystocele A hernia that is formed when the urinary bladder is pushed into the anterior vaginal wall

D

dandruff White or gray dead, scaly skin flakes of epidermal cells

decoding Process of searching through one's memory, experience, and knowledge base to determine the meaning of the intended message

deep somatic pain Pain that is diffuse and arises from ligaments, tendons, bones, blood vessels, and nerves, which tends to last longer than cutaneous pain

depression For the musculoskeletal system, this is the movement in which the elevated part is moved downward to its original position

dermatome An area of skin innervated by the cutaneous branch of one spinal nerve

dermis A layer of connective tissue that lies just below the epidermis

developmental dysplasia of the hip A congenital disorder that results from inadequate development of the hip socket

diaphoresis Profuse perspiration or sweating that may occur during exertion, fever, pain, and emotional stress and in the presence of some metabolic disorders such as hyperthyroidism

diastasis recti abdominis Condition in which the rectus abdominis muscles that run vertically down the midline of the abdomen separate during the third trimester and allow the abdominal contents to protrude

diastole The phase of ventricular relaxation in which the ventricles relax and are filled as the atria contract; also associated with the bottom number of a blood pressure reading

diastolic pressure The lowest arterial blood pressure of the cardiac cycle occurring when the heart is at rest

diet recall A remembrance of all food, beverages, and nutritional supplements or products consumed in a set period such as a 24-hour period

dilation Progressive opening of the cervix

diplopia Double vision

disability A physical or mental impairment that impacts one or more of a person's life activities. People with disabilities may be in need of healthcare services by reason of mental health, physical, sensory, developmental, age, or illness concerns

diversity The state of being different

documentation The recording of information about a patient. This is a legal document used to plan care, to communicate information between and among healthcare providers, and to monitor quality of care

dorsiflexion Flexion of the ankle so that the superior aspect of the foot moves in an upward direction

Down syndrome A chromosomal defect that causes varying degrees of mental retardation; its prominent facial features include slanted eyes, a flat nasal bridge, a flat nose, a protruding tongue, and a short neck

ductus arteriosus The third shunt in fetal circulation that shunts blood into the descending aorta

ductus venosus A shunt in fetal circulation that enables the fetus to maximize oxygenation from the maternal circulation

dullness A flat percussion tone that is soft and of short duration

dysphagia Difficulty swallowing

dyspnea Shortness of breath or difficulty getting one's breath

dysreflexia An alteration in urinary elimination that affects patients with spinal cord injuries at level T7 or higher

E

ecchymosis Bruising resulting from the escape of blood from a ruptured blood vessel into the tissues

eccrine glands Glands that produce a clear perspiration mostly made up of water and salts, which they release into funnel-shaped pores at the skin surface

ectropion Eversion of the lower eyelid and eyelashes; causes include muscle weakness, scarring, facial paralysis, eyelid growths, congenital disorders, surgery, radiation, and certain medications

edema Accumulation of fluid in the tissues or in a body cavity

edentulism Complete loss of one's natural teeth

effacement Thinning of the cervix occurring near the end of pregnancy in preparation for labor

egophony Ausculation of voice sounds; when patient says "E," normal lungs sound like "eeeeee"

electrocardiogram (ECG) Electrical representations of the cardiac cycle documented by deflections on recording paper

electronic health record (EHR) Digital patient chart

electronic medical record (EMR) Digital patient chart

elevation Lifting or moving superiorly along a frontal plane

embryo Child during any development stage of pregnancy prior to birth

emmetropia The normal refractive condition of the eye

empathy Understanding, being aware, being sensitive to the feelings, thoughts, and/or experiences of another

encoding The process of formulating a message for transmission to another person

endocardium The innermost layer of the heart, a smooth layer that provides an inner lining for the chambers of the heart

entropion Inversion of the eyelid and eyelashes; causes include muscle weakness, inflammation, infection, muscle spasm, or congenital or developmental complications

epicardium The outer layer of the heart wall that is also called the visceral pericardium

epidermis The outer layer of skin on the body

epididymis A comma- or crescent-shaped system of ductules emerging posteriorly from the testis that holds the sperm during maturation

epididymitis A common infection in males characterized by a dull, aching pain

epispadias A condition in which the urethral meatus is located on the superior aspect of the glans

epitrochlear nodes Lymph nodes located on the medial surface of the arm above the elbow that drain the ulnar surface of the forearm and the third, fourth, and fifth digits

esophagitis Inflammatory process of the esophagus, caused by a variety of irritants

esophoria Inward turning of the eye toward the nose

ethnicity The awareness of belonging to a group in which certain characteristics or aspects such as culture and biology differentiate the members of one group from another

ethnocentrism The tendency to believe one's way of life, values, beliefs, and customs are superior to those of others

eupnea The regular, even-depth, rhythmic pattern of inspiration and expiration; normal breathing

eustachian tube The bony and cartilaginous auditory tube that connects the middle ear with the nasopharynx; helps to equalize the air pressure on both sides of the tympanic membrane

eversion A movement in which the sole of the foot is turned laterally

exophoria Outward turning of the eye

extension A bending movement around a joint that increases the angle between the bone of the limb at the joint

F

false reassurance The patient is assured of a positive outcome with no basis for believing in it

febrile seizures Seizures caused by fever

femoral hernia A bulging over the area of the femoral artery in the groin caused by a weakening or tear in the abdominal wall

fetal alcohol syndrome (FAS) Congenital condition caused by exposure to high levels of alcohol during fetal development; fetal defects may include mental retardation, developmental delays, and physical deformities

fetoscope A specialized stethoscope for listening to fetal heart sounds, beginning at approximately 18 weeks of gestation

fetus The developing product of conception, usually from the eighth week until birth

fever blisters Lesions or blisters on the lips may be caused by the herpes simplex virus

fibrous joint Articulation of bones joined by fibrous tissue

flag sign Dyspigmentation of the mouth or a part of the mouth

flatness A dull percussion tone that is soft and has a short duration

flexion A bending movement that decreases the angle of the joint and brings the articulating bones closer together

focused interview An interview that enables the nurse to clarify points, to obtain missing information, and to follow up on verbal and nonverbal cues identified in the health history

follicular hyperkeratosis Goose bump flesh

food deserts Low-income, urban or rural areas that lack access to healthy, affordable food. When food is available, it is generally high-calorie food of poor nutritional quality, such as found in fast food restaurants and convenience stores

food frequency questionnaire A questionnaire that assesses intake of a variety of food groups on a daily, weekly, or longer basis

food security A parameter used in nutritional assessment, free access to adequate and safe food

foramen ovale The second shunt in fetal circulation prior to birth that connects the fetal right atrium to the fetal left atrium

fracture A partial or complete break in the continuity of the bone from trauma

fremitus The palpable vibration on the chest wall when the patient speaks

friction rub A rough, grating sound caused by the rubbing together of organs or an organ rubbing on the peritoneum

functional assessment An observation to gather data while the patient is performing common or routine activities

functional status Includes the ability of the individual to safely perform activities of daily living, instrumental activities of daily living, and advanced activities of daily living

fundal height Size of the fundus; after 20 weeks of pregnancy, the weeks of gestation equal the fundal height in centimeters

fundus The inner back surface of the internal eye; the top of the uterus

G

galactorrhea Lactation not associated with childbearing or breast feeding

gender identity Comprises the most significant aspects of an individual's sexual life, including sexual attractions, behaviors, and desires

genital warts Raised, moist, cauliflower-shaped papules

genitourinary system The urinary system and the reproductive organs

genogram Documentation of a family history in the form of a diagram

genuineness The ability to present oneself honestly and spontaneously

geography The country, region, section, community, or neighborhood in which one was born and raised or in which one currently resides or works

geriatric syndromes A group of conditions, not classified as a specific disease, that are commonly identified in older adults and are believed to significantly attribute to mortality

gestational age The age of the fetus, which can be referred to in weeks from the last normal menstrual period

glaucoma A group of eye conditions causing optic nerve damage, and the leading cause of blindness in the United States

gliding The simplest type of joint movement; one flat bone surface glides or slips over another similar surface; the bones are merely displaced in relation to one another

glomeruli Tufts of capillaries of the kidneys that filter more than 1 liter (1 L) of fluid each minute; plural: glomeruli

glossitis Inflammation or redness of the tongue. Often seen in malnutrition

goiter Enlargement of the thyroid gland, commonly visible as swelling of the anterior neck; cause is often lack of iodine intake

glycosuria Glucose in urine

Goodell's sign An increase in cervical vascularity that contributes to the softening of the cervix during pregnancy

guarding A tensing of the muscles of a particular area to protect from pain or agitation of sites impacted by injury or disease

gynecologic age The difference between one's current age and age at menarche

gynecomastia Benign temporary breast enlargement in one or both breasts in males

H

hair A thin, flexible, elongated fiber composed of dead, keratinized cells that grow out in a columnar fashion

hallux valgus The great toe is abnormally adducted at the metatarsophalangeal joint

health Absence of disease along with a state of physical, mental, and social well-being

health assessment A systematic method of collecting data about a patient for the purpose of determining the patient's current and ongoing health status, predicting risks to health, and identifying health-promoting activities

healthcare-associated infections (HAIs) An infection that results directly from the delivery of healthcare services in a facility such as a clinic, hospital, or long-term care facility

health disparities Preventable gaps in the quality of health and healthcare that mirror differences in socioeconomic status, racial and ethnic background, and levels of education

health equity The absence of avoidable or remediable differences among groups of people, whether those groups are defined socially, economically, demographically, or geographically

health history Information about the patient's health in his or her own words and based on the patient's own perceptions. Includes biographic data, perceptions about health, past and present history of illness and injury, family history, a review of systems, and health

health pattern A set of related traits, habits, or acts that affect a patient's health

health promotion Behavior motivated by the desire to increase well-being and actualize human potential

heart An intricately designed pump composed of a meticulous network of synchronized structures; is responsible for receiving unoxygenated blood from the body and returning oxygenated blood to the body

heart murmurs Atypical sounds of the heart often indicating a functional or structural abnormality

Heberden's nodes Hard, typically painless, bony enlargements associated with osteoarthritis

Hegar's sign The softening of the uterus and the region that connects the body of the uterus and cervix that occurs throughout pregnancy

helix The external large rim of the auricle of the ear

hematuria Blood in the urine

hepatitis An inflammatory process of the liver caused by viruses, bacteria, chemicals, or drugs

heritage A range of meanings, behaviors, and contemporary activities that are drawn from a combination of an individual's culture, inherited traditions, objects, and monuments

heritage consistency The extent to which one's lifestyle reflects one's traditional heritage, as well as the degree to which the individual identifies with his traditional heritage

heritage inconsistency The degree to which an individual adopts and implements beliefs and practices obtained by way of acculturation into a dominant or host culture

hernia A protrusion of an organ or structure through an abnormal opening or weakened area in a body wall

hirsutism Male-pattern hair growth in women; often associated with polycystic ovarian syndrome, Cushing's syndrome, congenital adrenal hyperplasia, androgen-secreting tumors, or certain medications

hydrocephalus The enlargement of the head caused by inadequate drainage of cerebrospinal fluid, resulting in abnormal growth of the skull

hydronephrosis An enlargement of the kidney caused by an obstruction, as in kidney stone or pregnancy

hydroureter An enlargement of the ureter caused by an obstruction, as in kidney stone or pregnancy

hymen A thin layer of skin within the vagina

hyoid A bone that is suspended in the neck approximately 2 cm (1 in.) above the larynx

hyperalgesia Excessive sensitivity to pain

hyperesthesia An increased sensation

hyperextension A bending of a joint beyond 180 degrees

hyperopia A condition in which the light rays focus behind the retina; also called farsightedness

hyperresonance Abnormally loud auscultatory tone that is low and of long duration

hyperthermia Body temperature that is greater than expected. Also called a fever, it may be caused by an infection, trauma, surgery, or a malignancy

hyperthyroidism The excessive production of thyroid hormones, resulting in enlargement of the gland, exophthalmos (bulging eyes), fine hair, weight loss, diarrhea, and other alterations

hypodermis A cellular layer of subcutaneous tissue consisting of loose connective tissue; stores approximately half of the body's fat cells, cushions the body against trauma, insulates the body from heat loss, and stores fat for energy

hypoesthesia A decreased but not absent sensation

hypospadias A condition in which the urethral meatus is located on the underside of the glans

hypothermia Body temperature that is less than expected. This is usually a response to prolonged exposure to cold

hypothyroidism Metabolic disorder causing enlarged thyroid due to iodine deficiency

hypoalgesia Decreased pain sensation

I

immunocompetence A biochemical assessment laboratory measurement used in nutritional assessment. A depressed immune status can result from malnutrition, disease, medication, or other disease treatments

incontinence The inability to retain urine; may be classified as functional, reflex, stress, urge, or total

infective endocarditis A condition caused by bacterial infiltration of the lining of the heart's chambers

inguinal hernia When a separation of the abdominal muscle exists, the weak points of these canals afford an area for the protrusion of the intestine into the groin region

inspection The skill of observing the patient in a deliberate, systematic manner

integumentary system Composed of skin, hair, and nails

interactional skills Actions that are used during the encoding/decoding process to obtain and disseminate information, develop relationships, and promote understanding of self and others

interdependent relationships Relationships in which the individual establishes bonds with others based on some single factor such as trust or a common goal

interpretation of findings The cognitive action of analyzing and prioritizing the data collected during the complete health assessment

interview Subjective data gathering, including the health history and focused interview, that include primary and secondary sources

intimate partner violence Physical, sexual, or psychological harm by a current or former partner or spouse that can occur among heterosexual or same-sex couples and does not require sexual intimacy

intractable pain Pain that is highly resistant to relief

introitus Vaginal opening

inversion A movement in which the sole of the foot is turned medially or inward

iris The circular, colored muscular aspect of the eye's middle layer located in the anterior portion of the eye

iritis Inflammation of the iris that is characterized by redness around the iris and cornea, decreased vision, and deep, aching pain; pupil is often irregular

J

jaundice Yellowing of the skin, sclera, and mucous membranes caused by deposition of bile pigments

joint (Articulation) The point where two or more bones in the body meet

K

keratin A fibrous protein that gives the epidermis its tough, protective qualities

kidneys Bean-shaped organs located in the retroperitoneal space on either side of the vertebral column

koilonychia A clinical finding of poor nutrition; spoon-shaped ridges in the cardia

kyphosis An exaggerated thoracic dorsal curve that causes asymmetry between the sides of the posterior thorax

L

labia A dual set of liplike structures lying on either side of the vagina

labial adhesions A condition common in preadolescent females that occurs when the labia minora fuse together

landmarks Thoracic reference points and specific anatomic structures used to help provide an exact location for the assessment findings and an accurate orientation for documentation of findings

lanugo A fine, downy hair in newborns that is most prominent on the upper chest, shoulders, and back

left atrium The left atrium of the heart is the chamber that receives oxygenated blood from the pulmonary system

left ventricle The most powerful of all heart chambers, pumps the oxygenated blood outward through the aorta to the periphery of the body

lens A flexible, transparent, biconvex (convex on both surfaces) structure situated directly behind the pupil that separates the anterior and posterior segments of the eye; responsible for fine focusing of images

Leopold's maneuvers A special palpation sequence of the pregnant female's abdomen used to determine the position of the fetus after 28 weeks' gestation

leukorrhea A profuse, nonodorous, nonpainful vaginal discharge that protects against infection

lightening The descent of the fetal head into the pelvis

linea nigra A dark line running from the umbilicus to the pubic area that may occur during pregnancy; often accompanied by increased pigmentation of the areolae and nipples

listening Paying undivided attention to what the patient says and does

lobule A small flap of flesh at the inferior end of the auricle of the ear

lordosis An exaggerated lumbar curve of the spine that compensates for pregnancy, obesity, or other skeletal changes

lunula A moon-shaped crescent that appears on the nail body over the thickened nail matrix

lymph Clear fluid that passes from the intercellular spaces of the body tissue into the lymphatic system

lymphedema Swelling that is caused by some degree of lymphatic system obstruction

lymphadenopathy The enlargement of lymph nodes that is often caused by infection, allergies, or a tumor

lymphatic vessels Vessels that extend from the capillaries to collect lymph in organs and tissues

lymph nodes Rounded lymphoid tissues that are surrounded by connective tissue; located along the lymphatic vessels in the body

M

macula Appears as a hyperpigmented spot on the temporal aspect of the retina and is responsible for central vision

macular degeneration Narrowed blood vessels with a granular pigment in the macula, resulting in a loss of central vision

malnutrition An imbalance, whether a deficit or excess, of the required nutrients of a balanced diet

mammary ridge "Milk line," which extends from each axilla to the groin

mammary souffle A murmur over the mammary vessel due to increased blood flow, occasionally heard during pregnancy

manubrium The superior or upper portion of the sternum

mapping The process of dividing the abdomen into quadrants or regions for the purpose of examination

mastalgia Breast pain

mastoiditis Inflammation of the mastoid that may occur secondary to a middle ear or a throat infection

McDonald's rule A method for estimating fetal growth that states that after 20 weeks in pregnancy, the weeks of gestation approximately equal the fundal height in centimeters

mediastinal space The area where the heart sits obliquely within the thoracic cavity between the lungs and above the diaphragm

mediastinum Part of the thorax, or thoracic cavity, that contains the heart, trachea, esophagus, and major blood vessels of the body

medulla The inner portion of the kidney, composed of structures called pyramids and calyces

melanin Skin pigment produced in the melanocytes in the stratum basale

menarche Age of first menstrual period

meninges Three connective tissue membranes that cover, protect, and nourish the central nervous system

menopause Occurs when the woman has not experienced a menstrual period in over a year

milia Harmless skin markings on newborns; areas of tiny white facial papules due to sebum that collects in the openings of hair follicles

miosis Excessive or prolonged constriction of the pupil of the eye

mixed-status family A family in which one or more family members are undocumented immigrants and other family members are citizens, lawful permanent residents, or immigrants with another form of temporary legal immigration status

Mongolian spots Gray, blue, or purple spots in the sacral and buttocks areas of newborns that fade during the first year of life

Montgomery's glands (tubercles) The sebaceous glands on the areola, which enlarge and produce a secretion that protects and lubricates the nipples

moral code Comprises the internalized values, virtues, and rules one learns from significant others

mucous plug A protective covering of the cervix that develops during pregnancy due to progesterone

multigravida A female who has been pregnant two or more times

mydriasis Excessive or prolonged dilation of the pupil of the eye

myocardium The second, thick, muscular layer of the heart, made up of bundles of cardiac muscle fibers reinforced by a branching network of connective tissue fibers called the fibrous skeleton of the heart

myopia (nearsightedness) A condition in which the light rays focus in front of the retina

N

Nägele's rule A formula that can be used to compute the fetus's expected date of birth (EDB) based on the mother's last menstrual period (LMP)

nails Thin plates of keratinized epidermal cells that shield the distal ends of the fingers and toes

nasal polyps Smooth, pale, benign growths found along the turbinates of the nose

neuropathic pain Pain resulting from current or past damage to the peripheral or central nervous system rather than a particular stimulus

neuropathy Nerve damage or dysfunction that may lead to weakness or numbness

nevus flammeus "Stork bites," which are irregular red or pink patches found most commonly on the back of the neck following birth

nociception The physiologic processes related to pain perception

nociceptors The receptors that transmit pain sensation

nocturia Nighttime urination

nonsuicidal self-injury (NSSI) Behaviors committed by and aimed at oneself that result in deliberate actual or potential self-harm

nuchal rigidity Stiffness of the neck as experienced when the meningeal membranes are irritated or inflamed

nursing diagnosis The second step of the nursing process, whereby the nurse uses critical thinking and applies knowledge from the sciences and other disciplines to analyze and synthesize the data

nursing process A systematic, rational, dynamic, and cyclic process used by the nurse for planning and providing care for the patient

nutritional health Using vitamins, foods, nutrients, or herbs to achieve or maintain good health

nystagmus Rapid fluttering or constant involuntary movement of the eyeball

O

obesity Weight of 20% or more above recommended body weight

obesity paradox The condition where both obesity and nutrient deficiencies occur simultaneously in a person

objective data Data observed or measured by the professional nurse, also known as overt data or signs since they are detected by the nurse. These data can be seen, felt, heard, or measured.

oliguria Diminished volume of urine

onycholysis Separation of the nail plate from the nail bed

opposition The movement of touching the thumb to the tips of the other fingers of the same hand

optic atrophy Degeneration of the optic nerve resulting in a change in the color of the optic disc and decreased visual acuity

optic disc The creamy yellow area on the retina of the eye where the optic nerve leaves the eye

orchitis Inflammation of the testicles

orthopnea Difficulty breathing (dyspnea) when supine that is relieved by sitting upright

orthostatic hypotension A sudden drop in systolic blood pressure of 20 mmHg or more or diastolic pressure of 10 mmHg within three minutes of moving from a lying down to a sitting or standing position

ossicles Bones of the middle ear: the malleus, the incus, and the stapes

otitis externa Swimmer's ear, infection of the outer ear or ear canal

otitis media Middle ear infection

ovaries Almond-shaped glandular structures that produce ova as well as estrogen and progesterone

overnutrition Excessive intake or storage of essential nutrients

overweight A weight of 10% to 20% in excess of recommended body weight

oxygen saturation The percentage of oxygen in the blood

P

pain A highly unpleasant sensation that affects a person's senses and emotions and is associated with real or potential tissue damage

pain rating scale Assessment of the intensity of pain using a standardized measurement tool. The tools, which may be numbers, words, or pictures, provide the patient the opportunity to describe the degree of discomfort

pain reaction Responses to pain, including the autonomic nervous system and behavioral responses to pain

pain sensation The acknowledgment of pain, often known as pain threshold

pain threshold The point at which the sensation of pain is perceived

pain tolerance The maximum amount and duration of pain that an individual is able to endure without relief

palate The anterior portion of the roof of the mouth formed by bones

palpation The skill of assessing the patient through the sense of touch to determine specific characteristics of the body

palpebrae The eyelid

palpebral fissure The opening between the upper and lower eyelids

papilledema Swelling and protrusion of the blind spot of the eye caused by edema

paranasal sinuses Mucus-lined, air-filled cavities that surround the nasal cavity and perform the same air-processing functions of filtration, moistening, and warming

paraphrasing Restating the patient's basic message to test whether it was understood

paraurethral glands (Skene's glands) Glands located just posterior to the urethra that open into the urethra and secrete a fluid that lubricates the vaginal vestibule during sexual intercourse

Parkinson disease A chronic, progressive movement disorder characterized by the malfunction and death of brain neurons and subsequent decrease in dopamine production; primarily affects neurons located in the substantia nigra, which is involved in motor control

paronychia An inflammation of the cuticle, sometimes caused by infection

patient portals Digital access to patient information

patient record A legal document used to plan care, to communicate information between and among healthcare providers, and to monitor quality of care

peau d'orange "Orange peel" appearance caused by edema from blocked lymphatic drainage in advanced cancer

pediculosis capitis Small parasitic insects that live on the scalp and neck, often called head lice

pedigree A graphic representation or diagram that depicts both medical history and genetic relationships. In a pedigree, each family member is represented by a symbol, using a circle for females and a square for males

pellagra A photosensitive symmetric rash caused by a diet that is deficient in niacin

penis The male organ used for both elimination of urine and ejaculation of sperm during reproduction

percussion "Striking through" a body part with an object, fingers, or reflex hammer, ultimately producing a measurable sound

pericardium A thin sac composed of a fibroserous material that surrounds the heart

perineum The space between the vaginal opening and anal area or between the scrotum and anus

periorbital edema Swollen, puffy eyelids

peripheral nervous system (PNS) System of the body that consists of the cranial nerves and spinal nerves

peripheral vascular system Blood vessels of the body that together with the heart and the lymphatic vessels make up the body's circulatory system

peritoneum A thin, double layer of serous membrane in the abdominal cavity

peritonitis A local or generalized inflammatory process of the peritoneal membrane of the abdomen

petechiae Pinpoint hemorrhages on the skin, can be related to vitamin C deficiency

Peyronie disease Disease that causes the shaft of the penis to be crooked during an erection

phantom pain Painful sensation experienced in a missing body part (amputation) or paralyzed area

phimosis Condition in which the foreskin of a penis cannot be fully retracted

physical assessment Hands-on examination of the patient; components are the survey and examination of systems

physiologic anemia Decrease in hemoglobin and hematocrit caused by plasma volume increase outpacing the increase in red blood cells (RBCs)

pica Abnormal craving for or eating of nonfood items such as chalk or dirt

pingueculae Yellowish nodules that are thickened areas of the bulbar conjunctiva caused by prolonged exposure to sun, wind, and dust; may be on either side of the pupil and cause no problems

pinna The external portion of the ear

Piskacek's sign The irregular shape of the uterus due to the implantation of the ovum

placenta A vascular organ that connects the developing fetus to the uterine lining; facilitates the delivery of oxygen and nutrients from mother to fetus, and allows for the release of fetal carbon dioxide and other metabolic waste products

plantar flexion Extension of the ankle (pointing the toes) away from the body

pleximeter The device (or finger) that accepts the tap or blow from a hammer (or tapping finger)

plexor A hammer or tapping finger used to strike an object

polypharmacy Concurrent use of multiple medications to treat one or more conditions and/or diseases

positive regard The ability to appreciate and respect another person's worth and dignity with a nonjudgmental attitude

posterior triangle A landmark area of the posterior neck bordered by the trapezius muscle, the sternocleidomastoid muscle, and the clavicle

preinteraction The period before first meeting with the patient in which the nurse reviews information and prepares for the initial interview

presbycusis High-frequency hearing loss that occurs over time; often associated with aging

presbyopia Decreased ability of the eye lens to change shape to accommodate for near vision

pressure ulcer Localized region of damaged or necrotic tissue caused by the exertion of pressure over a bony prominence

primary lesions The initial lesion of a disease

primary prevention Interventions that occur to promote health and well-being before a problem occurs

primary source The patient is the best source because he or she can describe personal symptoms, experiences, and factors leading to the current concerns

primigravida A female pregnant for the first time

proband The individual around whom a pedigree is created

prolapsed uterus Condition in which the uterus may protrude right at the vaginal wall with straining, or it may hang outside the vaginal wall without any straining

pronation Movement of the forearm so that the palm faces down, posteriorly or inferiorly

prostate gland Organ that borders the urethra near the lower part of the bladder; it lies just anterior to the rectum and is composed of glandular structures that continuously secrete a milky, alkaline solution

protein-calorie malnutrition A nutrient deficiency resulting from undernutrition

protraction A nonangular anterior movement in a transverse plane

pruritus Itching, usually due to dry skin, that may increase with age

psychosocial functioning The way a person thinks, feels, acts, and relates to self and other; it is the ability to cope and tolerate stress, and the capacity for developing a value and belief system

psychosocial health Being mentally, emotionally, socially, and spiritually well

pterygium An opacity of the bulbar conjunctiva that can grow over the cornea and block vision

ptosis One eyelid drooping

pulse Wave of pressure felt at various points in the body due to the force of the blood against the walls of the arteries

pupil Opening in the center of the iris that allows light to enter the eye

Purkinje fibers Fibers that fan out and penetrate into the myocardial tissue to spread the current into the tissues themselves

purpura Flat, reddish-blue, irregularly shaped extensive patches of varying size

Q

quickening The fluttery initial sensations of fetal movement perceived by the mother

R

race The identification of an individual or group by shared genetic heritage and biologic or physical characteristics

radiating pain Pain perceived at one location that then extends to nearby tissues

rales/crackles Discontinuous adventitious lung sounds that are intermittent, nonmusical, and brief

Raynaud disease A condition in which the arterioles in the fingers develop spasms, causing intermittent skin pallor or cyanosis and then rubor (red color)

rectocele A hernia that is formed when the rectum pushes into the posterior vaginal wall

referred pain Pain felt in a part of the body that is considerably removed or distant from the area actually causing the pain

reflecting A communication technique used in letting the patient know that the nurse empathizes with the thoughts, feelings, or experiences expressed

reflexes Automatic stimulus–responses that involve a nerve impulse passing from a peripheral nerve receptor to the spinal cord and then outward to an effector muscle without passing through the brain; the muscle typically contracts following stimulation of the nerve receptor

regurgitation Backflow of blood into the chambers of the heart

religion A specific fundamental set of beliefs and practices generally agreed upon by a number of persons or sects

resonance A long, low-pitched hollow sound elicited with percussion over the lungs

respiratory cycle Consists of an inspiratory and expiratory phase of breathing

respiratory rate The number of times the individual inhales and exhales during a 1-minute period

retina The third and innermost membrane, the sensory portion of the eye, a direct extension of the optic nerve

retraction A nonangular posterior movement in a transverse plane

retrobulbar neuritis An inflammatory process of the optic nerve behind the eyeball

rhonchi A range of whistling or snoring sounds heard during auscultation when there is some type of airway obstruction; types of rhonchi include sibilant wheezes, sonorous rhonchi, and stridor

rickets A clinical finding associated with poor nutritional health resulting in bowed legs

right atrium A thin-walled chamber located above and slightly to the right of the right ventricle that forms the right border of the heart; receives unoxygenated blood from the periphery of the body

right ventricle Part of the heart formed triangularly that comprises much of the anterior or sternocostal surface of the heart; pushes unoxygenated blood out to the pulmonary vessels, where oxygenation occurs

ripening Softening of the cervix near the end of pregnancy in anticipation of birth

role development The individual's capacity to identify and fulfill the social expectations related to the variety of roles assumed in a lifetime

Romberg's test A test that assesses coordination and equilibrium

rotation The turning movement of a bone around its own long axis

S

S1 The first heart sound (lub) heard when the atrioventricular (AV) valves close; closure of these valves occurs when the ventricles have been filled

S2 The second heart sound (dub) heard when the aortic and pulmonic valves close; they close when the ventricles have emptied their blood into the aorta and pulmonary arteries

SBAR Situation, Background, Assessment, and Recommendation format used to guide communication

sclera The outermost layer of the eye, an extremely dense, hard, fibrous membrane that helps to maintain the shape of the eye

scoliosis A lateral curvature of the lumbar or thoracic spine that is more common in children with neuromuscular deficits

scrotum A loosely hanging, pliable, pear-shaped pouch of darkly pigmented skin located behind the penis that houses the testes, which produce sperm

sebaceous glands Oil glands that secrete sebum, an oily secretion, which generally is released into hair follicles

secondary lesions Skin condition or changes to the skin that occur following a primary lesion

secondary prevention Focus on early diagnosis of health problems and prompt treatment with the restoration of health

secondary source A person or record beyond the patient that provides additional information about the patient

seizures Sudden and rapid physical manifestations (as convulsions or loss of consciousness) resulting from excessive discharges of electrical energy in the brain

self-concept The beliefs and feelings one holds about oneself

semilunar valves Valves that separate the ventricles from the vascular system

seminal vesicles A pair of saclike glands, located between the bladder and rectum, that are the source of 60% of the semen produced

serous layer of pericardium The inner layer of the parietal layer of the pericardium

sexual orientation An individual's predisposition toward affiliation, affection, bonding, thoughts, or sexual fantasies in relationship to members of the same sex, the other sex, both sexes, or neither sex

sexual orientation label Designation that may be used to describe an individual's sexual orientation—for example, straight (or heterosexual), gay, lesbian, and bisexual

sinoatrial (SA) node The node located at the junction of the superior vena cava and right atrium that initiates the electrical impulse; natural "pacemaker" of the heart

sinus arrhythmia (Heart period variability) Presents with heart rate increases during inspiration and decreases during expiration

smegma A white, cheesy sebaceous matter that collects between the glans of the penis and the foreskin

social determinants of health The situations in which a person is born, lives, works, and ages, as well as the systems in place to deal with illness

somatic protein Another term for muscle mass or skeletal muscle

spermatic cord A cord composed of fibrous connective tissue; its purpose is to form a protective sheath around the nerves, blood vessels, lymphatic structures, and muscle fibers associated with the scrotum

sphygmomanometer An instrument used to measure arterial blood pressure

spiritual care Defined as meeting patients' spiritual needs by way of recognizing and respecting these needs, facilitating participation in religious rituals, engaging in active listening, promoting hope, demonstrating empathy, and making referrals to other professionals

spiritual distress An interruption in one's value system or beliefs

spirituality Refers to the individual's sense of self in relation to others and a higher being, what one believes gives meaning to life, and what fosters hope for one's will to live

spiritual state Describes the person's feelings about their spirituality that can fluctuate along a continuum of well-being to spiritual distress

spinal cord A continuation of the medulla oblongata that has the ability to transmit impulses to and from the brain via the ascending and descending pathways

stenosis Prevents the heart valve(s) from opening properly, forcing the heart to work harder to pump blood through the valve(s)

sternum The flat, narrow center bone of the upper anterior chest

strabismus A condition in which the axes of the eyes cannot be directed at the same object

stress Perceived or physical response to environmental factors; the body's response to thoughts and feelings that may result in a behavioral or physiologic response

stress incontinence Involuntary leaking of urine caused from stress on the bladder related to pressures such as coughing, sneezing, running, or heavy lifting

striae (Stretch marks) A change in connective tissue resulting in silvery, shiny, irregular markings on the skin; often seen in obesity, pregnancy, and ascites

striae gravidarium Also known as stretch marks, these pinkish-purplish skin depressions in connective tissue develop in the second half of pregnancy

stridor Loud, high-pitched crowing heard without stethoscope due to obstructed upper airway

stroke volume The amount of blood that is ejected with every heartbeat

subcultures Groups that exist within a larger culture. Subcultures are composed of individuals who have a distinct identity based on some characteristic such as occupation, a medical problem, or a specific ethnic heritage

subjective data Information that the patient experiences and communicates to the nurse, known as covert data or symptoms

subluxation A partial dislocation of the bones in a joint, such as the head of the radius, which may occur when a child is dangled by his or her hands

substance use disorder (SUD) Recurrent use of drugs and/or alcohol that causes a significant life impairment, which results in a person's failure to meet work, school or family obligations

suicidal ideation Considering, planning, or thinking about committing suicide

summarizing Tying together the various messages that the patient has communicated throughout the interview

supination Movement of the forearm so that the palm faces up, anteriorly or superiorly

supine hypotension syndrome (vena cava syndrome) Occurs when pressure from the pregnant uterus compresses the aorta and the inferior vena cava when the female is in the supine position

suspensory ligaments (Cooper's ligaments) Ligaments that extend from the connective tissue layer, through the breast, and attach to the fascia underlying the breast

sutures Nonmovable joints that connect two bones

syncope Brief loss of consciousness, usually sudden

synovial joint Articulation of bones separated by a fluid-filled joint cavity

systole The phase of ventricular contraction in which the ventricles have been filled, then contract to expel blood into the aorta and pulmonary arteries; also associated with the top number of a blood pressure reading

systolic pressure The highest arterial blood pressure during the height of a ventricular contraction; the first number in a blood pressure reading

T

temperature The degree of hotness or coldness within the body as measured by a thermometer

tendons Tough fibrous bands that attach muscle to bone, or muscle to muscle

teratogen An agent that causes birth defects, such as a virus, a drug, a chemical, or radiation

terminal hair Dark, coarse, long hair that appears on eyebrows, the scalp, and the pubic region

tertiary prevention Activity aimed at restoring the individual to the highest possible level of health and functioning

testes Two firm, rubbery, olive-shaped structures that manufacture sperm and are thus the primary male sex organs

thalamus The largest subdivision of the diencephalon, which is the gateway to the cerebral cortex; the location where all input channeled to the cerebral cortex is processed

thelarche Breast budding, often the first pubertal sign in females

thrill A soft vibratory sensation assessed by palpation with either the fingertips or palm flattened to the chest

thyroid gland The largest gland of the endocrine system which is butterfly shaped and is located in the anterior portion of the neck

tophi Uric acid deposits that cause inflammation, pain, and swelling in the joint

torticollis A spasm of the sternocleidomastoid muscle on one side of the body, which often results from birth trauma

tracheal sounds Harsh, high-pitched sounds heard over the trachea when the patient inhales and exhales

tragus A small projection on the external ear that is positioned in front of the external auditory canal

transgender Also referred to as *gender nonconforming*, individuals who identify themselves and live as the gender that is not associated with their birth gender

trichotillomania Compulsive hair twisting or plucking

tympanic membrane Also called the eardrum, this membrane separates the external ear and middle ear

tympany A loud, high-pitched, drumlike tone of medium duration characteristic of an organ that is filled with air

U

ulcerative colitis A recurrent inflammatory process causing ulcer formation in the lower portions of the large intestine and rectum

umbilical hernia A protrusion at the umbilicus, visible at birth

undernutrition Insufficient intake or storage of essential nutrients; also referred to as malnutrition

uniform language The consistent use of accepted terminology by all individuals involved in documenting any aspect of the patient's care, including patient data that pertains to assessment and treatment

ureters Mucus-lined narrow tubes approximately 25 to 30 cm (10 to 12 in.) in length and 6 to 12 mm (0.25 to 0.5 in.) in diameter whose major function is transporting urine from the kidney to the urinary bladder

urethra A mucus-lined tube that transports urine from the urinary bladder to the exterior

urethral stricture Condition indicated by pinpoint appearance of the urinary meatus

urinary retention A chronic state in which the patient cannot empty his or her bladder

urinary system The kidneys, renal vasculature (blood vessels), ureters, bladder, and urethra

uterine tubes Ducts on either side of the uterus's fundus; also known as fallopian tubes

uterus A pear-shaped, hollow, muscular organ that is located centrally in the pelvis between the neck of the bladder and the rectal wall

uvula A fleshy pendulum that hangs from the edge of the soft palate in the back of the mouth; the uvula moves with swallowing, breathing, and phonation

V

vagina A long, tubular, muscular canal that extends from the vestibule to the cervix at the inferior end of the uterus; major function is serving as the female organ of copulation, the birth canal, and the channel for the exit of menstrual flow

varicocele A varicose enlargement of the veins of the spermatic cord causing a soft compressible mass in the scrotum; may lead to male infertility

varicosities Distended veins

vegan Dietary choice in which no animal products are consumed

veins Tubular, walled vessels that carry deoxygenated blood from the body periphery back to the heart

vellus hair Pale, fine, short hair that appears over the entire body except for the lips, nipples, palms of hands, soles of feet, and parts of external genitals

venous insufficiency Inadequate circulation in the venous system usually due to incompetent valves in deep veins or a blood clot in the veins

vernix caseosa A cheesy white substance that coats the skin surfaces at birth

vesicular sounds Soft and low-pitched breath sounds heard over the periphery; inspiration is longer than expiration

viability The point at which the fetus can survive outside the uterus

visceral layer of pericardium The innermost layer of the pericardium that lines the surface of the heart

visceral pain Pain that results from stimulation of pain receptors deep within the body such as the abdominal cavity, cranium, or the thorax

visual field Refers to the total area of vision in which objects can be seen while the eye remains focused on a central point

vital signs The systematic measurement of temperature, pulse, respirations, blood pressure, and pain status

vitiligo A skin condition identified by patchy, depigmented skin over various areas of the body

vitreous humor A refractory medium, a clear gel within the eye that helps maintain the intraocular pressure and the shape of the eye, and transmits light rays through the eye

vulnerable populations Groups that are not well integrated into the U.S. healthcare system because of racial, ethnic, cultural, economic, geographic, or health characteristics

W

wellness A state of life that is balanced, personally satisfying, and characterized by the ability to adapt and to participate in activities that enhance quality of life

wellness theories Describe ways the nurse may approach patient care

wheezes High-pitched squeaky or sibilant breath sounds heard on expiration

whispered pectoriloquy Auscultation of voice sounds; patient whispers "one, two, three," normal lung sounds will be faint, almost indistinguishable

X

xanthelasma Soft, yellow plaques on the lids at the inner canthus, which are sometimes associated with high cholesterolemia

xerophthalmia A clinical finding of poor nutrition, dry mucosa

Index

Page numbers followed by italic *f* indicate figures, italic *t* indicate tables, and italic *b* indicate boxes.